坎贝尔骨科手术学
关节外科

Campbell's Operative Orthopaedics

第 14 版
（影印版）

Frederick M. Azar, MD

James H. Beaty, MD

人民卫生出版社
·北 京·

图书在版编目（CIP）数据

坎贝尔骨科手术学 . 关节外科 : 英文 /（美）弗雷德里克·M. 阿扎尔（Frederick M. Azar），（美）詹姆斯·H. 比蒂（James H. Beaty）主编 . —影印本 . —北京：人民卫生出版社，2021.12

ISBN 978-7-117-32520-2

Ⅰ. ①坎… Ⅱ. ①弗… ②詹… Ⅲ. ①骨科学 – 外科手术 – 英文②关节 – 外科手术 – 英文 Ⅳ. ①R68

中国版本图书馆 CIP 数据核字（2021）第 241257 号

人卫智网	www.ipmph.com	医学教育、学术、考试、健康，购书智慧智能综合服务平台
人卫官网	www.pmph.com	人卫官方资讯发布平台

图字：01–2021–6747 号

坎贝尔骨科手术学
关 节 外 科
Kanbeier Guke Shoushuxue
Guanjie Waike

主　　编：Frederick M. Azar　James H. Beaty
出版发行：人民卫生出版社（中继线 010-59780011）
地　　址：北京市朝阳区潘家园南里 19 号
邮　　编：100021
E - mail：pmph @ pmph.com
购书热线：010-59787592　010-59787584　010-65264830
印　　刷：三河市宏达印刷有限公司（胜利）
经　　销：新华书店
开　　本：889×1194　1/16　印张：32
字　　数：1524 千字
版　　次：2021 年 12 月第 1 版
印　　次：2022 年 1 月第 1 次印刷
标准书号：ISBN 978-7-117-32520-2
定　　价：466.00 元

坎贝尔骨科手术学
关节外科

Campbell's Operative Orthopaedics

第 14 版
（影印版）

Frederick M. Azar, MD

Professor

Department of Orthopaedic Surgery and Biomedical Engineering University of Tennessee–Campbell Clinic

Chief of Staff, Campbell Clinic

Memphis, Tennessee

James H. Beaty, MD

Harold B. Boyd Professor and Chair

Department of Orthopaedic Surgery and Biomedical Engineering University of Tennessee–Campbell Clinic

Memphis, Tennessee

Editorial Assistance

Kay Daugherty *and* **Linda Jones**

人民卫生出版社
·北 京·

Elsevier (Singapore) Pte Ltd.
3 Killiney Road,
#08–01 Winsland House I,
Singapore 239519
Tel:（65）6349–0200; Fax:（65）6733–1817

ELSEVIER

This English Reprint of Parts Ⅱ, Ⅲ, Ⅳ, and Ⅴ from Campbell's Operative Orthopaedics, 14E by Frederick M. Azar and James H. Beaty was undertaken by People's Medical Publishing House and is published by arrangement with Elsevier (Singapore) Pte Ltd.

Parts Ⅱ, Ⅲ, Ⅳ, and Ⅴ from Campbell's Operative Orthopaedics, 14E by Frederick M. Azar and James H. Beaty由人民卫生出版社进行影印，并根据人民卫生出版社与爱思唯尔（新加坡）私人有限公司的协议约定出版。

Notice

Practitioners and researchers must always rely on their own experience and knowledge in evaluating and using any information, methods, compounds or experiments described herein. Because of rapid advances in the medical sciences, in particular, independent verification of diagnoses and drug dosages should be made. To the fullest extent of the law, no responsibility is assumed by Elsevier, authors, editors or contributors in relation to the adaptation or for any injury and/or damage to persons or property as a matter of products liability, negligence or otherwise, or from any use or operation of any methods, products, instructions, or ideas contained in the material herein.

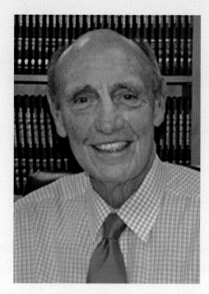

S. Terry Canale, MD

It is with humble appreciation and admiration that we dedicate this edition of *Campbell's Operative Orthopaedics* to Dr. S. Terry Canale, who served as editor or co-editor of five editions. He took great pride in this position and worked tirelessly to continue to improve "The Book." As noted by one of his co-editors, "Terry is probably the only person in the world who has read every word of multiple editions of *Campbell's Operative Orthopaedics.*" He considered *Campbell's Operative Orthopaedics* an opportunity for worldwide orthopaedic education and made it a priority to ensure that each edition provided valuable and up-to-date information. His commitment to and enthusiasm for this work will continue to influence and inspire every future edition.

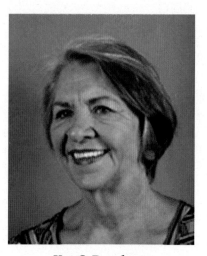

Kay C. Daugherty

It is with equal appreciation and regard that we dedicate this edition to Kay C. Daugherty, the managing editor of the last nine editions *Campbell's Operative Orthopaedics.* Over the last 40 years, she has faithfully and tirelessly edited, reshaped, and overseen all aspects of publication from manuscript preparation to proofing. She has a profound talent to put ideas and disjointed words into comprehensible text, ensuring that each revision maintains the gold standard in readability. Each edition is a testament to her dedication to excellence in writing and education. A favorite quote of Mrs. Daugherty to one of our late authors was, "I'll make a deal. I won't operate if you won't punctuate." We are grateful for her many years of continual service to the Campbell Foundation and for the publications yet to come.

CONTRIBUTORS

FREDERICK M. AZAR, MD
Professor
Director, Sports Medicine Fellowship
University of Tennessee–Campbell Clinic
Department of Orthopaedic Surgery and
    Biomedical Engineering
Chief-of-Staff, Campbell Clinic
Memphis, Tennessee

JAMES H. BEATY, MD
Harold B. Boyd Professor and Chair
University of Tennessee–Campbell Clinic
Department of Orthopaedic Surgery and
    Biomedical Engineering
Memphis, Tennessee

MICHAEL J. BEEBE, MD
Instructor
University of Tennessee–Campbell Clinic
Department of Orthopaedic Surgery and
    Biomedical Engineering
Memphis, Tennessee

CLAYTON C. BETTIN, MD
Assistant Professor
Director, Foot and Ankle Fellowship
Associate Residency Program Director
University of Tennessee–Campbell Clinic
Department of Orthopaedic Surgery and
    Biomedical Engineering
Memphis, Tennessee

TYLER J. BROLIN, MD
Assistant Professor
University of Tennessee–Campbell Clinic
Department of Orthopaedic Surgery and
    Biomedical Engineering
Memphis, Tennessee

JAMES H. CALANDRUCCIO, MD
Associate Professor
Director, Hand Fellowship
University of Tennessee–Campbell Clinic
Department of Orthopaedic Surgery and
    Biomedical Engineering
Memphis, Tennessee

DAVID L. CANNON, MD
Associate Professor
University of Tennessee–Campbell Clinic
Department of Orthopaedic Surgery and
    Biomedical Engineering
Memphis, Tennessee

KEVIN B. CLEVELAND, MD
Instructor
University of Tennessee–Campbell Clinic
Department of Orthopaedic Surgery and
    Biomedical Engineering
Memphis, Tennessee

ANDREW H. CRENSHAW JR., MD
Professor Emeritus
University of Tennessee–Campbell Clinic
Department of Orthopaedic Surgery and
    Biomedical Engineering
Memphis, Tennessee

JOHN R. CROCKARELL, MD
Professor
University of Tennessee–Campbell Clinic
Department of Orthopaedic Surgery and
    Biomedical Engineering
Memphis, Tennessee

GREGORY D. DABOV, MD
Assistant Professor
University of Tennessee–Campbell Clinic
Department of Orthopaedic Surgery and
    Biomedical Engineering
Memphis, Tennessee

MARCUS C. FORD, MD
Instructor
University of Tennessee–Campbell Clinic
Department of Orthopaedic Surgery and
    Biomedical Engineering
Memphis, Tennessee

RAYMOND J. GARDOCKI, MD
Assistant Professor
University of Tennessee–Campbell Clinic
Department of Orthopaedic Surgery and
    Biomedical Engineering
Memphis, Tennessee

BENJAMIN J. GREAR, MD
Instructor
University of Tennessee–Campbell Clinic
Department of Orthopaedic Surgery and
    Biomedical Engineering
Memphis, Tennessee

JAMES L. GUYTON, MD
Associate Professor
University of Tennessee–Campbell Clinic
Department of Orthopaedic Surgery and
    Biomedical Engineering
Memphis, Tennessee

JAMES W. HARKESS, MD
Associate Professor
University of Tennessee–Campbell Clinic
Department of Orthopaedic Surgery and
    Biomedical Engineering
Memphis, Tennessee

ROBERT K. HECK JR., MD
Associate Professor
University of Tennessee–Campbell Clinic
Department of Orthopaedic Surgery and
    Biomedical Engineering
Memphis, Tennessee

MARK T. JOBE, MD
Associate Professor
University of Tennessee–Campbell Clinic
Department of Orthopaedic Surgery and
    Biomedical Engineering
Memphis, Tennessee

DEREK M. KELLY, MD
Professor
Director, Pediatric Orthopaedic Fellowship
Director, Resident Education
University of Tennessee–Campbell Clinic
Department of Orthopaedic Surgery and
    Biomedical Engineering
Memphis, Tennessee

SANTOS F. MARTINEZ, MD
Assistant Professor
University of Tennessee–Campbell Clinic
Department of Orthopaedic Surgery and
    Biomedical Engineering
Memphis, Tennessee

ANTHONY A. MASCIOLI, MD
Assistant Professor
University of Tennessee–Campbell Clinic
Department of Orthopaedic Surgery and
    Biomedical Engineering
Memphis, Tennessee

BENJAMIN M. MAUCK, MD
Assistant Professor
Director, Hand Fellowship
University of Tennessee–Campbell Clinic
Department of Orthopaedic Surgery and
    Biomedical Engineering
Memphis, Tennessee

MARC J. MIHALKO, MD
Assistant Professor
University of Tennessee–Campbell Clinic
Department of Orthopaedic Surgery and
    Biomedical Engineering
Memphis, Tennessee

WILLIAM M. MIHALKO, MD PhD
Professor, H.R. Hyde Chair of Excellence in
    Rehabilitation Engineering
Director, Biomedical Engineering
University of Tennessee–Campbell Clinic
Department of Orthopaedic Surgery and
    Biomedical Engineering
Memphis, Tennessee

ROBERT H. MILLER III, MD
Associate Professor
University of Tennessee–Campbell Clinic
Department of Orthopaedic Surgery and
    Biomedical Engineering
Memphis, Tennessee

G. ANDREW MURPHY, MD
Associate Professor
University of Tennessee–Campbell Clinic
Department of Orthopaedic Surgery and
    Biomedical Engineering
Memphis, Tennessee

ASHLEY L. PARK, MD
Clinical Assistant Professor
University of Tennessee–Campbell Clinic
Department of Orthopaedic Surgery and
    Biomedical Engineering
Memphis, Tennessee

EDWARD A. PEREZ, MD
Associate Professor
University of Tennessee–Campbell Clinic
Department of Orthopaedic Surgery and
    Biomedical Engineering
Memphis, Tennessee

BARRY B. PHILLIPS, MD
Professor
University of Tennessee–Campbell Clinic
Department of Orthopaedic Surgery and
    Biomedical Engineering
Memphis, Tennessee

DAVID R. RICHARDSON, MD
Associate Professor
University of Tennessee–Campbell Clinic
Department of Orthopaedic Surgery and
    Biomedical Engineering
Memphis, Tennessee

MATTHEW I. RUDLOFF, MD
Assistant Professor
Co-Director, Trauma Fellowship
University of Tennessee–Campbell Clinic
Department of Orthopaedic Surgery and
    Biomedical Engineering
Memphis, Tennessee

JEFFREY R. SAWYER, MD
Professor
Co-Director, Pediatric Orthopaedic
    Fellowship
University of Tennessee–Campbell Clinic
Department of Orthopaedic Surgery and
    Biomedical Engineering
Memphis, Tennessee

BENJAMIN W. SHEFFER, MD
Assistant Professor
University of Tennessee–Campbell Clinic
Department of Orthopaedic Surgery and
    Biomedical Engineering
Memphis, Tennessee

DAVID D. SPENCE, MD
Assistant Professor
University of Tennessee–Campbell Clinic
Department of Orthopaedic Surgery and
    Biomedical Engineering
Memphis, Tennessee

NORFLEET B. THOMPSON, MD
Instructor
University of Tennessee–Campbell Clinic
Department of Orthopaedic Surgery and
    Biomedical Engineering
Memphis, Tennessee

THOMAS W. THROCKMORTON, MD
Professor
Co-Director, Sports Medicine Fellowship
University of Tennessee–Campbell Clinic
Department of Orthopaedic Surgery and
    Biomedical Engineering
Memphis, Tennessee

PATRICK C. TOY, MD
Associate Professor
University of Tennessee–Campbell Clinic
Department of Orthopaedic Surgery and
    Biomedical Engineering
Memphis, Tennessee

WILLIAM C. WARNER JR., MD
Professor
University of Tennessee–Campbell Clinic
Department of Orthopaedic Surgery and
    Biomedical Engineering
Memphis, Tennessee

JOHN C. WEINLEIN, MD
Assistant Professor
Director, Trauma Fellowship
University of Tennessee–Campbell Clinic
Department of Orthopaedic Surgery and
    Biomedical Engineering
Memphis, Tennessee

WILLIAM J. WELLER, MD
Instructor
University of Tennessee–Campbell Clinic
Department of Orthopaedic Surgery and
    Biomedical Engineering
Memphis, Tennessee

A. PAIGE WHITTLE, MD
Associate Professor
University of Tennessee–Campbell Clinic
Department of Orthopaedic Surgery and
    Biomedical Engineering
Memphis, Tennessee

KEITH D. WILLIAMS, MD
Associate Professor
University of Tennessee–Campbell Clinic
Department of Orthopaedic Surgery and
    Biomedical Engineering
Memphis, Tennessee

DEXTER H. WITTE III, MD
Clinical Assistant Professor in
    Radiology
University of Tennessee–Campbell Clinic
Department of Orthopaedic Surgery and
    Biomedical Engineering
Memphis, Tennessee

PREFACE

When Dr. Willis Campbell published the first edition of *Campbell's Operative Orthopaedics* in 1939, he could not have envisioned that over 80 years later it would have evolved into a four-volume text and earned the accolade of the "bible of orthopaedics" as a mainstay in orthopaedic practices and educational institutions all over the world. This expansion from some 400 pages in the first edition to over 4,500 pages in this 14th edition has not changed Dr. Campbell's original intent: "to present to the student, the general practitioner, and the surgeon the subject of orthopaedic surgery in a simple and comprehensive manner." In each edition since the first, authors and editors have worked diligently to fulfill these objectives. This would have not been possible without the hard work of our contributors who always strive to present the most up-to-date information while retaining "tried and true" techniques and tips. The scope of this text continues to expand in the hope that the information will be relevant to physicians no matter their location or resources.

As always, this edition also is the result of the collaboration of a group of "behind the scenes" individuals who are involved in the actual production process. The Campbell Foundation staff—Kay Daugherty, Linda Jones, and Tonya Priggel—contributed their considerable talents to editing often confusing and complex author contributions, searching the literature for obscure references, and, in general, "herding the cats." Special thanks to Kay and Linda who have worked on multiple editions of *Campbell's Operative Orthopaedics* (nine editions for Kay and six for Linda). They probably know more about orthopaedics than most of us, and they certainly know how to make it more understandable. Thanks, too, to the Elsevier personnel who provided guidance and assistance throughout the publication process: John Casey, Senior Project Manager; Jennifer Ehlers, Senior Content Development Specialist; and Belinda Kuhn, Senior Content Strategist.

We are especially appreciative of our spouses, Julie Azar and Terry Beaty, and our families for their patience and support as we worked through this project.

The preparation and publication of this 14th edition was fraught with difficulties because of the worldwide pandemic and social unrest, but our contributors and other personnel worked tirelessly, often in creative and innovative ways, to bring it to fruition. It is our hope that these efforts have provided a text that is informative and valuable to all orthopaedists as they continue to refine and improve methods that will ensure the best outcomes for their patients.

Frederick M. Azar, MD
James H. Beaty, MD

CONTENTS

PART I

RECONSTRUCTIVE PROCEDURES OF THE HIP IN ADULTS

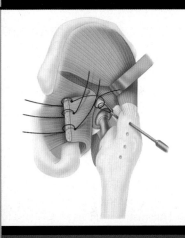

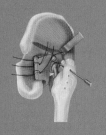

CHAPTER 1

ARTHROPLASTY OF THE HIP

James W. Harkess, John R. Crockarell Jr.

Total hip arthroplasty is the most commonly performed adult reconstructive hip procedure. This chapter discusses cemented and noncemented arthroplasties, bearing choices, and current trends in surgical approaches and less invasive techniques. In addition, revision hip arthroplasty, which comprises an enlarging segment of procedures performed, is reviewed.

The results of the Charnley total hip arthroplasty (THA) are the benchmark for evaluating the performance of other arthroplasties. The laboratory and clinical contributions of Charnley have improved the quality of life for many patients. Nevertheless, the history of hip arthroplasty has been dynamic, and research continues to improve results, especially in young patients. Investigation has proceeded along multiple paths, including (1) improvement in the durability of implant fixation, (2) reduction in the wear of the articulating surfaces, and (3) technical modifications in the operation to speed rehabilitation and reduce implant-positioning errors.

In response to the problem of loosening of the stem and cup based on the alleged failure of cement, press-fit, porous-coated, and hydroxyapatite-coated stems and cups have been investigated as ways to eliminate the use of cement and to use bone ingrowth or ongrowth as a means of achieving durable skeletal fixation. Although some initial cementless implant designs have proved very successful, others have been beset by premature and progressive failure because of inadequate initial fixation, excessive wear, and periprosthetic bone loss secondary to particle-induced osteolysis. As experience has accumulated, the importance of certain design parameters has become apparent and the use of cementless fixation for the femoral and acetabular components has become more common.

Many different techniques have evolved to improve cemented femoral fixation, including injection of low-viscosity cement, occlusion of the medullary canal, reduction of porosity, pressurization of the cement, and centralization of the stem. Similar techniques have been less successful in improving the results of acetabular fixation. Stem fracture has been largely eliminated by routine use of superalloys in their fabrication.

As technologic advances improve the longevity of implant fixation, problems related to wear of articulating surfaces have emerged. Highly crosslinked polyethylenes have demonstrated reduced wear and have now largely replaced conventional ultra-high-molecular-weight polyethylene. Ceramic-ceramic articulations have been used because of their low coefficient of friction and superior in vitro wear characteristics; these have also been successful. The initial enthusiasm for metal-on-metal articulations has been tempered by high failure rates caused by metal hypersensitivity reactions. The introduction of these more wear-resistant bearings has led to the use of larger component head sizes and modifications of postoperative regimens.

Consider the problems of previous materials and design modifications that did not become apparent until the results of a sufficient number of 5-year or more follow-up studies were available. There is little debate that the results of revision procedures are less satisfactory and that primary THA offers the best chance of success. Selection of the appropriate patient, the proper implants, and the technical performance of the operation are of paramount importance.

THA procedures require the surgeon to be familiar with the many technical details of the operation. To contend successfully with the many problems that occur and to evaluate new concepts and implants, a working knowledge of biomechanical principles, materials, and design also is necessary.

APPLIED BIOMECHANICS

The biomechanics of THA are different from those of the screws, plates, and nails used in bone fixation because these latter implants provide only partial support and only until the bone unites. Total hip components must withstand many years of cyclic loading equal to at least three times body weight. A basic knowledge of the biomechanics of the hip and of THA is necessary to perform the procedure properly, to manage the problems that may arise during and after surgery successfully, to select the components intelligently, and to counsel patients concerning their physical activities.

FORCES ACTING ON THE HIP

To describe the forces acting on the hip joint, the body weight can be depicted as a load applied to a lever arm extending from the body's center of gravity to the center of the femoral head (Fig. 1.1). The abductor musculature, acting on a lever arm extending from the lateral aspect of the greater trochanter to the center of the femoral head, must exert an equal moment to hold the pelvis level when in a one-legged stance and a greater moment to tilt the pelvis to the same side when

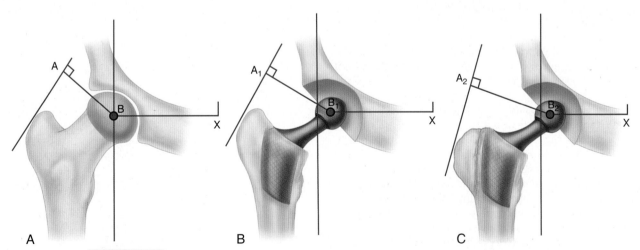

FIGURE 1.1 Lever arms acting on hip joint. **A,** Moment produced by body weight applied at body's center of gravity, X, acting on lever arm, B-X, must be counterbalanced by moment produced by abductors, A, acting on shorter lever arm, A-B. Lever arm A-B may be shorter than normal in arthritic hip. **B,** Medialization of acetabulum shortens lever arm B_1-X, and use of high offset neck lengthens lever arm A_1-B_1. **C,** Lateral and distal reattachment of osteotomized greater trochanter lengthens lever arm A_2-B_2 further and tightens abductor musculature.

walking. Because the ratio of the length of the lever arm of the body weight to that of the abductor musculature is about 2.5:1, the force of the abductor muscles must approximate 2.5 times the body weight to maintain the pelvis level when standing on one leg. The estimated load on the femoral head in the stance phase of gait is equal to the sum of the forces created by the abductors and the body weight and has been calculated to be three times the body weight; the load on the femoral head during straight-leg raising is estimated to be about the same.

An integral part of the Charnley concept of THA was to shorten the lever arm of the body weight by deepening the acetabulum and to lengthen the lever arm of the abductor mechanism by reattaching the osteotomized greater trochanter laterally. The moment produced by the body weight is decreased, and the counterbalancing force that the abductor mechanism must exert is decreased. The abductor lever arm may be shortened in arthritis and other hip disorders in which part or all of the head is lost or the neck is shortened. It also is shortened when the trochanter is located posteriorly, as in external rotational deformities, and in many patients with developmental dysplasia of the hip. In an arthritic hip, the ratio of the lever arm of the body weight to that of the abductors may be 4:1. The lengths of the two lever arms can be surgically changed to make their ratio approach 1:1 (see Fig. 1.1). Theoretically, this reduces the total load on the hip by 30%. Femoral rotational alignment also plays a role in these changes in moment arms. In a finite element model, Terrier et al. found that changes in moment arms with cup medialization were inversely correlated with femoral anteversion, such that hips with less femoral anteversion gained more in terms of muscle moments.

Understanding the benefits derived from medializing the acetabulum and lengthening the abductor lever arm is important; however, neither technique is currently emphasized. The principle of medialization has given way to preserving subchondral bone in the pelvis and to deepening the acetabulum only as much as necessary to obtain bony coverage for the cup. Because most total hip procedures are now done without osteotomy of the greater trochanter, the abductor lever arm is altered only relative to the offset of the head to the stem. These compromises in the original biomechanical principles of THA have evolved to obtain beneficial tradeoffs of a biologic nature; to preserve pelvic bone, especially subchondral bone; and to avoid problems related to reattachment of the greater trochanter.

Calculated peak contact forces across the hip joint during gait range from 3.5 to 5.0 times the body weight and up to six times the body weight during single-limb stance. Experimentally measured forces around the hip joint using instrumented prostheses generally are lower than the forces predicted by analytical models, in the range of 2.6 to 3.0 times the body weight during single-limb stance phase of gait. When lifting, running, or jumping, however, the load may be equivalent to 10 times the body weight. Excess body weight and increased physical activity add significantly to the forces that act to loosen, bend, or break the femoral component.

The forces on the joint act not only in the coronal plane but, because the body's center of gravity (in the midline anterior to the second sacral vertebral body) is posterior to the axis of the joint, also in the sagittal plane to bend the stem posteriorly. The forces acting in this direction are increased

when the loaded hip is flexed, as when arising from a chair, ascending and descending stairs or an incline, or lifting (Fig. 1.2). During the gait cycle, forces are directed against the prosthetic femoral head from a polar angle between 15 and 25 degrees anterior to the sagittal plane of the prosthesis. During stair climbing and straight-leg raising, the resultant force is applied at a point even farther anterior on the head. Such forces cause posterior deflection or retroversion of the femoral component. These so-called out-of-plane forces have been measured at 0.6 to 0.9 times body weight.

Implanted femoral components must withstand substantial torsional forces even in the early postoperative period. Consequently, femoral components used without cement must be designed and implanted so that they are immediately rotationally stable within the femur. Similarly, the shape of a cemented implant must impart rotational stability within its cement mantle.

The location of the center of rotation of the hip from superior to inferior also affects the forces generated around the implant. In a mathematical model, the joint reaction force was lower when the hip center was placed in the anatomic location compared with a superior and lateral or posterior position. Isolated superior displacement without lateralization produces relatively small increases in stresses in the periacetabular bone. This has clinical importance in the treatment of developmental dysplasia and in revision surgery when superior bone stock is deficient. Placement of the acetabular component in a slightly cephalad position allows improved coverage or contact with viable bone. Nonetheless, clinical studies have documented a higher incidence of progressive radiolucencies and migration of components in patients with protrusion, dysplasia, and revision situations when the hip center was placed in a nonanatomic position.

STRESS TRANSFER TO BONE

The quality of the bone before surgery is a determinant in the selection of the most appropriate implant, optimal method of fixation, response of the bone to the implant, and ultimate success of the arthroplasty. Dorr et al. proposed a

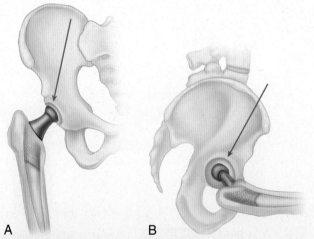

FIGURE 1.2 Forces producing torsion of stem. Forces acting on hip in coronal plane **(A)** tend to deflect stem medially, and forces acting in sagittal plane **(B)**, especially with hip flexed or when lifting, tend to deflect stem posteriorly. Combined, they produce torsion of stem.

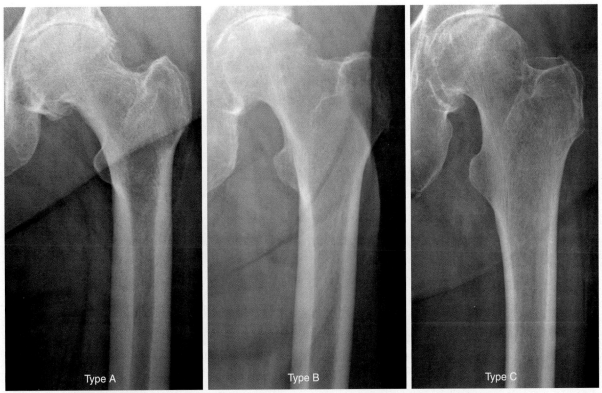

Type A   Type B   Type C

FIGURE 1.3   Dorr radiographic categorization of proximal femurs according to shape, correlation with cortical thickness, and canal dimension. (From Dorr LD, Faugere MC, Mackel AM, et al: Structural and cellular assessment of bone quality of proximal femur, *Bone* 14:231, 1993.)

radiographic categorization of proximal femurs based on their shape and correlated those shapes with measurements of cortical thickness and canal dimensions (Fig. 1.3). Type A femurs have thick cortices on the anteroposterior view and a large posterior cortex seen on the lateral view. The narrow distal canal gives the proximal femur a pronounced funnel shape or "champagne flute" appearance. The type A femur is more commonly found in men and younger patients and permits good fixation of either cemented or cementless stems. Type B femurs exhibit bone loss from the medial and posterior cortices, resulting in increased width of the intramedullary canal. The shape of the femur is not compromised, and implant fixation is not a problem. Type C femurs have lost much of the medial and posterior cortex. The intramedullary canal diameter is very wide, particularly on the lateral radiograph. The "stovepipe"-shaped type C bone is typically found in older postmenopausal women and creates a less favorable environment for cementless implant fixation.

The material a stem is made of, the geometry, length, and size of the stem, and the method and extent of fixation dramatically alter the pattern in which stress is transferred to the femur. Adaptive bone remodeling arising from stress shielding compromises implant support and predisposes to fracture of the femur or the implant itself. Stress transfer to the femur is desirable because it provides a physiologic stimulus for maintaining bone mass and preventing disuse osteoporosis. A decrease in the modulus of elasticity of a stem decreases the stress in the stem and increases stresses to the surrounding bone. This is true of stems made of metals with a lower modulus of elasticity, such as a titanium alloy, particularly if the cross-sectional diameter is relatively small. Larger-diameter stems made of the same material are stronger, but they also are stiffer or less elastic, and the increased cross-sectional diameter negates any real benefits of the lower modulus of elasticity. The bending stiffness of a stem is proportional to the fourth power of the diameter, and small increases in stem diameter produce much larger increments of change in flexural rigidity. When the stem has been fixed within the femur by bone ingrowth, load is preferentially borne by the stiffer structure and the bone of the proximal femur is relieved of stress.

Detailed examinations of stress shielding of the femur after cementless total hip replacement found that almost all femurs showing moderate or severe proximal resorption involved stems 13.5 mm in diameter or larger. With a press-fit at the isthmus and radiographic evidence of bone ingrowth, more stress shielding was evident. Extensive porous coating in smaller size stems does not seem to produce severe stress shielding. More recent follow-up with larger stem sizes shows greater stress shielding, however, with more extensively coated stems (Fig. 1.4). Localized bone hypertrophy can be seen in areas where an extensively porous-coated stem contacts the cortex. This is seen often at the distal end of the porous coating with an extensively coated stem. Such hypertrophy is less pronounced when the porous surface is confined to the proximal portion of the stem. In a meta-analysis of studies of femoral bone loss, Knutsen et al. found that cementless stems had more proximal bone loss than cemented implants and cobalt-chromium stems had nearly double the proximal bone loss seen with titanium alloy femoral stems.

Videodensitometry analysis of autopsy-retrieved femurs found that for cemented and cementless implants, the area

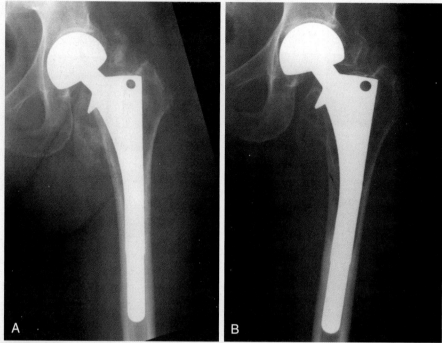

FIGURE 1.4 Response of bone to load. **A,** Postoperative radiograph of extensively porous-coated stem. **B,** Two years later, cortical and cancellous bone density in proximal femur has decreased as a result of stress shielding.

of greatest decrease in bone mineral density occurred in the proximal medial cortex. Dual energy x-ray absorptiometry scans show bone loss in the proximal femur progresses over a period of at least 5 years after surgery. This loss of mineral density does not occur with resurfacing arthroplasty. Shorter length stem designs also aim to load the proximal femoral bone in a more physiological manner to reduce bone loss in this area.

If a prosthesis has a collar that is seated on the cut surface of the neck, it is postulated that axial loading of the bone would occur in this area. It is technically difficult, however, to obtain this direct contact of a collar or cement with the cut surface of bone. Although the role of a collar in preventing loosening of a cemented femoral component has not been clearly established, any loading of the proximal medial neck is likely to decrease bone resorption and reduce stresses in the proximal cement. The presence of a collar on cementless femoral components is more controversial because it may prevent complete seating of the stem, making it loose at implantation.

Cementless stems generally produce strains in the bone that are more physiologic than the strains caused by fully cemented stems, depending on the stem size and the extent of porous coating. Proximal medial bone strains have been found to be 65% of normal with a collarless press-fit stem and 70% to 90% with a collared stem with an exact proximal fit. A loose-fitted stem with a collar can produce proximal strains greater than in the intact femur, although the consequences of a loose stem negate any potential benefits in loading provided by the collar. When a stem is loaded, it produces circumferential or hoop stresses in the proximal femur. Proximal wedging of a collarless implant may generate excessive hoop strains that cause intraoperative and postoperative fractures of the proximal femur. Prophylactic cerclage wire placement increases energy to failure and may reduce the

risk of periprosthetic fracture, particularly when the femur is osteopenic or bony defects are present.

Stem shape also seems to affect stress transfer to bone. In a review of three different types of titanium stems with tapered geometries, an overall incidence of radiographic proximal femoral bone atrophy of only 6% was found in the 748 arthroplasties studied. In no patient was the proximal bone loss as severe as that seen in patients with stems of a cylindrical distal geometry that filled the diaphysis.

Cadaver studies have identified a wide variability in the degree and location of bone remodeling between individuals in clinically successful arthroplasties with solid fixation. A strong correlation was shown, however, between the bone mineral density in the opposite femur and the percentage of mineral loss in the femur that had been operated on, regardless of the method of implant fixation; it seems that patients with diminished bone mineral density before surgery are at greatest risk for significant additional bone loss after cemented and cementless THA.

The amount of stress shielding that is acceptable in the clinical setting is difficult to determine. In a series of 208 hip arthroplasties followed for a mean 13.9 years, Engh et al. reported patients with radiographically evident stress shielding had lower mean walking scores but no increase in other complications and were less likely to require revision for stem loosening or osteolysis. Although proximal femoral stress shielding does not seem to affect adversely early or midterm clinical results, experience with failed cemented implants has also shown that revision surgery becomes more complex when femoral bone stock has been lost. Ongoing investigations into materials and stem design are likely to be beneficial in reducing adverse femoral remodeling.

On the pelvic side, finite analysis has indicated that with the use of a cemented polyethylene cup, peak stresses develop in the pelvic bone. A metal-backed cup with a polyethylene liner reduces the high areas of stress and distributes the stresses more evenly. Similar studies have indicated that increased peak stresses develop in the trabecular bone when the subchondral bone is removed and that decreased peak stresses develop when a metal-backed component is used. The highest stresses in the cement and trabecular bone develop when a thin-walled, polyethylene acetabular component is used and when the subchondral bone has been removed. Stress on the cement-bone interface may also be increased up to 9% when a larger diameter femoral head is utilized. A thick-walled polyethylene cup of 5 mm or more, as opposed to a thin-walled polyethylene cup, tends to reduce the stresses in the trabecular bone, similar to the effect of the metal-backed cup. The preservation of subchondral bone in the acetabulum and the use of a metal-backed cup or thick-walled polyethylene cup decrease the peak stress levels in the trabecular bone of the pelvis.

Favorable early results with metal-backed, cemented acetabular components led to their widespread use in the past. Longer follow-up has shown no sustained benefit, however, from the use of metal backing, and in some series survivorship of the cemented metal-backed acetabular components has been worse than that of components without metal backing. Using a thick-walled, all-polyethylene component and retaining the subchondral bone of the acetabulum are two steps that seem to provide a satisfactory compromise without excessive stress shielding or stress concentration.

When cementless acetabular fixation is used, metal backing is required for skeletal fixation. Ideally, the metal should contact acetabular subchondral bone over a wide area to prevent stress concentration and to maximize the surface area available for biologic fixation. The accuracy of acetabular preparation and the shape and size of the implant relative to the prepared cavity dramatically affect this initial area of contact and the transfer of stress from the implant to the pelvis. If a hemispherical component is slightly undersized relative to the acetabulum, stress is transferred centrally over the pole of the component, with the potential for peripheral gaps between the implant and bone. Conversely, if the component is slightly larger than the prepared cavity, stress transfer occurs peripherally, with the potential for fracture of the acetabular rim during implantation (see section on implantation of cementless acetabular components). Polar gaps also may remain from incomplete seating of the component.

The manner of stress transfer from a cementless acetabular component to the surrounding acetabular bone dictates its initial stability. As the cup is impacted into the acetabulum, forces generated by elastic recoil of the bone stabilize the implant. Peripheral strains acting on a force vector perpendicular to the tangent at the rim stabilize the cup. Strains medial to the rim generate a force vector that pushes laterally and destabilizes the cup (Fig. 1.5).

Stress shielding of the periacetabular bone by cementless implants has received less attention than with femoral components but does occur. Using a novel method of CT-assisted osteodensitometry, Mueller et al. assessed bone density around cementless titanium acetabular components at 10 days and 1 year postoperatively. Cortical bone density cephalad to the implant increased by 3.6%. Conversely, cancellous bone density decreased by 18%, with the area of greatest loss

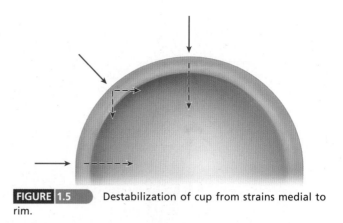

FIGURE **1.5**   Destabilization of cup from strains medial to rim.

anterior to the cup. The clinical importance of acetabular stress shielding has not been determined.

DESIGN AND SELECTION OF TOTAL HIP COMPONENTS

Total hip femoral and acetabular components of various materials and a multitude of designs are currently available. Few implant designs prove to be clearly superior or inferior to others. Certain design features of a given implant may provide an advantage in selected situations. Properly selected and implanted total hip components of most designs can be expected to yield satisfactory results in a high percentage of patients. No implant design or system is appropriate for every patient, and a general knowledge of the variety of component designs and their strengths and weaknesses is an asset to the surgeon. Selection is based on the patient's needs, the patient's anticipated longevity and level of activity, the bone quality and dimensions, the ready availability of implants and proper instrumentation, and the experience of the surgeon.

We routinely use many total hip systems from different manufacturers; we present here an overview of the available systems, emphasizing similar and unique features. Numerous investigators and manufacturers have changed their designs within a relatively short time to incorporate newer concepts, and this confuses many orthopaedic surgeons and patients. The surgeon's recommendations should be tempered by the knowledge that change does not always bring about improvement and that radical departure from proven concepts of implant design yields unpredictable long-term results.

Total hip femoral and acetabular components are commonly marketed together as a total hip system. While the practice is off-label, the variety of modular head sizes with most femoral components allows use with other types of acetabular components if necessary. Femoral and acetabular components are discussed separately.

FEMORAL COMPONENTS

The primary function of the femoral component is the replacement of the femoral head and neck after resection of the arthritic or necrotic segment. The ultimate goal of a biomechanically sound, stable hip joint is accomplished by careful attention to restoration of the normal center of rotation of the femoral head. This location is determined by three factors: (1) vertical height (vertical offset), (2) medial offset (horizontal offset or, simply, offset), and (3) version of the

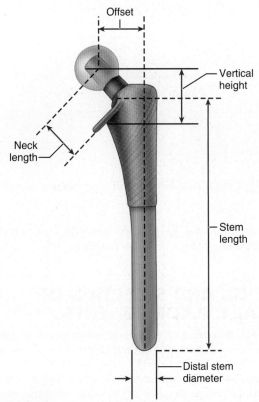

FIGURE 1.6 Features of femoral component. Neck length is measured from center of head to base of collar; head-stem offset, from center of head to line through axis of distal part of stem; stem length, from medial base of collar to tip of stem; and angle of neck, by intersection of line through center of head and neck with another along lateral border of distal half of stem.

femoral neck (anterior offset) (Fig. 1.6). Vertical height and offset increase as the neck is lengthened, and proper reconstruction of both features is the goal when selecting the length of the femoral neck.

In most modern systems, neck length is adjusted by using modular heads with variable internal bores that mate with a uniformly tapered trunnion on the femoral component (Fig. 1.7). The taper is commonly referred to as a Morse taper, although there is no defined standard across all manufacturers. A Morse taper is approximately 3 degrees on each side and the size is typically designated by the diameters at the upper and lower ends. The most common taper used presently is 12 mm/14 mm, but this has varied over time even within the implant offerings of a given manufacturer. It should also be noted that each manufacturer has unique specifications for their tapers and they vary by diameter at the smaller and larger ends, length, taper angle, and surface finish. Consequently, femoral heads from one manufacturer are not compatible with femoral trunnions of another even if the nominal size is the same. Toggling of the head on the trunnion, dissociation, material loss, and corrosion may result from such a mismatch.

Neck length typically ranges from 25 to 50 mm, and adjustment of 8 to 12 mm for a given stem size routinely is available. When a long neck length is required for a head diameter up to 32 mm, a skirt extending from the lower aspect of the head may be required to fully engage the Morse taper (Fig. 1.8). For heads larger than 32 mm a skirt is unnecessary even for longer neck lengths.

Vertical height (vertical offset) is determined primarily by the base length of the prosthetic neck plus the length gained by the modular head used. In addition, the depth the implant is inserted into the femoral canal alters vertical height. When cement is used, the vertical height can be adjusted further by variation in the level of the femoral neck osteotomy. This additional flexibility may be unavailable when a cementless femoral component is used because depth of insertion is determined more by the fit within the femoral metaphysis than by the level of the neck osteotomy.

Offset (i.e., horizontal offset) is the distance from the center of the femoral head to a line through the axis of the distal part of the stem and is primarily a function of stem design. Inadequate restoration of offset shortens the moment arm of the abductor musculature and results in increased joint reaction force, limp, and bone impingement, which may result in dislocation. Offset can be increased by simply using a longer modular neck, but doing so also increases vertical height, which may result in overlengthening of the limb. To address individual variations in femoral anatomy, many components are now manufactured with standard and high offset versions. This is accomplished by reducing the neck-stem angle (typically to about 127 degrees) or by attaching the neck to the stem in a more medial position (Fig. 1.9). Reduction of the neck-stem angle increases offset but also reduces vertical height slightly. When the neck is attached in a more medial position, offset is increased without changing height; leg length is therefore unaffected.

Version refers to the orientation of the neck in reference to the coronal plane and is denoted as *anteversion* or *retroversion*. Restoration of femoral neck version is important in achieving stability of the prosthetic joint. The normal femur has 10 to 15 degrees of anteversion of the femoral neck in relation to the coronal plane when the foot faces straight forward, and the prosthetic femoral neck should approximate this. Proper neck version usually is accomplished by rotating the component within the femoral canal. This presents little problem when cement is used for fixation; however, when press-fit fixation is used, the femoral component must be inserted in the same orientation as the femoral neck to maximize the fill of the proximal femur and achieve rotational stability of the implant. This problem can be circumvented by the use of a modular femoral component in which the stem is rotated independent of the metaphyseal portion. So-called anatomic stems have a slight proximal posterior bow to reproduce the contour of the femoral endosteum, predetermining the rotational alignment of the implant. Most such stems have a few degrees of anteversion built into the neck to compensate for this, and separate right and left stems are required. Finally, femoral components have been produced with dual modular necks in different geometries and lengths to allow the adjustment of length, offset, and version independently (Fig. 1.10). However, tribocorrosion at the taper junction between the neck and stem has been reported with these dual modular necks, and several of the designs have been either recalled or voluntarily withdrawn from the market. Consequently, their use has declined markedly over the past few years.

The size of the femoral head, the ratio of head and neck diameters, and the shape of the neck of the femoral component have a substantial effect on the range of motion of the hip,

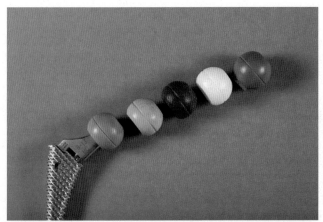

FIGURE 1.7 Modular heads for femoral components. Neck taper mates with modular femoral heads. Motion is absent between head and neck segments. Different diameter heads with various neck extensions are available. Extended neck, or "skirt," of longer components has larger diameter than neck of conventional components, and arc of motion of hip is decreased.

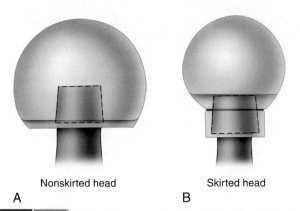

Nonskirted head   Skirted head
A   B

FIGURE 1.8 Head-to-neck ratio of implants. Large-diameter head with trapezoidal neck **(A)** has greater range of motion and less impingement than smaller diameter head and skirted modular neck **(B)**.

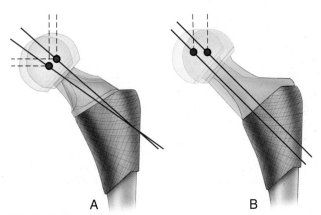

A   B

FIGURE 1.9 Variations in femoral component necks to increase offset. **A,** Neck-stem angle is reduced. **B,** Neck is attached at more medial position on stem. **SEE TECHNIQUE 1.5.**

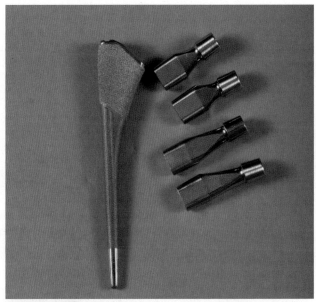

FIGURE 1.10 Modular femoral neck with taper junctions for stem body and femoral head. Multiple configurations allow independent adjustment of length and offset and version.

the degree of impingement between the neck and rim of the socket, and the stability of the articulation. This impingement can lead to dislocation, accelerated polyethylene wear, acetabular component loosening, and liner dislodgment or fracture. For a given neck diameter, the use of a larger femoral head increases the head-neck ratio and the range of motion before the neck impinges on the rim of the socket will be greater (Fig. 1.11). When this impingement does occur, the femoral head is levered out of the socket. The "jump distance" is the distance the head must travel to escape the rim of the socket and is generally approximated to be half the diameter of the head (Fig. 1.12). For both of these reasons, a larger-diameter head is theoretically more stable than a smaller one. In a large series of total hips performed with a head size of 36 mm or larger, Lombardi et al. reported a dislocation rate of only 0.05%. The introduction of advanced bearing surfaces has allowed the use of larger head sizes than those traditionally used in the past. In practical terms, the femoral head diameter is limited by the size of the acetabulum, regardless of the bearing materials used for the femoral head and acetabulum.

In a range-of-motion simulation with digitized implants and virtual reality software, Barrack et al. found an improvement of 8 degrees of hip flexion when head size was increased from 28 to 32 mm. Range of motion was dramatically reduced by the use of a circular neck, especially when combined with a skirted modular head, which increases the diameter of the femoral neck (Fig. 1.13). A trapezoidal neck yielded greater range of motion without impingement than a circular one (Fig. 1.14). In an experimental range-of-motion model with head sizes larger than 32 mm, Burroughs et al. found that impingement between prosthetic components could be largely eliminated. When a head size larger than 38 mm was used, however, the only impingement was bone on bone and was dependent on bony anatomy and independent of head size. The ideal configuration of the prosthetic head and neck segment includes a trapezoidal neck and a larger diameter head without a skirt.

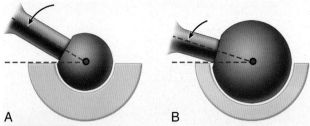

FIGURE 1.11 Range of motion with different head sizes. For given diameter neck, implant with smaller femoral head (**A**) will have lesser arc of motion than larger one (**B**).

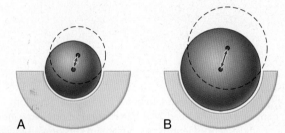

FIGURE 1.12 Jump distance. With subluxation, smaller head (**A**) has shorter distance to travel before escaping rim of acetabular component than larger one (**B**).

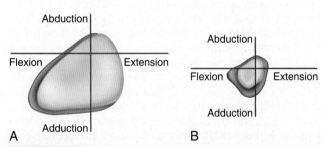

FIGURE 1.13 Effects of head size and neck geometry on range of motion. **A,** Changing from 28-mm head *(light shading)* to 32-mm head *(dark shading)* results in 8-degree increase in flexion before impingement. **B,** Large circular taper has dramatically decreased range of motion to impingement *(dark shading),* which is diminished even further by having skirted modular head *(light shading).* (From Barrack RL, Lavernia C, Ries M, et al: Virtual reality computer animation of the effect of component position and design on stability after total hip arthroplasty, *Orthop Clin North Am* 32:569, 2001.)

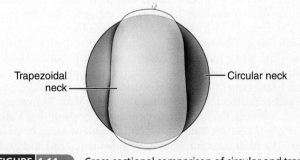

FIGURE 1.14 Cross-sectional comparison of circular and trapezoidal neck.

All total hip systems in current use achieve fixation of the femoral prosthesis with a metal stem that is inserted into the medullary canal. Much of the design innovation to increase prosthetic longevity has been directed toward improvement in fixation of the implant within the femoral canal. Many femoral stems have been in clinical use for variable periods since the 1990s. Recognition of the radiographic profile of a stem is often beneficial, however, in planning revision surgery. Readers are directed to previous editions of this text and other historical references for this information.

Femoral components are available in both cemented and cementless varieties.

■ CEMENTED FEMORAL COMPONENTS

With the introduction of the Charnley low-friction arthroplasty, acrylic cement became the standard for femoral component fixation. Advances in stem design and in the application of cement have dramatically improved the long-term survivorship of cemented stems. Despite these advances, the use of cement for femoral fixation has declined precipitously over the past decade and there has been little recent innovation in implant design. Nonetheless, worldwide registry data suggest that in patients older than 75 years outcomes are better with cemented femoral fixation, owing mainly to a lower risk of periprosthetic fracture.

Certain design features of cemented stems have become generally accepted. The stem should be fabricated of high-strength superalloy. Most designers favor cobalt-chrome alloy because its higher modulus of elasticity may reduce stresses within the proximal cement mantle. The cross section of the stem should have a broad medial border and preferably broader lateral border to load the proximal cement mantle in compression. Sharp edges produce local stress risers that may initiate fracture of the cement mantle and should be avoided. A collar aids in determining the depth of insertion at implantation.

Mounting evidence suggests that failure of cemented stems is initiated at the prosthesis-cement interface with debonding and subsequent cement fracture. Various types of surface macrotexturing can improve the bond at this interface (Figs. 1.15 to 1.17). The practice of precoating the stem with polymethyl methacrylate (PMMA) has been associated with a higher than normal failure rate with some stem designs and has largely been abandoned. Noncircular shapes, such as a rounded rectangle or an ellipse, and surface irregularities, such as grooves or a longitudinal slot, also improve the rotational stability of the stem within the cement mantle (see Fig. 1.17).

There is concern that even with surface modifications the stem may not remain bonded to the cement. If debonding does occur, a stem with a roughened or textured surface generates more debris with motion than a stem with a smooth, polished surface. Higher rates of loosening and bone resorption were found with the use of an Exeter stem with a matte surface than with an identical stem with a polished surface. Similar findings have been reported when comparing the original polished Charnley stem with its subsequent matte-finish modification. For this reason, interest has been renewed in the use of polished stems for cemented applications. Ling recommended a design that is collarless, polished, and tapered in two planes (Fig. 1.18) to allow a

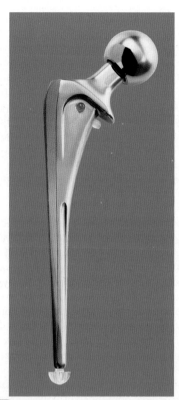

FIGURE 1.15 Summit stem. Integral proximal polymethyl methacrylate spacers and additional centralizer facilitate proper stem position and uniform cement mantle. (Courtesy DePuy Synthes Orthopaedics, Inc., Warsaw, IN.)

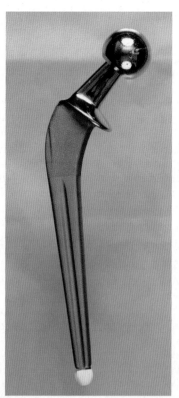

FIGURE 1.17 Spectron EF stem. Rounded rectangular shape and longitudinal groove improve rotational stability. (Courtesy Smith & Nephew, Memphis, TN.)

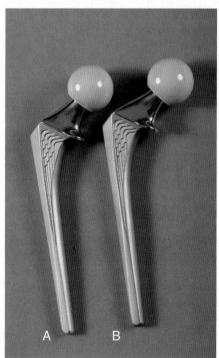

FIGURE 1.16 Omnifit EON stem. Normalized proximal texturing converts shear forces to compressive forces. **A,** Standard offset. **B,** Enhanced offset. (Courtesy Stryker Orthopaedics, Kalamazoo, MI.)

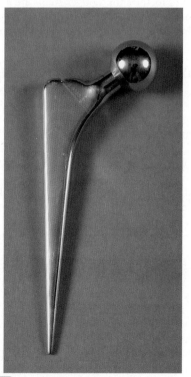

FIGURE 1.18 Collarless, polished, tapered (CPT) hip stem. CPT design allows controlled subsidence and maintains compressive stresses within cement mantle. (Courtesy Zimmer Biomet, Warsaw, IN.)

small amount of subsidence and to maintain compressive stresses within the cement mantle. Such implants are often referred to as taper-slip or force-closed devices. A collar on a polished stem is to be avoided since it may prevent this controlled subsidence. Registry data support a lower rate of loosening in the long term with polished stems than with matte finished stems.

Stems should be available in a variety of sizes (typically four to six) to allow the stem to occupy approximately 80% of the cross section of the medullary canal with an optimal cement mantle of approximately 4 mm proximally and 2 mm distally. Neutral stem placement within the canal lessens the chance of localized areas of thin cement mantle, which may become fragmented and cause loosening of the stem. Some designs have preformed PMMA centralizers that are affixed to the distal or proximal aspects, or both, of the stem before implantation to centralize the stem within the femoral canal and provide a more uniform cement mantle (see Fig. 1.15). The centralizers bond to the new cement and are incorporated into the cement mantle.

Finally, the optimal length of the stem depends on the geometry and size of the femoral canal. The stem of the original Charnley component was about 13 cm long. This was long enough to obtain secure fixation in the metaphysis and proximal diaphysis of the femur. A stem of longer length, which engages the isthmus, makes it more difficult to err and place the stem in a varus position. As a result of the normal anterior bow of the femoral canal, however, the tip of the stem may impinge on the anterior cortex or even perforate it when the cortex is thin. In addition, it is technically difficult to occlude the canal below the level of the isthmus adequately, and the result may be an inadequate column of cement around the stem and beyond the tip. The lengths of current stem designs range from 120 to 150 mm. Longer stems are available if the cortex has been perforated, fractured, or weakened by screw holes or other internal fixation devices and particularly for revision procedures.

■ CEMENTLESS FEMORAL COMPONENTS

In the mid-1970s, problems related to the fixation of femoral components with acrylic cement began to emerge. As a result, considerable laboratory and clinical investigations have been performed in an effort to eliminate cement and provide for biologic fixation of femoral components. The two prerequisites for biologic fixation are immediate mechanical stability at the time of surgery and intimate contact between the implant surface and viable host bone. To fulfill these requirements, implants must be designed to fit the endosteal cavity of the femur as closely as possible. Still, the femur must be prepared to some degree to match accurately the stem that is to be inserted. In general, the selection of implant type and size must be more precise than with their cemented counterparts. Current cementless stem designs differ in their materials, surface coating, and shape.

Experience has been confined largely to the use of two materials: (1) titanium alloy with one of a variety of surface enhancements and (2) cobalt-chromium alloy with a sintered beaded surface. Both materials have proved to be satisfactory. Titanium has been recommended by many designers because of its superior biocompatibility, high fatigue strength, and lower modulus of elasticity. Titanium is more notch-sensitive than cobalt-chrome alloy, however, predisposing it to

initiation of cracks through metallurgic defects and at sites of attachment of porous coatings. When the stem is of a titanium substrate, the porous surface must be restricted to the bulkier proximal portions of the stem and away from areas that sustain significant tensile stresses, such as on the lateral border of the stem. Titanium alloy has been recommended as the material of choice because its modulus of elasticity is approximately half that of cobalt-chromium alloy and therefore less likely to be associated with thigh pain. However, Lavernia et al. reported titanium alloy and cobalt-chromium alloy stems of an identical tapered design in 241 patients. Thigh pain was unrelated to the material composition of the stem but was more common in patients with a larger stem size.

A variety of surface modifications including porous coatings, grit blasting, plasma spraying, and hydroxyapatite coating have been used to enhance implant fixation. Many cementless femoral component designs feature combinations of these surface enhancements. Although the type and extent of coating necessary is controversial, most experts agree that it should be circumferential at its proximal boundary. Some early porous stem designs used patches or pads of porous coating with intervening smooth areas, which allowed joint fluid to transport particulate debris to the distal aspect of the stem. Schmalzried et al. referred to these extensions of joint fluid as the "effective joint space." This design feature has been associated with early development of osteolysis around the tip of the stem despite bone ingrowth proximally. Circumferential porous coating of the proximal aspect of the stem provides a more effective barrier to the ingress of particles and limits the early development of osteolysis around the distal aspect of the stem.

Bone ingrowth into a porous coating has demonstrated durable fixation for a multitude of cementless stem designs. Porous coatings have historically been created by either beads or fiber mesh (Fig. 1.19A and B) applied to the stem by sintering or diffusion bonding processes. Both processes require heating of the underlying substrate and can cause significant reduction in the fatigue strength of the implant. A considerable volume of research has determined the optimal pore size for bone ingrowth into a porous surface to be between 100 and 400 μm. Most porous-coated implants currently available have pore sizes in this range. Highly porous metals such as tantalum were initially utilized for cementless fixation of acetabular components but have more recently been applied to femoral stems also (Fig. 1.19C). Porous metals have higher porosity than traditional porous coatings, and their high coefficient of friction against cancellous bone may improve their initial stability. Porous tantalum closely resembles the structure of cancellous bone. Rapid and extensive bone ingrowth into this implant surface has been reported.

Bone ongrowth implies growth of bone onto a roughened (albeit nonporous) surface. Ongrowth surfaces are created by grit blasting or plasma spray techniques. Grit blasting involves the use of a pressurized spray of aluminum oxide particles to produce an irregular surface ranging from 3 to 8 μm in depth (Fig. 1.20A). Plasma spray techniques use high-velocity application of molten metal onto the substrate in a vacuum or argon gas environment and produce a highly textured surface (Fig. 1.20B). Heating of the implant is not required, and, consequently, there is little reduction in fatigue strength compared with the application of porous coatings. Hydroxyapatite

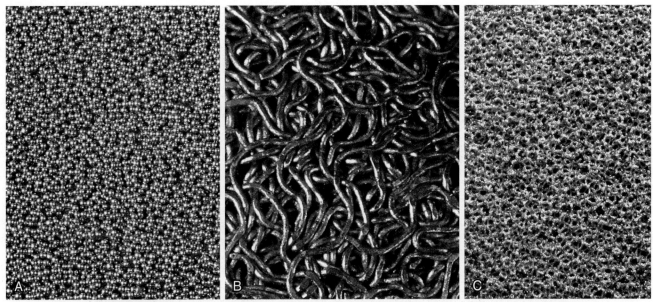

FIGURE 1.19 Types of bone ingrowth surfaces. Traditional surfaces produced from sintered beads (**A**) and diffusion bonded fiber mesh (**B**). **C,** Newer highly porous tantalum more closely resembles structure of trabecular bone. (**A** courtesy Smith & Nephew, Memphis, TN; **B** and **C** courtesy Zimmer Biomet, Warsaw, IN.)

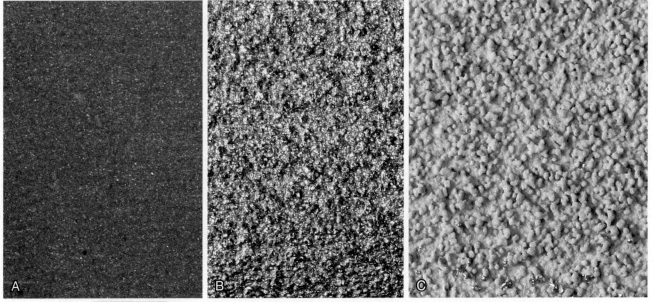

FIGURE 1.20 Types of bone ongrowth surfaces. **A,** Grit-blasted surface. More highly textured plasma-sprayed surfaces: titanium (**B**) and hydroxyapatite (**C**). (**A,** Courtesy Zimmer, Warsaw, IN; **B,** Courtesy Biomet Orthopedics, Warsaw, IN; **C,** Courtesy Stryker Orthopaedics, Mahwah, NJ.)

and other osteoconductive calcium phosphate coatings can also be applied to implants by plasma spray (Fig. 1.20C). The thickness of the coating is typically 50 to 155 μm. Although the literature reports mixed results with regard to whether hydroxyapatite coating improves outcomes, there is no evidence that it is deleterious.

The evolution of cementless femoral fixation has resulted in a variety of implants. The shape of a cementless stem determines the areas of the femoral canal where fixation is obtained and the surgical technique required for implantation. Outcomes are also generally more dependent on stem

geometry than on either materials or surface enhancements. Khanuja, Vakil, Goddard, and Mont proposed a classification system for cementless stems based on shape. Types 1 through 5 are straight stems, and fixation area increases with type. Type 6 is an anatomic shape.

Type 1 stems are so-called single-wedge stems. They are flat in the anteroposterior plane and tapered in the mediolateral plane (Fig. 1.21). Fixation is by cortical engagement only in the mediolateral plane and by three-point fixation along the length of the stem. The femoral canal is prepared by broaching alone, with no distal reaming. Consequently, it

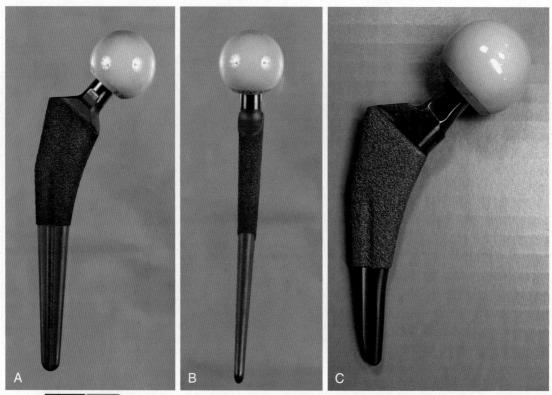

FIGURE 1.21 Taperloc stem. Single wedge design is tapered in medial-lateral plane **(A)** and flat in anteroposterior plane. **B,** Plasma-sprayed proximal surface. **C,** Shortened microplasty version. (Courtesy Zimmer Biomet, Warsaw, IN.)

is important to ensure that the stem is wedged proximally. In Dorr type A femurs, distal engagement alone risks fracture or rotational instability. Consequently, many of these designs have been modified with reduced distal sizing to avoid this problem. These stems have performed well in Dorr type B and C femurs.

Type 2 stems engage the proximal femoral cortex in both mediolateral and anteroposterior planes. So-called dual-wedge designs fill the proximal femoral metaphysis more completely than type 1 stems (Fig. 1.22). Femoral preparation typically requires distal reaming followed by broaching of the proximal femur. They can be used safely in Dorr type A femurs.

Type 3 represents a more disparate group of implants. These stems are tapered in two planes, but fixation is achieved more at the metaphyseal-diaphyseal junction than proximally as with types 1 and 2. Type 3A stems are tapered with a round conical distal geometry. Longitudinal cutting flutes are added to type 3B stems (Fig. 1.23). These implants have recently gained popularity in complex revision cases. Type 3C implants are rectangular and thus provide four-point rotational support (Fig. 1.24). Such implants have been used extensively in Europe with success.

Type 4 are extensively coated implants with fixation along the entire length of the stem. Canal preparation requires distal cylindrical reaming and proximal broaching (Fig. 1.25). Excellent long-term results have been achieved with these implants. Femoral stress shielding and thigh pain have been reported with various designs. Their use in Dorr type C femurs can be problematic because of the large stem diameter required.

Type 5 or modular stems have separate metaphyseal sleeves and diaphyseal segments that are independently sized and instrumented. Such implants often are recommended for patients with altered femoral anatomy, particularly those with rotational malalignment such as developmental dysplasia. Both stem segments are prepared with reamers, leading to a precise fit with rotational stability obtained both proximally and distally. This feature makes modular stems an attractive option when femoral osteotomy is required (Fig. 1.26). Modular stems can be used for all Dorr bone types, but increased cost and potential problems with modular junctions should be taken into account.

Type 6 or anatomic femoral components incorporate a posterior bow in the metaphyseal portion and variably an anterior bow in the diaphyseal portion, corresponding to the geometry of the femoral canal (Fig. 1.27). Right and left stems are required, and anteversion must be built into the neck segment. Anatomic variability in the curvature of the femur usually requires some degree of overreaming of the canal; if the tip of the stem is eccentrically placed, it impinges on the anterior cortex. This point loading has been suggested to be a source of postoperative thigh pain. The popularity of anatomic stems has declined over the past decade in favor of straight designs.

With cementless devices, the requirements for canal filling often mean the stem must be of sizable diameter. Because stiffness of a stem is proportional to the fourth power of the diameter, an increased prevalence of femoral stress shielding can be seen with larger stems. The mismatch in stiffness between implant and bone also has been cited as a cause of postoperative thigh pain. Current stem designs deal with this problem in

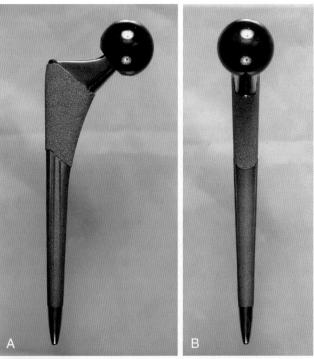

FIGURE 1.22 Synergy stem. Dual wedge design is tapered in medial-lateral **(A)** and anteroposterior **(B)** planes. Longitudinal flutes provide additional rotational stability. Shown with oxidized Zirconia head. (Courtesy Smith & Nephew, Memphis, TN.)

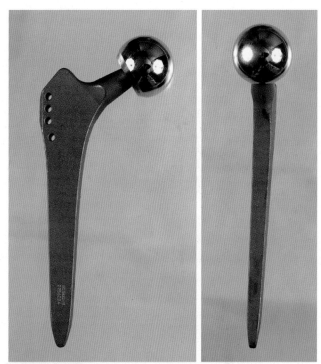

FIGURE 1.24 Alloclassic stem. Conical straight stem with rectangular cross-section and grit-blasted nonporous surface. (Courtesy Zimmer Biomet, Warsaw, IN.)

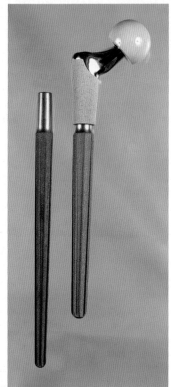

FIGURE 1.23 Restoration modular stem. Tapered round conical distal geometry with longitudinal cutting flutes are available in varying lengths for primary and revision indications. Proximal segments are available in various lengths and offsets for soft-tissue tensioning. (Courtesy Stryker Orthopaedics, Mahwah, NJ.)

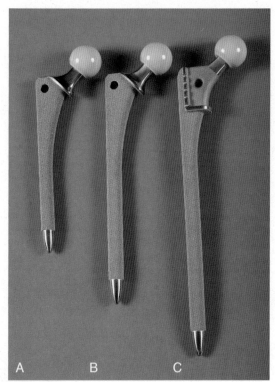

FIGURE 1.25 Extensively porous-coated stems. **A,** Anatomic medullary locking (AML) stem for primary and revision arthroplasties when isthmus is intact. **B,** Extensively coated solution long stem used for revisions when proximal bone loss is severe. **C,** Calcar replacement long stem. (Courtesy Depuy Synthes, Warsaw, IN.)

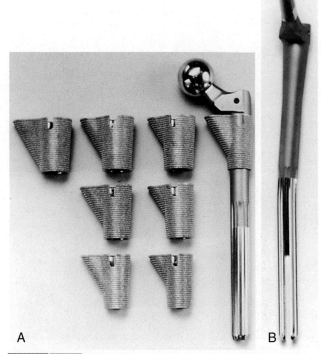

FIGURE 1.26   S-ROM modular stem. **A,** Multiple proximal sleeve sizes can be combined with given diameter stem. Stem can be rotated in relation to sleeve to correct rotational deformity of femur. Distal flutes improve rotational stability. **B,** Long curved stem. Distal part of stem is slotted in coronal plane to diminish bending stiffness. (Courtesy Depuy Synthes, Warsaw, IN.)

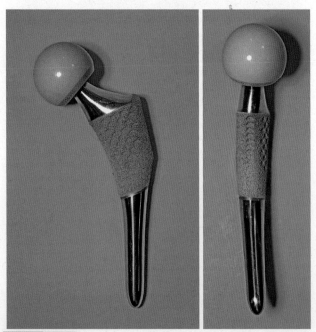

FIGURE 1.27   Anato anatomic stem. Asymmetric metaphyseal shape conforms more closely to proximal femoral geometry. Femoral neck is anteverted **7** degrees, and dedicated right and left stems are required. (Courtesy Stryker Orthopedics, Mahwah, NJ.)

several ways. The section modulus of the stem can be changed to allow greater flexibility while leaving the implant diameter unchanged so that stability is not compromised. The addition of deep, longitudinal grooves reduces bending and torsional stiffness. The bending stiffness in the distal third of the stem also can be reduced substantially by splitting the stem in the coronal plane, similar to a clothespin (see Fig. 1.26). Tapered distal stem geometries are inherently less stiff than cylindrical ones (see Fig. 1.22) and have been associated with minimal thigh pain.

A considerable amount of data supports a superiority of cementless femoral fixation in younger patients. Takenaga et al. reported a series of extensively porous-coated stems in patients 59 years of age or younger. At a minimum of 10 years after surgery no stems showed radiographic signs of loosening or had undergone revision for loosening. Survivorship was better than in a cohort of cemented stems from the same institution. McLaughlin and Lee reported a series of single-wedge design stems in patients younger than 50 years. At a minimum follow-up of 20 years, no stems were revised for aseptic loosening. Costa, Johnson, and Mont reported 96% survivorship at mean follow-up of 5 years in a series of patients who had arthroplasty at a mean age of 20 years. Using a stem fully coated with hydroxyapatite, Jacquot et al. reported a 30-year survival of 93.6% with stem revision as the endpoint. Evidence supporting the use of cementless femoral fixation in patients over the age of 75 is less compelling. Registry data and individual series both call attention to a higher rate of revision for periprosthetic fractures in this population.

■ SPECIALIZED AND CUSTOM-MADE FEMORAL COMPONENTS

The adoption of minimally invasive surgical techniques has generated interest in shorter bone-sparing femoral implants. Some are novel implants designed to fit within the intact ring of bone of the femoral neck (Fig. 1.28). Others are shortened versions of existing designs described previously (see Fig. 1.21C). These implants have been used most commonly in minimally invasive anterior approaches where access to the femoral canal is more difficult. A shorter stem also avoids the problem of proximal-distal mismatch encountered with conventional length stems in Dorr type A femurs. Ideally, short femoral stems should allow retention of a longer segment of the femoral neck and increased physiologic load transfer in the proximal femur to reduce bone loss. Data supporting the use of these implants are limited. The surgical technique must be more precise to avoid varus malalignment and undersizing. Subsidence has been reported more commonly with some designs.

Despite the large array of femoral components available, deformity or bone loss from congenital conditions, trauma, tumors, or previous surgery may make it impossible for any standard stem to fit the femur or restore adequately the position of the femoral head. Several types of calcar replacement femoral components (see Fig. 1.25C) are available for patients with loss of varying amounts of the proximal femur in lieu of the use of bone grafts. Limb salvage procedures for some malignant or aggressive benign bone and soft-tissue tumors may require a customized component. Modular segmental replacement stems also are used in patients with extensive femoral bone loss from multiple failed arthroplasty procedures and periprosthetic fractures (Fig. 1.29). Rarely, a

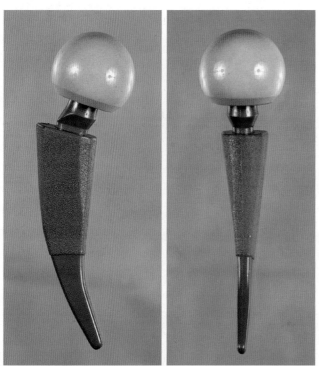

FIGURE 1.28 Metha short hip stem. Designed for less-invasive surgery with retention of femoral neck and metaphyseal fixation (shown with modular neck). (Courtesy Aesculap Implant Systems, LLC, Center Valley, PA.)

prosthesis may be required to replace the entire femur, incorporating hip and knee arthroplasties.

Customized, cementless, CT-generated computer-assisted design/computer-assisted manufacturing (CAD/CAM) prostheses have been recommended when preoperative planning indicates that an off-the-shelf prosthesis cannot provide optimal fit or when excessive bone removal would be required. Such implants require a carefully made preoperative CT scan of the acetabulum, hip joint, and femur. An identical broach is supplied with the implant to prepare the femur. Customized femoral components also have been recommended for revision surgery with proximal femoral osteolysis, congenital hip dislocation, excessively large femurs, and grossly abnormal anatomy and when a fracture has occurred below the tip of a femoral stem. With the proliferation of newer revision stem designs and techniques of femoral osteotomy for revision procedures, custom stems are seldom needed in our practice.

ACETABULAR COMPONENTS

Acetabular components can be broadly categorized as cemented or cementless. Acetabular reconstruction rings also are discussed in this section.

■ CEMENTED ACETABULAR COMPONENTS

The original sockets for cemented use were thick-walled polyethylene cups. Vertical and horizontal grooves often were added to the external surface to increase stability within the cement mantle, and wire markers were embedded in the plastic to allow better assessment of position on postoperative radiographs. Many of these designs are still in regular use.

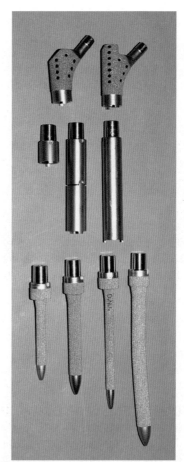

FIGURE 1.29 Specialized femoral components for replacement of variable length of proximal femur. Orthogenesis limb preservation system uses modular segmental replacement stem for replacement of large segment of proximal femur. Stem can be combined with total knee replacement to replace entire femur. (Courtesy Depuy Synthes, Warsaw, IN.)

More recent designs have modifications that ensure a more uniform cement mantle. PMMA spacers, typically 3 mm in height, ensure a uniform cement mantle and avoid the phenomenon of "bottoming out," which results in a thin or discontinuous cement mantle (Fig. 1.30). A flange at the rim of the component aids in pressurization of the cement as the cup is pressed into position.

Despite such changes in implant design, the long-term survivorship of cemented acetabular components has not substantially improved. Consequently, there has been a trend toward cementless fixation of acetabular components in most patients. The simplicity and low cost of all-polyethylene components make them a satisfactory option in older, low-demand patients.

At times, cement is also used as the means of fixation of a polyethylene insert into an acetabular component that lacks an intrinsic locking mechanism for the polyethylene or when a dedicated insert is not available for a cementless acetabular component that is to be retained during revision surgery. Cemented acetabular fixation also is used in some tumor reconstructions and when operative circumstances indicate that bone ingrowth into a porous surface is unlikely, as in revision arthroplasty in which extensive acetabular bone

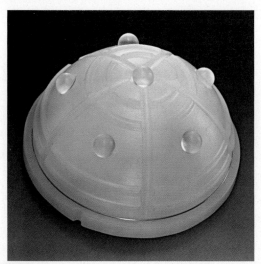

FIGURE 1.30 Acetabular component designed for cement fixation. Textured surface and polymethyl methacrylate spacers optimize cement mantle and cement-prosthesis interface. (Courtesy Smith & Nephew, Memphis, TN.)

grafting has been necessary. In these instances, a cemented acetabular component often is used with an acetabular reconstruction ring (see Fig. 1.36).

■ CEMENTLESS ACETABULAR COMPONENTS

Most cementless acetabular components are porous-coated over their entire circumference for bone ingrowth. Instrumentation typically provides for oversizing of the implant 1 to 2 mm larger than the reamed acetabulum as the primary method of press-fit fixation. Fixation of the porous shell with transacetabular screws has become commonplace but carries some risk to intrapelvic vessels and viscera and requires flexible instruments for screw insertion. Analyses of retrieved porous acetabular components showed that bone ingrowth occurs most reliably in the vicinity of the fixation devices, such as pegs or screws. The most extensive ingrowth has been reported in components initially fixed with one or more screws. Pegs, fins, and spikes driven into prepared recesses in the bone provide some rotational stability, but less than that obtained with screws. The use of these other types of supplemental fixation devices has declined as manufacturers have incorporated highly porous metal coatings with improved initial press-fixation (Figs. 1.31 and 1.32). Solid metal shells without screw holes have not proven beneficial in reducing the presence or size of osteolytic lesions; their use has consequently diminished.

Hydroxyapatite coating has been advocated in the past to enhance bone ingrowth into the porous coating of cementless acetabular components. The process has not demonstrated improved survivorship, and with the introduction of newer porous surfaces, the use of hydroxyapatite coating has declined.

Most systems feature a metal shell with an outside diameter of 40 to 75 mm that is used with a modular insert, also called a liner. With this combination, a variety of femoral head sizes, typically 22 to 40 mm, can be accommodated according to the patient's need and the surgeon's preference. The liner must be fastened securely within the metal shell. These mechanisms of fixation have been under increasing scrutiny

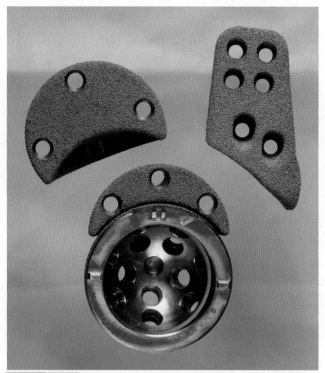

FIGURE 1.31 Zimmer trabecular metal acetabular component with various modular augments for bony deficiencies. (Courtesy Zimmer Biomet, Warsaw, IN.)

because in vivo dissociation of polyethylene liners from their metal backings has been reported. In addition, micromotion between the nonarticulating side of the liner and the interior of the shell may be a source of polyethylene debris generation, or "backside wear." Recognition of this problem has led to improvements in the fixation of the liner within the metal shell, and some designs also have included polishing the interior of the shell. Monoblock acetabular components with nonmodular polyethylene also have been produced to alleviate the problem of backside wear but have not proven to be superior to modular implants.

With the adoption of newer bearing surfaces and dual mobility implants (see Fig. 1.35), manufacturers have introduced acetabular components that will accept any of a variety of insert types. Newer locking mechanisms typically incorporate a taper junction near the rim for hard bearings. The polyethylene locking mechanism may be recessed within the shell where it is less susceptible to damage if impingement from the femoral neck occurs (Fig. 1.32B).

Finally, the issue of excessive wear of thin shells of polyethylene is a major concern. The metal backing must be of sufficient thickness to avoid fatigue failure, and there must be a corresponding decrease in thickness of the polyethylene insert for a component of any given outer diameter. High stresses within the polyethylene are likely when the thickness of the plastic is less than 5 mm, leaving the component at risk for premature failure as a result of wear. To maintain sufficient thickness of the polyethylene, a smaller head size must be used with an acetabular component that has a small outer diameter.

Most modern modular acetabular components are supplied with a variety of polyethylene insert choices. Some

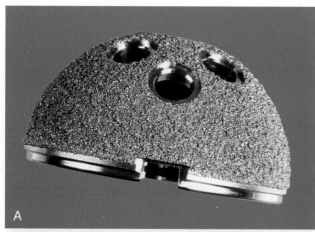

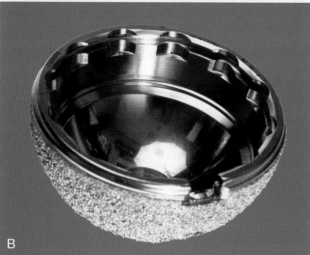

FIGURE 1.32 R3 acetabular component. **A,** Hemispherical shell with optional screw fixation and highly porous titanium coating. **B,** Locking mechanism is recessed to avoid thin polyethylene at rim and accept various bearing inserts. (Courtesy Smith & Nephew Orthopaedics, Memphis, TN.)

designs incorporate an elevation over a portion of the circumference of the rim, whereas others completely reorient the opening face of the socket up to 20 degrees. Still other designs simply lateralize the hip center without reorienting its opening face (Fig. 1.33). Lateralization also allows for the use of a larger-diameter head while maintaining adequate polyethylene thickness. Such designs can compensate for slight aberrations in the placement of the metal shell and improve the stability of the articulation; however, with elevated rim liners, motion can be increased in some directions but decreased in others. An improperly positioned elevation in the liner can cause impingement rather than relieve it, rendering the joint unstable. With larger-diameter femoral heads, elevated rim liners are being used less frequently.

A constrained acetabular component includes a mechanism to lock the prosthetic femoral head into the polyethylene liner. The tripolar-style mechanism features a small inner bipolar bearing that articulates with an outer true liner (Fig. 1.34A). The bipolar segment is larger than the introitus of the outer liner, preventing dislocation. Other designs use a liner with added polyethylene at the rim that deforms to capture the femoral head. A locking ring is applied to the rim to prevent

escape of the head (Fig. 1.34B). Other unique designs are also available from individual manufacturers. Indications for constrained liners include insufficient soft tissues, deficient hip abductors, neuromuscular disease, and hips with recurrent dislocation despite well-positioned implants. Constrained acetabular liners have reduced range of motion compared with conventional inserts. Consequently, they are more prone to failure because of prosthetic impingement. A constrained liner should not be used to compensate for an improperly positioned shell, and skirted femoral heads should be avoided in combination with constrained inserts.

A dual mobility acetabular component is an unconstrained tripolar design. The implant consists of a porous-coated metal shell with a polished interior that accepts a large polyethylene ball into which a smaller metal or ceramic head is inserted (Fig. 1.35). The two areas of articulation share the same motion center. The design effectively increases the head size and the head-neck ratio of the construct. Implant impingement is reduced and stability is improved without reducing the range of motion as with constrained implants. A modular metal shell and insert are available for cases in which screw fixation may be required. In a large series of primary total hip arthroplasties using a dual mobility implant, Combes et al. reported a dislocation rate of 0.88%. Wegrzyn et al. reported dislocations in 1.5% of revision cases. Also reported are intraprosthetic dislocations between the small head and polyethylene ball. As with constrained acetabular devices, dual mobility components cannot be relied on to compensate for technical errors in implant positioning.

Custom components for acetabular reconstruction rarely are indicated. Most deficient acetabula can be restored to a hemispherical shape, and a standard, albeit large, acetabular component can be inserted. In patients with a large superior segmental bone deficiency, the resulting acetabular recess is elliptical rather than hemispherical. A cementless acetabular component with modular porous metal augments (see Fig. 1.31) can be used instead of a large structural graft or excessively high placement of a hemispherical component. Augments of various sizes are screwed into bony defects to support the acetabular component. The augments are joined to the implant with the use of bone cement.

With the introduction of revision implants with augments, custom components for acetabular reconstruction rarely are indicated. When bony deficits are massive, a custom implant can be produced based on a CT scan with subtraction of the metal artifacts. The imaging requirements vary according to the manufacturer. Such implants typically have both superior and inferior flanges that rest on intact bone and provide for additional screw fixation. The placement of the flanges, screw locations, and trajectories can all be built into the plan. Typically, a detailed 3D-printed model of the bony pelvis (Fig. 1.36) and proposed implant are produced before the actual implant is manufactured (Fig. 1.37).

Historically, metal rings, wire mesh, and other materials have been used to improve acetabular fixation. These devices were intended to reinforce cement, and generally their long-term performance was poor. More recently, numerous acetabular reconstruction rings have been introduced to allow bone grafting of the deficient acetabulum behind the ring, rather than relying on cement on both sides of the device. (Cement is used only to secure an all-polyethylene acetabular component to the ring.) The reconstruction ring provides

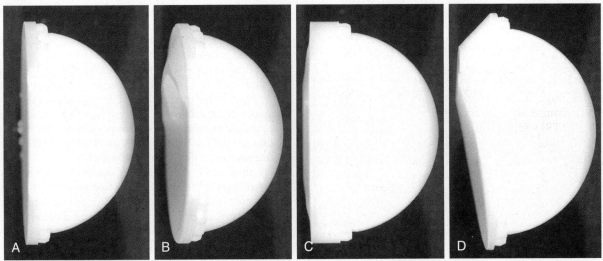

FIGURE 1.33 Array of liner options available with contemporary modular acetabular system: standard flat liner **(A)**, posterior lip without anteversion **(B)**, 4-mm lateralized flat **(C)**, and anteverted 20 degrees **(D)**. (Courtesy Smith & Nephew, Memphis, TN.) **SEE TECHNIQUE 1.3.**

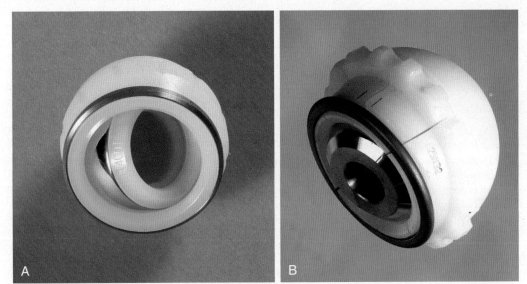

FIGURE 1.34 **A,** Tripolar design with small bipolar shell captured within outer liner. **B,** Peripheral locking ring design. (**A** courtesy Stryker Orthopaedics, Mahwah, NJ; **B** courtesy Zimmer Biomet, Warsaw, IN.)

immediate support for the acetabular component and protects bone grafts from excessive early stresses while union occurs. These devices are commonly referred to as *antiprotrusio rings* and *cages.*

The preferred devices are those with superior and inferior plate extensions that provide fixation into the ilium and the ischium (Fig. 1.38). Success with these devices depends on selection of the proper device and careful attention to technique. Implantation of the antiprotrusio cage requires full exposure of the external surface of the posterior column for safe positioning and screw insertion. Alternatively, the inferior plate can be inset into a prepared recess in the ischium without the need for inferiorly placed screws. For all types of devices, dome screws are placed before the plates are attached to the external surface of the ilium. Results to date seem to be

best when the device is supported superiorly by intact host bone rather than by bone grafts. These implants do not provide for long-term biologic fixation and are prone to fracture and loosening. The advent of highly porous metal implants has reduced the need for cages in current practice. Rarely, an antiprotrusio cage may be used in tandem with a revision acetabular shell. This "cup-cage" construct has greater potential for biologic fixation.

ALTERNATIVE BEARINGS

Osteolysis secondary to polyethylene particulate debris has emerged as a notable factor endangering the long-term survivorship of total hip replacements. Several alternative bearings have been advocated to diminish this problem, particularly in younger, more active patients who are at higher risk for rapid polyethylene wear. Newer highly crosslinked polyethylenes have now largely replaced traditional ultra-high molecular weight polyethylene (UHMWPE) in hip arthroplasty. The material is mated with a femoral head of either cobalt-chromium alloy or ceramic. This has become the dominant bearing couple used in hip arthroplasty today. Investigation continues on ceramic-on-ceramic bearings. The initial enthusiasm for large-head metal-on-metal bearings has waned with reports of adverse local tissue response (ALTR) with these implants, and their use has largely been abandoned. Metal-on-metal resurfacing arthroplasty remains a viable option in younger, male patients.

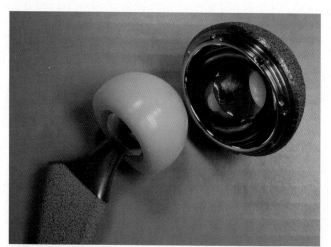

FIGURE 1.35 Dual mobility acetabular component. Porous-coated shell with polished interior, large polyethylene head, and smaller inner bearing. (Courtesy Stryker Orthopaedics, Mahwah, NJ.)

HIGHLY CROSSLINKED POLYETHYLENE

Historically, polyethylene implants have been sterilized by subjecting them to 2.5 Mrad of either electron-beam or gamma radiation. These processes produce free radicals in the material, however, predisposing the polyethylene to oxidation and rendering it more susceptible to wear. Higher doses of radiation can produce polyethylene with a more highly crosslinked molecular structure. Initial testing of this material has shown remarkable wear resistance. Crosslinking is accomplished by either gamma or electron-beam radiation at a dose between 5 and 10 Mrad. However, the radiation process also generates uncombined free radicals. If these are allowed to remain, the material is rendered more susceptible to severe oxidative degradation. The concentration of these free radicals can be reduced by a postirradiation heating process, either remelting or annealing. Remelting entails heating the material above its melting point (approximately 135°C). Free radicals are virtually eliminated with remelting, but the crystallinity of the resulting material is also reduced. The decrease in crystallinity diminishes the material properties of polyethylene, particularly fracture toughness and ultimate tensile strength. *Annealing* refers to a process of heating the material just below the melting point. This avoids the reduction in crystallinity and consequent reduction in mechanical properties, but annealing is less effective than remelting in extinguishing residual free radicals. Newer manufacturing methods have sought to mitigate the deleterious effects of remelting. Soaking the radiated polyethylene in vitamin E (or vitamin E "doping") appears to be effective in scavenging free radicals without a remelting stage. Another process applies the radiation in three smaller doses with annealing after each stage. Terminal sterilization is most commonly done with

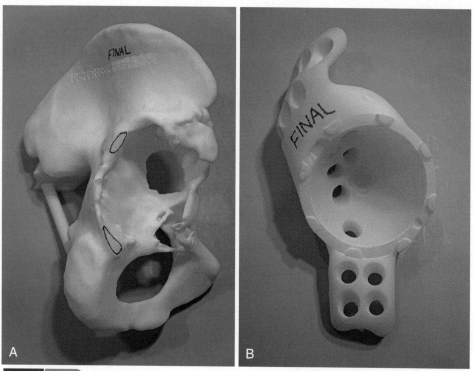

FIGURE 1.36 Custom triflange acetabular model. **A,** CT-based model showing large acetabular deficiencies. **B,** Custom acetabular component has intimate fit and flanges for multiple screw fixation.

either gas plasma or ethylene oxide because gamma radiation would generate additional free radicals. The processes used by individual manufacturers for production of highly cross-linked polyethylenes are proprietary and differ in the initial resin used, the amount and type of radiation used, the use of postirradiation thermal processing, and the method of terminal sterilization. Although early clinical results for all methods are encouraging, the long-term performance of these materials may vary and will need to be studied individually.

Test data from contemporary hip simulators have shown an 80% to 90% reduction in wear with highly crosslinked polyethylenes. When tested in conditions of third-body wear with abrasive particulates or against a roughened counterface, crosslinked polyethylene has improved wear performance substantially compared with conventional polyethylene. Muratoglu et al. showed that the wear rate of this material is not related to the size of the femoral head, within the range of 22 to 46 mm in diameter. Consequently, larger femoral head sizes can be used. Highly crosslinked polyethylenes remain within current American Society for Testing and Materials standards, but concerns have been raised over the potential for fatigue, delamination, and implant fracture when a thin liner is used to accommodate a large-diameter head. Prior attempts to improve the performance of polyethylene have universally failed. Carbon fiber reinforcement, heat pressing, and Hylamer (DePuy, Warsaw, IN) are notable examples.

Early clinical results have shown reductions in wear that are less dramatic than those predicted in hip simulators. The bedding-in process is similar with highly crosslinked and conventional polyethylenes and affects calculations of wear rates using short-term clinical studies. Longer follow-up is needed to assess the true wear reduction after the bedding-in process is complete and a steady state of wear is reached.

It also is important to view reports of wear "reduction" in the context of the quality and performance of the material used as the control.

There are now a sufficient number of studies with 10-year follow-up to conclude that the performance of highly crosslinked polyethylenes surpasses that of conventional polyethylene. Snir et al. found that after an initial bedding-in period, there was an annual mean wear rate of 0.05 mm/year with a first-generation highly crosslinked polyethylene. Using precision radiostereometric analysis, Glyn-Jones et al. measured steady-state wear of only 0.003 mm/year at 10 years. In a series of patients younger than 50 years, Rames et al. observed survivorship of 97.8% at 15 years with no wear-related revisions and a liner wear rate of 0.0185 mm/year. The available data indicate a wear rate for highly crosslinked polyethylenes as well below the generally accepted osteolysis threshold of 0.1 mm/year. Using data from the Australian Orthopaedic Association National Joint Replacement Registry, de Steiger found the 16-year cumulative percentage of revisions for all causes was 6.2% for highly crosslinked polyethylene compared to 11.7% for conventional polyethylene.

Femoral head size appears to have less of an effect on highly crosslinked polyethylene than on conventional material. Allepuz et al. published data aggregated from six national and regional registries that showed no difference in wear rates with 32-mm heads compared with smaller diameter sizes. Lachiewicz, Soileau, and Martell reported no difference in liner wear rates with 36- to 40-mm heads compared with smaller sizes; however, volumetric wear was higher in patients with larger diameter heads. Most of the published data involve head sizes of 32 mm and smaller. Tower et al. reported four fractures of a highly crosslinked polyethylene liner in a design with thin polyethylene at the rim and a relatively vertical position of the acetabular component. Using an

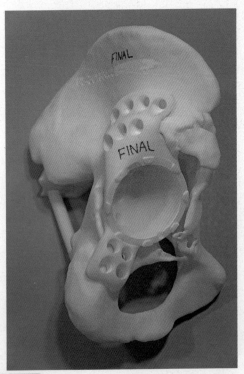

FIGURE 1.37 Implant trial and bone model can be sterilized for reference in surgery.

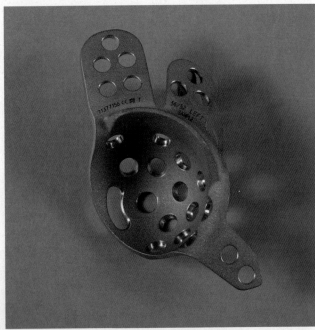

FIGURE 1.38 Contour antiprotrusio cage has titanium support ring fixed to ilium and ischium with screws. Alternatively, inferior fin can be impacted into ischium without screws. (Courtesy Smith & Nephew, Memphis, TN.)

excessively thin polyethylene liner purely to accommodate a larger head is still to be avoided.

Highly crosslinked polyethylene liners from most manufacturers are compatible with existing modular acetabular components. The liner can be replaced with the newer material without revising the shell in the event of reoperation for osteolysis, dislocation, or at the time of revision of the femoral component. An array of liner options is available as has been the case with conventional polyethylene (see Fig. 1.33).

CERAMIC-ON-CERAMIC BEARINGS

Alumina ceramic has many properties that make it desirable as a bearing surface in hip arthroplasty. Because of its high density, implants have a surface finish smoother than metal implants. Ceramic is harder than metal and more resistant to scratching from third-body wear particles. The liner wear rate of alumina-on-alumina has been shown to be 4000 times less than cobalt-chrome alloy-on-polyethylene. Hamadouche et al. measured ceramic wear at less than 0.025 mm/year in a series of patients with a minimum of 18.5 years' follow-up.

Early ceramic implants yielded disappointing clinical results because of flawed implant designs, inadequate fixation, implant fracture, and occasional cases of rapid wear with osteolysis. Numerous improvements have been made in the manufacture of alumina ceramics since the 1980s. Hot isostatic pressing and a threefold decrease in grain size have substantially improved the burst strength of the material. Refinements in the tolerances of the Morse taper have reduced the incidence of ceramic head fracture further. In addition, proof testing validates the strength of each individual implant before release. Ceramic head fracture is more common with smaller head sizes and shorter neck lengths. A 28 mm head with short neck length will have less material between the corner of the taper bore and articulating surface than a 36 mm head with longer neck length. Application of a ceramic femoral head onto a stem trunnion with wear or surface damage found at revision surgery can produce uneven load distribution within the head and contribute to fracture. Consequently, manufacturers have produced ceramic heads fitted with a metal sleeve for use in these circumstances.

Impingement between the femoral neck and rim of the ceramic acetabular component creates problems unique to this type of articulation. Impact loading of the rim can produce chipping or complete fracture of the acetabular insert. Repetitive contact at extremes of motion also can lead to notching of the metal femoral neck by the harder ceramic and initiate failure through this relatively thin portion of the implant. In past series, ceramic wear has been greater when the acetabular component has been implanted in an excessively vertical orientation. Ceramic-on-ceramic arthroplasties may be more sensitive to implant malposition than other bearings. "Stripe wear" has been reported on retrieved ceramic heads. This term describes a long, narrow area of damage resulting from contact between the head and the edge of the ceramic liner. Microseparation of the implants during the swing phase of gait is a recognized phenomenon. Walter et al. mapped the position of stripes on retrieved implants, however, and proposed they occur with edge loading when the hip is flexed, as with rising from a chair or stair climbing.

Enthusiasm for ceramic-on-ceramic implants has been somewhat tempered by reports of reproducible noise, particularly squeaking. The incidence is generally low but in some series has exceeded 10% and has been a source of dissatisfaction requiring revision. The onset of squeaking usually occurs more than 1 year after implantation, and the development of stripe wear has been implicated in noise generation. A specific cementless femoral component with unique metallurgy and taper size has been implicated in several reports. Vibrations generated at the articulating surfaces may be amplified by a more flexible stem, resulting in audible events. The etiology of squeaking has not been fully elucidated and is likely multifactorial.

Osteolysis has been reported around first-generation alumina ceramic implants in instances of high wear. Wear particles are typically produced in smaller numbers and are of smaller size than seen with polyethylene, however, and the cellular response to ceramic particles seems to be less. Alumina ceramic is inert, and ion formation does not occur. There have been no adverse systemic effects reported with ceramic bearings.

Ongoing investigation with composites of alumina and zirconia ceramic (BIOLOX delta, CeramTec GmbH, Plochingen, Germany) holds promise for further improvement in the material properties of these implants. Excellent wear properties and increased fracture toughness have been reported for this material. In a series of delta ceramic-on-ceramic total hips in patients younger than 50 years, Kim et al. found excellent survivorship, but 10% still experienced noise generation including squeaking. Blakeney et al. reported a 23% incidence of squeaking when a large-diameter (32 to 48 mm head) delta ceramic-on-ceramic couple was used. The incidence of head fracture with delta ceramic is approximately 1 in 100,000 (0.001%) compared to 1 in 5000 (0.0201%) with pure alumina ceramic.

Acetabular components include a ceramic insert that mates with a metal shell by means of a taper junction. Lipped and offset liners are unavailable. The locking mechanism for a given implant may not be compatible with other types of inserts. Chipping of the insert on implantation has been reported in multiple series. Special care should be taken during the operative assembly of the acetabular component to ensure that the insert is properly oriented before impaction. Metal backing of the insert has been advocated by one manufacturer to prevent insertional chips and protect the rim of the ceramic from impingement. Alumina ceramic femoral heads are manufactured with only a limited range of neck lengths, and skirted heads are unavailable. Careful preoperative planning with templates is required to ensure that the neck resection is made at an appropriate level for restoration of hip mechanics with the range of neck lengths available.

Oxidized zirconium (OXINIUM, Smith & Nephew, Memphis, TN) is a zirconium metal alloy that is placed through an oxidation process to yield an implant with a zirconia ceramic surface of approximately 5 μm in thickness. The enhanced surface is integral to the metal substrate and not a surface coating. So-called ceramicized metals have the same surface hardness, smoothness, and wettability of typical ceramics, but are not susceptible to chipping, flaking, or fracture. Compared with cobalt chromium alloy, the material contains no detectable nickel and has therefore been recommended for patients with demonstrated metal hypersensitivity. Oxidized zirconium is currently available only in femoral head components mated with polyethylene and not as a ceramic-on-ceramic couple. Reduced wear has been reported when oxidized zirconium is mated with a conventional polyethylene acetabular component. Aoude et al. found no difference in wear rates between cobalt chromium and oxidized zirconium when mated with highly crosslinked polyethylene. The material is more prone to surface damage than conventional ceramic heads after episodes of dislocation.

So-called trunnionosis describes the process of fretting corrosion that may occur between a femoral component trunnion and a cobalt-chrome alloy femoral head leading to adverse local tissue response. The factors contributing to this phenomenon have not been fully elucidated but appear to be more common than previously recognized. The emergence of this problem combined with the reduced fracture risk with newer ceramics has led to an increase in the use of ceramic and ceramicized metal heads worldwide. Some large database studies have also reported a lower risk of infection with ceramic bearings. The reason for this association is unclear.

INDICATIONS AND CONTRAINDICATIONS FOR TOTAL HIP ARTHROPLASTY

Originally, the primary indication for THA was the alleviation of incapacitating arthritic pain in patients older than age 65 years whose pain could not be relieved sufficiently by nonsurgical means and for whom the only surgical alternative was resection of the hip joint (Girdlestone resection arthroplasty) or arthrodesis. Of secondary importance was the improved function of the hip. After the operation had been documented to be remarkably successful, the indications were expanded to include the other disorders listed in Box 1.1.

Historically, patients 60 to 75 years old were considered the most suitable candidates for THA, but since the 1990s this age range has expanded. With an aging population, many older individuals are becoming candidates for surgery. In a meta-analysis reviewing the impact of advanced age on outcomes of lower extremity arthroplasty, Murphy et al. found that the most elderly patients were at higher risk for mortality, complications, and longer length of stay. Nonetheless, these patients experienced significant gains in pain relief, and activities of daily living and were satisfied with the outcome of arthroplasty surgery.

The 1994 National Institutes of Health Consensus Statement on Total Hip Replacement concluded that "THR [total hip replacement] is an option for nearly all patients with diseases of the hip that cause chronic discomfort and significant functional impairment." In younger individuals, THA is not the only reconstruction procedure available for a painful hip; the expanding field of hip preservation (see chapter 4) provides surgeons with a variety of options that may delay or obviate the need for arthroplasty.

Femoral or periacetabular osteotomy should be considered for young patients with osteoarthritis if the joint is not grossly incongruous and satisfactory motion is present. Periacetabular osteotomy in patients with dysplasia may decrease the need for structural bone grafting if later conversion to arthroplasty is needed. If an osteotomy relieves symptoms for 10 years or more, and then an arthroplasty is required, the patient will have been able to engage in more physical activity, bone stock will have been preserved, and patient will be older and less physically active and will need

the use of an arthroplasty for fewer years. Core decompression and osteotomy should be considered for patients with idiopathic osteonecrosis of the femoral head, especially when involvement is limited. Management of femoroacetabular impingement should be considered in suitable candidates. Arthrodesis is performed less frequently today, but is still a viable option for young, vigorous patients with unilateral hip disease and especially for young, active men with osteonecrosis or posttraumatic arthritis. If necessary at a later age, the arthrodesis can be converted to a THA. Finally, some designs of hip resurfacing (see chapter 2) have been successful and remain an alternative to THA in young, active men.

Before any major reconstruction of the hip is recommended, conservative measures should be advised, including weight loss, nonopioid analgesics, reasonable activity modification, low-impact exercise, and ambulatory aids. These measures may relieve the symptoms enough to make an operation unnecessary or at least delay the need for surgery for a significant period.

Surgery is justified if, despite these measures, pain at rest and pain with motion and weight bearing are severe enough to prevent the patient from working or from carrying out activities of daily living. Pain in the presence of a degenerative or destructive process in the hip joint as evidenced on imaging studies is the primary indication for surgery. In our opinion, patients with limitation of motion, limp, or leg-length inequality but with little or no hip pain are not candidates for THA.

In a study of a large inpatient database, Rasouli et al. found a higher risk of systemic complications with bilateral total hip procedures carried out under a single anesthetic. Stavrakis et al. found a higher rate of sepsis, but no difference in other complications. The major indication is a medically fit patient with bilateral severe involvement with stiffness or fixed flexion deformity because rehabilitation may be difficult if surgery is done on one side only. Elderly patients with other comorbidities are not suitable candidates for such a procedure. A documented patent ductus arteriosus or septal defect is an absolute contraindication. More intensive intraoperative monitoring, including an arterial line, pulmonary artery catheter, and urinary catheter, is recommended. The surgeon should decide in concert with the anesthesiologist as to whether the second procedure could be completed safely.

Absolute contraindications for THA include active infection of the hip joint or any other region and any unstable medical illnesses that would significantly increase the risk of morbidity or mortality. Asymptomatic bacteriuria has not been associated with postoperative surgical site infections and should not be considered a contraindication.

PREOPERATIVE PATIENT EVALUATION AND OPTIMIZATION

Hip arthroplasty for degenerative and traumatic conditions is a major cost center for payors. Over the past decade, a greater burden has been placed on both surgeons and institutions to reduce perioperative complications, minimize readmissions, and maintain favorable outcomes, all while reducing the cost of the episode of care.

A thorough general medical evaluation, including laboratory tests, is a recognized prerequisite that affords the

BOX 1.1

Disorders of the Hip Joint for Which Total Hip Arthroplasty May Be Indicated

Inflammatory arthritis
  Rheumatoid
  Juvenile idiopathic
  Ankylosing spondylitis
Osteoarthritis (degenerative joint disease, hypotrophic arthritis)
  Primary
  Secondary
    Developmental dysplasia of hip
    Coxa plana (Legg-Calvé-Perthes disease)
    Posttraumatic
    Slipped capital femoral epiphysis
    Paget disease
    Hemophilia
Osteonecrosis
  Idiopathic
  Post fracture or dislocation
  Steroid induced
  Alcoholism
  Hemoglobinopathies (sickle cell disease)
  Lupus
  Renal disease
  Caisson disease
  Gaucher disease
  Slipped capital femoral epiphysis
Failed reconstruction
  Osteotomy
  Hemiarthroplasty
  Resection arthroplasty (Girdlestone procedure)
  Resurfacing arthroplasty
Acute fracture, femoral neck and trochanteric
Nonunion, femoral neck and trochanteric fractures
Pyogenic arthritis or osteomyelitis
  Hematogenous
  Postoperative
  Tuberculosis
Hip fusion and pseudarthrosis
  Bone tumor involving proximal femur or acetabulum
  Hereditary disorders (e.g., achondroplasia)

clinician the opportunity to uncover and treat various problems before surgery. Comorbidities known to be inherent to elderly patients should be considered, especially cardiopulmonary disease, renal insufficiency, malnutrition, and the propensity for thromboembolism. Functional limitations from an arthritic hip may mask the symptoms of coronary or peripheral vascular disease. Various models of risk stratification have identified a number of potentially modifiable factors that may be addressed preoperatively in order to minimize the risk of complications.

Cardiovascular complications are one of the most common causes of perioperative mortality and hospital readmission. Patients with a known history of cardiac disease or the presence of new symptoms should prompt a cardiology consultation. Aspirin, clopidogrel, and other antiplatelet medications are best discontinued 7 to 10 days before surgery. The

presence of vascular stents presents a particular dilemma that should be managed in cooperation with a cardiac consultant. If clopidogrel is to be discontinued before surgery, then it is acceptable to continue aspirin and restart clopidogrel as soon as the bleeding risk at the surgery site permits. Oral anticoagulants such as warfarin and factor Xa inhibitors should be discontinued in sufficient time for coagulation studies to return to normal. A bridging program with a short-acting anticoagulant such as enoxaparin may be required when discontinuing warfarin.

The prevalence of obesity has increased dramatically in Western societies and has been repeatedly identified as a risk factor for delayed wound healing, deep infection, cardiac events, and kidney injury. The risk of infection increases gradually with elevation of body mass index (BMI). There is no definitive BMI at which surgery is contraindicated, but studies frequently stratify risk according to a BMI greater or less than 40 kg/m^2 (class III, morbid obesity). A delay in surgery with a structured weight reduction diet plan should be encouraged for these patients. The role of bariatric surgery before arthroplasty and its effect on outcomes remains undetermined.

Diabetes mellitus has consistently been recognized as a risk factor for postoperative complications, particularly infection. Preoperative screening for HbA1c elevation identifies patients with poor glycemic control over a period of 2 to 3 months. The literature is inconclusive regarding a threshold value of HbA1c that is predictive of subsequent infection. Cancienne et al. identified a HbA1c of more than 7.5% as a significant risk factor for postoperative joint infection. The Second International Consensus Meeting on Musculoskeletal Infection recommended that the upper threshold for HbA1c that may be predictive of subsequent joint infection is most likely to be within the range of 7.5% to 8%. Screenings finding a higher value should be referred for glycemic control prior to surgery.

Current tobacco use has been shown to increase the risk of wound complications in many types of surgery, including arthroplasty. Duchman et al. reported current smokers had a 1.8% incidence of wound complications compared to 1.1% in nonsmokers. Smoking cessation for at least 6 weeks before surgery is recommended to mitigate this risk. Compliance can be assessed by measuring the blood level of cotinine, a metabolite of nicotine.

Patients having nasal colonization with *Staphylococcus aureus* are at increased risk for infection following hip arthroplasty. Some institutions have instituted screening for nasal MSSA/MRSA colonization with polymerase chain reaction assays. Nasal administration of mupirocin, povidone-iodine, and chlorhexidine products have all been used for decolonization. Universal treatment without individual screening is the most cost-effective modality.

Preoperative anemia, defined by the World Health Organization (WHO) as a Hb level in men less than 13.0 g/dL and 12.0 g/dL for women has been identified as an independent predictor for complications including infection. Perioperative blood transfusion has also been associated with complications including mortality, sepsis, and thromboembolism. Preoperative iron supplementation and erythropoietin administration can decrease the need for allogeneic transfusion. The perioperative use of tranexamic acid and a comprehensive institutional blood management protocol are also important adjuncts for reducing transfusions.

A low BMI (less than 18.5 kg/m²) is associated with a higher risk for infection and may be a surrogate for poor nutritional status in the elderly. Low serum albumin, prealbumin, transferrin, and total lymphocyte count are indicative of poor nutrition and/or anemia.

Many herbal medications and nutritional supplements may cause increased perioperative blood loss, and we recommend that these medications be discontinued preoperatively. Pyogenic skin lesions should be eradicated, and preoperative skin preparation with chlorhexidine for several days should be considered. Dental problems, as well as urinary retention caused by prostatic or bladder disease, should be addressed before surgery.

If a patient has a history of previous surgery, purulent drainage from the hip, or other indications of ongoing infection, laboratory investigation including erythrocyte sedimentation rate (ESR) and C-reactive protein (CRP), nuclear scans, and a culture and sensitivity determination of an aspirate of the hip are advisable before surgery. Infection must be suspected if part of the subchondral bone of the acetabulum or femoral head is eroded or if bone has been resorbed around an internal fixation device.

The physical examination should include the spine and the upper and lower extremities. The soft tissues around the hip should be inspected for any inflammation or scarring where the incision is to be made. Gentle palpation of the hip and thigh may reveal areas of point tenderness or a soft-tissue mass. The strength of the abductor musculature should be determined by the Trendelenburg test. The lengths of the lower extremities should be compared, and any fixed deformity should be noted. Adduction contracture of the hip can produce apparent shortening of the limb despite equally measured leg lengths. Abduction contracture conversely produces apparent lengthening. Fixed flexion deformity of the hip forces the lumbar spine into lordosis on assuming an upright posture and may aggravate lower back pain symptoms. Conversely, fixed lumbar spine deformity from scoliosis or ankylosing spondylitis may produce pelvic obliquity, which must be taken into account when positioning the implants. When the hip and the knee are both severely arthritic, usually the hip should be operated on first. Hip arthroplasty may alter knee alignment and mechanics. Also, knee arthroplasty is technically more difficult when the hip is stiff, and rehabilitation would be hampered.

An alternative or additional diagnosis should be considered. The complaint of "hip pain" can be brought about by a variety of afflictions, and arthritis of the hip joint is one of the less common ones. True hip joint pain usually is perceived in the groin and lateral hip, sometimes in the anterior thigh, and occasionally in the knee. Arthritic pain usually is worse with activity and improves to some degree with rest and limited weight bearing. Pain in atypical locations and of atypical character should prompt a search for other problems. Pain isolated to the buttock or posterior pelvis often is referred from the lumbar spine, sacrum, or sacroiliac joint. Arthritis often coexists in the hip and lumbar spine. A THA done to relieve symptoms predominantly referred from the lumbar spine would do little to improve the patient's condition. Likewise, surgical intervention in the face of mild hip arthritis when the pain is actually caused by unrecognized vascular claudication, trochanteric bursitis, pubic ramus

---

BOX 1.2

Recommended Weight-Adjusted Doses of Antimicrobials for Prophylaxis of Hip and Knee Arthroplasty in Adults

Antimicrobial	Recommended Dose	Redosing Interval
Cefazolin	2 g (consider 3 g if patient weight is ≥129 kg*)	4 hr
Vancomycin	15-20 mg/kg*	Not applicable
Clindamycin	600-900 mg†	6 hr

*Actual body weight.
†No recommended adjustment for weight.
From Aboltins CA, Berdal JE, Casas F, et al: Hip and knee section, prevention, antimicrobials (systemic): Proceedings of International Consensus on Orthopedic Infections, *J Arthroplasty* 34:S279, 2019.

---

fracture, or an intraabdominal problem subjects the patient to needless risk.

The Harris, Iowa (Larson), Judet, Andersson, and d'Aubigné and Postel systems for recording the status of the hip before surgery are useful for evaluating postoperative results. Pain, ability to walk, function, mobility, and radiographic changes are recorded. As yet, no particular hip rating system has been uniformly adopted. The Harris system is the most frequently used (Box 1.2).

Adoption of a single rating system by the orthopaedic community would help standardize the reporting of results. Rating systems have been criticized as being subjective, for downgrading the importance of pain relief, and for emphasizing range of motion rather than functional capabilities as a result of hip motion. Improved motion in the hip is of little benefit if one is still unable to dress the foot and trim the toenails. The Western Ontario and McMaster Universities Osteoarthritis Index (WOMAC) considers the functional abilities of patients with hip arthritis in greater depth than specific hip rating systems. The 36-item short-form health survey (SF-36) is a more generic survey of health and well-being. These two tools often are used in addition to a hip rating score in reporting results. Finally, patient reported outcome measures (PROMs) have become increasingly important in evaluating outcomes by hospital administrators, insurance carriers, and policymakers. The Hip Disability and Osteoarthritis Outcome Score (HOOS), Jr is a six-question survey of pain, function, and daily living derived from the HOOS. The survey is efficient to administer and has been validated and endorsed by major orthopaedic societies. The Veterans RAND 12-Item Health Survey (VR-12) and the Patient-Reported Outcomes Measurement Information System (PROMIS Global-10) are both short-form instruments to measure general physical and mental health apart from the hip.

General inhalation anesthesia or regional anesthesia can be used for the surgery. The choice should be made in collaboration with the anesthesiologist and may be based on institutional protocols or the specific needs of the patient. The introduction of multimodal pain management protocols has been an important adjunct to the surgical anesthetic. Preemptive analgesia including lumbar plexus blockade, periarticular injection of long-acting local anesthetics, cele-coxib, gabapentin, intravenous or oral acetaminophen, and long-acting oral analgesics such as tramadol have helped reduce the need for more potent opioids.

Finally, preoperative education classes and institutional rehabilitation protocols have proven to be useful adjuncts in shortening hospital stays and reducing readmissions. With careful patient selection, proactive management of comorbidities, preoperative education, and the use of preemptive analgesia, we have reduced length of stay for most patients to a single hospital day. In carefully selected younger patients, we are now performing THA as an outpatient procedure in both hospital and surgery center settings. As payers, including CMS (Centers for Medicare & Medicaid Services) and private insurers, transition to bundled payment methodologies, strategies to reduce cost while maintaining patient safety will become even more important for maintaining surgeon compensation for hip arthroplasty procedures.

PREOPERATIVE RADIOGRAPHS

Before surgery, radiographs of the hips are reviewed and, if indicated, radiographs of the spine and knees are obtained. An anteroposterior view of the pelvis showing the proximal femur and a lateral view of the hip and proximal femur are the minimal views required. Radiographs of the pelvis should be reviewed specifically to evaluate the structural integrity of the acetabulum, to estimate the size of the implant required and how much reaming would be necessary, and to determine whether bone grafting would be required. In patients with developmental dysplasia, the pelvis should be evaluated with special care to determine the amount of bone stock present for fixation of the cup. In patients with previous acetabular fractures, obturator and iliac oblique views are obtained, in addition to the routine anteroposterior view of the hip, because a significant defect may be present in the posterior wall. A three-dimensional CT scan also is helpful in evaluating the acetabulum in these complex cases.

The width of the medullary canal also is noted because it may be narrow, especially in patients with dysplasia or dwarfism. In these instances, a femoral component with a straight stem may be needed. In Paget disease, old fractures of the femoral shaft, or congenital abnormalities, a lateral radiograph of the proximal femur may reveal a significant anterior bowing that may make preparation of the canal more difficult. If excessive bowing or a rotational deformity is present, femoral osteotomy may be required before or in addition to the arthroplasty. Appropriate instruments must be available to remove any internal fixation devices implanted during previous surgery (see the section on failed reconstructive procedures); otherwise, the procedure may be unduly prolonged.

Preoperative planning should include the use of templates supplied by the prosthesis manufacturer. Careful templating before surgery removes much of the guesswork during surgery and can shorten operative time by eliminating repetition of steps. The wide array of implant sizes and femoral neck lengths allows precise fitting to the patient, but it also allows for major errors in implant sizing and limb length when used without careful planning. Templating aids in selecting the type of implant that would restore the center of rotation of the hip and provide the best femoral fit and in judging the level

of bone resection and selection of the neck length required to restore equal limb lengths and femoral offset.

PREOPERATIVE TEMPLATING FOR TOTAL HIP ARTHROPLASTY
TECHNIQUE 1.1

(CAPELLO)
- Make an anteroposterior pelvic radiograph and a lateral view of the affected hip. The pelvic film must include the upper portion of both femurs and the entire hip joint.
- Position the hips in 15 degrees of internal rotation to delineate better femoral geometry and offset. Femoral offset will be underestimated when the hips are positioned in external rotation.
- On the lateral view, place the femur flat on the cassette to avoid distortion and include the upper portion of the femur.
- On each view, tape a magnification marker (with lead spheres 100 mm apart) to the thigh so that the marker is parallel to the femur and is the same distance from the film as the bone.
- Tape the marker to the upper medial thigh for the anteroposterior view and move it to the anterior thigh for the lateral view.
- Measure the distance between the centers of the spheres to estimate the amount of magnification of the radiograph. For a standard pelvic radiograph, magnification is approximately 20%.
- Templates are marked as to their degree of magnification. Take any discrepancy into account when templating.
- Draw a line at the level of and parallel to the ischial tuberosities that intersects the lesser trochanter on each side and compare the two points of intersection and measure the difference to determine the amount of limb shortening.
- Place the acetabular overlay templates on the film and select the size that matches the contour of the patient's acetabulum without excessive removal of subchondral bone. The medial position of the acetabular template is at the teardrop and the inferior margin at the level of the obturator foramen. Mark the center of the acetabular component on the radiograph; this corresponds to the new center of rotation of the hip.
- Place the femoral overlay templates on the film and select the size that most precisely matches the contour of the proximal canal and fills it most completely. Make allowance for the thickness of the desired cement mantle if cement is to be used.
- Select the appropriate neck length to restore limb length and femoral offset. If no shortening is present, match the center of the head with the previously marked center of the acetabulum. If a discrepancy exists, the distance between the femoral head center and the acetabular center should be equal to the previously measured limb-length discrepancy.

■ When the neck length has been selected, mark the level of anticipated neck resection and measure its distance from the top of the lesser trochanter to use as a reference intraoperatively. Template the femur on the lateral view in a similar manner to ascertain whether the implant determined on the anteroposterior film can be inserted without excessive bone removal.

■ Measure the diameter of the canal below the tip of the stem to determine the size of the medullary plug if cement is to be used.

■ If a fixed external rotation deformity of the hip is present, templating is inaccurate.

■ If the opposite hip is without deformity, template the normal hip and transpose the measurements to the operative side as a secondary check.

Many modifications of this technique are commonly used. For determining leg-length discrepancy, a line between the inferior edge of the acetabular teardrop (interteardrop line) or the bottom of the obturator foramen (interobturator line) can be used as the reference line. Perpendicular measurements to the proximal corner of each lesser trochanter are compared to compute the leg-length discrepancy. Meerman et al. found measurements from the interteardrop line to be more accurate than those from the ischium.

Digital radiographs are now commonplace in orthopaedic practice. Templating digital images requires specialized software and a library of precision templates supplied by each manufacturer that can be manipulated on a high-resolution computer monitor in a manner similar to that described for conventional films. A number of software packages are commercially available and may be integral to a picture archiving and communication system (PACS) or acquired as a separate module. Magnification is assessed in a manner similar to that used for conventional radiographs with a marker of known size placed at the level of the hip joint. The software then calibrates the image, and the digital templates are scaled to the correct degree of magnification. The subsequent steps are specific to the software package but generally mimic the process described for acetate templates used on printed radiographs. Iorio et al. and Whiddon et al. found acceptable accuracy with digital templating. Eliminating the cost of printing films and having a permanent archive of the preoperative plan are clear advantages of digital methods. Archibeck et al. concluded that placement of a magnification marker did not improve the accuracy of digital templating compared to assuming a standard 20% magnification as has been used in the past for acetate templates with film radiographs. Sershon et al. found that accuracy of templating did not vary by BMI for either femoral or acetabular sizing. Shin et al. described a technique using acetate templates on a digital monitor with radiographs adjusted for magnification. The technique avoids the need for costly software and was accurate for both implant sizing and correction of leg length and offset.

THE HIP-SPINE RELATIONSHIP

A recent meta-analysis by An et al. found that a history of spinal fusion imparted a twofold risk of early hip dislocation and over threefold risk for revision. Additionally, most early dislocations occur with acetabular components that have been placed in the so-called safe zone as described by Lewinnek. The findings have led to questions regarding the acceptance of a universal guideline for acetabular component placement and a recognition that altered spinopelvic motion may put the acetabular component in a functionally unsafe orientation with changes of posture.

In normal patients, the lower lumbar spine is flexible in the sagittal plane. When moving from standing to sitting position, the pelvis tilts posteriorly to accommodate flexion of the hip joint. For each 1 degree of increased pelvic tilt, acetabular anteversion increases from 0.7 to 0.8 degrees. This translates to a change of acetabular anteversion of approximately 15.6 degrees when moving from standing to sitting position and reduces anterior impingement as the hip flexes. Acetabular inclination also increases with pelvic tilt and may be protective of anterior impingement with hip flexion. Deformity and stiffness of the lumbar spine from degenerative processes or lumbar fusion can prevent this normal accommodation and lead to excessive anterior impingement with sitting or posterior impingement when standing.

For patients with a history of spinal fusion, deformity, or stiffness, it may be necessary to obtain additional radiographs to assess spinopelvic kinematics and make adaptations to the surgical plan for proper component positioning. A lateral view of the lumbar spine and pelvis in both standing and sitting positions is the minimum required. Some have also recommended obtaining a standing anteroposterior (AP) view of the pelvis. A number of new terms have been defined to assist hip surgeons in addressing the needs of "hip-spine" patients.

The anterior pelvic plane (APP) is defined by the points of the two anterior superior iliac spines (ASIS) and the pubic symphysis on a lateral radiograph of the pelvis. Anterior and posterior pelvic tilt describe the direction of motion of the upper portion of the ilium (Fig. 1.39). Sacral slope (SS) is the angle between the superior endplate of the S1 vertebra and a horizontal reference, typically the inferior border of the radiograph. Both APP and SS can be used to assess spinopelvic motion with changes in posture.

Moving from a standing to sitting position normally results in posterior pelvic tilt with a concomitant reduction in lumbar lordosis and flattening of SS (Fig. 1.40). The normal change in SS from standing to sitting is between 11 and 30 degrees. Spinopelvic stiffness is defined as a change in SS of ≤10 degrees. When this is the case, the hip joint must flex further to assume a seated position, with a greater risk of anterior impingement (Fig. 1.41). In these patients, more anteversion of the acetabular component will be needed to compensate for the reduced posterior pelvic tilt imposed by the stiff spine.

The term *pelvic incidence* (PI) refers to the angle between a line drawn from the center of the femoral heads to the center of the superior endplate of S1 and a second line drawn perpendicular to the S1 endplate (Fig. 1.42). It is a measurement of the anterior to posterior relationship of the femoral head to the lower lumbar spine. PI is a fixed value and does not change with posture. When combined with measures of the lumbar lordosis (typically the angle between superior endplates of L1 and S1), it may identify patients with a flat-back spinal deformity. These patients may have excessive posterior pelvic tilt while standing. This increases the functional anteversion of the acetabulum upon standing, with resulting risk of anterior instability. Therefore, acetabular component anteversion may need to be reduced in these patients.

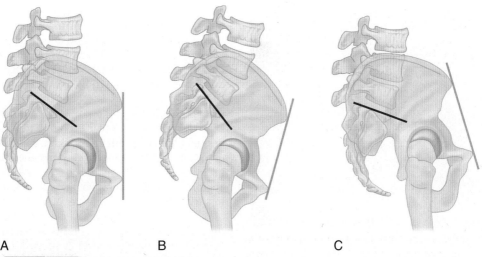

A   B   C

FIGURE 1.39   Anterior pelvic plane (*orange lines*) and effect on sacral slope (*purple lines*). Neutral (**A**), anterior (**B**), and posterior (**C**) pelvic tilt.

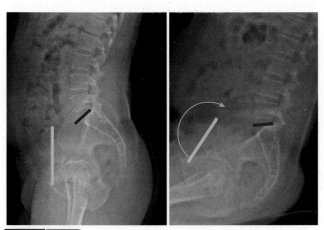

FIGURE 1.40   Standing and sitting lateral radiographs of a patient with normal spinal pelvic mobility. When the patient sits, lumbar lordosis decreases and the pelvis "rolls back," which is demonstrated by an increase in posterior pelvic tilt (*yellow line*) and a flattening of the sacral slope (*red line*). (From Luthringer TA, Vigdorchik JM: A preoperative workup of a "hip-spine" total hip arthroplasty patient: a simplified approach to a complex problem, *J Arthroplasty* 34[7S]:S57, 2019.)

When patients have alterations in spinopelvic mechanics, the so-called safe zone for acetabular component position can be altered in terms of anteversion and also significantly narrowed. In addition to adjustments in implant positioning, dual mobility components (see Fig. 1.35) have proven useful in reducing the rate of instability. Innovative new modalities such as EOS imaging (EOS Imaging, Paris) may also simplify the evaluation of these complex cases.

PREPARATION AND DRAPING

An operating table that tilts easily is recommended, especially if the patient is placed in the lateral position. If the patient is not anchored securely, the proper position in which to place the acetabular component is difficult to determine. A variety of pelvic positioning devices are commercially available for this purpose. Positioning devices should be placed so as not to impede the motion of the hip intraoperatively; otherwise, assessing stability is difficult. Also, the positioning devices should be placed against the pubic symphysis or the ASIS so that no pressure is applied over the femoral triangles, or limb ischemia or compression neuropathy may result. We have previously used suction-deflated beanbags for this purpose. Dedicated hip positioning devices are more secure, but errors in positioning may still occur, even with these devices, resulting in misjudgment of acetabular component anteversion. Bony prominences and the peroneal nerve should be padded, especially if a lengthy procedure is expected. If the patient is to be operated on in the supine position, a small pad is placed beneath the buttock of the affected hip; this is especially helpful in obese patients because it tends to allow the loose adipose tissue to drop away from the site of the incision.

The adhesive edges of a U-shaped plastic drape are applied to the skin to seal off the perineal and gluteal areas, and the hip and entire limb are prepared with a suitable bactericidal solution. The foot preferably is covered with a stockinette, and the final drapes should be of an impervious material to allow abundant irrigation without fear of contaminating the field. If anterior dislocation of the hip is anticipated in the lateral position, a draping system that incorporates a sterile pocket suspended across the anterior side of the operating table is helpful; this allows the leg to be placed in the bag while the femur is being prepared and delivered back onto the table without contaminating the sterile field.

SURGICAL APPROACHES AND TECHNIQUES

Many variations have evolved in the surgical approaches and techniques used for THA. This is in keeping with the natural tendency of surgeons to individualize operations according to their own clinical and educational experiences. The surgical approaches differ chiefly as to whether the patient is operated on in the lateral or the supine position and whether the hip is dislocated anteriorly or posteriorly.

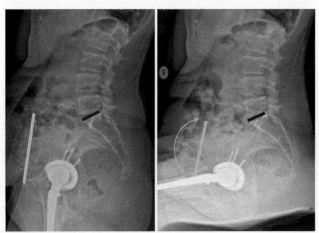

FIGURE 1.41 Standing and sitting lateral radiographs of a patient with a stiff spine who underwent revision of the shown construct for asymmetric polyethylene wear, osteolysis, and posterior instability. Note the lack of "pelvic rollback" in the seated position (no change in sacral slope, *red*) and the proximity of the flexing proximal femur to the anterior acetabular rim *(yellow)*. (From Luthringer TA, Vigdorchik JM: A preoperative workup of a "hip-spine" total hip arthroplasty patient: a simplified approach to a complex problem, *J Arthroplasty* 34[7S]:S57, 2019.)

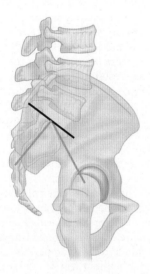

FIGURE 1.42 Pelvic incidence is the angle between line drawn from center of femoral head to center of sacral endplate and second line perpendicular to sacral endplate *(orange lines)*.

The choice of specific surgical approach for THA is largely a matter of personal preference and training. The surgical protocol for a given total hip system may advocate a certain approach, as reflected in the technique manual. In reality, virtually all total hip femoral and acetabular components can be properly implanted through numerous approaches, provided that adequate exposure is obtained. Each approach has relative advantages and drawbacks.

The original Charnley technique used the anterolateral surgical approach with the patient supine, osteotomy of the greater trochanter, and anterior dislocation of the hip. This approach is used much less commonly now as a result of problems related to reattachment of the greater trochanter. Amstutz advocated the

anterolateral approach with osteotomy of the greater trochanter, but with the patient in the lateral rather than the supine position. The Müller technique also uses the anterolateral approach with the patient in the lateral position but includes release of only the anterior part of the abductor mechanism. The Hardinge direct lateral approach is done with the patient supine or in the lateral position. A muscle-splitting incision through the gluteus medius and minimus allows anterior dislocation of the hip and affords excellent acetabular exposure. Residual abductor weakness and limp after this approach may be the result of avulsion of the repair of the anterior portion of the abductors or of direct injury to the superior gluteal nerve. The Dall variation of this approach involves removal of the anterior portion of the abductors with an attached thin wafer of bone from the anterior edge of the greater trochanter to facilitate their later repair. Abductor function is better after bony reattachment of the anterior portions of these muscles. Head et al. used a modification of the direct lateral approach, in which the patient is in the lateral position and the vastus lateralis is reflected anteriorly in continuity with the anterior cuff of the abductors. This approach allows much greater exposure of the proximal femur than the Hardinge approach, and is more appropriate for revision surgery. Keggi described a supine anterior approach through the medial border of the tensor fascia lata (TFL) muscle; variations of this approach have become popular recently and are advocated for a reduced risk of posterior dislocation. Femoral exposure is more difficult through this so-called direct anterior approach, and injury to the lateral femoral cutaneous nerve (LFCN) can be problematic. The posterolateral approach with posterior dislocation of the hip requires placing the patient in the lateral position and has proven satisfactory for primary and revision surgery. Exposure of the anterior aspect of the acetabulum can be difficult, and historically the postoperative dislocation rate is higher with the posterolateral approach than with the anterolateral or direct lateral approaches.

The specific technique for implantation of a given total hip system varies according to the method of skeletal fixation; the preparation for ancillary fixation devices for the acetabulum; the shape of the femoral component; the length of the stem; and the assembly of modular portions of the acetabular component, the femoral head, and, with some systems, the femoral component itself. The instrumentation supplied with a system is specific for that system and always should be used. The manufacturer supplies a technique manual with the system that gives a precise description of the instruments and the manner in which they are to be used for correct implantation of the components. Although instruments in various systems serve similar purposes, there may be substantial differences in their configurations and in the way they are assembled and used. The surgeon and scrub nurse should become thoroughly familiar with all of the instrumentation before proceeding with the operative procedure. A practice session with plastic bone models or a cadaver is useful before using a new prosthesis for the first time.

Considering the number of total hip systems in current use, this text cannot discuss the particular points of all or any one of them. A general technical guideline is presented for exposure and insertion of cemented and cementless femoral and acetabular components, along with points germane to many types of implants. Additional steps are required for preparation and insertion of certain implants, and the manufacturer's technique must always be followed in these instances. The techniques presented here are for the posterior and direct anterior approaches; the preparation

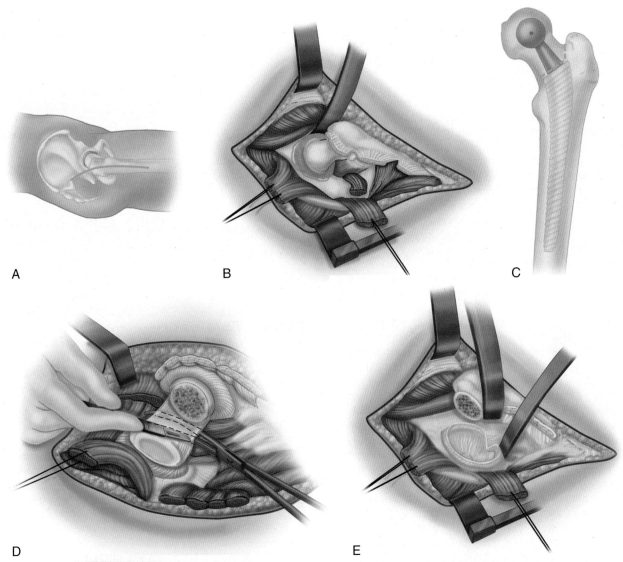

A

B

C

D

E

FIGURE 1.43   **A,** Skin incision for posterolateral approach to hip. **B,** Completed posterior soft-tissue dissection. **C,** Neck cut planned at appropriate level and angle by using trial components of templated size. **D,** Anterior capsule divided along course of psoas tendon sheath. **E,** Femur retracted well anteriorly to allow unimpeded access to acetabulum. (**A, B,** and **E** redrawn from Capello WN: Uncemented hip replacement, Tech Orthop 1:11, 1986; also Courtesy Indiana University School of Medicine.)
SEE TECHNIQUES 1.2 AND 1.4.

of the femur and acetabulum is similar for other approaches. A traditional approach is presented here. Although a less extensile exposure may be appropriate in most cases (see section "Minimally Invasive Techniques"), it is important for surgeons to understand the full array of soft-tissue releases that may be needed in stiff hips and more complex procedures.

TOTAL HIP ARTHROPLASTY THROUGH POSTEROLATERAL APPROACH

POSTEROLATERAL APPROACH WITH POSTERIOR DISLOCATION OF THE HIP

The posterolateral approach is a modification of posterior approaches described by Gibson and by Moore. The approach

can be extended proximally by osteotomy of the greater trochanter with anterior dislocation of the hip (see section on trochanteric osteotomy). The approach can be extended distally to allow a posterolateral approach to the entire femoral shaft. We use the posterolateral approach for primary and revision THA.

TECHNIQUE 1.2

- With the patient firmly anchored in the straight lateral position, make a slightly curved incision centered over the greater trochanter. Begin the skin incision proximally at a point level with the ASIS along a line parallel to the posterior edge of the greater trochanter. Extend the incision distally to the center of the greater trochanter and along the course of the femoral shaft to a point 10 cm distal to the greater trochanter (Fig. 1.43A). Adequate extension of the upper portion of the incision is required for reaming of the femoral canal from a superior direction, and the distal extent of the exposure is required for preparation and insertion of the acetabular component from an anteroinferior direction.

- Divide the subcutaneous tissues along the skin incision in a single plane down to the fascia lata and the thin fascia covering the gluteus maximus superiorly.
- Dissect the subcutaneous tissues from the fascial plane for approximately 1 cm anteriorly and posteriorly to make identification of this plane easier at the time of closure.
- Divide the fascia in line with the skin wound over the center of the greater trochanter.
- Bluntly split the gluteus maximus proximally in the direction of its fibers and coagulate any vessels within the substance of the muscle.
- Extend the fascial incision distally far enough to expose the tendinous insertion of the gluteus maximus on the posterior femur.
- Bluntly dissect the anterior and posterior edges of the fascia from any underlying fibers of the gluteus medius that insert into the undersurface of this fascia. Suture moist towels or laparotomy sponges to the fascial edges anteriorly and posteriorly to exclude the skin, prevent desiccation of the subcutaneous tissues, and collect cement and bone debris generated during the operation.
- Insert a Charnley or similar large self-retaining retractor beneath the fascia lata at the level of the trochanter. Take care not to entrap the sciatic nerve beneath the retractor posteriorly.
- Divide the trochanteric bursa and bluntly sweep it posteriorly to expose the short external rotators and the posterior edge of the gluteus medius. The posterior border of the gluteus medius is almost in line with the femoral shaft, and the anterior border fans anteriorly.
- Maintain the hip in extension as the posterior dissection is done. Flex the knee and internally rotate the extended hip to place the short external rotators under tension.
- Palpate the sciatic nerve as it passes superficial to the obturator internus and the gemelli. Complete exposure of the nerve is unnecessary unless the anatomy of the hip joint is distorted.
- Palpate the tendinous insertions of the piriformis and obturator internus and place tag sutures in the tendons for later identification at the time of closure.
- Divide the short external rotators, including at least the proximal half of the quadratus femoris, as close to their insertion on the femur as possible. Maintaining length of the short rotators facilitates their later repair. Coagulate vessels located along the piriformis tendon and terminal branches of the medial circumflex artery located within the substance of the quadratus femoris. Reflect the short external rotators posteriorly, protecting the sciatic nerve.
- Bluntly dissect the interval between the gluteus minimus and the superior capsule. Insert blunt cobra or Hohmann retractors superiorly and inferiorly to obtain exposure of the entire superior, posterior, and inferior portions of the capsule.
- Divide the entire exposed portion of the capsule immediately adjacent to its femoral attachment. Retract the capsule and preserve it for later repair (Fig. 1.43B).

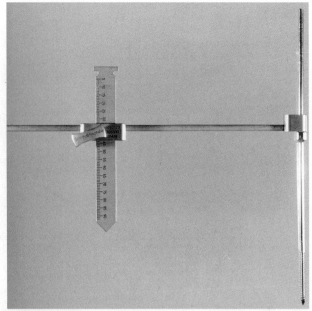

FIGURE 1.44 Device for intraoperative leg-length measurement. Sharp pin is placed in pelvis above acetabulum or iliac crest, and measurements are made at fixed point on greater trochanter. Adjustable outrigger is calibrated for measurement of leg length and femoral offset. **SEE TECHNIQUE 1.2.**

- To determine leg length, insert a Steinmann pin into the ilium superior to the acetabulum and make a mark at a fixed point on the greater trochanter. Measure and record the distance between these two points to determine correct limb length after trial components have been inserted. Make all subsequent measurements with the limb in the identical position. Minor changes in abduction of the hip can produce apparent changes in leg-length measurements. We currently use a device that enables the measurements of leg length and offset (Fig. 1.44).
- Dislocate the hip posteriorly by flexing, adducting, and gently internally rotating the hip.
- Place a bone hook beneath the femoral neck at the level of the lesser trochanter to lift the head gently out of the acetabulum. The ligamentum teres usually is avulsed from the femoral head during dislocation. In younger patients, however, it may require division before the femoral head can be delivered into the wound.
- If the hip cannot be easily dislocated, do not forcibly internally rotate the femur because this can cause a fracture of the shaft. Instead, ensure that the superior and inferior portions of the capsule have been released as far anteriorly as possible. Remove any osteophytes along the posterior rim of the acetabulum that may be incarcerating the femoral head. If the hip still cannot be dislocated without undue force (most often encountered with protrusio deformity), divide the femoral neck with an oscillating saw at the appropriate level and subsequently remove the femoral head segment with a corkscrew or divide it into several pieces.
- After dislocation of the hip, deliver the proximal femur into the wound with a broad, flat retractor.
- Excise residual soft tissue along the intertrochanteric line and expose the upper edge of the lesser trochanter.

- Mark the level and angle of the proposed osteotomy of the femoral neck with the electrocautery or with a shallow cut with an osteotome. Many systems have a specific instrument for this purpose. If not, plan the osteotomy by using a trial prosthesis (see Fig. 1.43C). Use the stem size and neck length trials determined by preoperative templating.
- Align the trial stem with the center of the femoral shaft and match the center of the trial femoral head with that of the patient. The level of the neck cut should be the same distance from the top of the lesser trochanter as determined by preoperative templating.
- Perform the osteotomy with an oscillating or a reciprocating power saw. If this cut passes below the junction of the lateral aspect of the neck and greater trochanter, a separate longitudinal lateral cut is required. Avoid notching the greater trochanter at the junction of these two cuts because this may predispose to fracture of the trochanter.
- Remove the femoral head from the wound by dividing any remaining soft-tissue attachments. Keep the head on the sterile field because it may be needed as a source of bone graft.

EXPOSURE AND PREPARATION OF THE ACETABULUM

- Isolate the anterior capsule by passing a curved clamp within the sheath of the psoas tendon.
- Retract the femur anteriorly with a bone hook to place the capsule under tension.
- Carefully divide the anterior capsule between the jaws of the clamp (Fig. 1.43D).
- Place a curved cobra or Hohmann retractor in the interval between the anterior rim of the acetabulum and the psoas tendon (Fig. 1.43E). Erroneous placement of this retractor over the psoas muscle can cause injury to the femoral nerve or adjacent vessels. The risk increases with a more inferior placement of the retractor. The safest position is near the level of the anterosuperior iliac spine. Place an additional retractor beneath the transverse acetabular ligament to provide inferior exposure.
- Retract the posterior soft tissues with a right-angle retractor placed on top of a laparotomy sponge to avoid compression or excessive traction on the sciatic nerve. As an alternative, place Steinmann pins or spike retractors into the posterior column. Avoid impaling the sciatic nerve or placing the pins within the acetabulum, where they would interfere with acetabular preparation.
- Retract the femur anteriorly and medially and rotate it slightly to determine which position provides the best acetabular exposure. If after complete capsulotomy the femur cannot be fully retracted anteriorly, divide the tendinous insertion of the gluteus maximus, leaving a 1-cm cuff of tendon on the femur for subsequent reattachment.
- Complete the excision of the labrum. Draw the soft tissues into the acetabulum and divide them immediately adjacent to the acetabular rim. Keep the knife blade within the confines of the acetabulum at all times to avoid injury to important structures anteriorly and posteriorly.
- Expose the bony margins of the rim of the acetabulum around its entire circumference to facilitate proper placement of the acetabular component.
- Use an osteotome to remove any osteophytes that protrude beyond the bony limits of the true acetabulum.
- Begin the bony preparation of the acetabulum. The procedure for cartilage removal and reaming of the acetabu-

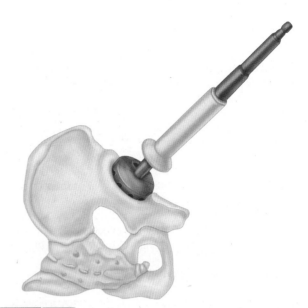

FIGURE 1.45 Reaming of acetabulum. **SEE TECHNIQUES 1.2 AND 1.7.**

lum is similar for cementless and cemented acetabular components.

- Excise the ligamentum teres and curet any remaining soft tissue from the region of the pulvinar. Brisk bleeding from branches of the obturator artery may be encountered during this maneuver and require cauterization.
- Palpate the floor of the acetabulum within the cotyloid notch. Occasionally, hypertrophic osteophytes completely cover the notch and prevent assessment of the location of the medial wall. Remove the osteophytes with osteotomes and rongeurs to locate the medial wall. Otherwise, the acetabular component can be placed in an excessively lateralized position.
- Prepare the acetabulum with power reamers (Fig. 1.45). Begin with a reamer smaller than the anticipated final size and direct it medially down to, but not through, the medial wall. Make frequent checks of the depth of reaming to ensure that the medial wall is not violated. This allows a few millimeters of deepening of the acetabulum with improved lateral coverage of the component.
- Direct all subsequent reamers in the same plane as the opening face of the acetabulum.
- Retract the femur well anteriorly so that reamers can be inserted from an anteroinferior direction without impingement. If the femur is inadequately retracted anteriorly, it may force reamers posteriorly, and excessive reaming of the posterior column occurs. Use progressively larger reamers in 1- or 2-mm increments.
- Irrigate the acetabulum frequently to assess the adequacy of reaming and to adjust the direction of the reaming to ensure that circumferential reaming occurs. Reaming is complete when all cartilage has been removed, the reamers have cut bone out to the periphery of the acetabulum, and a hemispherical shape has been produced.
- Expose a bleeding subchondral bone bed but maintain as much of the subchondral bone plate as possible.
- Curet any remaining soft tissue from the floor of the acetabulum and excise any overhanging soft tissues around the periphery of the acetabulum. Search for subchondral

- cysts within the acetabulum and remove their contents with small curved curets.
- Fill the cavities with morselized cancellous bone obtained from the patient's femoral head or acetabular reamings and impact the graft with a small punch.
- Before insertion of the acetabular component, ensure that the patient remains in the true lateral position. If the pelvis has been rotated anteriorly by forceful anterior retraction of the femur, the acetabular component can easily be placed in a retroverted position, which may predispose to postoperative dislocation. Most systems have trial acetabular components that can be inserted before final implant selection to determine the adequacy of fit, the presence of circumferential bone contact, and the adequacy of the bony coverage of the component; using the trial components also allows the surgeon to make a mental note of the positioning of the component before final implantation.
- Proceed with implantation of either a cementless or cemented acetabular component.

COMPONENT IMPLANTATION

IMPLANTATION OF CEMENTLESS ACETABULAR COMPONENT

The size of the implant is determined by the diameter of the last reamer used. An acetabular component that is the same size as the last reamer has intimate contact with bone but no intrinsic stability. Fixation must be augmented with fins, spikes, or screws. A component that is oversized by 1 to 2 mm can be press-fit into position to provide a greater degree of initial stability. Attempts to impact a much larger component into position results in diminished congruency between the bone and porous surface and incomplete seating of the component against the medial wall. It also might fracture the acetabulum.

Major intrapelvic and extrapelvic vessels and nerves are at risk for injury with erroneously placed transacetabular screws. Wasielewski et al. devised a clinically useful system for determining safe areas for placement of the screws. The system is based on two lines, one drawn from the ASIS through the center of the acetabulum and the other drawn perpendicular to the first, creating four quadrants: anterosuperior, anteroinferior, posterosuperior, and posteroinferior (Fig. 1.46). Screws placed through the anterosuperior quadrant emerge within the pelvis dangerously close to the external iliac artery and vein. Screws passing through the anteroinferior quadrant may injure the obturator nerve and vessels. Screws placed through the posterosuperior and posteroinferior quadrants do not emerge within the pelvis, but they may pass into the sciatic notch and endanger the sciatic nerve and superior gluteal vessels. The drill bit and screw threads can be palpated in the vicinity of the sciatic notch, however, as they emerge so that injury of these structures can be avoided. The

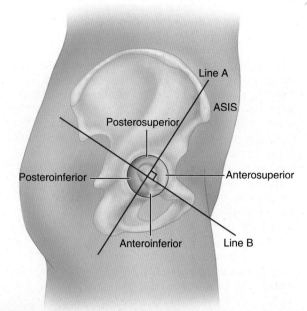

FIGURE 1.46 Acetabular quadrant system described by Wasielewski et al. for determining safe screw placement (see text). Quadrants are formed by intersections of lines A and B. Line A extends from anterior superior iliac spine (ASIS) through center of acetabulum to posterior aspect of fovea, dividing acetabulum in half. Line B is drawn perpendicular to line A at midpoint of acetabulum, dividing it into quadrants: anterosuperior, anteroinferior, posterosuperior, and posteroinferior. (Redrawn from Wasielewski RC, Cooperstein LA, Kruger MP, et al: Acetabular anatomy and the transacetabular fixation of screws in total hip arthroplasty, J Bone Joint Surg 72A:501, 1990.)

posterosuperior quadrant is the safest, and screws longer than 25 mm frequently can be placed through strong bone in this area. The anterosuperior quadrant should be avoided if possible. In a subsequent study, Wasielewski et al. found that only the peripheral halves of the posterior quadrants were safe for screw placement when the acetabular component was implanted with a high hip center.

TECHNIQUE 1.3

- Place the operating table in a completely level position and ensure that the patient remains in the true lateral position.
- Expose the acetabulum circumferentially and retract or excise any redundant soft tissues that may be drawn into the acetabulum as the component is inserted.
- Prepare the appropriate recesses for any ancillary fixation devices present on the component as specified by the manufacturer's technique.
- Attach the acetabular component to the positioning device included with the system instrumentation. Be certain of the means by which the positioning device orients the socket. Usually a rod emerging from the positioning device is oriented either parallel or perpendicular to the floor to determine the proper angle of abduction (or inclination) (Fig. 1.47A). An additional extension from the alignment device determines anteversion (or forward flexion) in relation to the axis of the trunk of the patient (Fig. 1.47B). The optimal inclination of the component is 40

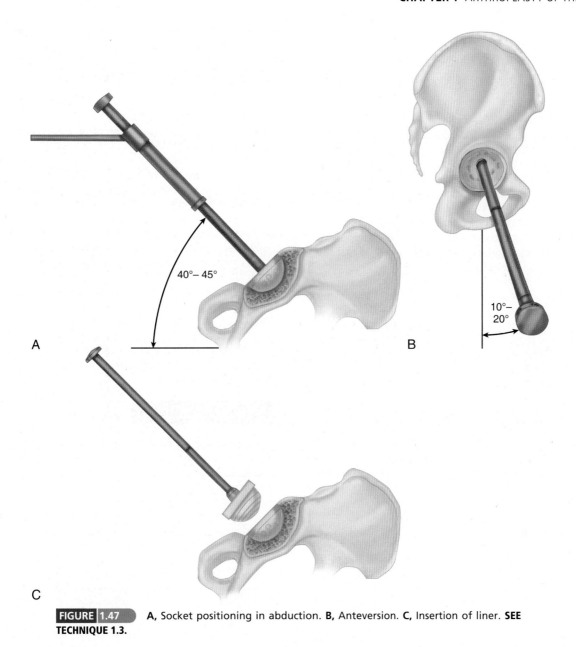

FIGURE 1.47 **A,** Socket positioning in abduction. **B,** Anteversion. **C,** Insertion of liner. **SEE TECHNIQUE 1.3.**

to 45 degrees. The optimal degree of anteversion is 20 degrees.

- The transverse acetabular ligament also is a useful anatomic reference for component positioning. Place the component parallel and just superior to the ligament.
- If the femur demonstrates excessive anteversion or the femoral component is of an anatomic design with anteversion already built in the femoral neck, position the socket in a lesser degree of anteversion. Excessive anteversion of the socket in this case may result in anterior dislocation. Plan for combined anteversion of the femur and acetabulum between 25 and 40 degrees. Carefully reassess the positioning of the implant before impaction because it may be difficult to extricate or change if malpositioned. The edges of the component should match the position of the trial implant fairly closely. If they do not,

carefully reassess the positioning of the patient and the insertion device.

- Maintain the alignment of the positioning device as the component is impacted into position. A change in pitch is heard as the implant seats against subchondral bone. Reassess the positioning; if it is satisfactory, remove the positioning device.
- Examine the subchondral bone plate through any available holes in the component to confirm intimate contact between implant and bone. If a gap is present, impact the component further.
- If screws are to be used for ancillary fixation, place them preferably in the posterosuperior quadrant. Use a flexible drill bit and a screwdriver with a universal joint to insert the screws from within the metal shell. Use a drill sleeve to center the drill hole within the hole of the metal shell.

If the drill hole is placed eccentrically or at too steep an angle, as the screw is inserted its threads may engage the edge of the hole in the metal shell and lift it away from the bone as the screw is advanced; this requires repositioning and reimpaction of the implant. Additionally, if a screw is placed eccentrically, the edge of the head may sit proud within the screw hole and prevent insertion of the liner. Bicortical purchase usually can be obtained with screws in the posterior quadrants.

- Confirm screw length with an angled depth gauge. Self-tapping 6.5-mm screws are preferred. Use a screw-holding clamp to maintain alignment of the screw as the self-tapping threads become engaged. Screw alignment cannot be maintained by a screwdriver with a universal joint. Ensure that the screw head seats completely and is recessed below the inner surface of the shell so that the liner can be fully seated.
- If screws are inserted in the posterior quadrants, palpate along the posterior wall and place a finger within the sciatic notch to protect the sciatic nerve.
- If the drill bit exits in close proximity to the sciatic nerve, use a screw slightly shorter than the measured length or choose a different hole.
- After insertion of one or two screws, test the stability of the component. There should be no detectable motion between implant and bone. If the fixation is unstable, place additional screws.
- With a curved osteotome, remove any osteophytes that protrude beyond the rim of the acetabular component. Pay particular attention to the anteroinferior rim. Retained osteophytes in this region cause impingement on the femur in flexion and internal rotation, reducing motion and predisposing to dislocation.
- Irrigate any debris from within the metal shell.
- Insert the polyethylene liner ensuring that no soft tissue becomes interposed between the polyethylene liner and its metal backing because this would prevent complete seating and engagement of the locking mechanism (Fig. 1.47C). If the system has a variety of liner options available (see Fig. 1.33), a set of trial liners usually accompanies the instrumentation. Final selection of the degree of rim elevation and the position of rotation of the offset within the metal shell can be delayed until the time of trial reduction. The center of the offset usually is placed superiorly or posterosuperiorly. Use the smallest offset that provides satisfactory stability.

Intraoperative changes in the position of the pelvis can affect the accuracy of orientation of the acetabular component. Abduction of the hip or traction on the limb may rotate the pelvis in the craniocaudal plane and lead to errors in the abduction angle. Forceful anterior retraction of the femur rotates the pelvis forward with the tendency to position the acetabular component with inadequate anteversion if the surgeon relies solely on a positioning guide affixed to the insertion device. The surgeon also should evaluate component position relative to bony landmarks. In the ideal position, the inferior edge of the implant should lie just within and parallel to the transverse ligament. The degree of lateral coverage of the implant should also be compared with the amount estimated by preoperative templating.

IMPLANTATION OF CEMENTED ACETABULAR COMPONENT

The design features of cemented acetabular components are discussed in the earlier section on cemented acetabular components. Many components incorporate numerous preformed PMMA pods that ensure a uniform 3-mm cement mantle (see Fig. 1.31). Although some designs incorporate an offset or rim elevation in the polyethylene, the components are not modular and must be inserted as a single unit. The position of rotation of the offset must be selected before cementing the component. All-polyethylene implants usually are available in relatively few sizes. There may be some variability in the thickness of the cement mantle depending on the size of the acetabulum. The size of the implant can be denoted by either the outer diameter of the polyethylene or the outer diameter of the polyethylene plus the additional size provided by the PMMA spacers. Typically, this adds 6 mm to the outer diameter of the implant. The size of the reamed acetabulum should be equal to the outer diameter of the component including the spacers. Otherwise, the component cannot be completely seated.

TECHNIQUE 1.4

- Place the operating table completely level.
- Obtain circumferential exposure of the bony rim of the acetabulum.
- Retract the femur well anteriorly to allow unobstructed passage of the implant into the acetabulum.
- Check the component positioning device again to be certain of its mechanism for orienting the component in proper position. Also, ensure that the positioner can be easily released from the component such that it does not tend to pull the component away from the cement as it is polymerizing. Use a trial component to evaluate the fit and the bony coverage of the component when placed in the optimal position (see Fig. 1.43). Also note the relationship of the edges of the trial component to the bony rim so that this can be reproduced when the final implant is cemented.
- Place the implantable component on the positioner so that it is immediately available when the cement is mixed. Do not contaminate the surface of the implant with blood or debris because this would compromise the cement-prosthesis interface.
- Drill multiple 6-mm holes through the subchondral bone plate of the ilium and ischium for cement intrusion (Fig. 1.48). As an alternative, 12-mm holes can be drilled in the ilium and ischium with additional 6-mm holes between them. Do not drill through the medial wall because this would allow cement intrusion into the pelvis.
- Obturate any penetration of the medial wall with bone grafts or a small wire mesh.
- Curet any loose bone from the drill holes and remove debris and bone marrow from the surface of the acetabulum with pulsatile lavage.
- Thoroughly dry the acetabulum and promote hemostasis with multiple absorbable gelatin sponge (Gelfoam) pledgets or gauze soaked in topical thrombin or 1:500,000 epinephrine solution.

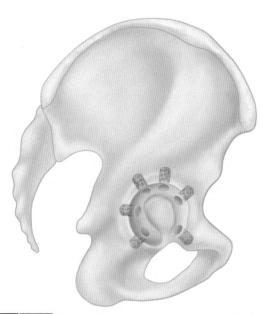

FIGURE 1.48   Fixation holes for cement in acetabulum. **SEE TECHNIQUE 1.4.**

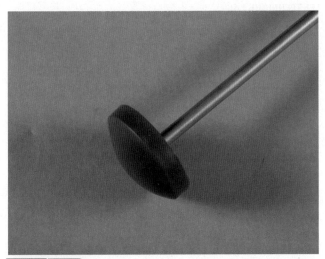

FIGURE 1.49   Acetabular cement pressurizer. Flexible Silastic dam seals rim of acetabulum while manual pressure is applied. **SEE TECHNIQUE 1.4.**

- Mix one package of cement for a smaller patient and two packages for a larger size acetabulum or if an injecting gun is used for cement delivery. Reduce the porosity of the cement by vacuum mixing. Inject the cement in an early dough phase. If the cement is chilled or injected in a very low-viscosity state, it runs out of the acetabulum and pressurization is difficult.
- Dry the acetabulum and suction the fixation holes with a small catheter immediately before cement injection. Inject each of the fixation holes first. Use a cement injection nozzle, which has a small occlusive seal that allows pressurization of each of the holes. Fill the remainder of the acetabulum with cement injected from the gun. Pressurize the major portion of the acetabular cement with a rubber impactor (Fig. 1.49).

- After removing the pressurizing device, carefully dry any blood or fluid that may have accumulated over the surface of the cement.
- Some types of cement, such as Palacos, do not pass through a low-viscosity state and are not easily injected through a gun. Such cements may be used in dough form and inserted manually. Change to a new pair of outer gloves before handling the cement. The bolus of cement is placed into the acetabulum after it ceases to stick to the dry gloves and its surface becomes slightly wrinkled.
- Finger pack a smaller bolus of cement into each of the previously prepared fixation holes. Distribute the remainder of the cement uniformly over the surface of the acetabulum and pressurize it. Remove any blood on the surface of the cement with a dry sponge.
- Insert the acetabular component using the appropriate positioning device. Place the apex of the cup in the center of the cement mass to distribute the cement evenly. Note the relationship of the rim of the component to the bony margins of the acetabulum to verify that the position of the trial component has been reproduced. If no spacers are used, avoid excessive pressure because the cup can be bottomed out against the floor of the acetabulum, producing a discontinuity in the cement mantle.
- Hold the positioner motionless as the cement begins to polymerize. When the cement becomes moderately doughy, carefully remove the positioning device. Stabilize the edge of the component with an instrument as the positioner is removed.
- Replace the device with a ball-type pusher inserted into the socket to maintain pressure as the cement hardens.
- Trim the extruded cement around the edge of the component and remove all cement debris from the area.
- After the cement has hardened completely, test the stability of the newly implanted socket by pushing on several points around the circumference with an impactor. If any motion is detected or blood or small bubbles extrude from the interface, the component is loose and must be removed and replaced (see the section on removal of the cup and cement from the acetabulum).
- Remove any residual osteophytes or cement projecting beyond the rim of the implant because they may cause impingement and postoperative dislocation.
- Long-term outcomes with cemented acetabular components are correlated with the presence of radiolucencies on immediate postoperative radiographs, emphasizing the importance of technique and obtaining a dry bed for cement penetration into cancellous bone.

EXPOSURE AND PREPARATION OF THE FEMUR

- Place a laparotomy sponge in the depths of the acetabulum to protect the acetabular component and prevent the introduction of debris during preparation and insertion of the femoral component.
- Expose the proximal femur by markedly internally rotating the femur so that the tibia is perpendicular to the floor (Fig. 1.50). Allow the knee to drop toward the floor, and push the femur proximally.
- To deliver the proximal femur from the wound, place a broad, flat retractor deep to it and lever it upward. Retract the posterior edge of the gluteus medius and minimus to expose the piriformis fossa and to avoid injuring the

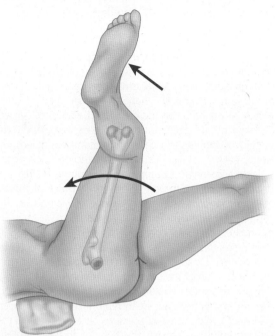

FIGURE 1.50   Positioning of femur for reaming, with patient in lateral position (looking down on patient). Hip is internally rotated, flexed, and adducted until tibia is vertical and axis of knee joint is horizontal. Femoral neck now points downward 15 to 20 degrees, and consequently table is tilted to opposite side for reaming of canal. (From Eftekhar NS: *Principles of total hip arthroplasty*, St. Louis, 1978, Mosby.) **SEE TECHNIQUE 1.4.**

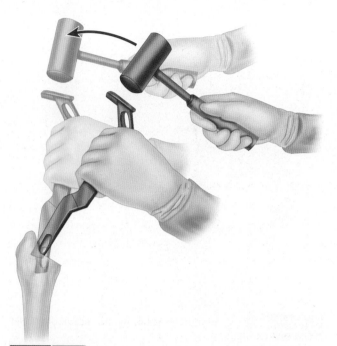

FIGURE 1.51   Removal of remaining lateral edge of femoral neck and medial portion of greater trochanter with box osteotome. **SEE TECHNIQUE 1.4.**

former during preparation and insertion of the femoral component.

■ Excise any remaining soft tissue from the posterior and lateral aspect of the neck. Use a box osteotome or a specialized trochanteric router to remove any remaining portions of the lateral aspect of the femoral neck and the medial portion of the greater trochanter to allow access to the center of the femoral canal (Fig. 1.51).

■ If inadequate bone is removed from these areas, the stem may be placed in varus and may be undersized, the lateral femoral cortex may be perforated, or the femoral shaft or greater trochanter may be fractured.

■ If the proximal femoral cortex is thin, or if stress risers are present because of previous internal fixation devices or disease, place a cerclage wire around the femur above the level of the lesser trochanter to prevent inadvertent fracture.

IMPLANTATION OF CEMENTLESS FEMORAL COMPONENT

The design features of relevant implants are reviewed in the earlier section on cementless femoral components. Younger patients with good quality femoral bone are the best candidates for cementless femoral fixation. Straight femoral

components require straight, fully fluted reamers, but anatomic-type components may require femoral preparation with flexible reamers to accommodate the slight curvature of the stem. Some designs of tapered stems require only broaching for canal preparation. Reaming can be done by hand or with low-speed power reamers. Only the instrumentation supplied by the manufacturer should be used to machine the femur to match precisely the femoral stem shape being implanted. The preoperative plan should be reviewed for the anticipated stem size, as determined by templating.

TECHNIQUE 1.5

■ Expose the proximal femur as described in Technique 1.2.

■ Insert the smallest reamer at a point corresponding to the piriformis fossa. The insertion point is slightly posterior and lateral on the cut surface of the femoral neck. An aberrant insertion point does not allow access to the center of the medullary canal.

■ After the point of the reamer has been inserted, direct the handle laterally toward the greater trochanter (Fig. 1.52). Aim the reamer down the femur toward the medial femoral condyle. If this cannot be accomplished, remove additional bone from the medial aspect of the greater trochanter, or varus positioning of the femoral component results. Generally, a groove must be made in the medial aspect of the greater trochanter to allow proper axial reaming of the canal. Insert the reamer to a predetermined point. Most reamers are marked so as to be referenced against the tip of the greater trochanter or the femoral neck cut to determine the proper depth of insertion.

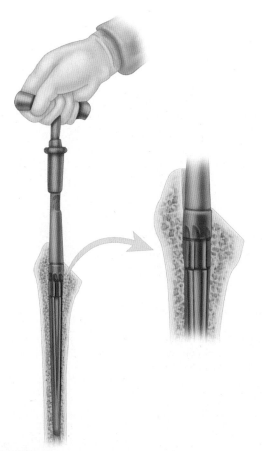

FIGURE 1.52 Reaming of femoral canal. Hand or power reamers must be lateralized into greater trochanter to maintain neutral alignment in femoral canal. (Redrawn courtesy Smith & Nephew, Memphis, TN.) **SEE TECHNIQUES 1.5 AND 1.6.**

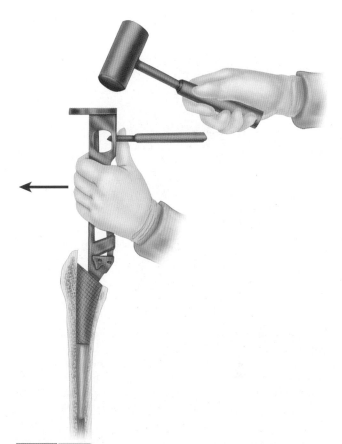

FIGURE 1.53 Femoral broaching. Progressively larger broaches are inserted, lateralizing each one to maintain neutral alignment. (Redrawn courtesy Smith & Nephew, Memphis, TN.) **SEE TECHNIQUE 1.5.**

- Proceed with progressively larger reamers until diaphyseal cortical reaming is felt. Assess the stability of the axial reamer within the canal. No deflection of the tip of the reamer in any plane should be possible.
- If an extensively porous-coated straight stem is used, ream the femoral diaphysis so that 10 to 40 mm of the stem fits tightly in the diaphysis, but underream the canal 0.5 mm smaller than the cylindrical distal portion of the stem so that a tight distal fit can be achieved.
- Proceed with preparation of the proximal portion of the femur. Remove the residual cancellous bone along the medial aspect of the neck with precision broaches. Begin with a broach at least two sizes smaller than the anticipated stem. Never use a broach larger than the last straight or flexible reamer used.
- Place the broach precisely in the same alignment as the axial reamers.
- Push the broach handle laterally during insertion to ensure that enough lateral bone is removed and avoid varus positioning of the stem (Fig. 1.53).
- Rotate the broach to control anteversion. From the posterior approach, the medial aspect of the broach must be rotated toward the floor.
- Align the broach to match precisely the axis of the patient's femoral neck. Do not attempt to place the broach in additional anteversion because this would lead to un-

dersizing of the stem and insufficient rotational stability (Fig. 1.54). Maintain precise control over anteversion as the broach is gently impacted down the canal. Seat the cutting teeth of the broach at least to the level of the cut surface of the neck.
- Proceed with progressively larger broaches, maintaining the identical alignment and rotation. Use even blows with a mallet to advance the broach. The broach should advance slightly with each blow of the mallet. If motion ceases, do not use greater force to insert the broach. Reassess the broach size, adequacy of distal reaming, and alignment and rotation of the broach.
- If a broach sized smaller than that anticipated by templating cannot be fully inserted, the broach may be in varus. Lateralize farther into the greater trochanter with reamers to achieve neutral alignment in the femoral canal and proceed with broaching.
- Seat the final broach to a point where it becomes axially stable within the canal and would not advance farther with even blows of the mallet. The cutting teeth should be seated at or just below the level of the preliminary neck cut to allow precision machining of the remaining neck if a collared stem is to be used.
- Assess the fit of the broach within the canal. The broach should be in intimate contact with a large portion of the endosteal cortex, especially posteriorly and medially.
- When a straight stem is used, there may be a thin rim of remaining cancellous bone anteriorly. Conversely, an ana-

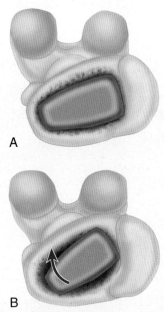

FIGURE 1.54 Femoral component anteversion (as viewed from posterior approach). **A,** Stem placed in same axis as femoral neck. Largest possible stem size fills metaphysis well and obtains rotational stability. **B,** Stem placed in excessive anteversion. Largest possible stem size does not completely fill metaphysis and tends to retrovert when femur is loaded. **SEE TECHNIQUES 1.5 AND 1.6.**

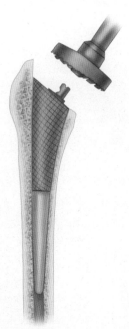

FIGURE 1.55 Planing of calcar with precision reamer placed over broach trunnion. (Redrawn courtesy Smith & Nephew, Memphis, TN.) **SEE TECHNIQUES 1.5 AND 1.6.**

tomic stem often fills this area. If the broach seems to fill the canal completely, with little remaining cancellous bone, assess the rotational stability of the broach. Manually attempt to rotate the broach into a retroverted position. Carefully observe the broach for any motion within the femoral canal. If rotational motion is evident, proceed to the next largest stem size. Proceed one size at a time with distal axial reaming and subsequent broaching until the broach fills the proximal femur as completely as possible and adequate axial and rotational stability has been achieved.

- When adequate stability has been obtained, make the final adjustment of the neck cut. Most systems have a precision calcar planer that fits onto a trunnion on the implanted broach (Fig. 1.55). Precise preparation of the neck is essential if a collared stem is to be used; this step is optional when a collarless stem design is employed. The final level of the neck cut should correspond with the measured distance above the lesser trochanter determined by preoperative templating. If different, adjust the component neck length accordingly.
- Select the trial neck component determined through preoperative templating. In most systems, the trial head and neck components fit onto the trunnion used for attachment of the broach handle (Fig. 1.56). Evaluate the center of the femoral head relative to the height of the tip of the greater trochanter and compare the level with the templated radiographs.
- If the neck length seems satisfactory, irrigate any debris out of the acetabulum.
- Apply traction to the extremity with the hip in slight flexion. Gently lift the head over the superior lip of the acetabulum and any elevation in the polyethylene liner that may have been inserted. If the reduction is difficult, check

for any remaining tight capsule, especially anteriorly, and incise it. If reduction is still impossible, use a shorter neck length, rotate the elevation in the liner to a different position, or remove it entirely.

- As an alternative, use a plastic-covered pusher that fits over the head of the femoral component to push the head into the socket. Do not use excessive force or place excessive torsion on the femur as the hip is reduced, or femoral fracture may occur.
- Reassess the limb length and femoral offset by the previously placed pin near the acetabulum and make changes accordingly.
- Move the hip through a range of motion. Note any areas of impingement between the femur and pelvis or between the prosthetic components with extremes of positioning. Impingement can occur with flexion, adduction, and internal rotation if osteophytes have not been removed from the anterior aspect of the acetabulum, greater trochanter, or femoral neck. Likewise, impingement during external rotation may require removal of bone from the posterior aspect of the greater trochanter, the rim of the acetabulum, or the ischium.
- If prosthetic neck impingement occurs on an elevated polyethylene liner, rotate it to a slightly different position or remove it entirely.
- The hip should be stable (1) in full extension with 40 degrees of external rotation; (2) in flexion to 90 degrees with at least 45 degrees of internal rotation; and (3) with the hip flexed 40 degrees with adduction and axial loading (the so-called position of sleep). If the hip dislocates easily and the head can be manually distracted from the socket more than a few millimeters (the so-called shuck test), use a longer neck length.
- If excessive lengthening of the extremity would result from a longer neck length, use a stem design with a greater

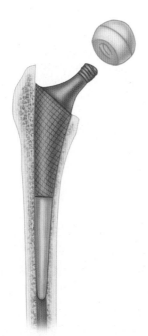

FIGURE 1.56 Assembly of trial head and neck segments determined from preoperative templating. (Redrawn courtesy Smith & Nephew, Memphis, TN.) **SEE TECHNIQUE 1.5.**

degree of offset, if available (see Fig. 1.9). This change would reduce bony impingement and improve soft-tissue tension without additional lengthening of the limb. Slight lengthening of the limb is preferable, however, to the risk of instability.

■ If the hip cannot be brought into full extension, use a shorter neck length, or, if a severe flexion contracture was present preoperatively, release any remaining tight anterior capsular tissues.

■ If there is uncertainty regarding appropriateness of implant size and position or of limb length, then make an intraoperative radiograph for confirmation.

■ If stability is acceptable, note the position of any elevation of the trial polyethylene liner, redislocate the hip by flexion and internal rotation, and gently lift the head out of the acetabulum. Remove the trial components and broach.

■ If a modular trial polyethylene liner has been used, place the final component at this time.

■ Regain exposure of the proximal femur and remove any loose debris within the femoral canal, but do not disturb the bed that has been prepared.

■ Insert the appropriate-size femoral component. Insert the stem to within a few centimeters of complete seating by hand. Reproduce the precise degree of anteversion determined by the broach.

■ Gently impact the stem down the canal. Use the driving device provided with the system or a plastic-tipped pusher. Use blows of equal force as the component is seated. As the component nears complete seating, it advances in smaller increments with each blow of the mallet. Do not use progressively increasing force to insert the component, or femoral fracture can result. Insertion is complete when the stem no longer advances with each blow of the mallet. An audible change in pitch usually can be detected as the stem nears final seating.

■ Occasionally, it is impossible to seat the prosthesis to the level of the cut surface of the neck. If a collared prosthesis has been used and the collar has not made full contact with bone, leave the collar slightly proud rather than risk femoral fracture. When a collarless prosthesis is used, occasionally the prosthesis may advance a few millimeters past the level achieved with the broach. In these instances, the neck length can be changed and an additional trial reduction is necessary to confirm the final neck length and the stability of the joint.

■ Test the stability of the implanted stem to rotational and extraction forces. If the stem is deemed unstable, decide whether it can be impacted further or whether a larger stem size can be inserted.

■ Carefully inspect the femoral neck and greater trochanter for any fractures that may have occurred during stem insertion.

■ If a fracture is produced as the stem is being seated, immediately stop the insertion procedure. Completely expose the fracture to its distal extent and then remove the stem. Otherwise, the extent of the fracture may be underestimated.

■ If an incomplete fracture occurs with extension only to the level of the lesser trochanter, place a cerclage wire around the femur above the lesser trochanter. Reinsert the stem and ensure the cerclage wire tightens as the stem is seated into position. Reassess the stability of the implanted stem.

■ If the fracture extends below the level of the lesser trochanter, a longer stem with greater distal fixation is required (see later). If the greater trochanter is fractured and unstable, proceed with fixation as for a trochanteric osteotomy (see section on trochanteric osteotomy).

■ Wipe any debris from the Morse taper segment of the prosthetic neck and carefully dry it.

■ Place the prosthetic head of appropriate size and neck length onto the trunnion and affix it with a single blow of a mallet over a plastic-capped head impactor. Use only femoral heads specifically designed to mate with the stem and ensure that the femoral head and acetabular component are of a corresponding size.

■ Remove any debris from the acetabulum and again reduce the hip. Ensure no soft tissues have been reduced into the joint.

■ Confirm the stability of the hip through a functional range of motion.

IMPLANTATION OF CEMENTED FEMORAL COMPONENT

Improvements in preparation of the femur and the mixing and delivery of cement and modifications in component design have yielded dramatic improvements in the survivorship of cemented femoral components. Cement fixation is indicated especially when the femoral cortex is thin or osteoporotic and secure press-fit fixation is less predictably achieved. Design features of femoral components used with cement are reviewed in the earlier section on femoral stems used with cement.

TECHNIQUE 1.6

- Expose the proximal femur as described. Use rongeurs, a box osteotome, or a trochanteric reamer to remove residual portions of the lateral aspect of the neck and gain access to the center of the canal.
- Insert a small, tapered reamer to locate the medullary canal. Insert the tip of the reamer into the lateralmost aspect of the cut surface of the neck and swing it into the greater trochanter to point it toward the medial femoral condyle (see Fig. 1.52). This maneuver ensures neutral positioning of the femoral component.
- Review the preoperative plan for the templated stem size. Begin with the smallest size broach. Insert the broaches in 10 to 15 degrees of anteversion in relation to the axis of the flexed tibia. From the posterior approach, this means that the medial aspect of the broach must be rotated toward the floor (see Fig. 1.54). Maintain correct axial alignment as the broach is inserted.
- Alternatively, impact and extract the broach to facilitate its passage. Use progressively larger broaches to crush and remove cancellous bone in the proximal femur. Because fixation is achieved with cement, the requirements for absolute stability of the broach are not as rigorous as with cementless techniques. Nonetheless, a stem that fills the femoral canal with an adequate cement mantle is still desirable.
- Use the largest size broach that can be easily inserted proximally. If resistance is felt during insertion of the broach, the area of impingement is most likely distal within the diaphysis. The broach cannot be used to prepare cortical bone in the diaphysis. Do not attempt to impact the broach further because a femoral fracture can occur, or the broach can become incarcerated.
- A narrow canal can be anticipated easily by preoperative templating. Use graduated-sized reamers to enlarge the canal sufficiently to allow insertion of a broach that is appropriately sized proximally. Because removal of all cancellous bone from the canal leaves a smooth cortical surface not amenable to microinterlock with cement, avoid excessive reaming of the medullary canal. Canal preparation is distinctly different with this procedure than for a cementless stem, even though many contemporary total hip systems use the same instrumentation for the two applications.
- In most current systems, the broach is larger than the corresponding stem size, although the amount of oversizing varies. The channel prepared allows insertion of an appropriate-size stem with an adequate surrounding cement mantle. A cement mantle thickness of 2 to 4 mm proximally and 2 mm distally is satisfactory.
- If a stem with a collar is to be used, countersink the final broach slightly below the provisional femoral neck cut. Precisely prepare the femoral neck to receive the collar by using a planer (see Fig. 1.55). If a collarless stem is used, mark the height of the shoulder of the broach on the greater trochanter in order to reproduce this position when the final stem is implanted.

- Select the templated neck length and assemble a trial component. Note the relationship of the trial collar to the cut surface of the femoral neck for axial and rotational positioning of the final stem as it is implanted. The medial edge of the collar may sit flush with the medial cortex or may protrude slightly beyond it; either is acceptable. Reproduction of this degree of overhang helps prevent varus or valgus positioning of the stem as the final component is inserted.
- Perform a trial reduction, as described in Technique 1.5, to determine limb length, range of motion, and stability of the arthroplasty.
- If the limb has been excessively lengthened, use a shorter trial neck. Alternatively, seat the broach further and recut the femoral neck to reduce limb length while maintaining the same degree of femoral offset. A smaller broach size may be required to accomplish this.
- Because the stem is to be fixed with cement, the depth of insertion of the component is predetermined at this point. This is in contrast to a cementless implant, which may achieve stability at a slightly different depth of insertion than did the corresponding broach.
- When final component sizes have been selected and limb length and stability have been assessed, dislocate the hip and remove the trial components.
- Regain exposure of the proximal femur.
- Remove remaining loose cancellous bone from the femur using a femoral canal brush or curets. Retain a few millimeters of dense cancellous bone for cement intrusion.
- Occlude the femoral canal distal to the anticipated tip of the stem to allow pressurization of the cement and to prevent extrusion of the cement distally into the femoral diaphysis. This is accomplished by use of a plastic, flexible canal plug or a bone block fashioned to fit the canal or by injecting a small plug of cement distally. A preformed flexible plastic plug is the easiest to use, but it must be of a large enough size to prevent its distal migration during cement pressurization (Fig. 1.57).
- Determine the canal diameter by using sounds. Insert the cement restrictor to a depth of approximately 1 to 2 cm below the anticipated tip of the stem. Determine the depth of insertion by comparing the insertion device with the broach or the actual stem. Account for any additional length required by the use of a distal stem centralizer. Gently tap the restrictor into place, or it may be forced distal to the isthmus.
- After insertion of the cement restrictor, reinsert the broach or trial stem to ensure that the restrictor has been placed sufficiently distal to allow the stem to be fully seated.
- As an alternative, fashion a plug of bone removed from the femoral head or neck. This plug should be slightly larger than the diameter of the canal. Impact it into position with a punch.
- Occlusion of the canal with a small bolus of PMMA requires more preparation but is more reliable when the canal is excessively large or when the canal must be occluded below the level of the isthmus to insert a longer length stem. To occlude the canal with a PMMA plug, mix a single package of cement. Insert the cement when it is in the early dough phase because extremely low-viscosity cement runs down the canal and does not completely occlude it. Inject a small bolus of cement at the prede-

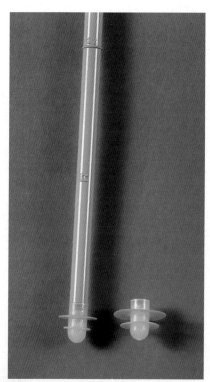

FIGURE 1.57   Occlusion of medullary canal. Plastic plug with flexible, thin flanges can be inserted to occlude medullary canal; plugs of several different diameters are available. They are screwed to end of calibrated rod for insertion to correct depth. **SEE TECHNIQUE 1.6.**

termined level using a cement injecting gun or a cement syringe, or introduce the cement through a small chest tube, using a plunger to maintain the cement bolus in proper position as the chest tube is extracted. Rotate the injecting gun in all directions to disperse the cement uniformly. Reinsert the trial component and gently tamp the cement before it hardens to ensure that the final component can be fully seated.

- After occluding the femoral canal, thoroughly irrigate it to remove loose debris, bone marrow, and blood. This is best accomplished by using a pulsatile lavage system with a long, straight tip and radially directed spray. Thoroughly irrigate all debris and bone marrow out of the residual trabeculae of cancellous bone so that maximal cement intrusion can be obtained. Thorough lavage of the canal also reduces the amount of marrow embolization that can occur during cement pressurization and stem insertion.
- Dry the canal with a tampon sponge with a suction attachment or with sponges soaked in 1:500,000 epinephrine solution to diminish bleeding while the cement is being prepared.
- Open the previously determined implants. Do not touch the stem or allow it to become contaminated with blood or debris because this may compromise the cement-implant interface after implantation.
- Assemble any modular PMMA spacers that can be used to centralize the stem within the canal.
- Do not leave unfilled any holes in the stem intended for centralizers because entrapped air would expand with the

heat of cement polymerization, producing a void in the cement mantle. Fill such holes with cement before introducing the implant, or use the centralizers provided with the system. Centralizers also can be fixed to the implant with a small amount of cement to ensure an adequate interface between the two. This distal stem centralizer size is determined by the canal diameter previously determined from sounds. Ideally, the centralizer should be at least 4 mm larger than the diameter of the distal end of the stem to ensure a 2-mm circumferential cement mantle.

- Change the outer gloves. Mix two batches of cement for a standard-size femur and three batches for a larger femur or if a long-stem component is to be used. Current pressurization techniques require a greater volume of cement than has been used in the past. Prepare the cement with a porosity reduction technique such as vacuum mixing.
- If internal fixation devices have been removed from the femoral shaft during the same procedure, the holes left in the femoral cortex must be occluded to allow pressurization of the cement and to prevent its egress into the soft tissues. Have an assistant place fingers over the holes before cement injection, or use a small amount of cement to occlude them before the remainder of the femur is filled with cement.
- Use a cement-injecting gun for the most reliable cement delivery. Plan to inject the cement as it enters a dough phase, or when it no longer sticks to a gloved finger. This typically is about 4 minutes after the start of mixing for Simplex cement, although it can vary significantly with the type of cement used, the room temperature, humidity, and whether the monomer component or stem was heated before mixing. If the cement is injected in an excessively low-viscosity state, it tends to run out of the femur during pressurization, making it more susceptible to the introduction of blood and debris, thus weakening the mantle and compromising the cement-bone interface. If injected late or in a high viscosity state, then it may be difficult to fully insert the stem before cement polymerization occurs.
- Pack a sponge within the acetabulum and shield the surrounding soft tissues with sponges to prevent the escape of cement.
- Immediately before introduction of the cement injecting gun, remove any packing sponges and suction the distal aspect of the canal to remove any blood that has pooled there.
- Pump the trigger of the cement injecting gun to deliver cement to the tip of the nozzle so that no air is introduced. Insert the nozzle to the level of the cement restrictor, and use smooth, sequential compressions of the trigger to deliver the cement in a uniform manner (Fig. 1.58). Allow the pressure of the injected cement to push the nozzle out of the canal as the canal is filled in a retrograde fashion. Do not pull the nozzle back too quickly or voids would be created in the cement column. Fill the canal to the level of the cut surface of the femoral neck.
- Pressurize the cement by one of many methods. Preferably, use an occlusive nozzle that allows the injection of more cement through it (Fig. 1.59). Ensure that an adequate seal is maintained and slowly inject more cement

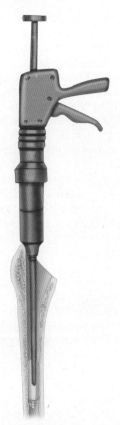

FIGURE 1.58 Retrograde injection of cement with gun. Cement gun with long nozzle can be used to inject semiliquid cement. Distal part of canal is filled first, and tip is slowly withdrawn as cement is injected. Injection is continued until canal is completely filled and tip of nozzle is clear of canal. (Redrawn courtesy Smith & Nephew, Memphis, TN.) **SEE TECHNIQUE 1.6.**

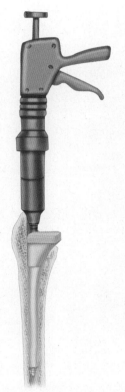

FIGURE 1.59 Cement pressurization. Flexible pressurizing nozzle is placed over end of cement gun to seal proximal femur, and firm pressure is applied as additional cement is injected. (Redrawn Courtesy Smith & Nephew, Memphis, TN.) **SEE TECHNIQUE 1.6.**

over approximately 30 seconds to produce intrusion of cement into remaining cancellous bone bed. As an alternative, use a plastic impactor or mechanical plunger-type device placed over a glove or rubber sheet. Cement and bone marrow can be seen extruding from the small vascular foramina along the femoral neck during pressurization.

- Remove the pressurization device; if a void has been left in the proximal cement by the device, refill it with cement.
- Have the femoral component immediately available for insertion and insert the component when the cement has entered a medium dough phase, typically at about 6 minutes after the start of mixing for Simplex cement. The optimal time may be considerably less for other types of cement.
- Determine the desired amount of anteversion and the mediolateral position of the stem before insertion. Changes in alignment and rotation of the stem as it is inserted introduce voids into the cement.
- Hold the stem by the proximal end and insert it manually at first. Insert the tip of the stem within the center of the cement mantle. Use firm, even pressure to insert the stem. When the cement has been pressurized, it can be difficult to seat the stem completely by hand; have a plastic-tipped head impactor and a mallet immediately available to complete the seating of the stem. Most

contemporary systems have an insertion device for this purpose.

- Reproduce the position of the trial collar in relation to the cut surface of the femoral neck to aid in aligning the stem properly. Remove the cement from the region of the collar to ensure that the stem has been fully inserted; if not, impact it farther. If a collarless stem is used, reproduce the height of the shoulder with the previously made mark on the greater trochanter.
- Maintain firm pressure on the proximal end of the component as the cement hardens. Hold the stem motionless. This is best accomplished with a plastic-tipped pusher or dedicated stem inserter that is not rigidly fixed to the component. Insertion devices that screw into the femoral component or are rigidly fixed to it cause any small amount of motion between the surgeon and the assistant holding the leg to be transmitted to the cement-prosthesis interface.
- As the cement enters a late dough phase, cut the cement around the edges of the prosthesis and carefully remove it from the operative field. Do not pull the cement from beneath the component, or proximal support may be lost.
- After the cement has fully hardened, use a small osteotome to remove any additional fragments of cement and carefully inspect the anterior aspect of the neck for retained cement.
- Meticulously remove all cement debris from the wound. Irrigate and inspect carefully the acetabular component and remove any cement that may have entered it during femoral cementing.

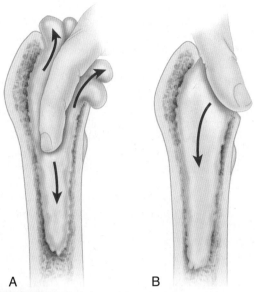

FIGURE 1.60 Manual cement packing. **A,** When cement is inserted manually, it must be packed firmly in canal with finger before stem is introduced. **B,** After canal has been filled, cement is pressed with thumb, preventing its escape and increasing pressure within canal. **SEE TECHNIQUE 1.6.**

- Carefully clean and dry the taper, and assemble the modular femoral head with a single blow using a plastic-capped impactor.
- The preferred method for filling the canal with cement is to use an injecting gun with the cement in a medium viscosity state. Some cements, such as Palacos, exist primarily in a dough phase, however, and are not easily injected. Under these circumstances, the cement can be inserted manually. To insert cement into the femoral canal manually, mold the cement into the shape of a sausage and hold it in the palm of one hand or in an open plastic container. Push the cement into the canal with the index finger or thumb of the opposite hand as far distally as the finger reaches (Fig. 1.60A). If the cement is still sticky, pack it by short strokes with the fingertip. Avoid mixing blood with the cement and keep the bolus of cement intact. Lamination of the cement or incorporation of blood weakens it.
- After the cavity has been filled, press the cement with the thumb (Fig. 1.60B). A mechanical impactor or plunger can be used. Two packages usually suffice, but additional cement may be necessary for larger medullary canals. A small plastic suction tube can be placed in the femoral canal to allow air and blood to escape while the cement is being inserted. If a suction tube is used, place it into the canal before the cement is introduced; remove it after about two thirds of the cement has been inserted.

SOFT-TISSUE REPAIR AND CLOSURE
- After reduction of the hip, proceed with repair of the posterior soft-tissue envelope. Repair the preserved portion of the posterior capsule with heavy nonabsorbable sutures placed through holes in the posterior edge of the greater trochanter. Reattach the previously tagged tendons of the short external rotator muscles.
- Repair any portion of the gluteus maximus insertion and quadratus femoris that has been divided.
- Careful reconstruction of the posterior soft-tissue envelope greatly reduces the risk of postoperative dislocation.
- If desired, place a closed-suction drain deep to the fascia. Abduct the hip 10 degrees while closing the fascial incision with closely approximated sutures. Tight closure of this layer helps stabilize the hip and may prevent a superficial inflammatory process from extending to a deeper level. Loosely approximate the subcutaneous layer with interrupted, absorbable sutures.
- Close the skin in routine fashion.

TOTAL HIP ARTHROPLASTY THROUGH THE DIRECT ANTERIOR APPROACH

DIRECT ANTERIOR APPROACH WITH ANTERIOR DISLOCATION OF THE HIP

The direct anterior approach uses the distal half of the traditional Smith-Petersen approach to the hip. Initially described by Light and Keggi in 1980, modifications of the approach have become considerably more popular over the last decade. The interval is both intermuscular and internervous, so little muscular dissection is required. Performed with the patient supine, the procedure can be done on a conventional radiolucent table or a specialized table similar to those used in fracture surgery. An accessory hook mounted on the side of the table can be used to aid in elevating the femur for preparation and component implantation. Intraoperative fluoroscopy can also be used to check the progress of reaming, the positioning of implants, and restoration of limb length. The position of the pelvis is also more reliable when the patient is supine than in the lateral decubitus position.

The approach traverses anatomy that may be unfamiliar even to experienced hip surgeons. The learning curve for the procedure can be improved by cadaver laboratory instruction sponsored by orthopaedic societies and industry or by personal visitation with surgeons already experienced in the procedure. Acetabular preparation and component implantation generally are straightforward. Access to the femur is more difficult, leading many surgeons to use shorter or curved femoral components to simplify the procedure (see Figs. 1.21C and 1.28).

Certain patient factors make the approach more complex. The interval cannot be safely extended distally, so a separate exposure is required to access the femur in patients with deformity requiring osteotomy, removal of previously placed implants, or placement of femoral cerclage. Access to the femoral canal can be more difficult in patients with a wide iliac crest and those with a short, varus femoral neck. In obese patients the subcutaneous layer about the anterior aspect of the hip tends to be thinner than the lateral aspect, and with the patient supine gravity displaces the tissues away from the incision. In patients with a large panniculus, however, the inguinal crease is prone to dermatitis and chronic fungal infection leading to problems with wound healing.

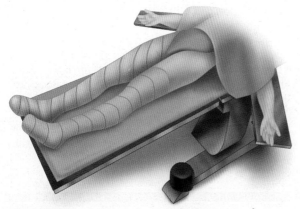

FIGURE 1.61 Direct anterior approach. Patient positioned supine with anterior superior iliac spine placed at level of table break. (Redrawn from Biomet.) **SEE TECHNIQUE 1.7.**

The anterior approach also has been advocated because of a low incidence of dislocation, although this difference has diminished with the use of larger femoral heads and soft-tissue repair. Some investigators have also reported faster functional recovery with the direct anterior approach, including shorter hospitalization, less narcotic use, and less reliance on ambulatory aids at 2 weeks. Few report any differences past 6 weeks postoperatively.

TECHNIQUE 1.7

- Position the patient supine on a radiolucent table with the ASIS at the level of the table break such that the operated limb can be positioned in marked hyperextension (Fig. 1.61). Place a small bolster under the operative hip to aid in elevating the femur. If fluoroscopy is to be used, ensure that the pelvis is level and that both hips can be adequately imaged.
- Prepare the skin of both lower limbs above the level of the ASIS and drape the limbs separately such that the operated limb can be crossed beneath the opposite limb in a figure-of-four position. An additional padded and draped Mayo stand is useful for supporting the opposite limb during preparation of the femur.
- Place the skin incision lateral to the interval between the tensor fascia lata (TFL) and sartorius to avoid injury to the fibers of the lateral femoral cutaneous nerve (LFCN), which may be variable in its course. Begin the incision approximately 3 cm distal and 3 cm lateral to the ASIS. Extend the incision distal and slightly lateral for 8 to 12 cm.
- Divide the fascia over the muscle belly of the TFL fibers to stay lateral to the LFCN (Fig. 1.62A).
- Now bluntly dissect medially with an index finger in the interval between the TFL and sartorius (Fig. 1.62B). If uncertain of the correct plane, expose proximally to ascertain that the dissected interval is lateral to the ASIS.
- The femoral neck can be palpated through a thin layer of fat overlying the anterior capsule. Within this fat layer in the distal extent of the interval, locate the ascending branches of the lateral circumflex vessels and cauterize them with electrocautery or a bipolar sealer (Fig. 1.62C). Brisk bleeding may be encountered if these vessels are divided and allowed to retract.
- Place blunt curved retractors superior and inferior to the femoral neck. Elevate the fibers of the rectus femoris from the anterior hip capsule and place a pointed retractor over the anterior rim of the acetabulum just distal to the direct head of the rectus (Fig. 1.62D). Release the fibers of the reflected head of the rectus to allow improved medial retraction of the direct head. Slight flexion of the hip also relaxes the rectus. Take care in the placement of the retractor beneath the rectus to avoid injury to the femoral nerve and vessels.
- Divide the anterior hip capsule in a T-shaped or H-shaped fashion for later repair, or alternatively excise the capsule. Release the inferior capsule to the level of the lesser trochanter. Now replace the superior and inferior curved retractors inside the capsule to completely expose the femoral neck.
- Perform an in situ osteotomy of the femoral neck at the level determined by preoperative templating. Measure the osteotomy from the lesser trochanter or by use of fluoroscopy. It may be necessary to make a second parallel osteotomy at the subcapital region producing a "napkin ring" of bone, which is secured with a threaded Steinmann pin for removal (Fig. 1.63A).
- Extract the femoral head with a corkscrew, which can be placed before the neck osteotomy is made. Take care to protect the TFL from sharp bone edges when removing the femoral head. Recheck the neck osteotomy height. If the femoral neck is left excessively long, acetabular exposure will be more difficult.
- To expose the acetabulum, place curved retractors distal to the transverse acetabular ligament and along the posterior rim of the acetabulum to displace the femur posteriorly (Fig. 1.63). An additional retractor can be placed over the anterior acetabular rim if needed. Excise the labrum and prepare the acetabulum with reamers (see Fig. 1.45). Specialized offset reamers and cup positioners are available for this purpose. The progress of acetabular reaming and cup positioning can be verified using fluoroscopy. There is a tendency to place the cup in excessive abduction and anteversion with the patient supine.
- Elevation of the femur is the most difficult step with the patient supine. To expose the proximal femur, place the operated limb in figure-of-four position beneath the opposite limb. Adduct the femur slightly and externally rotate 90 degrees. Avoid excessive knee flexion because this position tightens the rectus femoris, making femoral elevation more difficult.
- Now "break" the table to position the operated hip in hyperextension. Raise the table and place it in the Trendelenburg position to prevent the lower end from approaching the floor. Support the opposite leg on a padded sterile Mayo stand or arm board (Fig. 1.64A).
- Elevate the femur laterally and upward with a bone hook placed within the femoral canal or around the lateral aspect of the femur. Take care that the femur is not trapped behind the acetabulum during this maneuver; elevation of the femur will be more difficult, or fracture of the greater trochanter may occur. A sterile hook mounted on a table attachment can be used during this step (Fig. 1.64B). Place the hook just distal to the vastus ridge. Position a curved retractor beneath the posteromedial femoral neck to retract the medial soft tissues. Place an additional pronged retractor over the tip of the greater trochanter to protect the abductor musculature and lift the femur anteriorly.

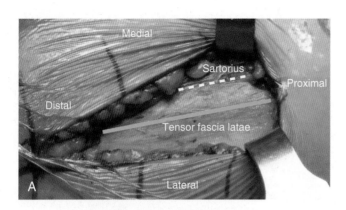

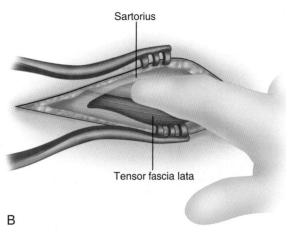

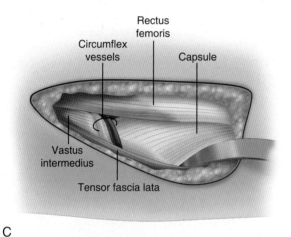

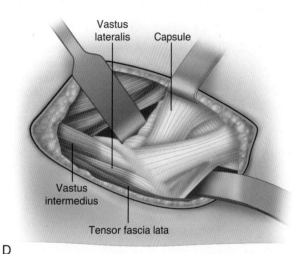

FIGURE 1.62   **A,** Fascial incision *(green line)* is positioned over the tensor fascia latae (TFL) muscle and lateral to the interval between TFL and sartorius *(dashed white line)*. **B,** Blunt dissection medially beneath fascia leads to interval between TFL and sartorius. **C,** Within the fat layer at distal extent of interval are branches of the lateral femoral circumflex vessels that must be identified and carefully cauterized. **D,** Extracapsular placement of retractors superiorly and inferiorly before capsulotomy. An additional retractor may be placed medially beneath rectus femoris. (**A** from Post ZD, Orozco F, Diaz-Ledezma C, et al: Direct anterior approach for total hip arthroplasty: indications, technique, and results, *J Am Acad Orthop Surg* 22:595-603, 2014. **B-D** redrawn from Depuy.) **SEE TECHNIQUE 1.7.**

- Additional soft-tissue release often is required at this stage to avoid excess retraction force, which may result in femoral fracture. Patients with fixed external rotation deformity typically require a greater amount of release to deliver the femur anteriorly. First, release the superior capsule from the greater trochanter from anterior to posterior, completely exposing the trochanteric fossa or "saddle" (Fig. 1.65). In more difficult cases, release the piriformis and conjoined tendons to allow elevation of the femur without undue traction (Fig. 1.66).
- Prepare the femur and implant the femoral component (see Technique 1.5). It is technically easier to implant a femoral component using a broach-only technique because it may be difficult to pass straight reamers down the femoral canal even with satisfactory femoral exposure. Specialized angled broach handles and stem insertion devices also simplify the procedure (Fig. 1.67). A canal sound or guide pin is useful to judge the alignment of the femoral canal and avoid varus stem positioning or perforation of the lateral femoral cortex.
- During the trial reduction of implants, take special care to assess the stability of the hip in extension and external rotation, particularly if a complete anterior capsulectomy has been performed during the initial exposure. Use fluoroscopy to assess position of the implants and restoration of limb length and offset. Limb length also can be assessed directly by comparison with the opposite limb.
- If the anterior capsule has been retained, perform a secure closure of the capsular flaps. When closing the fascial layer, take small bites on the medial edge to avoid entrapment of the LFCN in the repair.

Some proponents of the supine intermuscular approach have advocated the use of a dedicated surgical table similar to those used in lower extremity fracture care. Both feet are secured in compression boots attached to mobile spars that

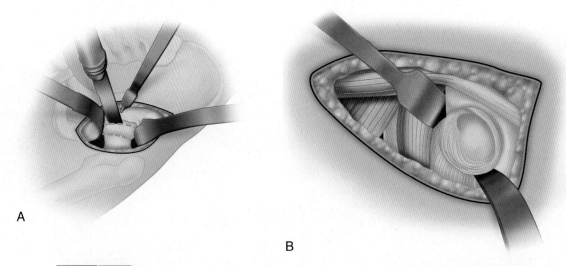

FIGURE 1.63   **A,** Femoral neck osteotomy. Two parallel cuts made *(dashed lines)* and "napkin ring" segment removed with a threaded pin. Femoral head is then removed with corkscrew. **B,** Retractors placed inferior to transverse ligament and also posteriorly to retract femur. (**A** redrawn from Biomet. **B** redrawn from Depuy.) **SEE TECHNIQUE 1.7.**

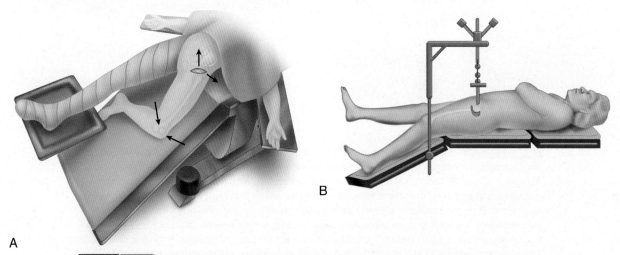

FIGURE 1.64   **A,** Table position for exposure of femur. Operated limb is placed in figure-of-four position beneath opposite lower limb, and lower end of table is dropped to place hip in hyperextension. Proximal femur must be retracted laterally and upward. **B,** Accessory hook mounted to table aids femoral elevation. (**A** redrawn from Biomet; **B** courtesy Innomed, Inc. Savannah, GA.) **SEE TECHNIQUE 1.7.**

allow traction, rotation, and angulation of the limb in any direction (Fig. 1.68). An integral hook is used to aid in femoral elevation, and intraoperative fluoroscopic imaging is easily obtained. Because both feet are secured in boots, however, it is more difficult to manually assess the stability of the hip and directly compare limb lengths. The use of such a table requires a significant institutional financial investment, and the use of strong traction and limb rotation also introduces a risk of traction nerve palsy and fractures.

Matta et al. reported a series of 494 primary arthroplasties performed on a dedicated table. Clinical and radiographic results were excellent, but there was one femoral nerve palsy, three greater trochanteric fractures, two femoral shaft fractures, and three ankle fractures. The complications underscore the importance of obtaining exposure by judicious soft-tissue releases rather than by forceful traction and limb rotation.

The results using intraoperative fluoroscopy have been mixed. Hamilton et al. reported no excessively abducted cups (over 55 degrees) using fluoroscopy with the direct anterior approach. Leucht et al. found that fluoroscopy reduced the incidence of limb length discrepancy of more than 1 cm but did not improve the precision of cup positioning. In a large series from the Rothman Institute, Tischler et al. found no difference in acetabular inclination angle, leg length, or offset using fluoroscopy and concluded that the increased operative time and cost were not justified at a high-volume arthroplasty institution. Careful attention must be paid to both the

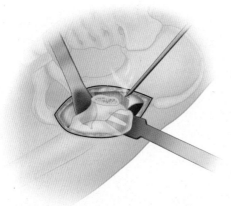

FIGURE 1.65 Soft-tissue release for femoral elevation. Superior capsule is released from anterior to posterior to completely expose trochanteric fossa and allow elevation of femur without undue force. (Redrawn from Biomet.) **SEE TECHNIQUE 1.7.**

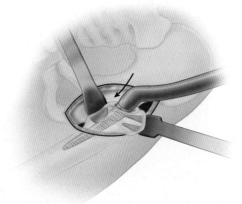

FIGURE 1.67 Femoral instrumentation. After adequate elevation of femur, preparation is facilitated by instruments with offset handles. (Redrawn from Biomet.) **SEE TECHNIQUE 1.7.**

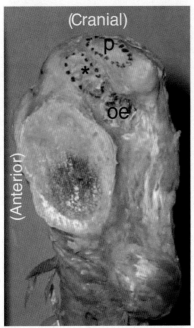

FIGURE 1.66 Insertions of short external rotators as viewed from medial. Piriformis (*p*) inserts near cephalad extent of greater trochanter. Conjoined tendon (*asterisk*) and obturator externus (*oe*) insert more distal. (From Ito Y, Matsushita I, Watanabe H, Kimura T: Anatomic mapping of short external rotators shows the limit of their preservation during total hip arthroplasty, *Clin Orthop Relat Res* 470:1690, 2012.) **SEE TECHNIQUE 1.7.**

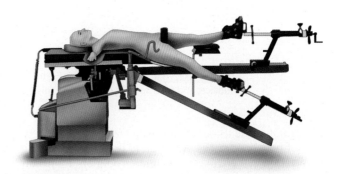

FIGURE 1.68 Dedicated table for positioning during direct anterior approach. Surgeon controls elevation of femur with integral hook. (ProFx table, courtesy Mizuho OSI, Union City, CA.)

tilt and rotation of the pelvis in relation to the x-ray beam to maximize the utility of intraoperative fluoroscopy. Standard protection in the form of a lead apron and thyroid shield are recommended for those in proximity to the beam. McArthur et al. reported radiation dose and fluoroscopy times that were comparable to other fluoroscopically guided hip procedures.

MINIMALLY INVASIVE TECHNIQUES

Hip arthroplasty has been performed through small incisions by Kennon et al. since the 1980s. More recently, minimally invasive techniques have been introduced to the orthopaedic community and have received widespread media attention. The term *minimally invasive total hip replacement* does not describe a single operation but rather a group of procedures performed through various incisions of smaller dimensions than traditionally described.

The introduction of these techniques has generated considerable controversy in the orthopaedic community. Advocates of these techniques have advanced the position that minimally invasive hip replacement has the potential to reduce soft-tissue injury, postoperative pain, operative blood loss, and hospital length of stay; increase speed of the patient's postoperative rehabilitation; and produce a more cosmetically acceptable surgical scar. Adoption of minimally invasive techniques has revolutionized other procedures, such as meniscectomy, cruciate ligament reconstruction, rotator cuff repair, discectomy, and others. Critics of these new techniques cite the excellent results of current methods with regard to pain relief, functional improvement, and long-term durability, with a remarkably low complication rate. The potential benefits of smaller incisions must be weighed against the pitfalls of poor exposure and the learning curve associated with any new procedure. There is the potential for implant loosening from suboptimal bone preparation, dislocation from malpositioned implants, infection and delayed wound healing from trauma to the skin, unrecognized fractures, neurovascular

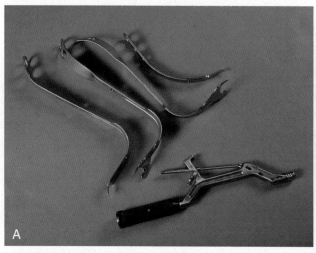
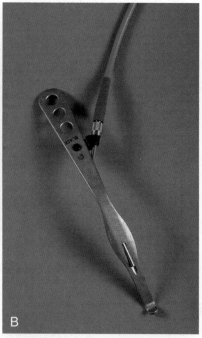

FIGURE 1.69   **A** and **B,** Array of retractors with long handles, angulated acetabular insertion device, and fiberoptic lighting **(B)** for minimally invasive hip surgery. (Courtesy Zimmer, Warsaw, IN.)

compromise, and leg-length inequality from the lack of exposure of bony landmarks. All of these problems may require reoperation and are likely to be more common in the hands of surgeons performing fewer procedures. Surgeons must decide whether the potential risks in adopting minimally invasive techniques are justifiable given the scope of their individual practices.

There is general consensus that a minimally invasive hip arthroplasty is done through an incision of 10 cm or less. A single posterior incision is currently the most commonly used approach, followed by single-incision direct anterior approaches. We have gradually adopted minimally invasive techniques and now perform hip arthroplasty in most patients through a single posterior incision of 8 to 10 cm (Video 1.1). We have more recently adopted the direct anterior approach in selected primary procedures.

Thin patients are ideal for minimally invasive approaches. The operation is more difficult in muscular males and obese patients (BMI > 30 kg/m^2). Although a longer incision may be needed in these individuals, the same principles can be applied. Patients requiring revision surgery and patients with dysplasia, prior reconstructive procedures, or very stiff hips require larger incisions. As a basic tenet, there should never be any hesitation to lengthen the incision if exposure is inadequate. An operation done well through a larger incision is preferable to an unsatisfactory result with a small incision.

At a given time, only a portion of the hip is exposed. A variety of specialized instruments are helpful in gaining exposure and viewing the acetabulum and femur while protecting the surrounding soft tissues (Fig. 1.69). A long Charnley retractor blade is needed to avoid excessive stretching of the wound corners. Acetabular retractors with long handles and blades narrower than usual reduce clutter within the wound. Some systems have incorporated fiberoptic lighting into acetabular retractors. Angulated acetabular reamer

shafts and component positioning devices reduce the retraction required on the inferior soft tissues. Reamers with side cutouts are more easily inserted into the acetabulum and appear to be acceptably accurate. It is particularly helpful to have an assistant to position the limb for femoral preparation and implant placement. Exposure also is enhanced by the use of hypotensive regional anesthesia to reduce intraoperative bleeding.

Sculco and Jordan advocated a posterolateral approach to the hip through a 6- to 10-cm incision. The incision is placed in line with the femur along the posterior edge of the greater trochanter with approximately one third of the incision proximal to the tip of the greater trochanter and two thirds distal. The gluteus maximus is split for only a short distance, the incision of the fascia lata is limited, and the quadratus femoris is left mostly intact but retracted to expose the lesser trochanter and resect the femoral neck. The incision may be easily extended in either direction to approximate a more traditional posterior approach if needed. In a prospective randomized study by this group, Chimento et al. showed that patients with an 8-cm posterolateral approach had less intraoperative and total blood loss and limped less at 6 weeks' follow-up than patients with a standard approach. There were no differences in operative time, transfusion requirements, narcotic use, hospital stay, or other rehabilitation milestones. Complications were similar in the two groups, and a 5-year follow-up on the same cohort showed no radiographic loosening. Radiographic measures of cup and stem position and cement technique were not compromised in the minimally invasive group. DiGioia et al. found that patients in the mini-incision group walked with less of a limp and had better stair-climbing ability at 3 months and improvement in the limp, distance walking, and stair-climbing at 6 months. There were no differences at 1 year. In a prospective, randomized series, Dorr et al. found that a group that had minimally invasive surgery had shorter hospital stays, less in-hospital pain, and less need for assistive devices. There were no differences after hospital discharge.

Other investigators have not shown any benefit to the use of a smaller incision. In a prospective, randomized, controlled trial, Ogonda et al. found that a minimally invasive approach was safe and reproducible but offered no benefit compared with a traditional approach. The trial was done after the senior author had gained considerable experience with less invasive techniques, and the learning curve was not included in this series. In another study from the same institution, Bennett et al. found no difference in any gait analysis parameter at 2 days after surgery. Goldstein et al. likewise were unable to show any differences between a standard and minimally invasive posterolateral approach. In another prospective series with 5-year follow-up, Wright et al. found no difference other than patients' enthusiasm regarding the cosmetic appearance of the scar.

Minimally invasive anterior incisions are modifications of the Smith-Petersen approach. Although the acetabular exposure is superior, it can be difficult to place the femur in a position where the stem can be inserted in line with the shaft. Several manufacturers have introduced shorter stems with curved broaches to simplify femoral component placement (see Fig. 1.28). Although a claim of the anterior approach is that no muscle or tendon is transected, multiple authors recommend release of the posterior capsule and short external rotators to deliver the femur into the wound. Problems related to injury to the lateral femoral cutaneous nerve (LFCN) have led many to place the skin incision slightly lateral to the intermuscular plane of the deeper dissection.

Parratte and Pagnano evaluated tissue injury with various approaches and concluded that it is not possible to routinely perform minimally invasive THA without causing some measurable degree of muscle damage. Rather, the location and extent of muscle damage is specific to the approach. Tissue damage in the anterior approach involved the anterior part of the gluteus medius, the TFL, and the external rotators. The posterior approach was associated with substantial damage to the short external rotators and gluteus minimus and a small amount of damage to the gluteus medius. Bergin et al. measured serum inflammatory markers in patients undergoing hip arthroplasty through minimally invasive posterior and anterior approaches. Serum creatine kinase levels in the posterior group were 5.5 times higher than the anterior group in the postanesthesia unit. The clinical significance of the finding was not delineated.

Advocates frequently describe enhanced recovery after minimally invasive hip arthroplasty. However, multimodal pain management and accelerated rehabilitation protocols have been introduced simultaneously, and these factors also influence the speed of recovery. In a series of 100 patients, Pour et al. found that at the time of hospital discharge, patient satisfaction and walking ability were better in patients who had received an accelerated preoperative and postoperative rehabilitation regimen regardless of the size of the incision. Poehling-Monaghan et al. found no systematic advantage of a direct anterior approach over a mini-posterior approach when using the same rapid rehabilitation protocols with no hip positioning precautions.

Minimally invasive techniques and instrumentation continue to evolve. Refinements in surgical approaches and the integration of computer-assisted navigation may ultimately improve outcomes and surpass the excellent results of standard hip arthroplasty procedures. Rigorous scientific study of these new methods must precede widespread adoption in clinical practice.

COMPUTER-ASSISTED SURGERY

Improper positioning of acetabular and femoral components may compromise the outcome of the arthroplasty because of impingement, dislocation, increased wear, and leg-length discrepancy. Patient size, the presence of deformity, limited surgical exposure, intraoperative movement of the pelvis, inaccuracies in conventional instrumentation, and surgeon experience are all variables that may negatively affect the accuracy of component positioning. Surgeons' assessments of intraoperative position of both femoral and acetabular components are inaccurate when compared with postoperative CT scans. Strategies such as computer-assisted surgical navigation are being investigated to improve the accuracy of the operation.

Computer-assisted navigation provides the surgeon with real-time information regarding the positioning of the femur and pelvis relative to each other and to the surgical instrumentation. The tracking of these positions is by infrared stereoscopic optical arrays that must be visible to a camera. Navigation of the acetabular component requires registration of anatomic landmarks to allow the computer to determine the position of the pelvis in space. Although individual navigation systems vary in both durable equipment and software algorithms, there are three general types of systems: imageless, fluoroscopic, and CT based.

Imageless navigation is based only on landmarks that are digitized at the time of surgery without confirmation by imaging studies. A reference frame is attached to the pelvis, and an optical pointer is then used to reference the ASIS and pubic symphysis by palpation or by small percutaneous incisions. The registration process is performed with the patient supine to allow access to the opposite anterior spine. If the operation is to be done with the patient in the lateral position, the optical tracker is mounted to the pelvis and must be prepared and draped into the surgical field after the patient is repositioned. In larger patients, inaccurate digitization of pelvic landmarks can introduce errors. Computer screen images are of standardized bone models and do not reflect the patient's individual anatomy. Using imageless navigation, Hohmann et al. demonstrated a significant decrease in deviation of acetabular component placement with respect to both inclination and anteversion compared with conventional techniques. Ellapparadja et al. found restoration of both leg length and offset within 6 mm in over 95% of cases. Conversely, Brown et al. found no difference in acetabular inclination angle or leg-length discrepancy between imageless navigation and conventional techniques.

When fluoroscopic navigation is used, reference frames are again applied to the bones. Fluoroscopic images made at multiple angles are combined to yield three-dimensional information. The referencing process can be performed with the patient in the lateral position. If there is a change during the procedure, then new images may be acquired. A radiolucent operating table is required, and protective lead aprons must be worn by the surgical team. Bulky fluoroscopic equipment must remain available during the procedure, and time has to be allotted for acquisition of images. Fluoroscopic navigation has been more reliable for limiting variability of cup abduction than for anteversion. No preoperative planning or imaging is required. Consequently, the technique provides no information about the requirements for restoration of proper hip mechanics.

CT-based navigation provides detailed, patient-specific information compared with imageless and fluoroscopic techniques. Information from the preoperative CT scan is used to produce a virtual bone model which is then coupled to the patient's bony anatomy by the process of registration. Intraoperative registration requires digitization of multiple points on the bony surface of the acetabulum using an instrumented pointer that are then mapped onto the computer model. The process can be done with the patient in the lateral position without the need for repositioning. The accuracy of the mapping and navigation can be confirmed in real time. Detailed information is available preoperatively regarding component size, positioning, leg length, offset, and range of motion. Preoperative imaging and planning are required, but no intraoperative imaging is needed, and the surgical procedure is consequently faster than with imageless navigation.

Beckmann et al., in a meta-analysis of the use of navigation to improve acetabular component position, found that whereas mean cup inclination and anteversion angles were not significantly different, navigation reduced the variability in cup position and the risk of placing the acetabular component beyond the safe zone. Long-term outcomes and cost utility data were not available. Moskal and Capps drew similar conclusions and found fewer dislocations in hips with navigated acetabular component placement. To assess the accuracy of navigation in correcting leg length, Manzotti et al. compared 48 navigated hip arthroplasties with a matched cohort of procedures using a traditional freehand alignment method. Restoration of limb length was significantly better in the computer-assisted group. Dorr et al. reported using navigation to optimize restoration of offset: offset was restored within 6 mm of the contralateral hip in 78 of 82 hips.

Interest in robotic technologies has increased over the past decade, although to a lesser degree than in knee arthroplasty. Robotics complement surgical navigation with the addition of both bone preparation and component implantation being assisted by a sterile draped robotic arm. Current systems are CT based and require intraoperative placement of tracking arrays and bony registration. Typically, the femur is prepared first and femoral version assessed. Acetabular version can then be adjusted to obtain correct combined anteversion. Acetabular reaming is carried out with visual and tactile feedback from the computer, and bone removal outside of the planned resection is effectively prevented. The acetabular component is then implanted with precision guidance from the robotic arm according to the preoperative plan. Kanawade et al. found a contemporary robotic system achieved precision in acetabular inclination, anteversion, and center of rotation in over 80% of cases.

There has been little development of patient-specific instrumentation in THA compared with knee procedures. In one study, Small et al. found that such instruments improved accuracy of acetabular anteversion but not abduction angle.

Computer-assisted navigation appears effective in reducing outliers in component positioning and can be beneficial in restoring optimal hip mechanics. Whether these advances

in accuracy will translate to improvements in outcomes and implant survivorship remains to be validated. The cost of necessary equipment, software, and imaging studies may be prohibitive for many institutions.

TROCHANTERIC OSTEOTOMY

Although osteotomy of the trochanter for exposure and lateral reattachment to lengthen the lever arm of the abductors was an integral part of Charnley's concept of THA, most total hip procedures are done now without osteotomy. The advocates of osteotomy believe that in addition to the opportunity to advance the trochanter laterally and distally at the time of surgery, dislocation of the hip is easier, exposure of the acetabulum is better, preparation of the femoral canal is complicated by fewer penetrations, cement can be inserted more optimally, and components can be inserted more easily and more accurately. The disadvantages of osteotomy are increased blood loss, a higher incidence of hematoma formation, longer operating time, technical difficulty with fixation of the trochanter, nonunion, wire breakage, bursitis, greater postoperative pain, and delayed rehabilitation.

In most patients, adequate exposure can be obtained with the posterolateral, anterior, anterolateral, or direct lateral approach without osteotomy of the trochanter. Although leaving the trochanter intact has many advantages, osteotomy may be necessary if the anatomy of the hip is markedly distorted, such as in cases of ankylosis or fusion, severe protrusio acetabuli, or developmental dysplasia with high dislocation of the hip. Occasionally, residual laxity of the abductor musculature results in hip instability despite proper restoration of length and offset. In this instance, trochanteric osteotomy with distal reattachment can render the hip more stable without lengthening the limb excessively. In revision procedures, trochanteric osteotomy facilitates exposure of the femur and acetabulum and may be required to extract the femoral component without excessive risk of fracturing the femur.

Three basic types of trochanteric osteotomies are currently used in hip arthroplasty: (1) the standard or conventional type, (2) the so-called trochanteric slide, and (3) the extended trochanteric osteotomy (Fig. 1.70). Various modifications have been described for each type. The various types are suitable for specific purposes and should be tailored to the procedure being contemplated. Finally, the fixation method must be adapted to the type of osteotomy.

The standard trochanteric osteotomy is indicated when extensile exposure of the acetabulum is needed for complex revisions of the acetabular component, placement of an antiprotrusio cage, or a large structural bone graft. Superior retraction of the greater trochanter and abductor musculature yields unparalleled exposure of the ilium with less tension on the superior gluteal neurovascular bundle than would be experienced with the trochanteric slide technique. When a standard trochanteric osteotomy is done, the vastus lateralis first should be detached subperiosteally from the lateral aspect of the femur distal to the vastus tubercle. The osteotomy may be made with a power saw or an osteotome. The osteotomy is initiated just distal to the vastus tubercle and directed proximally and medially at an angle of approximately 45 degrees to the shaft of the femur. It should not extend into the femoral neck, and special care must be taken not to injure the sciatic nerve. In general, a large piece of bone should be removed, with all of the tendinous attachments of the gluteus

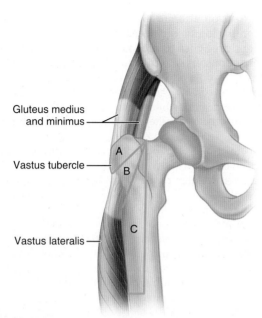

Gluteus medius and minimus

Vastus tubercle

Vastus lateralis

FIGURE 1.70 Types of trochanteric osteotomy and their relationships to muscular attachments. *A,* Standard trochanteric osteotomy with only superior abductor attachment. *B,* Trochanteric slide with abductors and vastus lateralis attached to trochanteric fragment; *C,* Extended trochanteric osteotomy.

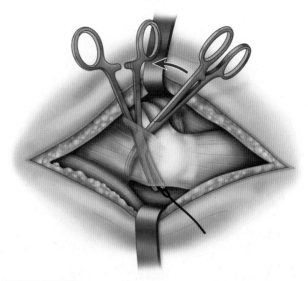

FIGURE 1.71 Gallbladder clamp is inserted into joint and pushed through capsule posterior to insertion of gluteus medius to grasp Gigli saw (see text).

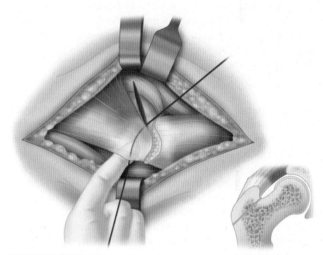

FIGURE 1.72 Before trochanter is osteotomized, finger is used to ensure that Gigli saw is sufficiently posterior and sciatic nerve is not trapped between saw and bone. *Inset,* Direction of osteotomy is first distal and then lateral to detach trochanter just proximal to abductor tubercle.

medius and underlying gluteus minimus muscles. Other soft-tissue attachments, including the short external rotators, are released as necessary to allow superior retraction of the trochanteric fragment. The osteotomy also can be made with a Gigli saw passed deep to the abductor muscles and directed laterally (Figs. 1.71 and 1.72). Charnley emphasized keeping the "strap" of the lateral capsule from the superior aspect of the acetabulum to the base of the trochanter intact to make reattachment more stable than pulling on muscle fibers alone.

Excessive tension on the trochanter by the abductors can be lessened by maintaining the distal soft-tissue attachments on the trochanter. Glassman, Engh, and Bobyn described a technique of osteotomy that maintains an intact musculoosseous sleeve composed of the gluteus medius, greater trochanter, and vastus lateralis. This technique has been termed the *trochanteric slide technique* (Fig. 1.73). Although nonunion rates for this procedure were similar to the rates for other techniques, superior migration of more than 1 cm occurred in only 11% of the nonunions, and the incidence of abductor insufficiency and limp was significantly lower than in similar series. Neither a standard osteotomy nor a trochanteric slide is ideal when the bed for reattachment has been compromised, such as when the greater trochanter has been filled with cement.

More recently, various techniques of extended trochanteric osteotomy have been introduced. In essence, these are proximal femoral osteotomies in which a segment of the lateral femoral cortex of variable length is raised in continuity with the greater trochanter. These techniques are of greatest benefit in removing well-fixed implants in revision surgery and when the bony bed for reattachment of a standard osteotomy would be compromised. Because a large segment of the lateral femoral cortex is removed, and cementing techniques are rendered imperfect, extended trochanteric osteotomies

are used only when a cementless femoral reconstruction is anticipated (see Technique 1.5). Lakstein et al. described a modified technique in which the posterior capsule and short external rotators are left intact to reduce the risk of dislocation.

The lever arm of the abductors is lengthened according to the amount of lateral placement of the osteotomized trochanter. The hip should not be abducted more than 10 to 15 degrees while the trochanter is being reattached, or excess strain on the fixation would result when the hip is adducted, and avulsion and nonunion of the trochanter may follow. The position of reattachment of the greater trochanter has been found to affect the rate of union. Anatomic reduction or a slight distal overlap of the trochanter results in trochanteric union within 6 months. Fixation of the trochanter with

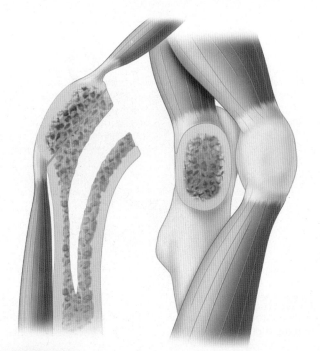

FIGURE 1.73 Trochanteric slide technique described by Glassman, Engh, and Bobyn. Osteotomy is oriented in sagittal plane and includes origin of vastus lateralis. (Redrawn from Glassman AH, Engh CA, Bobyn JD: A technique of extensile exposure for total hip arthroplasty, *J Arthroplasty* 2:11, 1987.)

residual superior and medial tilt invariably led to delayed union or nonunion. For union to occur reliably, compression must be applied across the osteotomy. Fixation should stabilize the trochanteric fragment to vertical and anterior displacement. Displacement in the anteroposterior plane occurs when the hip is loaded in flexion, and fixation failure is more complex than the abductors simply pulling the trochanteric fragment superiorly. A biplanar or chevron osteotomy yields greater resistance to anteroposterior displacement than a uniplanar osteotomy. Such an osteotomy is useful in complex primary procedures but is impractical in most revisions because of the loss of bone needed not only to perform but also to repair the osteotomy.

Various wire fixation techniques using two, three, or four wires have been described and are illustrated in Figures 1.74 and 1.75. No. 16, 18, or 20 wire can be used, and because spool wire is more malleable, it is easier to tighten and tie or twist. A Kirschner wire spreader or wire tightener is used to tighten the wire. Stainless steel, cobalt-chrome alloy, or titanium alloy wire may be used, depending on the metal of the femoral component. Also, multiple filament wire or cable is available; the ends are pulled through a short metal sleeve, which is crimped after the wire has been tightened. Special care should be taken not to kink or nick the wire.

In our experience, wire fixation techniques do not predictably provide rigid fixation of the trochanter. Trochanteric nonunion rates of 25% have been reported using wiring techniques. With the trend toward cementless femoral revision, techniques requiring intramedullary passage of wires and screws have become difficult. In most cases, we prefer an extramedullary cable fixation device instead (Figs. 1.76 and 1.77). A variety of new devices featuring proximal hooks with

a plate extension also are available (Fig. 1.78). Full weight bearing on the hip should be delayed for 4 to 6 weeks if fixation is not rigid. When fixation is less stable (i.e., with a small piece of bone or soft bone, difficulty in pulling the bone down to the femur, or loss of the bony bed for reattachment of the trochanteric fragment), the hip may be maintained in abduction in a spica cast or orthosis for 6 weeks. (See the section on complications for trochanteric nonunion and wire breakage problems.)

Dall described a modification of the direct lateral approach that involves osteotomy of the anterior portion of the greater trochanter rather than division of the anterior portion of the abductor insertion from the trochanter. Head et al. used a similar osteotomy in conjunction with an extensile direct lateral approach for revision arthroplasty (Fig. 1.79). This approach detaches only the internal rotational component of the abductors and leaves the important abductor portion of the gluteus medius intact. Reattachment of the anterior trochanteric fragment allows for primary bony union and is easier than direct repair of the abductor tendon to bone.

SURGICAL PROBLEMS RELATIVE TO SPECIFIC HIP DISORDERS

Much information has been accumulated since the 1970s concerning the various entities for which THA has been performed. In some instances, the routine surgical techniques must be modified to meet the needs of the various conditions. For this reason, the following entities are discussed relative to THA. Revision surgery for failed THA is discussed in a separate section.

ARTHRITIC DISORDERS
▥ OSTEOARTHRITIS (PRIMARY OR SECONDARY HYPERTROPHIC ARTHRITIS OR DEGENERATIVE ARTHRITIS)

Osteoarthritis is the most common indication for THA; it can be primary or secondary to femoroacetabular impingement, to previous trauma, or to childhood disorders of the hip. The extremity often is shortened slightly, although the discrepancy can be greater than 1 cm if erosion or deformation of the femoral head or acetabulum has occurred. The hip often is flexed, externally rotated, and adducted, and there is additional apparent shortening of the limb because of the deformity. Less commonly, the limb may appear lengthened because of a fixed abduction contracture. Removal of the osteophytes from the anterior or posterior margin of the acetabulum may be necessary to dislocate the hip safely. The subchondral bone of the acetabulum is thick and hard, and considerable reaming may be required before a bleeding surface satisfactory for bone ingrowth is reached. Osteophytes may completely cover the pulvinar and obscure the location of the medial wall.

If the femoral head has been displaced laterally, intraarticular osteophytes inferiorly may thicken the bone considerably and require deepening of the acetabulum to contain the cup fully (Fig. 1.80). Failure to medialize the acetabulum in this instance may leave the superior portion of the cup unsupported or supported primarily by osteophytes rather than native bone. Careful attention to the removal of

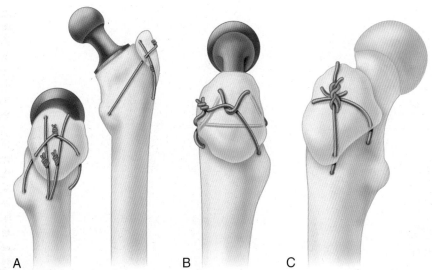

FIGURE 1.74 Wire fixation of trochanter. **A,** Two vertical wires are inserted in hole drilled in lateral cortex below abductor tubercle; they emerge from cut surface of neck, and one is inserted in hole in osteotomized trochanter. Two vertical wires are tightened and twisted, and transverse wire that was inserted in hole drilled in lesser trochanter and two holes in osteotomized trochanter is tightened and twisted. **B,** One-wire technique of Coventry. After component has been cemented in femur, two anteroposterior holes are drilled in femur beneath osteotomized surface and two holes are drilled in osteotomized trochanter. One end of wire is inserted through lateral loop before being tightened and twisted. **C,** Oblique interlocking wire technique of Amstutz for surface replacement. (**A** modified from Smith & Nephew, Memphis, TN; **B** and **C** redrawn from Markolf KL, Hirschowitz DL, Amstutz HC: Mechanical stability of the greater trochanter following osteotomy and reattachment by wiring, *Clin Orthop Relat Res* 141:111, 1979.)

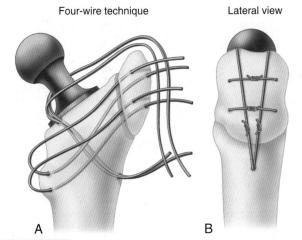

Four-wire technique   Lateral view

A   B

FIGURE 1.75 Harris four-wire technique of reattachment of trochanter. **A,** Two vertical wires are inserted through hole drilled in lateral cortex and come out in groove cut in neck of femur so as not to interfere with seating of collar. Two transverse wires are inserted in holes in lesser trochanter and in two holes in osteotomized greater trochanter. **B,** Two transverse wires are tied over two tied vertical wires. One transverse wire can be used instead of two. (Redrawn from Harris WH: Revision surgery for failed, nonseptic total hip arthroplasty: the femoral side, *Clin Orthop Relat Res* 170:8, 1982.)

acetabular osteophytes is necessary to avoid impingement, decreased range of motion, and dislocation. Trochanteric osteotomy usually is unnecessary, but often the greater trochanter is enlarged, and some bone must be removed from its anterior or posterior surface to prevent impingement during rotation.

■ INFLAMMATORY ARTHRITIS

THA often is indicated to relieve pain and increase range of motion in patients with inflammatory arthritis and other collagen diseases, such as rheumatoid arthritis, juvenile idiopathic arthritis, juvenile rheumatoid arthritis or Still disease, psoriatic arthritis, and systemic lupus erythematosus, especially when involvement is bilateral. Arthroplasties of the knees and other joints may be necessary. Often these patients are generally disabled, having varying degrees of dermatitis, vasculitis, fragile skin, osteopenia, and poor musculature. In addition, they have been or are receiving corticosteroids and other immunosuppressive drugs; consequently, the risks of fracture during surgery and infection after surgery are greater. The femoral head may be partially absent because of erosion or osteonecrosis, and some degree of acetabular protrusion may be present.

Limitation of motion of the cervical spine, upper extremities, and temporomandibular joints complicates the anesthesia, and fiberoptic techniques may be required to intubate the patient safely. Preoperative flexion and extension radiographs of the cervical spine to rule out subluxation are advisable if endotracheal intubation is planned. Additional corticosteroids also may be required in the perioperative period.

Special handling of the limb is necessary so as not to fracture the femur or acetabulum or damage the skin. Preparation of the femur usually is easy because the canal is wide, but the cortex is thin and easily penetrated or fractured. Similarly,

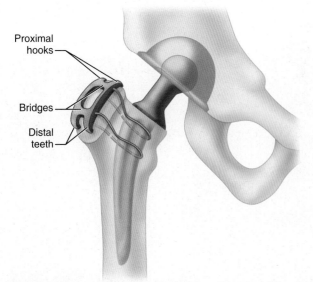

Proximal hooks

Bridges

Distal teeth

FIGURE 1.76   Dall-Miles cable grip device for reattachment of trochanter. (Redrawn from Dall DM, Miles AW: Reattachment of the greater trochanter: the use of the trochanter cable-grip system, *J Bone Joint Surg* 65B:55, 1983.)

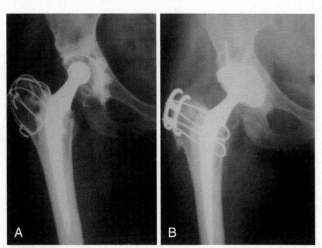

A   B

FIGURE 1.77   **A,** Fifteen years after Charnley total hip replacement, acetabular loosening and wear are apparent, but there is no evidence of femoral loosening. **B,** Exposure for acetabular revision was improved by trochanteric slide osteotomy, leaving femoral component intact. Reattachment was secured with cable fixation device (Dall-Miles). Wires are completely extramedullary and do not violate femoral cement mantle. Union was complete at 3 months.

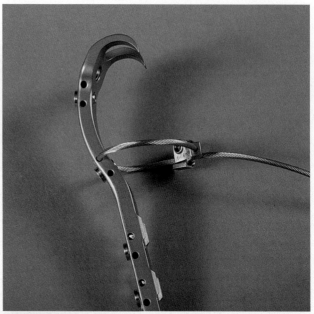

FIGURE 1.78   Accord trochanteric fixation plate. Trochanteric fragment is captured by proximal hooks. Plate extension is fixed to femur with cerclage cables and can be used to stabilize standard or extended trochanteric osteotomy. (Courtesy Smith & Nephew, Memphis, TN.)

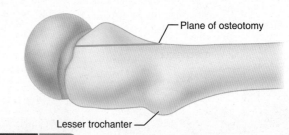

Plane of osteotomy

Lesser trochanter

FIGURE 1.79   Osteotomy of anterior trochanter in direct lateral approach (see text). (Redrawn from Head WC, Mallory TH, Berklacich FM, et al: Extensile exposure of the hip for revision arthroplasty, *J Arthroplasty* 2:265, 1987.)

the acetabulum is soft and easily reamed, and the medial wall is easily penetrated. Care must be taken not to fracture the anterior margin of the acetabulum or the femoral neck with a retractor used to lever the femur anteriorly. Severe osteopenia often makes cementless fixation more difficult, although successful use of cementless femoral and acetabular components has been reported in several series. Small components may be necessary, especially in patients with juvenile idiopathic arthritis, because the bones often are underdeveloped. Excessive femoral anteversion and anterior bowing of the proximal femur also are common in patients with juvenile

idiopathic arthritis. Extreme deformity may require femoral osteotomy.

When operations on the hip and the knee are indicated, opinions vary concerning which joint should be treated first. Total knee replacement can be technically difficult in the presence of a markedly stiff arthritic hip joint. Conversely, a severe flexion contracture of the knee may predispose to dislocation of a total hip replacement. If involvement is equal, the hip arthroplasty probably should be done first.

Most patients with rheumatoid arthritis, including young patients, have excellent pain relief and increased mobility after THA. Functional improvement as evidenced by hip scores may be limited, however, by other involved joints. Because these patients are relatively inactive, they are not physically demanding of the hip. Although the incidence of radiolucencies at 10 years is high, patients continue to function well with their reduced demands. In most series, radiolucencies and demarcation are more common around the acetabulum than the femur for cemented and cementless fixation.

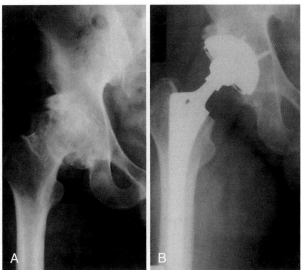

FIGURE 1.80 Inadequate deepening of acetabulum. **A** and **B**, Degenerative arthritis with intraarticular osteophyte formation and lateral subluxation. Medial osteophytes were not removed, and socket remains in lateralized position. Superior coverage is provided only by large osteophyte.

OSTEONECROSIS

Osteonecrosis of the femoral head remains a challenge for diagnosis and for treatment. In some instances, the cause of the osteonecrosis can be identified as being associated with alcoholism, corticosteroids, systemic lupus erythematosus, renal disease, caisson disease, and various other diseases (sickle cell disease and Gaucher disease are discussed separately). Osteonecrosis may also be associated with coagulopathies and human immunodeficiency virus (HIV). In many patients with osteonecrosis of the femoral head, no disease process can be identified, however, and in these patients the osteonecrosis is classified as idiopathic. Up to 75% of patients with atraumatic osteonecrosis have radiographic or MRI evidence of bilateral hip disease at presentation.

In the so-called idiopathic group and in patients with corticosteroid-related osteonecrosis without subchondral collapse or significant arthritic changes in the hip (stages I and II), symptoms can be relieved by core decompression, as advocated by Hungerford; by vascularized fibular grafting; or by valgus osteotomy with or without bone grafting (see chapter 4). Hip fusion is not recommended because the involvement often is bilateral. Resurfacing arthroplasty is recommended only if the avascular segment constitutes a small segment of the femoral head (usually <50%).

With osteonecrosis, the capsule and synovial tissue proliferation frequently is quite hyperemic; and on entering the capsule, a considerable amount of bleeding may be encountered. Often a large synovial effusion is present and may raise suspicion of infection, although this is uncommon. If cortical bone grafting of the femoral head was done previously, such as with a vascularized fibular graft, careful attention must be paid to removing the intramedullary portion of the graft completely. Conventional reamers and broaches are ineffective in this regard. Fehrle et al. found that undersizing and varus placement of the femoral component were common because of inadequate graft removal, especially in the trochanteric

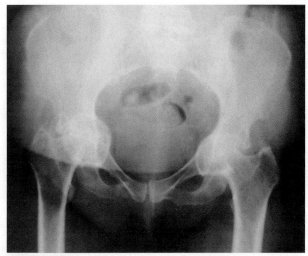

FIGURE 1.81 Primary protrusio acetabuli. Otto pelvis in 52-year-old woman. Femoral head has migrated medial to ilioischial (Kohler) line. Hip motion is severely limited.

fossa. They recommended removing the graft remnants with a high-speed burr and using intraoperative radiographs with the broach in place to ensure adequate removal of the graft and a good femoral fit.

Many patients with osteonecrosis are young, and total hip procedures have not been as satisfactory in this group as in older patients or those with osteoarthritis. Many reports of unsatisfactory results were based on patients who were operated on with first-generation cementing techniques, however, and the results may prove more favorable with improved methods, materials, and designs. Improved results have been reported with the use of an alumina ceramic head with highly crosslinked polyethylene. At average 8.5 years' follow-up, wear was low and no hip had aseptic loosening or osteolysis. The use of advanced bearings appears particularly warranted in this young population.

Patients with osteonecrosis potentially are at greater risk of complications because of the previously noted comorbidities. Stavrakis, SooHoo, and Lieberman found a higher risk of both sepsis and readmission based on information from a statewide hospital database. In a study of patients in the National Surgical Quality Improvement Program (NSQIP) database, Lovecchio et al. found a higher risk of both transfusion and readmission for patients with osteonecrosis.

PROTRUSIO ACETABULI

Protrusio acetabuli can be primary or secondary. The primary form, arthrokatadysis (Otto pelvis), involves both hips, occurs most often in younger women, and causes pain and limitation of motion at a relatively early age (Fig. 1.81). The secondary form can be caused by migration of an endoprosthesis, septic arthritis, or prior acetabular fracture. It can be present bilaterally in Paget disease, arachnodactyly (Marfan syndrome), rheumatoid arthritis, ankylosing spondylitis, and osteomalacia. The radiographic hallmark of protrusio acetabuli is the medial migration of the femoral head beyond the ilioischial (Kohler) line. The deformity may progress until the greater trochanter impinges on the side of the pelvis. Frequently, there is an associated varus deformity of the femoral neck.

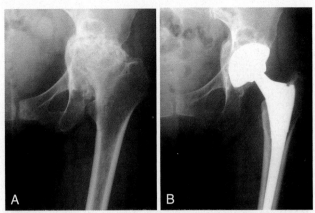

FIGURE 1.82 Reconstruction for protrusio acetabuli deformity. **A,** Protrusio deformity in 52-year-old woman with lupus. **B,** After total hip arthroplasty. Hip center was restored to more lateral and inferior position. Large acetabular component allowed rim fixation without need for screws, and medial deficits were grafted with cancellous autograft from femoral head with excellent incorporation. Low neck resection and high-offset stem design helped avoid overlengthening of limb.

The principles of reconstruction of a protrusion deformity are as follows: (1) the hip center must be placed in an anatomic location to restore proper joint biomechanics; (2) the intact peripheral rim of the acetabulum should be used to support the acetabular component; and (3) the remaining cavitary and segmental defects in the medial wall must be reconstructed, preferably with bone grafting (Fig. 1.82). Determining the anatomic location of the hip center and the degree of migration caused by progressive protrusion can be difficult. Variations in the amount of flexion and rotation of the pelvis may distort radiographic measurements. Ranawat, Dorr, and Inglis proposed a method of determining the hip center by the radiographic relationships of the Kohler and Shenton lines and the height of the pelvis. Although this method is useful for radiographic measurement, it offers no assistance in correcting the hip center to the anatomic location during surgery. Generally, the relationship of the prosthetic socket to the remaining acetabular rim and the measurement of the remaining medial and superior bony deficits in comparison to the preoperative templating assist in bringing the hip center to a more lateral and inferior position. The adequacy of correction of the deformity correlates with long-term prosthetic survivorship.

Often, because of the medial migration of the femur, the sciatic nerve is nearer the joint than normally, and consequently it should be identified early in the operation and protected. Trochanteric osteotomy occasionally may be required for exposure. Dislocation of the hip can be extremely difficult, and removal of a small overhanging portion of the posterior acetabular wall may facilitate dislocation. In severe cases, the femoral head is incarcerated within the acetabulum and dislocation is impossible. In this instance, the femoral neck must be osteotomized in situ at the appropriate angle. Considerable capsular release is necessary to deliver the proximal end of the femur out of the depth of the wound. The femoral head is removed from the acetabulum with a corkscrew or a threaded pin. If it is more firmly fixed in the acetabulum, it is sectioned and removed piecemeal. The medial wall of the acetabulum

usually is thin or may be partly membranous, and it should not be penetrated. Medial reaming is unnecessary; instead, the cartilage and soft tissues are removed with a curet. The smooth, sclerotic floor is roughened with a curet or chisel, but penetrating into the pelvis is avoided.

The peripheral rim of the acetabulum is intact when a protrusio deformity occurs. This rim can be relied on to provide stability for a cementless socket but must be prepared carefully. When the femoral head has protruded into the pelvis, an "hourglass" deformity is created and the walls of the periphery of the acetabulum diverge (Fig. 1.83A). If only the periphery of the acetabulum is reamed to a larger size, the walls can be made to converge. The acetabular component is stabilized on the reshaped rim, and the thin or deficient medial wall is not relied on to prevent recurrent deformity. Reaming is begun with the largest size reamer that fits comfortably into the opening of the acetabulum. The reamer is advanced only until it is flush with the rim, and the medial wall is not reamed. Progressively larger reamers are inserted in the same manner until a convergent rim is created that is wide enough to support the acetabular component (Fig. 1.83B). The anterior and posterior walls are palpated frequently during reaming to avoid excessive bone removal or the creation of a complete segmental defect in the anterior or posterior wall. Any segmental or cavitary deficit that remains medially is grafted with particulate cancellous bone, wafers, or a solid graft from the femoral head and impacted by using the last reamer, turning it in the reverse direction for a few turns. A component 1 to 2 mm larger than the final reamer size improves stability on the prepared rim (Fig. 1.83C).

Sloof et al. popularized the technique of impaction grafting of the acetabulum for correction of protrusio associated with rheumatoid arthritis and revision procedures. Particulate cancellous bone grafts measuring 0.5 to 1.0 cm are tightly impacted into the medial acetabular defects, and a segment of wire mesh is placed on top of the bone graft. A conventional acetabular component is cemented into the construct. Weight bearing is limited for 3 months. In a series of 36 hips with protrusio caused by rheumatoid arthritis, Sloof et al. reported a survival rate of 90% at 12 years with the impaction grafting technique. Although this technique has not been widely used, Sloof's approach has been adapted for use in the femur in revision procedures and has gained more widespread acceptance (see Technique 1.31). In a series of 20 hips with protrusion deformity due to rheumatoid arthritis, Zhen et al reported no acetabular fractures with this technique despite the thin, osteopenic acetabular rim.

Surgical correction of protrusio acetabuli often entails significant lengthening of the limb. Patients with bilateral deformity should be advised of this before surgery. The lengthening occurs on both sides of the joint; the center of the acetabulum is brought to a more inferior and lateral position, and the femoral side is lengthened because of the prior varus deformity of the femoral neck. We have found a low-level femoral neck resection coupled with a femoral component with enhanced offset (see Fig. 1.16) to be helpful in minimizing limb lengthening while maintaining adequate joint stability (see Fig. 1.82).

DEVELOPMENTAL DYSPLASIA

In surgery for developmental dysplasia of the hip, proper patient selection is crucial. Pelvic or periacetabular osteotomy

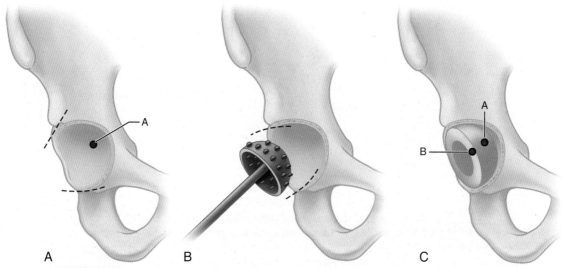

FIGURE 1.83 Insertion of acetabular component for protrusio. **A,** Peripheries of acetabular walls are divergent, and hip center is displaced superiorly and medially. **B,** Peripheral reaming creates new rim with convergent walls. **C,** Implanted component is stable on prepared rim. Hip center shifted from point A to point B and is now in more anatomic location.

should be considered in young patients with retained cartilage space on radiographs. THA still is often required for patients with symptomatic arthritis secondary to dysplasia.

The complexity of the reconstruction is influenced by the degree of anatomic abnormality (Fig. 1.84). The classification of Crowe et al. has been used to describe the degree of dysplasia and is based on the magnitude of proximal femoral migration relative to the acetabulum as measured on an anteroposterior radiograph of the pelvis. The migration is calculated by measuring the vertical distance between the interteardrop line and the medial head-neck junction of the involved hip. The degree of subluxation is the ratio of this distance to the vertical diameter of the opposite femoral head. If the distance from the medial head-neck junction to the interteardrop line is half the vertical diameter of the opposite femoral head, the degree of subluxation is 50%. In patients in whom the opposite femoral head also is deformed, the vertical diameter of the femoral head is estimated as 20% of the height of the entire pelvis as measured from the top of the iliac crest to the bottom of the ischial tuberosities. Dysplastic hips are classified by the amount of subluxation: type I, less than 50%; type II, 50% to 75%; type III, 75% to 100%; and type IV, greater than 100% subluxation.

In addition to the proximal migration of the femur, several deformities of the bone and soft tissues are of surgical importance. The femoral head is small and deformed; the femoral neck is narrow and short, with varying but often marked anteversion. The greater trochanter usually is small and often located posteriorly. The femoral canal is narrow; Dunn and Hess found its average width 2 cm inferior to the lesser trochanter to be only 1.5 cm. The narrowness of the femur and the increased anterior bowing of the proximal third make canal preparation difficult. If the femoral head has subluxated and migrated proximally, the acetabulum is oblong and its roof is eroded. In high and intermediate dislocations, the impingement of the femoral head on the ilium stimulates the formation of a false acetabulum that usually is not deep or wide enough for containment of the cup. The

thickest bone available usually is in the true acetabulum, and the cup should be implanted there if possible (Fig. 1.85).

The abductor muscles frequently are poorly developed and oriented more transversely than normal. The adductors, psoas, hamstrings, and rectus femoris muscles usually are shortened. The capsule is elongated and redundant. Extensive capsulectomy and tenotomy of the psoas, rectus femoris, and adductors may be required to correct the deformity. The sciatic nerve has never assumed its normal length and is susceptible to stretch injury when the bony and soft-tissue deformities are corrected.

Before surgery, anteroposterior radiographs of the pelvis and proximal femur and a lateral view of the femur must be studied carefully to determine the amount of bone available in which to fix the cup, the level at which it should be fixed, the problems likely to be encountered in reaming the femoral canal because of the anterior bowing and narrow width, the need for a femoral osteotomy, and the size and type of components to be used. In patients with unilateral dislocations, lengthening of the affected extremity during surgery is desirable to correct some or all of the discrepancy in limb lengths. No more than 3 to 4 cm of lengthening should be planned. The leg lengthening often is offset to some extent by the necessity of shortening the femur to place the femoral head in the true acetabulum.

The shallow dysplastic acetabulum may require a very small acetabular component (≤40 mm). Implants of this size are not typically part of the standard implant sets and may need to be specially ordered. A 22-mm femoral head size should be used because it can be difficult to maintain adequate polyethylene thickness when a larger head size is used with a small cup. Charnley and Feagin warned that no more than 5 mm of the cup should protrude beyond the bone. If possible, the entire cup should be confined within the bone, and the medial wall of the acetabulum should be left intact. Intentional fracture of the medial wall or penetration of the medial wall with reamers to obtain lateral coverage has been proposed, but this is not universally accepted.

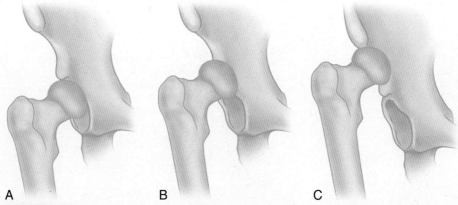

A   B   C

FIGURE 1.84 Developmental subluxation or dislocation. **A,** Dysplastic hip with defect in superior aspect of acetabulum. **B,** Intermediate congenital dislocation with false acetabulum above true acetabulum, usually with shallow groove connecting two acetabula. **C,** High dislocation of hip, with some reactive bone on side of ilium where head impinges on cortex.

Most authors recommend placement of the acetabular component within the true acetabulum (see Fig. 1.85), rather than leaving the center of rotation in a superiorly displaced position with the cup in a false acetabulum (Fig. 1.86). This medial and inferior location diminishes joint contact forces compared with the superior and laterally displaced position of a false acetabulum. In addition, placement in the true acetabulum facilitates limb lengthening, improves abductor function, and in most cases places the acetabular component in the best available bone stock. Long-term studies have found the frequency of loosening to be two to three times higher when the cup is placed outside the true acetabulum than when it is initially positioned within the true acetabulum.

With Crowe type I hips, there is relatively little bony deformity, and the acetabular component can be placed in the true acetabulum without difficulty. Medialization to the floor of the acetabulum provides adequate containment of a standard component. In Crowe type II and type III hips, when the socket is placed within the true acetabulum, a large superior segmental deficit remains with a lack of superior coverage of the component (Fig. 1.87). In most patients, grafting is not required if the acetabular component is placed in a slightly high location as long as it is not also lateralized.

Although early reports of acetabular grafting showed acetabular loosening in as many as 47%, other reports of bulk acetabular bone grafting in developmental dysplasia of the hip have been more positive, with loosening in approximately 15%.

Technique is most important in achieving success with solid acetabular bone grafts. All cartilage and soft tissue are removed from the contact areas between donor and host bone. The fit of the graft to the host is crucial; the head is placed in the defect in its most congruous position. The graft should be positioned beneath a buttress of host bone that is capable of supporting weight bearing, and the trabeculae of the graft should be oriented in line with the weight-bearing forces. The graft is provisionally fixed with smooth Kirschner wires. Definitive fixation is achieved with two or three cancellous lag screws with washers. The screws should be oriented in parallel and along lines of weight-bearing forces. Screws must be inserted with careful interfragmentary technique, and the graft should be overdrilled to allow this if necessary.

Initial shaping of the graft is done with a high-speed burr. Final shaping of the graft and remaining host acetabulum is done with hemispherical reamers. Caution must be exercised during reaming to avoid excessive torque on the graft. For this reason, we prefer to prepare and ream the graft before definitive screw fixation (Fig. 1.88). In this way, the final sites for screw fixation are selected after the graft has been prepared and are not compromised during the reaming process. Final shaping of the lateral aspect of the graft also can be done at this point with a trial acetabular component in place before final screw fixation. If a portion of the graft is left prominent beyond the lateral edge of the cup, the unstressed portion likely will be resorbed over time (Fig. 1.89).

The rate of union and resorption and the long-term viability of acetabular grafts are concerns. Sanzén et al. found no incorporation of cortical bone grafts. Limited resorption of the lateral aspect of the graft occurred in 20 of 32 hips, but resorption involving bone supporting the socket occurred in only three hips (see Fig. 1.89). Radioisotope scanning did not correlate with bone resorption, nonunion, or loss of bone structure. In most reported cases of acetabular loosening after bulk acetabular bone grafting, the graft was viable and revision was accomplished without the need for additional bone grafting.

There is no potential for bone ingrowth from bulk acetabular grafts. The amount of the component that must be placed in contact with viable host bone for long-term stability remains to be determined. This problem and the failure of large bulk grafts led Harris to advocate placement of a small, porous acetabular component at a superiorly displaced position. Isolated superior displacement or superomedial displacement results in only limited increase in joint contact forces. In reconstructing a hip with a so-called high hip center, a larger amount of the porous surface can be placed against viable host bone. When a small socket is placed in a superior and medial position, however, femoral-pelvic impingement and instability become problems. Resection of a large amount of bone from the anterior column adjacent to the superior pubic ramus and from the ischium often is required to allow motion and reduce the risk of dislocation. Some degree of superior displacement of the hip center is acceptable. Nawabi et al. found

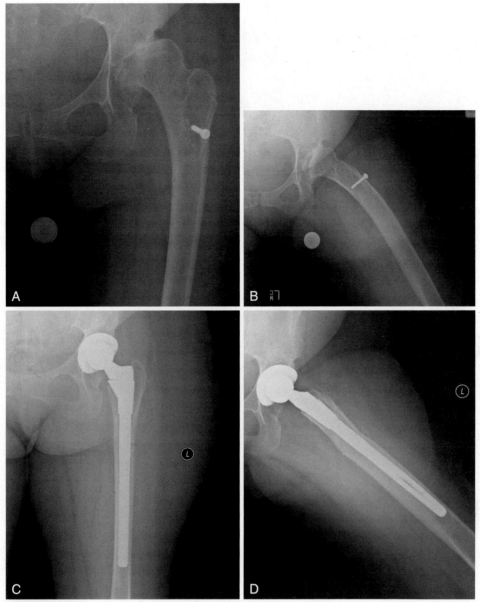

FIGURE **1.85**   Developmental dysplasia. **A** and **B,** Thirty-year-old woman with prior femoral and acetabular osteotomies. There is residual Crowe type 1 dysplasia. Femur is excessively anteverted with anterior bow and retained hardware. **C** and **D,** Small acetabular component placed at level of true acetabulum. Femoral osteotomy was needed to correct angular and rotational deformities.

no loosening when the hip center was approximately 1 cm higher than the anatomic position, but found a higher wear rate in hips in which the center was left in a lateralized position. Utilizing highly crosslinked polyethylene, Galea et al. found no acetabular loosening and low wear in 123 hips with a high hip center.

With a high dislocation, as in Crowe type IV, the acetabulum is hypoplastic, but its superior rim has not been eroded by the femoral head. The reconstruction usually can be done with a conventional, albeit very small acetabular component placed within the true acetabulum and without structural bone grafting. When the hip is initially exposed, the femoral head is dislocated from a false acetabulum and the site of the true acetabulum may not be immediately apparent. A ledge of bone usually separates the true acetabulum from the false

one, and it should be used as a landmark from which dissection is carried inferiorly. The transverse acetabular ligament usually can be located along with the cotyloid fossa, retaining some atrophic fat from the pulvinar. A retractor placed inferior to the transverse ligament and into the obturator foramen ensures that the dissection has been carried far enough inferior to place the component in the true acetabulum. The depth of the acetabulum often is deceptive because it is filled with bone. Removal of the pulvinar exposes the depth of the cotyloid fossa and the medial wall of the acetabulum, allowing the surgeon to determine the amount of medialization that can be safely accomplished by reaming. If the cotyloid fossa is not apparent, a hole can be drilled and a depth gauge used to determine the thickness of the available bone. The anterior wall of the acetabulum often is thin and can be

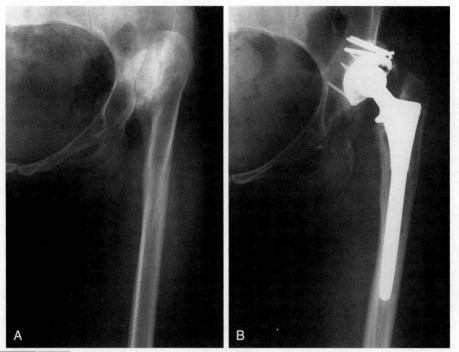

FIGURE 1.86 Placement of cup in false acetabulum. **A,** Dislocation in 35-year-old woman. **B,** Cup was implanted in false acetabulum with high hip center. Limb remains 4 cm short, and abductor function is poor.

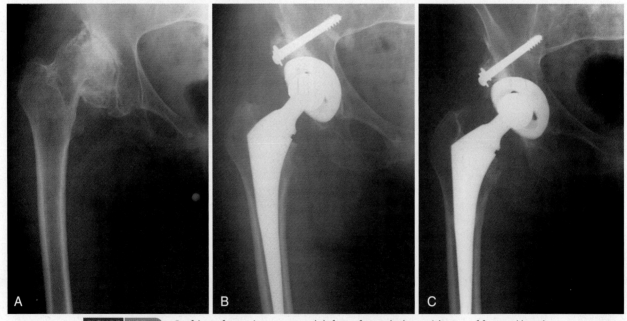

FIGURE 1.87 Grafting of superior segmental defect of acetabulum with part of femoral head. **A,** Sequelae of dysplasia in 54-year-old woman. **B,** Cementless socket is placed in true acetabulum. Autogenous graft is fixed with cancellous screws and covers about 30% of implant. **C,** At 5 years, graft has united and socket is stable.

penetrated easily, but the posterior wall usually is adequately thick. When enlargement of the acetabulum from anterior to posterior is necessary, more bone is resected from the posterior wall than from the anterior wall. Any reaming must be done with care so as not to compromise the rim of the acetabulum or penetrate the medial wall. The bone is often very

soft, and the final reamers may be used in reverse to enlarge the acetabulum by impaction rather than removal of bone.

Transacetabular screw fixation of the acetabular component usually is required because of rim deficiencies and osteopenia. Liu et al. used three-dimensional CT to simulate placement of the acetabular component within the

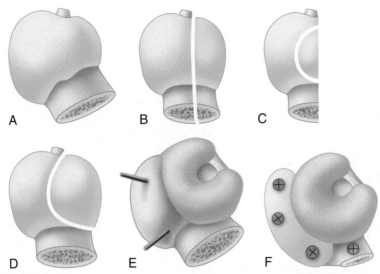

FIGURE 1.88 Bone graft, superior and posterior aspect of acetabulum. Large bone bank femoral head with some neck attached **(A)** is cut in coronal plane **(B)** so that upper part is slightly more than half of head. **C,** Full-thickness elliptical piece of bone is cut out with end-cutting reciprocating saw. This concave surface of graft is placed on convex surface of pelvis above and posterior to acetabulum. **D,** Graft is rotated 90 degrees, and another elliptical cut is made that is slightly smaller than diameter of acetabulum. Several fittings are necessary for graft to have maximal contact with underlying bone. **E,** Graft is temporarily fixed to underlying bone with two Kirschner wires. **F,** Four lag screws fix graft to pelvis. High-speed burr and reamers are used to finish contouring graft.

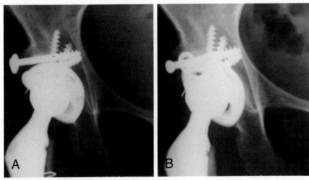

FIGURE 1.89 Resorption of femoral head autograft. **A,** After total hip arthroplasty with femoral head autograft for superior and posterior segment deficits. Graft is united at 6 months. Portion of graft protrudes beyond edge of component. **B,** Two years after surgery, unstressed lateral portion of graft has resorbed. Note medial migration of washers. Function is excellent, component shows no migration, and there is no resorption of graft that supports socket.

true acetabulum in hips with Crowe type IV dysplasia and found that the center of rotation shifted anteroinferiorly. Consequently, the "safe zone" for screw placement (see Fig. 1.46) is narrower. Screws placed in the medial portion of the posterosuperior quadrant risk injury to the obturator vessels.

When the center of the acetabulum has changed little, as with Crowe type I and type II dysplasias, femoral length is not problematic and the femoral reconstruction generally is straightforward. Small-diameter cemented or cementless stems generally are satisfactory. The femoral component must be placed in neutral or slight anteversion in relation to the axis of the knee joint. Marked anteversion of the femoral neck

can be misleading when positioning the femoral component, and anterior instability may occur, particularly if the acetabular component has been placed in additional anteversion. Excessive femoral anteversion can be corrected with a modular cementless femoral component that can be rotated into any degree of version (see Fig. 1.26). This does not correct the posterior displacement of the greater trochanter, however, which may cause impingement in external rotation.

For Crowe type III and type IV hips, femoral length is more problematic. When the prosthetic socket has been placed in the true acetabulum, the femur must be translated distally several centimeters to reduce the prosthetic femoral head into the acetabulum. Often the tissues most limiting this distal translation are the hamstrings and rectus femoris rather than the abductors. In such cases, a femoral shortening osteotomy allows reduction of the femoral head into the true acetabulum without extensive soft-tissue release. Osteotomy of the greater trochanter and resection of 2 to 3 cm from the proximal femoral metaphysis may be necessary to permit reduction of the joint without causing undue tension on the sciatic nerve or fracture of the femoral shaft (Fig. 1.90). As described by Dunn and Hess, the bone should be resected 0.5 cm at a time, and trial reductions are repeated until enough shortening is obtained to reduce the hip without undue soft-tissue tension. The narrow canal and the resection of the metaphyseal flare of the femur often require the use of a component with a small, straight stem.

Sponseller and McBeath described a technique of subtrochanteric femoral shortening using the femoral component for intramedullary fixation. This approach allows correction of excessive femoral anteversion along with the posterior displacement of the greater trochanter while avoiding trochanteric osteotomy and the potential for nonunion. The

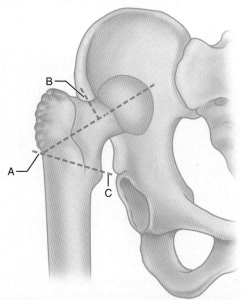

FIGURE 1.90   Dunn and Hess osteotomy of greater trochanter and resection of proximal femoral metaphysis (see text). Trochanter is resected along lines *A* and *B* for large fragment to facilitate reattachment and to increase abductor lever arm. Metaphysis is divided at about line *C*. (From Dunn HK, Hess WE: Total hip reconstruction in chronically dislocated hips, *J Bone Joint Surg* 58A:838, 1976.)

architecture of the proximal femoral metaphysis is preserved, and the orientations of the greater trochanter and abductors are corrected to restore hip mechanics and prevent instability and limp. A standard stem design also can be used. Additionally, the level of the femoral osteotomy provides excellent exposure of the acetabulum if structural bone grafting is required (Fig. 1.91). The femur is provisionally prepared with reamers and broaches before the femoral osteotomy. The depth of reaming of the distal canal should take into account the length of the segment of femur that will be removed in the shortening. The osteotomy is made just distal to the lesser trochanter, and the two fragments are retracted anteriorly for acetabular preparation and implantation. A trial reduction is then carried out with the femoral component in the proximal fragment alone. Traction is applied to the distal femoral fragment, and the overlapping portion is resected from the distal fragment. Final preparation of the distal fragment is then carried out. A larger diameter stem may be required to obtain a tight fit after removing the segment from the femur. The two fragments are reduced, the proximal fragment is derotated to 10 to 15 degrees of anteversion, and the osteotomy site trimmed for optimal apposition. The final stem is implanted, maintaining the proper rotation of the fragments and the implant. The stem must be rotationally stable within both fragments to ensure union. Prophylactic cerclage wiring of the distal fragment (or both fragments) helps prevent fractures, because a very tight fit is required. The resected portion of femur can be bivalved and placed over the osteotomy as onlay grafts. Becker and Gustilo reported using a chevron-shaped osteotomy to improve rotational stability. A short oblique or step-cut osteotomy fixed with cerclage wires also provides greater rotational stability than a transverse osteotomy but adds a degree of technical difficulty. Muratli et al.

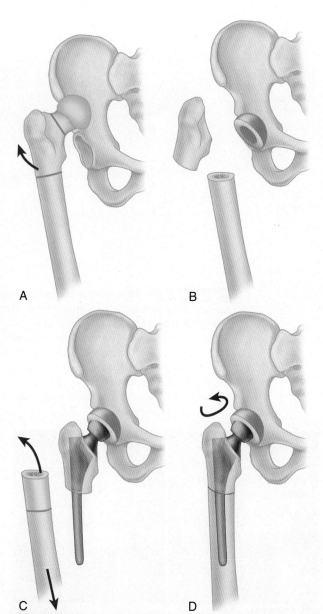

FIGURE 1.91   Subtrochanteric femoral shortening osteotomy. **A,** Initial femoral osteotomy is made at subtrochanteric level. **B,** Proximal femur is retracted to expose level of true acetabulum, and socket is placed in anatomic location. **C,** Proximal femoral fragment is prepared, and trial reduction is done with femoral component placed only in proximal fragment. Traction is applied to distal femoral fragment, and overlapping portion of femur is resected. **D,** Femoral fragments are reduced, and excessive femoral anteversion is corrected. Femoral component provides intramedullary fixation of osteotomy.

investigated multiple osteotomy configurations in composite femurs. None proved superior in stability and the application of strut grafts did not make a significant contribution to stability. Sofu et al. reported nonunion in 4 of 73 patients when a cable plate was used for osteotomy stabilization in conjunction with a tapered femoral component. We have used a modular stem with distal flutes to gain rotational stability with a simple transverse osteotomy, and union has been reliable (Fig. 1.92).

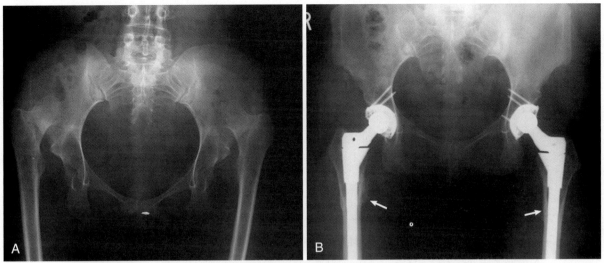

FIGURE 1.92 Subtrochanteric femoral shortening osteotomy. **A,** Bilateral high congenital dislocations and progressive pain in 35-year-old woman. **B,** After bilateral, staged, total hip arthroplasties. Both sides were lengthened about 3 cm despite removal of 6-cm segment of femur. Femoral osteotomies *(arrows)* united uneventfully by 3 months with modular, fluted femoral components.

In most cases, THA can be performed without osteotomy of the trochanter, but if at the end of trial reduction the trochanter impinges on the pelvis when the hip is abducted, it should be osteotomized and reattached distally. In addition, if the trochanter is posterior and impinges on the posterior aspect of the acetabulum during external rotation, it must be osteotomized and reattached more laterally. Abduction is improved when a stem with greater offset is used; there is less tendency for impingement (Fig. 1.93).

The results of THA in selected patients with dysplastic or intermediate dislocation of the hip have been satisfactory for stability, mobility, and pain relief. With high dislocations, a Trendelenburg gait and some limitation of motion usually persist, however. The survivorship of cemented arthroplasty in dysplastic hips is inferior to that of other groups because of the young age of the patients and the complexity of the procedures. Early and midterm cementless results seem more promising. In a series of 28 Crowe IV hips requiring femoral shortening osteotomy, Ollivier et al. reported 10-year survivorship free of revision for aseptic loosening of 89%. The chief complications in most series have been intraoperative femur fracture, dislocation, and sciatic nerve injury (see the section on complications).

LEGG-CALVÉ-PERTHES DISEASE

The potential for Legg-Calvé-Perthes disease (LCPD) to cause symptomatic secondary osteoarthritis has long been recognized. Froberg et al. found that 13% of patients with LCPD eventually required hip arthroplasty; the prevalence was highest in patients with more severe head involvement.

The sequelae of LCPD include anatomic abnormalities that may impact the performance of hip arthroplasty. The acetabulum often is dysplastic and may be retroverted, although grafting is seldom required as with developmental dysplasia. The limb is shortened due to coxa vara deformity, and the greater trochanter is increased in height. Femoral neck version abnormalities may result from the disease process or prior reconstructive surgery. Often there is a size

mismatch between the metaphyseal and diaphyseal regions of the femur, which makes fixation more difficult with conventional cementless femoral components.

Hanna et al. carried out a meta-analysis of 245 hips operated for sequelae of LCPD. The revision rate at a mean of 7.5 years was 7% and complications included intraoperative fracture and sciatic nerve palsy with lengthening. Fractures were less common when a modular stem design (see Fig. 1.26) was used.

SLIPPED CAPITAL FEMORAL EPIPHYSIS

Patients with adolescent slipped capital femoral epiphysis (SCFE) may develop secondary osteoarthritis due to femoroacetabular impingement with abnormal hip mechanics. Arthroplasty also may be required due to osteonecrosis or chondrolysis following surgery for fixation of the neck. Deformity of the femoral neck with retroversion may occur because of the disease process. Antiquated fixation devices placed in adolescence may become completely encased in cortical bone, making their extraction difficult.

In a report from the New Zealand National Joint Registry, Boyle, Frampton, and Crawford found no difference in outcomes between patients with SCFE and primary osteoarthritis undergoing hip arthroplasty.

DWARFISM

Dwarfism is typically defined as having a height of less than 147 cm (4 ft 10 in) and can result from a variety of endocrine disorders such as growth hormone deficiency, achondroplasia, and skeletal dysplasias. Premature osteoarthritis of the hip often is seen in skeletal dysplasias because of abnormalities of articular cartilage, arrested joint development, and altered mechanics. The problems encountered in THA in short-statured individuals (Fig. 1.94) are similar to those encountered in persons with hip dysplasia. Excessive femoral bowing is common, and the femoral canal may be wide proximally but narrow distally, creating a mismatch. Many patients have had prior surgery, including osteotomy that may complicate

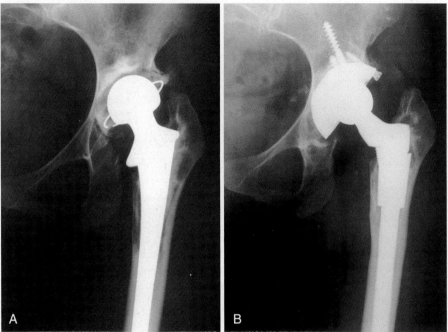

FIGURE 1.93   Trochanteric impingement. **A,** Total hip replacement in patient with congenital hip dislocation. Valgus neck with little offset produced trochanteric impingement in abduction. Motion was severely limited. **B,** After revision for loosening with progressive osteolysis. Stem with greater offset restored adequate abduction.

arthroplasty further. Thorough preoperative planning is imperative. Often, special miniature femoral components are necessary because of the narrow canal and femoral osteotomy or customized short stems may be required to accommodate femoral bowing. Cups with small outside diameters are necessary. CT of the pelvis and femur is helpful in delineating abnormal bony anatomy and size and in determining whether custom implants would be necessary.

Many syndromes that cause short stature involve other joints, including the cervical spine, which may be unstable. Lumbar deformities also may cause referred pain in the hip and should be investigated before hip surgery. Knee instability also may bring about the need for future knee arthroplasty with stemmed implants; therefore, a long-stem femoral component for the hip arthroplasty should be avoided if possible.

Survivorship in this challenging group of patients is worse than in those with osteoarthritis. In a series of 102 hips in patients with dwarfism, Modi et al. found 10-year survivorship of 80.7%. Failures were related to postoperative femoral and acetabular fracture and wear of noncrosslinked polyethylene.

TRAUMATIC AND POSTTRAUMATIC DISORDERS
■ ACUTE FEMORAL NECK FRACTURES
Conventional fracture fixation techniques and hemiarthroplasty traditionally have been recommended for displaced, acute fractures of the femoral neck. THA has been perceived as excessively costly, with a higher risk of dislocation. Recent evidence suggests the management of acute femoral neck fractures should be reevaluated.

A number of randomized controlled trials are available comparing internal fixation, hemiarthroplasty, and THA. In a multicenter study of 450 patients, Rogmark et al. reported 43% failures with internal fixation compared with 6% with arthroplasty. Arthroplasty patients also had better walking ability and less pain, but dislocation occurred in 8%. Blomfeldt et al. randomized 120 cognitively normal patients to either hemiarthroplasty or THA. Blood loss and operative time were higher in the total hip group, but there were no differences in complication rates or mortality. Harris hip scores were higher in the total hip group at both 4 and 12 months. All patients had the same anterolateral approach, and there were no dislocations in either group. In a 4-year follow-up of this same series of patients, Hedbeck et al. found that these differences persisted and increased, favoring total hip replacement. Macaulay et al. compared results of 40 patients randomized to hemiarthroplasty and total hip replacement. Operative time was only 7 minutes longer in the total hip group, although all participating surgeons were specialized in hip arthroplasty. At 24 months, total hip patients had significantly less pain than those with hemiarthroplasties and had significantly better SF-36 mental health and WOMAC function scores. Only one patient with a THA (5.8%) experienced dislocation requiring revision. Iorio et al. carried out a cost-effectiveness analysis of treatment methods for displaced femoral neck fractures accounting for initial hospital costs, rehabilitation, and costs of reoperations and complications. They concluded that cemented total hip replacement was the most cost-effective and that internal fixation was the most expensive. In a review of data from The Swedish Hip Arthroplasty Register, Hansson et al. found THA patients had significantly reduced risk of revision and reoperation compared to hemiarthroplasty.

Although this topic remains controversial, THA is an acceptable option for treatment of acute, displaced fractures of the femoral neck in patients who are living independently,

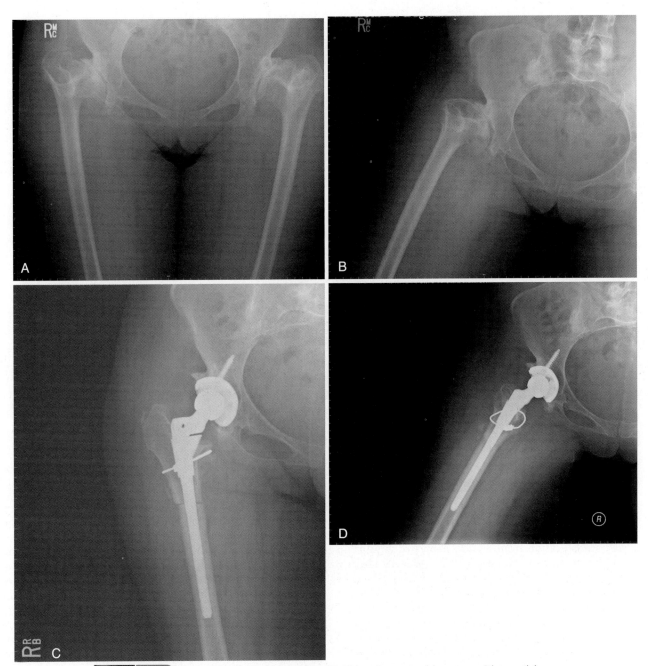

FIGURE 1.94 Painful hip in dwarfism. **A** and **B,** Thirty-five-year-old woman with spondyloep-iphyseal dysplasia. Femoral canal measures only 7 mm. **C** and **D,** After reconstruction with miniature components and 22-mm head. Femoral shortening and derotational osteotomy were required to correct deformity.

fully ambulatory, mentally lucid, and living an active life-style. Those who are less healthy, institutionalized, cognitively impaired, or require assistive devices for ambulation are better suited for hemiarthroplasty. The selection process also depends on availability of experienced personnel at a given institution.

The risk of complications in patients with acute femoral neck fractures is higher than in patients with osteoarthritis. Using information from the National Hospital Discharge Survey (NHDS) over the years 1990 to 2007, Sassoon et al. found that patients having total hip replacement for acute fracture had higher rates of mortality and pulmonary embolism (PE) compared with osteoarthritis patients. Rates were also higher for hematoma formation, infection, and dislocation, although these differences decreased over time. There was no difference in dislocation rate between groups during the most recent period. Fracture patients had a longer length of stay and discharge to a rehabilitation facility at all time periods. Schairer et al. evaluated a large number of patients receiving THA for femoral neck fracture in the NSQIP database. Having a femoral neck fracture vs. osteo-arthritis was associated with greater rates of medical complications, longer hospitalization, discharge to inpatient care facility, and unplanned readmission.

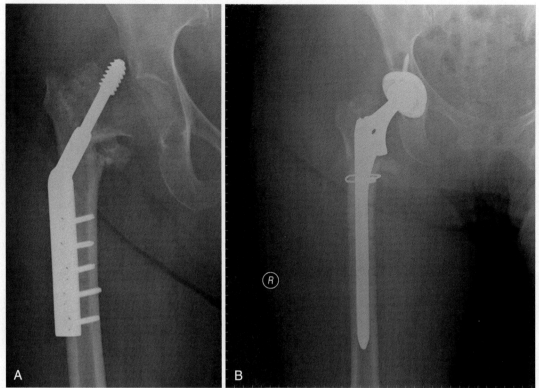

FIGURE 1.95 Nonunion of trochanteric fracture. **A,** Eight weeks after internal fixation, lag screw was cut out, creating large cavitary defect in head and neck. Repeat fixation is unlikely to succeed. **B,** Calcar replacement femoral component was required to restore length. Long stem bypasses screw holes by two bone diameters.

Specific measures can be taken to reduce the incidence of dislocation in this population. In a series of 372 acute femoral neck fractures, Sköldenberg et al. reduced the risk of dislocation from 8% to 2% by switching from the posterolateral to the anterolateral approach. The use of anterior approaches appears justified. If a posterior approach is used, consideration should be given to use of a larger-diameter head and careful repair of the posterior capsule and short external rotators. Using such an approach, Konan et al. had no dislocations in a series of 20 patients. Cementless dual-taper femoral components were used in this series with no stem loosening and no fractures reported. Using a single taper cementless stem in 85 patients, Klein et al. reported two intraoperative fractures requiring cerclage cables and one postoperative fracture requiring revision of the femoral component. The utility of modern cementless femoral components in this population is not well established. Registry data support the use of cemented femoral components in this population.

Other indications are displaced fractures of the femoral neck in patients with Paget disease (see later under Paget Disease) and displaced neck or trochanteric fractures in patients with a preexisting painful arthritic hip. Femoral neck fractures are uncommon in most patients with arthritis of the hip, however, except for patients with rheumatoid arthritis. These patients usually have osteoporosis, and internal fixation of displaced fractures often is unsatisfactory. For this reason, a THA may be considered.

◾ FAILED HIP FRACTURE SURGERY

Internal fixation of proximal femoral fractures may fail because of implant breakage, nonunion, malunion, osteonecrosis, or posttraumatic osteoarthritis. Patients with pain caused by destruction of the femoral head and acetabulum as a result of intrusion of an internal fixation device are best treated with THA. This is common in nonunion of trochanteric and femoral neck fractures (Fig. 1.95). THA for painful posttraumatic osteonecrosis of the femoral head or nonunion usually is possible, but certain technical points are noteworthy. Bleeding may be more extensive than usual because of the increased vascularity of the subsynovial tissue, which is part of a reactive process secondary to the avascular bone in the head. Considerable soft-tissue release may be necessary for exposure and restoration of limb length. Proprietary instruments for extraction of fracture fixation devices and broken screws should be available. The possibility of infection should always be considered, and ESR and CRP should be obtained as with revision procedures. Finally, intraoperative fluoroscopy should be available to aid in finding and removing previous fixation devices. It is generally advisable to remove fixation devices after the hip has been dislocated to reduce the risk of femoral fracture with dislocation maneuvers.

With nonunion of a femoral neck fracture, a portion of the femoral neck may be eroded but reconstruction usually can be accomplished easily using a standard femoral component with a long neck. In contrast, with trochanteric nonunions, the length of the femur generally cannot be restored

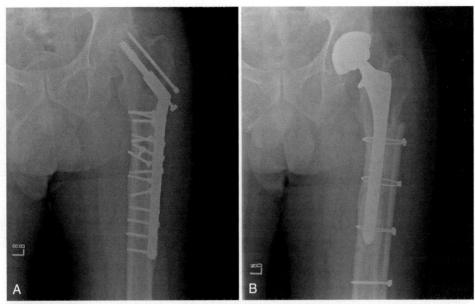

FIGURE 1.96 Femoral strut grafting. **A,** A 52-year-old man 25 years after plating of comminuted trochanteric fracture with shaft extension. Multiple screws were intracortical and difficult to remove. Lateral femoral cortex under plate was thin with multiple defects from screw removal. **B,** Long allograft cortical strut was used to avoid an excessively long stem.

with a standard implant, and a calcar replacement stem often is required (see Fig. 1.25C). Because a calcar replacement stem simplifies the operation, allows early weight bearing, and obviates the need for union at a graft-host junction, it is preferable to bone grafting.

Plates and screws in the proximal femur may be covered with bone and difficult to remove. Removal of broken screws may leave a large defect in the femoral cortex that can give rise to fracture. In these cases, a longer stem is required to bypass screw holes by approximately two bone diameters (Fig. 1.95). Cortical bone beneath a femoral side plate may become markedly porotic and easily perforated by reamers and broaches. We have used cortical strut grafts over the site of the plate in these cases for protection from fracture (Fig. 1.96). When a cemented stem is used, an attempt should be made to occlude femoral screw holes during cementation. Still, the cement mantle quality is typically inferior compared with intact femurs. Additionally, with previously unstable trochanteric fractures, malunion with medial displacement at the fracture site may produce distortion of the proximal femur and make preparation of the femur more hazardous. When a cephalomedullary nail has been used for fracture fixation, the endosteal surface becomes sclerotic and cement interdigitation is less reliable. We prefer cementless femoral fixation in these cases also (Fig. 1.97). Prior intramedullary nail placement also leaves a variably sized defect in the abductor mechanism and may have produced fragmentation of the greater trochanter, requiring fixation.

Hospitalization and subsequent rehabilitation of patients with THA for sequelae of failed fixation of a hip fracture are more prolonged than for similar patients with arthroplasty for arthritic conditions. Many patients with hip fractures have been nonambulatory for a period after the initial fracture and become very debilitated. Complications are more common, and the overall mortality is higher than for patients who undergo THA for arthritic conditions. Archibeck et al.

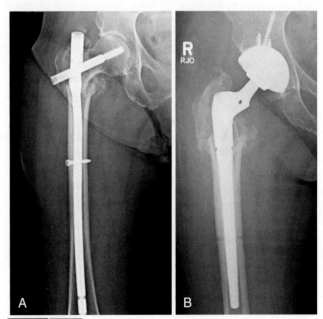

FIGURE 1.97 Broken intramedullary nail. **A,** Six months after cephalomedullary fixation of trochanteric fracture, nail has broken with fracture nonunion. **B,** Tapered cementless femoral component. Greater trochanter was united although with defect in abductor mechanism from prior surgery.

reported an early complication rate of 11.8% including dislocations and periprosthetic fractures. Conversion surgery from prior intertrochanteric fracture fixation is associated with higher complication rates and worse outcomes than for prior femoral neck fractures. Haidukewych and Berry reported a series of 60 patients with prior intertrochanteric fracture fixation. Surgical time was prolonged with blood loss of more than 1000 mL. Medical complications arose in 20%

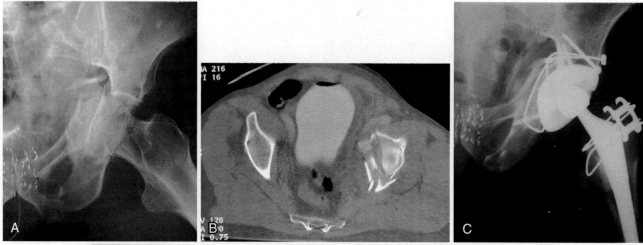

FIGURE 1.98 Primary total hip with acute acetabular fracture. **A,** Elderly man with mild preexisting arthritis of hip had moderately comminuted T-type fracture of acetabulum. **B,** CT scan showing comminution of weight-bearing area of acetabular dome. **C,** Fracture was fixed with lag screws and figure-of-eight braided cable. Primary total hip accomplished with cementless acetabular component fixed with multiple screws. Fracture is united, implants are well positioned, and fixation is stable.

and survival was 87.5% at 10 years. In a series of 59 cases, Morice et al. reported an intraoperative femoral fracture in 17% and dislocation in 6.8%. There were significantly more intraoperative fractures and medical complications in those with prior intertrochanteric fractures. Pui et al. also reported a multi-institutional series of 60 patients comparing conversion from cephalomedullary devices and sliding hip screws. The complication rate in converted nail patients was significantly higher, at 41.9% versus 11.7% with sideplate devices. In contrast, Hernandez reported a series of 62 patients converted from in situ fixation of intracapsular femoral neck fractures. There was a low rate of complications, and survival free of any reoperation was 97% at 5 years.

■ ACETABULAR FRACTURES

Fractures of the acetabulum with or without dislocation of the hip, although they can become painful later, usually are treated initially by open reduction and internal fixation. A united fracture provides better bone for support of the acetabular component if arthroplasty should become necessary. Occasionally, primary arthroplasty is indicated in an older osteoporotic patient who has an acetabular fracture combined with an unreconstructable fracture of the femoral head or neck, marked articular surface impaction or comminution, or a previously arthritic joint (Fig. 1.98). Both the fracture reduction and arthroplasty can be carried out though a single approach. Mears and Shirahama reported a technique of acetabular fracture fixation with braided cables combined with acute THA. Fracture union occurred in 19 patients, and there were no loose implants. In a larger series of elderly patients with acute acetabular fractures treated with arthroplasty, Mears and Velyvis found good or excellent outcomes in 79% of cases. Small degrees of acetabular component migration occurred within the first 6 weeks, but no acetabular component had evidence of late radiographic loosening. Weaver et al. reported a series of elderly patients treated with either open reduction

internal fixation (ORIF) or acute hip arthroplasty. Those treated with ORIF had a 30% rate of reoperation compared to 14% in the arthroplasty group. Pain scores were also better in the arthroplasty group.

High rates of blood transfusion and prolonged operative times have been reported in several series. Chakravarty et al. described a technique of percutaneous column fixation combined with THA to reduce operative time and blood loss associated with traditional acetabular fracture fixation techniques. This procedure is best accomplished with collaboration of surgeons familiar with techniques of open reduction of acetabular fractures and of complex hip arthroplasty.

In old fractures of the acetabulum treated nonoperatively, residual pelvic deformity and areas of nonunion are common. A significant bony defect may be present posteriorly, especially if there has been a previous fracture of the posterior wall. Judet views of the acetabulum and a CT scan show the extent of the defect and detect areas of nonunion not identified on plain radiographs. Failure to recognize these posterior deficiencies often leads to placement of the acetabular component in retroversion, with subsequent dislocation. At the time of arthroplasty, either the acetabulum must be deepened so that the posterior edge of the cup is supported by bone or the posterior wall must be extended by a graft consisting of part of the excised femoral head and neck or an allograft anchored with several screws or a buttress plate. For smaller contained defects, morselized autograft from the femoral head is adequate. In patients with nonunion of a displaced transverse acetabular fracture or patients with extremely irregularly shaped defects, an antiprotrusio cage may be used along with a hemispherical acetabular component (cup-cage construct).

If open reduction of the acetabulum has been done previously, extensive soft-tissue scarring can be expected and exposure may be difficult. Heterotopic ossification complicates exposure further and can cause impingement after the components are placed. Excision of heterotopic bone is laborious and increases operative time and blood loss. Efforts to prevent recurrence of heterotopic bone are warranted (see section on heterotopic ossification).

Previously placed internal fixation devices can be exposed during the process of reaming the acetabulum, and it may be necessary to remove them to implant the acetabular component properly. Considerable additional exposure may be required to remove screws and plates, risking injury to the sciatic nerve within scarred soft tissues. The ready availability of metal-cutting tools and screw removal instruments facilitates extraction of previously placed implants from the interior of the acetabulum without added extraarticular exposure. The acetabular component often can be implanted with removal of only a portion of the hardware, leaving the remainder undisturbed.

Makridis et al. conducted a meta-analysis of published series of total hip replacement in patients with acetabular fractures. Heterotopic ossification, infection, dislocation, and nerve injuries were the most commonly reported complications. Acetabular component survival was only 76% at 10 years. Yuan, Lewallen, and Hanssen reported no aseptic loosening with a highly porous metal acetabular component (see Fig. 1.31), but failures related to infection were reported. In a case-control study of patients undergoing hip arthroplasty after prior acetabular fracture compared to those with osteoarthritis or avascular necrosis, Morison et al. found the prior fracture patients had a markedly inferior 10-year survivorship and higher rates of infection, dislocation, and heterotopic ossification.

FAILED RECONSTRUCTIVE PROCEDURES
■ PROXIMAL FEMORAL OSTEOTOMY AND DEFORMITY

Several problems may be encountered in inserting the femoral stem for arthroplasty after proximal femoral osteotomy or when the proximal femur is otherwise deformed. Anatomic distortion and scarring from previous surgery make the surgical exposure more hazardous. The displacement of the fragments and the dense, cancellous bone in the femoral canal at the level of the healed osteotomy require careful reaming to broach the obstruction and to avoid cortical perforation or fracture. A high-speed burr may be required to remove dense intramedullary bone. Implant malposition and bony impingement resulting from the distorted femoral architecture can lead to hip instability. Previously placed internal fixation devices often are covered with bone, and their removal alone constitutes a significant operation. Broken screws are common, and the femur is prone to fracture after their removal. The femoral cement-bone interface often is imperfect when there are multiple cortical perforations, and the durability of fixation is compromised. If removal of implants is complex, a staged procedure is appropriate, with the arthroplasty being done after the soft tissues and any femoral cortical defects have healed.

Deformity may be present either in the proximal metaphyseal area or distally in the diaphysis. The location, type, and degree of deformity are important factors in preoperative planning. A metaphyseal valgus deformity produces a femur with a straight medial border, and conventional metaphyseal-filling cementless implants are unsuitable. We have used modular stems (Fig. 1.99) effectively in this situation (also see Fig. 1.23). Alternatively, the deformed neck segment may be

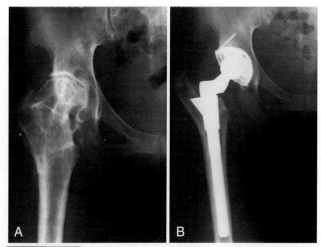

FIGURE 1.99 Femoral osteotomy. **A,** Prior valgus femoral osteotomy for posttraumatic osteonecrosis in 42-year-old woman. Mild deformity of proximal femur is present. **B,** After reconstruction with modular stem with sleeve reversed. Repeat osteotomy was avoided.

resected and replaced with a calcar-replacement type of stem (see Fig. 1.25C). When there has been a previous metaphyseal varus osteotomy, conventional implants generally can be used, although overhang of the greater trochanter may require trochanteric osteotomy to avoid fracture or varus stem alignment. Metaphyseal rotational deformities usually can be managed by cementing a slightly smaller stem in the proper rotational alignment or by use of a cementless stem with diaphyseal fixation alone. Repeat osteotomy at the metaphyseal level should be avoided because the proximal fragment would be small, and it would be difficult to achieve stability at the osteotomy site. The application of supplemental plates and strut grafts to the metaphysis often is technically unsatisfactory, and the added bulk increases the risk of bony impingement and dislocation. If repeat osteotomy is required to manage a metaphyseal deformity, it generally should be done at the subtrochanteric level where fixation is more reliable.

Diaphyseal deformities generally have a more substantial effect on implant placement. For deformities in the distal part of the diaphysis, a short stem can be used and the deformity need not be directly treated. If the deformity is in the subtrochanteric area, however, careful preoperative planning is mandated. Minor angular and translational deformities usually can be negotiated with a cemented stem of a size smaller than usual to preserve an adequate circumferential cement mantle. If angular deformity is significant, however, or translation of greater than 50% is present, repeat osteotomy is needed (Fig. 1.100). Surgery can be done in two stages, although the introduction of cementless stems has simplified the operation and made union predictable with a single-stage procedure. Osteotomy also provides direct access to dense intramedullary bone at the previous surgical site, simplifying its removal. Stable fixation must be obtained at the osteotomy site for union to occur. A fluted or extensively porous-coated stem is needed to achieve distal fixation, and a precise fit in both fragments must be obtained to provide rotational stability. If this cannot be achieved with the stem alone, a cortical strut or a plate must be added. An oblique or step-cut osteotomy is intrinsically more stable than a transverse one, although the procedure is

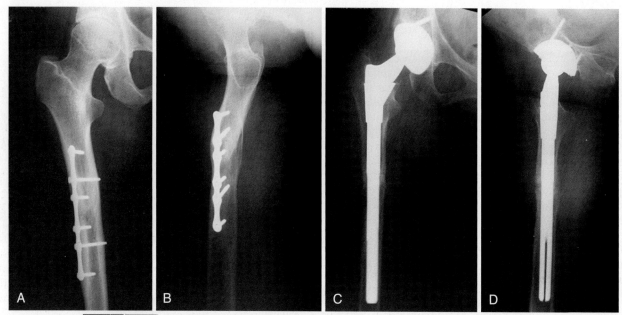

FIGURE 1.100 Femoral osteotomy. **A** and **B,** Significant anterior angulation with rotational malunion and canal stenosis in 68-year-old woman after femoral osteotomy in childhood. **C** and **D,** Repeat osteotomy was required for correction of deformity before femoral component could be implanted.

more challenging from a technical standpoint. This is particularly true if there is rotational malalignment that must be corrected. Cement can be used for stem fixation, but the cement inevitably extrudes into the osteotomy site and jeopardizes union. For this reason, we prefer cementless femoral components when a femoral osteotomy is necessary. Mortazavi et al. reported a series of 58 patients with proximal femoral deformity who had hip arthroplasty. Nonprimary femoral components were used in 25%, and 23% required femoral osteotomy. Cementless fixation provided reliable fixation in this technically challenging situation.

■ ACETABULAR OSTEOTOMY

With a resurgence of interest in pelvic and periacetabular osteotomy, the need for later hip arthroplasty in these patients is likely to become more common. Parvizi, Burmeister, and Ganz reported results in 41 patients undergoing total hip procedures after prior periacetabular osteotomy. Because the initial osteotomies were performed through a Smith-Petersen approach, the procedures were done through virgin lateral soft tissues. There were no acetabular column defects, but retroversion of the acetabulum was a common finding. The prior osteotomy was not thought to compromise the results of the arthroplasty. Shigemura et al. conducted a meta-analysis of hip arthroplasties following pelvic osteotomy. They found less cup anteversion, but no difference in cup abduction, operative time, or blood loss between cases with or without prior pelvic osteotomy. Therefore, careful attention is needed when positioning the acetabular component. In a series of patients with prior Chiari osteotomy, Hashemi-Nejad et al. found less acetabular augmentation was needed compared with dysplastic hips without prior osteotomy.

■ ARTHRODESIS AND ANKYLOSIS

With widespread media attention to the success of hip replacement, patients often are unwilling to accept arthrodesis as a

primary treatment option and likewise request conversion of an existing arthrodesis to restore motion. The effects of hip fusion on other joints are significant. Often the ipsilateral knee is limited in motion, with a variable degree of ligamentous laxity, and has a tendency for valgus malalignment. Pain caused by arthritis or other conditions of the lumbar spine can increase significantly when sitting with the spine partially flexed because of a fused hip. Care must be taken, however, to determine whether back and leg pain may be caused by a herniated lumbar disc or some other condition that may not be improved by THA. If the hip is fused in poor position (i.e., flexed >30 degrees, adducted >10 degrees, or abducted to any extent), osteotomy to correct the position may be considered, especially in younger patients. Arthrodesis of one hip also applies greater mechanical stress to the opposite hip. THA may be indicated if a fused hip causes severe, persistent low back pain or pain in the ipsilateral knee or contralateral hip or if a pseudarthrosis after an unsuccessful fusion is sufficiently painful (Fig. 1.101).

The history of the initial reason for the arthrodesis is important. Patients with prior infection require a thorough evaluation to rule out persistence. A careful assessment of the function of other joints, especially the lumbar spine, should be done, and leg-length discrepancy should be measured. Preoperative metal-subtraction CT can be helpful in determining the adequacy of bone stock and the presence of a pseudarthrosis.

Function of the abductors is difficult to evaluate before surgery, but in some patients active contraction of these muscles can be palpated. Examination of the hip with the knee flexed helps differentiate the TFL from the abductor muscles. If the hip has been fused since childhood, and the trochanter appears relatively normal, the abductor muscles are probably adequate. If the bone around the hip has been grossly distorted by disease or by one or more fusion operations, the abductor muscles may be inadequate. The utility of electromyographic

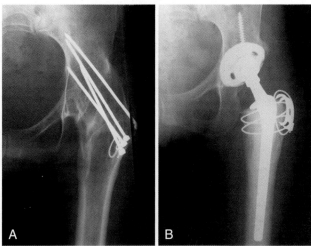

FIGURE 1.101 **A,** Arthrodesis in 61-year-old woman who developed disabling back pain four decades after successful arthrodesis of hip. **B,** After conversion to hybrid total hip arthroplasty. Trochanteric osteotomy provided excellent exposure. Patient had persistent Trendelenburg limp after surgery, but back pain had diminished.

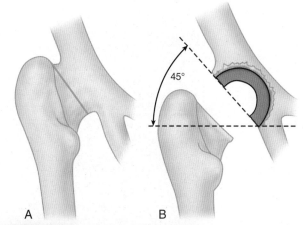

FIGURE 1.102 Osteotomy of neck in conversion of fusion to total hip arthroplasty. **A,** Neck usually is short and should be osteotomized proximally at base of trochanter. **B,** Sufficient bone is left on pelvic side for full coverage of cup at inclination of approximately 45 degrees and without penetrating medial cortex of pelvis.

testing of abductor function or imaging modalities such as MRI has not been established. Weak abductor musculature is associated with poorer functional outcome.

At surgery, a variety of screwdrivers, metal cutters, and other extraction instruments should be available to remove antiquated fixation devices. The conversion of a fused hip to a THA is safer and easier if the trochanter is osteotomized. Complete mobilization of the femur without trochanteric osteotomy is difficult, and the resulting inadequate exposure predisposes to component malposition, errors in femoral reaming, and fractures. In addition, the limb often is fixed in external rotation, and consequently the trochanter is posterior, overhanging the hip joint. Osteotomy of the neck can be difficult through a posterior approach unless the trochanter is osteotomized. The sciatic nerve often is displaced closer to the hip because the head-neck length is shorter than normal and the nerve may be fixed in scar tissue; for this reason, special care is taken to avoid damage to the nerve. Careful monitoring of tension on the nerve is necessary, and neurolysis may be indicated if the extremity is significantly lengthened.

After the femoral neck has been exposed, it is divided with a saw. The location of the osteotomy is determined from bony landmarks or the position of previous fixation devices. The neck should not be divided flush with the side of the ilium because sufficient bone must be left to cover the superior edge of the cup (Fig. 1.102). After the neck has been divided, release of the psoas tendon, gluteus maximus insertion, and capsulotomy are necessary to mobilize the proximal femur.

Usually the pelvic bone is sufficiently thick to cover the cup adequately if the site for acetabular preparation is chosen carefully. Distortion of the normal bony architecture may cause difficulty in locating the appropriate site for acetabular placement. Usually the anterior inferior iliac spine (AIIS) remains intact and serves as a landmark. Additionally, a retractor can be placed in the obturator foramen. Acetabular preparation is performed with conventional reamers, centering within the available bone to preserve the anterior and

posterior columns. Intraoperative fluoroscopy or radiograph is helpful early in the acetabular preparation to ensure that the position of the reamer is as expected.

The femoral canal is prepared in the usual manner, taking into account any deformity from prior disease or femoral osteotomy. Trochanteric fixation is accomplished by standard techniques (see Figs. 1.74 to 1.76). If the abductors are markedly atrophic or deficient, a constrained (see Fig. 1.34) or dual mobility (see Fig. 1.35) acetabular component should be considered.

After the procedure has been completed, the patient is placed supine. If the hip cannot be abducted 15 degrees because the adductors are tight, a percutaneous adductor tenotomy is done through a separate small medial thigh incision. The extremity usually is lengthened by the procedure and corrects prior flexion deformity. Lengthening usually is desirable because in most instances the limb has been shortened by the original disease, by the procedure for fusing the hip, or by the flexion deformity.

The postoperative treatment is routine, but the hip should be protected for at least 3 months by use of crutches and then by use of a cane while the hip abductors and flexors are being rehabilitated. Patients rarely regain flexion to 90 degrees, but they achieve sufficient motion to relieve back symptoms and permit sitting and walking and tying shoes. Walking ability usually is improved, but in patients with inadequate abductor function the gait pattern may worsen, and the support of a cane or walker may be required even if the patient did not use one before conversion to arthroplasty. Most patients have some degree of residual abductor weakness and limp, although this tends to improve over several years.

The complication rate for conversion of an arthrodesis to an arthroplasty is high. In the Mayo Clinic series of Strathy and Fitzgerald, 33% of patients experienced failure within 10 years because of loosening, infection, or recurrent dislocation. Patients with a spontaneous ankylosis fared much better than patients who had a prior surgical arthrodesis. Jauregui et al. conducted a meta-analysis of 1104 hip fusion conversions and reported 5.3% had infection, 2.6% developed instability, 6.2% had loosening, 4.7% with nerve complications, and

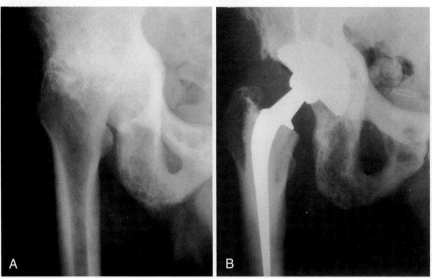

FIGURE 1.103 **A,** Extensive Paget disease of acetabulum and proximal femur in 82-year-old man. Note protrusio deformity and varus femoral neck. **B,** After total hip replacement. Acetabulum required autogenous bone graft from femoral head. Considerable blood loss occurred during acetabular preparation. Cementless acetabular component appears bone ingrown 5 years after surgery.

13.1% experienced abductor-related complications. Celiktas et al. reported a series of 28 patients operated through a posterior approach without trochanteric osteotomy. Although their procedures were technically feasible, five patients had intraoperative trochanteric fracture.

METABOLIC DISORDERS
■ PAGET DISEASE
Patients with Paget disease may have degenerative arthritis in one or both hips, varying degrees of protrusio acetabuli, varus deformity of the neck and proximal femur, and anterolateral bowing of the shaft (Fig. 1.103). In addition, incomplete (stress) fractures may develop on the convex side of the femoral shaft. These fractures, the metabolic disease alone, secondary sarcoma formation, and radicular problems referable to the lumbar spine all can cause hip pain, in addition to the hip arthritis, and it may be difficult to differentiate the sources of pain. Preoperative medical management with bisphosphonates and calcitonin can help control pain and decrease perioperative blood loss. If the disease is active, the administration of calcitonin before and after surgery is advisable to decrease the osteoclastic activity and possibly to reduce the risk of loosening as a result of postoperative bone resorption.

The deformed proximal femoral bone may be osteoporotic or markedly dense, and these changes can cause technical difficulties. Consequently, anteroposterior and lateral radiographs of the hip and femoral shaft should be evaluated carefully before surgery to determine the extent of bowing and the presence of lytic or dense lesions. Usually the anterolateral bowing is not a problem in reaming the canal or positioning the stem because the medullary canal is wide. If the deformity is considerable, however, a femoral osteotomy may be needed for stem placement. The presence of dense intramedullary bone can make identification and opening of the canal difficult. A high-speed burr and intraoperative use of

fluoroscopy are helpful when this is recognized on preoperative radiographs.

Bleeding can be excessive, especially in patients with osteoporotic bone. The lack of a dry bone bed can reduce cement interdigitation in the femur and the acetabulum and compromise fixation. Conversely, cementless fixation has proven durable despite concerns that altered bone morphology may prevent osseointegration.

The results of THA for painful arthritis and for displaced femoral neck fractures in Paget disease are encouraging, with a reported 7- to 10-year survival rate of 86%. The results of internal fixation of these fractures and of endoprostheses for fractures or arthritis in this disease have been unsatisfactory. THA has become the procedure of choice. Heterotopic bone formation has been reported as a common postoperative complication, and prophylactic measures to reduce its formation seem warranted.

■ GAUCHER DISEASE
Patients with the chronic nonneuropathic form of Gaucher disease may have osteonecrosis of the femoral head bilaterally, and if it is sufficiently painful, they may require a THA. Osteonecrosis of the femoral head may produce the first symptoms that suggest the diagnosis of Gaucher disease. The disease is characterized, however, by osteopenia, with areas in which the trabeculae have a moth-eaten appearance and patchy areas of sclerosis; much of the bone marrow may be replaced by Gaucher cells. Because the medullary canal usually is wide, implant fixation even with cement is difficult, and the femur can be fractured easily. The disease often is characterized by recurring, nonspecific bone pain, making evaluation of some postoperative symptoms difficult. Anemia and thrombocytopenia may complicate surgical interventions. Many patients have required splenectomy, and infections are a common complication of Gaucher disease. Other complications include excessive intraoperative and postoperative

hemorrhage and a high incidence of loosening because of the continued Gaucher cell proliferation and erosion of bone. Enzyme replacement therapy may ameliorate the osseous problems associated with the disease.

■ SICKLE CELL ANEMIA

Patients with sickle cell anemia and sickle cell trait may develop painful osteonecrosis of the femoral head. The process can be bilateral. Radiographs may reveal a large collapsed avascular area or an arthritic process caused by small focal areas of osteonecrosis near the articular surface.

In the past, the life expectancy of patients with the SS form of sickle cell anemia was thought to be short (approximately 30 years), but with improvements in medical management and antibiotics, they may live much longer. Although patients with sickle cell trait also develop osteonecrosis, they do so less often than patients with sickle cell disease. Many more patients have the trait than the disease, however.

Patients with sickle cell anemia may require transfusions before surgery, and transfusion reactions owing to alloimmunization are more frequent. Many patients are chronically dependent on narcotic analgesics, and epidural anesthesia and multimodal pain management techniques are advisable. Cardiopulmonary care must be aggressively managed, and perioperative hypoxia, acidosis, and dehydration must be avoided. A multidisciplinary approach to the medical management of sickle cell patients reduces morbidity.

Acetabular bone quality may be poor and a variable degree of protrusio deformity may be present, making hip dislocation more difficult. Bone grafting of acetabular defects may be required (see section on protrusio acetabuli). Areas of femoral intramedullary sclerosis from prior infarction may be manifest as "femur within femur" on preoperative radiographs. In our experience, this problem is underestimated by preoperative radiographs, and at surgery the canal may be completely obstructed by very dense bone. Major technical problems in reaming the canal must be anticipated, and the risk of femoral fracture and cortical perforation is high. Use of fluoroscopy is helpful for centering instruments in the femoral canal, and reaming over a guidewire is inherently safer. Preliminary removal of sclerotic bone with a high-speed burr also makes broaching easier.

Although these patients are more susceptible to *Salmonella* infections, the literature does not support this as being a pathogen in postoperative sepsis of hip arthroplasty. Specific prophylaxis for *Salmonella* does not seem to be warranted. Because of functional asplenia, patients with sickle cell anemia are prone to developing hematogenous infection of the hip after surgery. Aggressive antibiotic management is indicated when the possibility of hematogenous infection exists. The ESR is of no value in determining whether a patient with sickle cell disease has an inflammatory process. Pain resulting from a sickle cell crisis caused by vascular occlusion often presents a problem in determining whether a particular pain is caused by infection.

Complications such as excessive bleeding, hematoma formation, and wound drainage are common after arthroplasty in patients with sickle cell disease; complications have been reported in nearly 50% of THAs in sickle cell patients. Because no other option yields consistently superior results, the procedure is still justified in patients with severe pain and disability. Patients should be advised, however, of the increased

risk of complications imposed by their disease. Recent series using cementless fixation have been somewhat more encouraging. Ilyas et al. reported 10-year survivorship of 98% using cementless femoral and acetabular components, with deep infection in 6.77%.

■ CHRONIC RENAL FAILURE

Osteoporosis, osteonecrosis, and femoral neck fracture are common sequelae of chronic renal failure. With the institution of hemodialysis and the success of renal transplantation, an increasing number of these patients are becoming candidates for hip arthroplasty. Poor wound healing, infection, and an array of general medical complications related to the disease process can be anticipated. Sakalkale, Hozack, and Rothman reported THA in 12 patients on long-term hemodialysis. There was an early complication rate of 58%, and infection developed in 13%. Longevity was limited after surgery, and the authors recommended limiting the procedure to patients with a longer life expectancy. Lieberman et al. reported their results after THA in 30 patients who had renal transplants and 16 who were being treated with hemodialysis. Patients with transplants had postoperative courses similar to other patients with osteonecrosis, whereas in the patients who were being treated with hemodialysis 81% had poor results and 19% developed infection. These authors recommended limiting hip arthroplasty to patients who are expecting renal transplant or who have already had successful transplantation. In contrast, a series from the Mayo Clinic found a higher cumulative revision rate in transplant patients, with complications in 61%. A high rate of loosening of cemented femoral components was noted. More encouraging results have been reported with cementless, extensively porous-coated implants. Nagoya found predictable bone ingrowth with no infections in 11 patients on long-term hemodialysis with average follow-up of more than 8 years.

■ HEMOPHILIA

Hemophilic arthropathy involves the hip joint far less often than the knee and elbow. Consequently, there is a paucity of information specific to hip arthroplasty. When hip involvement develops before skeletal maturity, valgus deformity of the femoral neck, flattening of the femoral head, and a variable degree of acetabular dysplasia are present. The radiographic appearance is similar to that of LCPD.

A multidisciplinary approach is essential for surgical treatment of hemophilic arthropathy. Ready access to a well-managed blood bank and an experienced hematology staff are requisites; for this reason, arthroplasty in hemophilic patients generally is done only in specialized centers. Patients with circulating antibodies to clotting factor replacements (inhibitors) are not considered suitable candidates for surgery because of the risk of uncontrollable hemorrhage. In a study of the Nationwide Inpatient Sample, Kapadia et al. reported transfusions in 15.06% of hemophiliacs compared to 9.84% in matched controls following lower extremity arthroplasty.

Complications occur frequently in these patients. In a multicenter study, Kelley et al. reported that 65% of cemented acetabular components and 44% of cemented femoral components had radiographic evidence of failure at a mean follow-up of 8 years. Nelson et al. found similar failure rates in a long-term study of patients from a single center. Results have been better with modern cementless implants. Carulli et al. reported no failures or complications at mean follow-up of 8.1 years in 23 patients with a mean age of 40.6 years.

Late hematogenous infection may be a significant problem, and the risk increases if patients previously exposed to HIV through factor replacements develop clinical manifestations of acquired immunodeficiency syndrome. Enayatollahi et al. reported infection in 10.98% of patients with both HIV and hemophilia versus 2.28% in patients with HIV only.

INFECTIOUS DISORDERS
■ PYOGENIC ARTHRITIS

Most patients with a history of pyogenic arthritis of the hip who are considered candidates for THA had the hip joint infection in childhood and had either a spontaneous or surgical hip fusion or developed a pseudarthrosis of the hip. Pyogenic arthritis of the hip in adults is rare except after internal fixation of fractures.

Arthroplasty may be considered in an adult whose hip was fused by a childhood pyogenic infection and in whom inflammation has not been evident for many years. A solid fusion with a uniform trabecular pattern crossing the joint usually indicates the absence of residual infection. Focal areas of decreased density and some sclerosis and irregularity of the trabeculae crossing the joint line may signify a residual focus of infection, however. Tang et al. found MRI to be 100% sensitive in showing the presence of active infection in patients with prior osteomyelitis. Determination of ESR and CRP levels, hip joint aspiration, bone biopsy, and radionuclide scanning all may play a role in the preoperative evaluation. Intraoperative frozen sections of periarticular tissues also should be obtained. When any of these studies points to residual infection around the hip, a two-stage procedure is appropriate.

Often the limb is shortened as a result of partial destruction of the femoral head and neck and the acetabulum. The flexed and adducted position of the hip adds to the apparent shortening. The femur may be hypoplastic with anteversion of the femoral neck and variable degrees of resorption of the femoral head. Deep scarring may be present as a result of multiple incision and drainage procedures and sinuses around the hip. If present, previous incisions should be used, and prior sinus tracks should be completely excised. Lack of subcutaneous tissues over the trochanter and in the area of the proposed incision may require rotation of a skin flap before the THA.

In a group of 44 patients who underwent THA after pyogenic arthritis in childhood, Kim found no reactivations of infection despite the use of acetabular allografts in 60% of the patients. Perioperative femoral fracture was common because many of these patients had a small, deformed proximal femur. In a larger series of 170 patients from the same institution, there were no recurrent infections when the period of quiescence had been at least 10 years. Operative difficulties were frequent, however, and polyethylene wear and implant loosening were common late complications. Similarly, Park et al. reported that poor results in this population were attributed to anatomic abnormalities that had developed as a result of infection rather than recurrence of infection following arthroplasty.

■ TUBERCULOSIS

The hip is the second most common site of osseous involvement of tuberculosis following the spine, resulting in severe cartilage and bone destruction, limb shortening, and instability. The diagnosis should be considered in patients who come from a country in which the disease is prevalent, in patients with a history of having been in a spica cast as a child, in patients being treated for acquired immunodeficiency syndrome, and in patients with undiagnosed arthritis of the hip. Tuberculous bacilli are fewer in number in bone infections than in infected sputum, making the diagnosis of tuberculous osteomyelitis difficult.

A longer period of chemotherapy has been recommended when hip arthroplasty is performed in the presence of active tuberculous arthritis. *Mycobacterium tuberculosis* has little biofilm and adheres poorly to implants. Many patients with reactivation of tuberculous infections after THA can be treated with debridement and drug therapy with retention of the prosthesis. Because of the emergence of drug-resistant strains of tuberculosis, preoperative tissue biopsy with culture and sensitivity are helpful in selecting the optimal chemotherapeutic agents.

Most patients are candidates for a single-stage procedure. In a systematic review of the available literature, Tiwari et al. identified 226 patients in whom antituberculosis treatment was administered for 2 weeks preoperatively and continued for 6 to 18 months following hip arthroplasty. Only three patients had reactivation of infection at mean follow-up of 5.48 years. The presence of a sinus track often is indicative of superinfection with *S. aureus,* and a two-stage procedure is indicated in these patients. Radical debridement of all infected tissue is required in either scenario. Both cemented and cementless fixation have been successful at mid-term follow-up.

TUMORS

Possible candidates for THA include patients with (1) metastatic tumors with a reasonable life expectancy, (2) some low-grade tumors, such as chondrosarcoma and giant cell tumor, and (3) benign destructive lesions, such as pigmented villonodular synovitis. For patients with primary lesions, curing the disease, and not restoration of function, should be the goal of surgery. Consequently, careful planning to determine the amount of tissue to be resected may require a bone scan, CT, and MRI. The surgical approach must be more extensive than usual to ensure complete excision of the tumor. A conventional THA may suffice, however, if only a limited amount of the acetabulum or the femoral head and neck must be resected to excise the tumor and a margin of normal tissue. If the greater trochanteric and subtrochanteric areas are resected, the hip may be unstable because reattaching the abductor muscles is difficult. An extra-long femoral component may be necessary because of other lesions more distal in the femoral shaft. A custom-made component or segmental replacement stem can be used (see Fig. 1.29); the gluteal muscles are sutured to holes made in the component for this purpose. An allograft-prosthesis composite with a long stem is an option in young patients. Cement fixation within the graft and a step-cut at the junction of the graft and host bone provide stability. The acetabulum can be reconstructed with cement, with additional support provided by a reinforcement ring or cage (see Fig. 1.36) or by threaded Steinmann pins inserted through the iliac wing into the acetabulum.

NEUROMUSCULAR DISORDERS

Patients with chronic neuromuscular disorders who come to hip arthroplasty usually have increased muscle tone or spasticity. Spasticity may be congenital, as with cerebral palsy, or acquired through brain or spinal cord injury. Acquired spasticity may be complicated by the presence of heterotopic ossification about the hip. Patients become candidates for THA because of fracture, end-stage hip arthritis, or painful subluxation. Although this group encompasses a broad range of congenital and acquired diseases and syndromes, certain management principles are applicable to all.

Patients with generalized neurologic problems are at greater risk for complications, and careful attention must be paid to care of the skin, pulmonary function, and urinary tract to prevent sepsis at these sites. Early mobilization, at least to a chair and preferably to weight-bearing status, prevents further muscular deterioration. Patients with retained motor function and intact cognition have better potential for recovery of mobility.

Combined flexion and adduction contractures are common, but their presence may not be appreciated when a patient has an acute fracture. This combination of deformities predisposes to postoperative dislocation, especially when surgery is performed through a posterior approach. A direct anterior or anterolateral approach may be preferable, although these approaches are less extensile when excision of heterotopic ossification is needed. Release of the anterior capsule and psoas and percutaneous adductor tenotomy all may be required. The degree of contractures usually is more severe in patients with congenital neurologic disorders. Placement of the acetabular component in additional anteversion also makes the hip more stable. If the stability of the hip during surgery is unsatisfactory, or if the patient's muscular control of the hip is insufficient to maintain appropriate postoperative precautions, a hip spica cast probably should be worn for 4 to 6 weeks until the soft tissues have healed sufficiently to stabilize the joint. Occasionally, a constrained acetabular component may be necessary to prevent postoperative dislocation. Other tenotomies may be required to achieve knee extension and a plantigrade foot. In a series of 39 patients with cerebral palsy, Houdak et al. reported no difference in the rate of reoperation, survivorship, and complications compared to patients with osteoarthritis. Dislocations occurred in 7%.

Patients with paralytic conditions, such as the residuals of poliomyelitis, may develop hip arthritis in either the affected limb or a normal contralateral hip. Dysplasia may be present on the paralytic side, and overuse degenerative arthritic changes predominate on the nonparalytic side. Yoon et al. found that polio patients often had some residual pain after hip arthroplasty, possibly caused by muscular weakness inherent to the disease.

COMPLICATIONS

Medical and surgical complications can occur after THA and exert a significant effect on patient satisfaction and overall outcome of the procedure. Prevention of complications should be a consistent focus of all involved stakeholders.

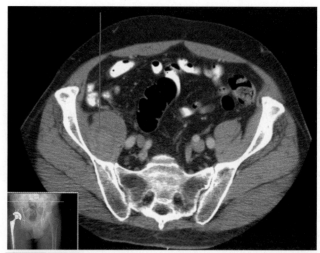

FIGURE 1.104 CT scan shows fluid within the iliopsoas muscle sheath consistent with hematoma secondary to impingement from acetabular component. (From Bartelt RB, Sierra RJ: Recurrent hematomas within the iliopsoas muscle caused by impingement after total hip arthroplasty, *J Arthroplasty* 26:665, 2011.)

Prompt diagnosis and effective treatment are critical for a successful result.

MORTALITY

According to a 2014 meta-analysis, the 30-day mortality rate was 0.3% for primary THA and the 90 day rate was 0.65%. Increased mortality rates were associated with advanced age, male gender, and medical comorbidities, particularly cardiovascular disease. Although careful preoperative medical evaluation is warranted in all patients, special attention should be directed to patients with these risk factors.

HEMATOMA FORMATION

Careful preoperative screening should identify patients with known risk factors for excessive hemorrhage, including antiplatelet, antiinflammatory, or anticoagulant drug therapy; herbal medication use; blood dyscrasias and coagulopathies; and family or patient history of excessive bleeding with previous surgical procedures.

The most important surgical factor in preventing hematoma is careful hemostasis. Common sources of bleeding are (1) branches of the obturator vessels near the ligamentum teres, transverse acetabular ligament, and inferior acetabular osteophytes, (2) the first perforating branch of the profunda femoris deep to the gluteus maximus insertion, (3) branches of the femoral vessels near the anterior capsule, and (4) branches of the inferior and superior gluteal vessels. The iliac vessels are at risk from penetration of the medial wall of the acetabulum and removal of a medially displaced cup. Bleeding from a large vessel injury usually becomes apparent during the operation (see section on vascular injuries). Late bleeding (1 week postoperatively) may occur from a false aneurysm or from iliopsoas impingement (Fig. 1.104). Arteriography may be required for identification of a false aneurysm along with possible embolization. Acetabular revision may likewise be necessary to correct iliopsoas impingement.

Excessive hemorrhage leading to hematoma formation uncommonly requires surgical intervention. Most patients can be managed by dressing changes, discontinuation of anticoagulants, treatment of coagulopathy, and close observation of the wound. Indications for surgical treatment of hematoma include wound dehiscence or marginal necrosis, associated nerve palsy, and infected hematoma. Evacuation of the hematoma and achievement of meticulous hemostasis should be accomplished in the operating room. The hematoma should be cultured to assess possible bacterial contamination, and antibiotics should be continued until these culture results become available. Debridement of necrotic tissue as needed and watertight closure also are required. Closed suction drainage seems warranted in this setting to avoid a recurrence.

HETEROTOPIC OSSIFICATION

Heterotopic ossification varies from a faint, indistinct density around the hip to complete bony ankylosis. Calcification can be seen radiographically by the third or fourth week; however, the bone does not mature fully for 1 to 2 years. The classification of Brooker et al. is useful in describing the extent of bone formation:

Grade I: islands of bone within soft tissues
Grade II: bone spurs from the proximal femur or pelvis with at least 1 cm between opposing bone surfaces
Grade III: bone spurs from the proximal femur or pelvis with less than 1 cm between opposing bone surfaces
Grade IV: ankylosis

Risk factors for heterotopic ossification include history of heterotopic ossification, diagnosis of hypertrophic osteoarthritis, ankylosing spondylitis, diffuse idiopathic skeletal hyperostosis (DISH), or Paget disease, male gender, and African-American ethnicity.

Surgical technique may play a role in the development of heterotopic ossification. Anterior and anterolateral approaches carry a higher risk of heterotopic ossification than transtrochanteric or posterior approaches.

Most who develop heterotopic ossification are asymptomatic; however, restricted range of motion and pain may occur in patients with more severe Brooker grade III or IV ossification. Routine prophylaxis against heterotopic ossification is not recommended for all patients but is warranted in high-risk groups.

Prophylaxis may include low-dose radiation and nonsteroidal antiinflammatory drugs (NSAIDs). Preoperative and postoperative radiation regimens with doses as low as 500 cGy have been successful. In a multicenter evaluation of radiation prophylaxis, failures occurred more commonly in patients treated more than 8 hours preoperatively or more than 72 hours postoperatively. Preoperative treatment should result in less patient discomfort than in the early postoperative period. Radiation exposure is limited to the soft tissues immediately around the hip joint, and ingrowth surfaces must be appropriately shielded (Fig. 1.105).

NSAIDs reduce the formation of heterotopic bone in many studies. Historically, nonselective cyclooxygenase-1 (COX-1) and cyclooxygenase-2 (COX-2) inhibitors for 6 weeks have been recommended, although courses of administration of 7 days are successful. Compliance is limited by medical contraindications to these drugs and patient intolerance. Multiple meta-analyses comparing COX-1 and COX-2 inhibitors showed no difference in efficacy in preventing heterotopic ossification. In light of a more favorable safety profile

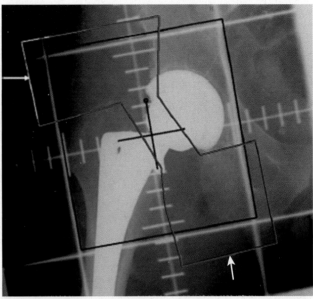

FIGURE 1.105 Anteroposterior radiograph showing radiation portals for total hip arthroplasty. Potential ingrowth portions of femoral and acetabular components were spared. (From Hashem R, Tanzer M, Rene M, et al: Postoperative radiation therapy after hip replacement in high-risk patients for the development of heterotopic bone formation, *Cancer Radiother* 15:261, 2011.)

for the COX-2 inhibitors, they have been recommended for HO prophylaxis.

An operation to remove heterotopic bone is rarely indicated because associated pain usually is not severe and excision is difficult, requiring extensile exposure. The ectopic bone obscures normal landmarks and is not easily shelled out of the surrounding soft tissues. Substantial blood loss can be anticipated. Decreased technetium bone scan activity indicates that the heterotopic bone is mature, allowing for reliable excision. Radiation and NSAIDs have been used successfully to prevent recurrence. Range of motion should improve, but pain may persist.

THROMBOEMBOLISM

Thromboembolic disease is one of the more common serious complications following THA. In early reports of hip arthroplasty without routine prophylaxis, venous thrombosis occurred in 50% of patients, and fatal pulmonary embolism occurred in 2% (Johnson et al.). More recently, a meta-analysis of studies including patients who were anti-coagulated prophylactically after surgeries between 1995 and 2015 found an estimated PE rate of 0.21%, which remained consistent across this time period.

Thromboembolism can occur in vessels in the pelvis, thigh, and calf. Of all thromboses, 80% to 90% occur in the operated limb. The temporal relationship of deep vein thrombosis (DVT) and PE to surgery is controversial. The peak prevalence of DVT varies among studies, with a range of 4 to 17 days after surgery reported. With shorter hospital stays, more thromboembolic events occur after discharge.

The best method of prophylaxis for thromboembolism is debatable. Currently, mechanical and pharmacologic modalities are used. For patients undergoing elective THA, the American College of Chest Physicians (ACCP) recommends one of the following anticoagulant agents: low molecular-weight heparin (LMWH), fondaparinux, apixaban, dabigatran, rivaroxaban, low-dose unfractionated heparin, adjusted-dose warfarin, aspirin, or intermittent pneumatic compression. For patients with high risk of bleeding, mechanical prophylaxis with intermittent pneumatic compression or no prophylaxis should be used. A minimum of 10 to 14 days of prophylaxis is preferred, with a period of up to 35 days also being suggested.

In 2011, the American Academy of Orthopaedic Surgeons (AAOS) published a revised clinical practice guideline regarding the prevention of venous thromboembolic disease after hip or knee arthroplasty. These recommendations stratify patients based on their risk of thromboembolism and major bleeding. Previous venous thromboembolism (VTE) is considered a risk factor for recurrence, whereas bleeding disorders or active liver disease are associated with increased risk for bleeding complications. After assessment of these risk factors, prophylactic measures are tailored accordingly. Patients who are not at increased risk for VTE or bleeding complications should receive pharmacologic and/or mechanical prophylaxis. Those with a history of VTE require combined pharmacologic and mechanical prophylactic measures, whereas patients with increased bleeding risk are covered with mechanical devices only.

The continuation of prophylaxis after the patient has been discharged presents a dilemma. With the ongoing emphasis on cost containment and reducing the length of hospitalization, many patients are discharged at a time when they remain at elevated risk for developing DVT. If anticoagulants are to be continued after discharge, preparation must be made for monitoring their effects. Routine clinical evaluation for wound issues and patient education regarding signs and symptoms of DVT, PE, and bleeding complications are required. Our current practice includes the use of aspirin along with mechanical compression devices during the initial stay for low-risk patients. Aspirin is continued for up to 5 weeks postoperatively. High-risk patients, particularly those with previous history of thromboembolism, are treated with LMWH or apixaban for up to 5 weeks.

NEUROLOGIC INJURIES

An analysis of the literature by Goetz et al. determined the risk of nerve palsy after primary THA for arthritis to be 0.5%, for hip dysplasia 2.3%, and 3.5% for revision surgery. The sciatic, femoral, obturator, lateral femoral cutaneous, and superior gluteal nerves can be injured by direct trauma, traction, pressure, positioning, ischemia, and thermal injury.

The sciatic nerve is particularly susceptible to injury during revision surgery because it may be bound within scar tissue, which places it at risk during the exposure. Injudicious retraction of firm, noncompliant soft tissues along the posterior edge of the acetabulum can cause a stretch injury or direct contusion of the nerve. Exposure of the sciatic nerve during a posterior approach is not necessary routinely but may be advisable if the anatomy of the hip is distorted. The nerve may be displaced from its normal position and tethered by scar tissue along the posterior column. If so, it is carefully exposed, mobilized, and protected during the remainder of the operation. Usually it can be identified more easily in the normal tissue proximal or distal to the scar by the characteristic loose fatty tissues that surround it. When the soft tissues from the posterior aspect

of the femur are being released, the dissection must remain close to the femur, especially in revision procedures. If an anchoring hole for a cemented acetabular component penetrates the medial or posterior cortex, a wire mesh retainer or bone graft should be inserted to prevent extrusion of the cement into the sciatic notch. Careful retractor placement during femoral and acetabular preparation is also mandatory.

The association between limb lengthening and sciatic nerve palsy has been studied with varying conclusions. Edwards et al. correlated the amount of lengthening with the development of sciatic palsy. Injury to the peroneal branch occurred with lengthenings of 1.9 to 3.7 cm. In comparison, complete sciatic palsy occurred with lengthenings of 4 to 5.1 cm. Other authors have questioned the importance of lengthening alone in relation to postoperative sciatic nerve palsy. Nercessian, Piccoluga, and Eftekhar reported 1284 Charnley THAs with lengthening of up to 5.8 cm. Laceration of the sciatic nerve accounted for the only nerve palsy in this group. Eggli, Hankemayer, and Müller reviewed 508 total hip arthroplasties performed for congenital dysplasia of the hip and found no correlation between the amount of lengthening and nerve palsy. They concluded that these palsies were the result of mechanical trauma rather than lengthening alone.

Modular head exchange and/or femoral shortening have been used to treat sciatic palsy attributed to overlengthening. Silbey and Callaghan reported one patient with postoperative sciatic nerve palsy that resolved with early exchange of a modular head to one with a shorter neck length. Sakai et al. similarly noted complete resolution of postoperative sciatic nerve palsy after shortening of the calcar and modular femoral neck.

Sciatic nerve palsy also has been reported as a result of subgluteal hematoma formation, which may occur in association with prophylactic or therapeutic anticoagulation. Subgluteal hematoma should be suspected in patients with pain, tense swelling, and tenderness in the buttock and thigh, along with evidence of a sciatic nerve deficit. Early diagnosis and prompt surgical decompression are imperative.

Dislocation in the perioperative period may injure the sciatic nerve by direct contusion or by stretch. The status of the sciatic nerve always should be documented before any reduction maneuvers are performed. Reduction requires gentle techniques with general anesthesia if necessary.

Postoperative positioning can cause isolated peroneal nerve palsy. Triangular abduction pillows that are secured to the lower extremities with straps can cause peroneal nerve compression if applied tightly over the region of the fibular neck. Such straps should be applied loosely and positioned to avoid this area.

Patients with persistent sciatic or peroneal palsy should have the foot supported to prevent fixed equinus deformity. In most patients, partial function returns, although complete recovery is uncommon. Studies with follow-up of more than 1 year show complete recovery in 20% to 50% of patients.

Late exploration of the sciatic nerve may be considered if some recovery is not present in 6 weeks, or if direct compression is suspected. CT of the acetabulum is helpful in delineating the position of an offending object. Chughtai et al. found improved outcomes with sciatic nerve decompression compared to nonoperative management in both a series of

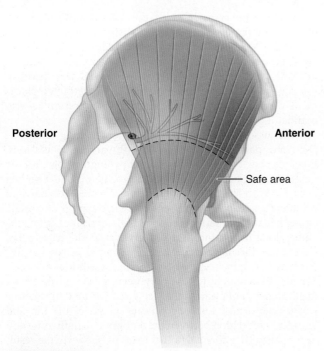

Posterior

Anterior

Safe area

FIGURE **1.106** Safe zone for splitting of the gluteus medius muscle 5 cm proximal to greater trochanter. (Redrawn from Jacobs LG, Buxton RA: The course of the superior gluteal nerve in the lateral approach to the hip, *J Bone Joint Surg* 71A:1239, 1989.)

19 patients treated at their institution and in a review of the literature.

Because injury to the femoral nerve is less common and is easily overlooked in the early postoperative period, diagnosis often is delayed. The femoral nerve lies near the anterior capsule of the joint and is separated from it only by the iliopsoas muscle and tendon. It can be injured by retractors placed anterior to the iliopsoas or during anterior capsulectomy. Hematoma within the iliacus muscle, extruded acetabular cement, and correction of severe flexion contracture are other known causes of femoral nerve palsy. Fleischman et al. reported femoral nerve palsy in 0.21% of patients, with a 14.8-fold increased incidence in patients operated on through an anterior approach, either direct anterior or anterolateral. While significant recovery did not begin until greater than 6 months postoperatively, 75% had complete resolution of motor involvement.

Affected patients should wear a knee immobilizer or hinged knee brace with drop-locks for walking to prevent knee buckling while the quadriceps remains weak.

Similarly, obturator nerve injury may occur with extruded cement, mechanical injury secondary to retractors, or prominent implants such as screws placed in the anteroinferior quadrant (see section on vascular injuries). Persistent groin pain may be the only symptom.

The superior gluteal nerve is most susceptible to injury with anterolateral approaches that split the gluteus medius muscle. A safe zone has been described for splitting the muscle 5 cm proximal to the greater trochanter (Fig. 1.106). Other maneuvers that may injure the superior gluteal nerve include vigorous acetabular retraction for component insertion and extreme leg positioning for femoral preparation. Abductor weakness with a Trendelenburg gait may result from superior gluteal nerve injury.

The LFCN is vulnerable to injury when the direct anterior approach is utilized, as it lies in the subcutaneous tissue of the anterolateral thigh after emerging from under the inguinal ligament. Starting the skin incision 3 cm distal and lateral to the ASIS and incising the tensor sheath with lateral retraction of the TFL muscle may protect the nerve somewhat. Nonetheless, the incidence of LFCN injury has been reported in up to 81% of cases using the direct anterior approach.

VASCULAR INJURIES

Vascular complications as a result of THA are rare (0.04% primary THA, 0.2% revision); however, they can pose a threat to the survival of the limb and the patient. Mortality rates after these injuries range from 7% to 9%, with 15% risk of amputation and 17% chance of permanent disability. Risk factors for vascular injury include revision surgery and intrapelvic migration of components. Vessels can be injured by laceration, traction on the limb, retraction of the surrounding soft tissues, or direct trauma by components such as screws, cement, cables, antiprotrusio cages or rings, threaded acetabular components, or structural allografts.

In general, the measures taken to avoid injury to the femoral nerve also protect the accompanying femoral artery and vein. An anterior retractor should be blunt tipped, carefully placed on the anterior rim, and not allowed to slip anteromedial to the iliopsoas. Care must be taken in releasing the anterior capsule, especially in the presence of extensive scarring, or in the correction of a flexion contracture.

Removal of soft tissue and osteophytes from the inferior aspect of the acetabulum can cause bleeding from the obturator vessels. Penetration of the medial wall of the acetabulum while reaming or intrusion of cement into the pelvis may injure the iliac vessels. These vessels usually are separated from the medial cortex of the pelvis by the iliopsoas muscle, but in some patients this muscle is thin.

The use of transacetabular screws for socket fixation places the pelvic vessels at risk for injury. Wasielewski et al. described the acetabular quadrant system for guidance in the placement of these screws. A line drawn from the ASIS through the center of the acetabulum and a second line perpendicular to the ASIS line divide the acetabulum into four quadrants (see Fig. 1.46). The external iliac vein lies adjacent to the bone of the anterosuperior quadrant, and the obturator vessels and nerve are in close proximity to the pelvic bone in the anteroinferior quadrant. Thinner bone, lack of soft-tissue interposition, and relative immobility of the vessels make them more susceptible to injury. The use of a short drill bit and meticulous technique are mandatory whenever screws are placed in the anterior quadrants. Screw placement should be limited to the posterior quadrants whenever possible. The posterosuperior quadrant, which roughly corresponds to the superior acetabulum between the ASIS and greater sciatic notch, allows for the longest screws and contains the best bone for fixation. The posteroinferior quadrant requires shorter screws. Although the superior gluteal vessels and sciatic nerve are potentially at risk from screws placed through the posterosuperior quadrant, the drill bit and screw tip can be palpated through the sciatic notch to protect these structures from injury. Excessive bleeding encountered during placement of the acetabular component or screw

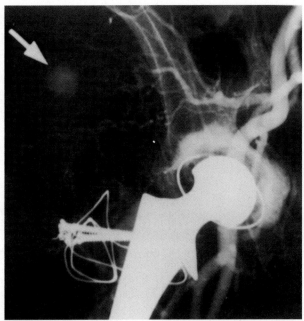

FIGURE 1.107   False aneurysm in 67-year-old woman who had two total hip revisions and continued to bleed intermittently from operative site for approximately 32 weeks after surgery. Arteriogram showed false aneurysm *(arrow).* Suture inserted to close fascia had penetrated wall of branch of superior gluteal artery. Aneurysm was ligated proximally and distally and excised.

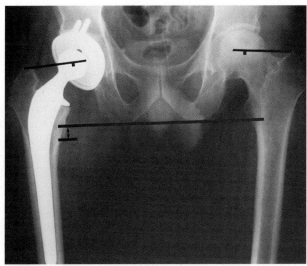

FIGURE 1.108   Total hip arthroplasty for osteonecrosis in 47-year-old man. Femoral head was reconstructed level with tip of trochanter. Oversized acetabular component brought hip center more inferior and overlengthened limb 1 cm despite correct positioning of femoral head.

insertion may require retroperitoneal exposure and temporary clamping of the iliac vessels to prevent additional blood loss. Emergent vascular surgical consultation may be required intraoperatively. Arteriography and transcatheter embolization also have been used to control excessive postoperative intrapelvic bleeding.

Late vascular problems include thrombosis of the iliac vessels, arteriovenous fistula, and false aneurysms. False aneurysms have been reported especially in patients with postoperative hip infections, after migration of threaded acetabular components, and from the use of pointed acetabular retractors. This diagnosis should be considered in patients who have persistent bleeding from the incision or a pulsatile mass (Fig. 1.107).

Because of the risk of vascular injury associated with removal of a markedly protruded acetabular component, arteriography, contrast-enhanced CT scan, or both may be considered before undertaking this type of revision. In addition, the patient's abdomen should be prepared for surgery, and the assistance of a vascular surgeon may be required.

The contralateral limb is at risk for vascular injury because of errors in positioning and pelvic immobilization. Pelvic positioning devices should apply pressure to the pubic symphysis or iliac spines, and pressure over the femoral triangle should be avoided.

LIMB-LENGTH DISCREPANCY
Ideally, the leg lengths should be equal after THA, but it may be difficult to determine this accurately at the time of surgery. Lengthening may result from insufficient resection of bone from the femoral neck, use of a prosthesis with a neck that is too long, or inferior displacement of the center of rotation

of the acetabulum (Fig. 1.108). Proximal femoral morphology can also play a role, as patients with a high femoral cortical index have increased incidence of lengthening, while low femoral cortical index is associated with shortening (Fig. 1.109).

In a survey of 1114 primary THA patients, 30% reported a perceived limb length discrepancy. Of these, only 36% were radiographically confirmed.

The functional significance of leg-length inequality after THA is not well defined. In a study of 101 patients who had primary THA and were studied postoperatively with standing 3D imaging, anatomical leg length, anatomical femoral length, and functional leg length did not correlate with patient perception of limb length discrepancy. Other variables, including pelvic obliquity, difference in knee flexion/recurvatum, and difference in tibial plafond to ground height, did correlate with perceived limb length discrepancy, however. Innmann et al. found that both restoration of hip offset and minimization of limb length discrepancy had an additive positive effect on clinical outcome.

The risk of excessive leg lengthening can be minimized by a combination of careful preoperative planning and operative technique. Edeen et al. found that clinical measurements of leg lengths correlated with radiographic measurements to within 1 cm in only 50% of patients. Flexion and adduction contractures produce apparent shortening of the extremity, and abduction contracture, although less common, produces apparent lengthening. True bony discrepancies sometimes require surgical correction, whereas apparent discrepancies arising from contracture must be recognized, but seldom require operative intervention. A history of previous lower extremity trauma should be sought, and the extremities should be examined for differences below the level of the hip. Good-quality radiographs and templates of known magnification (see discussion of preoperative templating in the section on preoperative radiographs) are used to select a

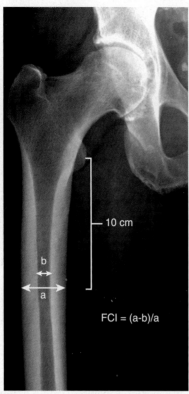

FIGURE 1.109 Femoral cortical index (FCI) ratio, 10 cm below lesser trochanter, measures ratio of cortical diameter (*a-b*) to total femoral diameter (*a*). (From Lim YW, Huddleston JI 3rd, Goodman SB, et al: Proximal femoral shape changes the risk of a leg length discrepancy after primary total hip arthroplasty, *J Arthroplasty* 33:3699, 2018.)

$$FCI = (a-b)/a$$

10 cm

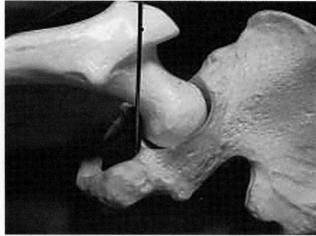

FIGURE 1.110 Steinmann pin in position to mark greater trochanter on initial exposure of hip. Subsequent measurements reference distance from pin to this trochanteric reference line. (From Ranawat CS, Rao RR, Rodriguez JA, et al: Correction of limb-length inequality during total hip arthroplasty, *J Arthroplasty* 16:715, 2001.)

prosthesis that allows intraoperative restoration of leg length and femoral offset.

Several clinical methods for determining leg length have been described. One involves intraoperative evaluation of soft-tissue tension around the hip, commonly referred to as the "shuck test." When traction is applied to the limb with the hip in extension, distraction of 2 to 4 mm usually occurs. The extent of soft-tissue release, the type of anesthesia, and the degree of muscular relaxation may change the surgeon's appreciation of tissue laxity. In addition, soft-tissue tension depends not only on the height of the femoral head but also on the femoral offset (see Fig. 1.6). If femoral offset has been reduced and is not appreciated at surgery, tissue tension has to be restored by inadvertent overlengthening of the limb; in effect, height is substituted for offset to place the soft tissues under tension. Careful preoperative templating should alert the surgeon to this possibility, and arrangements should be made for implants that allow reproduction of the patient's natural offset and appropriate soft-tissue tensioning without overlengthening of the limb. Although the assessment of soft-tissue tension is a useful maneuver, it alone should not be relied on to determine limb length equality.

Multiple methods of limb-length determination have been described using transosseous pins placed above and below the hip joint and a measuring device. Ranawat et al. used a pin below the infracotyloid groove and measured the distance between it and a mark on the greater trochanter. This technique resulted in an average limb-length discrepancy of 1.9 mm, with no patient requiring a shoe lift (Fig. 1.110).

These techniques depend on precise repositioning of the limb in the same degree of flexion, abduction, and rotation for each measurement.

Currently, the most reliable method of equalizing leg lengths is the combination of preoperative templating and intraoperative measurement. Using this approach in a series of 84 hips, Woolson et al. reported that only 2.5% of patients had legs that were lengthened more than 6 mm. In a study of the usefulness and accuracy of preoperative planning, Knight and Atwater concluded that femoral and acetabular component size could not be predicted reliably by templating; however, when templating was combined with operative measurement, the postoperative leg length was within 5 mm of the planned degree of lengthening in 92% of patients.

Computer-assisted techniques may hold promise in achieving limb-length equality after THA. A recent meta-analysis found increased accuracy of limb-length restoration with computer-assisted surgery but no benefit in clinical outcomes. Increased cost and longer operative times have limited the widespread adaptation of computer-assisted techniques.

If both hips are diseased and bilateral staged surgery is expected, length is determined by the stability of the hip, and leg lengths are equalized by making the same bony resections and using the same implants on both sides. The patient should be advised that a shoe lift may be required between surgeries. Occasionally, arthroplasty may be indicated in a hip that is already longer than the contralateral side. Shortening of the limb by excessive neck resection or use of a prosthesis with a neck that is too short poses the risk of dislocation because of inadequate soft-tissue tension or impingement. In this instance, distal transfer of the greater trochanter or shortening by a subtrochanteric osteotomy may be considered.

The main objectives of THA are, in order of priority, pain relief, stability, mobility, and equal leg length. The patient should be informed before surgery that no assurance can be given that the limb lengths will be equal. If lengthening of the limb provides a substantially more stable hip, the discrepancy is preferable to the risk of recurrent dislocation. Discrepancies of less than 1 cm generally are well tolerated, and the perception of the discrepancy tends to diminish with time. Apparent leg-length inequality and pelvic obliquity caused by residual soft-tissue contracture usually respond to physical therapy with appropriate stretching.

Patients with an unacceptable limb-length discrepancy must be evaluated carefully to determine the cause of the discrepancy if surgical treatment is to be successful. Pelvic radiographs are evaluated for component placement that may cause limb-length discrepancy, such as an inferiorly placed acetabular component below the teardrop or a proximally placed femoral component with insufficient neck resection. Parvizi et al. described limb-length discrepancy caused by acetabular component malpositioning and subsequent instability, which had been accommodated by overlengthening with the modular femoral head. In their group of patients surgically treated for limb-length discrepancy, most required revision of a maloriented acetabular component. Limb lengths were equalized in 15 of the 21 patients, with the average limb-length discrepancy decreasing from 4 cm to 1 cm. Only one patient developed recurrent instability, whereas three patients with pain secondary to neuropraxia had complete resolution of their symptoms.

DISLOCATION

The historical prevalence of dislocation after THA is approximately 3%. Anatomic, surgical, and epidemiologic factors may increase this risk. Trochanteric nonunion, abductor muscle weakness, and increased preoperative range of motion are anatomic features that increase the risk of instability. Component malposition, bony and/or component impingement, inadequate soft-tissue tension, and smaller head size are variables under the surgeon's control that have also been implicated. Previous hip surgery, including revision hip replacement, female sex, advanced age, and American Society of Anesthesiologists (ASA) score, prior hip fracture, cervical myelopathy, spinopelvic imbalance, Parkinson disease, dementia, depression, chronic lung disease, and preoperative diagnosis of osteonecrosis or inflammatory arthritis are patient-specific factors that negatively affect hip stability.

Postoperative dislocation is more common when there has been previous surgery on the hip and especially with revision total hip replacement. A recent meta-analysis reported an incidence of 9.04% after 4656 revision surgeries. Contributing factors included increased age at surgery, small femoral head size, history of dislocation, two or more previous revisions, and the use of nonelevated liners.

The choice of surgical approach may affect the rate of postoperative dislocation. There is a tendency to retrovert the socket when THA is done through a posterolateral approach, especially if inadequate anterior retraction of the femur forces the acetabular positioning device posteriorly during component insertion. Division of the posterior capsule is another factor, and meticulous repair of the posterior soft-tissue envelope improves stability. Various soft-tissue repair techniques are advocated for improving hip stability after the posterolateral approach, with dislocation rates ranging from 0% to 0.85%. A meta-analysis comparing posterior approaches with and without soft-tissue repair showed an almost 10-fold reduction in dislocation rates from 4.46% to 0.4% in favor of soft-tissue repair. Our preference includes repair of the posterior capsule and short external rotators to the greater

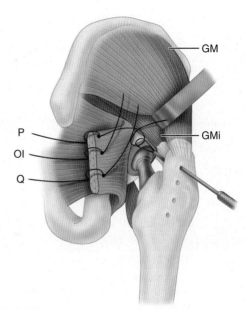

FIGURE **1.111**   Sutures passed through trochanteric drill holes using suture passer. External rotators and hip capsule are incorporated into repair. *GM*, Gluteus maximus; *GMi*, gluteus minimus; *OI*, obturator internus; *P*, piriformis; *Q*, quadratus femoris. (From Osmani O, Malkani A: Posterior capsular repair following total hip arthroplasty: a modified technique, *Orthopedics* 27:553, 2004.)

trochanter and/or abductor tendons with nonabsorbable sutures (Fig. 1.111).

A theoretical advantage to direct lateral, anterolateral, and direct anterior approaches is the preservation of the posterior capsule and short external rotators. Recent studies comparing anterior and posterior approaches with current postoperative protocols have questioned this advantage. A meta-analysis by Wang et al. found no difference in dislocation rates in level I studies comparing direct anterior and posterior approaches.

In fixing the cup in the proper position the surgeon must be able to judge the position of the patient's pelvis in the horizontal and vertical planes. Errors in positioning the patient on the operating table are a common source of acetabular malposition, and secure stabilization of the patient in the lateral position is crucial. When in the lateral position, women with broad hips and narrow shoulders are in a relative Trendelenburg position, and the tendency is to implant the cup more horizontally than is planned. In men with a narrow pelvis and broad shoulders, the reverse is true. With reference to anteversion, the pelvis flexes upward by 35 degrees in the lateral position, and with extension in the supine position it becomes relatively retroverted. Also, forceful anterior retraction of the femur for acetabular exposure often tilts the patient forward. In this instance, placement of the acetabular component in the usual orientation relative to the operating table produces inadvertent retroversion relative to the pelvis. Acetabular insertion devices may provide a false sense of security, and the true position of the pelvis must always be taken into account. Circumferential acetabular exposure that allows observation of bony landmarks is essential. When an acetabular insertion device is used, the angle at which it holds the cup must be known. The trial cup should be placed in the position in which the final cup is to be inserted, and its relationship to the periphery of the acetabulum and the

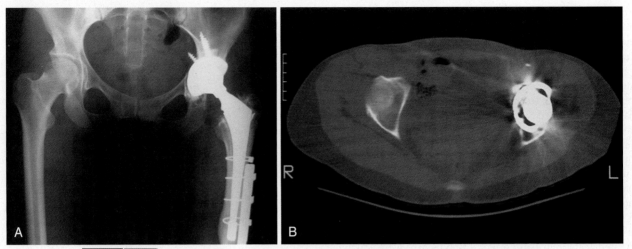

FIGURE 1.112 Determination of angle of anteversion (or retroversion) of cup by CT. **A,** Acetabular component appears well positioned in 39-year-old nurse who had multiple revisions and was referred for femoral loosening with recurrent subluxation. **B,** CT scan shows acetabular retroversion of 20 degrees.

TABLE 1.1

Ideal Cup Position by Spinopelvic Mobility*

	INCLINATION	ANTEVERSION	COMBINED ANTEVERSION
Normal	35°-45°	15°-25°	25°-45°
Stiff	45°-50°†	20°-25°	35°-45°
Kyphotic	35°-40°	15°-20°	25°-35°
Hypermobile	35°-40°	12°-20°	25°-35°

*Cup anteversion is dependent on combined anteversion, which must be higher for stiff imbalance and lower for hypermobile hips to keep sitting ante-inclination within its normal range. In hips that are retroverted, it is difficult to achieve cup anteversion exceeding 12 to 15 degrees, so combined anteversion becomes critical in achieving stability for those hips. The range for each of these patterns is within 10 degrees, and it is difficult to achieve this precision at surgery without some form of navigation. However, these would be the ideal coronal cup angles for these patterns to keep the sagittal ante-inclination in its normal range. Total hip replacement has done so well for so many years because these cup angle numbers are within the cup positions that most surgeons strive to achieve at surgery.
†Inclination of 50 degrees is reserved for elderly patients.
From Ike H, Dorr LD, Trasolini N, et al: Spine-pelvis-hip relationship in the functioning of a total hip replacement, *J Bone Joint Surg Am* 100:1606, 2018.

transverse acetabular ligament should be carefully noted. This orientation is precisely reproduced on placement of the final implant.

Quantifying the degree of anteversion of the cup by plain radiographic examination is difficult. McLaren reported a mathematic method of determining the degree of anteversion whereby the relative positions of the anterior and posterior halves of the circumferential wire in a cemented cup are considered. Similarly, the anteversion of a cementless acetabular component can be estimated by comparing its anterior and posterior margins. Superimposition of the two margins suggests little or no anteversion. If they form an ellipse, some degree of anteversion or retroversion is present. A cross-table lateral view of the affected hip also is helpful in assessing acetabular anteversion, but CT can be used to assess the degree of anteversion of the cup more accurately (Fig. 1.112). The inclination or abduction of the acetabular component can be measured more directly from plain radiographs, although flexion or extension of the pelvis relative to the beam may distort this relationship.

Cup position correlates somewhat with dislocation risk. Lewinnek et al. reviewed radiographs of 300 total hip replacements and proposed a "safe" range of 15 ± 10 degrees anteversion and inclination of 40 ± 10 degrees. More recently, other authors have challenged the safety of these parameters for cup positioning due to the fact that many dislocations occur despite acetabular components being within the "safe" zone. Patients with spinopelvic imbalance, in particular, may require cup positioning outside of the Lewinnek zone to achieve hip stability. A stiff lumbosacral junction requires relatively increased inclination and combined anteversion. Kyphotic or hypermobile patients are better served with lesser degrees of inclination and anteversion (Table 1.1). Other factors, such as femoral component offset, neck length, and soft-tissue balance also contribute to hip stability and must be carefully addressed intraoperatively.

If the cup is excessively anteverted, anterior dislocation can occur during hip extension, adduction, and external rotation. If the cup is overly retroverted, dislocation occurs posteriorly with flexion, adduction, and internal rotation. Excessive inclination of the cup can lead to superior dislocation with adduction, especially if there is a residual adduction contracture, or if the femur impinges on osteophytes left along the inferior margin of the acetabulum (Fig. 1.113). Conversely, if the cup is inclined almost horizontally, impingement occurs

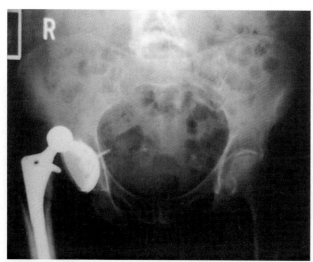

FIGURE 1.113 Excessive inclination of acetabulum. Recurrent dislocation is caused by 65-degree inclination of socket. Hip dislocated with adduction when patient was standing. Revision was required.

early in flexion and the hip dislocates posteriorly. This tendency is accentuated if the cup also is in less anteversion.

Femoral component anteversion is estimated intraoperatively by comparing the axis of the prosthetic femoral neck with the shaft of the tibia when the knee is in 90 degrees of flexion. Neutral version is defined by the prosthetic neck aligned perpendicular to the tibia. Relative anteversion occurs when this angle is greater than 90 degrees and retroversion when it is less (Fig. 1.114). Generally, the femoral component should be implanted with the neck in 5 to 15 degrees of anteversion. Severe anteversion of the anatomic femoral neck is seen in developmental dysplasia or juvenile rheumatoid arthritis, whereas retroversion may be encountered with previous slipped capital femoral epiphysis, proximal femoral malunion, or low levels of neck resection. If the neck of the component is in more than 15 degrees of anteversion, anterior dislocation is more likely (Fig. 1.115). Conversely, retroversion of the femoral component tends to make the hip dislocate posteriorly, especially during flexion and internal rotation.

Amuwa and Dorr described the concept of combined anteversion, in which the anteversion of the femoral component is determined by femoral preparation first. The acetabular component is then placed and the sum of the anteversion of the cup and stem is determined, with the goal of 35 degrees total and an acceptable range of 25 to 50. Computer navigation is required to precisely determine these values.

Impingement may occur because of prominences on the femoral side, acetabular side, or both sides of the joint. Bone or cement protruding beyond the flat surface of the cup must be removed after the cup has been fixed in place; otherwise, it serves as a fulcrum to dislocate the hip in the direction opposite its location. Residual osteophytes, especially located anteriorly, cannot be seen well on standard radiographs but are easily shown by CT scan (Fig. 1.116). After a shallow acetabulum is deepened to provide coverage of the superior part of the cup, excess bone may need to be removed anteriorly, posteriorly, or inferiorly. If the greater trochanter is enlarged or distorted because of previous surgery or as

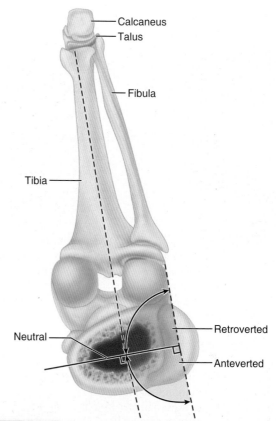

FIGURE 1.114 Anteversion of femoral component is estimated by comparing tibial axis with prosthetic femoral neck axis. Ninety degrees represents neutral anteversion. Acute angles (<90 degrees) are consistent with relative retroversion and obtuse angles (>90 degrees) with increasing anteversion.

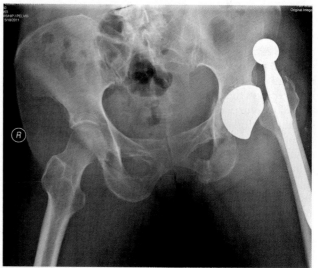

FIGURE 1.115 Dislocation caused by malrotation of femoral component. Component was malrotated into 70 degrees of anteversion. Hip dislocated anteriorly several times and was revised.

a result of the underlying disease process, some bone often must be removed from its anterior or posterior margin to prevent impingement. Finally, bony impingement is much more likely if femoral offset has not been adequately restored. The

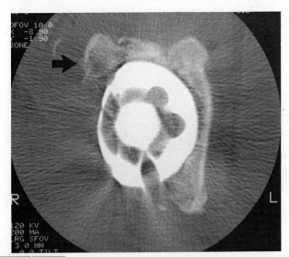

FIGURE 1.116 Recurrent posterior dislocation after arthroplasty after fracture of acetabulum. Acetabular component had been placed in inadequate degree of anteversion because of deficiency of posterior wall. Retained anterior osteophyte *(arrow)* produced impingement in flexion and internal rotation and contributed to dislocation. Revision was required.

use of a femoral component with enhanced offset can be very beneficial in this situation (see Fig. 1.9).

The ratio of the head diameter to that of the neck of the prosthesis is important, as smaller heads have a lower "jumping distance" required for dislocation (see Fig. 1.12). Larger head size is a stabilizing factor reported in some series of primary and revision total hip arthroplasties. Modular femoral head components that have an extension, or "skirt," to provide additional neck length reduce the head-to-neck diameter ratio because the neck of the component is fitted over a tapered trunnion that must be of sufficient diameter (see Fig. 1.8). The range of motion to impingement is decreased compared with a shorter neck that does not use a skirt. Although lengthening the prosthetic neck may improve soft-tissue tension and increase offset, the range of prosthetic motion and ultimate stability of the hip may be diminished if the longer neck requires the addition of a skirted head.

Many current acetabular components have modular liners with elevations that can be rotated into a variety of positions to reorient the face of the acetabulum to a slight degree to provide greater coverage of the prosthetic head (see Fig. 1.35). Such components may improve stability, but they may have the opposite effect if an excessively large elevation is used, or if it is rotated into an inappropriate orientation. Careful assessment of impingement of the prosthetic neck on the liner elevation during trial reduction is mandatory.

Dual mobility acetabular components have their proponents, especially in patients at high risk for dislocation. By providing an increased head-to-neck ratio without a metal-on-metal articulation, they allow greater range of motion to impingement and jumping distance compared to standard components (see Fig. 1.35). De Martino et al. reviewed the literature regarding these components and reported a 0.9% dislocation rate in primary arthroplasties and 1.3% in revisions. Their use does involve additional modularity and the risk of intraprosthetic dislocation.

The adequacy of soft-tissue tension across the hip joint often is suggested as a cause of postoperative dislocation. In a series of 1318 patients, dislocation was significantly less frequent when cup position was appropriate and abductor tension was restored. Trochanteric nonunion, with resultant diminished abductor tension, also is associated with an increased incidence of dislocation. Woo and Morrey found a dislocation rate of 17.6% in patients with displaced trochanteric nonunions compared with 2.8% when the trochanter healed by osseous or fibrous union without displacement.

Physical therapists, nurses, and other caregivers should be aware of the positions likely to cause dislocation. These positions may differ from patient to patient, depending on the surgical approach and other factors. Above all, the patient should be able to voice the appropriate precautions before discharge, and instructions should be reiterated at follow-up office visits. Specialized devices for reaching the floor and dressing the feet are helpful for maintaining independence while avoiding extremes of positioning in the early postoperative period. The efficacy of postoperative hip precautions is debated in the literature. A recent meta-analysis including three randomized controlled trials concluded that very low quality evidence was available on this topic and could not recommend for or against functional restrictions after hip replacement.

Most dislocations occur within the first 3 months after surgery. The dislocation often is precipitated by malpositioning of the hip at a time when the patient has not yet recovered muscle control and strength. Late dislocations can be caused by progressive improvement in motion after surgery or later onset of spinopelvic imbalance. Impingement caused by component malposition or retained osteophytes may not become manifest until extremes of motion are possible. Late dislocations are more likely to become recurrent and require surgical intervention. Von Knoch et al. reported that 55% of late dislocations were recurrent, with 61% of the recurrent dislocators requiring surgery.

All attending personnel, including nurses and physical therapists, should be aware that excessive pain, limited range of motion, rotational deformity, or shortening of the limb is suggestive of dislocation. If these symptoms are noted, radiographs of the hip should be obtained. Reduction usually is not difficult if dislocation occurs during the early postoperative period and a timely diagnosis is made. If the dislocation is not discovered for more than a few hours, reduction may be more difficult because of additional swelling and muscle spasm. Intravenous sedation and analgesia often are sufficient, but sometimes a general anesthetic is required to assist with reduction of the hip. Reduction techniques should always be gentle to minimize damage to the articulating surfaces. The use of image intensification sometimes is valuable in reducing the hip. Reduction is accomplished by longitudinal traction and slight abduction when the head is at the level of the acetabulum. The Allis or Stimson maneuver also can be used. Radiographs should be repeated to confirm the adequacy of reduction. Modular polyethylene liners may dissociate from their metal backings when dislocation occurs, or when reduction is attempted. Incongruous placement of the femoral head within the metal backing indicates such an occurrence. Open reduction with replacement of the liner or revision of the acetabular component is required (Fig. 1.117).

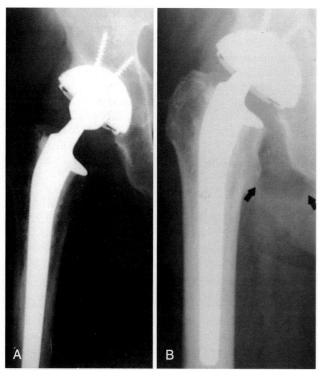

FIGURE 1.117 Dissociation of modular polyethylene liner. **A,** After placement of metal-backed acetabular component with modular polyethylene liner. **B,** Six weeks after surgery, hip dislocated while patient was sitting in low chair. After reduction maneuver, femoral head is eccentrically located in metal backing. Radiolucent shadow of displaced polyethylene liner is visible in soft tissues inferiorly (arrows). Reoperation was required to replace liner.

If the components are in satisfactory position, closed reduction is followed by a period of bed rest. After posterior dislocation, mobilization is accomplished in a prefabricated abduction orthosis that maintains the hip in 20 degrees of abduction and prevents flexion past 60 degrees. Immobilization for 6 weeks to 3 months has been recommended. The efficacy of abduction bracing was challenged in a retrospective review by DeWal et al., who found no difference in the risk of subsequent dislocation between groups of patients treated with or without an abduction brace.

Wera et al. published a series of 75 revision THAs performed for recurrent dislocation according to a proposed algorithmic classification. The six etiologies were:

Type I: acetabular component malposition
Type II: femoral component malposition
Type III: abductor deficiency
Type IV: impingement
Type V: late wear
Type VI: unresolved

Types I and II are treated by revision of the malpositioned component(s). Abductor deficiency and those without known etiology for dislocation (types III and VI) are revised to a constrained acetabular liner or dual mobility construct. When impingement is the causative factor (type IV), sources of impingement are removed, offset is restored, and head size is increased. Late wear (type V) associated with instability requires modular head and liner exchange, including a larger

femoral head. In their series, repeat dislocation occurred in 14.6% of patients, with the highest risk of recurrence in those with abductor deficiency.

If no component malposition or source of impingement is identifiable, distal advancement of the greater trochanter was recommended by Kaplan, Thomas, and Poss to improve soft-tissue tension. In their series, 17 of 21 patients had no additional dislocations. Ekelund reported similar results.

Constrained liner designs offer higher resistance to dislocation than do unconstrained components because the femoral head is mechanically captured into the socket. Callaghan et al. reported the best results with constrained acetabular components. They used a tripolar liner in combination with a new uncemented acetabular component (6% failure rate) or cemented into a well-fixed existing shell (7% failure rate). They did not report increased wear or osteolysis with this device. In a literature review of constrained components, Williams, Ragland, and Clarke found an average recurrent dislocation rate of 10% and an average reoperation rate for reasons other than instability of 4%.

If a constrained component is used, the range of motion of the hip is reduced, and correct positioning of the component is crucial to minimize impingement of the neck on the rim of the liner. Excessive prosthetic impingement with constrained components can disrupt the liner locking mechanism or lever the entire component out of the acetabulum if fixation is not rigid. Guyen, Lewallen, and Cabanela categorized the various modes of failure of a tripolar constrained liner in 43 patients. Failures occurred at the bone/implant interface (type I), at the liner/shell interface (type II), at the locking mechanism (type III), by dislocation of the inner bearing from the bipolar femoral head (type IV), and as a result of infection (type V). They recommended the use of these devices only as a last resort because of their complexity and multiple modes of mechanical failure.

Finally, some patients are not candidates for reconstruction. Noncompliant individuals; alcohol and drug abusers; elderly, debilitated patients; and patients with several previous failed attempts to stop recurrent dislocation are best treated by removal of the components without further reconstruction.

FRACTURES

Fractures of the femur or acetabulum can occur during and after THA. While periprosthetic femoral fractures are more common and often require some form of treatment, acetabular fractures probably occur more frequently than recognized. According to the Mayo Clinic Total Joint Registry, intraoperative femoral fractures occur in 1.7% of primary total hip arthroplasties and in 12% of revision procedures. Primary total hip patients at risk for intraoperative periprosthetic fracture include females, elderly patients, and those treated with uncemented stems.

Femoral fracture is likely to occur during one of several stages in the procedure. Fracture can occur early while attempting to dislocate the hip. Elderly patients and those with rheumatoid arthritis or disuse osteoporosis can be fractured by a moderate rotational force. Cortical defects from previous surgery or fixation devices increase the risk further. If resistance is met in attempting dislocation in these patients, more of the capsule must be released. Osteophytes extending from the margin of the acetabulum must be resected before dislocation; otherwise, the femur or the posterior wall of the acetabulum may be fractured. In some patients with intrapelvic protrusion of the acetabulum, the neck should be divided and the head removed from the acetabulum in a piecemeal fashion. Complex deformities of the proximal femur also increase the risk of fracture, especially when the medullary canal is narrowed. Revision surgery carries a substantially higher risk of fracture than primary procedures because of the presence of thin cortices from implant migration and osteolysis.

Fractures of the femur can occur during broaching or insertion of the femoral component. Broaches are designed to crush and remove cancellous bone and do not remove cortical endosteal bone safely from the diaphysis. The need to remove cortical bone distally can be anticipated from preoperative templating. A straight or flexible reamer must be used to remove this bone before insertion of the broach, or a major fracture extending into the femoral shaft may occur.

Intraoperative femoral fractures occur more commonly in cementless THAs. Abdel et al. reported intraoperative fractures of the proximal femur in 3.0% of cementless primary arthroplasties and in 19% of cementless revision procedures.

The Vancouver classification of periprosthetic femoral fractures has been altered to include intraoperative fractures and perforations (Fig. 1.118). Type A fractures are confined to the proximal metaphysis. Type B fractures involve the proximal diaphysis but can be treated with long-stem fixation. Type C fractures extend beyond the longest revision stem and may include the distal femoral metaphysis. Each type is subdivided into simple perforations (subtype 1), nondisplaced (subtype 2), or displaced (subtype 3). Treatment options include bone grafting, cerclage, long-stem revision, or open reduction and internal fixation depending on the level and displacement of the fracture.

If a femoral fracture occurs during cementless total hip surgery, it must be completely exposed to its most distal extent. This is done with the broach or actual component in place because the fracture gap may close when the implant is removed, and the extent of the fracture may be underestimated. Once the fracture is exposed, the implant is removed, and cerclage wires or cables are placed around the femoral shaft. A trial broach one size smaller can be inserted in the canal to prevent overtightening and potential collapse or overlap of the fracture fragments. One cable should be placed distal to the fracture to prevent its propagation during final component insertion. As the final component is reinserted, the cables come under increased tension, and further expansion of the fracture is prevented. There is a tendency to underestimate such fractures and to regard them as stable. We know of no objective method for determining whether such fractures are in fact stable and recommend cerclage fixation in all cases. Prophylactic placement of cerclage wires should be considered when the cortex is thin or weakened by internal fixation devices or other stress risers. Cobalt chrome cables and hose clamps have the advantage of superior stiffness compared with other cerclage systems.

Postoperative femoral shaft fractures can occur months or years after surgery. Most of these injuries result from low-energy trauma, with high-energy mechanisms reported in

less than 10%. Larsen, Menck, and Rosenklint identified massive heterotopic bone formation around the hip as a potential risk factor. Decreased motion in the hip joint transfers stress to the femoral shaft, similar to a hip arthrodesis. Cortical defects, stem loosening, and osteolysis also can predispose to late postoperative fracture.

The treatment of periprosthetic femoral fracture depends primarily on the location and stability of the fracture, fixation of the indwelling femoral component, quality of the remaining bone, and medical condition and functional demands of the patient. Treatment options include nonoperative management, open reduction and internal fixation of the fracture while leaving the stem *in situ*, and femoral revision with or without adjunctive internal fixation.

Duncan and Masri proposed a classification system for postoperative periprosthetic femoral fractures. It provides a straightforward, validated system that provides guidance in making treatment decisions. The factors considered include the location of the fracture, the fixation of the stem, and the quality of the remaining bone stock (Table 1.2).

Type A fractures involve the trochanteric area and are divided into fractures involving the lesser or greater trochanter. Most type A fractures are stable and can be managed conservatively with a period of protected weight bearing. Greater trochanteric fractures with significant displacement may be treated with trochanteric fixation. Surgical treatment of lesser trochanteric fractures should be reserved for those that involve the medial cortex of the femur and cause instability of the femoral stem.

Type B fractures occur at the tip of the stem or just distal to it. These are the most common fractures in large series and the most problematic. In type B1 fractures, the stem remains well fixed, whereas in type B2 fractures, the stem is loose. In type B3 fractures, the stem is loose, and the proximal femur is deficient because of osteolysis, osteoporosis, or fracture comminution. Primary open reduction and internal fixation with the prosthesis left in situ is most appropriate for type B1 fractures in which the stem remains solidly fixed. Fixation must be rigid; treatment with simple cerclage wiring, bands, or isolated screws is associated with high failure rates. Plate fixation has evolved from the Ogden plate, fixed with screws distally and Parham bands proximally, to cable-plate systems such as the Dall-Miles plate, with incorporated sites for cable attachment proximally and screws distally, to locking plates using unicortical screws proximally and bicortical screws distally, placed with percutaneous techniques (Fig. 1.119). Biomechanical studies show greater mechanical stability for constructs with proximal and distal screw fixation in comparison with those fixed proximally with cables only. Allograft struts, used alone or in combination with plate fixation, also show promise in the fixation of periprosthetic femoral fractures (Fig. 1.120).

If the stem is loose, as in type B2 fractures, revision with a long-stem femoral component is preferable. This approach not only restores stability to the femoral component but also provides reliable intramedullary fixation of the fracture. Current treatment of these injuries typically involves the use of cementless long-stem femoral components. In a series of 118 periprosthetic femoral fractures, Springer, Berry, and Lewallen reported improved outcomes using extensively porous-coated cementless femoral components. We have used proximally porous coated modular uncemented stems, distally fluted tapered stems, and extensively porous coated stems with good success (Fig. 1.121). Supplemental internal fixation with cerclage or onlay cortical allograft struts is sometimes required to restore rotational stability at the fracture site. Additional bone grafting at the fracture site is recommended by most authors.

In type B3 fractures, the proximal femur is so deficient that it cannot be treated with open reduction and internal fixation or support a new femoral component. The femur can be reconstructed with an allograft prosthesis composite (see Technique 1.32) to restore bone stock. Alternatively, the revision can be done with a proximal femoral replacement prosthesis, such as that used for tumor reconstructions (see Fig. 1.28). Distally fluted tapered stems are enjoying increasing popularity in treating some B3 fractures (Fig. 1.122). Fracture union, implant stability, and some restoration of proximal femoral bone stock have been observed.

Type C fractures occur well below the tip of the stem with no stem loosening. These can be treated with internal fixation, leaving the femoral component undisturbed (Fig. 1.123). As in B1 fractures, locked plates and less invasive techniques are gaining popularity. Areas of stress concentration between fixation devices and the femoral stem should be avoided.

Duncan and Haddad added type D fractures, which involve the femur and ipsilateral hip and knee arthroplasties to this classification.

These challenging injuries are treated similarly to those described above based on implant fixation and residual bone stock. With stable implants above and below and reasonable bone for fixation, ORIF with locking and non-locking plates has been used (Fig. 1.124). Comminuted fractures with unreconstructable bone stock and/or loose implants may require revision surgery of the adjacent implant(s) with modular proximal, distal, or total femoral replacement prostheses.

Fracture of the acetabulum seldom occurs intraoperatively in primary arthroplasties, although fragile portions of the posterior wall can be fractured easily during revision surgery. Haidukewych et al., in a review of 7121 primary total hip arthroplasties, found a 0.4% prevalence of intraoperative acetabular fracture. All of these occurred in uncemented components, most commonly with a single monoblock elliptical design. Most of the fractures were stable, and the original acetabular component was retained. Components that were thought to be unstable were converted to a different component that allowed supplemental screw fixation. All fractures united, and no revisions were necessary.

Hickerson et al. described a periprosthetic acetabular fracture treatment algorithm based on the extent of the fracture and stability of the implant. Intraoperative fracture

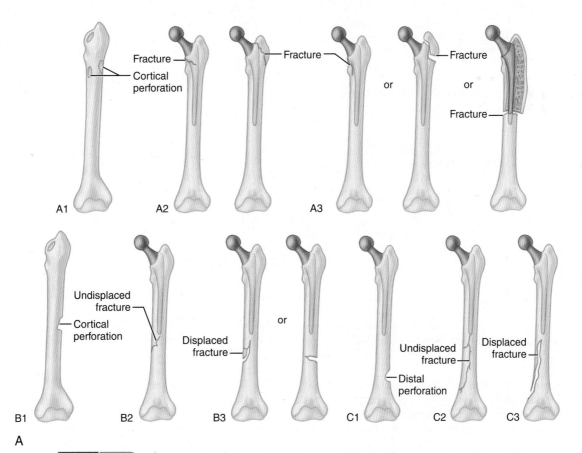

FIGURE 1.118 Intraoperative periprosthetic fractures of femur. (Redrawn from Greidanus NV, Mitchell PA, Masri BA, et al: Principles of management and results of treating the fractured femur during and after total hip arthroplasty, *Instr Course Lect* 52:309, 2003.)

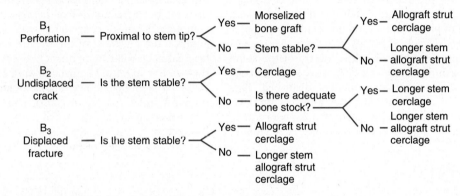

**Proximal
metaphyseal**

A_1
Perforation —— Morselized bone graft

A_2
Undisplaced —— Cerclage ± bone graft
crack

A_3
Unstable —— Diaphyseal fitting stem and cerclage
fracture

Diaphyseal

B_1
Perforation —— Proximal to stem tip? —< Yes —— Morselized bone graft —< Yes —— Allograft strut cerclage
                                         No —— Stem stable? —— No —— Longer stem allograft strut cerclage

B_2
Undisplaced —— Is the stem stable? —< Yes —— Cerclage
crack   No —— Is there adequate bone stock? —< Yes —— Longer stem cerclage
                                                                              No —— Longer stem allograft strut cerclage

B_3
Displaced —— Is the stem stable? —< Yes —— Allograft strut cerclage
fracture   No —— Longer stem allograft strut cerclage

**Distal diaphyseal/
metaphyseal**

C_1
Perforation —— Morselized bone graft

C_2
Undisplaced crack
extending into —— Cerclage/strut
distal metaphysis

C_3
Displaced —— ORIF
distal fracture

B

FIGURE 1.118 Cont'd

treatment recommendations are based on wall or column involvement and cup stability. Postoperative fractures are similarly managed based on cup stability and fracture displacement (Fig. 1.125).

We agree with the authors that if reasonable fracture stability is achieved, then an uncemented hemispherical component with additional screw fixation should suffice. If implant stability is questionable despite fracture fixation, however, consideration should be given to the use of an antiprotrusio cage with proximal and distal fixation through the flanges of or a cup/cage construct (Fig. 1.126). (See Acetabular Revision section.)

TROCHANTERIC NONUNION

Trochanteric osteotomy is seldom necessary in primary THA. Exceptions include some patients with congenital hip dysplasia, protrusio acetabuli, or conversion of an arthrodesis. If the femur has been shortened, distal advancement of the trochanter may be required to restore appropriate myofascial tension to the abductor mechanism. Trochanteric osteotomy is also sometimes necessary for the extensile exposure of the acetabulum and femur required for revision surgery.

Avoiding nonunion of the greater trochanter requires careful attention to the technical details of the osteotomy and

TABLE 1.2

Vancouver Classification of Fractures of the Femur After Total Hip Arthroplasty

TYPE	LOCATION	SUBTYPE
A	Trochanteric region	A_G: greater trochanter A_L: lesser trochanter
B	Around or just distal to stem	B_1: prosthesis stable B_2: prosthesis unstable B_3: bone stock inadequate
C	Well below stem	

From Duncan CP, Masri BA: Fracture of the femur after hip replacement, *Instr Course Lect* 44:293, 1995.

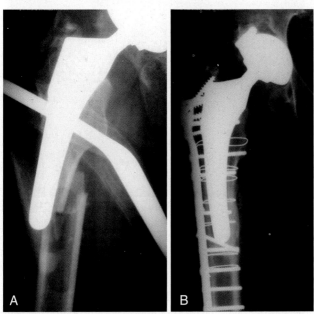

FIGURE 1.119 Type B1 femoral fracture. **A,** Preoperative radiograph shows well-fixed stem and spiral femoral fracture. **B,** Postoperative radiograph demonstrates anatomic reduction and fixation with lateral plate, locking and nonlocking screws, and cable. (From Pike J, Davidson D, Grabuz D, et al: Principles of treatment for periprosthetic femoral shaft fractures around well-fixed total hip arthroplasty, *J Am Acad Orthop Surg* 17:677, 2009.)

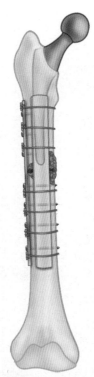

FIGURE 1.120 Lateral plate and anterior cortical strut graft used for fixation of type B1 femoral fracture; cancellous allograft also is placed at fracture site.

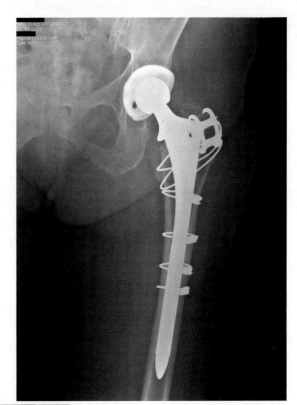

FIGURE 1.121 Type B2 femoral fracture. Loose femoral component was revised to extensively porous coated stem. Cerclage cables were used to assist with fixation and restoration of rotational stability.

its reattachment. Factors contributing to trochanteric nonunion include a small trochanteric fragment, poor-quality bone, inadequate fixation, excessive abductor tension, prior radiation therapy, and patient noncompliance. The most significant problems of trochanteric nonunion are related to proximal migration of the trochanteric fragment. Failure of trochanteric fixation and proximal migration are not caused simply by the abductors pulling the fragment off superiorly. Charnley proposed that anterior and posterior motion of the trochanter occurs first as the hip is loaded in flexion, as during rising from a chair or stair-climbing. This produces shear forces between the trochanter and its underlying bed. Subsequent fatigue failure of the fixation device allows proximal migration.

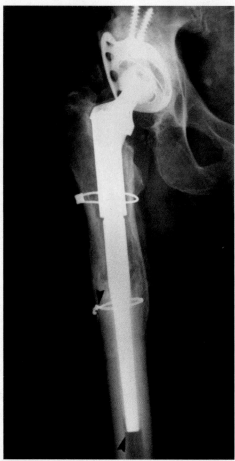

FIGURE 1.122 Type B3 femoral fracture. Femoral component was revised to modular tapered fluted stem. Note restoration of proximal bone stock and solid fracture union. (From Mulay S, Hassan T, Birtwistle S, Power R: Management of types B2 and B3 femoral periprosthetic fractures by a tapered, fluted, and distally fixed stem, *J Arthroplasty* 20:751, 2005.)

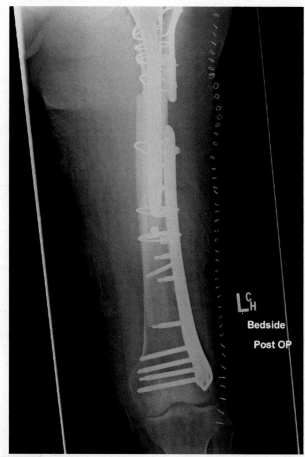

FIGURE 1.123 Type C fracture of distal femur. Fracture was fixed with lateral plate using locking screws and cables. (From Davidson D, Pike J, Grabuz D, et al: Intraoperative fractures during total hip arthroplasty. Evaluation and management, *J Bone Joint Surg* 90A:2000, 2008.)

The incidence of nonunion in primary surgery varies from approximately 3% to 8%, but revision surgery carries greater risk. Nonunion rates of 9% to 13% have been reported in revision surgeries using trochanteric wiring, wire plus mesh, trochanteric bolt, cable-grip, and cable-plate techniques.

McCarthy et al. found that union was more likely when a trochanteric slide osteotomy was used, cables were placed circumferential to the femur rather than intramedullary, and good bone-to-bone apposition was achieved.

Although stable fibrous union without proximal migration usually produces good functional results with little pain (Fig. 1.127), trochanteric nonunion and/or trochanteric migration are typically associated with gait abnormalities and worsened functional outcomes. According to Amstutz and Maki, migration of more than 2 cm significantly impairs abductor function even if union eventually occurs (Fig. 1.128).

Trochanteric nonunion also is associated with an increased incidence of dislocation. Woo and Morrey found a dislocation rate of 17.6% in patients with displaced trochanteric nonunions compared with 2.8% when the trochanter healed by osseous or fibrous union without displacement.

Prominent or broken trochanteric implants often are a source of lateral hip pain. Injection of a local anesthetic may be helpful in establishing the diagnosis. Local steroid injections often relieve such symptoms. Removal of the hardware occasionally is indicated, but Bernard and Brooks found that less than 50% of patients obtain substantial relief from simple wire removal.

Broken trochanteric wires or cables can migrate with untoward effects (Fig. 1.129). Cases of delayed sciatic nerve symptoms associated with migrated wires impinging upon the nerve have been reported. Fragmentation of braided cables may generate a large amount of intraarticular metal debris that damages the articulating surfaces. Complete excision of this type of wire debris at revision is almost impossible, and subsequent revisions may be at risk for accelerated wear. Altenburg et al. found higher rates of acetabular wear, osteolysis, and acetabular revision in patients who underwent cemented THA via trochanteric osteotomy repaired with braided cables in comparison to those who had wire fixation. They recommended cable removal if fretting or trochanteric nonunion occurs.

Trochanteric repair occasionally is indicated for a displaced trochanteric nonunion with a painful pseudarthrosis or significant abductor weakness with Trendelenburg limp. Established pseudarthrosis is suspected if a patient has pain with resisted hip abduction, local tenderness to palpation, and relief of pain by injection of local anesthetic into the area

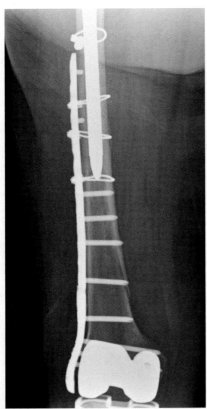

FIGURE 1.124 Interprosthetic fracture (type D) in elderly patient treated with locking plate, unicortical screws and cables proximally, bicortical screws distally.

of the pseudarthrosis. Surgery should be approached cautiously, and patients should be informed that union may not be obtained with a second operation. Wire fixation alone has met with poor results; therefore, augmented techniques are warranted. Hodgkinson, Shelley, and Wroblewski obtained bony union in 81% of patients using a double crossover wire with a compression spring, and Hamadouche et al. reported successful union in 51 of 72 patients with previous trochanteric nonunion treated with a claw plate combined with wire fixation.

Careful preparation and contouring of the trochanteric fragment are essential to obtain maximal stability. An attempt must be made to place the trochanter against bone. It must not be reattached under excessive tension, and the hip should be abducted no more than 10 to 15 degrees for approximation. Autogenous bone grafting seems prudent. Weight bearing and active abduction exercises are delayed until there is early radiographic evidence of bony union. A period of bracing in abduction or spica cast application reduces tension on the repair.

Chin and Brick described a technique to facilitate reattachment of a severely migrated greater trochanter whereby the abductor muscles are advanced by subperiosteal release from their origin on the iliac wing. Union was achieved in four of four patients.

If the direct lateral approach has been used, avulsion of the repaired abductor mechanism can occur and presents many of the same problems as trochanteric migration: pain, abductor weakness, and hip instability. A few small series of patients treated with late abductor tendon repair have shown mixed results in terms of pain relief and overall patient satisfaction, probably caused by chronic degeneration of the abductor mechanism. Augmented repair techniques using a gluteus maximus muscle flap or an Achilles tendon allograft have shown promise in small case series.

GLUTEUS MAXIMUS AND TENSOR FASCIA LATA TRANSFER FOR PRIMARY DEFICIENCY OF THE ABDUCTORS OF THE HIP

TECHNIQUE 1.8

- Perform a standard posterior approach to the hip through a skin incision that parallels the gluteus maximus in its middle third proximally and in line with the femur for 10 cm distal to the greater trochanter.
- Split the gluteus maximus in line with its fibers in its middle third for about half the length of the muscle.
- Split the fascia lata longitudinally well below the distal extent of the TFL muscle belly.
- Release the anterior edge of the gluteus maximus flap from the fascia lata anteriorly, leaving a fascial cuff distally and anteriorly. Release the gluteus maximus fascia from the fascia lata up to the iliac crest.
- Make a transverse incision in the anterior gluteus maximus fascia to allow proper tensioning (Fig. 1.130A).
- Elevate the gluteus maximus flap off of the underlying remnants of the gluteus medius and minimus.
- Incise the distal fascia lata transversely and separate it from the sartorius anteriorly, leaving a cuff of fascia at least 1 cm wide.
- Use a half-inch osteotome to make a 4-cm long trough in the lateral cortex of the greater trochanter.
- Split the proximal vastus lateralis longitudinally.
- Drill holes in the edges of the trochanteric trough for later suture fixation.
- With the hip in neutral abduction, suture the gluteus maximus flap to the trough in the greater trochanter with No. 5 nonabsorbable sutures (Fig. 1.130B).
- Transfer the fascia lata flap over the greater trochanter and gluteus maximus flap and suture it distally under the vastus lateralis.
- Suture the edges of the transferred flaps to each other with absorbable and nonabsorbable sutures.
- Intermittently check for appropriate tension of each flap by slight adduction of the hip.
- Close the proximal split in the gluteus maximus with absorbable sutures.
- Repair the anterior and posterior portions of the fascia lata flap with absorbable sutures to the sartorius and distal gluteus maximus, respectively (Fig. 1.130C).
- Postoperatively, 6 weeks of touch-down weight bearing is allowed with two-handed support.

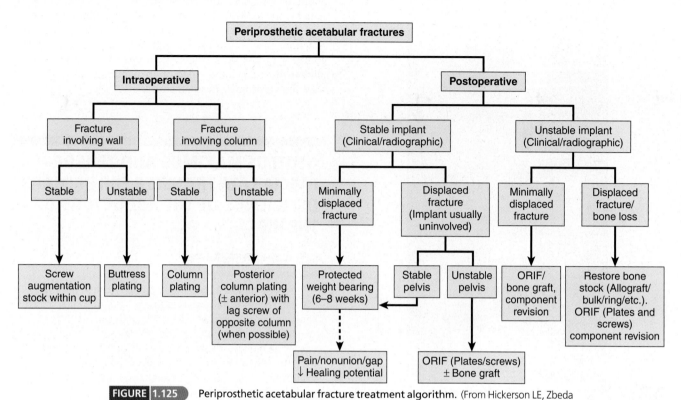

FIGURE **1.125** Periprosthetic acetabular fracture treatment algorithm. (From Hickerson LE, Zbeda RM, Gadinsky NE, et al: Outcomes of surgical treatment of periprosthetic acetabular fractures, *J Orthop Trauma* 33 [Suppl 2]:s48, 2019.)

- Standing abduction exercises and full weight bearing are initiated at 6 weeks.
- Side-lying abduction exercises begin at 8 weeks, and the patient is allowed to use one crutch in the opposite hand. Further abductor strengthening and gait training begin at 3 months postoperatively.
- Cane use is encouraged for a full year.

INFECTION

Postoperative infection is a difficult complication affecting THA. It is painful, disabling, costly, often requiring removal of both components, and is associated with reported survival rates of 88.7% and 67.2% at one and 5 years after diagnosis. Consistent efforts at prevention are mandatory. Treatment of infection requires appropriate assessment of its chronicity and causative factors, the status of the wound, and the overall health of the patient.

After the introduction of modern hip arthroplasty, septic complications threatened the continued viability of the procedure. Charnley reported infection in 6.8% of the first 683 procedures. The experience of Wilson et al. in the United States was even more ominous, with 11% of 100 arthroplasties becoming infected. Advances in understanding of patient selection, the operating room environment, surgical technique, and the use of prophylactic antibiotics have dramatically reduced the risk of this devastating complication.

Currently, approximately 1% to 2% of hip arthroplasties become infected. The incidence of sepsis is higher in patients with various comorbidities. Risk calculators are available with relative weightings for these medical and surgical factors (Table 1.3).

Additional risk factors include prolonged operative time and wound healing complications, such as necrosis of the skin and postoperative hematoma.

Bacterial infections can occur by one of four mechanisms: (1) direct contamination of the wound at the time of surgery, (2) local spread of superficial wound infection in the early postoperative period, (3) hematogenous spread of distant bacterial colonization or infection from a separate site, or (4) reactivation of latent hip infection in a previously septic joint. Strict attention to surgical technique and the operating room environment is essential in preventing infection by direct contamination. Water-repellent gowns and drapes are recommended. Double gloves also are recommended to protect the patient and operating team from contamination, as glove puncture is common. It is especially important to handle tissues gently and to minimize dead space and hematoma formation. The level of airborne bacteria can be reduced by limiting traffic through the operating room.

■ ANTIBIOTIC PROPHYLAXIS

Most total hip infections are caused by gram-positive organisms, particularly coagulase-negative staphylococci and *S. aureus*. Although the relative percentages of infections with

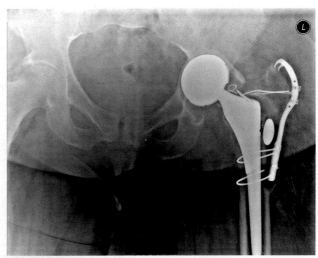

FIGURE 1.128 Trochanteric nonunion with marked proximal migration and hardware failure. Revision was necessary for acetabular loosening as well.

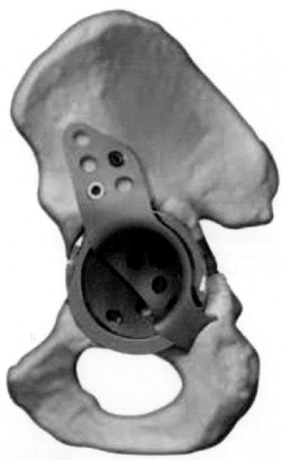

FIGURE 1.126 Trabecular metal acetabular revision system: cup-cage construct. (See section on acetabular revision.) (Courtesy Zimmer Biomet, Warsaw, IN.)

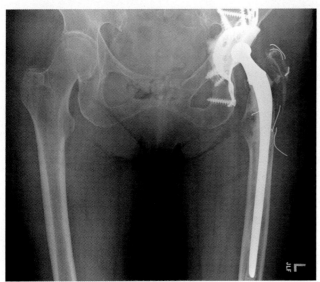

FIGURE 1.127 Trochanteric nonunion without migration usually produces little pain and only mild functional limitation.

these organisms have remained roughly stable, their virulence has increased. Methicillin resistance has become common in many medical centers, and the elaboration of glycocalyx by *Staphylococcus* and *Pseudomonas* is recognized as a marker for higher virulence. Gram-negative organisms are encountered more frequently in hematogenous infections, especially those emanating from the urinary tract. Mixed infections typically occur when a draining sinus has developed, with superinfection by one or more additional organisms (Table 1.4).

It is generally recognized that the most important factor in reducing perioperative sepsis is routine use of antibiotic prophylaxis. The second International Consensus Meeting on Musculoskeletal Infection recently made recommendations regarding antibiotic prophylaxis for hip and knee arthroplasty. First- or second-generation cephalosporins such as cefazolin or cefuroxime continue to be the antibiotics of choice. Vancomycin is preferred in patients who are carriers of resistant *S. aureus* or who are at high risk for colonization with this organism. Clindamycin is recommended for patients allergic to cephalosporins (see Box 1.2).

■ CLASSIFICATION

Appropriate initial treatment of an infection depends on its extent and chronicity, implant stability, and the patient's medical status. Although the treatment of deep infection after THA is typically surgical, the decision of whether to remove or retain the components may partially be guided by the chronicity of the infection. Tsukayama classified periprosthetic infections into four categories:

1. Early postoperative infection: onset within the first month after surgery
2. Late chronic infection: onset more than 1 month after surgery, insidious onset of symptoms
3. Acute hematogenous infection—onset more than 1 month after surgery, acute onset of symptoms in previously well-functioning prosthesis, distant source of infection
4. Positive intraoperative cultures: positive cultures obtained at the time of revision for supposedly aseptic conditions

The classification described by Trampuz and Zimmerli extends the definition of an early infection to 3 months postoperatively. Delayed infections occur between 3 and 24 months from the index surgery, and late infections occur after 24 months.

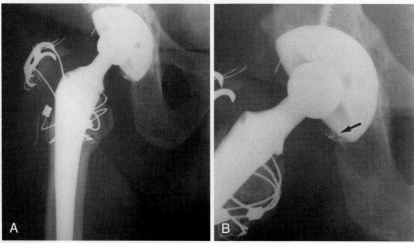

FIGURE 1.129 Trochanteric nonunion with wire in joint. **A,** Wire breakage after fixation of trochanteric nonunion with braided cables. **B,** Fragmentation of braided cables, with voluminous debris in vicinity of articulation *(arrow).*

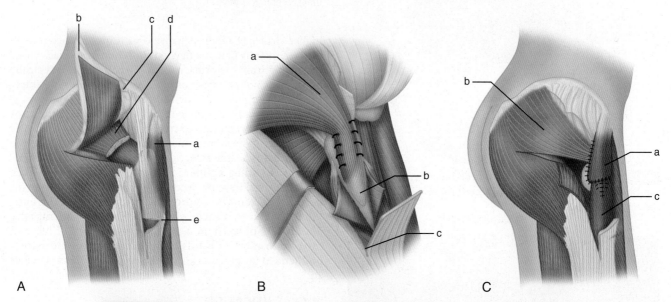

FIGURE 1.130 Gluteus maximus and tensor fascia lata transfer for primary deficiency of the hip abductors. **A,** Partial transverse incision in anterior portion of gluteus maximus flap. Gluteus maximus and fascia lata split split (a). Gluteus maximus flap released (b). Anterior edge of gluteus maximus flap released and transverse incision made in fascia (c). Gluteus maximus flap elevated (d). Anterior fascia lata incised to edge of sartorius. **B,** Gluteus maximus flap sutured into trough in greater trochanter. Gluteus maximus flap (a) sutured to edges of decorticated greater trochanter. Fascia lata extension (b) placed on cortical bone under elevated vastus lateralis (c). **C,** Fascia lata flap repaired to sartorius and distal gluteus maximus. Tensor fascia lata (a) transferred over greater trochanter and gluteus maximus flap (b). Inferior edge sutured under vastus lateralis flaps (c). (Redrawn from Whiteside LA: Surgical technique: gluteus maximus and tensor fascia lata transfer for primary deficit of the abductors of the hip, *Clin Orthop Relat Res* 472:645, 2014.) **SEE TECHNIQUE 1.8.**

■ DIAGNOSIS

A careful history and physical examination are crucial in making the diagnosis of total hip infection. Although the diagnosis of early postoperative infection or acute hematogenous infection is often not difficult, late chronic infections can be challenging to distinguish from other causes of pain in a patient with a previous THA. Early or late acute infections may be characterized by pain, fever, or erythema. Pain unrelieved by a seemingly well-functioning arthroplasty may be a clue towards chronic infection. A history of excessive wound drainage after the initial arthroplasty, multiple episodes of wound erythema, and prolonged antibiotic treatment by the operating surgeon also are worrisome. Physical examination focuses on the presence of painful hip range of motion, swelling, erythema, sinus formation, or fluctuance.

Often radiographs of the affected hip are normal or at best may be indistinguishable from aseptic loosening of the prosthesis. Progressive radiolucencies or periosteal reaction occasionally may be seen, indicating possible infection.

TABLE 1.3A

Institutional Risk Calculation for Any Periprosthetic Joint Infection

RISK FACTOR	POINTS
BMI	$(0.0865 \times BMI^2) - (5.072 \times BMI) + 74.35$
Male	18
Government insurance	7
Surgical factors:	
▪ THA, primary	18
▪ THA, revision	50
▪ TKA, primary	28
▪ TKA, revision	81
▪ Both THA and TKA, revision	87
▪ 1 prior procedure	60
▪ 2 prior procedures	87
▪ ≥3 prior procedures	100
Comorbidities:	
▪ Drug abuse	62
▪ HIV/AIDS	49
▪ Coagulopathy	38
▪ Renal disease	35
▪ Psychosis	31
▪ Congestive heart failure	31
▪ Rheumatologic disease	30
▪ Deficiency anemia	19
▪ Diabetes mellitus	19
▪ Liver disease	17
▪ Smoker	10

AIDS, Acquired immunodeficiency syndrome; *BMI*, body mass index; *HIV*, human immunodeficiency virus; *THA*, total hip arthroplasty.
From Tan TL, Maltenfort MG, Chen AE, et al: Development and evaluation of a preoperative risk calculator for periprosthetic joint infection following total joint arthroplasty, *J Bone Joint Surg Am* 100:777, 2018.

TABLE 1.3B

Cumulative Point Values and Corresponding Estimated Periprosthetic Joint Infection Rate for Any Periprosthetic Joint Infection

CUMULATIVE POINT VALUE	ESTIMATED PJI RATE* (%)
0	0.36 (0.30-0.43)
10	0.47 (0.40-0.55)
20	0.61 (0.52-0.70)
30	0.79 (0.69-0.90)
40	1.02 (0.90-1.15)
50	1.32 (1.18-1.47)
60	1.70 (1.54-1.88)
70	2.19 (2.01-2.41)
80	2.83 (2.61-3.08)
90	3.64 (3.38-3.93)
100	4.67 (4.36-5.02)
110	5.97 (5.59-6.41)
120	7.60 (7.13-8.17)
130	9.65 (9.03-10.38)
140	12.16 (11.34-13.14)
150	15.22 (14.13-16.52)
160	18.89 (17.46-20.58)

*The 95% CI is given in parentheses.
PJI, Periprosthetic joint infection.
From Tan TL, Maltenfort MG, Chen AE, et al: Development and evaluation of a preoperative risk calculator for periprosthetic joint infection following total joint arthroplasty, *J Bone Joint Surg Am* 100:777, 2018.

TABLE 1.4

Breakdown of Bacteria Found in Infected Arthroplasties

	UNITED STATES	UNITED KINGDOM	AUSTRALIA
S. aureus	35	29	40
Coag (-) staph	31	36	13
Streptococci	11	7	3
Enterococci	7	9	1.5
Gram negative	5	12	5
Other	11	7	37

Data from Fulkerson E, Valle CJ, Wise B, et al: Antibiotic susceptibility of bacteria infecting total joint arthroplasty sites, *J Bone Joint Surg* 88:1231–7, 2006; Peel TN, Cheng AC, Choong PF, Buising KL: Early onset prosthetic hip and knee joint infection: treatment and outcomes in Victoria, Australia, *J Hosp Infect* 82:248–253, 2012.

Laboratory evaluation includes ESR, CRP, and D-dimer. Peripheral white blood cell (WBC) count is rarely elevated in late chronic infection and is not a sensitive screening tool. ESR greater than 30 mm/h and CRP greater than 10 mg/L are reasonably sensitive and specific for the diagnosis of chronic infection. The threshold for a positive D-dimer test has been reported to be 850 ng/mL.

Hip aspiration is warranted if the one of the three previously mentioned lab values are elevated, or if the index of suspicion for infection is high despite normal values. Aspiration should not be undertaken until at least 2 weeks after discontinuation of antibiotic therapy. This is done in an outpatient setting with the patient under local anesthesia. Fluoroscopy or ultrasonography are useful for accurate insertion of the needle. The aspiration is done with the same attention to sterile technique as a surgical procedure, with a full surgical scrub and preparation. Skin flora may be introduced into the cultures and confuse the results, or, worse, they may be introduced into the joint. An 18-gauge spinal needle is inserted from anterior at a point just lateral to the femoral artery along a line from the symphysis pubis to the ASIS. As an alternative, the needle is inserted laterally, just superior to the greater trochanter. The tip of the needle must enter the joint and must be seen and felt to come in contact with the metal of the neck of the femoral component. Gentle rotation of the extremity helps bring fluid toward the needle if none is easily withdrawn after entering the joint. Aerobic and anaerobic cultures, and cell count with differential, are obtained from the aspirant. Leukocyte esterase test strip and alpha-defensin testing are additional synovial fluid markers for infection that have shown high sensitivity and specificity; they should be obtained if sufficient fluid is available.

The International Consensus Meeting criteria for the diagnosis of periprosthetic hip or knee infection include both preoperative and intraoperative measures (Box 1.3).

Major criteria (diagnostic of infection if at least one is present)
- Two positive periprosthetic cultures with phenotypically identical organisms
- A sinus track communicating with the joint or visualization of the prosthesis

Minor criteria
- Elevated serum CRP or D-dimer
- Elevated ESR
- Elevated synovial fluid WBC count *or* ++change on leukocyte esterase test strip or positive alpha-defensin
- Elevated synovial fluid polymorphonuclear neutrophil percentage (PMN%)
- Positive histologic analysis of periprosthetic tissue
- A single positive culture
- Positive intraoperative purulence

■ MANAGEMENT

The treatment of infected THA consists of one or more of the following:

1. Antibiotic therapy
2. Debridement and irrigation of the hip with component retention
3. Debridement and irrigation of the hip with component removal
4. One-stage or two-stage reimplantation of THA
5. Amputation

Management choices are made based on the chronicity of the infection, the virulence of the offending organism(s), the status of the wound and surrounding soft tissues, and the physiologic status of the patient.

▌ EARLY POSTOPERATIVE INFECTION

Early infections may range in severity from superficial cellulitis that can be managed with antibiotics alone to deep infections that require surgical management. Superficial infections causing wound dehiscence or purulent drainage and infections associated with wound necrosis or infected hematoma often require surgical debridement. Thorough inspection should be made for subfascial extension of the infection, which requires a more extensive procedure.

If an infection is thought to be superficial, preoperatively the joint is not aspirated to avoid contaminating it. Once medical comorbidities are optimized, arrangements are made to take the patient to the operating room, and the hip is prepared and draped in the routine manner. The previous skin incision and surgical approach are used. The wound is opened down to the deep fascia, and the structures are examined carefully to determine whether the infection extends beneath it and into the hip joint. If this fascial layer was closed carefully at the time of surgery, it may have acted as a barrier and prevented extension of the infection into the deeper tissues. If there is any question at the time of surgery as to whether the infection is deep, it is wiser to insert a needle into the hip joint to determine the presence or absence of a deep infection than to risk not draining an infected joint. If the infection is superficial, the wound is thoroughly irrigated with large quantities of a physiologic solution or an aqueous iodophor solution, and all necrotic subcutaneous tissue and skin are excised. The skin edges are approximated with interrupted monofilament sutures.

If the infection extends to the hip joint, the wound is thoroughly debrided and irrigated. The hip must be dislocated to perform this procedure thoroughly, and if modular components have been implanted, the liner and femoral head are exchanged to limit the number of previously contaminated

---

BOX 1.3

Proposed 2018 International Consensus Meeting Criteria for Periprosthetic Joint Infection

MAJOR CRITERIA (AT LEAST ONE OF THE FOLLOWING)				DECISION	
Two positive growths of the same organism using standard culture methods				Infected	
Sinus track with evidence of communication to the joint or visualization of the prosthesis				Infected	

	THRESHOLD			
Minor Criteria	Acute	Chronic	Score	Decision
Serum CRP (mg/L)	100	10		
or			2	
D-dimer (µg/L)	Unknown	860		
Elevated serum ESR (mm/h)	No role	30	1	
Elevated synovial WBC (cells/µL)	10,000	3000		Combined preoperative and postoperative score: ≥6 Infected
or				3-5 Inconclusive
Leukocyte esterase	++	++	3	<3 Not infected
Positive alpha-defensin (signal/cutoff)	1.0	1.0		
Elevated synovial PMN (%)	90	70	2	
Single positive culture			2	
Positive histology			3	
Positive interoperative purulence			3	

CRP, C-reactive protein; *ESR*, erythrocyte sedimentation rate; *WBC*, white blood cells; *PMN*, polymorphonuclear neutrophils.
From Shobat N, Bauer T, Buttaro M, et al: Hip and knee section, What is the definition of a periprosthetic joint infection (PJI) of the knee and the hip? Can the same criteria be used for both joints? Proceedings of International Consensus on Orthopedic Infections, *J Arthroplasty* 34:S325, 2019.

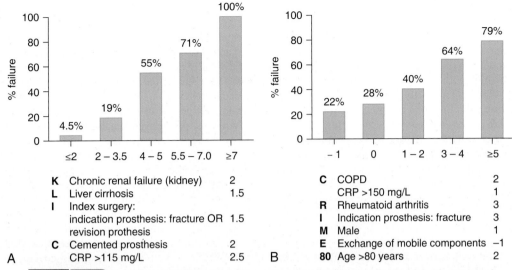

FIGURE 1.131 KLIC and CRIME80 scoring systems estimate failure rates for debridement and component retention in the early postoperative and acute hematogenous settings, respectively. (From Argenson JN, Arndt M, Babis G, et al: Hip and knee section, treatment, debridement and retention of implant: Proceedings of International Consensus on Orthopedic Infections, *J Arthroplasty* 334:S399, 2019.)

foreign bodies and allow for more thorough debridement. Implants should be tested carefully for stability and should be left *in situ* only if there is no evidence of loosening. Cultures of joint fluid or other fluid collections encountered along with tissue cultures from the superficial, deep, and periprosthetic layers are sent for analysis of the offending organism and antibiotic sensitivities. The appropriate antibiotic, as determined by the cultures and sensitivity tests, is given intravenously most commonly for 6 weeks, preferably under the direction of an infectious disease consultant. Continued oral antibiotic therapy for suppression may be considered in patients unable to tolerate further surgical procedures.

Success rates for patients with early postoperative or acute hematogenous infections treated with debridement, irrigation, and implant retention range from 20% to 100%. The KLIC and CRIME80 scoring systems are available to estimate the chance of success with debridement and component retention in these settings (Fig. 1.131).

LATE CHRONIC INFECTION

Surgical debridement and component removal are required for late chronic infection if eradication of the infection is to be reasonably expected. Poor results are documented after debridement and component retention in patients with late chronic infections.

The joint is approached through the previous incision. Narrow skin bridges between previous scars should be avoided to minimize the risk of marginal wound necrosis. Sinus tracks are debrided, and previously placed nonabsorbable sutures and trochanteric implants are removed. The hip is dislocated, and all infected and necrotic material is excised. Joint fluid and tissue specimens from the acetabular and femoral regions are sent for cultures for a total of at least three specimens. Intraoperative Gram stains are not helpful at this stage because of poor sensitivity. The femoral and acetabular components and any other foreign material, including cement, cement restrictors, cables, or wires, are removed to

eliminate all surfaces that could harbor bacteria (see section on revision of THA). One possible exception to the recommended complete removal of implants is a well-fixed component whose removal would cause significant bone loss.

After all cultures are taken, the joint is irrigated copiously with saline or dilute povidone-iodine solution using pulsatile lavage. After irrigation, the joint should be carefully inspected again for retained foreign bodies or infected or necrotic tissue. Intraoperative radiographic or image intensifier inspection is indicated if complete implant removal is in doubt. If this inspection proves satisfactory, the fascia is closed with a running, absorbable, monofilament suture, and the skin is closed with interrupted nonabsorbable monofilament sutures. Antibiotic-impregnated methacrylate beads and temporary articulating antibiotic spacers are discussed in the section on reimplantation after infection.

ACUTE HEMATOGENOUS INFECTION

Some patients have no history suggestive of perioperative sepsis, yet the hip becomes acutely painful long after the index operation. In these instances, the infection may have been caused by hematogenous spread from a remote site of infection or from transient bacteremia caused by an invasive procedure. Patients with total hip arthroplasties should be advised to request antibiotic management immediately if they have a pyogenic infection, and they must be observed carefully for any evidence of hip infection.

Transient bacteremia occurs after dental procedures, including simple cleaning; however, the role of antibiotic prophylaxis in this setting has been questioned. In 2012, the AAOS and American Dental Association published recommendations for antibiotic prophylaxis for patients with total joint arthroplasties undergoing dental procedures.

1. The practitioner might consider discontinuing the practice of routinely prescribing prophylactic antibiotics for patients with hip and knee prosthetic joint implants undergoing dental procedures. *Grade of Recommendation: Limited*

2. We are unable to recommend for or against the use of topical oral antimicrobials in patients with prosthetic joint implants or other orthopaedic implants undergoing dental procedures. *Grade of Recommendation: Inconclusive*

3. In the absence of reliable evidence linking poor oral health to prosthetic joint infection, it is the opinion of the work group that patients with prosthetic joint implants or other orthopaedic implants maintain appropriate oral hygiene. *Grade of Recommendation: Consensus*

Pain on weight bearing, with motion of the hip, and at rest is the chief symptom of acute hematogenous infection. The patient may be febrile and have an elevated peripheral WBC count; the ESR and CRP level also usually are elevated. The diagnosis usually can be established by aspirating the hip and obtaining appropriate studies as previously described. While reports on cultures are being completed, broad-spectrum antibiotics effective against gram-positive and gram-negative organisms are administered intravenously. If acute hematogenous infection is confirmed, debridement and component retention may be attempted as in early postoperative infection. The acceptable amount of time between onset of symptoms and debridement is controversial, ranging from 5 days to 3 months. Other factors, such as the virulence of the infecting organism, medical status of the patient, and overall quality and integrity of the surrounding soft tissues, also must be considered. Alternatively, some authors have pursued a more aggressive approach to patients with acute hematogenous infection by complete removal of components and immediate reimplantation with primary cementless components. Hansen et al. treated 27 patients in this manner, along with 6 weeks of intravenous antibiotics and varying courses of oral antibiotics; 70% retained their implants although repeat debridement was required in four. Regardless of the timing of the infection and other variables, if the prosthesis is loose, debridement should be combined with complete component removal as for late chronic infection.

■ RECONSTRUCTION AFTER INFECTION

The results of modified Girdlestone resection arthroplasty after a total hip replacement in general are not as satisfactory as the results after hip joint infections that have required less bone and soft-tissue resection. Almost all patients require some sort of assistive device to walk. Functional outcomes are poor in elderly patients, females, and patients with more extensive resection of bone from the proximal femur. Most patients are unwilling to live with the constraints of a resection arthroplasty and will elect to undergo reimplantation of their prosthesis.

Reconstruction after infection of a THA is problematic. The functional impairment of the patient, the infecting organism(s), the adequacy of debridement, and evidence of control of local and distant sites of infection all are factors in the decision to implant a new prosthesis.

Another dilemma involves the decision to proceed with reimplantation of the hip prosthesis at the time of the initial debridement, so-called one-stage exchange, or to wait to reimplant the arthroplasty at a second operation. Two-stage or delayed reimplantation, commonly done in North America for chronic infections, is advantageous for a number of reasons: (1) the adequacy of debridement is ensured because repeat debridement of soft tissues, necrotic bone, and retained cement can be done before reimplantation; (2) the infecting organisms are identified, their sensitivities are determined, and appropriate antibiotic management is instituted for a prolonged period

before reimplantation; (3) diagnostic evaluation for foci of persistent infection can be done; (4) distant sites of infection responsible for hematogenous spread can be eradicated; and (5) an informed decision can be made as to whether the degree of disability from the resection arthroplasty would justify the risks inherent in the implantation of another prosthesis. The disadvantages of a two-stage reconstruction include (1) the prolonged period of disability, (2) the sizable cost, including lost wages, (3) delayed rehabilitation, and (4) technical difficulty of the procedure owing to shortening and scarring.

According to the International Consensus on Musculoskeletal Infection, one-stage exchange is reasonable when effective antibiotics are available and systemic symptoms of sepsis are absent. Other relative contraindications to single-stage treatment include lack of preoperative identification of the infecting organism, patients with multiple medical comorbidities, presence of sinus track(s), and soft-tissue compromise possibly requiring flap coverage. The committee also recognized the importance of antibiotic-containing cement or bone graft in the reconstruction to achieve success. Conversely, two-stage exchange arthroplasty is indicated for septic or medically compromised patients, unidentified organisms, virulent/drug-resistant bacteria, sinus tracts, and compromised surrounding soft tissues.

Delayed reconstruction is associated with lower rates of recurrent infection in most studies. In a review of 168 patients treated with two-stage exchange, infection-free survival was 87.5% at 7 years average follow-up. Femoral component fixation method, with or without cement, had no effect on reinfection or mechanical complication rates. The decision regarding cemented or cementless reimplantation should be guided by the available femoral bone stock and the physiologic age and expected longevity of the patient, in addition to the reported infection cure rates with each technique. Two-stage exchange does carry a significant risk of mortality. An administrative database study of over 10,000 patients treated with prosthesis removal and spacer placement found 90-day mortality rate to be 2.6%, significantly higher than carotid endarterectomy, prostatectomy, and kidney transplantation.

Duncan and Beauchamp described a technique of two-stage reimplantation in which a prosthesis of antibiotic-loaded acrylic cement (PROSTALAC) is implanted at the time of the initial debridement. The prosthesis is constructed intraoperatively by molding antibiotic-laden cement around a simplistic femoral component and an all-polyethylene acetabular component. The custom-made components are implanted with an interference fit without any attempt to achieve cement intrusion, simplifying extraction during the second stage. In the interim, the articulated spacer maintains leg length and improves control of the limb and mobilization. At 10- to 15-year follow-up, Biring et al. reported an overall 89% success rate with the PROSTALAC technique. Others have described similar interval spacers of various types, with 77% to 100% eradication of the infection reported (Fig. 1.132). Complications other than recurrent or persistent infection include dislocation or fracture of the interval prosthesis.

The optimal timing for reimplantation of another prosthesis has not been determined. Numerous authors have reported series of patients in whom reimplantation was undertaken in periods of less than 1 year, with an incidence of recurrent infection similar to that in patients in whom reconstruction was delayed further. Currently, we continue

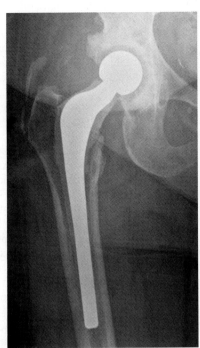

FIGURE 1.132 Prosthesis of antibiotic loaded acrylic cement (PROSALAC) after original component removal, debridement, and irrigation.

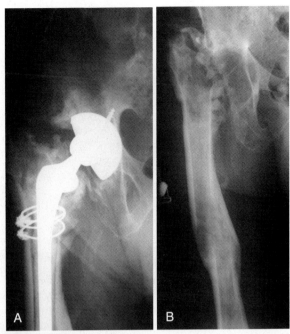

FIGURE 1.133 **A** and **B,** Elderly, minimally ambulatory man with infected total hip arthroplasty and draining sinuses. Treatment with resection arthroplasty and intravenous antibiotics was successful.

parenteral antibiotics for 6 weeks. Reconstruction is performed at approximately 3 months if the ESR and CRP are improving, and repeat aspiration of the hip (if performed because of concern of persistent infection) is negative.

Reimplantation of a total hip can be difficult because of extensive scarring of the soft tissues and disuse osteoporosis. Restoration of limb length and full motion of the hip may not be achieved, and dislocation after surgery is not uncommon. The sciatic nerve may be encased in scar tissue near the posterior margin of the acetabulum and should be protected. Complete capsulectomy, along with release of the iliopsoas and gluteus maximus tendons may be necessary to reduce the hip. The superior margin of the acetabulum may be deficient, and augmentation in this area may be required. The bone usually is soft, and the acetabular bed can be prepared easily, but care must be taken not to penetrate the medial wall of the acetabulum. If the anterior or posterior wall is thin, it may be fractured if an oversized acetabular component is press-fitted into place. The femoral canal must be prepared carefully to avoid fracture or penetration of the cortex. Placement of one or more prophylactic cerclage wires helps prevent shaft fracture. Before the femoral component is permanently seated, a trial reduction of the hip is absolutely necessary. Using a femoral component with a short neck or shortening the femur by removing more bone from the neck may be necessary before the hip can be reduced.

Aerobic and anaerobic tissue cultures are taken from at least three sites, along with tissue specimens for histologic examination. If eradication of the infection is in doubt, frozen sections of tissue can be examined by the pathologist for evidence of residual inflammatory change. If large numbers of polymorphonuclear cells are present (10/high-power field), the hip is debrided again, and reimplantation is delayed. If cultures taken at the time of surgery are positive, the appropriate antibiotics are continued, although the optimal duration and method of administration are unknown in this setting.

Recurrence of infection after two-stage reimplantation of an infected total hip is a particularly difficult situation and seldom results in a satisfactory outcome. Repeated two-stage exchange can be attempted if the infection is controlled after the first stage, the patient is able to tolerate subsequent surgery, and adequate soft tissues are available for coverage. A 36% to 40% success rate has been reported in these circumstances. Resection arthroplasty is more effective in resolving the infection but is associated with poor function and residual pain (Fig. 1.133).

Treatment of the infection takes precedence over reconstruction of the hip. In rare cases, disarticulation of the hip may be indicated as a lifesaving measure because of uncontrollable infection, severe soft-tissue compromise, or vascular complications. This drastic procedure should be considered in the presence of a persistent, painful, untreatable infection that is debilitating to the patient and a limb that hinders walking and sitting.

LOOSENING

Femoral and acetabular loosening are some of the most serious long-term complications of THA and commonly lead to revision. (The treatment of component loosening is discussed in the section on revision of THA.) In all patients suspected of having loosening of one or both components, the possibility of infection must be considered. In this section, noninfected (aseptic) loosening is discussed (loosening as a result of sepsis is discussed in the section on infection).

Criteria for the diagnosis of loosening of either the femoral or acetabular component have not been universally accepted. This complicates the comparison of available studies in the literature of loosening and long-term performance of THA. Some studies define failure as radiographic evidence of loosening despite continued satisfactory clinical performance. Others stress survivorship and define the end point as revision or removal of the prosthesis.

At each postoperative visit, radiographs should be inspected for changes in the components, the cement

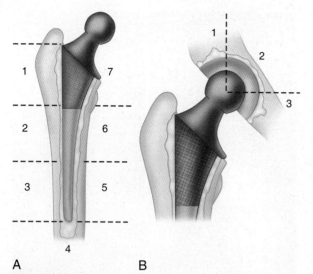

FIGURE 1.134 Zones around cement mass in femur **(A)**, as described by Gruen, and in pelvis **(B)**, as described by DeLee and Charnley. (Redrawn from Amstutz HC, Smith RK: Total hip replacement following failed femoral hemiarthroplasty, *J Bone Joint Surg* 61A:1161, 1979.)

(if present), the bone, and the interfaces between them. Anteroposterior and lateral radiographs must include the entire length of the stem and must be inspected carefully and compared with previous films for changes. It is helpful to record the specific zones around acetabular and femoral components in which changes develop (Fig. 1.134). The femoral component and associated interfaces are divided into seven zones, as described by Gruen et al. The acetabular component and surrounding bone are divided into three zones, as described by DeLee and Charnley.

■ FEMORAL LOOSENING

To compare radiographs made at various intervals after surgery, standardized technique and positioning of the limb should be used. Albert et al. found apparent changes in the position of the femoral component with 10 degrees of rotation of the extremity. Such changes may be interpreted incorrectly as component migration or mask real changes in component position.

▌ CEMENTED FEMORAL COMPONENTS

Following is a list of changes in the stem and the cement around it suggestive of loosening of the femoral component.
1. Radiolucency between the superolateral one third of the stem (Gruen zone 1) and the adjacent cement mantle, indicating debonding of the stem from the cement and possible early stem deformation
2. Radiolucency between the cement mantle and surrounding bone
3. Subsidence of the stem alone or in combination with the surrounding cement mantle
4. Change of the femoral stem into a more varus position
5. Fragmentation of the cement, especially between the superomedial aspect of the stem and the femoral neck (Gruen zone 7)
6. Fracture of the cement mantle, most commonly near the tip of the stem (Gruen zone 4)

7. Deformation of the stem
8. Fracture of the stem

Harris, McCarthy, and O'Neill defined femoral component loosening radiographically in three gradations: definite loosening, when there is migration of the component or cement; probable loosening, when a complete radiolucency is noted around the cement mantle; and possible loosening, when an incomplete radiolucency surrounding more than 50% of the cement is seen.

Subsidence may not be appreciated unless the relationship of the stem and cement mantle to the proximal femur is carefully evaluated with serial radiographs. The stem may subside in the cement, in which case there usually is a fracture of the cement near the tip of the stem, or the entire cement mantle and stem may subside. Subsidence may be quantified by measuring the distance between a fixed point on the stem and another radiographic landmark, such as a trochanteric wire or cable or a bony prominence such as the lesser or greater trochanter.

The following are technical problems that contribute to stem loosening:
1. Failure to remove the soft cancellous bone from the medial surface of the femoral neck; consequently, the column of cement does not rest on dense cancellous or cortical bone and support the stem. The cement is subjected to greater forces and fractures more easily.
2. Failure to provide a cement mantle of adequate thickness around the entire stem; a thin column cracks easily. The tip of the stem should be supported by a plug of cement because this part of the stem is subjected to axial loading.
3. Removal of all trabecular bone from the canal, leaving a smooth surface with no capacity for cement intrusion or failure to roughen areas of smooth neocortex that surrounded previous implants.
4. Inadequate quantity of cement and failure to keep the bolus of cement intact to avoid lamination.
5. Failure to pressurize the cement, resulting in inadequate flow of cement into the interstices of the bone.
6. Failure to prevent stem motion while the cement is hardening.
7. Failure to position the component in a neutral alignment (centralized) within the femoral canal.
8. The presence of voids in the cement as a result of poor mixing or injecting technique.

Barrack, Mulroy, and Harris described a grading system for the femoral component cement mantle. Complete filling of the medullary canal without radiolucencies ("white-out") is termed grade A. Slight radiolucency at the bone-cement interface (<50%) is grade B. Lucency surrounding 50% to 99% of the interface or any cement mantle defect constitutes grade C. Complete lucency on any projection or a defect of the mantle at the tip of the stem is considered grade D. Grade C and D mantles have been associated with increased risk of loosening, as reported by Malik et al. and Chambers et al. (Fig. 1.135).

▌ CEMENTLESS FEMORAL COMPONENTS

Engh et al. proposed a simple classification system for uncemented femoral component fixation based on radiographic inspection. Fixation is classified as (1) bone ingrowth, (2) stable fibrous fixation, or (3) unstable.

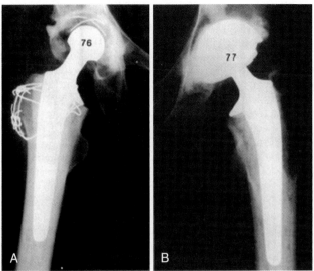

FIGURE 1.135   **A,** Postoperative radiograph shows excellent cement distribution ("white out"). **B,** Postoperative radiograph shows slight radiolucencies at cement-bone interface. (From Barrack RL, Mulroy RD, Harris WH: Improved cementing techniques and femoral component loosening in young patients with hip arthroplasty: a 12-year radiographic review, *J Bone Joint Surg* 74B:385, 1992. Copyright British Editorial Society of Bone and Joint Surgery.)

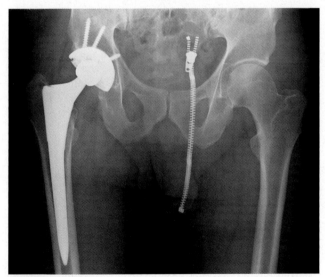

FIGURE 1.136   Cementless stem with bone ingrowth. No radiolucent lines are present. Trabeculae directed toward porous surface indicate stable fixation. Note calcar atrophy.

Fixation by bone ingrowth is defined as an implant with no subsidence and minimal or no radiopaque line formation around the stem. Most of the bone-implant interface seems stable. Cortical hypertrophy may be present at the distal end of the porous surface, and "spot welds" may be evident between the stem and endosteum. Variable degrees of proximal stress shielding can be seen (Fig. 1.136).

An implant is considered to have stable fibrous ingrowth when no progressive migration occurs, but an

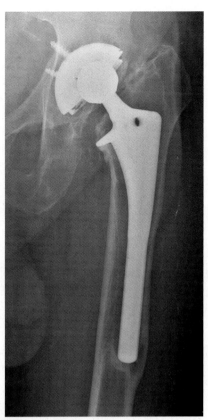

FIGURE 1.137   Unstable cementless stem. Stem has subsided over time. Radiolucencies surround entire stem, revealing lack of bone ingrowth.

extensive radiopaque line forms around the stem. These lines surround the stem in parallel fashion and are separated from the stem by a radiolucent space 1 mm wide. The femoral cortex shows no signs of local hypertrophy, suggesting that the surrounding shell of bone has a uniform load-carrying function.

An unstable implant is defined as one with definite evidence of progressive subsidence or migration within the canal and is at least partially surrounded by divergent radiopaque lines that are more widely separated from the stem at its extremities. Increased cortical density and thickening typically occur beneath the collar (if present) and at the end of the stem, indicating regions of local loading and lack of uniform stress transfer (Fig. 1.137).

Subsidence of a cementless femoral component early in the postoperative course may allow the stem to attain a more stable position within the femoral canal. Bone ingrowth may still occur, and early subsidence is still compatible with durable implant fixation. Subsidence seen months or years after surgery implies that the implant fixation is unstable. A bony pedestal often develops in zone 4 at the stem tip and is evidence of pistoning of the stem (Fig. 1.138). The determination of small amounts of subsidence is difficult because of differences in magnification and positioning on serial films and stress-related rounding and atrophy of the calcar.

Separation of metallic beads from the substrate material may occur as the stem is impacted into position, and loose beads may be identified on immediate postoperative

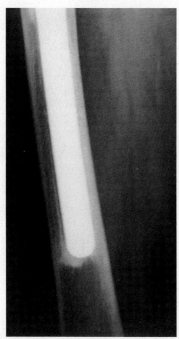

FIGURE 1.138 Formation of bony pedestal. Three years after cementless femoral revision, formation of bony pedestal at tip of stem indicates pistoning.

radiographs. If bead shedding is progressive on serial radiographs, it may indicate micromotion at the bone-implant interface.

■ ACETABULAR LOOSENING

Serial radiographs should be inspected for changes in the acetabular bone, the component itself, and the three zones of the bone-implant interface (see Fig. 1.134).

■ CEMENTED ACETABULAR COMPONENTS

Changes in the pelvis and acetabular component that can be observed in serial radiographs include the following:
1. Absorption of bone from around part or all of the cement mantle and an increase in the width of the area of absorption, which is especially significant if more than 2 mm wide and progressive 6 months or more after surgery.
2. Cephalad translation combined with sagittal plane rotation, which correlates highly with aseptic loosening.
3. Wear of the cup, as indicated by a decrease in the distance between the surface of the head and the periphery of the cup.
4. Fracture of the cup and cement (both rare).
5. A radiolucency 2 mm wide with or without a surrounding fine line of density, which may develop in one or more of the three zones around the cement mass in the pelvis (see Fig. 1.134). As in the femur, this is produced by the dense, fibrous membrane that forms around the surface of the cement and the surrounding shell of reactive bone.

Although femoral loosening commonly occurs at the stem-cement interface, acetabular loosening rarely occurs at the cup-cement interface. In autopsy-retrieved specimens, Schmalzried et al. determined that acetabular loosening occurs by three-dimensional resorption of bone adjacent to the cement mantle. The process is initiated at the periphery of the cup and progresses toward the dome. This finding explains the frequent appearance of early radiolucencies at the periphery of the implant that later involve all three zones. The mechanical stability of the implant is determined by the overall degree of bone resorption at the cement-bone interface.

Technical problems encountered during surgery that may result in loosening of the cup include the following:
1. Inadequate support of the cup by the surrounding bone and cement, especially superiorly and posteriorly, because bone stock is insufficient, or the acetabulum is not reamed deeply enough. The entire cement mantle and the cup may rotate and be extruded from the pelvis if the acetabulum is not deep enough, or if the posterior wall is deficient. The cup may migrate medially into the pelvis if the bone on the medial wall of the acetabulum is inadequate, or if it is reamed too much or fractured during the preparation of the acetabulum.
2. Failure to remove all of the cartilage, loose bone fragments, fibrous tissue, and blood, and failure to make a sufficient number of holes in the acetabulum so that the surface is irregular enough to secure a good cement-bone bond.
3. Failure to pressurize the cement adequately to obtain an optimal cement-bone bond. It is more difficult to pressurize cement in the acetabulum than in the femur because the cement tends to leak out of the acetabulum. Mechanical devices are available to pressurize cement, and cups with flanges tend to pressurize the cement more adequately.
4. Failure to distribute the cement around the entire outer surface of the cup, which may occur if the cup is pressed too firmly into the acetabulum while the cement is still doughy, or if the amount of cement is insufficient, so that part of the cup is in direct contact with bone. This can be prevented by using spacers or pods fixed to the surface of the cup.
5. Movement of the cup or cement mantle while the cement is hardening, which may occur while removing the positioning device.
6. Movement of a relatively undersized cup while it is held in a large cement mantle within the acetabulum. A small-diameter cup would not pressurize the cement adequately in this situation.
7. Malpositioning of the cup, so that the neck of the femoral component impinges on the margin of the socket, transferring excessive force to the cup. Impingement may occur while the hip is being flexed if the cup is relatively horizontal and not anteverted.

It is generally agreed that the acetabular component is loose if a radiolucency of 2 mm or more in width is present in all three zones. The significance of partial acetabular lucencies is determined by their width and the presence or absence of associated symptoms. Hodgkinson, Shelley, and Wroblewski correlated the extent of radiolucencies at the bone-cement interface with intraoperative assessment of loosening of the socket; 94% of sockets with demarcation in all three zones were loose at revision. When two zones of the bone-cement interface showed radiolucency, 71% were loose, and only 7% were unstable when demarcation was present only in one zone. The extent of radiolucent line formation was more important than the width of the lucency in determining loosening.

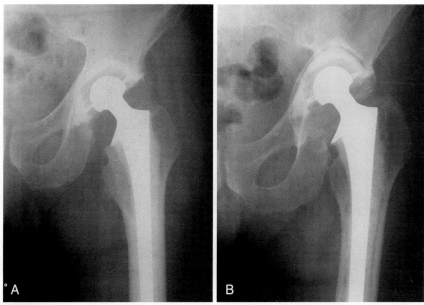

FIGURE 1.139   Change in position of cemented cup in a 59-year-old woman. **A,** Immediately after surgery. **B,** Seven years later, pain developed. Complete radiolucency has developed, and cup has migrated proximally and become more horizontal. Change in position of cup is definite evidence of loosening.

A change in the position of the cup in inclination, anteversion, or retroversion, as seen on the anteroposterior radiograph, is definite evidence of loosening (Fig. 1.139). Because of the difficulty in obtaining serial comparable radiographic views, however, a change in the position of the cup is sometimes difficult to verify. Using a consistent bony landmark such as the acetabular teardrop may be helpful.

CEMENTLESS ACETABULAR COMPONENTS

Radiographic criteria for loosening of cementless acetabular components are similar to those for uncemented femoral fixation. Engh, Griffin, and Marx classified these components as stable, probably unstable when progressive radiolucencies are present, and definitely unstable when measurable migration occurs. Loosening of cementless, porous-coated acetabular components is an uncommon finding with follow-up of 10 years. Most series report variable incidences of radiolucencies around porous acetabular components, although the significance of these findings remains to be determined. Leopold et al. found nonprogressive radiolucencies in one or more zones in more than 50% of revision acetabular components that were performing well clinically.

Other types of cementless acetabular components have been less successful. Threaded components and some hydroxyapatite-coated, nonporous components had excessively high early failure rates. These implants typically show migration on serial radiographs, although they form narrower radiolucencies than loose cemented acetabular components (Fig. 1.140).

DIAGNOSIS

Establishing whether symptoms are the result of loosening or some other process can be problematic. In many instances, it is difficult to determine whether a radiolucent area around the cement mantle of the femur or acetabulum represents a nonprogressive finding, loosening, or infection. Often aseptic loosening can be verified only by observing a patient over time to determine whether symptoms develop and whether radiographs show progressive changes. Some radiographic evidence of loosening most often appears before the onset of symptoms. Careful review of previous radiographs of a patient with symptoms often reveals changes that may have been overlooked or were thought to be insignificant when the patient was asymptomatic.

Loosening usually produces pain on weight bearing, which may be present in the thigh or groin. So-called "start-up" pain refers to pain that is worst with the first few steps and improves to some degree with further ambulation. This pain suggests a loose implant that moves but settles into a relatively stable position with weight bearing. Usually the pain is relieved by rest and aggravated by rotation of the hip. An antalgic gait may develop, and sometimes a patient volunteers that the limb is becoming shorter and increasingly externally rotated. Although most patients with loosening have an asymptomatic period postoperatively, some complain of pain from the time of surgery. Early postoperative pain should suggest that an infection has developed, that one or both components was not fixed securely, or that the pain is referred from a source extraneous to the hip joint.

The diagnosis of loosening is accepted in most instances if progressive radiolucency or implant migration occurs, and a patient has symptoms on weight bearing and motion that are relieved by rest. If a patient is asymptomatic, making the diagnosis of loosening is less urgent, unless a considerable amount of bone has been destroyed. If destruction of bone is progressive, even if symptoms are absent, revision usually is indicated because with delay, additional bone may be lost, making revision much more difficult and the results less satisfactory.

Migration of a component can be shown by placing small metal markers in the bone adjacent to the femoral and acetabular components and subsequently making radiographs in two planes. This roentgen stereophotogrammetric analysis

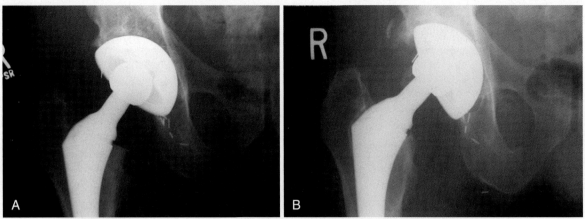

FIGURE 1.140 Change in position of cementless cup in 62-year-old man. **A,** Immediately after implantation of cementless hydroxyapatite-coated cup. **B,** Four years after surgery, hip became painful. Acetabular component has migrated into more vertical position without excessive wear. Revision was required.

(RSA) method requires computer software for interpretation of the data and is highly sensitive to small changes in implant position. It can be used to predict early failure but is not practical for routine clinical use.

OSTEOLYSIS

Osteolysis has been reported in association with numerous loose and well-fixed cemented and cementless components of several designs. Although increased fluid pressure and implant motion may play a role, the final pathway is effected by the host response to particulate debris of all types. It is now recognized that particles of metal, cement, and polyethylene can produce periprosthetic osteolysis, either alone or in concert. Osteolysis also has been reported in conjunction with metal-on-metal and ceramic-on-ceramic bearing surfaces.

The mechanism of production of osteolysis (and its prevention and treatment) can be viewed from three perspectives: (1) the generation of wear particles, (2) the access of these particles to the periprosthetic bone, and (3) the cellular response to the particulate debris. Most polyethylene particles are produced by abrasive, adhesive, microfatigue, and third-body wear mechanisms. The number of particles actually present in periprosthetic membranes vastly exceeds what has previously been estimated from light microscopy. Maloney, Smith, and Schmalzried examined the membranes from failed cementless femoral components with electron microscopy and automated particle analysis and found that particles (metal and polyethylene) were predominantly less than 1 micron in size and were present in amounts of more than 1 billion per gram of tissue. Macrophages are the predominant cell line involved in the response to particulate debris. Surface interaction between macrophages and wear debris can incite an inflammatory response whether phagocytosis occurs or not. Multiple cytokines and chemokines are produced as a result of this interaction. These mediators ultimately result in bone loss by activation of osteoclast production and inhibition of osteoblast formation from mesenchymal stem cells (Fig. 1.141).

Particles of polyethylene and other debris are dispensed through the joint fluid. Fluid flows according to pressure gradients, and any area of bone accessed by joint fluid is a potential site for deposition of debris. It is now recognized that segments of the femoral and acetabular components that are not contiguous with the articulating surfaces still may come in contact with joint fluid. Schmalzried, Jasty, and Harris described these areas of access as the "effective joint space," which is defined by the intimacy of contact between the implants and bone. This concept explains the development of osteolysis at the tip of a well-fixed femoral component with noncircumferential porous coating or over the dome of an acetabular component with holes in the metal backing.

The pattern of osteolysis depends on the implant design. Femoral components with limited or noncircumferential porous coating are subject to early development of distal cortical lesions because debris may gain access to the distal parts of the implant-bone interface by way of channels between areas of bone ingrowth (Fig. 1.142). Circumferential and more extensive porous coating seems to prevent distal osteolysis, but proximal lesions in the greater and lesser trochanters may be seen. Although the overall incidences of osteolysis may be equal, the confinement of bone loss to the proximal portion of the femur lessens the likelihood of implant loosening.

Acetabular components with thin polyethylene, incongruent or poorly supported liners, and poor fixation of the liner within its metal backing have higher rates of pelvic osteolysis. Lesions may be detected at the periphery of the acetabular component or in retroacetabular areas (Fig. 1.143). Peripheral lesions probably result from ingress of debris from the articulating surfaces, similar to the process that occurs with cemented acetabular components. Retroacetabular lesions may result from wear of the back side of the liner, with migration of debris through holes in the metal backing, although osteolytic defects of this type have been reported in implants without screw holes. The design of implants, the manufacturing and quality of polyethylene, and the measurement and reduction of wear are discussed in other sections of this chapter.

The progressive nature of particle-induced bone loss underscores the importance of continuing radiographic follow-up of patients after hip arthroplasty, especially if an implant considered at high risk for wear has been used. Many patients with osteolytic changes remain asymptomatic until catastrophic failure occurs from gross implant migration or periprosthetic fracture. Serial radiographs must be scrutinized carefully for progressive wear and for the development of osteolysis, and osteolytic changes must be differentiated from stress shielding and other forms of bone loss. Finally, radiographs provide only a two-dimensional picture of a three-dimensional problem. The degree of bone loss encountered at surgery, especially in the acetabulum, often is greater than is apparent radiographically.

When femoral or pelvic osteolysis has been detected, more frequent follow-up is advisable. Radiographs should be made at 6- to 12-month intervals. Loose implants and large lytic lesions are clear indications for surgery. Progressive osteolysis is another cause for reoperation, even in the absence of symptoms. If allowed to progress, revision becomes more complex or impossible. If the fixation of the implant has been compromised by the lytic process, complete revision of the component is unavoidable. If the implant remains stable despite periprosthetic bone loss, some investigators recommend bone grafting of the defect(s) with retention of the implant.

Grafting of proximal femoral deficits with retention of a stable femoral component is straightforward. In three series of patients who had femoral bone grafting of osteolytic lesions around well-fixed stems, no stems loosened and lesions generally showed graft incorporation at 3- to 5-year follow-up.

Options for treatment of acetabular osteolysis around a well-fixed cementless component include liner and femoral head exchange alone, liner and head exchange combined with bone grafting of osteolytic lesions, and complete acetabular revision of the liner and modular shell with or without bone grafting. Isolated liner and head exchange has the advantage of a simpler procedure and retention of well-fixed components that should minimize iatrogenic bone loss.

Narkbunnam et al. developed a scoring system to help determine acetabular component loosening in the setting of osteolysis based on the location and size of lytic lesions in the three Delee and Charnley zones. With increasing diameter of osteolysis, thickness of radiolucencies, and number of zones involved, the chances of implant loosening increase (Table 1.5).

Hamilton et al. detailed their experience with this technique over a 17-year period encompassing several acetabular designs. They reported an approximately 10% re-revision rate, mainly for recurrent dislocation and acetabular loosening. They continue to use this technique but recommend complete acetabular revision for cups with notoriously poor designs, careful assessment of cup stability at the time of liner exchange, and consideration of converting to a larger femoral head size to reduce the chance of dislocation. New Zealand Joint Registry data are more ominous for head and liner exchange, with 75% survivorship at 10 years' follow-up.

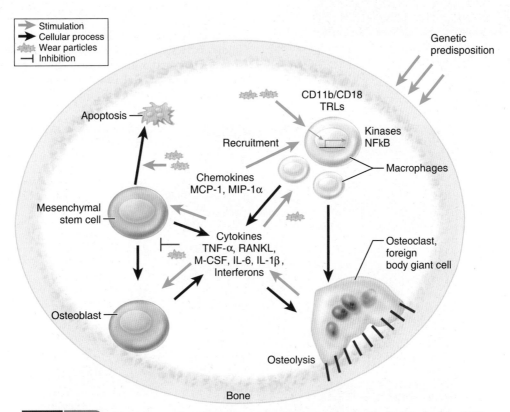

FIGURE 1.141 Biologic reactions between wear debris and host cells. *IL,* Interleukin; *MCP,* monocyte chemoattractant protein; *M-CSF,* macrophage colony-stimulating factor; *MIP,* macrophage inflammatory protein; *NFκB,* nuclear factor κB; *RANKL,* receptor activator of nuclear factor κB ligand; *TLR,* Toll-like receptor; *TNF,* tumor necrosis factor. (From Tuan RS, Lee FY, T Konttinen Y, et al: Implant Wear Symposium 2007 Biologic Work Group. What are the local and systemic biologic reactions and mediators to wear debris, and what host factors determine or modulate the biologic response to wear particles? *J Am Acad Orthop Surg* 16[Suppl 1]:S42, 2008.)

Approximately half of the re-revisions were for instability and 20% for acetabular loosening.

Curettage and grafting of retroacetabular defects present more of a technical challenge. Some of these deficits may be accessible from the periphery of the acetabulum

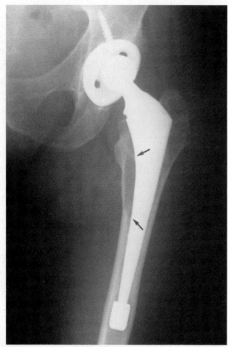

FIGURE 1.142   Distal femoral osteolysis. Five years after cementless reconstruction for osteonecrosis. Femoral component was not circumferentially porous coated. Large lytic defects have developed around middle and distal portions of stem *(arrows)*.

if complete circumferential exposure is obtained. Others can be debrided and grafted through screw holes in the retained shell. Small curets and suction tips facilitate removal of membrane via the holes. Caution must be taken during the debridement because a complete medial bony defect may be present. Bone grafting of large defects through screw holes is a time-consuming and tedious process, but probably less so than complete revision with significant bone loss. This approach presupposes that (1) the metal backing remains well fixed within the acetabulum; (2) the implant is a modular type and the locking mechanism remains competent; (3) a replacement liner of adequate thickness and acceptable design can still be obtained; and (4) the lytic areas are accessible for grafting without removal of the metal shell. Maloney et al. reported the results of this technique in a series of 35 patients. At a minimum of 2 years, all of the acetabular components remained radiographically stable, and all lytic lesions regressed in size or remained the same size. In a retrospective comparison of patients with acetabular osteolysis treated with either liner exchange and bone grafting versus complete acetabular revision, Restrepo et al. found a 10% rate of loosening of retained acetabular shells. They recommended complete revision in cups with broken locking mechanisms, complete wear-through of the acetabular liner, or malpositioned components, which could predispose to dislocation.

Cementing a new liner into the existing shell has been described in cases in which the locking mechanism is incompetent or a replacement liner is not available. Biomechanical studies have shown similar mechanical stability of such constructs compared with standard liner locking mechanisms. Springer, Hanssen, and Lewallen found no liner dissociation or acetabular loosening with this technique. To be technically

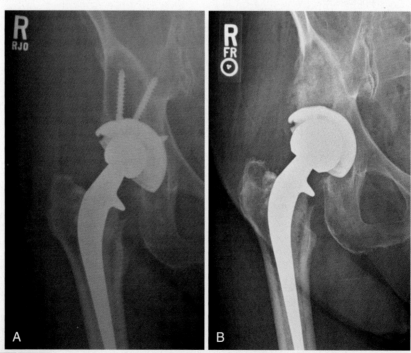

FIGURE 1.143   **A** and **B,** Painful osteolysis and acetabular wear with well-fixed components. Patient was treated with liner and femoral head exchange along with bone grafting through supra-acetabular defect.

TABLE 1.5		
Scoring System for Osteolytic Lesions		
LOCATION	**SCORE**	**DESCRIPTION**
Zone I	0	No lesion
	1	Small lesion size <1 cm
	2	Lesion size ≥1 cm, superolateral rim intact ≥1 cm or radiolucent line at bone <2 mm thick
	3	Superolateral rim intact <1 cm or radiolucent line ≥2 mm thick
	4	Lesion/radiolucent line invades entire superolateral rim or rim fracture
Zone II	0	No lesion
	1	Small lesion size <1 cm or radiolucent line <2 mm thick
	2	Lesion size ≥1 cm or radiolucent line ≥2 mm thick
	3	Lesion invades ilioischial line
Zone III	0	No lesion
	1	Radiolucent line <2 mm thick
	2	Loculated lesion at teardrop/ischium or radiolucent line ≥2 mm thick
	3	Lesion invades ilioischial line or significant ischial lysis

Total possible score of 10. Optimal cutoff score for loosening ≥5.
From Narkbunnam R, Amanatullah DE, Electricwalla AJ, et al: Radiographic scoring system for the evaluation of stability in cementless acetabular components in the presence of osteolysis, *Bone Joint J* 99-B:601, 2017.

feasible, the shell must be large enough to permit the insertion of a liner of acceptable thickness, allowing for a 2-mm cement mantle. Some authors recommend scoring the back of the new liner to improve fixation and scoring the metal shell if screw holes are not present. One biomechanical study demonstrated superior loads to failure with liners designed for cementation with integrated pods that provide for a uniform cement mantle compared with scored liners originally designed for cementless components.

ADVERSE LOCAL TISSUE REACTION

Modular components offer intraoperative flexibility when choosing the type of bearing surface desired and when fine-tuning the patient's anatomy in terms of offset, length, and anteversion, while limiting the chance of postoperative instability. With these choices, some significant drawbacks to modularity arise, including the production of metal ions and metal particles, which can cause tissue damage and even necrosis, commonly referred to as adverse local tissue reaction (ALTR). Such reactions have been noted in three major settings in the recent era of THA: metal-on-metal bearings, modular neck femoral components, and stems with modular femoral heads. These scenarios overlap in some patients who have been treated with components with two or three of these features.

The diagnosis of ALTR should be included in the differential of any patient presenting with a persistently painful THA. As with any patient, the workup begins with a detailed history and physical examination and considers both intraarticular and extraarticular sources of hip pain. Laboratory evaluation initially includes serum values (as described in the section on infection), including ESR, CRP, and D-dimer tests. It is well known that ESR and CRP may be elevated in the setting of ALTR alone. Serum cobalt and chromium levels also are used when evaluating patients with any of the previously mentioned "at risk" components and in whom infection and other sources of pain have been excluded. The various

scenarios have yielded metal ion levels and ratios that correlate fairly well with the presence of tissue damage necessitating surgical intervention (Table 1.6).

While metal ion levels are very useful in raising suspicion of ALTR, advanced imaging with either ultrasound or metal artifact reduction sequence magnetic resonance imaging (MARS MRI) is often used to confirm the diagnosis and aid in preoperative planning. Joint aspiration adds value as well by confirming the diagnosis based on the fluid's gross appearance and by ruling out infection. A manual cell count and differential are recommended, as automated counts may be falsely positive due to the cellular debris present. Likewise, alpha-defensin testing in the setting of ALTR has a relatively high false-positive rate at 31%. Once the diagnosis is made, surgical planning involves addressing the modular components to be revised and the soft-tissue damage to be debrided and/or reconstructed (Fig. 1.144).

REVISION AFTER ADVERSE LOCAL TISSUE REACTION

TECHNIQUE 1.9

- Expose the hip through an approach familiar to the surgeon that allows extensile exposure of both sides of the joint if necessary and adequate access to components requiring removal.
- Send joint fluid for culture.
- Send at least three soft-tissue samples for culture and for frozen section analysis intraoperatively if the diagnosis of infection is still being considered.

TABLE 1.6		
Metal Ion Levels and Risk of Adverse Local Tissue Reaction		
COBALT	**CHROMIUM**	**COBALT/CHROMIUM RATIO (SENSITIVITY/SPECIFICITY)**
METAL-ON-POLYETHYLENE TAPER		
1 (95/94)		2 (83/72)
1 (100/90)	0.15 (100/50)	1.4 (93/70)
METAL-ON-METAL THA (ASR)		
3.2 (68/71)		
2.4 (78/46)		1.4 (80/49)
MODULAR NECK		
2.8 (88/32)		3.8 (70/50)

ASR, Articular Surface Replacement System.

- Debride the pseudotumor and any other necrotic tissue as encountered, keeping in mind the concurrent goals of avoiding neurovascular compromise and hip instability.
- Remove the modular femoral head and assess the femoral taper for corrosion and material loss.
- If the femoral component does not require revision due to loosening or malposition, it may be retained if the taper does not have visible material loss or corrosion that cannot be acceptably removed. We have used a Bovie scratch pad or wet and dry laparotomy sponges for this purpose.
- Modular neck femoral components may also need removal to rid the patient of a modular neck/stem junction and may require an extended trochanteric osteotomy if the component is well fixed with sclerotic host bone.
- If revising a femoral component with a fixed neck and modular head mated with a polyethylene liner, revise the head to a ceramic femoral head and titanium sleeve of appropriate length, head size, and offset to ensure stability. Revise the liner to a polyethylene liner optimized for stability.
- If revising a modular acetabular component with a metal liner, the acetabular shell may be retained if it is appropriately positioned for stability. Revise the liner to a polyethylene liner optimized for stability.
- If revising a monoblock acetabular component, the surgeon may consider converting to a dual mobility construct on the femoral side if the acetabular component is appropriately positioned, not visibly damaged on its surface, and well fixed.
- Retain as much capsule as is feasible for exposure and repair the capsule as anatomically as possible.
- If abductor tendon damage is encountered, primary repair or secondary reconstructive procedures such as a gluteus maximus transfer may be necessary (see Technique 1.8).

The results of surgery for ALTR generally are poor, with relatively high rates of infection, instability, and reoperation. Patients should be referred to surgeons and hospitals with the required levels of implant availability, diagnostic methods, and surgical expertise if unavailable in their local setting.

REVISION OF TOTAL HIP ARTHROPLASTY

Because increasing numbers of primary THAs are being performed in younger and more active patients, the number of revision procedures has increased. Between 1990 and 2002, 17.5% of all hip arthroplasties performed in the United States were revision procedures. Because of expected increases in both primary and revision procedures, this percentage was predicted to remain fairly steady at 16.3% in 2005 and 14.5% in 2030.

Revision of THA usually is much more difficult, and the results typically are not as satisfactory as after a primary THA. Revision requires more operative time and blood loss, and the incidences of infection, thromboembolism, dislocation, nerve palsy, and fracture of the femur are higher. The complexities of revision surgery underscore the importance of technical precision in primary arthroplasty. A well-done index procedure provides the patient with the best opportunity for long-term success.

INDICATIONS AND CONTRAINDICATIONS

In determining the need for revision of painful THA, the patient first must be evaluated to determine whether their symptoms are the result of failed THA or other problems, including spinal disease, tumor, vascular occlusion, stress fracture, or complex regional pain syndrome. If the symptoms are caused by a failed THA, the decision must be made as to whether the patient has sufficient disabling pain to warrant a major operation. Activity modification, weight loss, use of external support, and analgesic medications may be more appropriate. Many patients are elderly, not physically active, and their general condition may be such that revision surgery would be ill advised. In debilitated patients in whom reconstruction would be exceedingly complex, a modified Girdlestone resection arthroplasty may be a more suitable alternative. It may be difficult, however, for a patient with a painful, disabling hip problem to accept the decision that another operation should not be done.

Pain is the major indication for revising a THA. Sometimes the operation is performed in the absence of disabling pain to prevent progression of structural abnormalities that, with delay, would make the operation more difficult. A recent query of the National Inpatient Sample database found the following most common indications for revision hip replacement: (1) dislocation, (2) mechanical loosening, (3) other mechanical problems, (4) infection, (5) osteolysis, (6) periprosthetic fracture, (7) wear, (8) and implant failure or breakage.

One of the more common indications for revision is painful loosening of one or both components, and this usually can be substantiated by serial radiographic findings (see section on loosening). It is vital that mechanical loosening be differentiated from septic loosening based on the clinical and radiographic presentation, as well as screening laboratory values as described in the section on infection. The hip should be aspirated if there is clinical suspicion of infection based on a history of delayed wound healing, radiographic changes, or abnormal laboratory values. The routine aspiration of all hips before revision has been largely abandoned, mainly because of poor sensitivity and positive predictive value.

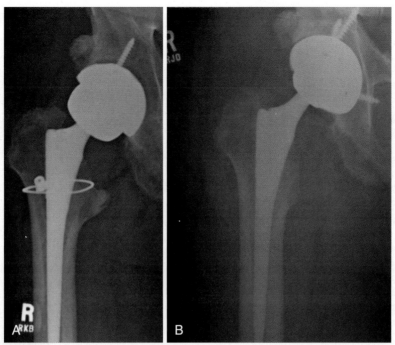

FIGURE 1.144 **A,** Painful metal-on-metal total hip arthroplasty. **B,** Acetabular component revised to trabecular metal multi-hole socket with polyethylene liner.

Pain associated with loose total hip components typically occurs with the first few steps a patient takes (so-called start-up pain). A loose acetabular component usually produces pain in the groin, whereas a loose femoral component may cause pain in the thigh or knee. Ancillary studies are seldom required, but comparison of previous radiographs often is helpful. If bone loss associated with loosening or osteolysis is severe or progressive, revision should be considered because symptoms are likely to worsen, and further resorption of bone would make the procedure more difficult and the result less favorable.

Revision is indicated for progressive stem deformation or incomplete fracture. Left untreated, the stem ultimately fractures completely, and revision is much more difficult because the distal segment must be retrieved from the medullary canal. Complete stem fracture, failure of a Morse taper junction, or disengagement of a modular liner locking mechanism typically requires revision.

Revision surgery is not often indicated for some functional problems, such as painless loss of motion in the hip or limb lengthening. In the absence of substantial heterotopic bone formation, reoperation to increase motion is unlikely to be successful. Shortening of the operated limb may result in recurrent dislocation, which is a significantly greater problem. Likewise, surgery to diminish limp is inadvisable unless a known mechanical source is identifiable and surgically correctable.

When pain similar to that present before the primary arthroplasty continues postoperatively, reevaluation is necessary to determine whether the hip abnormality was the cause of pain. In patients who continue to have pain after surgery and who have had no significant period of pain relief, technical problems or infection should be suspected. Every effort should be made to determine the cause of pain before considering exploration or revision. Occasionally, no source for

the pain can be determined, yet the patient is insistent that "something must be done." The results of revision surgery in this setting are unpredictable, and the patient's condition may be worsened if complications occur.

PREOPERATIVE PLANNING

Planning for a complex revision THA requires more time than for a routine primary procedure. All points in the preoperative planning for primary surgery (see section on preoperative evaluation) are applicable to the formulation of a general plan for a revision procedure; however, intraoperative findings and complications often require changes in the basic plan. Anticipation of potential complications and the formulation of numerous contingency plans to deal with them require additional equipment and expedite their management.

High-quality radiographs of the pelvis and entire femur must be obtained. Poor-quality films may lead to underestimation of bone loss because areas of thinned cortex cannot be distinguished from adjacent cement. Magnification markers are helpful in precision templating and identify the need for extra-small or extra-large components. Lateral views of the femur should be obtained to estimate the bow of the femur and to assist in choosing femoral components of appropriate diameter, length, and overall geometry. Femoral osteotomy can be anticipated if significant angular or rotational deformity is present. The presence of intrapelvic cement or a markedly protruded acetabular component may require further evaluation with vascular studies. Finally, acetabular deficiencies can be assessed further by CT. Useful information about bone stock can be gained even in the presence of a metal-backed acetabular component (see Fig. 1.116).

Radiographic identification of the type of prosthesis and a review of the operative notes often are helpful, especially if one component is to be left in situ. A mental note of the stem shape and any peculiarities in its surface can aid in determining the sites of cement removal necessary for extraction. In addition, the head size must be determined. Revision of the opposite component may be required for mismatch, malposition, or incorrect neck length, and the required implant inventory and equipment must be available.

Substantially more equipment is needed for revision surgery than for primary THA. Many hospitals do not have this expensive equipment readily available, and it must be brought in as needed. If the prosthesis to be revised is a contemporary design, arrangements should be made to have the instruments specific to that system available. Unique extraction tools, screwdrivers, and head disassembly instruments can make the procedure much easier. In addition, inventory specific to that system (e.g., modular heads and polyethylene liners to accommodate anticipated head sizes and offset requirements) may eliminate the need to revise both components. Additional equipment and materials often needed during revision surgery include the following:

- Image intensifier and radiolucent operating table
- Stem and cup extraction instruments
- Hand instruments for cement removal
- Motorized or ultrasonic cement removal instruments
- Motorized metal-cutting instruments
- Flexible intramedullary reamers
- Flexible thin osteotomes for cementless stem removal
- Trephine reamers
- Curved osteotomes or modular blades for cementless socket removal
- Fiberoptic lighting
- Pelvic reconstruction plates, screws, and instruments
- Trochanteric fixation device and cerclage wires or cables
- Allograft bone (cancellous chips, femoral head, struts, and segmental allograft)

In addition to equipment, a large prosthetic inventory must be available. A variety of short- and long-stem femoral components, calcar replacement stems, or stems with extended neck lengths are necessary to correct limb-length discrepancy, bone loss, and intraoperative femoral fracture. Most manufacturers have available sets of femoral components that are specifically designed to meet the needs of revision procedures. Acetabular components of 70 to 75 mm sometimes are needed to fill large acetabular deficiencies. Rarely, deficits are so massive that a custom-made component is the only solution (Fig. 1.145).

SURGICAL APPROACH

Many different skin incisions already may be present from previous surgery. If possible, a previous incision should be used. Skin necrosis between incisions is less of a problem than in the knee, but the possibility should not be ignored. All approaches used for primary THA can be used for revision surgery. The requirement for extensile exposure becomes even more important, however, in the revision setting. Straightforward acetabular revisions are performed through an anterior, anterolateral, direct lateral, or posterolateral approach. Access to the posterior column of the acetabulum is difficult through an anterior approach, however, as is extensile exposure of the femur. Also, the superior gluteal nerve is at risk if the exposure

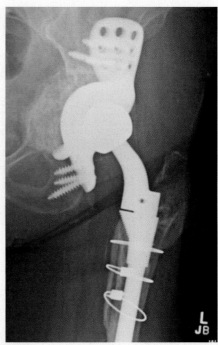

FIGURE 1.145 Custom triflange acetabular component for pelvic discontinuity. Note large amount of bone graft for medial segmental defect.

is extended more than 5 cm above the superior rim of the acetabulum.

The posterolateral approach with elevation of the vastus lateralis provides excellent exposure of the posterior column of the acetabulum and of the femoral shaft, but the risk of dislocation is higher than with anterior approaches. Anterior acetabular exposure is difficult from the posterolateral approach, especially if a femoral component with a fixed head is left in situ. In this case, the abductors must be stripped off the ilium superiorly and anteriorly and the prosthetic femoral head placed in this recess superior and anterior to the acetabulum. Complete release of the anterior capsule and sometimes the gluteus maximus insertion is required to allow adequate anterior translation of the femur.

The transtrochanteric approach provides the most complete exposure of the femur and the acetabulum and is utilized for complex revision procedures. Reattachment of the greater trochanter may be a problem, however, especially if the leg is lengthened or the fragment is osteoporotic. Trochanteric osteotomy can be done easily by a standard method or trochanteric slide technique (see section on trochanteric osteotomy) at any stage of the procedure if required for exposure or for removal and reimplantation of the components. If problems are anticipated with extraction of the femoral component or adjacent cement, an extended trochanteric osteotomy is preferable (Fig. 1.146). If a standard-sized trochanteric fragment is sufficient for exposure, we prefer to perform a trochanteric slide and leave the vastus lateralis attached if at all possible to avoid proximal migration of the fragment. The vastus origin can be released if necessary for further exposure, but this may render reattachment of the trochanter more difficult.

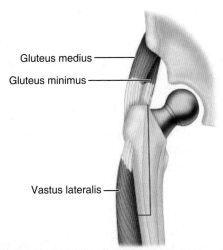

FIGURE 1.146 Extended trochanteric osteotomy. (Modified from Jando VT, Greidnaus NV, Masri BA, et al: Trochanteric osteotomies in revision total hip arthroplasty: contemporary techniques and results, *Instr Course Lect* 54:143, 2005.)

Gluteus medius

Gluteus minimus

Vastus lateralis

TRANSTROCHANTERIC APPROACH FOR REVISION TOTAL HIP ARTHROPLASTY

TECHNIQUE 1.10

- If a trochanteric nonunion exists, use it to improve exposure, and attempt to obtain union by improving fixation.
- Carefully remove previously placed wires and other internal fixation devices to avoid fragmenting soft areas of bone.
- The sciatic nerve usually does not need to be exposed, but if the limb is to be lengthened significantly, expose the nerve or palpate it to ensure it is not placed under undue tension. Posteriorly placed retractors should have smooth edges and must be placed carefully against bone, without soft-tissue interposition.
- Divide soft tissues immediately adjacent to the trochanter to minimize the risk of injury to the sciatic nerve.
- If any tendons of the short external rotators can be identified, tag them for later reattachment. More commonly, the short external rotators are absent; the pseudocapsule should be tagged for repair at the time of closure.
- The thickness of the residual hip capsule varies. Often, proliferative synovium on its articular surface contains large amounts of particulate polyethylene and cement debris.
- The pseudocapsule can be thinned if its overall thickness limits exposure or produces impingement.
- Release portions of the gluteus maximus insertion, if necessary.
- Elevate the vastus lateralis muscle belly from posterior to anterior while preserving its origin at the vastus tubercle.
- Osteotomize the greater trochanter from posterior to anterior using an oscillating saw, leaving the anterior cortex intact.

- Complete the osteotomy with a broad, flat osteotome.

See also Videos 1.2 and 1.3.

■ REMOVAL OF THE FEMORAL COMPONENT

REMOVAL OF CEMENTED FEMORAL COMPONENT

TECHNIQUE 1.11

- Occasionally, the femoral component is so grossly loose that it can be removed simply by hand. "Loose" does not always equate with "easily removed," however. In most cases, the stem must be forcibly disimpacted from the femur by some means.
- If the stem has a fixed head, use a commercially available extraction device with an attached slap hammer or driving platform. Several devices are available that pass over the head and hook around the neck of the implant (Fig. 1.147).
- If the stem is a contemporary design with a modular head, standard extraction devices simply pull the head off and cannot be used. Most systems with modular heads have a specific stem extraction device that is part of the system instrumentation. Typical designs have a hook that is inserted through a hole in the stem, a threaded device that screws into the stem, or a clamp-like device that is secured to some irregularity on the neck. Identify the stem design and contact the manufacturer's representative to have the extraction device available in the operating room. An extraction device is available that bolts onto the modular neck and may be useful if an implant-specific extractor is not available (Fig. 1.148).
- If no extraction device is available, use the collar as a driving platform. Tap the stem out from below with a mallet and punch. If the collar does not protrude beyond the medial cortex of the neck, remove a small amount of bone from the neck to expose a portion of the collar.
- Extraction of early design cemented stems usually presents no major problems. Most of these designs are smooth and tapered with few surface irregularities. Before attempting to extract the stem, remove overhanging bone from the greater trochanter that may impede stem removal. If the stem has a proximal curvature, remove the lateral cement that lies over the shoulder of the implant (Fig. 1.149); otherwise, the stem cannot move proximally without fracturing the femoral metaphysis.
- Removal of cemented stems that have been precoated with PMMA or are porous-coated can be difficult. If the stem is not loose, it is unlikely that it can be extracted without first removing some of the cement or porous coating.
- Use a motorized instrument with a long, thin burr to separate the proximal cement or porous surface from the stem.
- Do not use osteotomes for cement removal at this point because they may create a wedge effect that would split the femur. Use osteotomes only after the stem has been

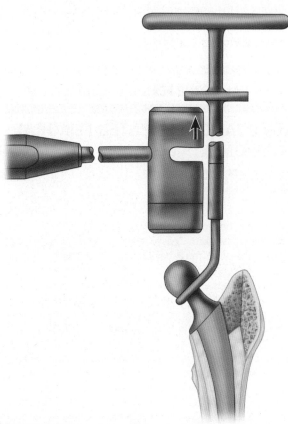

FIGURE 1.147 Moreland femoral component extractor. (Redrawn from Johnson & Johnson, DePuy, Warsaw, IN.) **SEE TECHNIQUE 1.11.**

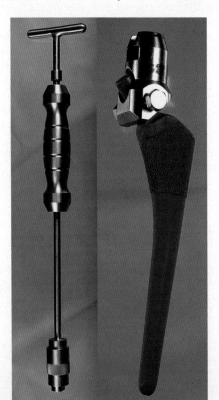

FIGURE 1.148 Femoral component extractor for modular femoral component. Bolts are tightened around modular femoral neck, and device is attached to slap hammer for component removal. (Courtesy Smith & Nephew, Memphis, TN.) **SEE TECHNIQUE 1.11.**

safely extracted and a central space has been opened into which the fragmented cement can displace.

- Pass the cutting burr circumferentially around the stem until the precoated or porous surface has been completely exposed.
- Insert the burr at an angle to remove the medial cement from beneath the collar.
- Remove the collar from the stem with a metal-cutting, carbide-tipped burr if necessary to gain access to the medial surface of the implant. If the stem is composed of a modern high-strength alloy, this may take an excessive amount of time.
- After removal of the proximal cement, attempt to extract the stem.
- If it cannot be removed with forceful blows on the extractor and the proximal cement has been removed as completely as possible, do an extended trochanteric osteotomy (see Fig. 1.153 and Technique 1.14) to gain access to a larger portion of the cement-prosthesis interface or make a small window in the femoral cortex. Place the window just distal to the level exposed by proximal cement removal and not at the tip of the stem. Remove additional cement through the window until the stem can be extracted.

REMOVAL OF CEMENTLESS FEMORAL COMPONENT

TECHNIQUE 1.12

- The extraction of cementless stems varies in complexity, depending on the extent of the porous coating, the amount of bone ingrowth, and the degree to which the stem fills the medullary canal. A loose-fitting, nonporous, cementless stem can be extracted without intervention at the bone-implant interface. A well-ingrown, fully porous-coated stem that fills the canal presents a significant problem for removal. Such a situation may arise when the stem is being removed because of infection or dislocation. Identify the stem type on preoperative radiographs, and determine the amount of porous surface. Evaluate the bone-implant interface to estimate the probability of bone ingrowth (see section on loosening of cementless femoral components).
- If the porous coating is limited to the proximal aspect of the stem, disrupt the areas of bone ingrowth using specialized thin, flexible osteotomes (Fig. 1.150). Standard osteotomes usually are too thick for this purpose and may split the femur if they are inserted adjacent to a stem that fills the canal. Insert the thin osteotomes immediately adjacent to the porous surface to avoid penetration of the femoral cortex. Direct them at various angles to gain access to all aspects of the porous surface.

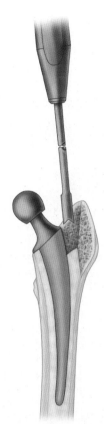

FIGURE 1.149 Moreland V osteotome for removal of lateral cement over shoulder of implant for stems with proximal curvature. (Redrawn from Johnson & Johnson, DePuy, Warsaw, IN.) **SEE TECHNIQUE 1.11.**

- Alternatively, disrupt the areas of ingrowth with a long, thin, high-speed burr inserted immediately adjacent to the stem. Carefully monitor the line and depth of insertion to avoid cortical penetration.
- Extract the stem after disruption of the bone ingrowth. Areas of purely fibrous ingrowth sometimes can be loosened by forceful attempts at stem extraction without the use of osteotomes.
- An extensively porous-coated implant may be considerably more difficult to remove. Osteotomes are effective in disrupting ingrowth into the flat areas of the proximal stem, but the area of greatest bone ingrowth often is at the distal extent of the porous coating. The stem is round at this level and fills the canal. Osteotomes cannot be directed into this interface without excessive risk of femoral fracture.
- After disrupting areas of proximal ingrowth with osteotomes or a thin burr, attempt to extract the stem using moderate force. If the stem cannot be extracted without risk of fracturing the femur, an alternative means must be used to disrupt areas of distal bone ingrowth.

Glassman and Engh described a technique for removal of implants with extensive distal bone ingrowth. Specialized trephine reamers and high-speed, metal-cutting instruments are required.

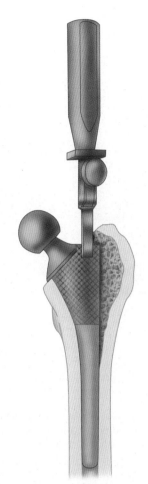

FIGURE 1.150 Moreland specialized, thin, flexible osteotome for disrupting bone ingrowth at proximal end of porous-coated stem. (Redrawn from Johnson & Johnson, DePuy, Warsaw, IN.) **SEE TECHNIQUE 1.12.**

REMOVAL OF IMPLANTS WITH EXTENSIVE DISTAL BONE INGROWTH

TECHNIQUE 1.13

(GLASSMAN AND ENGH)
- Disrupt areas of bone ingrowth proximally with thin osteotomes.
- Using a high-speed burr, make a small transverse window in the femoral cortex at the level of the junction of the triangular and cylindrical portions of the stem.
- Transect the prosthesis at this level using a carbide-tipped, metal-cutting burr (Fig. 1.151A). Avoid notching or dividing the opposite cortex.
- Remove the proximal portion of the stem.
- Remove the distal cylindrical portion of the stem by reaming over it with a trephine reamer (Fig. 1.151B). Determine the proper size of the trephine reamer by measuring the distal end of the removed proximal portion of the stem. Irrigate the trephine frequently to avoid burning

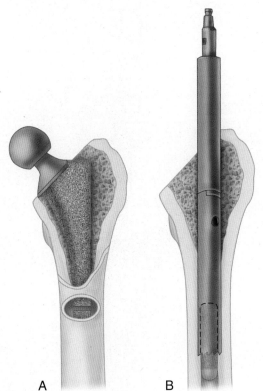

FIGURE 1.151 Removal of implants with extensive distal bone ingrowth (Glassman and Engh). **A,** Prosthesis is transected with carbide-tipped, metal-cutting burr. **B,** Distal cylindrical portion of stem is removed by reaming over it with trephine reamer. (Redrawn from Johnson & Johnson, DePuy, Warsaw, IN.) **SEE TECHNIQUES 1.13 AND 1.14.**

the bone. More than one set of reamers may be required. After the distal ingrowth has been disrupted, withdraw the trephine from the canal with the distal stem fragment inside it.

Younger et al. described a technique of extended trochanteric osteotomy for difficult femoral revisions. The greater trochanter is removed along with an attached segment of the lateral femoral cortex, minimizing the risk of trochanteric fracture and avoiding the problems of reattachment of a smaller trochanteric fragment. The technique is ideally suited for removal of well-fixed cementless or cemented stems after dislocation of the hip. Other indications include varus remodeling of the femur and removal of loose femoral components with well-fixed cement mantles. The osteotomy also can be done before dislocation if difficulty is anticipated with dislocation, or after removal of the stem. This osteotomy provides direct access to the distal portion of the femoral canal for safe, expedient removal of cement and insurance of proper reaming of the distal femur for neutral stem alignment. Extensile exposure of the acetabulum can be achieved as with other methods of trochanteric osteotomy. Distal translation of the osteotomized segment allows precise tensioning of the abductors to improve the stability of the joint. The procedure is most appropriately used when a cementless

femoral revision is planned because cement intrusion into the osteotomy site may inhibit union. Union rates of 98% to 99% with this osteotomy have been reported.

EXTENDED TROCHANTERIC OSTEOTOMY

TECHNIQUE 1.14

(YOUNGER ET AL.)

- Plan the length of the osteotomy so that the distal extent of the well-fixed cemented or cementless prosthesis is maximally exposed, leaving enough of the femoral isthmus intact to allow endosteal cortical contact by the revision prosthesis over a distance of 5 to 6 cm (Fig. 1.152).
- Expose the hip by a posterolateral approach with circumferential exposure of both implants.
- Protect the sciatic nerve throughout the procedure.
- Dislocate the hip, or, alternatively, perform the osteotomy before dislocation if the procedure is complicated by stem subsidence, acetabular protrusion, or stiffness of the hip.
- Position the thigh in internal rotation.
- Incise the vastus lateralis along its posterior edge to the level of the distal extent of the planned osteotomy.
- Mark the osteotomy longitudinally just lateral to the linea aspera, extending distally to the level determined by preoperative radiographs (Fig. 1.153A).
- With a thin, high-speed burr, make multiple perforations in the posterior femoral cortex and connect them with the burr. Skirt the lateral edge of the underlying femoral component.
- Divide the lateral cortex transversely at the predetermined level.
- Perforate the anterior cortex with the burr at multiple sites, attempting to create an osteotomy fragment constituting approximately one third the circumference of the femur. Leave as much of the vastus lateralis attached to the fragment as possible.
- Divide the superior portion of the anterior cortex with an oscillating saw because the burr may not be long enough in the trochanteric region.
- Insert two or more broad osteotomes into the posterior limb of the osteotomy and gently create a controlled fracture through the perforated anterior cortex, leaving the anterior soft-tissue attachments undisturbed (Fig. 1.153B).
- With the osteotomy fragment reflected anteriorly, the lateral portion of the femoral component is visible, and the anterior and posterior surfaces are accessible. Remove cement from the interfaces under direct vision to allow extraction of the stem.
- If a well-fixed cementless stem is in place, pass a Gigli saw blade beneath the collar and direct it distally, following the medial edge of the femoral component (Fig. 1.153C). Control the blade so that additional bone is not removed from the anterior or posterior cortex.

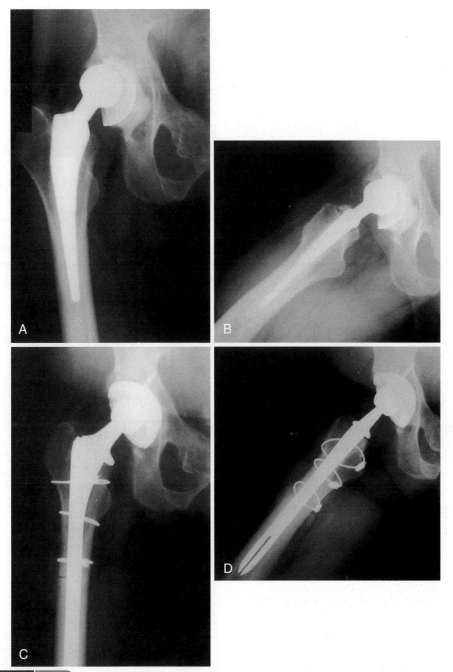

FIGURE 1.152 Extended trochanteric osteotomy. **A** and **B,** Acetabular loosening with damage to femoral head. Porous femoral component has been cemented and remains well fixed, but femoral revision is required because head is not modular. **C** and **D,** Extended trochanteric osteotomy greatly simplified removal of femoral component and cement without bone loss and facilitated acetabular exposure. Note formation of callus around osteotomy at 3 months. **SEE TECHNIQUE 1.14.**

- Divide the interface down to the distal extent of the porous surface. Several Gigli saw blades may be required.
- Alternatively, make the osteotomy shorter and divide the femoral component with a high-speed, metal-cutting burr at the junction of the triangular and cylindrical portions of the stem.
- Remove the distal segment of the stem with a trephine reamer (see Fig. 1.151B). Remove any remaining cement

or distal pedestal under direct vision through the osteotomy site.
- Place a prophylactic cable or wire around the femoral shaft and distal to the osteotomy to prevent propagation of a nondisplaced fracture.
- After placement of the revision femoral component, repair the osteotomy with multiple cerclage wires.
- Shape the undersurface of the osteotomy fragment to fit the revision prosthesis.

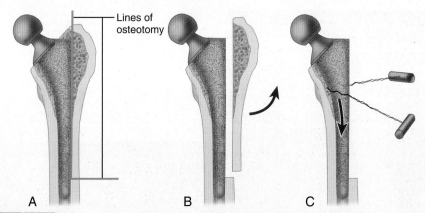

Lines of osteotomy

A **B** **C**

FIGURE 1.153 Extended trochanteric osteotomy for difficult stem removal. **A,** Longitudinal portion of osteotomy follows lateral border of stem and extends distally to predetermined level. **B,** Anterior cortex is divided, and entire lateral cortical segment, with trochanter, is retracted anteriorly, exposing lateral surface of stem. **C,** Bone ingrowth is disrupted with Gigli saw passed down medial side of stem. **SEE TECHNIQUES 1.11 AND 1.14.**

- Remove the distal edge of the osteotomy fragment and advance it distally to adjust the soft-tissue tension around the hip joint if necessary.
- Supplement the posterior edge of the osteotomy site with cancellous bone graft. If the osteotomized fragment is thin and fragile, reinforce it with a cortical allograft strut.

REMOVAL OF A BROKEN FEMORAL COMPONENT

Extraction of a fractured femoral stem is a difficult problem. The proximal portion usually is loose and easily removed along with any fragmented proximal cement. In contrast, the distal portion of the stem remains firmly fixed in the femur. Most stems fracture in the proximal or middle third and are accessible from above. A fiberoptic light usually is necessary to view the fractured end of the stem and make preparations for removal. Numerous techniques have been described for removal of broken stems. Some of these require specialized instrumentation for removal of the broken fragment from above (see Technique 1.13 and Fig. 1.151B), and others require the creation of a femoral cortical window to give direct access to the stem.

Techniques for removal of the broken fragment from above may be time-consuming and may fail. In these cases, a femoral window is required to allow access to the broken fragment directly. Window techniques have the disadvantage of weakening the femur, especially if the window is made at the distal aspect of the stem. Moreland, Marder, and Anspach devised a technique for broken stem removal using a tungsten carbide punch inserted through a small proximal window. They reported successful extraction of 10 broken stems by this technique, with no failures. The technique is attractive because only a small window is required, and the window usually is bypassed a satisfactory distance by a standard length revision stem.

REMOVAL OF A BROKEN STEM—PROXIMAL WINDOW

TECHNIQUE 1.15

(MORELAND, MARDER, AND ANSPACH)

- Remove the proximal fragment of the prosthesis and proximal cement.
- Measure the distance from the opening of the femur to the top of the broken prosthesis. Make the window just distal to this level, not at the tip of the prosthesis.
- Spread the fibers of the vastus lateralis to expose a small area of the anterior femoral cortex at this level.
- Use a small burr to make a longitudinal window 4 mm wide and 10 mm long.
- Remove bone and cement to expose the proximal end of the retained stem fragment.
- Introduce a narrow carbide-tipped punch into the distal aspect of the window and direct it cephalad (Fig. 1.154).
- Make a small divot in the surface of the prosthesis and drive it proximally.
- As the stem moves proximally, reposition the punch progressively more distally and continue driving it proximally until it becomes loose and can be removed from above.
- If the punch does not gain adequate purchase, use a metal-cutting burr to make a larger divot.

Occasionally, the above-described method is not successful, and a more extensive femoral window is necessary. This may occur when the stem has a complex geometry that cannot move proximally without bringing the cement mantle with it. An I-beam configuration that tapers distally is an example. Cement must be removed from around the stem before it can be extracted.

REMOVAL OF A BROKEN STEM—DISTAL WINDOW

TECHNIQUE 1.16

- Remove a cortical window from the anterolateral aspect of the femur 0.8 cm in diameter and extending about 3 cm proximal and distal to the tip of the prosthesis. Preserve the cortical fragment in a single piece.
- Remove all cement visible within the medullary canal with small burrs and osteotomes.
- Insert an offset driver through the window and drive the stem proximally through the residual cement mantle. Ensure that the window is large enough, or the driver may impinge on the edge and produce a complete fracture of the femur.
- After the broken stem fragment has been removed, use the window to remove additional cement and to guide cement removal instruments down the center of the canal.
- Replace the cortical fragment in its bed and secure it with multiple cerclage wires.
- Use a stem of sufficient length to bypass the defect by a distance of two cortical diameters. In our opinion, creating a large cortical window in the femur should be reserved as a last resort.

Fracture of cementless femoral components has not been a significant problem, although the incidence may escalate as the length of follow-up in young, active patients increases. The difficulty in removal of the distal portion of such a stem is determined by the extent of the porous surface, the amount of bone ingrowth, and the degree to which the stem fills the medullary canal. For a fracture to occur, it is likely the distal portion of the stem is well fixed and the stem has been subjected to cantilever bending. The proximal fragment is likely to be loose and can be removed after the residual bone-implant interface is disrupted with thin osteotomes. A trephine drill is used to core out the distal fragment (see Fig. 1.151B).

■ REMOVAL OF FEMORAL CEMENT

Removal of the femoral cement mantle usually is the most time-consuming and hazardous part of revision total hip surgery. This task is delayed until after the acetabular component has been revised because persistent bleeding from the femoral canal obstructs the view of the acetabulum and adds to the operative blood loss. As such, this sometimes arduous task begins late in the operation, when the surgeon already may be fatigued from a difficult exposure and acetabular reconstruction. Femoral fracture, cortical penetration, and further destruction of femoral bone stock sometimes result from hurried attempts to remove femoral cement.

Femoral cement removal requires a wide array of instruments, including a fiberoptic light source; a long, straight suction catheter; cement removal osteotomes with various configurations; a long pituitary rongeur for removal of loose cement fragments; long, hooked instruments for retrograde cement removal; a high-speed burr with long attachments; and reamers of graduated diameters. Many manufacturers supply the aforementioned instruments in sets specifically designed for this purpose. A radiolucent operating table and image intensification to view the hip and femur are often necessary.

The most appropriate technique for removal of femoral cement depends on the quality of the surrounding bone and the depth of cement within the femoral canal. The proximal cement is easily accessible, and the bone-cement interface is relatively easily viewed without additional lighting. The surrounding cortex often is thin and fragile, however, because of osteolysis. If this is the case, one or more cerclage wires are placed around the femur to diminish the risk of fracture. The cement from the midportion to the tip of the stem is more difficult to see, as is the bone-cement interface. Fiberoptic lighting is essential. We have used a combination device containing a fiberoptic light and irrigation and suction ports to see the interface better. The cement distal to the tip of the previous stem often fills the canal completely and extends a variable distance down the shaft, depending on whether a cement restrictor was used. The distal cement is the most difficult portion to see and remove. If cement removal seems exceedingly difficult, an extended trochanteric osteotomy may be appropriate.

REMOVAL OF FEMORAL CEMENT

TECHNIQUE 1.17

- To remove the proximal cement, clear soft tissue and overhanging cement away from the proximal femur to expose the proximal edge of the bone-cement interface.
- Remove any cement and overhanging bone from the greater trochanter first to allow unobstructed passage of instruments directly down the canal. This is especially important if the previous stem was placed in varus. If the trochanter blocks passage of instruments directly down the canal, the instruments are likely to exit through a perforation created in the posterolateral cortex (Fig. 1.155). Osteotomize the greater trochanter if necessary.
- Make numerous longitudinal radial splits in the proximal cement column (Fig. 1.156).
- Insert osteotomes into the bone-cement interface and fracture the fragments of cement into the open central area (Fig. 1.157). Do not attempt to wedge instruments into the bone-cement interface before making the radial splits, or a femoral fracture is likely to occur.
- Removal of cement from around the middle and distal segments of the stem is more difficult, although it still can be accomplished with hand tools. Adequate lighting, irrigation, and suction become more important to show the bone-cement interface. The available space centrally narrows because of the taper of the

stem. Narrow, angled cement osteotomes are often required.

- Small cement fragments may occlude the central space. Remove them with a pituitary rongeur or curet.
- Review the preoperative radiographs to determine the relative thickness of areas of cement to be removed and to determine any deviation of the tip of the stem that may direct instruments out through the cortex rather than centrally in the canal. Also take into account the normal anterolateral bow of the femur. Sometimes this segment of the cement mantle can be removed en masse by passing a large threaded tap into the defect left by the stem and extracting it with a slap hammer.
- Removal of the distal cement mass usually is the most difficult. If the plug of cement is thin and not tightly adherent to the cortex, it occasionally can be driven distally in the canal and left. This should not be done in the presence of infection.
- If the plug is thin and does not fill the canal completely, it often can be extracted with a hook. Pass the hook between the cortex and cement through any apparent gaps on the preoperative radiographs (Fig. 1.158A). Turn the hook 90 degrees to engage the cement and gently tap the hook with a mallet to withdraw the cement plug (Fig. 1.158B).
- Fragmentation of solid distal cement with cruciate-shaped osteotomes can be attempted, but this technique is slow and unrealistic if the distal cement extends more than 1 cm.
- If the cement plug fills the canal and is firmly fixed, perforate it with a drill and use reamers to enlarge the hole. Carefully drill the initial hole in the center of the distal cement plug and align the drill with the femoral canal. Use a centering sleeve to position the drill bit precisely (Fig. 1.159). Enlarge the hole with masonry drills specially designed for this purpose. After a hole of sufficient size has been made, remove the remaining cement adherent to the cortex with a reverse cutting hook. Alternatively, insert a tap into the hole and extract the cement plug with a mallet.

REMOVAL OF DISTAL CEMENT WITH A HIGH-SPEED BURR

Turner et al. recommended the use of a high-speed burr for removal of distal cement. We have used this technique with success, but meticulous attention to technique is mandatory to prevent femoral cortical perforation. The high-speed burr can be deflected easily from the hard cement to the softer bone, which is removed preferentially. Careful monitoring of the path of the burr under biplane image intensification is necessary.

TECHNIQUE 1.18

(TURNER ET AL.)
- Orient the C-arm either horizontally or vertically, and rotate the leg to obtain two-plane views of the femur.

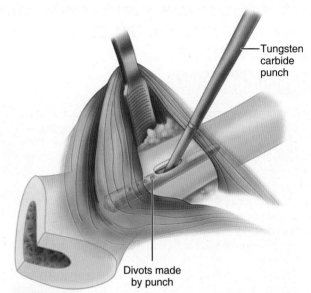

FIGURE 1.154 Method of removal of broken stem described by Moreland, Marder, and Anspach. Small window is made in anterior femoral cortex just distal to break in stem. Carbide punch is used to push prosthesis proximally. (Redrawn from Moreland JR, Marder R, Anspach WE Jr: The window technique for the removal of broken femoral stems in total hip replacement, *Clin Orthop Relat Res* 212:245, 1986.) **SEE TECHNIQUE 1.15.**

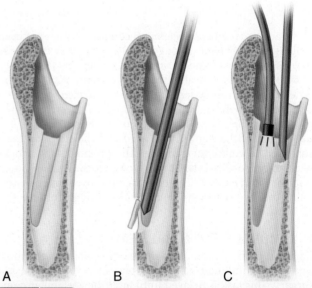

FIGURE 1.155 Removal of cement from femoral canal. **A** and **B,** After removal of varus stem, channel in cement is such that drill or osteotome tends to follow channel and penetrate cortex. **C,** Cement must be removed from medial wall to prevent penetration; fiberoptic light is helpful in this procedure. **SEE TECHNIQUE 1.17.**

Repeated manipulation of the C-arm increases the risk of contamination of the field.
- Insert the cutting tool with short strokes. The burr cuts cement on the forward stroke and removes debris as it is withdrawn.
- Irrigate the canal continuously to remove debris and cool the burr. If the burr becomes too hot, the cement can melt

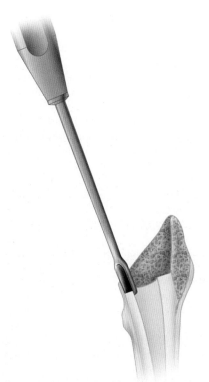

FIGURE 1.156 Removal of cement from femoral canal. Longitudinal radial splits are made in proximal cement column. (Redrawn from Johnson & Johnson, DePuy, Warsaw, IN.) **SEE TECHNIQUE 1.17.**

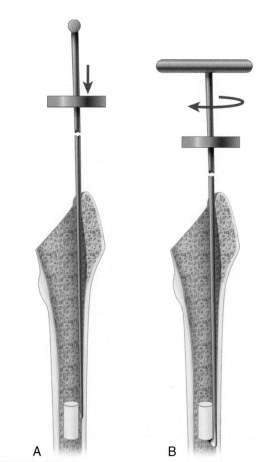

A   B

FIGURE 1.158 Removal of solid cement below tip of prosthesis. **A,** Thin, curved hook is inserted between cortex and cement plug. **B,** Hook is turned 90 degrees and used to pull up cement. (Redrawn from Johnson & Johnson, DePuy, Warsaw, IN.) **SEE TECHNIQUE 1.17.**

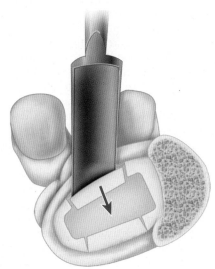

FIGURE 1.157 Fragmentation of proximal cement. After longitudinal radial splits have been made in cement column, curved osteotome is inserted into bone-cement interface and cement fragment is fractured into central vacancy. **SEE TECHNIQUE 1.17.**

and reform behind the cutting end, which makes extraction difficult.
- Frequently monitor the path of the burr in two planes under the image intensifier. Follow a path down the center of the canal, not along the course of the previous stem.
- After the cement column has been perforated, use a larger side-cutting burr to remove additional cement along each area of the cortex.

- Continue to monitor the path of the burr under biplane image intensification. Never use this technique without radiographic guidance.
- If resistance suddenly decreases as a burr or reamer is being advanced, cortical penetration is likely. Insert a ball-tipped guidewire, such as that used for flexible medullary reaming, into the canal and move it in various directions. Sometimes the movement of the rod can be palpated in the soft tissues of the distal thigh if perforation has occurred. Obtain intraoperative radiographs, or view the rod under the image intensifier.
- If cortical perforation is evident, expose the area of the femur.
- Elevate and preserve any segments of cortex that may have been fractured off.
- Use the window created to remove additional cement and subsequently to guide the burr or reamer in the correct path down the center of the medullary canal.
- Reconstruct the area of cortical perforation with cortical strut grafts and/or use a stem of sufficient length to bypass the defect by a distance of at least two cortical diameters.

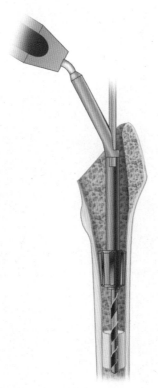

FIGURE 1.159 Centering sleeve is used as drill guide to position drill bit precisely in center of cement plug. (Redrawn from Johnson & Johnson, DePuy, Warsaw, IN.) **SEE TECHNIQUE 1.17.**

Even with experienced surgeons, Turner et al. reported femoral cortical perforation in 10% of cases using high-speed cement removal instruments. Mallory stated that when such aggressive instrumentation is used, perforation is almost expected. Such perforations occur in an uncontrolled manner, producing large gaps in the cortex. They often occur anteriorly and laterally, where they render the femur susceptible to fracture and are difficult to reconstruct. Mallory recommended a technique using "controlled perforations" for safe, rapid removal of femoral cement using a high-speed burr.

REMOVAL OF DISTAL CEMENT WITH A HIGH-SPEED BURR AND CORTICAL WINDOW

TECHNIQUE 1.19

(MALLORY)
- Obtain extensile exposure of the femoral shaft by elevation of the vastus lateralis.
- After removal of the prosthesis, create a 9-mm hole in the anterior or anterolateral cortex of the femur using a high-speed burr. Use the prosthesis as a template to determine the most beneficial site for placement of the hole.

- Usually the first hole is placed 8 to 10 cm distal to the vastus lateralis ridge.
- Use the portal to guide the burr visually down the center of the femoral shaft.
- Shine a fiberoptic light through the perforation to illuminate the femoral canal. Irrigate the canal through the hole to remove cement debris generated by the burr.
- Place a second or occasionally a third perforation with a distance of at least 5 cm separating the portals. Make the most distal portal at the level of the distal cement mantle.
- Reconstruct the femur with a long stem prosthesis that extends a distance of twice the diameter of the femur past the most distal perforation.

In a related biomechanical study, Dennis et al. found no significant changes in stress patterns of the femur around anteriorly placed holes. In addition, no cumulative stress concentrations were seen when multiple holes were located at least 5 cm apart. In contrast, tensile strain increased 40% after a hole was drilled through the lateral femoral cortex. Careful placement of perforations in the anterior cortex, with adequate spacing between them, is essential.

Ultrasonically driven tools for cement removal are also commercially available. Ultrasonic instruments are of greatest value in removing cement distal to the tip of the prosthesis (Fig. 1.160). The incidence of cortical perforation with ultrasonic techniques has been low, but ultrasonic tools rarely suffice for removal of all of the cement and usually are used along with standard hand tools.

If the revision femoral prosthesis is to be recemented, it is acceptable to leave some of the cement in the femur, provided that it is firmly bonded to the femur with no radiolucency on radiographs and there is no evidence of infection. If enough cement is removed to allow placement of the new prosthesis in proper alignment with an adequate cement mantle, the new cement bonds to the old cement. If a cementless revision prosthesis is to be used, it is preferable to remove all of the cement to facilitate bone grafting and biologic fixation. Retained cement also may deflect reamers used for canal preparation and lead to femoral perforation. If infection is present, all of the cement must be removed. Regardless of the type of revision prosthesis, all of the membrane from the bone-cement interface must be removed because it impairs fixation. Curets and reverse cutting hooks are used to remove the membrane. In addition, the smooth surface of any neocortex must be removed to allow fixation to true cortical bone. A high-speed burr, flexible reamers, and curets are used to remove this bone from the femoral canal.

■ REMOVAL OF THE ACETABULAR COMPONENT
▌CEMENTED ACETABULAR COMPONENT

To remove the cup and cement from the acetabulum, the surgical exposure must provide direct access to the entire circumference of the cup. We have found the posterolateral approach (see Technique 1.2) satisfactory, usually without osteotomizing the trochanter. The trochanter should be osteotomized if needed, however, to gain the necessary exposure. The capsule is released from the anterior edge of

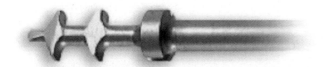

FIGURE 1.160 Ultrasonic attachment for removal of loose cement plug from distal femoral canal. With ultrasonic device turned on, tool is advanced into center of cement plug. When the device is off, cement hardens onto the attachment. The attachment and associated cement plug are removed with a slap hammer.

the acetabulum, and a retractor is inserted in this region to lever the proximal femur anteriorly (see Fig. 1.43D and E). If the femoral component is not being revised and the femoral head is modular, the head is removed to improve exposure. If the head is not modular, the abductors and capsule are elevated from the anterosuperior aspect of the acetabulum, and the femur is rotated to place the head into this recess.

The following technique can be used to remove a loose all-polyethylene cup.

REMOVAL OF A LOOSE ALL-POLYETHYLENE CUP

TECHNIQUE 1.20

- If the cup has a flange, remove it with an osteotome or rongeur to expose the cement-cup and cement-bone interfaces.
- Starting superiorly, remove cement from between the cup and surrounding bone with a thin osteotome, minimizing damage to the bone.
- Drive a thin, curved osteotome between the cup and cement in numerous places around the cup and carefully pry the cup partially out of the cement (Fig. 1.161A). Avoid doing this with the instrument between the cement and bone because this may damage the remaining acetabular bone or fracture the rim of the acetabulum.
- Place a small punch in one of the grooves along the edge of the component and tap it out from behind with a mallet, or use a commercially available extraction device that engages the polyethylene from within the recess to extract it (Fig. 1.161B).
- If the cup is more securely fixed in the acetabulum or if removal is not successful by the aforementioned method, divide the cup into quarters with a saw or burr and remove it in segments. The amount of polyethylene debris generated with this technique is of concern and should be carefully removed (Fig. 1.162).

De Thomasson et al. described removal of well-fixed all-polyethylene components with acetabular reamers to thin the polyethylene and allow easier extraction. They reported no fractures or acetabular defects with this technique (Fig. 1.163).

REMOVAL OF A METAL-BACKED, CEMENTED ACETABULAR COMPONENT

TECHNIQUE 1.21

- Use curved osteotomes to fragment the cement and disrupt as much of the cement-prosthesis interface as possible.
- Insert an impactor into a surface irregularity or groove along the superolateral edge of the prosthesis and attempt to tap it out from behind.
- If the metal backing cannot be loosened by external dissection, remove the polyethylene liner. Use a metal-cutting, high-speed burr to remove a quarter section of the metal backing.
- The apex of the cement mantle and cement-prosthesis interface is now exposed. Disrupt this interface with curved osteotomes and remove the remainder of the metal backing.
- When extracting a cup and cement that are appreciably displaced into the acetabulum, especially if there has been an infection, vascular damage is possible. For this reason, preoperative advanced imaging may be advisable to determine how close the cement mass is to the vascular structures. Prepare and drape the patient so that, if necessary, a lower abdominal incision can be made for retroperitoneal exposure of the pelvic vessels, and preoperatively make arrangements to have personnel available for vascular repair if necessary (see section on vascular injuries).
- Usually a moderate amount of cement remains in the acetabulum after removal of the cup, unless bone resorption was marked, or the loosening was caused by infection, in which case most or all of the cement is extracted with the cup.
- Remove the cement from the floor of the acetabulum by lifting the edge of the cement with a curet and cracking it gently with an osteotome; do not damage the medial wall of the acetabulum or drive the cement into the pelvis.
- If a metal mesh or plastic disc restrainer has been used to cover a centering hole or defect, it usually comes out with the cement.
- The fibrous membrane covering the cement mantle may be thick, and most often it remains adherent to the bone rather than the cement. Completely remove the fibrous tissue with a curet or Cobb elevator. A high-speed burr can be used to remove firmly adherent fibrous tissue that remains.
- Remove plugs of cement from the anchoring holes if possible.
- Except in the presence of infection, removing pieces of cement that have been displaced into the pelvis is unnecessary, difficult, and may cause excessive bleeding.

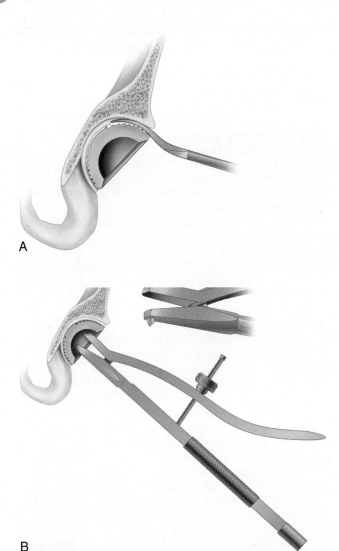

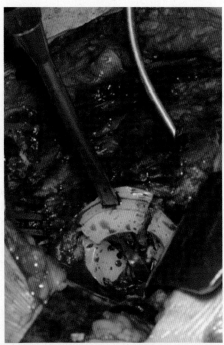

FIGURE 1.162 Well-fixed, cemented polyethylene component has been divided into quarters and is being removed in segments from the underlying cement. (From Burgess AG, Howie CR: Removal of a well fixed cemented acetabular component using biomechanical principles, *J Orthop* 14:302, 2017.)

FIGURE 1.161 Removal of polyethylene cup. **A,** Curved, thin osteotome or gouge is used to disrupt interface between implant and cement. **B,** Cup is removed by prying it gently from cement with extraction device. (Redrawn from Smith & Nephew, Memphis, TN.) **SEE TECHNIQUE 1.20.**

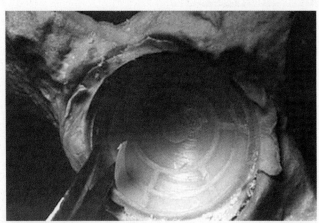

FIGURE 1.163 Acetabular reamer reams cup until cement is visible through transparent polyethylene. Remaining polyethylene and cement are removed with curved osteotomes or gouges. (From de Thomasson E, Mazel C, Gagna G, et al: A simple technique to remove well-fixed, all-polyethylene cemented acetabular component in revision hip arthroplasty, *J Arthroplasty* 16:538, 2001.)

CEMENTLESS ACETABULAR COMPONENT

Removal of a well-fixed, porous, cementless acetabular component is difficult and may result in removal of additional bone stock with the need for a larger implant for reconstruction. When the prior implant has been placed against the medial wall of the acetabulum, it is possible that a complete medial segmental bony deficit would result from the extraction. If the reason for revision of the component is malposition with recurrent dislocation, exchanging the polyethylene liner for one with a larger lip or degree of offset may suffice. If not, revision of the ingrown metal backing is done. Our preferred technique for removal of well-fixed porous acetabular components involves an acetabular centering device attached to a rotating handle and blades of varying diameters to disrupt the bone-implant interface. Mitchell et al. reported 31 revisions with this technique, resulting in minimal bone loss and 5 minutes of operative time for cup removal.

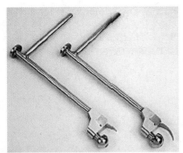

FIGURE 1.164 Explant System (Zimmer Orthopaedics, Warsaw, IN) used to remove well-fixed, acetabular, cementless components. (From Mitchell PA, Masri BA, Garbuz DS, et al: Removal of well-fixed, cementless, acetabular components in revision hip arthroplasty, *J Bone Joint Surg* 85B:949, 2003. Copyright British Editorial Society of Bone and Joint Surgery.) **SEE TECHNIQUE 1.22.**

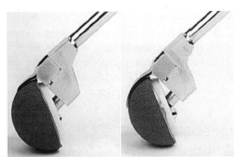

FIGURE 1.165 Two blades used by Explant System. Short blade *(left)* and full-radius blade *(right)*. (From Mitchell PA, Masri BA, Garbuz DS, et al: Removal of well-fixed, cementless, acetabular components in revision hip arthroplasty, J Bone Joint Surg 85B:949, 2003. Copyright British Editorial Society of Bone and Joint Surgery.) **SEE TECHNIQUE 1.22.**

TECHNIQUE 1.22

(MITCHELL)
- If no screws are present, leave the liner in place; otherwise, remove the liner to allow screw removal and replace it to accommodate the centering device. If the liner is excessively worn or damaged, a trial liner can be used. A trial bipolar head that matches the inner diameter of the cup may be used to center the blade in a resurfacing acetabular component for which appropriately sized trial liners are not available.
- Employing a centering device of a diameter matching the internal diameter of the liner, use a short blade initially to disrupt the interface between the implant and bone by rotating the handle of the device (Fig. 1.164). The outer diameter of the implant must be known to choose the appropriate blade.
- After the short blade has made a channel circumferentially, use a longer blade in the same manner to disrupt any remaining bone ingrowth at the dome of the implant.
- Lift the implant out between the blade and centering device (Fig. 1.165).

RECONSTRUCTION OF ACETABULAR DEFICIENCIES

Deficiency of acetabular bone stock is one of the major problems in revision THA and may result from numerous factors, including the following: (1) osteolysis caused by wear, loosening, or infection; (2) excessive bone resection at the time of previous surgery, especially if the patient has had a resurfacing procedure or previous acetabular revision; (3) preexisting bone deficit from acetabular fracture or dysplasia that was not corrected at the time of previous surgery; and (4) inadvertent destruction of bone during removal of a previous component or cement.

■ CLASSIFICATION

The development of guidelines for management of acetabular deficiencies has been hindered by a lack of standard nomenclature to describe them. The AAOS Committee on the Hip devised a clinically useful classification system for acetabular deficiencies (Table 1.7). The system is equally applicable to primary arthroplasties, however. Description of acetabular deficits makes preoperative planning easier and simplifies operative management (Fig. 1.166).

Acetabular deficits are of two basic types: segmental and cavitary. A segmental deficiency is a complete loss of bone in the supporting rim of the acetabulum, including the medial wall. A cavitary deficiency is a volumetric loss in the bony substance of the acetabular cavity. Segmental and cavitary deficits are subdivided according to their location: anterior, superior, posterior, or central. These deficiencies may be isolated or may exist in combinations. A protrusio deformity represents a central cavitary deficit. When a loose socket migrates into the pelvis, a combined central segmental and cavitary deficit is produced. Previous cement fixation holes produce combined superior and posterior cavitary deficits. Superior segmental and superior cavitary deficits occur in congenital hip dysplasia or with superior migration of an endoprosthesis or loosened socket.

Pelvic discontinuity describes a fracture traversing the anterior and posterior columns with separation of the superior and inferior portions of the acetabulum. Arthrodesis implies no actual deficiency of acetabular bone stock, although the site of the true acetabulum may be difficult to locate.

Although the AAOS classification is helpful in describing acetabular defects, the various types may be difficult to appreciate on plain radiographs. Paprosky et al. developed a classification system based on preoperative radiographs and intraoperative findings with the various classes determined by the relative position of the acetabular component to the host acetabulum, and the status of the host bone defined by bony landmarks. This system is helpful in preoperative planning because the defects encountered at surgery can often be predicted by the class of deficiency (Fig. 1.167 and Table 1.8).

Anteroposterior and lateral radiographs, Judet views, and CT scans are often helpful in evaluating the acetabular deficits preoperatively. Ultimately, the degree of deficiency is determined intraoperatively when components are removed, and complete acetabular exposure is achieved. Preoperative templating is useful to anticipate the size of the component(s) required and the need for structural augmentation when the new component is placed in the proper location.

■ MANAGEMENT

The objectives of acetabular reconstruction are to (1) restore the center of rotation of the hip to its anatomic location, (2) establish normal joint mechanics, (3) reestablish the structural integrity of the acetabulum, and (4) obtain rigid fixation of the revision prosthesis to host bone. Currently, most acetabular revisions are done with cementless components.

MANAGEMENT OF ACETABULAR CAVITARY DEFICITS

TECHNIQUE 1.23

- Cavitary deficiencies are the easiest to manage. If the deficits are very small, ream to a slightly larger size to increase the area of host bone in contact with the implant surface. Insert the revision socket using the same techniques as for primary replacement (see Technique 1.3).
- If the deficits are larger, significant additional reaming would compromise the rim of the acetabulum and create a segmental deficiency.
- Fill larger cavitary deficiencies with morselized autogenous or allograft cancellous bone grafts and impact them into place by using the last-sized reamer, turning in reverse or by impaction with an acetabular trial component of appropriate size. A larger-than-average final acetabular component may be required (Fig. 1.168).
- Large superior and central cavitary deficiencies require more extensive bone grafting. Use morselized graft or a solid bulk graft for large defects, with additional particulate bone graft to fill any smaller cavitary deficits (Fig. 1.169). In either case, use the bone graft only as filler material and not as a structural support for the new implant. The intact peripheral rim of the acetabulum should be able to provide implant stability before the addition of any bone grafts.
- Through judicious reaming and careful implant sizing, place as much of the porous surface of the implant as possible against viable host bone. Use an implant oversized 1 to 2 mm relative to the last reamer to achieve rim fixation, especially if large medial deficits have been grafted.

TABLE 1.7

American Academy of Orthopaedic Surgeons Classification of Acetabular Deficiencies

TYPE I: SEGMENTAL DEFICIENCIES
Peripheral
Superior
Anterior
Posterior
Central (medial wall absent)

TYPE II: CAVITARY DEFICIENCIES
Peripheral
Superior
Anterior
Posterior
Central (medial wall intact)

TYPE III: COMBINED DEFICIENCIES

TYPE IV: PELVIC DISCONTINUITY

TYPE V: ARTHRODESIS

From D'Antonio JA, Capello WN, Borden LS, et al: Classification and management of acetabular abnormalities in total hip arthroplasty, *Clin Orthop Relat Res* 243:126–137, 1989.

- Use ancillary screw fixation if the stability of the implant is in question with press-fit fixation alone.
- Insert an acetabular liner that will accommodate a femoral head 32 mm or larger, if possible, to enhance stability.

■ SEGMENTAL DEFICITS

Many segmental acetabular deficits involve only a small area of the rim. These deficits seldom compromise prosthetic stability and usually can be disregarded. Segmental deficits in the anterior column usually do not require reconstruction (Fig. 1.170). If the prosthesis is contained by bone posteriorly and superiorly, the center of rotation of the hip is restored, and component stability is achieved, structural augmentation of the acetabulum is not required. In addition, central segmental deficits can be managed similarly to central cavitary deficits. Particulate bone grafts are contained by intact soft tissues over the medial wall defect and incorporate readily. Structural medial wall bone grafts are seldom necessary. Some isolated superior segmental deficits can be managed with an oblong-shaped revision acetabular component. This prosthetic solution allows restoration of the hip center to an anatomic location without the need for additional structural augmentation (Fig. 1.171). Implantation of these devices requires special instruments and is technically more challenging than for hemispherical implants. There is a tendency to place such implants in an excessively vertical position. A few small series have reported successful use of these implants in carefully selected patients. In our practice, they have been replaced by modular augments combined with hemispherical components.

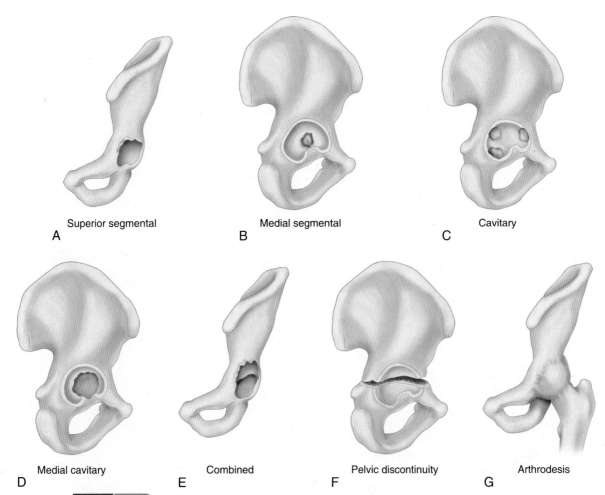

Superior segmental

A

Medial segmental

B

Cavitary

C

Medial cavitary

D

Combined

E

Pelvic discontinuity

F

Arthrodesis

G

FIGURE 1.166 **A,** Superior segmental defect violates superior supporting rim and part of anterior supporting rim of acetabulum. **B,** Medial segmental defect violates medial supporting rim. **C,** Three cavitary defects involve excavation of bone without violation of superior, posterior, or anterior rim. **D,** Medial cavitary. Excavation of medial wall of acetabulum occurred without violation of medial rim (contained bone defect). **E,** Combined segmental cavitary defects. Superior, anterior segmental lesion combined with superior, anterior, and medial cavitary defects. **F,** Pelvic discontinuity. Interruption of anterior and posterior columns creates rare but unstable defect. **G,** Arthrodesis. Acetabular cavity filled with bone.

Structural augmentation is needed most commonly for a large posterior or superior segmental deficiency that compromises the stability of the implant or that requires superior displacement of the center of rotation of the hip more than 2.5 cm to place the implant against intact bone. Segmental defects of this type may be managed with structural allografts or, more recently, with modular metal augments. In most reported series, results of structural bone grafting for segmental deficiencies have been best when at least 50% of the support of the revision acetabular component was provided by host bone rather than graft. Modular augments are advantageous because rigid initial fixation of the augment can be achieved, resorption of the augment is not a concern (unlike with allograft), and multiple augment sizes and configurations are available to accommodate complex bone loss and deformity (see Fig. 1.31). Mid-term follow-up on porous tantalum cups with modular augments shows good results with reliable fixation except in the setting of pelvic discontinuity.

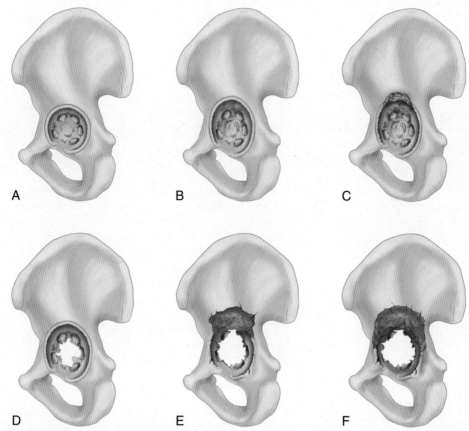

FIGURE 1.167 **A,** Type I defect has minimal bone loss and negligible component migration. **B,** Type 2A defect with less than 2 cm superomedial migration. **C,** Type 2B defect with less than 2 cm superolateral migration. **D,** Type 2C defect with medial migration only. **E,** Type 3A defect with more than 2 cm component migration and bone loss from 10-o'clock to 2-o'clock position. **F,** Type 3B defect with more than 2 cm migration and bone loss from 9-o'clock to 5-o'clock position. (Redrawn from Paprosky WG, Perona PG, Lawrence JM: Acetabular defect classification and surgical reconstruction in revision arthroplasty: a 6-year follow-up evaluation, *J Arthroplasty* 9:33, 1994.)

TABLE 1.8

Paprosky Classification of Acetabular Deficiencies

Type I	Supportive rim with no bone lysis or migration
Type II	Distorted hemisphere with intact supportive columns and <2-cm superomedial or superolateral migration
	a. Superomedial
	b. Superolateral (no dome)
	c. Medial only
Type III	Superior migration >2-cm and severe ischial and medial osteolysis
	a. Kohler's line intact, 30%-60% of component supported by graft (bone loss: 10 o'clock to 2 o'clock position)
	b. Kohler's line not intact, >60% of component supported by graft (bone loss: 9.00 o'clock to 5.00 o'clock position)

From Paprosky WG, Perona PG, Lawrence JM. Acetabular defect classification and surgical reconstruction in revision arthroplasty. A 6-year follow-up evaluation. *J Arthroplasty* 9:33–44, 1994.

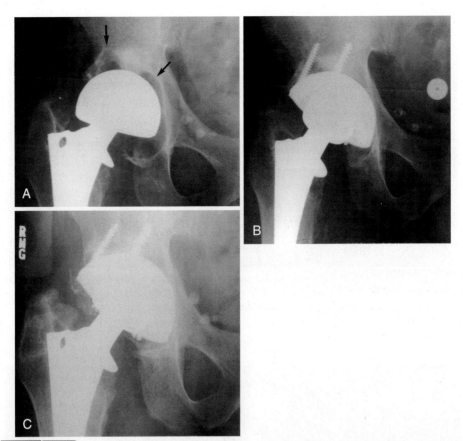

FIGURE 1.168 **A,** Cavitary deficiencies *(arrows)* in 42-year-old postal worker with groin pain 13 years after bipolar hemiarthroplasty. Polyethylene wear has produced large superior and medial cavitary deficiencies. **B,** Defects were filled with cancellous allograft with placement of porous revision implant. Hip center accurately restored. **C,** At 4 years, bone grafts have remodeled and appearance is that of a primary arthroplasty. **SEE TECHNIQUE 1.23.**

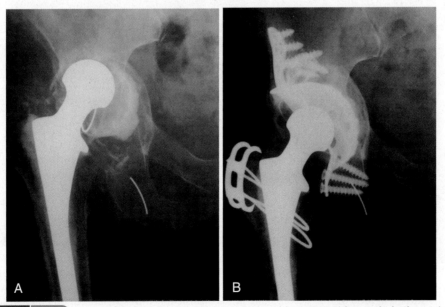

FIGURE 1.169 **A,** Large cavitary deficiencies in 85-year-old woman with acetabular loosening 18 years after primary cemented arthroplasty. Large superior and medial cavitary deficiencies combined with poor bone stock. Fixation is unlikely with conventional porous-coated implants. **B,** Extensive bone grafting with cancellous allograft combined with antiprotrusio cage. Implant is stable at 2 years, and bone graft is incorporated. **SEE TECHNIQUE 1.23.**

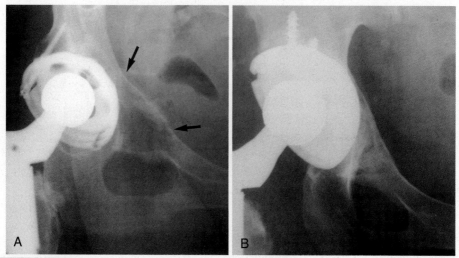

FIGURE 1.170 Anterior segmental deficiency in young woman. **A,** Polyethylene wear produced this segmental deficiency *(between arrows)* in anterior column of acetabulum. Posterior column is intact. **B,** Revision accomplished with large-diameter porous implant and cancellous bone grafting. No structural graft was required.

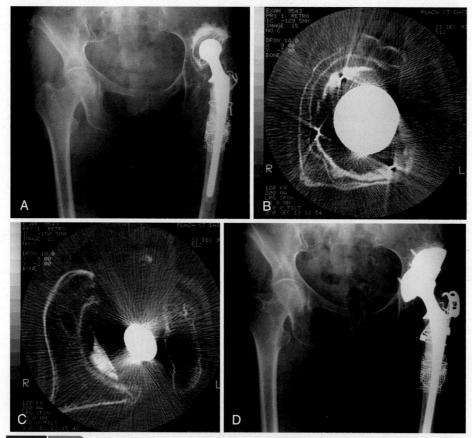

FIGURE 1.171 Superior segmental deficiency. **A,** Elderly woman with two previous revisions for developmental dysplasia. Residual high hip center with superior segmental deficit can be seen. **B,** CT scan shows deficient posterior bone stock at high location. **C,** Best available posterior bone stock is at level of true acetabulum. **D,** Reconstruction with specialized, oblong revision acetabular component. No structural bone grafts were required, and early weight bearing was facilitated.

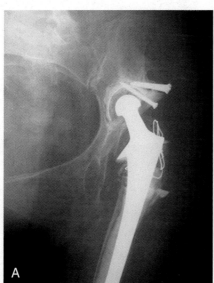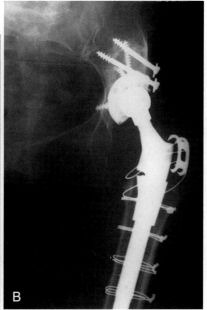

FIGURE 1.172 Superior segmental deficiency. **A,** Multiple previous revisions had been done for sequelae of congenital hip dysplasia. Socket previously was placed in false acetabulum with high hip center. Large superior segmental defect is above true acetabulum. **B,** Five years after revision with structural bone grafting of superior segmental deficit and cementless acetabular component, no migration is seen but bone ingrowth is unlikely. **SEE TECHNIQUE 1.24.**

MANAGEMENT OF SEGMENTAL ACETABULAR DEFICIT WITH FEMORAL HEAD ALLOGRAFT

TECHNIQUE 1.24

- If a segmental deficit is limited to the superior or the posterior rim of the acetabulum, a femoral head allograft usually is sufficient. Use bone from an osteoarthritic femoral head. Osteoporotic bone from a patient with a femoral neck fracture is inadequate.
- With a high-speed burr or matching male and female reamers, prepare the surfaces of the graft and the recipient bed to match or leave the graft slightly larger than the deficit so that an interference fit can be obtained to enhance stability.
- Use rigid internal fixation to secure the graft to host bone. Most superior segmental deficits have a residual shelf of bone that supports the graft, and lag screws alone are sufficient for fixation (Fig. 1.172). Because bony support of posteriorly placed structural grafts often is not achieved, fixation with a buttress plate is required.
- Provisionally fix the graft with Kirschner wires.
- Ream the acetabulum to contour the inner surface of the graft along with the host acetabular bed for the final acetabular component.
- Contour a pelvic reconstruction plate along the posterior column and fix it with multiple screws. Remove the Kirschner wires.

- After placement of the revision socket, use ancillary screws to fix the implant to host bone. Screws fixing the socket to the bone graft do little to increase the stability of the construct.

MANAGEMENT OF SEGMENTAL ACETABULAR DEFICIT WITH METAL AUGMENT

TECHNIQUE 1.25

(JENKINS ET AL., MODIFIED)
- Ream the native acetabulum in 1-mm increments until two points of fixation are found.
- Place an acetabular trial one size larger than the last reamer and assess stability.
- If stability is questionable, acetabular augments are used to improve stability by filling bony defects.
- Using trial augments as guide for sizing the defect, ream the defect line to line or use a high-speed burr to accommodate the augment while minimizing host bone removal.
- Place the acetabular component first and fix it provisionally with two screws.
- Back out the screws two or three turns and place the augment in the desired position and fix it provisionally with screws.
- Remove the augment screws and augment.

- Place doughy cement at the interface of the augment and acetabular component; replace the augment into position. Tighten the provisional acetabular component screws and fix the augment definitively with screws placed through the previously placed screw holes.
- Add screws through the acetabular component as needed for stability with the goal of achieving fixation in the superior and inferior hemispheres of the acetabulum (Fig. 1.173).

■ COMBINED DEFICITS

Combined superior and either posterior or anterior segmental deficits usually are too large to be managed with a femoral head allograft. Distal femoral allografts, modular metal augments, cancellous allograft combined with an antiprotrusio cage, acetabular allografts, custom triflanged acetabular components, and hemispherical components placed at a high hip center all have been used to reconstruct these massive segmental deficiencies. Cementless hemispherical components have shown better results when more than 50% of their surface is in contact with host bone. A tantalum metal revision socket has been developed, which may require less than 50% host bone available for stability, but long-term results are unavailable. Antiprotrusio cages have been combined with structural allografts and cancellous impaction grafting for combined defects where less than 50% host bone is available for fixation.

Sporer et al. described a technique of structural grafting using a distal femoral or proximal tibial allograft fashioned in the shape of the numeral 7. The technique is recommended when superior migration of the hip center of more than 3 cm has occurred while the anterior and posterior columns are mostly intact (Paprosky IIIA). At 10 years' follow-up, 17 of 23 uncemented hemispherical cups combined with distal femoral allografts were successful without radiographic loosening or revision of the acetabular component. Historically, this technique was considered for younger patients to improve bone stock, but most patients currently are treated with modular metal augmentation of hemispherical acetabular components with or without an antiprotrusio cage.

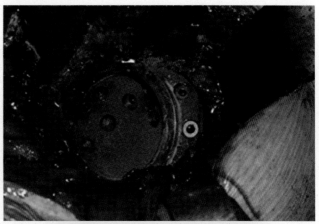

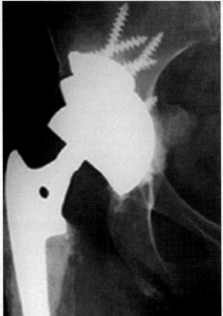

FIGURE 1.173 Combined deficiency including superior segmental defect treated with modular augment, tantalum revision socket, and cancellous autograft. (From Jenkins DR, Odland AN, Sierra RF, et al: Minimum five-year outcomes with porous tantalum acetabular cup and augment construct in complex revision total hip arthroplasty, *J Bone Joint Surg Am* 99:49, 2017.)

MANAGEMENT OF COMBINED DEFICITS WITH STRUCTURAL GRAFTING

TECHNIQUE 1.26

(SPORER ET AL.)
- Select a distal femoral allograft of appropriate size to fill the defect. Shape the condylar portion of the graft with female reamers so that the size of the graft is approximately 2 mm larger than the defect. Fashion the graft in the shape of an inverted 7.
- Make a diaphyseal cut in the coronal plane, leaving the anterior cortex thick enough for screw fixation.

- Make an oblique cut through the posterior cortex, exiting just proximal to the posterior condyles (Fig. 1.174A).
- Place the graft over the defect in the superior portion of the acetabulum and gently impact it into place with the cut portions of the graft buttressed against the superior portion of the acetabulum and ilium.
- Secure the graft to the ilium with multiple screws or a plate. Place the screws in a staggered fashion and tap the drill holes to avoid fracturing the graft (Fig. 1.174B).
- Ream the graft and remaining portions of the acetabulum with standard acetabular reamers to a size that leaves the anterior and posterior columns intact while maximizing contact for bone ingrowth for the revision prosthesis (Fig. 1.174C).

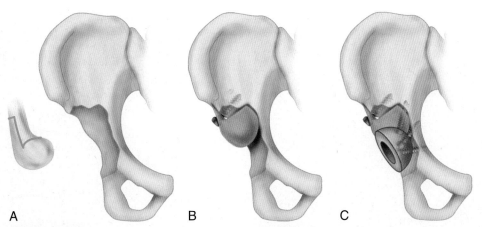

FIGURE 1.174 Paprosky "7" graft for segmental acetabular deficiency. **A,** Distal femoral allograft is shaped to resemble numeral 7. **B,** Graft is shaped to fit acetabular deficiency and fixed as shown, with several screws placed above acetabulum through remaining cortical portion of graft. **C,** Graft is reamed, and revision component is implanted. **SEE TECHNIQUE 1.26.**

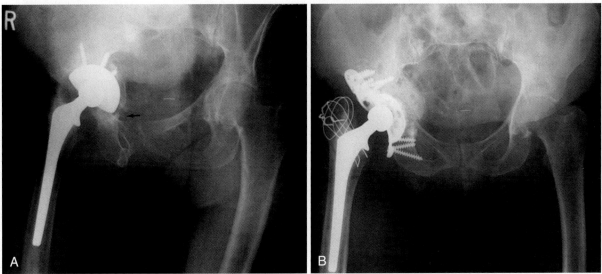

FIGURE 1.175 Pelvic discontinuity. **A,** Four years after total hip replacement in 70-year-old woman with history of pelvic irradiation for cervical carcinoma; acetabular component failed. Large deficiency of anterior column with fracture through posterior column *(arrow)*. **B,** Acetabular reconstruction done with antiprotrusio cage and extensive bone grafting.

- Impact the acetabular component in the appropriate position and fix it to the host bone with multiple screws.

  When segmental and cavitary deficits occur simultaneously, the segmental defect is reconstructed first to restore the rim. Any remaining cavitary deficits are filled with particulate cancellous graft.

PELVIC DISCONTINUITY

Pelvic discontinuity results from a transverse fracture of the acetabulum with complete separation between the superior and inferior halves (Fig. 1.175). Abdel et al. recommended posterior column plating and uncemented hemispherical components for patients with acute pelvic discontinuity or in chronic pelvic discontinuity with bone stock of sufficient quantity and quality for healing.

Paprosky et al. developed an algorithm for treating pelvic discontinuity based on its perceived healing potential. If such potential exists, the discontinuity is treated in compression with plating of the posterior column and a structural allograft or with a tantalum revision socket used as a hemispherical plate. If healing potential is insufficient, as in the setting of previous pelvic irradiation, the discontinuity is placed in distraction and the acetabulum reconstructed with a highly porous metal socket. Other options in this setting include a tantalum metal socket combined with an antiprotrusio cage (so-called cup-cage construct), or a custom triflanged acetabular component (Fig. 1.176, Fig. 1.145).

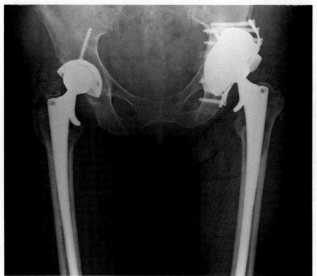

FIGURE 1.176 Cup-cage construct. Pelvic discontinuity and large superior segmental defect required tantalum hemispherical acetabular component with superior augment, antiprotrusio cage, and cemented polyethylene liner.

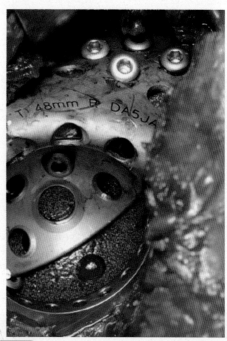

FIGURE 1.178 Cup-cage construct with transverse screws through the ilium along with dome and ischial screws. Note unitization of construct with dome screws through the cage and cup. (From Abdel MP, Trousdale RT, Berry DJ: Pelvic discontinuity associated with total hip arthroplasty: evaluation and management, *J Am Acad Orthop Surg* 25:330, 2017.) **SEE TECHNIQUE 1.28.**

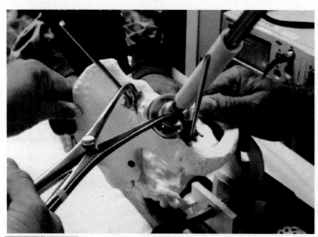

FIGURE 1.177 Acetabular distraction. Acetabular reamer in place while discontinuity is tensioned with distraction device. (From Sheth NP, Melnic CM, Paprosky WG: Acetabular distraction: an alternative for severe acetabular bone loss and chronic pelvic discontinuity, *Bone Joint J* 96-B[11 Suppl A]:36, 2014.) **SEE TECHNIQUE 1.27.**

ACETABULAR DISTRACTION FOR MANAGEMENT OF PELVIC DISCONTINUITY

TECHNIQUE 1.27

(SHETH ET AL.)

- Expose the failed acetabular component via a posterolateral approach and remove it along with the fibrous membrane from the floor of the acetabulum.

- Stress the inferior half of the acetabulum to confirm the presence of a discontinuity.
- Place acetabular augments as needed for anterosuperior or posteroinferior segmental defects.
- Temporarily distract the acetabulum with a large lamina spreader to assess the mobility of the discontinuity.
- Place a large Kirschner wire or Steinmann pin in the dome and ischium and place a distractor over the pins.
- Ream the acetabulum on reverse to shape the remaining bone into a hemispherical shape without removing a significant amount (Fig. 1.177).
- Insert an acetabular trial of the same size as the last reamer and check for stability.
- Remove the final trial and reverse ream cancellous allograft into any remaining cavitary defects.
- Insert the acetabular component into place and fix it with multiple screws, ideally using the sciatic buttress and ischium for screw fixation.
- After the appropriate liner and head size are determined by trialing, insert the definitive liner and femoral head.
- Postoperatively, the patient should remain touch-down weight bearing for 6 to 12 weeks and progress to weight bearing to tolerance with a cane by 3 months.

CUP-CAGE TECHNIQUE FOR MANAGEMENT OF PELVIC DISCONTINUITY

TECHNIQUE 1.28

(ABDEL ET AL., MODIFIED)

- Expose the failed acetabular component through a posterolateral approach and remove it along with the fibrous membrane from the floor of the acetabulum.
- Stress the inferior half of the acetabulum to confirm the presence of a discontinuity.
- Place acetabular augments as needed for anterosuperior or posteroinferior segmental defects.
- Ream the acetabulum on reverse to shape the remaining bone into a hemispherical shape without removing a significant amount.
- Insert an acetabular trial of the same size as the last reamer and check for stability.
- Remove the final trial and reverse ream cancellous allograft into any remaining cavitary defect.
- Insert the acetabular component into place and fix it with multiple screws.
- Place the cage over the acetabular component.
- Distally the inferior flange of the cage can be fixed onto the ischium with screws or into a slot in the ischium; alternatively, the inferior flange can be removed before placement of the cage, for a so-called half-cage construct.
- Unitize the cage to the acetabular component by placing at least one screw through the cage and cup into the dome of the acetabulum.
- Place screws through the iliac flange of the cage superiorly.
- Proceed with trialing and acetabular liner and femoral head placement (Fig. 1.178).

In rare instances, the acetabulum is so deficient that a whole acetabular allograft or a custom triflanged component is the only option. Garbuz, Morsi, and Gross found that 45% of massive acetabular allograft revisions required revision at minimum 5-year follow-up. Their best results were obtained when the allograft was augmented with an acetabular reinforcement ring. DeBoer et al. reviewed a group of 20 hips in 18 patients with pelvic discontinuity treated with a custom, triflanged component. At average 10-year surveillance, no components were revised and none were radiographically loose. Dislocation was the most common complication, occurring in five hips. Procedures of this degree of complexity are best referred to a major center with surgeons skilled in revision surgery.

MANAGEMENT OF PELVIC DISCONTINUITY WITH ALLOGRAFTING AND CUSTOM COMPONENT

TECHNIQUE 1.29

(DEBOER ET AL.)

- Expose the failed acetabular component through a posterolateral approach and remove it along with any residual cement and fibrous membrane.
- Trace the sciatic nerve up to the greater sciatic notch to avoid injury during ischial dissection and cup implantation.
- Perform limited dissection in the sciatic notch region and avoid abductor tension by abduction and proximal translation of the femur.
- Elevate the gluteus medius subperiosteally off of the ilium for placement of the iliac flange of the component.
- Release part of the hamstring origin from the ischium before placement of the ischial flange.
- Place cancellous allograft bone along the area of the discontinuity.
- Fix the ischial flange first with multiple screws.
- Insert iliac screws second, reducing this flange to host bone.
- Place the desired acetabular liner, giving consideration to a dual mobility construct or constrained liner if the abductor muscles are deficient.

RECONSTRUCTION OF FEMORAL DEFICIENCIES

Femoral bone stock is deficient to some degree in most revisions, a condition that may result from (1) osteolysis caused by loosening, wear, or infection, (2) perforation or creation of windows during removal of the previous stem or other implant, (3) stress shielding from an excessively stiff implant, or (4) preexisting osteoporosis. Reconstruction may be complicated further by femoral deformity or fracture.

■ CLASSIFICATION

The AAOS Committee on the Hip proposed a system for the classification of femoral deficiencies in THA (Table 1.9). Although the system is most commonly used in reference to revision surgery, it also is applicable to primary arthroplasties. The essential terminology from the acetabular classification has been maintained to promote continuity. Accurate description of deficiencies simplifies preoperative planning (Fig. 1.179).

Femoral bony deficiencies are of two basic types: segmental and cavitary. A segmental deficit is defined as any loss of

American Academy of Orthopaedic Surgeons Classification of Femoral Deficiencies

Type I	Segmental deficiencies
	Proximal
	Partial
	Complete
	Intercalary
	Greater trochanter
Type II	Cavitary deficiencies
	Cancellous
	Cortical
	Ectasia
Type III	Combined deficiencies
Type IV	Malalignment
	Rotational
	Angular
Type V	Femoral stenosis
Type VI	Femoral discontinuity

From D'Antonio J, McCarthy JC, Barger WL, et al: Classification of femoral abnormalities in total hip arthroplasty. *Clin Orthop* 296:133–139. 1993.

bone in the supporting cortical shell of the femur. A cavitary deficit is a contained lesion representing an excavation of the cancellous or endosteal cortical bone without violation of the cortical shell of the femur. Involvement can be categorized as level I, proximal to the inferior border of the lesser trochanter; level II, from the inferior margin of the lesser trochanter to 10 cm distally; or level III, distal to level II.

Segmental femoral deficiencies can be divided further into deficiencies that are partial or complete and by their involvement of the anterior, medial, or posterior cortex. When a segmental deficit has intact bone above and below, such as with a cortical window, it is referred to as an *intercalary deficit.* The greater trochanter is treated as a separate segmental deficit because of the special problems of trochanteric nonunion and abductor insufficiency.

Cavitary deficits are subdivided according to the degree of bone loss present within the femur. *Cancellous deficits* represent loss of only the cancellous medullary bone. *Cortical cavitary deficits* are more extensive and involve loss of cancellous and endosteal cortical bone stock. Ectasia is a specialized cavitary deficit in which the femur is dilated in addition to loss of cancellous bone, with thinning of the cortex. Combined segmental and cavitary deficits often are encountered in revision surgery, such as when a loose stem subsides or migrates into varus or retroversion, and there is concomitant osteolysis.

Distortion of the femoral canal is described separately. *Malalignment* refers to a distortion of the femoral architectural geometry and can be either angular or rotational. Developmental diseases of the hip, fracture malunion, previous osteotomy, and the process of loosening all may contribute to malalignment. *Stenosis* describes a partial or complete occlusion of the femoral canal resulting from previous trauma, fixation devices, or bony hypertrophy. *Femoral discontinuity* refers to a loss of femoral integrity, from either an acute fracture or an established nonunion.

Della Valle and Paprosky developed a femoral defect classification along with guidelines for treatment of each type of deficiency. Type I femurs have minimal metaphyseal cancellous bone loss with an intact diaphysis. This type of defect occurs with uncemented, non–porous-coated, press-fit stems. Most type I femurs can be reconstructed with cemented or uncemented primary length components. Type II femurs have extensive cancellous metaphyseal bone loss down to the level of the lesser trochanter with an intact diaphysis. Calcar replacement stems are often required to restore limb length. Cementless stems with diaphyseal fixation from extensive porous coating, tapered fluted stems, and proximally porous-coated modular stems have been used successfully in this setting. Type IIIA defects are characterized by extensive metaphyseal cancellous bone loss with some diaphyseal bone loss as well, but with more than 4 cm of diaphyseal bone available for distal fixation. Extensively porous-coated stems 8 inches or longer and tapered fluted stems are recommended for type IIIA femurs. Type IIIB defects are differentiated by less than 4 cm of intact diaphysis with extensive metaphyseal and diaphyseal bone loss. Extensively porous-coated cylindrical stems have performed poorly in this setting. Impaction grafting of the femur may be considered in this situation, along with tapered fluted stems. Type IV femurs have a widened femoral canal and no diaphyseal bone of sufficient quality for cementless fixation. Impaction grafting or proximal femoral replacement with an allograft-prosthetic composite construct or modular tumor prosthesis may be used in this extreme bone deficiency (Fig. 1.180).

■ MANAGEMENT

High-quality anteroposterior and lateral radiographs of the femur are prerequisites for femoral revision. When significant proximal deficits are present, films showing the distal portion of the femur are necessary to evaluate bone stock for distal fixation. Preoperative templating is helpful in evaluating leg-length discrepancy and for selecting the correct implant diameter, length, neck length, and offset. The need for specialized implants and bone grafts also can be anticipated. The objectives of femoral revision surgery are to (1) maintain femoral integrity and bone stock, (2) achieve rigid prosthetic fixation, (3) restore hip biomechanics to promote efficient abductor function, and (4) equalize leg lengths.

■ SEGMENTAL DEFICITS

Segmental deficits, such as femoral cortical windows, create stress risers in bone that predispose to postoperative fracture. Biomechanical studies have shown that the stress pattern of a tubular bone returns to normal at a distance of two bone diameters distant to a defect. A revision stem of sufficient length to pass at least this distance beyond cortical defects is used. If the ratio of the diameter of the perforation to that of the femur is less than 30%, the decrease in strength is not appreciably different for holes of varying size. For perforations less than one third the diameter of the bone, particulate graft can be used.

For larger cortical windows, an onlay cortical allograft strut is used (Fig. 1.181). Allograft cortical struts typically are harvested from the proximal or distal femur or from the tibia. The endosteal surface of the allograft strut is contoured to match the outer diameter of the host femur and is secured with multiple cerclage wires (Fig. 1.182). The interfaces are augmented with autogenous or allograft cancellous bone graft. Cortical strut grafts reliably unite to the femoral cortex when fixation of the

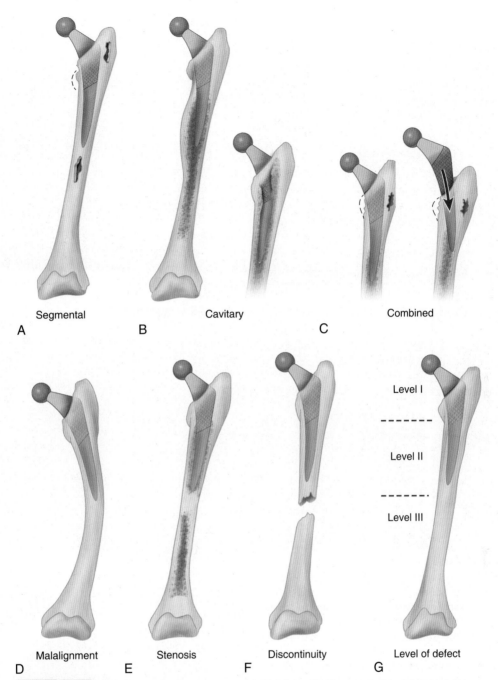

FIGURE 1.179 Femoral defects. **A,** Segmental defect: loss of femoral cortical bony support. It may be partial and proximal involving loss of bone through level of femur, or it may be intercalary lesion with intact bone above and below or involve greater trochanter. Most severe degree of segmental bone loss is complete proximal circumferential loss of bone. **B,** Cavitary defect: loss of cancellous or endosteal cortical bone without violation of outer cortical shell. Ectasia is severe form of cavitary defect in which femoral cavity is expanded. **C,** Combined defects: combination of segmental and cavitary bone loss in femur. It can occur in combination through any of three levels of femur. **D,** Malalignment: distortion of femoral architectural geometry in either rotational or angular plane. **E,** Femoral stenosis: partial or complete occlusion of femoral intramedullary canal. **F,** Femoral discontinuity: interruption of integrity of femoral shaft, usually as result of fracture or nonunion, with or without presence of implant. **G,** Femoral levels. (Redrawn from D'Antonio JA: Classification of femoral bony abnormalities. In Galante JO, Rosenberg AG, Callaghan JJ, editors: *Total hip revision surgery*, New York, 1995, Raven Press.)

graft and the implant is rigid. Lim et al. showed radiographic union in 96% of patients at an average of 5.4 years after surgery.

Segmental loss of cortical bone from the proximal femur is common in revision surgery. The medial neck frequently is absent down to and including the lesser trochanter. Femoral length must be restored for proper leg length and abductor tension.

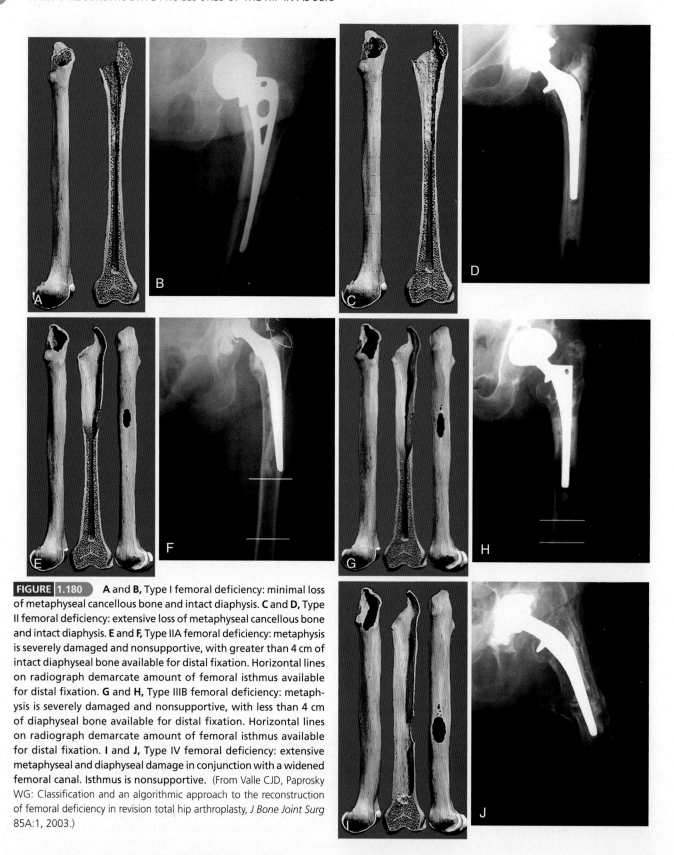

FIGURE 1.180 **A** and **B,** Type I femoral deficiency: minimal loss of metaphyseal cancellous bone and intact diaphysis. **C** and **D,** Type II femoral deficiency: extensive loss of metaphyseal cancellous bone and intact diaphysis. **E** and **F,** Type IIA femoral deficiency: metaphysis is severely damaged and nonsupportive, with greater than 4 cm of intact diaphyseal bone available for distal fixation. Horizontal lines on radiograph demarcate amount of femoral isthmus available for distal fixation. **G** and **H,** Type IIIB femoral deficiency: metaphysis is severely damaged and nonsupportive, with less than 4 cm of diaphyseal bone available for distal fixation. Horizontal lines on radiograph demarcate amount of femoral isthmus available for distal fixation. **I** and **J,** Type IV femoral deficiency: extensive metaphyseal and diaphyseal damage in conjunction with a widened femoral canal. Isthmus is nonsupportive. (From Valle CJD, Paprosky WG: Classification and an algorithmic approach to the reconstruction of femoral deficiency in revision total hip arthroplasty, *J Bone Joint Surg* 85A:1, 2003.)

A calcar replacement or extended neck prosthesis is a relatively simple option for restoring femoral length (Fig. 1.183). The opposite femur is templated to determine the size necessary to restore femoral length and offset. Rotational stability is achieved by using cement or a stem with distal flutes, extensive porous coating, or a curved stem. Reattachment of a trochanteric osteotomy fragment is difficult when a calcar replacement stem design has been used. Generally, no bony bed remains for reattachment, and although many such stem designs may provide for fixation of the trochanteric fragment to the stem, this is prone to failure. If trochanteric osteotomy is required for exposure, an extended-type osteotomy (see Fig. 1.153) is preferable when a calcar replacement stem is to be used.

When partial segmental deficits extend below the level of the lesser trochanter into zone II or III, a calcar replacement stem alone is insufficient, and distal fixation of the femoral component is required. The revision prosthesis must be supported predominantly by host bone; strut grafts are not reliable to provide primary support for the femoral component.

CAVITARY DEFICITS

Cavitary deficits are always present in the proximal femur to some degree after removal of the previous femoral component. If deficits are limited to cancellous bone and areas of intact trabecular bone remain adjacent to the cortex, sufficient cement interdigitation may occur to provide long-term fixation with a cemented revision prosthesis. Using second-generation cement technique, Mulroy and Harris found that 20% of stems had been revised again at 15.1 years, and an additional 6% were radiographically loose. Katz et al. found a similar failure rate

of 26% for cemented revision stems followed for more than 10 years. Third-generation cement technique has not improved the results with cemented femoral revisions. Hultmark et al. reported 85% survivorship at 10 years in 109 hips treated with second-generation or third-generation technique.

The loss of bone stock in the femur is a major factor in the failure of cemented femoral revisions. Often the trabecular surface of the bone is lost with a loosened prosthesis, leaving a smooth interface with few crevices for cement interdigitation. The mechanical interlock that is integral to cement fixation becomes difficult to obtain in this setting. In a cadaver study, Dohmae et al. measured femoral bone-cement interface shear strength at only 20.6% of primary strength after a single revision and 6.8% after a second cemented revision.

Particulate cancellous bone graft is useful for filling small deficits adjacent to a cementless revision stem that is mechanically stable by virtue of its fit within the canal. After obtaining the stem size that achieves stability, areas that require grafting are determined. The stem is inserted partially to occlude the canal and prevent the distal egress of particulate graft material. Cancellous

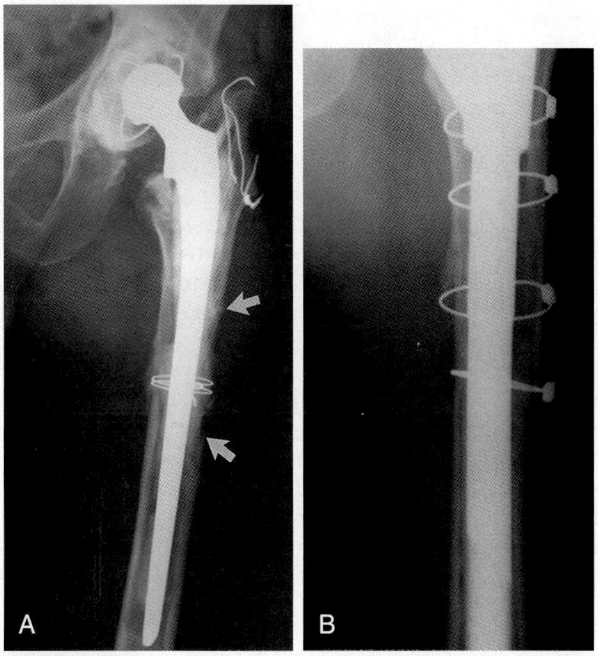

FIGURE 1.181 **A,** Patient was referred with failed long-stem cemented revision prosthesis. Large anterolateral cortical window had been created during previous surgery and was filled with cement *(arrows).* **B,** Window was used for cement removal. Femur was reconstructed with cementless long stem and allograft cortical strut to restore lateral cortex. Note restoration of bone stock at 3 years.

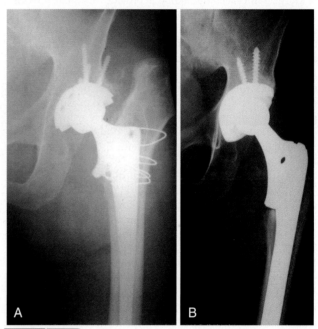

FIGURE 1.183 Restoration of femoral length with calcar replacement prosthesis. **A,** Severe stem subsidence produced this proximal segmental deficiency. Limb was 5 cm short. **B,** Length was easily restored, and stable fixation was achieved with calcar replacement stem.

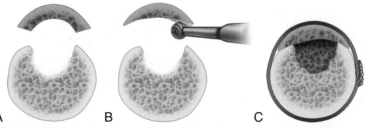

FIGURE 1.182 Placement of cortical allograft strut for femoral cortical defect. **A,** Mismatch between inner diameter of allograft strut and outer diameter of femur produced poor contact with host bone. **B,** Endosteal surface of graft is contoured with burr to produce matching curvatures. **C,** Graft is fixed securely with multiple cerclage wires.

bone graft is inserted into cavitary deficits as the stem is inserted so that the bone graft is impacted into position. Particulate bone grafting cannot be relied on, however, to provide axial or rotational stability to a cementless femoral component.

When more extensive cavitary deficits or ectasia is present proximally, a size mismatch occurs between the proximal and distal aspects of the femur. This mismatch can be accommodated in several ways:

1. Reaming the canal to a larger size to allow insertion of a larger implant that fills the metaphysis more completely
2. Use of a specialized revision femoral component that is intentionally oversized proximally compared with primary stems
3. Reliance on distal fixation of an extensively porous coated or tapered fluted component with cancellous grafting of proximal cavitary deficits or a reduction osteotomy of the proximal femur
4. Use of cancellous impaction bone grafting combined with a cemented femoral component

Reaming of the distal portion of the canal to allow insertion of a larger femoral component that provides adequate proximal fit sacrifices host bone unnecessarily. A larger diameter stem is more likely to produce stress shielding of the femur with additional bone loss. Larger, stiffer stems also have been implicated as a cause of postoperative thigh pain. To alleviate this problem, many implant systems now include modular revision femoral components with two or more proximal stem sizes for each distal diameter. These implants are oversized proximally compared with implants typically used in primary arthroplasties.

Cameron advocated the use of a modular stem to allow individual sizing of the proximal and distal portions of the femoral canal so that deficiencies can be managed without the need for additional removal of distal bone (see Fig. 1.26). Precise reaming of the remaining proximal bone stock allows a stem with limited porous coating to be used while restoring proximal loading of the femur. Using this approach, Cameron reported a 1.4% rate of aseptic loosening in a group of 320 revision arthroplasties at a mean follow-up of 7 years. McCarthy and Lee found 60% survivorship at 14-year follow-up using the same type of implant. Their series showed reliable fixation in Paprosky type II and IIIA femurs, but they recommended other forms of fixation for type IIIB and IV deficiencies. The version of this implant with hydroxyapatite sleeves has had excellent results in a series of predominantly type I through IIIA femoral defects, with 90.5% survivorship at 15-year follow-up and 0.7% rate of aseptic loosening.

MANAGEMENT OF FEMORAL DEFICIT WITH MODULAR FEMORAL COMPONENT

TECHNIQUE 1.30

(CAMERON)
- Perform the neck resection at the appropriate level, based on preoperative templating and/or intraoperative use of the neck resection guide. The neck resection is made per-

pendicular to the long axis of the femur. In the revision setting, further neck resection may not be necessary.
- Ream the diaphysis of the femur with straight rigid reamers until cortical contact is achieved. Final reamer diameter should be equal to or 0.5 mm larger than the minor diameter of the proposed femoral component.
- Ream the metaphysis with the appropriate conical reamer until cortical contact occurs within the metaphysis.
- Prepare the calcar region by milling with the triangle reamer to accommodate the triangular portion of the metaphyseal sleeve.
- Impact the trial metaphyseal sleeve.
- Assemble the remainder of the diaphyseal portion of the stem along with the proximal body and neck. Place this portion down the femoral canal in the desired amount of anteversion. This can be adjusted independent of the orientation of the metaphyseal sleeve.
- After trial reduction ensures adequate length and stability, place the final components as described previously for the trial components. Consider placing a prophylactic cable or wire around the proximal femur if it is osteopenic to prevent fracture.

Extensively porous-coated stems (see Fig. 1.25) achieve stability through distal fixation when proximal bone stock is deficient. Some of the longest follow-up studies of cementless femoral revisions have used this technique. At a mean 7.4 years, Lawrence, Engh, and Macalino found that 5.7% of stems required repeat revision. Weeden and Paprosky reported an overall mechanical failure rate of only 4.1% of extensively porous-coated revision stems with distal fixation at 14.2 years. Emerson, Head, and Higgins reported similarly favorable results with a 40% porous-coated calcar replacement stem. At average 11.5 years' follow-up, 94% remained in situ with only 3% mechanical failure rate leading to revision. These results surpass the results of most cemented femoral revision series with comparable follow-up.

REVISION WITH EXTENSIVELY POROUS-COATED FEMORAL STEM

TECHNIQUE 1.31

(MALLORY AND HEAD)
- Perform the neck resection at the appropriate level, based on preoperative templating and/or intraoperative use of the neck resection guide or a trial prosthesis. Approximately two thirds of the proximal femoral component should be supported by host bone.
- Ream the diaphysis of the femur with flexible reamers if a bowed component is desired. Reaming continues until cortical contact occurs. Rigid cylindrical reamers are used if a straight femoral component is chosen. Bowed stems require overreaming by one millimeter, whereas straight stems are reamed "line-to-line," in that the stem matches the size of the last reamer.

- Broach the proximal femur with appropriately sized broaches attached to a distal pilot of the same size as the last reamer. Broaching may be unnecessary or even impossible if the proximal femur is osteopenic.
- Assemble a trial component of the correct size and perform a trial reduction to ensure appropriate limb length, stability, and offset.
- Place the final femoral component, carefully maintaining the desired amount of anteversion while remaining vigilant for fractures.

- Thread the reamer adapter to the distal portion of the stem and ream the metaphysis.
- Perform a trial reduction with a provisional proximal segment. Adjust leg length, anteversion, and offset as needed for stability.
- Place the definitive proximal portion of the femoral component and reduce the hip.
- If an extended trochanteric osteotomy was performed, reduce the osteotomy and repair it with cerclage wiring. Preserve blood supply to the proximal femur as much as possible.

Unreliable fixation occurs with extensively porous coated stems when less than 4 cm of diaphyseal bone remains (Paprosky IIIB). Impaction grafting techniques and tapered fluted stems are recommended in this setting. Tapered fluted stems historically suffered from high rates of subsidence and problems with dislocation. Modular designs, which allow independent sizing of the distal and proximal portions, allow for more reliable distal fixation with lower rates of subsidence and improved restoration of offset and limb length (see Fig. 1.122). Often these components are combined with various types of femoral osteotomy to allow "straight-shot" access to the distal femur and to reduce the risk of femoral perforation or fracture. Mechanical failure of the modular taper has been reported and has led several authors to recommend some structural support to the proximal body of the prosthesis by cabling the host bone around the stem or by allograft augmentation with struts or more substantial grafts. In a retrospective multicenter series of 143 patients treated with the same modular fluted tapered stem, survivorship was 97% with 2.1-mm mean subsidence at average 40 months, follow-up. Another series of patients treated with modular tapered fluted stems for aseptic loosening with longer follow-up, including patients with Paprosky III or IV femoral defects, found 96% survivorship at 10 years.

When diaphyseal fixation is used, large gaps may remain between the femoral component and the remaining proximal femoral cortical shell. Kim and Franks described the use of a longitudinal wedge osteotomy of the posterolateral femoral cortex to reduce the size of the proximal femur. After removal of the cortical wedge, the remaining segments of cortex are carefully compressed, and cerclage wires are placed around the proximal portion of the revision stem. A reduction osteotomy restores some degree of proximal support of the prosthesis and improves the apposition of bone to the porous surface of the implant, improving the chances for bone ingrowth in difficult revisions.

Gie et al. described a technique for management of proximal femoral deficiencies that combines impaction bone grafting with a cemented revision stem (Fig. 1.184). The authors reported 98.8% survivorship for aseptic loosening and 87.7% survivorship for revision at 20 years with 705 femoral revision arthroplasties using this technique. Most of the complications were caused by dislocation (4.1%) or femoral fracture (5.4%). Similarly, a Swedish study of 1305 impaction grafting femoral revisions found 94% survivorship for all causes of failure at 15 years.

Collarless polished stems and collared stems with various finishes have been used successfully with impaction grafting in multiple studies. Longer-term follow-up is necessary to assess the effect of surface finish on the success of this technique. Impaction grafting requires specialized instrumentation and the availability of large amounts of cancellous bone graft. We have used this approach in some patients and been impressed by the degree of restoration of proximal femoral bone stock.

MANAGEMENT OF PROXIMAL FEMORAL BONE LOSS WITH MODULAR TAPERED FLUTED STEM

TECHNIQUE 1.32

(KWONG ET AL.)
- Expose and remove the previous femoral component by a posterolateral approach. Use an extended trochanteric osteotomy if necessary.
- Ream the diaphysis of the femur into a tapered shape with the appropriate reamers. Ream to the depth established by preoperative templating.
- Impact the distal portion of the stem into the prepared distal femur. Seat the stem only as far as reaming has occurred, based on preoperative templating. Place the stem initially with the bow directed laterally. Rotate the stem, moving the bow anteriorly as the stem is driven down the femoral shaft.

MANAGEMENT OF PROXIMAL FEMORAL DEFICIENCIES WITH IMPACTION BONE GRAFTING AND CEMENTED REVISION STEM

TECHNIQUE 1.33

(GIE, MODIFIED)
- Expose and remove the previous femoral component.
- Debride any residual cement or fibrous membrane from the canal. A well-fixed cement plug may be retained to support the bone graft and cement column.

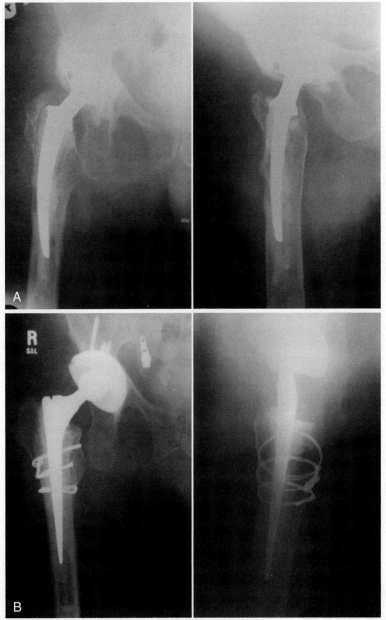

FIGURE 1.184 Impaction grafting. **A,** Failed cemented femoral component with large cavitary deficiencies and ectasia. **B,** One year after impaction grafting and cemented revision with collarless, polished, tapered stem. Small degree of subsidence has occurred.

- Inspect the femur for segmental defects. If present, occlude these with wire mesh or allograft struts.
- Occlude the canal 3 cm below the lowest cavitary defect or below the planned tip of the stem.
- After placing the centering guide, pack the canal with cancellous chips using progressively sized cylindrical packers.
- When the canal is two thirds full, shape the canal with the appropriately sized tamps. Tamping continues until rotational stability of the last tamp is achieved.
- Perform a trial reduction and assess leg length and stability.
- Remove the tamp and inject cement into the canal with a cement gun, followed by the definitive femoral prosthesis.

◼ MASSIVE DEFICITS

Occasionally, bone loss in the proximal femur is so extensive that the remaining bone cannot support a new prosthesis. Most patients with this problem have had multiple previous operations on the hip, and the femur may have been fractured or perforated. The cortex in the proximal femur is thin and fragile and may be completely absent in several areas, requiring a massive proximal femoral allograft or modular proximal femoral replacement prosthesis for reconstruction of the femur. Large segment allografts usually must be purchased from a regional tissue bank, and careful preoperative planning is required to ensure a graft of adequate size and length is obtained. Calibration markers are placed on preoperative radiographs of the allograft to ensure the graft spans the

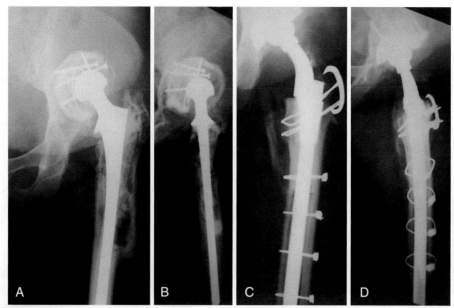

FIGURE 1.185 Proximal femoral allograft. **A** and **B,** Extensive ectasia and osteolysis of proximal femoral cortex in 42-year-old woman with three previous failed revisions. Distal portion of stem remained well fixed and required slotting of femur for removal of cement and stem. **C** and **D,** Reconstruction with proximal femoral allograft. Long step-cut in graft covered cortical slot and improved rotational stability between graft and host bone. Stem was cemented to graft only and not distally.

length of the bony deficit, and the canal of the graft is templated to ensure a prosthesis of adequate size can be placed through the graft. A large discrepancy between the diameter of the graft and the host femur makes the reconstruction more difficult.

Cement provides the best fixation between the prosthesis and allograft because bone ingrowth cannot be expected to occur. Most authors recommend fixation of the prosthesis into the distal host bone without cement if technically feasible. Whatever the means of fixation, axial and rotational stability must be achieved at the allograft-host junction. This can be accomplished by making a step-cut osteotomy (Fig. 1.185), by press-fitting the allograft into the host femur, or by using a plate or an additional onlay cortical strut.

Proximal femoral allograft reconstructions are technically demanding and are associated with higher complication rates than other revision procedures. Union at the graft-host junction often requires months, and unprotected weight bearing should be delayed until there is radiographic evidence of union. Despite incorporation at the interface, the greater substance of the graft persists as dead bone throughout the duration of implantation. Dislocation rates are high, and numerous authors advocate the prophylactic use of an abduction orthosis or spica cast. Fracture is common with unsupported load-bearing allografts, and these grafts should be supported by an intramedullary stem crossing the allograft-host junction. Because of the length of the procedure and the degree of soft-tissue dissection, infection is more common than in other revision arthroplasties, and these infections usually result in failure because of the large segment of dead bone. Most surgeons advocate the use of antibiotic-impregnated cement in procedures requiring large-segment allografts, although no long-term studies are available to support this practice.

Sternheim et al. published the longest follow-up study of allograft-prosthetic composites. They followed 28 patients for an average of 15 years and reported 75% survivorship. At similar long-term follow-up, Babis et al. reported a 69% success rate at 12 years.

MANAGEMENT OF MASSIVE DEFICITS WITH PROXIMAL FEMORAL ALLOGRAFT-PROSTHESIS COMPOSITE

TECHNIQUE 1.34

- Preferably, two separate surgical teams are available for the procedure. After appropriate measurements are taken, one team prepares the allograft while the other completes the surgical exposure, removes the components and cement, and prepares the distal femur.
- Expose the hip and femoral shaft through a transtrochanteric approach.
- Osteotomize the trochanter as a large fragment so that it can be rigidly reattached to the allograft later.
- Place a pin in the pelvis and measure the length of the femur to a fixed point distally so that limb length can be accurately restored.

- Dislocate the hip and remove the femoral component by previously described techniques.
- Evaluate the extent of bony deficiency and determine if an allograft is necessary for reconstruction. If so, divide the femoral shaft at the distal extent of the bony deficiency. Often the deficiency is more pronounced on one side of the bone than the other.
- Make a step-cut, oblique, or transverse osteotomy of the femur, preserving the best bone on the host distal femur.
- Split the remaining proximal femur longitudinally, preserving as much of the soft-tissue attachment as possible.
- Remove residual cement and membrane from the proximal fragments.
- Take cultures of the femoral allograft.
- Measure the length of the proximal femur that must be replaced and fashion the allograft to match the femoral osteotomy.
- Maintain proper rotational alignment between the allograft and host bone by aligning the linea aspera.
- Prepare the allograft at a separate workstation while cement is being removed from the remainder of the distal femur. Stabilize the allograft in a vise and use reamers and broaches to prepare it in standard fashion. Avoid excessive reaming of the allograft in an attempt to place a larger sized stem because the graft would be weakened.
- Place the trial femoral prosthesis within the allograft in the correct degree of anteversion and insert the composite into the distal femur.
- Trim the bone as necessary to produce a precise fit at the allograft-host junction.
- Provisionally fix the junction with bone-holding forceps or with a heavy plate held with forceps at each end.
- Measure the limb length, evaluate the stability of the joint, and make any necessary adjustments. Several trial reductions may be necessary to adjust the length of the limb and to contour precisely the junction between the allograft and the remaining host bone.
- Select a femoral prosthesis long enough to bypass the junction and achieve distal stability. Cement the prosthesis into the allograft first.
- Clean the graft with pulsed lavage and use cement mixed with porosity reduction techniques (see Technique 1.6).
- Remove cement from the distal portions of the stem and allograft. Pay special attention to the removal of cement from the distal end of the graft because it may impair union at the allograft-host junction.
- After the cement has hardened, insert the prosthesis-allograft composite into the distal femur. Often the size of the femoral component precludes a secure press-fit into the distal fragment. Axial and rotational stability usually still can be achieved by fixing the step-cut with multiple heavy cerclage wires or by placing supplemental allograft struts and cables.
- If cement is to be used for distal fixation, occlude the canal with a PMMA plug or plastic restrictor.
- Cement the stem into the distal femur as a separate step and carefully remove cement from the interface between the allograft and host bone.
- Augment the junction with additional morselized cancellous bone graft.

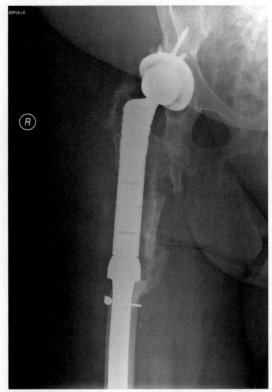

FIGURE 1.186 Modular proximal femoral replacement stem. Massive osteolysis caused by loose cemented stem with unreconstructable proximal femur required proximal femoral replacement. Remaining proximal femoral fragments were wrapped around prosthesis to enhance soft tissue attachment and leg control.

- Use the remaining fragments of the proximal femur to form a vascularized envelope around the allograft-host junction and use additional cerclage wires to fix them in position.
- Resect a portion of the greater trochanter from the allograft and prepare a bed for stable fixation of the host trochanteric fragment.
- Use wires or a trochanteric fixation device to secure the greater trochanter under appropriate tension.

Proximal femoral replacement traditionally has been limited to elderly, low-demand patients with severely compromised femoral bone not appropriate for other reconstructive techniques. Modular prostheses with proximal porous coating for improved reattachment of soft tissue and bone have been developed to improve restoration of limb length and instability issues that plagued previous megaprostheses (Fig. 1.186). In an analysis of the available literature regarding these implants in the treatment of nonneoplastic conditions, Korim et al. studied 356 hips followed for an average of 3.8 years. The implant retention rate was 83%, with a 23% reoperation rate, most commonly due to instability (16%). With longer-term follow-up, survivorship rates worsen, not surprisingly. Another series of 44 patients treated with proximal femoral replacement for Paprosky IIIB or IV femoral defects showed 86% survivorship without any revision or implant removal at 5 years and 66% at 10 years.

The relatively poor results must be balanced against the desperate circumstances surrounding these operations in multiply operated and often medically compromised patients.

MANAGEMENT OF MASSIVE DEFICITS WITH MODULAR MEGAPROSTHESIS

TECHNIQUE 1.35

(KLEIN ET AL.)

- Remove the previous femoral component through the desired approach. Exposure and removal of the femoral component is facilitated by the extreme bone loss already present.
- If necessary, split the femur in the coronal plane to expedite stem removal.
- Remove metal debris, cement, or other retained foreign material from around the femur.
- Expose and inspect the acetabular component. If it is well positioned and stable, it can be retained; otherwise, revise it as needed, being mindful that a constrained liner may be necessary.
- Perform a transverse femoral osteotomy at the most proximal level with intact circumferential bone.
- Prepare the distal femur by broaching, preserving available cancellous bone to allow better cement interdigitation.
- Place trial components and assess limb length, soft-tissue tension, and stability. Mark the distal femur with electrocautery to ensure proper rotational alignment of the final prosthesis.
- Insert a cement restrictor to the appropriate level and cement the femoral component into place. Make sure that the proximal flare of the prosthesis rests directly against the distal femoral segment, without intervening cement.
- Approximate the proximal femoral fragments to the proximal body of the prosthesis with wire or nonabsorbable suture. With the leg abducted, reattach the greater trochanter to the proximal body with nonabsorbable sutures through the holes in the prosthesis. If the trochanter is absent, the abductors may be sutured to the vastus lateralis or TFL.
- Reduce the hip and assess stability. If the hip is unstable despite restored limb lengths and appropriate component position, place a constrained liner, either by snap-fit or cementation, depending on the type of acetabular component in place.

■ FEMORAL DEFORMITY

Occasionally, femoral revision is complicated by residual angular malalignment of the femoral canal, so a revision prosthesis with a straight lateral border cannot be inserted without fracturing the femur. This is most common when a loose, cemented stem migrates into varus (Fig. 1.187). Other causes include malunion of fractures and previous femoral

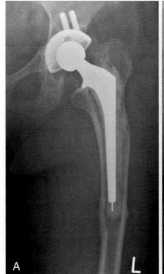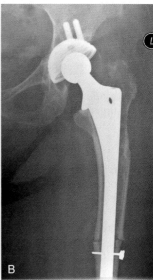

FIGURE 1.187   **A,** Osteotomy for femoral deformity. Loose cemented femoral component and osteolysis caused excessive varus and anterior bow. Standard long-stem prosthesis cannot accommodate deformity without fracture of femur. **B,** Transverse femoral osteotomy corrected deformity. Extensively porous coated stem gave excellent axial and rotational stability at osteotomy. No external immobilization was necessary.

osteotomies. In these cases, a femoral osteotomy must be done before a revision prosthesis can be safely inserted. The site and orientation of the osteotomy must be carefully planned by templating preoperative radiographs. An osteotomy to correct deformity in two planes may be required. The greatest difficulty involves obtaining rotational stability at the osteotomy site. Augmentation at the osteotomy site with allograft struts or a cable-plate may be necessary. Extensively porous-coated, distally tapered, fluted, and proximally porous-coated modular implants with flutes have been used successfully in combination with femoral osteotomy.

POSTOPERATIVE MANAGEMENT OF TOTAL HIP ARTHROPLASTY

There is no universally accepted postoperative rehabilitation program after THA. Although a pain-free hip can be restored with the most limited of efforts, a well-constructed rehabilitation program speeds the recovery of motion and function, diminishes limp, and aids the return to independent living.

Ideally, rehabilitation should begin before the operation. A patient who is motivated, informed, and has appropriate goals is a better participant in the rehabilitation process. A preoperative session may be used to teach the appropriate mechanisms for transfers, the use of supportive devices, how to negotiate steps, dislocation precautions, and the anticipated schedule for recuperation and hospital discharge.

In the immediate postoperative period, the hip is positioned in approximately 15 degrees of abduction while the patient is recovering from the anesthetic. For patients treated with a posterior approach, we use a triangular pillow to maintain abduction and prevent extremes of flexion (Fig. 1.188). This device aids rolling onto the opposite side in the early postoperative period but limits independent motion to some degree. Straps used to secure this device to the limb must be positioned carefully to avoid undue pressure on the peroneal nerve. For patients in whom a direct anterior approach is used, a pillow may be used instead.

If patient discomfort and anesthesia recovery allow, bed exercises and limited mobilization may be initiated on the day of surgery. Deep breathing, ankle pumps, quadriceps and gluteal isometrics, and gentle rotation exercises are begun. Straight leg raising, although beneficial after total knee surgery, is not helpful after THA. Groin pain often results, and this exercise places unnecessary rotational stress on the femoral component in the early postoperative period. Patients are instructed to exercise for a few minutes each hour they are awake.

When anesthetic recovery and pain allow, the patient can sit on the side of the bed or in a chair in a semirecumbent position. One or two pillows in the seat of the chair helps prevent excessive flexion. An additional pillow between the thighs limits adduction and internal rotation.

Gait training usually can begin on the day of surgery. Most elderly patients require a walker for balance and stability. Many younger patients require a walker for only a few days and progress more rapidly. The amount of weight bearing allowed on the operated limb depends on the means of fixation of the components, the presence of structural bone grafts, stress risers in the femur, and trochanteric osteotomy. If the components were cemented, early weight bearing to tolerance is permitted. With cementless, porous ingrowth implants, many authors recommend limited weight bearing for 6 to 8 weeks, whereas others encourage early weight bearing as comfort allows. In a literature review involving cementless implants and weight-bearing restrictions, Hol et al. found no adverse effects on subsidence and osseointegration with unrestricted weight bearing. They did recommend protected weight bearing during stair climbing for the first weeks after surgery because of high torsional loads. All implants and patients may not be the same in this regard, and the decision must be individualized according to the implant and experience of the surgeon. When the patient is able to walk far enough to reach the bathroom with supervision, bathroom privileges with an elevated toilet seat are allowed. A bedside commode may be used initially.

A few periods of instruction by an occupational therapist are useful. Patients who live alone can return to independent living sooner if they are able to dress, put on shoes, pick up objects from the floor, and carry out other activities of daily living in a safe manner. Many simple appliances are available to assist in these activities.

The patient can be discharged when able to get in and out of bed independently, walk over level surfaces, and climb a few steps. Printed instructions reviewing the home exercise program and precautions to prevent dislocation are helpful. The necessity of hip precautions has been questioned recently. A meta-analysis including 1122 patients from six studies concluded that unrestricted patients were more satisfied and resumed activity quicker without an increase in dislocation rate.

Initiatives to control the cost of THA have led to shortened hospital stays, and even same-day discharge from outpatient surgery centers in increasing numbers of cases. Outpatient or home health physical therapy historically has

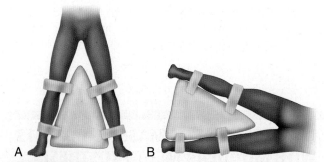

FIGURE 1.188 Triangular pillow splint used to keep hip abducted and neutrally rotated (see text). **A,** Anterior view with patient supine. **B,** Posterior view with patient in lateral position.

been recommended for all patients after discharge from the hospital. Recently, internet-based, self-directed physical therapy has grown in popularity in some centers. Klement et al. studied 941 patients initially managed with self-directed physical therapy after discharge and found that approximately one third were prescribed outpatient physical therapy because of slow recovery.

Patients with multiple joint involvement, preexisting weakness, or lack of social support may require an additional period of inpatient care at an inpatient facility before they can return safely to independent living. Carefully constructed protocols for exercise regimens, dislocation precautions (if desired), medical management, and anticoagulation make the transfer of care from one facility to another much easier.

For the first 6 weeks after surgery, patients may use an elevated toilet seat and one or two ordinary pillows between the knees when lying on the nonoperative side. Showers but not baths are allowed when wound healing is satisfactory. Sexual activity can be resumed in the supine position.

The patient is seen in the outpatient clinic approximately 2 weeks after surgery, and radiographs are made. If the procedure was an uncomplicated primary arthroplasty, two-handed support can be discontinued and the patient instructed in the use of a cane when strength and balance allow. The timing of this transition is usually best determined between the patient and their supervising physical therapist. If structural bone grafting was required, or the procedure was a revision, crutches can be continued for 3 months or longer, depending on radiographic incorporation of bone grafts. We encourage use of a cane until pain and limp have resolved. In patients who have had revision procedures, continued use of a cane is advisable. Strengthening exercises for the abductor muscles help eliminate limp. Stretching exercises are continued until the patient is able to reach the foot for dressing and nail care. The feet are dressed by placing the ankle of the operated limb on the opposite knee. Patients with uncomplicated hip procedures usually can resume driving at approximately 2 to 4 weeks. This decision should be individualized, depending on the return of strength, leg control, and reaction time.

Gait analysis and force-plate data suggest that recovery of strength in the musculature around the hip is a prolonged process. Foucher et al. reported persistent abductor weakness at 1 year postoperatively, supporting the need for a prolonged, supervised exercise regimen.

Many patients with sedentary occupations can return to work after 4 weeks. At 2 to 3 months, patients can return to occupations requiring limited lifting and bending. We do not encourage patients to return to manual labor after THA.

Limited athletic activity is permitted. Swimming, cycling, and golfing are acceptable. Jogging, racquet sports, and other activities requiring repetitive impact loading or extremes of positioning of the hip are unwise, and patients should be warned that such activities may increase the risk of failure of the arthroplasty.

After arthroplasty, cardiovascular fitness usually improves. Ries et al. found significant improvement in exercise duration, maximal workload, and peak oxygen consumption in hip arthroplasty patients compared with controls treated medically.

Follow-up visits are made at 6 weeks, 3 months, 1 year, and periodically thereafter. Routine radiographs are made at 2-year intervals and compared with previous films for signs of loosening, migration, wear, and implant failure. Regular follow-up is advised because loosening, wear, and osteolysis may occur in the absence of clinical symptoms, and revision is more difficult if the diagnosis is delayed until symptoms occur.

REFERENCES

GENERAL

Adelani MA, Keeney JA, Palisch A, et al.: Has total hip arthroplasty in patients 30 years or younger improved? A systematic review, *Clin Orthop Relat Res* 471:2595, 2013.

Huo MH, Dumont GD, Knight JR, Mont MA: What's new in total hip arthroplasty, *J Bone Joint Surg* 93:1944, 2011.

Huo MH, Stockton KG, Mont MA, Bucholz RW: What's new in total hip arthroplasty, *J Bone Joint Surg* 94:1721, 2012.

Khanuja HS, Vakil JJ, Goddard MS, Mont MA: Cementless femoral fixation in total hip arthroplasty, *J Bone Joint Surg* 93A:500, 2011.

Murphy BPD, Dowsey MM, Choong PFM: The impact of advanced age on the outcomes of primary total hip and knee arthroplasty for osteoarthritis: a systematic review, *J Bone Joint Rev* 6(e6), 2018.

Murphy BPD, Dowsey MM, Spelman T, et al.: What is the impact of advancing age on the outcomes of total hip arthroplasty? *J Arthroplasty* 33(4):1101, 2018.

Ninomiya JT, Dean JC, Incavo SJ: What's new in hip replacement, *J Bone Joint Surg* 97:1543, 2015.

Russell RD, Estrera KA, Pivec R, et al.: What's new in total hip arthroplasty, *J Bone Joint Surg* 95:1719, 2013.

Shershon RA, Diaz A, Bohl DD, et al.: Effect of body mass index on digital templating for total hip arthroplasty, *J Arthroplasty* 32(3):1024, 2017.

BIOMECHANICS, MATERIALS, IMPLANT DESIGN

BIOMECHANICS

Berry DJ: Utility of modular implants in primary total hip arthroplasty, *J Arthroplasty* 29:657, 2014.

Elkins JM, Callaghan JJ, Brown TD: The "landing zone" for wear and stability in total hip arthroplasty is smaller than we thought: a computational analysis, *Clin Orthop Relat Res* 473:441, 2015.

Gustke K: Short stems for total hip arthroplasty. Initial experience with the Fitmore™ stem, *J Bone Joint Surg* 94(Suppl A):47, 2012.

Howie DW, Holubowycz OT, Middleton R, The Large Articulation Study Group: Large femoral heads decrease the incidence of dislocation after total hip arthroplasty. A randomized controlled trial, *J Bone Joint Surg* 94:1095, 2012.

Jamieson ML, Russell RD, Incavo SJ, Noble PC: Does an enhanced surface finish improve acetabular fixation in revision total hip arthroplasty? *J Arthroplasty* 26:644, 2011.

Kawanabe K, Akiyama H, Goto K, et al.: Load dispersion effects of acetabular reinforcement devices used in revision total hip arthroplasty, *J Arthroplasty* 26:1061, 2011.

Kosashvili Y, Omoto D, Backstein D, et al.: Acetabular alignment and primary arc of motion for minus, skirtless, and skirted 28-, 32-, 36-, and 40-mm femoral heads, *J Arthroplasty* 28:279, 2013.

Kwon DG, Lee TJ, Kang JS, Moon KH: Correlation between stress shielding and clinical outcomes after total hip arthroplasty with extensively porous coated stems, *J Arthroplasty* 28:1728, 2013.

Kwon YM, Fehring TK, Lombardi AV, et al.: Risk stratification algorithm for management of patients with dual modular taper total hip arthroplasty: consensus statement of the American Association of Hip and Knee Surgeons, the American Academy of Orthopaedic Surgeons and the Hip Society, *J Arthroplasty* 29:2060, 2014.

Lachiewicz PF, Soileau ES: Low early and late dislocation rates with 36- and 40-mm heads in patients at high risk for dislocation, *Clin Orthop Relat Res* 471:439, 2013.

Lam L, Drew T, Boscainos P: Effect of acetabular orientation of stress distribution of highly cross-linked polyethylene liners, *Orthopedics* 36:e1346, 2013.

Lombardi Jr AV, Skeels MD, Berend KR, et al.: Do large heads enhance stability and restore native anatomy in primary total hip arthroplasty? *Clin Orthop Relat Res* 469:1547, 2011.

Molloy DO, Munir S, Cross MB, et al.: Fretting and corrosion in modular-neck total hip arthroplasty femoral stems, *J Bone Joint Surg* 96:488, 2014.

Moussa ME, Esposito CI, Elpers ME, et al.: Hip dislocation increases roughness of oxidized zirconium femoral heads in total hip arthroplasty: an analysis of 59 retrievals, *J Arthroplasty* 30:713, 2015.

Moyer R, Lanting B, Marsh J, et al.: Postoperative gait mechanics after total hip arthroplasty: systematic review and meta-analysis, *JBJS Rev* 6:e1, 2018.

Munro JT, Vioreanu MH, Masri BA, Duncan CP: Acetabular liner with focal constraint to prevent dislocation after THA, *Clin Orthop Relat Res* 471:3883, 2013.

Nam D, Barrack RL, Clohisy JC, et al.: Proximal femur bone density decreases up to 5 years after total hip arthroplasty in young, active patients, *J Arthroplasty* 31:2825, 2016.

Skendzel JG, Blaha JD, Urquhart AG: Case report. Total hip arthroplasty modular neck failure, *J Arthroplasty* 26:338, 2011, e1.

Terrier A, Florencio FL, Rüdiger HA: Benefit of cup medialization in total hip arthroplasty is associated with femoral anatomy, *Clin Orthop Relat Res* 472:3159, 2014.

Torelsen A, Makhau E, Sillesen N, Malchau H: A review of current fixation use and registry outcomes in total hip arthroplasty: the uncemented paradox, *Clin Orthop Relat Res* 471:2052, 2013.

von Lewinski G, Floerkemeier T: 10-year experience with short stem total hip arthroplasty, *Orthopedics* 38(Suppl 3):S51, 2015.

Waligora AC, Owen JR, Wayne JS, et al.: The effect of prophylactic cerclage wires in primary total hip arthroplasty: a biomechanical study, *J Arthroplasty* 32:2023, 2017.

Wegrzyn J, Tebaa E, Jacquel A, et al.: Can dual mobility cups prevent dislocation in all situations after revision total hip arthroplasty? *J Arthroplasty* 30:631, 2015.

ACETABULAR COMPONENT DESIGN

Akbari A, Roy ME, Whiteside LA, et al.: Minimal backside surface changes observed in retrieved acetabular liners, *J Arthroplasty* 26:686, 2011.

Catelli DS, Kowalski E, Beaulé PE, et al.: Does the dual-mobility hip prosthesis produce better joint kinematics during extreme hip flexion task? *J Arthroplasty* 32:3206, 2017.

Darrith B, Courtney PM, Della Valle CJ: Outcomes of dual mobility components in ttal hip arthroplasty: a systematic review of the literature, *Bone Joint J* 100-B:11, 2018.

De Martino I, D'Apolito R, Soranoglou VG, et al.: Dislocation following total hip arthroplasty using dual mobility acetabular components: a systematic review, *Bone Joint J* 99-B(1 Supple A):18, 2017.

Hiuguera Rueda CA, Ferguson DF, Scholl L, et al.: Influence of acetabular shell position and component design on hip dynamic dislocation, *J Arthroplasty* 34:766, 2019.

Jones CW, De Martino I, D'Apolito R, et al.: The use of dual-mobility bearings in patients at high risk of dislocation, *Bone Joint J* 101-B(1 Supple A):41, 2019.

Kurdziel MD, Ennin KA, Baker KC, et al.: Increasing liner anteversion decreases the interfacial strength of polyethylene liners cemented into titanium-alloy acetabular shells, *J Arthroplasty* 31:2922, 2016.

Van der Merwe JM: Comprehensive review of current constraining devices in total hip arthroplasty, *J Am Acad Orthop Surg* 26:479, 2018.

FEMORAL COMPONENT DESIGN

Allepuz A, Havelin L, Barber T, et al.: Effect of femoral head size on metal-on-HXLPE hip arthroplasty outcome in a combined analysis of six national and regional registries, *J Bone Joint Surg* 96(Suppl 1E):12, 2014.

Alonso-Rasgado T, Dell-Valle-Mojica JF, Jiminez-Cruz D, et al.: Cement interface and bone stress in total hip arthroplasty: relationship to head size, *Int J Orthop Res* 36:2966, 2018.

Knutsen AR, Lau N, Longjohn DB, et al.: Periprothetic femoral bone loss in total hip arthroplasty: systematic analysis of the effect of stem design, *Hip Ing* 27:26, 2017.

Lanting B, Naudie DDR, McCalden RW: Clinical impact of trunnion wear after total hip arthroplasty, *JBJS Rev* 4:e4, 2016.

Mueller U, Panzram B, Braun S, et al.: Mixing of head-stem components in total hip arthroplasty, *J Arthroplasty* 33:945, 2018.

Triantafyllopoulos GK, Elpers ME, Burket C, et al.: Large heads to not increase damage at the head-neck taper of metal-on-polyethylene total hip arthroplasties, *Clin Orthop Relat Res* 474:330, 2016.

BEARINGS

Amanatullah DF, Landa J, Strauss EJ, et al.: Comparison of surgical outcomes and implant wear between ceramic-ceramic and ceramic-polyethylene articulations in total hip arthroplasty, *J Arthroplasty* 26(Suppl 1):72, 2011.

Aoude AA, Antoniou J, Epure LM, et al.: Midterm outcomes of the recently FDA approved ceramic on ceramic bearing in total hip arthroplasty in patients under 65 years of age, *J Arthroplasty* 30:1388, 2015.

Babovic N, Trousdale RT: Total hip arthroplasty using highly cross-linked polyethylene in patients younger than 50 years with minimum 10-year follow-up, *J Arthroplasty* 28:815, 2013.

Baek SH, Kim SY: Cementless total hip arthroplasty with alumina bearings in patients younger than fifty with femoral head osteonecrosis, *J Bone Joint Surg* 90:1314, 2008.

Banzhof JA, Robbins CE, van der Ven A, et al.: Case report. Femoral head dislodgement complicating use of a dual mobility prosthesis for recurrent instability, *J Arthroplasty* 28(543):e1, 2013.

Beaulé PE, Mussett SA, Medley JB: Metal-on-metal bearings in total hip arthroplasty, *Instr Course Lect* 59:17, 2010.

Blakeney WG, Beaulieu Y, Puliero M, et al.: Excellent results of large-diameter ceramic-on-ceramic bearings in total hip arthroplasty. Is squeaking related to head size? *Bone Joint J* 100-B:1434, 2018.

Cogan A, Nizard R, Sedel L: Occurrence of noise in alumina-on-alumina total hip arthroplasty. A survey on 284 consecutive hips, *Orthop Traumatol Surg Res* 97:206, 2011.

Combes A, Migaud H, Girard J, et al.: Low rate of dislocation of dual-mobility cups in primary total hip arthroplasty, *Clin Orthop Relat Res* 471:3891, 2013.

D'Antonio JA, Capello WN, Naughton M: High survivorship with a titanium-encases alumina ceramic bearing for total hip arthroplasty, *Clin Orthop Relat Res* 472:611, 2014.

de Steiger R, Lorimer M, Graves SE: Cross-linked polyethylene for total hip arthroplasty markedly reduces revision surgery at 16 years, *J Bone Joint Surg Am* 100:1281, 2018.

FDA: Concerns about metal-on-metal hip implants. https://www.fda.gov/medical-devices/metal-metal-hip-implants/concerns-about-metal-metal-hip-implants, February 15, 2019.

Finkbone PR, Severson EP, Cabanela ME, Trousdale RT: Ceramic-on-ceramic total hip arthroplasty in patients younger than 20 years, *J Arthroplasty* 27:213, 2012.

Glyn-Jones S, Thomas GER, Garfjeld-Roberts P, et al.: Highly crosslinked polyethylene in total hip arthroplasty decreases long-term wear: a double-blind randomized trial, *Clin Orthop Relat Res* 473:432, 2015.

Hallows RK, Pelt CE, Erickson JA, Peters CL: Serum metal ion concentration: comparison between small and large head metal-on-metal total hip arthroplasty, *J Arthroplasty* 26:1176, 2011.

Haq RU, Park KS, Seon JK, Yoon TR: Squeaking after third-generation ceramic-on-ceramic total hip arthroplasty, *J Arthroplasty* 27:909, 2012.

Ki SC, Kim BH, Ryu JH, et al.: Squeaking sound in total hip arthroplasty using ceramic-on-ceramic bearing surfaces, *J Orthop Sci* 16:21, 2011.

Kim YH, Park JW, Kim JS: Alumina delta-on-alumina delta bearing in cementless total hip arthroplasty in patients aged <50 years, *J Arthroplasgty* 32:1048, 2017.

Kleeman LT, Bala A, Penrose CT, et al.: Comparison of postoperative complications following metal-on-metal total hip arthroplasty with other bearings in Medicare population, *J Arthroplasty* 33:1826, 2018.

Kurtz SM, Lau E, Baykal D, et al.: Outcomes of ceramic bearings after total hip arthroplasty in the Medicare population, *J Arthroplasty* 32:743, 2017.

Kurtz SM, MacDonald DW, Mont MA, et al.: Retrieval analysis of sequentially annealed highly crosslinked polyethylene used in total hip arthroplasty, *Clin Orthop Relat Res* 473:962, 2015.

Lachiewicz PF, Soileau ES, Martell JM: Wear and osteolysis of highly crosslinked polyethylene at 10 to 14 years: the effect of femoral head size, *Clin Orthop Relat Res* 474:365, 2016.

Latteier MJ, Berend KR, Lombardi Jr AV, et al.: Gender is a significant factor for failure of metal-on-metal total hip arthroplasty, *J Arthroplasty* 26(Suppl 1):19, 2011.

Lee GC, Kim RH: Incidence of modern alumina ceramic and alumina matrix composite femoral head failures in nearly 6 million hip implants, *J Arthroplasty* 32:546, 2017.

Lombardi Jr AV, Berend KR, Morris MJ, et al.: Large-diameter metal-on-metal total hip arthroplasty: dislocation infrequent but survivorship poor, *Clin Orthop Relat Res* 473:509, 2015.

Malviya A, Ramaskandhan J, Holland JP, Lingard EA: Current concepts review. Metal-on-metal total hip arthroplasty, *J Bone Joint Surg* 92:1675, 2010.

Migaud H, Putman S, Kern G, et al.: Do the reasons for ceramic-on-ceramic revisions differ from other bearings in total hip arthroplasty? *Clin Orthop Relat Res* 474:2190, 2016.

Morison ZA, Patel S, Khan HA, et al.: A randomized controlled trial comparing oxinium and cobalt-chrome on standard and cross-linked polyethylene, *J Arthroplasty* 29(Suppl 2):164, 2014.

Nam D, Barrack T, Johnson SR, et al.: Hard-on-hard bearings are associated with increased noise generation in young patients undergoing hip arthroplasty, *Clin Orthop Relat Res* 474:2115, 2016.

Park KS, Seon JK, Toon TR: The survival analysis in third-generation ceramic-on-ceramic total hip arthroplasty, *J Arthroplasty* 30:1976, 2015.

Paxton EW, Inacio MCS, Namba RS, et al.: Metal-on-conventional polyethylene total hip arthroplasty bearing surfaces have a higher risk of revision than metal-on-highly crosslinked polyethylene: results from a US registry, *Clin Orthop Relat Res* 473:1011, 2015.

Rames RD, Stambough JB, Pashos GE, et al.: Fifteen-year results of total hip arthroplasty with cobalt-chromium femoral heads on highly cross-linked polyethylene in patients 50 years and less, *J Arthroplasty* 34:1143, 2019.

Restrepo C, Post ZD, Kai B, Hozack WJ: The effect of stem design on the prevalence of squeaking following ceramic-on-ceramic bearing total hip arthroplasty, *J Bone Joint Surg* 92:550, 2010.

Schroder D, Bornstein L, Bostrom MPG, et al.: Ceramic-on-ceramic total hip arthroplasty, *Clin Orthop Relat Res* 469:437, 2011.

Snir N, Kaye ID, Klifto CS, et al.: 10-year follow-up wear analysis of first-generation highly crosslinked polyethylene in primary total hip arthroplasty, *J Arthroplasty* 29:630, 2014.

Stanat SJC, Capozzi JD: Squeaking in third- and fourth-generation ceramic-on-ceramic total hip arthroplasty. Meta-analysis and systematic review, *J Arthroplasty* 27:445, 2012.

Swanson TV, Peterson DJ, Seethala R, et al.: Influence of prosthetic design on squeaking after ceramic-on-ceramic total hip arthroplasty, *J Arthroplasty* 25(Suppl 1):36, 2010.

Tai SM, Munir S, Walter WL, et al.: Squeaking in large diameter ceramic-on-ceramic bearings in total hip arthroplasty, *J Arthroplasty* 30:282, 2015.

Wyles CC, Jimenez-Almonte JH, Murad MH, et al.: There are no differences in short- to mid-term survivorship among total hip-bearing surface options: a network meta-analysis, *Clin Orthop Relat Res* 473:2031, 2015.

CEMENTED FEMORAL COMPONENT

Bedard NA, Callaghan JJ, Steff MD, Liu SS: Systematic review of literature of cemented femoral components: what is the durability at minimum 20 years followup? *Clin Orthop Relat Res* 473:563, 2015.

Cooper HJ, Urban RM, Wixson RL, et al.: Adverse local tissue reaction arising from corrosion at the femoral neck-body junction in a dual-taper stem with a cobalt-chromium modular neck, *J Bone Joint Surg* 95:865, 2013.

Ghanem E, Ward DM, Robbins CE, et al.: Corrosion and adverse local tissue reaction in one type of modular neck stem, *J Arthroplasty* 30:1787, 2015.

Goyal N, Hozack WJ: Neck-modular femoral stems for total hip arthroplasty, *Surg Technol Int* 20:309, 2010.

Hoskins W, van Bavel D, Lorimer M, et al.: Polished cemented femoral stems have a lower rate of revision than matt finished cemented stems in total hip arthroplasty: an analysis of 96,315 cemented femoral stems, *J Arthroplasty* 33:1472, 2018.

Scanelli JA, Reiser GR, Sloboda JF, et al.: Cemented femoral component use in hip arthroplasty, *J Am Acad Orthop Surg* 27:119, 2019.

Westerman RW, Whitehouse SL, Hubble MJ, et al.: The Exeter V40 cemented femoral component at a minimum 10-year follow-up: the first 50 cases, *Bone Joint J* 100-B:1002, 2018.

UNCEMENTED FEMORAL COMPONENT

Amendola RL, Goetz DD, Liu SS, et al.: Two- to 4-year followup of a short stem THA construct: excellent fixation, thigh pain a concern, *Clin Orthop Relat Res* 475:375, 2017.

Banerjee S, Pivec R, Issa K, et al.: Outcomes of short stems in total hip arthroplasty, *Orthopedics* 36:700, 2013.

Costa CR, Johnson AJ, Mont MA: Use of cementless, tapered femoral stems in patients who have a mean age of 20 years, *J Arthroplasty* 27:497, 2012.

Ferguson RJ, Broomfield JA, Malak TT, et al.: Primary stability of a short bone-conserving femoral stem: a two-year randomized controlled trial using radiostereometric analysis, *Bone Joint J* 100-B:1148, 2018.

Freitag T, Hein MA, Wernerus D, et al.: Bone remodeling after femoral short stem implantation in total hip arthroplalsty: 1-year results from a randomized DEXA study, *Arch Orthop Trauma Surg* 136:125, 2016.

Hossain F, Konan S, Volpin A, et al.: Early performance-based and patient-reported outcomes of a contemporary taper fit bone-conserving short stem femoral component in total hip arthroplasty, *Bone Joint J* 99-B(4 Supple B):49, 2017.

Jacquot L, Bonnin MP, Machenaud A, et al.: Clinical and radiographic outcomes t 25-30 years of a hip stem fully coated with hydroxylapatite, *J Arthroplasty* 33:482, 2018.

Khanuja HS, Banerjee S, Jain D, et al.: Current concepts review. Short bone-conserving stems in cementless hip arthroplasty, *J Bone Joint Surg* 96:1742, 2014.

Khanuja HS, Vakil JJ, Goddard MS, Mont MA: Current concepts review. Cementless femoral fixation in total hip arthroplasty, *J Bone Joint Surg* 93:500, 2011.

Kim YH, Kim JS, Joo JH, Park JW: A prospective short-term outcome study of a short metaphyseal fitting total hip arthroplasty, *J Arthroplasty* 27:88, 2012.

Kolb A, Grübl A, Schneckener CD, et al.: Cementless total hip arthroplasty with the rectangular titanium Zweymüller stem. A concise follow-up, at a minimum of twenty years, of previous reports, *J Bone Joint Surg* 94:1681, 2012.

McGrory BJ, MacKenzie J, Babikian G: A high prevalence of corrosion at the head-neck taper with contemporary Zimmer non-cemented femoral hip components, *J Arthroplasty* 30:1266, 2015.

McLaughlin JR, Lee KR: Total hip arthroplasty with an uncemented tapered femoral components in patients younger than 50 years of age: a minimum 20-year follow-up study, *J Arthroplasty* 31:1275, 2016.

McLaughlin JR, Lee KR: Total hip arthroplasty with uncemented tapered femoral component in patients younger than 50 years, *J Arthroplasty* 26:9, 2011.

Meftah M, John M, Lendhey M, et al.: Safety and efficacy of non-cemented femoral fixation in patients 75 years of age and older, *J Arthroplasty* 28:1378, 2013.

Molli RG, Lombardi Jr AV, Berend KR, et al.: A short tapered stem reduced intraoperative complications in primary total hip arthroplasty, *Clin Orthop Relat Res* 470:450, 2012.

Pairon P, Haddad FS: Stem size in hip arthroplasty: could shorter be better and when will we know? *Bone Joint J* 100-B:1133, 2018.

Riley SA, Spears JR, Smith LS, et al.: Cementless tapered femoral stems for total hip arthroplasty in octogenarians, *J Arthroplasty* 31:2810, 2016.

Streit MR, Innmann MM, Merle C, et al.: Long-term (20- to 25-year) results of an uncemented tapered titanium femoral component and factors affecting survivorship, *Clin Orthop Relat Res* 471:3262, 2013.

Takenaga RK, Callaghan JJ, Bedard NA, et al.: Cementless total hip arthroplasty in patients fifty years of age or younger: a minimum ten-year follow-up, *J Bone Joint Surg* 94:2153, 2012.

Tudor FS, Donaldson JR, Rodriguez-Elizalde SR, Cameron HU: Long-term comparison of porous versus hydroxyapatite coated sleeve of a modular cementless femoral stem (SROM) in primary total hip arthroplasty, *J Arthroplasty* 30:1777, 2015.

Wechter J, Comfort TK, Tatman P, et al.: Improved survival of uncemented versus cemented femoral stems in patients aged <70 years in a community total joint registry, *Clin Orthop Relat Res* 471:3588, 2013.

UNCEMENTED ACETABULAR COMPONENT

Blakeney WG, Khan H, Khan RJK: Cluster hole versus solid cup in total hip arthroplasty: a randomized control trial, *J Arthroplasty* 30:223, 2015.

Halma JJ, Vogely C, Dhert WJ, et al.: Do monoblock cups improve survivorship, decrease wear, or reduce osteolysis in uncemented total hip arthroplasty? *Clin Orthop Relat Res* 471:3572, 2013.

Howard JL, Kremers HM, Loechler YA, et al.: Comparative survival of uncemented acetabular components following primary total hip arthroplasty, *J Bone Joint Surg* 93:1597, 2011.

Jauregui JJ, Banerjee S, Cherian JJ, et al.: Early outcomes of titanium-based highly-porous acetabular components in revision total hip arthroplasty, *J Arthroplasty* 30:1187, 2015.

Naudie DDR, Somerville L, Korczak A, et al.: A randomized trial comparing acetabular component fixation of two porous ingrowth surfaces using RSA, *J Arthroplasty* 28(Suppl 8):148, 2013.

Pang HN, Naudie DDR, McCalden RW, et al.: Highly crosslinked polyethylene improves wear but not surface damage in retrieved acetabular liners, *Clin Orthop Relat Res* 473:463, 2015.

Sato T, Nakashima Y, Komiyama K, et al.: The absence of hydroxyapatite coating on cementless acetabular components does not affect long-term survivorship in total hip arthroplasty, *J Arthroplasty* 31:1228, 2016.

Teusink MJ, Callagham JJ, Warth LC, et al.: Cementless acetabular fixation in patients 50 years and younger at 10 to 18 years of follow-up, *J Arthroplasty* 27:1316, 2012.

Toossi N, Adeli B, Timperley AJ, et al.: Acetabular components in total hip arthroplasty: is there evidence that cementless fixation is better? *J Bone Joint Surg* 95:168, 2013.

PREOPERATIVE EVALUATION

Akesson P, Chen AF, Deirmengian GK, et al.: General Assembly, prevention, risk mitigation, local factors: Proceedings of International Consensus on Orthopedic Infections, *J Arthroplasty* 34:S49, 2019.

An VVG, Phan K, Sivakumar BS, et al.: Prior lumbar spinal fusion is associated with an increased risk of dislocation and revision in total hip arthroplasty: a meta-analysis, *J Arthroplasty* 33:297, 2018.

Belmont PJ, Goodman GP, Hamilton W, et al.: Morbidity and mortality in the thirty-day period following total hip arthroplasty: risk factors and incidence, *J Arthroplasty* 29:2025, 2014.

Bozic KJ, Lau E, Kurtz S, et al.: Patient-related risk factors for periprosthetic joint infection and postoperative mortality following total hip arthroplasty in Medicare patients, *J Bone Joint Surg* 94:794, 2012.

Browne JA, Adib F, Brown TE, et al.: Transfusion rates are increasing following total hip arthroplasty: risk factors and outcomes, *J Arthroplasty* 28(Suppl 8):34, 2013.

Cancienne JM, Werner BC, Browne JA: Is there a threshold value of hemoglobin A1c that predicts risk of infection following primary total hip arthroplasty? *J Arthroplasty* 32:S236, 2017.

Cordero-Ampuero J, González-Fernández E, Martínez-Velez D, Esteban J: Are antibiotics necessary in hip arthroplasty with asymptomatic bacteriuria? Seeding risk with/without treatment, *Clin Orthop Relat Res* 471:3822, 2013.

Duchman KR, Gao Y, Pugely AJ, et al.: The effect of smoking on short-term complications following total hip and knee arthroplasty, *J Bone Joint Surg Am* 97:1049, 2015.

Elson LC, Barr CJ, Chandran SE, et al.: Are morbidly obese patients undergoing total hip arthroplasty at an increased risk for component malpositioning? *J Arthroplasty* 28(Suppl 1):41, 2013.

Greenky M, Gandhi K, Pulido L, et al.: Preoperative anemia in total joint arthroplasty: is it associated with periprosthetic joint infection? *Clin Orthop Relat Res* 470:2695, 2012.

Higuera CA, Elsharkawy K, Klika AK, et al.: Predictors of early adverse outcomes after knee and hip arthroplasty in geriatric patients, *Clin Orthop Relat Res* 469:1391, 2011.

Huddleston JL, Wang Y, Uquillas C, et al.: Age and obesity are risk factors for adverse events after total hip arthroplasty, *Clin Orthop Relat Res* 470:490, 2012.

Iorio R, Williams KM, Marcantonio AJ, et al.: Diabetes mellitus, hemoglobin A1C, and the incidence of total joint arthroplasty infection, *J Arthroplasty* 27:726, 2012.

Kapadia BH, Issa K, Pivec R, et al.: Tobacco use may be associated with increased revision and complication rates following total hip arthroplasty, *J Arthroplasty* 29:777, 2014.

Kapadia BH, Johnson AJ, Daley JA, et al.: Pre-admission cutaneous chlorhexidine preparation reduced surgical site infections in total hip arthroplasty, *J Arthroplasty* 28:490, 2013.

Klatte TO, Meinicke R, O'Loughlinn P, et al.: Incidence of bacterial contamination in primary THA and combined hardware removal. Analysis of preoperative aspiration and intraoperative biopsies, *J Arthroplasty* 28:1677, 2013.

Lombardi Jr AV, Berend KR, Adams JB, et al.: Smoking may be a harbinger of early failure with ultraporous metal acetabular reconstruction, *Clin Orthop Relat Res* 471:486, 2013.

Lyman S, Lee YY, Franklin PD, et al.: Validation of the HOOS, JR: a short-form hip replacement survey, *Clin Orthop Relat Res* 474:1472, 2016.

McKnight BM, Trasolini NA, Dorr LD: Spinopelvic motion and impingement in total hip arthroplasty, *J Arthroplasty* 37(7S):S53, 2019.

Meerman G, Malik A, Witt J, Haddad F: Preoperative radiographic assessment of limb-length discrepancy in total hip arthroplasty, *Clin Orthop Relat Res* 469:1677, 2011.

Poehling-Monaghan KL, Kamath AF, Taunton MJ, et al.: Direct anterior versus mini posterior THA with the same advanced perioperative protocols: surprising early clinical results, *Clin Orthop Relat Res* 473(2):623, 2015.

Rasouli MR, Maltenfort MG, Ross D, et al.: Perioperative morbidity and mortality following bilateral total hip arthroplasty, *J Arthroplasty* 29:142, 2014.

Shin JK, Son SM, Kim TW, et al.: Accuracy and reliability of preoperative onscreen templating using digital radiographs for total hip arthroplasty, *Hip Pelvis* 28(4):201, 2016.

Stavrakis AI, SooHoo NF, Lieberman JR: Bilateral total hip arthroplasty has similar complication rates to unilateral total hip arthroplasty, *J Arthroplasty* 30:1211, 2015.

Tripuraneni KR, Archibeck MJ, Junick DW, et al.: Common errors in the execution of preoperative templating for primary total hip arthroplasty, *J Arthroplasty* 25:1235, 2010.

Ward DT, Metz LN, Horst PK, et al.: Complications of morbid obesity in total joint arthroplasty: risk stratification based on BMI, *J Arthroplasty* 30(Suppl 9):42, 2015.

Wei W, Wei B: Comparison of topical and intravenous tranexamic acid on blood loss and transfusion rates in total hip arthroplasty, *J Arthroplasty* 29:2113, 2014.

Whiddon DR, Bono JV, Lang JE, et al.: Accuracy of digital templating in total hip arthroplasty, *Am J Orthop* 40:395, 2011.

SURGICAL TECHNIQUE

Alvarez AM, Suarez J, Patel P, Benton EG: Fluoroscopic imaging of acetabular cup position during THA through a direct anterior approach, *Orthopedics* 36:776, 2013.

Barrett WP, Turner SE, Leopold JP: Prospective randomized study of direct anterior vs postero-lateral approach for total hip arthroplasty, *J Arthroplasty* 28:1634, 2013.

Bergin PF, Doppelt JD, Kephart DJ, et al.: Comparison of minimally invasive direct anterior versus posterior total hip arthroplasty based on inflammation and muscle damage, *J Bone Joint Surg* 93:1392, 2011.

Berstock JR, Blom AW, Beswick AD: A systematic review and meta-analysis of the standard versus mini-incision posterior approach to total hip arthroplasty, *J Arthroplasty* 29:1970, 2014.

Brown ML, Reed JD, Drinkwater CJ: Imageless computer-assisted versus conventional total hip arthroplasty: one surgeon's initial experience, *J Arthroplasty* 29:1015, 2014.

Chakravarty R, Toossi N, Katsman A, et al.: Percutaneous column fixation and total hip arthroplasty for the treatment of acute acetabular fracture in the elderly, *J Arthroplasty* 29:817, 2014.

Christensen CP, Karthikeyan T, Jacobs CA: Greater prevalence of wound complications requiring reoperation with direct anterior approach total hip arthroplasty, *J Arthroplasty* 29:1839, 2014.

Cidambi KR, Barnett SL, Mallette PR, et al.: Impact of femoral stem design on failure after anterior approach total hip arthroplasty, *J Arthroplasty* 33:800, 2018.

Dastane M, Door LD, Tarwala R, Wan Z: Hip offset in total hip arthroplasty: quantitative measurement with navigation, *Clin Orthop Relat Res* 469:429, 2011.

Dorr LD, Jones JE, Padgett DE, et al.: Robotic guidance in total hip arthroplasty: the shape of things to come, *Orthopedics* 34:e652, 2011.

Ellapparadja P, Mahajan V, Deakin AH, Deep K: Reproduction of hip offset and leg length in navigated total hip arthroplasty: how accurate are we? *J Arthroplasty* 30:1002, 2015.

Epstein NJ, Woolson ST, Giori NJ: Acetabular component positioning using the transverse acetabular ligament. Can you find it and does it help? *Clin Orthop Relat Res* 469:412, 2011.

Ezzet KA, McCauley JC: Use of intraoperative x-rays to optimize component position and leg length during total hip arthroplasty, *J Arthroplasty* 29:580, 2014.

Goosen JHM, Kollen BJ, Castelein RM, et al.: Minimally invasive versus classic procedures in total hip arthroplasty. A double-blind randomized controlled trial, *Clin Orthop Relat Res* 469:200, 2011.

Grammatopoulos G, Gofton W, Cochran M, et al.: Pelvic positioning in the supine position leads to more consistent orientation of the acetabular component after total hip arthroplasty, *Bone Joint J* 100-B:1280, 2018.

Grob K, Monahan R, Gilbey H, et al.: Distal extension of the direct anterior approach to the hip poses risk to neurovascular structures. An anatomical study, *J Bone Joint Surg* 97:126, 2015.

Hamilton WG, Parks NL, Huynh C: Comparison of cup alignment, jump distance, and complications in a consecutive series of anterior approach and posterior approach total hip arthroplasty, *J Arthroplasty* 30:1959, 2015.

Hohmann E, Bryant A, Tetsworth K: A comparison between imageless navigated and manual freehand technique acetabular cup placement in total hip arthroplasty, *J Arthroplasty* 26:1078, 2011.

Innmann MM, Maier MW, Streit MR, et al.: Additive influence of hip offset and leg length reconstruction on postoperative improvement in clinical outcome after total hip arthroplasty, *Arthroplasty* 33:156, 2018.

Ito Y, Matsushita I, Watanabe H, Kimura T: Anatomic mapping of short external rotators shows the limit of their preservation during total hip arthroplasty, *Clin Orthop Relat Res* 470:1690, 2012.

Jameson SS, Mason JM, Baker PN, et al.: A comparison of surgical approaches for primary hip arthroplasty: a cohort study of patient reported outcome measures (PROMs) and early revision using linked national databases, *J Arthroplasty* 26:1248, 2014.

Kanawade V, Dorr LD, Banks SA, et al.: Precision of robotic guided instrumentation for acetabular component positioning, *J Arthroplasty* 30:392, 2015.

Lakstein D, Backstein DJ, Safir O, et al.: Modified trochanteric slide for complex hip arthroplasty: clinical outcomes and complication rates, *J Arthroplasty* 25:363, 2010.

Lakstein D, Kosashvili Y, Backstein D, et al.: Modified extended trochanteric osteotomy with preservation of posterior structures, *Hip Int* 20:102, 2010.

Lam L, Drew T, Boscainos P: Effect of acetabular orientation of stress distribution of highly cross-linked polyethylene liners, *Orthopedics* 36:e1346, 2013.

Leucht P, Huddleston HG, Bell MJ, Huddleston JL: Does intraoperative fluoroscopy optimize limb length and the precision of acetabular positioning in primary THA? *Orthopedics* 38:e380, 2015.

Lin F, Lim D, Wixson RL, et al.: Limitations of imageless computer-assisted navigation for total hip arthroplasty, *J Arthroplasty* 26:596, 2011.

Manzotti A, Cerveri P, De Momi E, et al.: Does computer-assisted surgery benefit leg length restoration in total hip replacement? Navigation versus conventional freehand, *Int Orthop* 35:19, 2011.

Martin CT, Pugely AJ, Gao Y, Clarke CR: A comparison of hospital length of stay and short-term morbidity between the anterior and the posterior approaches to total hip arthroplasty, *J Arthroplasty* 28:849, 2013.

Minoda Y, Ohzono K, Aihara M, et al.: Are acetabular component alignment guides for total hip arthroplasty accurate? *J Arthroplasty* 25:986, 2010.

Moskal JT, Capps SG: Acetabular component positioning in total hip arthroplasty: an evidence-based analysis, *J Arthroplasty* 26:1432, 2011.

Moskal JT, Capps SG: Is limited incision better than standard total hip arthroplasty? A meta-analysis, *Clin Orthop Relat Res* 471:1283, 2013.

Nam D, Sculco P, Su EP, et al.: Acetabular component positioning in primary THA via an anterior, posterolateral, or posterolateral-navigated surgical technique, *Orthopedics* 36:e1482, 2013.

Nam D, Sculco PK, Abdel MP, et al.: Leg-length inequalities following THA based on surgical technique, *Orthopedics* 36:3395, 2013.

Post ZD, Orozco F, Diaz-Ledezma C, et al.: Direct anterior approach for total hip arthroplasty: indications, technique, and results, *J Am Acad Orthop Surg* 22:595, 2014.

Queen RM, Butler RJ, Watters TS, et al.: The effect of total hip arthroplasty surgical approach on postoperative gait mechanics, *J Arthroplasty* 26(Suppl 1):66, 2011.

Queen RM, Schaeffer JF, Butler RJ, et al.: Does surgical approach during total hip arthroplasty alter gait recovery during the first year following surgery? *J Arthroplasty* 28:1639, 2013.

Rathod PA, Orishimo KF, Kremenic IJ, et al.: Similar improvement in gait parameters following direct anterior & posterior approach total hip arthroplasty, *J Arthroplasty* 29:1261, 2014.

Russo MW, Macdonell JR, Paulus MC, et al.: Increased complications in obese patients undergoing direct anterior total hip arthroplasty, *J Arthroplasty* 30(8):1384, 2015.

Sheth D, Cafri G, Inacio MCS, et al.: Anterior and anterolateral approaches for THA are associated with lower dislocation risk without higher revision risk, *Clin Orthop Relat Res* 473:3401, 2015.

Shubert D, Madoff S, Milillo R, Nandi S: Neurovascular structure proximity to acetabular retractors in total hip arthroplasty, *J Arthroplasty* 30:145, 2015.

Small T, Krebs V, Molloy R, et al.: Comparison of acetabular shell position using patient specific instruments vs. standard surgical instruments: a randomized clinical trial, *J Arthroplasty* 29:1030, 2014.

Taunton MJ, Mason JB, Odum SM, Springer BD: Direct anterior total hip arthroplasty yields more rapid voluntary cessation of all walking aids: a prospective, randomized clinical trial, *J Arthroplasty* 29(Suppl 2):169, 2014.

Tischler EH, Orozco F, Aggarwal VK, et al.: Does intraoperative fluoroscopy improve component positioning in total hip arthroplasty? *Orthopedics* 38:e1, 2015.

Üzel M, Akkin SM, Tanyeli E, Koebke J: Relationships of the lateral femoral cutaneous nerve to bony landmarks, *Clin Orthop Relat Res* 469:2605, 2011.

van Oldenrijk J, Hoogland PV, Tuijthof GJ, et al.: Soft tissue damage after minimally invasive THA. A comparison of 5 approaches, *Acta Orthop* 81:696, 2010.

Varin D, Lamontagne M, Beaulé PE: Does the anterior approach for THA provide closer-to-normal lower-limb motion? *J Arthroplasty* 28:1401, 2013.

Yi C, Agudelo JF, Dayton MR, Morgan SJ: Early complications of anterior supine intermuscular total hip arthroplasty, *Orthopedics* 36:e276, 2013.

Zawadsky MW, Paulus MC, Murray PJ, Johansen MA: Early outcome comparison between the direct anterior approach and the mini-incision posterior approach for primary total hip arthroplasty; 150 consecutive cases, *J Arthroplasty* 29:1256, 2014.

SPECIFIC DISORDERS

ARTHRITIC DISORDERS

Swarup I, Lee YY, Christoph EI, et al.: Implant survival and patient-reported outcomes after total hip arthroplasty in young patients with juvenile idiopathic arthritis, *J Arthroplasty* 30:398, 2015.

Zhen P, Li X, Zhou S, et al.: Total hip arthroplasty to treat acetabular protrusions secondary to rheumatoid arthritis, *J Orthop Surg Res* 13:92, 2018.

OSTEONECROSIS

Kim YH, Choi Y, Kim JS: Cementless total hip arthroplasty with alumina-on-highly cross-linked polyethylene bearing in young patients with femoral head osteonecrosis, *J Arthroplasty* 28:218, 2011.

Lovecchio FC, Manalo J, Demzik A, et al.: Avascular necrosis is associated with increased transfusions and readmission following primary total hip arthroplasty, *Orthopedics* 40:171, 2017.

Osawa Y, Seki T, Takegami Y, et al.: Cementless total hip arthroplasty for osteonecrosis and osteoarthritis produce similar results at ten years follow-up when matched for age and gender, *Int Orthop* 42:1683, 2018.

Stavrakis AI, SooHoo NF, Lieberman JR: A comparison of the incidence of complications following total hip arthroplasty in patients with or without osteonecrosis, *J Arthroplasty* 30:114, 2015.

Sternheim A, Abolghasemian M, Safir OA, et al.: A long-term survivorship comparison between cemented and uncemented cups with shelf grafts in revision total hip arthroplasty after dysplasia, *J Arthroplasty* 28:303, 2013.

DEVELOPMENTAL DYSPLASIA

Galea VP, Laaksonen I, Donahue GS, et al.: Developmental dysplasia treated with cementless total hip arthroplasty utilizing high hip center reconstruction: a minimum 13-year follow-up study, *J Arthroplasty* 33:2899, 2018.

Greber EM, Pelt CE, Gililland JM, et al.: Challenges in total hip arthroplasty in the setting of developmental dysplasia of the hip, *J Arthroplasty* 32:538, 2017.

Guenther D, Kendoff D, Omar M, et al.: Total hip arthroplasty in patients with skeletal dysplasia, *J Arthroplasty* 30:1574, 2015.

Kawai T, Tanaka C, Ikenaga M, Kanoe H: Cemented total hip arthroplasty with transverse subtrochanteric shortening osteotomy for Crowe group IV dislocated hip, *J Arthroplasty* 26:229, 2011.

Krych AJ, Howard JL, Trousdale RT, et al.: Total hip arthroplasty with shortening subtrochanteric osteotomy in Crowe type-IV developmental dysplasia: surgical technique, *J Bone Joint Surg* 92(Suppl 1, Part 2):176, 2010.

Nawabi DH, Meftah M, Nam D, et al.: Durable fixation achieved with medialized, high hip center cementless THAs for Crowe II and III dysplasia, *Clin Orthop Relat Res* 472:630, 2014.

Ollivier M, Abdel MP, Krych AJ, et al.: Long-term results of total hip arthroplasty with shortening subtrochanteric osteotomy in Crowe IV developmental dysplasia, *J Arthroplasty* 31:1756, 2016.

Sofu H, Kockara N, Gursu S, et al.: Transverse subtrochanteric shortening osteotomy during cementless total hip arthroplasty in Crowe type-III or IV developmental dysplasia, *J Arthroplasty* 30:1019, 2015.

Watts CD, Martin JR, Fehring KA, et al.: Inferomedial hip center decrease failure rates in cementless total hip arthroplasty for Crowe II and III hip dysplasia, *J Arthroplasty* 33:2177, 2018.

Zha GC, Sun JY, Guo KJ, et al.: Medial protrusio technique in cementless total hip arthroplasty for developmental dysplasia of the hip: a prospective 6- to 9-year follow-up of 43 consecutive patients, *J Arthroplasty* 31:1761, 2016.

LEGG-CALVÉ-PERTHES DISEASE

Al-Khateeb H, Kwok IHY, Hanna SA, et al.: Custom cementless THA in patients with Legg-Calve-Perthes disease, *J Arthroplasty* 29:792, 2014.

Baghdadi YMK, Larson AN, Stans AA, Mabry TM: Total hip arthroplasty for the sequelae of Legg-Calvé-Perthes disease, *Clin Orthop Relat Res* 471:2980, 2013.

Froberg L, Christensen F, Pedersen NW, Overgaard S: The need for total hip arthroplasty in Perthes disease: a long-term study, *Clin Orthop Relat Res* 469:1134, 2011.

Hanna SA, Sarraf KM, Ramachandran M, et al.: Systematic review of the outcome of total hip arthroplasty in patients with sequelae of Legg-Calvé-Perthes disease, *Arch Orthop Trauma Surg* 137:1149, 2017.

Suefert CR, McGrory BJ: Treatment of arthritis associated with Legg-Calve-Perthes disease with modular total hip arthroplasty, *J Arthroplasty* 30:1743, 2015.

SLIPPED CAPITAL FEMORAL EPIPHYSIS

Boyle MJ, Frampton CM, Crawford HA: Early results of total hip arthroplasty in patients with slipped upper femoral epiphysis compared with patients with osteoarthritis, *J Arthroplasty* 27(6):1003, 2012.

POSTTRAUMATIC DISORDERS

Archibeck MJ, Carothers JT, Gripuraneni KR, White Jr RE: Total hip arthroplasty after failed internal fixation of proximal femoral fractures, *J Arthroplasty* 28:168, 2013.

Callaghan JJ, Liu SS, Haidukewych GJ: Subcapital fractures: a changing paradigm, *J Bone Joint Surg* 94:19, 2012.

Dimitriou D, Helmy N, Hasler J, et al.: The role of total hip arthroplasty through the direct anterior approach in femoral neck fracture and factors affecting the outcome, *J Arthroplasty* 34:82, 2019.

Hansson S, Nemes S, Kärrholm J, et al.: Reduced risk of reoperation after treatment of femoral neck fractures with total hip arthroplasty: a matched pair analysis, *Acta Orthop* 88:500, 2017.

Hedbeck CJ, Enocson A, Lapidus G, et al.: Comparison of bipolar hemiarthroplasty with total hip arthroplasty for displaced femoral neck fractures: a concise four-year follow-up of a randomized trial, *J Bone Joint Surg* 93A:445, 2011.

Hernandez NM, Chalmers BP, Perry KI, et al.: Total hip arthroplasty after in situ fixation of minimally displaced femoral neck fractures in elderly patients, *J Arthroplasty* 33:44, 2018.

Herscovici Jr D, Lindvall E, Bolhofner B, Scaduto JM: The combined hip procedure: open reduction internal fixation combined with total hip arthroplasty for the management of acetabular fractures in the elderly, *J Orthop Trauma* 24:291, 2010.

Kahlenberg CA, Richarson SS, Schairer WW, et al.: Rates and risk factors of conversion hip arthroplasty after closed reduction percutaneous hip pinning for femoral neck fractures—a population analysis, *J Arthroplasty* 33:771, 2018.

Lee YK, Kim JT, Alkitaini AA, et al.: Conversion hip arthroplasty in failed fixation of intertrochanteric fracture: a propensity score matching study, *J Arthroplasty* 32:1593, 2017.

Lu M, Phillips D: Total hip arthroplasty for posttraumatic conditions, *J Am Acad Orthop Surg* 27:275, 2019.

Makridis KG, Obakponovwe O, Bobak P, Giannoudis PV: Total hip arthroplasty after acetabular fracture: incidence of complications, reoperation rates and functional outcomes: evidence today, *J Arthroplasty* 29:1983, 2014.

Morice A, Ducellier F, Bizot P, et al.: Total hip arthroplasty after failed fixation of a proximal femur fracture: analysis of 59 cases of intra- and extracapsular fractures, *Orthop Traumatol Surg Res* 104:681, 2018.

Morison Z, Moojen DJF, Nauth A, et al.: Total hip arthroplasty after acetabular fracture is associated with lower survivorship and more complications, *Clin Orthop Relat Res* 474:392, 2016.

Noticewala M, Murtaugh TS, Danoff J, et al.: Has the risk of dislocation after total hip arthroplasty performed for displaced femoral neck fracture improved with modern implants? *J Clin Orthop Trauma* 9:281, 2018.

Pui CM, Bostrom MP, Westrich GH, et al.: Increased complication rate following conversion total hip arthroplasty after cephalomedullary fixation for intertrochanteric hip fractures: a multi-center study, *J Arthroplasty* 28(Suppl 8):45, 2013.

Sassoon A, D'Apuzzo M, Sems S, et al.: Total hip arthroplasty for femoral neck fracture. Comparing in-hospital mortality, complications, and disposition to an elective patient population, *J Arthroplasty* 28:1659, 2013.

Schairer WW, Lane JM, Halsey DA, et al.: Total hip arthroplasty for femoral neck fracture is not a typical DRG 470: a propensity-matched cohort study, *Clin Orthop Relat Res* 475:353, 2017.

Sköldenberg O, Ekman A, Salemyr A, Bodén H: Reduced dislocation rate after hip arthroplasty for femoral neck fractures when changing from posterolateral to anterolateral approach, *Acta Orthop* 81:583, 2010.

Stambough JB, Nunley RM, Spraggs-Hughes AG, et al.: Clinical practice guidelines in action: differences in femoral neck fracture management by trauma and arthroplasty training, *J Am Acad Orthop Surg* 27:287, 2019.

Swart E, Roulette P, Leas D, et al.: ORIF or arthroplasty for displaced femoral neck fractures in patients younger than 65 years old: an economic decision analysis, *J Bone Joint Surg Am* 99:65, 2017.

Weaver MJ, Smith RM, Lhowe DW, et al.: Does total hip arthroplasty reduce the risk of secondary surgery following the treatment of displaced acetabular fractures in the elderly compared to internal fixation? A pilot study, *J Orthop Traum* 43:S40, 2018.

Woon CYL, Moretti VM, Schwartz BE, et al.: Total hip arthroplasty and hemiarthroplasty: US national trends in the treatment of femoral neck fractures, *Am J Orthop (Belle Mead NJ)* 46:E474, 2017.

Yuan BJ, Lewallen DG, Hanssen AD: Porous metal acetabular components have a low rate of mechanical failure in THA after operatively treated acetabular fracture, *Clin Orthop Relat Res* 473:536, 2015.

FAILED RECONSTRUCTIVE PROCEDURES

Celiktas M, Kose O, Turan A, et al.: Conversion of hip fusion to total hip arthroplasty: clinical, radiological outcomes and complications in 40 hips, *Arch Orthop Trauma Surg* 137:119, 2017.

Duncan S, Wingerter S, Keith A, et al.: Does previous osteotomy compromise total hip arthroplasty? A systematic review, *J Arthroplasty* 30:79, 2015.

Jain S, Giannoudis PV: Arthrodesis of the hip and conversion to total hip arthroplasty: a systematic review, *J Arthroplasty* 28:1596, 2013.

Jauregui JJ, Kim JK, Shield 3rd WP, et al.: Hip fusion takedown to a total hip arthroplasty—is it worth it? A systematic review, *Int Orthop* 41:1535, 2017.

Mortazavi SMJ, Restrepo C, Kim PJW, et al.: Cementless femoral reconstruction in patients with proximal femoral deformity, *J Arthroplasty* 26:354, 2011.

Muratli KS, Karatosun V, Uzun B, Celik S: Subtrochanteric shortening in total hip arthroplasty: biomechanical comparison of four techniques, *J Arthroplasty* 29:836, 2014.

Richards CJ, Duncan CP: Conversion of hip arthrodesis to total hip arthroplasty: survivorship and clinical outcome, *J Arthroplasty* 26:409, 2011.

Shigemura T, Yamamoto Y, Murata Y, et al.: Total hip arthroplasty after a previous pelvic osteotomy: a systematic review and meta-analysis, *Orthop Traumatol Surg Res* 104:455, 2018.

METABOLIC DISORDERS

Carulli C, Felici I, Martini C, et al.: Total hip arthroplasty in haemophilic patients with modern cementless implants, *J Arthroplasty* 30:1757, 2015.

Colgan G, Baker JF, Donlon N, et al.: Total hip arthroplasty in patients with haemophilia—What are the risks of bleeding in the immediate peri-operative period? *J Orthopaedics* 13:389, 2016.

Farook MZ, Awogbade M, Somasundaram K, et al.: Total hip arthroplasty in osteonecrosis secondary to sickle cell disease, *Int Orthop* 43:293, 2019.

Ilyas I, Alrumaih HA, Rabbani S: Noncemented total hip arthroplasty in sickle-cell disease: long-term results, *J Arthroplasty* 33:477, 2018.

Imbuldeniya AM, Tai SM, Aboelmagd T, et al.: Cementless hip arthroplasty in Paget's disease at long-term follow-up (average of 12.3 years), *J Arthroplasty* 29:1063, 2014.

Kapadia BH, Boylan MR, Elmallah RK, et al.: Does hemophilia increase the risk of postoperative blood transfusion after lower extremity total joint arthroplasty? *J Arthroplasty* 31:1578, 2016.

Modi RM, Kheir MM, Tan TL, et al.: Survivorship and complications of total hip arthroplasty in patients with dwarfism, *Hip Int* 27:460, 2017.

INFECTIOUS DISORDERS

Enayatollahi MA, Murpy D, Maltenfort MG, et al.: Human immunodeficiency virus and total joint arthroplasty: the risk for infection is reduced, *J Arthroplasty* 31:2146, 2016.

Li L, Chou K, Deng j, et al.: Two-stage total hip arthroplasty for patients with advanced active tuberculosis of the hip, *J Orthop Surg Res* 11:38, 2016.

Tiwari A, Karkhur Y, Maini L: Total hip replacement in tuberculosis of the hip: a systematic review, *J Clin Orthop* 9:54, 2018.

NEUROMUSCULAR DISORDERS

Alosh H, Kamath AF, Baldwin KD, et al.: Outcomes of total hip arthroplasty in spastic patients, *J Arthroplasty* 29:1566, 2014.

Houdek MT, Watts CD, Wyles CC, et al.: Total hip arthroplasty in patients with cerebral palsy: a cohort study matched to patients with osteoarthritis, *J Bone Joint Surg Am* 99:488, 2017.

Raphael BS, Dines JS, Akerson M, Root L: Long-term follow-up of total hip arthroplasty in patients with cerebral palsy, *Clin Orthop Relat Res* 468:1845, 2010.

Yoon BH, Lee YK, Yoo JJ, et al.: Total hip arthroplasty performed in patients with residual poliomyelitis: does it work? *Clin Orthop Relat Res* 472:933, 2014.

COMPLICATIONS

GENERAL

Bartelt RB, Sierra RJ: Recurrent hematomas within the iliopsoas muscle caused by impingement after total hip arthroplasty, *J Arthroplasty* 26:665, 2011.

Belmont Jr PJ, Goodman GP, Hamilton W, et al.: Morbidity and mortality in the thirty-day period following total hip arthroplasty: risk factors and incidence, *J Arthroplasty* 29:2025, 2014.

Berstock JR, Beswick AD, Lenguerrand E, et al.: Mortality after total hip replacement surgery: a systematic review, *Bone Joint Res* 3:175, 2014.

Healy WL, Iorio R, Clair AJ, et al.: Complications of total hip arthroplasty: standardized list, definitions, and stratification developed by The Hip Society, *Clin Orthop Relat Res* 474:357–364, 2016.

Shearer DW, Youm J, Bozic KJ: Short-term complications have more effect on cost-effectiveness of THA than implant longevity, *Clin Orthop Relat Res* 473:1702, 2015.

HETEROTOPIC OSSIFICATION

Biz C, Pavan D, Frizziero A, et al.: Heterotopic ossification following total hip arthroplasty: a comparative radiographic study about its development with the use of three different kinds of implants, *J Orthop Surg Res* 10:176, 2015.

Cai L, Wang Z, Luo X, et al.: Optimal strategies for the prevention of heterotopic ossification after total hip arthroplasty: a network meta-analysis, *Int J Surg* 62:74, 2019.

Hug KT, Alton TB, Gee AO: Classifications in brief: brooker classification of heterotopic ossification after total hip arthroplasty, *Clin Orthop Relat Res* 473:2154, 2015.

Joice M, Basileiadis GI, Amantullah DF: Non-steroidal anti-inflammatory drugs for heterotopic ossification prophylalxis after total hip arthroplasty, *Bone Joint J* 100-B:915, 2018.

Kan SL, Yang B, Ning GZ, et al.: Nonsteroidal anti-inflammatory drugs as prophylaxis for heterotopic ossification after total hip arthroplasty: a systematic review and meta- analysis, *Medicine (Baltimore)* 94:e828, 2015.

Newman EA, Holst DC, Bracey DN, et al.: Incidence of heterotopic ossification in direct anterior vs posterior approach to total hip arthroplasty: a retrospective radiographic view, *Int Orthop* 40:1967, 2016.

Oni JK, Pinero JR, Saltzman BM, Jaffe FF: Effect of a selective COX-2 inhibitor, celecoxib, on heterotopic ossification after total hip arthroplasty: a case-controlled study, *Hip Int* 24:256, 2014.

Pakos EE, Papadopoulos DV, Gelalis ID, et al.: Is prophylaxis for heterotopic ossification with radiation therapy after THR associated with early loosening or carcinogenesis? *Hip Int*, 2019 Apr 16. [Epub ahead of print].

Pavlou G, Salhab M, et al.: Risk factors for heterotopic ossification in primary total hip arthroplasty, *Hip Int* 22:50, 2012.

Thilak J, Panakkal JJ, Kim TY, et al.: Risk factors of heterotopic ossification following total hip arthroplasty in patients with ankylosing spondylitis, *J Arthroplasty* 30:2304, 2015.

Tippets DM, Zaryanov AV, Bruke WV, et al.: Incidence of heterotopic ossification in direct anterior total hip arthroplasty: a retrospective radiographic review, *J Arthroplasty* 29:1835, 2014.

Vasileiadis GI, Amanatullah DF, Crendhaw JR, et al.: Effect of heterotopic ossification on hip range of motion and clinical outcome, *J Arthroplasty* 30:361, 2015.

Vasileiadis G, Sioutis I, Mavrogenis A, et al.: COX-2 inhibitors for the prevention of heterotopic ossification after THA, *Orthopedics* 346:467, 2011.

Xue D, Zheng Q, Li H, et al.: Selective COX-2 inhibitor versus nonselective COX-1 and COX-2 inhibitor in the prevention of heterotopic ossification after total hip arthroplasty: a meta-analysis of randomised trial, *Int Orthop* 35:3, 2011.

THROMBOEMBOLISM

Colwell Jr CW, Froimson MI, Mont MA, et al.: Thrombosis prevention after total hip arthroplasty: a prospective, randomized trial comparing a mobile compression device with low-molecular-weight heparin, *J Bone Joint Surg* 92A:527, 2010.

Falck-Ytter Y, Francis CW, Johanson NA, et al.: Prevention of VTE in orthopedic surgery patients: Antithrombic Therapy and Prevention of Thrombosis, 9th ed: American College of Chest Physicians Evidence-Based Clinical Practice Guidelines, *Chest* 141(Suppl 2):e278S, 2012.

Gage BF, Bass AR, Lin H, et al.: Effect of low-intensity vs standard-intensity warfarin prophylaxis on venous thromboembolism or death among patients undergoing hip or knee arthroplasty: a randomized clinical trial, *JAMA* 322:834, 2019.

Ghosh A, Best AJ, Rudge SJ, et al.: Clinical effectiveness of aspirin as multimodal thromboprophylaxis in primary total hip and knee arthroplasty: a review of 6078 cases, *J Arthroplast* 34:1359, 2019.

Horlocker T, Wedel D, Rowlingson J, et al.: Regional anesthesia in the patient receiving antithrombotic or thrombolytic therapy: American Society of Regional Anesthesia and Pain Medicine Evidence-Based Guidelines (ed 3), *Reg Anesth Pain Med* 35:64, 2010.

Kapoor A, Chuang W, Radhakrishnan N, et al.: Cost effectiveness of venous thromboembolism pharmacological prophylaxis in total hip and knee replacement: a systematic review, *Pharmacoeconomics* 28:521, 2010.

Lieberman JR, Cheng V, Cote MP: Pulmonary embolism rates following total hip arthroplasty with prophylactic anticoagulation: some pulmonary emboli cannot be avoided, *J Arthroplasty* 32:980, 2017.

Mont M, Jacobs J: AAOS clinical practice guideline: preventing venous thromboembolic disease in patients undergoing elective hip and knee arthroplasty, *J Am Acad Orthop Surg* 19:777, 2011.

Mont M, Jacobs JJ, Boggio LN, et al.: Preventing venous thromboembolic disease in patients undergoing elective hip and knee arthroplasty, *J Am Acad Orthop Surg* 19:768, 2011.

Mostafavi Tabatabaee R, Rasouli M, et al.: Cost-effective prophylaxis against venous thromboembolism after total joint arthroplasty: warfarin versus aspirin, *J Arthroplasty* 30:159, 2015.

Pedersen AB, Andersen IT, Overgaard S, et al.: Optimal duration of anticoagulant thromboprophylaxis in total hip arthroplasty: new evidence in 55,540 patients with osteoarthritis from the Nordic Arthroplasty Register Association (NARA) group, *Acta Orthop* 90:298, 2019.

Pierce T, Cherian J, Jauregui J, et al.: A current review of mechanical compression and its role in venous thromboembolic prophylaxis in total knee and total hip arthroplasty, *J Arthroplasty* 30:2279, 2015.

Trivedi NN, Fitzgerald SJ, Schmaier AH, et al.: Venous thromboembolism chemoprophylaxis in total hip and knee arthroplasty: a critical analysis review, *JBJS Rev* 7:e2, 2019.

Warren JA, Sundaram K, Anis HK, et al.: Have venous thromboembolism rates decreased in total hip and knee arthroplasty? *J Arthroplasty*, 2019 Aug 29. [Epub ahead of print].

Zahir U, Sterling R, Pellegrini V, Forte M: Inpatient pulmonary embolism after elective primary total hip and knee arthroplasty in the United States, *J Bone Joint Surg* 95:e175, 2013.

HEMATOMA

Ando W, Yamamoto K, Koyama T, et al.: Chronic expanding hematoma after metal-on-metal total hip arthroplasty, *Orthopedics* 40:e1103, 2017.

Bartelt RB, Sierra RJ: Recurrent hematomas within the iliopsoas muscle caused by impingement after total hip arthroplasty, *J Arthroplasty* 26:665, e1-5, 2011.

Mortazavi SM, Hansen P, Zmistowski B, et al.: Hematoma following primary total hip arthroplasty: a grave complication, *J Arthroplasty* 28:498–503, 2013.

INFECTION

Aggarwal VK, Weintraub S, Klock J, et al.: A comparison of prosthetic joint infection rates between direct anterior and non-anterior approach total hip arthroplasty, *Bone Joint J* 101-B(6_Supple_B):2, 2019.

American Academy of Orthopaedic Surgery: Prevention of orthopaedic implant infection in patients undergoing dental procedures: evidence-based guideline and evidence report, December 7, 2012. www.aaos.org/research/guidelines/PUDP/PUDP_guideline.pdf.

Berbari E, Mabry T, Tsaras G, et al.: Inflammatory blood laboratory levels as markers of prosthetic joint infection: a systematic review and meta-analysis, *J Bone Joint Surg* 92A:2102, 2010.

Berend KR, Lombardi Jr AV, Morris MJ, et al.: Two-stage treatment of hip periprosthetic joint infection is associated with a high rate of infection control but high mortality, *Clin Orthop Relat Res* 471:510, 2013.

Bingham J, Clarke H, Spangehl M, et al.: The alpha defensin-1 biomarker assay can be used to evaluate the potentially infected total joint arthroplasty, *Clin Orthop Relat Res* 472:4006, 2014.

Bozic KJ, Lau E, Kurtz S, et al.: Patient-related risk factors for periprosthetic joint infection and postoperative mortality following total hip arthroplasty in Medicare patients, *J Bone Joint Surg* 94:794, 2012.

Bravo T, Budhiparama N, Flynn S, et al.: Hip and Knee Section, Prevention, Postoperative Issues: Proceedings of International Consensus on Orthopedic Infections, *J Arthroplasty* 34(Supple 2):323, 2019.

Browne JA, Cancienne JM, Novicoff WM, et al.: Removal of an infected hip arthroplasty is a high-risk surgery: putting morbidity into context with other major nonorthopedic operations, *J Arthroplasty* 32:2834, 2017.

Ekpo TE, Berend KR, Morris MJ, et al.: Partial two-stage exchange for infected total hip arthroplasty: a preliminary report, *Clin Orthop Relat Res* 472:437, 2014.

Hansen E, Tetreault M, Zmistowski B, et al.: Outcome of one-stage cementless exchange for acute postoperative periprosthetic hip infection, *Clin Orthop Relat Res* 471:3214, 2013.

Hernandez NM, Hart A, Tauton MJ, et al.: Use of povidone-iodine irrigation prior to wound closure in primary total hip and knee arthroplasty: an analysis of 11, 738 cases, *J Bone Joint Surg Am* 101:1144, 2019.

Hoberg M, Konrads C, Engelien J, et al.: Similar outcomes between two-stage revisions for infection and aseptic hip revisions, *Int Orthop* 40:459, 2016.

Jevsevar DS, Abt E: The new AAOS-ADA clinical practice guideline on Prevention of Orthopaedic Implant Infection in Patients Undergoing Dental Procedures, *J Am Acad Orthop Surg* 21:195, 2013.

Jiménez-Garrido C, Gómez-Palomo JM, Rodriguez-Delourme I, et al.: The Kidney, Liver, Index surgery and C reactive protein score is a predictor of treatment response in acute prosthetic joint infection, *Int Orthop* 42:33, 2018.

Kalra KP, Lin KK, Bozic KJ, Ries MD: Repeat 2-stage revision for recurrent infection of total hip arthroplasty, *J Arthroplasty* 25:880, 2010.

Kosashvili Y, Backstein D, Safir O, et al.: Dislocation and infection after revision total hip arthroplasty: comparison between the first and multiply revised total hip arthroplasty, *J Arthroplasty* 26:1170, 2011.

Kurtz SM, Lau EC, Son MS, et al.: Are we winning or losing the battle with periprosthetic joint infection: trends in periprosthetic joint infection and mortality risk for the Medicare population, *J Arthroplasty* 33:3238, 2018.

Li C, Renz N, Trampuz A, et al.: Twenty common errors in the diagnosis and treatment of periprosthetic joint infection, *Int Orthop*, 2019 Oct 22. [Epub ahead of print].

Mortazavi SM, O'Neil JT, Zmistowski B, et al.: Repeat 2-stage exchange for infected total hip arthroplasty: a viable option? *J Arthroplasty* 27:923, 2012.

Pedersen AB, Mehnert F, Johnsen SP, Sørensen HT: Risk of revision of a total hip replacement in patients with diabetes mellitus: a population-based follow-up study, *J Bone Joint Surg* 92B:929, 2010.

Pedersen AB, Svendsson JE, Johnsen SP, et al.: Risk factors for revision due to infection after primary total hip arthroplasty: a population-based study of 80,756 primary procedures in the Danish Hip Arthroplasty Registry, *Acta Orthop* 81:542, 2010.

Peng KT, Kuo LT, Hsu WH, et al.: The effect of endoskeleton on antibiotic impregnated cement spacer for treating deep hip infection, *BMC Musculoskelet Disord* 12:10, 2011.

Romanò CL, Romanò D, Albisetti A, Meani E: Preformed antibiotic-loaded cement spacers for two-stage revision of infected total hip arthroplasty. Long-term results, *Hip Int* 22(Suppl 8):S46, 2012.

Rosinsky PJ, Greenberg A, Amster-Khan H, et al.: Selective comoponent retainment in the treatment of chronic periprosthetic infection after total hip arthroplasty: a systematic review, *J Am Acad Orthop Surg*, 2019 Oct 24. [Epub ahead of print].

Senneville E, Joulie D, Legout L, et al.: Outcome and predictors of treatment failure in total hip/knee prosthetic joint infections due to Staphylococcus aureus, *Clin Infect Dis* 53(4):334, 2011.

Shahi A, Kheir MM, Tarabichi M, et al.: Serum D-dimer test is promising for the diagnosis of periprosthetic joint infection and timing of reimplantation, *J Bone Joint Surg Am* 99:1419, 2017.

Tan TL, Maltenfort MG, Chen AF, et al.: Development and evaluation of a preoperative risk calculator for periprosthetic joint infection following total joint arthroplasty, *J Bone Joint Surg Am* 100:777, 2018.

Triantafyllopoulos GK, Poultsides LA, Sakellariou VI, et al.: Irrigation and debridement for periprosthetic infections of the hip and factors determining outcome, *Int Orthop* 39:1203, 2015.

Urquhart DM, Hanna FS, Brennan SL, et al.: Incidence and risk factors for deep surgical site infection after primary total hip arthroplasty: a systematic review, *J Arthroplasty* 25:1216, 2010.

NEUROVASCULAR INJURIES

Chughtai M, Khlopas A, Gwam CU, et al.: Nerve decompression surgery are total hip arthroplasty: what are the outcomes? *J Arthroplasty* 32:1335, 2016.

Fleischman AN, Rothman RH, Parvizi J: Femoral nerve palsy following total hip arthroplasty: incidence and course of recovery, *J Arthroplasty* 33:1194, 2018.

Gala L, Kim PR, Beaulé PE: Natural history of lateral femoral cutaneous nerve neuropraxia after anterior approach total hip arthroplasty, *Hip Int* 29:161, 2019.

Goetz MB, Seybold D, Gossé F, et al.: The risk of nerve lesions in hip alloarthroplasty, *Z Orthop Unfall* 148:163, 2010.

Goulding K, Beaulé PE, Kim PR, et al.: Incidence of lateral femoral cutaneous nerve neuropraxia after anterior approach hip arthroplasty, *Clin Orthop Relat Res* 468:2397, 2010.

Grob K, Manestar M, Ackland T, et al.: Potential risk to the superior gluteal nerve during the anterior approach to the hip joint: an anatomical study, *J Bone Joint Surg* 97:1426, 2015.

Grob K, Monahan R, Gilbey H, et al.: Distal extension of the direct anterior approach to the hip poses risk to neurovascular structures: an anatomical study, *J Bone Joint Surg* 97:126, 2015.

Park J, Hozack B, Kim P, et al.: Common peroneal palsy following total hip arthroplasty: prognostic factors for recovery, *J Bone Joint Surg* 95:e551, 2013.

Shubert D, Madoff S, Milillo R, Nandi S: Neurovascular structure proximity to acetabular retractors in total hip arthroplasty, *J Arthroplasty* 30:145, 2015.

Sullivan CW, Banerjee S, Desai K, et al.: Safe zones for anterior acetabular retractor placement in direct anterior total hip aarthroplasty: a cadaveric study, *J Am Acad Orthop Surg* 27:e969, 2019.

Wolfe M, Bäumer P, Pedro M, et al.: Sciatic nerve injury related to hip replacement surgery: imaging detection by MR neurography despite susceptibility artifacts, *PLoS One* 9:e89154, 2014.

Zappe B, Glauser PM, Majewski M, et al.: Long-term prognosis of nerve palsy after total hip arthroplasty: results of two-year-follows-ups and long-term results after a mean time of 8 years, *Arch Orthop Trauma Surg* 134:1477, 2014.

LEG-LENGTH DISCREPANCY

Harwin SF, Pivec R: Limb-length discrepancy after total hip arthroplasty, *Orthopedics* 37:78, 2014.

Lazeenec JY, Folinais D, Florequin C, et al.: Does patients' perception of leg length after total hip arthroplasty correlate with anatomical leg length? *J Arthroplasty* 33:1562, 2018.

Licini DJ, Burnikel DJ, Meneghini RM, Ochsner JL: Comparison of limb-length discrepancy after THA: with and without computer navigation, *Orthopedics* 36:e543, 2013.

Lim YW, Huddleston 3rd JI, Goodman SB, et al.: Proximal femoral shape changes the risk of leg length discrepancy after primary total hp arthropasty, *J Arthroplasty* 33:3699, 2018.

Manzotti A, Cerveri P, De Momi E, et al.: Does computer-assisted surgery benefit leg length restoration in total hip replacement? Navigation versus conventional freehand, *Int Orthop* 35:19, 2011.

Nam D, Sculco PK, Abdel MP, et al.: Leg-length inequalities following THA based on surgical technique, *Orthopedics* 36:e395, 2013.

Ng VY, Kean JR, Glassman AH: Limb-length discrepancy after total hip arthroplasty, *J Bone Joint Surg* 95:1426, 2013.

Rajpaul J, Rasool MN: Leg length correction in computer assisted primary total hip arthroplasty: a collective review of the literature, *J Orthop* 15:442, 2018.

Rice IS, Stowell RL, Biswanath PC, Cortina GJ: Three intraoperative methods to determine limb-length discrepancy in THA, *Orthopedics* 37:e488, 2014.

Sykes A, Hill J, Orr J, et al.: Patients' perceptions of leg length discrepancy post total hip arthroplasty, *Hip Int* 25:452, 2015.

Tipton SC, Sutherland JK, Schwarzkopf R: The assessment of limb length discrepancy before total hip arthroplasty, *J Arthroplasty* 31(4):888–892, 2016.

DISLOCATION

Blizzard DJ, Klement MR, Penrose CT, et al.: Cervical myelopathy doubles the rate of dislocation and fracture after total hip arthroplasty, *J Arthroplaslty* 31(Suppl 9):242, 2016.

Brown ML, Ezzet KA: Relaxed hip precautions do not increase early dislocation rate following total hip arthroplasty, *J Am Acad Orthop Surg*, 2019 Sep 25. [Epub ahead of print].

De Martino I, D'Apolito R, Soranoglo VG, et al.: Dislocation following total hip arthroplasty using dual mobility components: a systematic review, *Bone Joint J* 99-B(ASuppl 1):18, 2017.

Garcia-Rey E, Garcia-Cimbrelo E: Abductor biomechanics clinically impact the total hip arthroplasty dislocation rate: a prospective long-term study, *J Arthroplasty* 31:484, 2016.

Gaudsen EB, Parhar HS, Popper JE, et al.: Risk factors for early dislocation following primary elective total hip arthroplasty, *J Arthroplasty* 33:1567, 2018.

Heckmann N, McKnight B, Stefl M, et al.: Late dislocation following total hip arthroplasty: spinopelvic imbalance as a causative factor, *J Bone Joint Surg Am* 100:1845, 2018.

Ike H, Dorr LD, Trasolini N, et al.: Spine-pelvis-hip relationship in the functioning of a total hip replacememt, *J Bone Joint Surg Am* 100:1606, 2018.

Krenzel BA, Berend ME, Malinzak RA, et al.: High preoperative range of motion is a significant risk factor for dislocation in primary total hip arthroplasty, *J Arthroplasty* 25(Suppl 6):31, 2010.

Saiz AM, Lum ZC, Pereira GC: Etiology, evaluation, and management of dislocation after primary total hip arthroplasty, *JBJS Rev* 7:e7, 2019.

Seagrave KG, Troelsen A, Madsen BG, et al.: Can surgeons reduce the risk for dislocation after primary total hip arthroplasty performed using the posterolateral approach? *J Arthroplasty* 32:3146, 2017.

Smith TO, Jepsen P, Beswick A, et al.: Assistive devices, hip precautions, environmental modifications and training to prevent dislocation and improve function after hip arthroplasty, *Cochrane Database Syst Rev* 7:CD010815, 2016.

Takao M, Otake Y, Fukuda N, et al.: The posterior capsular ligamentous complex contributes to hip joint stability in distraction, *J Arthroplasty* 33:919, 2018.

Wang Z, Hou JZ, Wu CH, et al.: A systemati review and meta-analysis of direct anterior approach versus posterior approach in total hip arthroplasty, *J Orthop Surg Res* 13:299, 2018.

Wera GD, Ting NT, Moric M, et al.: Classification and management of the unstable total hip arthroplasty, *J Arthroplasty* 27:710, 2012.

FRACTURE

Abdel MP, Houdek MT, Watts CD, et al.: Epidemiology of periprosthetic femoral fractures in 5427 revision total hip arthroplasties; a 40-year experience, *Bone Joint J* 98-B:468, 2016.

Abdel MP, Lewallen DG, Berry DJ: Periprosthetic femur fractures treated with modular fluted, tapered stems, *Clin Orthop Relat Res* 472:599, 2014.

Abdel MP, Watts CD, Houdek MT, et al.: Epidemiology o periprosthetic fracture of the femur in 32 644 primary total hip arthroplasties: a 40-year experience, *Bone Joint J* 98-B:461, 2016.

Corton K, Macdonald SJ, McCalden RW, et al.: Results of cemented femoral revisions for periprosthetic femoral fractures in the elderly, *J Arthroplasty* 27:220, 2012.

Ehlinger M, Adam P, Moser T, et al.: Type C periprosthetic fractures treated with locking plate fixation with a mean follow up of 2.5 years, *Orthop Traumatol Surg Res* 96:44, 2010.

Frisch NB, Charters MA, Sikora-Klak J, et al.: Intraoperative periprosthetic femur fracture: a biomechanical analysis of cerclage fixation, *J Arthroplasty* 30:1449, 2015.

Hickerson LE, Zbeda RM, Gadinsky NE, et al.: Outcomes of surgical treatment of periprosthetic acetabular fractures, *J Orthop Trauma* 33(Suppl 2):S49, 2019.

Lever JP, Zdero R, Housiainen MT, et al.: The biomechanical analysis of three plating fixation systems for periprosthetic femoral fracture near the tip of a total hip arthroplasty, *J Orthop Surg Res* 5:45, 2010.

Maury AC, Pressman A, Cayen B, et al.: Proximal femoral allograft treatment of Vancouver type-B3 periprosthetic femoral fracture after total hip arthroplasty, *J Bone Joint Surg* 88A:953, 2006.

Mayle RE, Della Valle CJ: Fractures about the hip. Intra-operative fractures during THA, *J Bone Joint Surg* 94(Suppl A):26, 2012.

Rayan F, Konan S, Haddad FS: Uncemented revision hip arthroplasty in B2 and B3 periprosthetic femoral fractures—a prospective analysis, *Hip Int* 20:38, 2010.

Sidler-Maier CC, Waddell JP: Incidence and predisposing factors of periprosthetic proximal femoral fractures: a literature review, *Int Orthop* 39:1673, 2015.

Singh JA, Jensen MR, Harmsen SW, Lewallen DG: Are gender, comorbidity, and obesity risk factors for postoperative periprosthetic fractures after primary total hip arthroplasty? *J Arthroplasty* 28:126, 2013.

Singh JA, Jensen MR, Lewallen DG: Patient factors predict periprosthetic fractures after revision total hip arthroplasty, *J Arthroplasty* 27:1507, 2012.

Unified Classification System for Periprosthetic Fractures (UCPF), *J Orthop Trauma* 32(Suppl 1):S141, 2018.

TROCHANTERIC NONUNION

Fehm MN, Huddleston JI, Burke DW, et al.: Repair of a deficient abductor mechanism with Achilles tendon allograft after total hip replacement, *J Bone Joint Surg* 92A:2305, 2010.

Hartofilakidis G, Babis GC, Georgiades G, Kourlaba G: Trochanteric osteotomy in total hip replacement for congenital hip disease, *J Bone Joint Surg* 93B:601, 2011.

Mei XY, Gong YJ, Safir OA, et al.: Fixation options following greater trochanteric osteotomies and fractures in total hip arthroplasty: a systematic review, *JBJS Rev* 6:e4, 2018.

Miozzari HH, Dora C, Clark JM, Nötzli HP: Late repair of abductor avulsion after the transgluteal approach for hip arthroplasty, *J Arthroplasty* 25:450, 2010.

Whiteside LA: Surgical technique: gluteus maximus and tensor fascia lata transfer for primary deficiency of the abductors of the hip, *Clin Orthop Relat Res* 472:645, 2014.

LOOSENING/OSTEOLYSIS

Albert C, Frei H, Duncan C, Fernlund G: Mechanisms of stem subsidence in femoral impaction allografting, *Crit Rev Biomed Eng* 39(6):493, 2011.

Dimitriou D, Liow MH, Tsai TY, et al.: Early outcomes of revision surgery for taper corrosion of dual taper total hip arthroplalsty in 187 patients, *J Arthroplasty* 31:1549, 2016.

Fillingham YA, Della Valle CJ, Bohl DD, et al.: Serum metal levels for diagnosis of adverse local tissue reactions secondry to corrosion in metal-on-polyethylene total hip arthroplasty, *H Arthroplasty* 32:S277, 2017.

Galea VP, Laaksonen I, Connell JW, et al.: What is the clinical presentation of adverse local tissue reaction in metal-on-metal hip arthroplasty? An MRI study, *Clin Orthop Relat Res* 477:353, 2019.

Hamilton WG, Hopper Jr RH, Engh Jr CA, Engh CA: Survivorship of polyethylene liner exchanges performed for the treatment of wear and osteolysis among porous-coated cups, *J Arthroplasty* 26(Suppl 6):75, 2010.

Harris B, Owen JR, Wayne JS, Jiranek WA: Does femoral component loosening predispose to femoral fracture? An in vitro comparison of cemented hips, *Clin Orthop Relat Res* 468:497, 2010.

Heijnens LJ, Schotanus MG, Kort NP, et al.: Results of cemented anatomically adapted total hip arthroplasty: a follow-up longer than 10 years, *J Arthroplasty* 31:194, 2016.

Kwon YM, MacAulifffe J, Arauz PG, et al.: Sensivity and specificity of metal ion level in predicting adverse local tissue reactions due to head-neck taper corrosion in primary metal-on-polyethylene total hip arthroplast, *J Arthroplasty* 33:3025, 2018.

Kwon YM, Rossi D, MacAuliffe J, et al.: Risk factors associated with early complications of revision surgery for head-neck taper corrosion in metal-on-polyethylene total hip arthroplasty, *J Arthroplasty* 33:3231, 2018.

Kwon YM, Tsai TY, Leone WA, et al.: Sensitivity and specificity of metal ion levels in predicting "pseudotumors" due to taper corrosion in patients with dual taper modular total hip arthroplaty, *J Arthroplasty* 32:996, 2017.

Matharu GS, Judge A, Pandit HG, et al.: Which factors influence the rate of failre following metal-on-metal hip arthroplasty revision surgery performed for adverse reactions to metal debris? An analysis from the National Joint Registry for England and Wales, *Bone Joint J* 99-B:1020, 2017.

McGrory BJ, Jorgensen AH: High early major complication rate after revision for mechanically assisted crevice corrosion in metal-on-polyethylene total hip arthroplasty, *J Arthroplasty* 32:3704, 2017.

Narkbunnam R, Amanatullah DF, Electricwala AJ, et al.: Radiographic scoring system for the evaluation of stability of cementless acetabular components in the presence of osteolysis, *Bone Joint J* 99-B:601, 2017.

Nieuwenhuijse MJ, Valstar ER, Kaptein BL, Nelissen RG: Good diagnostic performance of early migration as a predictor of late aseptic loosening of acetabular cups: results from ten years of follow-up with Roentgen stereophotogrammetric analysis (RSA), *J Bone Joint Surg* 94:874, 2012.

Okroj KT, Calkins TE, Kayupov E, et al.: The alpha-defensin test for diagnosing periprosthetic joint infection in the setting of an adverse local tissue reaction secondary to a filed metal-on-metal bearing or corrosion at the head-neck junction, *J Arthroplasty* 33:1896, 2018.

Patel AR, Sweeney P, Ochenjele G, et al.: Radiographically silent loosening of the acetabular component in hip arthroplasty, *Am J Orthop (Belle Mead NJ)* 44:406, 2015.

Teng S, Yi C, Krettek C, Jagodzinski M: Smoking and risk of prosthesis-related complications after total hip arthroplasty: a meta-analysis of cohort studies, *PLoS ONE* 10:e0125294, 2015.

Vadei L, Kieser DC, Frampton C, et al.: Survivorship of total hip replacements following isolated liner exchange for wear ALTR, *J Arthroplasty* 32:3484, 2017.

REVISION

Abdel MP, Cottino U, Larson DR: Modular fluted tapered stems in aseptic revision total hip arthroplasty, *J Bone Joint Surg Am* 99:873, 2017.

Abdel MP, Trousdale RT, Berry DJ: Pelvis discontinuity associated with total hip arthroplasty: evaluation and management, *J Am Acad Orthop Surg* 25:330, 2017.

Amanatullah DF, Howard JL, Siman H, et al.: Revision total hip arthroplasty in patients with extensive proximal femoral bone loss using a fluted tapered modular femoral component, *Bone Joint J* 97-B:312, 2015.

Babis GC, Sakellariou VI, Chatziantoniou AN, et al.: High complication rate in reconstruction of Paprosky type IIIa acetabular defects using an oblong implant with modular side plates and a hook, *J Bone Joint Surg* 93A:1592, 2011.

Babis GC, Sakellariou VI, O'Connor MI, et al.: Proximal femoral allograft-prosthesis composites in revision hip replacement: a 12-year follow-up study, *J Bone Joint Surg* 92B:349, 2010.

Blumenfeld TJ: Removing a well-fixed nonmodular large-bearing cementless acetabular component: a simple modification of an existing removal device, *J Arthroplasty* 25:498, 2010.

Bongers J, Smulders K, Nijhof MW: Severe obesity increases risk of infection after revision total hip arthroplasty, *J Arthroplasty*, 2019 Jul 27. [Epub ahead of print].

Flecher X, Paprosky W, Grillo JC, et al.: Do tantalum components provide adequate primary fixation in all acetabular revisions? *Orthop Traumatol Surg Res* 96:235, 2010.

Gwam CU, Mistry JB, Mohamed NS, et al.: Current epidemiology of revision total hip arthroplasty in the United States: National Inpatient Sample 2009 to 2013, *J Arthroplasty* 32:2088, 2017.

Harris B, Owen JR, Wayne JS, Jiranek WA: Does femoral component loosening predispose to femoral fracture? An in vitro comparison of cemented hips, *Clin Orthop Relat Res* 468:497, 2010.

Imbuldeniya AM, Walter WK, Zicat BA, Walter WL: The S-ROM hydroxyapatite proximally-coated modular femoral stem in revision hip replacement: results of 397 hips at a minimum ten-year follow-up, *Bone Joint J* 96-B:730, 2014.

Jenkins DR, Odland AN, Sierra RJ, et al.: Minimum five-year outcomes with porous tantalum acetabular cup and augment construct in complex revision total hip arthroplasty, *J Bone Joint Surg Am* 99:e49, 2017.

Korim MT, Esler CN, Ashford RU: Systematic review of proximal femoral arthroplasty for non-neoplastic conditions, *J Arthroplasty* 29:2117, 2014.

Lachiewicz PF, Soileau ES: Tantalum components in difficult acetabular revisions, *Clin Orthop Relat Res* 468:454, 2010.

Lamberton TD, Kenny PJ, Whitehouse SL, et al.: Femoral impaction grafting in revision total hip arthroplasty: a follow-up of 540 hips, *J Arthroplasty* 26:2254, 2011.

Lim CT, Ananatullah DF, Huddleston 3rd JI, et al.: Cortical strut allograft support of modular femoral junctions during revision total hip arthroplasty, *J Arthroplasty* 32:1586, 2017.

Megas P, Georgiou CS, Panagopoulos A, et al.: Removal of well-fixed components in femoral revision arthroplasty with controlled segmentation of the proximal femur, *J Orthop Surg Res* 9:137, 2014.

Schmidt A, Batailler C, Fary C, et al.: Dual mobility cups in revision total hip arthroplasty: efficient strategy to decrease dislocation risk, *J Arthroplasty*, 2019 Sep 5. [Epub ahead of print].

Sternheim A, Rogers BA, Kuzyk PR, et al.: Segmental proximal femoral bone loss and revision total hip replacement in patients with developmental dysplasia of the hip: the role of allograft prosthesis composite, *J Bone Joint Surg* 94:762, 2012.

Talmo CT, Robbins CE, Siddiqi A, et al.: Revision of a dual-modular stem in patients with adverse tissue reaction, *Hip Int*, 2019 Aug 7. [Epub ahead of print].

Trumm BN, Callaghan JJ, George CA, et al.: Minimum 20-year follow-up results of revision total hip arthroplasty with improved cementing technique, *J Arthroplasty* 29:236, 2014.

Viste A, Perry KI, Taunton MJ, et al.: Proximal femoral replacement in contemporary revision total hip arthroplasty for severe femoral bone loss: a review of outcomes, *Bone Joint J* 99-B:325, 2017.

Wilson MJ, Hook S, Whitehouse SL, et al.: Femoral impaction bone grafting in revision hip arthroplasty:705 cases from the originating centre, *Bone Joint J* 98-B:1611, 2016.

POSTOPERATIVE MANAGEMENT

Eannucci EF, Barlow BT, Carroll KM, et al.: A protocol of pose avoidance in place of hip precautions after posterior-approach total hip arthroplasty may not increase risk of post-operative dislocation, *HSS J* 15:247, 2019.

Foucher KC, Wimmer MA, Moisio KC, et al.: Time course and extent of functional recovery during the first postoperative year after minimally invasive total hip arthroplasty with two different surgical surgical approaches—a randomized controlled trial, *J Biomech* 44:372, 2011.

Haynes JA, Stambough JB, Sassoon AA, et al.: Contemporary surgical indications and referral trends in revision total hip arthroplasty: a 10-year review, *J Arthroplasty* 31:622, 2016.

Hernandez VH, Ong A, Orozco F, et al.: When is it safe for patients to drive after right total hip arthroplasty? *J Arthroplasty* 30:627, 2015.

Hio AM, van Grinsven S, Lucas C, et al.: Partial versus unrestricted weight bearing after an uncemented femoral stem in total hip arthroplasty: recommendation of a concise rehabilitation protocol from a systematic review of the literature, *Arch Orthop Trauma Surg* 130:547, 2010.

Hol AM, van Grinsven S, Lucas C, et al.: Partial versus unrestricted weight bearing after an uncemented femoral stem in total hip arthroplasty: recommendation of a concise rehabilitation protocol from a systematic review of the literature, *Arch Orthop Trauma Surg* 130:547, 2010.

Kornuijt A, Das D, Sijbesma T, et al.: The rate of dislocation is not increased when minimal precautions are used after total hip arthroplasty using the posterolateral approach: a prospective, comparative safety study, *Bone Joint J* 98-B:589, 2016.

Rondon AJ, Tan TL, Goswami K, et al.: When can I drive? Predictors of returning to driving after total joint arthroplasty, *J Am Acad Orthop Surg*, 2019 Sep 18. [Epub ahead of print].

van der Weegen W, Kornuijt A, Das D: Do lifestyle restrictions and precautions prevent dislocation after total hip arthroplasty? A systematic review and meta-analysis of the literature, *Clin Rehabil* 30:329, 2016.

Watts CD, Houdek MT, Wagner ER, et al.: Morbidly obese vs nonobese aseptic revision total hip arthroplasty: surprisingly similar outcomes, *J Arthroplasty* 31(4):842–845, 2016.

The complete list of references is available online at ExpertConsult.com.

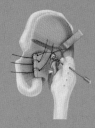

CHAPTER 2

SURFACE REPLACEMENT HIP ARTHROPLASTY

Marcus C. Ford

Currently, younger patients make up the fastest growing group of total hip arthroplasty (THA) patients; however, American Academy of Hip and Knee Surgeons (AAHKS) surveys have demonstrated that younger patients report decreased satisfaction and less frequent return to high-level activities than older THA patients. Surface replacement arthroplasty (SRA) is a potential treatment option for this group of younger, high-demand, hip arthroplasty patients.

Hip resurfacing is not a new concept. Early designs for SRA, beginning in the 1950s through 1970s, often used polyethylene components that produced unacceptable wear with excess acetabular bone loss and implant failure. Retrieval data from the Wagner and Amstutz implants demonstrated especially high rates of wear and osteolysis, leading to decreased interest in SRA by the early 1980s. The technique remained appealing, however, especially in younger patients, because SRA allows greater preservation of bone stock (on the femoral side) and more anatomic restoration of the hip joint compared to THA.

Metal-on-metal THA implants were used in Europe for many years but were not commonly accepted in the United States. First-generation European metal-on-metal components, including the McKee-Farrar and Ring designs, demonstrated low wear rates on retrieval analysis. Using metallurgy and technology from the successful metal-on-metal THAs, McMinn and Treacy introduced the modern SRA, the Birmingham Hip Resurfacing (BHR) System (Smith and Nephew Memphis, TN) (Fig. 2.1) in 1997. Early SRA issues due to thin polyethylene components and acetabular bone loss were eliminated by solid metal ingrowth acetabular components. Manufacturing techniques were developed for the BHR to mimic the high carbide content, low tolerances, and high implant stiffness that were successful in the McKee-Farrar and Ring THA designs.

With over 20 years of use outside the United States, SRA use received Food and Drug Administration (FDA) approval in 2006. Although many modern SRA designs have been used, the BHR remains the only SRA currently approved and available for use in the United States. Additionally, the BHR is one of two SRA implants to receive a 10A or better rating from the Orthopaedic Device Evaluation Panel (ODEP) and remains the only SRA implant to receive the maximum 10A* ODEP rating.

RESULTS

SRA remains a technically challenging procedure with increased implant costs. Thus, compared to THA, SRA must demonstrate similar revision and complication rates along with clinical advantages to warrant its continued use.

According to Australian Orthopaedic Association National Joint Replacement Registry (AOANJRR) data, the overall revision rate for SRA is greater than that of THA at 5 and 8 years; however, certain patient factors equalize revision rates: primary diagnosis, age, gender, and component size. Osteoarthritis has the lowest early revision rate, with other diagnoses such as osteonecrosis, dysplasia, and inflammatory arthritis showing significantly higher revision rates. For men younger than 55 years old with a primary diagnosis of osteoarthritis, SRA has equivalent or superior survivorship to THA at 8 years. The BHR has shown superior survivorship to other SRA designs in the registry.

Surgeons from Oxford, England, have demonstrated greater than 98% BHR survivorship at 12 to 15 years in appropriately selected patients. In a more recent report from a single American institution, 10-year survivorship was 98% for men younger than 60 years old with a diagnosis of osteoarthritis and femoral head sizes of at least 48 mm. Another North American multi-center study demonstrated equivalent complication and revision rates at 2-year follow-up compared to published THA results, and a recent systematic review found similar revision and complication rates.

There also is evidence to suggest that SRA patients have superior activity scores and faster return to sport than THA patients. Studies have demonstrated that SRA more accurately restores leg lengths and femoral offset; 100% restoration of femoral neck bone density also is achieved by 6 months after surgery, which may play a part in the reported decrease in thigh pain for SRA patients compared to THA patients.

Cobalt and chromium ion debris causing adverse local soft-tissue reactions or systemic toxicity remains a major concern with SRA. Current AAHKS guidelines recommend cobalt and chromium blood level checks on any SRA patient demonstrating symptoms of adverse tissue reaction or metal toxicity. For patients with bilateral BHR, a maximal threshold value of 5.5 µg/L for both cobalt and chromium is sensitive for identifying patients at risk for metallosis. An asymptomatic increase in metal ion levels also has been reported between early and mid-term follow-up in patients with unilateral SRA. If elevated blood cobalt and chromium levels are found, advanced imaging with either metal-subtraction sequence MRI or ultrasound is recommended to evaluate for local soft-tissue reaction. Certain SRA implants have demonstrated substantial issues with metallosis and soft-tissue reactions, but the BHR has demonstrated a less than 1% rate of adverse soft-tissue reaction secondary to metallosis in appropriately selected patients. Appropriate component positioning plays an important role in decreasing the potential for edge wear and the development of metallosis.

INDICATIONS AND PATIENT SELECTION

Currently, SRA is most often indicated for young (<65 years old), highly active males with femoral head sizes greater than or equal to 48 mm who have a diagnosis of osteoarthritis. Near-perfect proximal femoral anatomy is required; patients with large femoral head cysts or osteonecrosis are

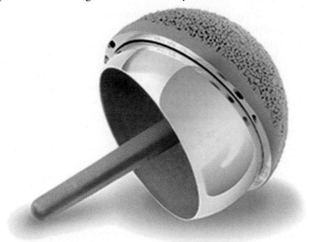

FIGURE 2.1 Birmingham Hip Resurfacing System (Smith & Nephew, Memphis TN).

not considered SRA candidates. Preoperative leg-length discrepancy is a relative contraindication to SRA. Patients with pre-existing renal disease also are not considered candidates for SRA because of the potential for metallosis. At our institution, we also no longer consider patients with significant acetabular dysplasia to be arthroplasty candidates.

PREOPERATIVE RADIOGRAPHIC EVALUATION AND TEMPLATING

As with all arthroplasty surgery, careful preoperative templating, radiographic evaluation, and planning are critical to success (Fig. 2.2). The femoral head and neck bone quality should be normal. Significant cystic change within the femoral head is a contraindication for SRA. If the femoral neck is enlarged by remodeling, there may not be a clear delineation between the head and neck, with the head being larger than the neck. If the neck and head are of the same width, especially along the superior neck as seen on an anteroposterior radiograph, then removing bone from the head will risk notching the femoral neck and thus risk neck fracture.

The first step in templating is to measure the size of the femoral component. A template is laid over a radiograph of the proximal femur. The width of the opening of the femoral component should be wider than the femoral neck by 2 to 4 mm total. If not, the next larger template should be used. Then, the center post of the implant is aligned over the center of the femoral neck on radiograph. The line from the top of the greater trochanter to where the line on the template intersects the lateral cortex is measured and documented (Fig. 2.2A). This distance will be used when measuring the valgus angle of the implant intraoperatively (Fig. 2.2B).

POSTOPERATIVE MANAGEMENT

Anteroposterior and cross-table lateral radiographs are taken in the recovery room to confirm component position (Fig. 2.3). Periarticular injections, hypotensive spinal anesthesia, tranexamic acid, and multimodal pain medication regimens are used perioperatively to allow same-day mobilization.

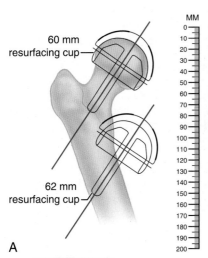

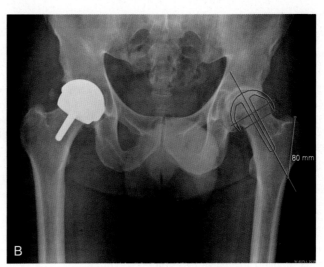

FIGURE 2.2 Templating of femoral component. Measurement will be used intraoperatively to measure valgus angle.

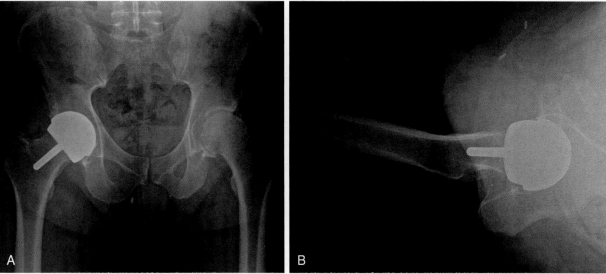

FIGURE 2.3 Postoperative anteroposterior and cross-table radiographs obtained to confirm component position.

Patients are allowed to bear weight as tolerated immediately after surgery. Because of the low risk of dislocation (0.3% in the Australian registry), hip precautions are not required for SRA patients.

Patients typically are evaluated at 4 to 6 weeks for clinical progress and radiographic evaluation. Patients can participate in low-impact exercise beginning at 6 weeks and are released to high-impact activities and sports 6 months after surgery.

HIP RESURFACING TECHNIQUE— BIRMINGHAM HIP REPLACEMENT

Currently, only one hip resurfacing product is available for use in the United States: Birmingham Hip Resurfacing System (Smith and Nephew, Memphis, TN).

TECHNIQUE 2.1

POSITIONING

- Position the patient laterally with the affected hip up. Stabilize the pelvis with a pelvic clamp or pegboard, with the pelvis oriented straight up and down. If the pelvis is leaning forward, the acetabular component may be placed in retroversion; if it is leaning backward, the acetabular component may be placed in excessive anteversion.

APPROACH AND EXPOSURE

- To resurface the hip, extensive exposure is necessary to view the acetabulum without removal of the femoral head. Therefore, steps must be taken to achieve exposure not routinely used in THA surgery.
- Make a curved posterolateral skin incision over the greater trochanter, angling the proximal portion posteriorly, pointing toward the posterior superior iliac spine (Fig.

2.4A). Carry the incision over the center of the greater trochanter and then distally over the shaft of the femur to end over the attachment of the gluteus maximus on the linea aspera.
- Divide the subcutaneous tissue in a single plane over the fascia of the gluteus maximus proximally and the fascia of the iliotibial band distally. Make a longitudinal incision over the middle to posterior third of the fascia over the greater trochanter and extend it distally over the femoral shaft. Extend the proximal end of the incision through the thin fascia over the gluteus maximus in the same direction as the skin incision. Bluntly split the fibers of the gluteus maximus muscle, taking care to find and cauterize any bleeding.
- Release the tendinous attachment of the gluteus maximus from the linea aspera to maximally internally rotate the femur to provide satisfactory exposure of the proximal femur and femoral head. If the gluteus maximus is not released, the sciatic nerve may be at risk of compression at the time of preparation of the femoral head. Place a hemostat under the gluteus maximus tendon as the tendon is divided to avoid injuring branches of the medial femoral circumflex artery and the first perforating artery. Leave a centimeter of tendon attached to the linea aspera and femoral shaft for later repair.
- Widely spread the fascial plane just divided using a Charnley or self-retaining retractor. The posterior greater trochanter and gluteus medius should be easily seen. Remove the trochanteric bursa.
- Retract the gluteus medius muscle and tendon anteriorly. A hooked instrument such as a Hibbs retractor is useful. Under the gluteus medius is the piriformis, which is exposed. Release the piriformis tendon from the femur. With an elevator, raise the gluteus minimus off the capsule of the hip to expose the posterosuperior hip capsule. Use of a narrow cobra retractor is helpful to see this area when it is placed under the gluteus minimus and medius.
- Expose the plane distally between the capsule and the short external rotator muscles. Release the short external

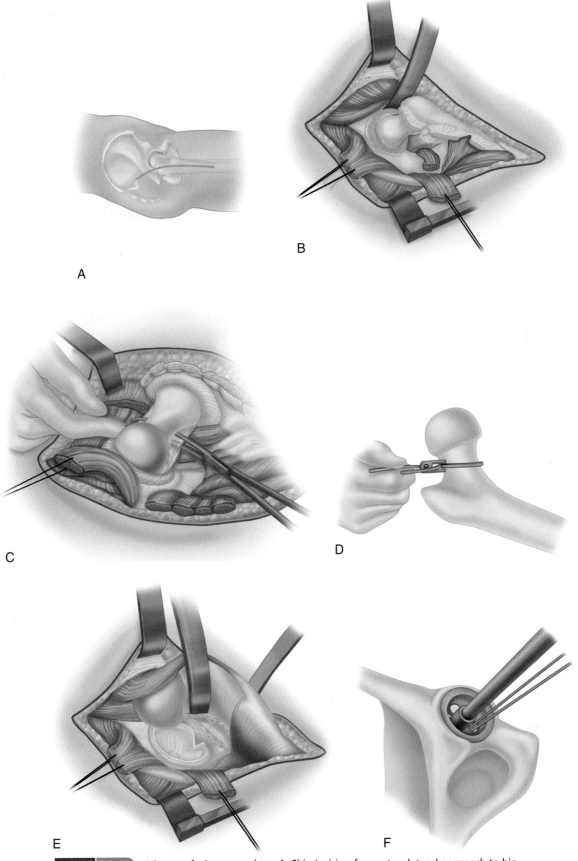

FIGURE 2.4 Hip resurfacing procedure. **A,** Skin incision for posterolateral approach to hip. **B,** Completed soft-tissue dissection. **C,** Anterior capsule divided along course of psoas tendon sheath. **D,** Measurement of femoral neck diameter. **E,** Femur retracted well anteriorly to allow access to acetabulum. **F,** Cup trial used to determine correct implant positioning.

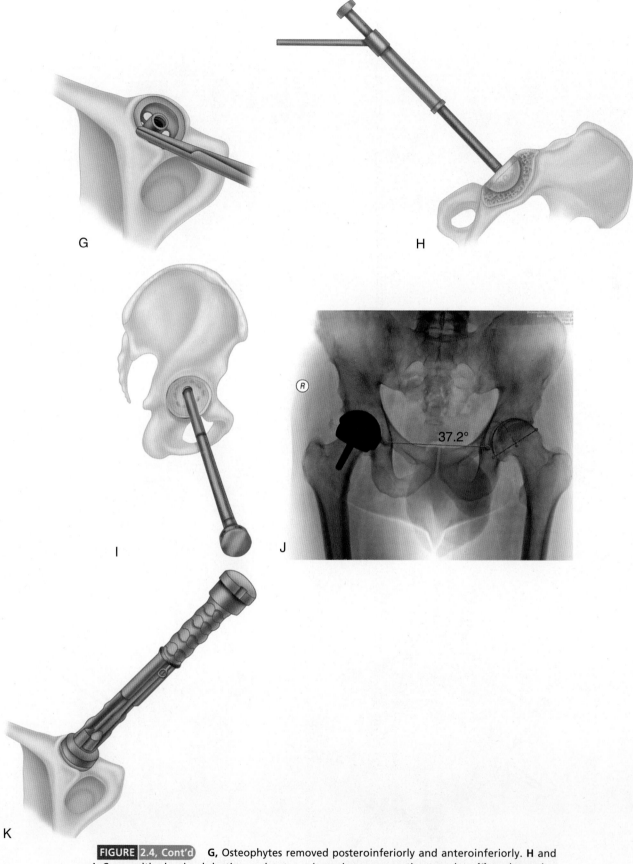

FIGURE 2.4, Cont'd G, Osteophytes removed posteroinferiorly and anteroinferiorly. **H** and **I,** Cup positioning in abduction and anteversion using preoperative template (**J**) to determine correct angle. **K,** Acetabular component fully impacted in 10 to 20 degrees anteversion and 35 to 45 degrees abduction. **SEE TECHNIQUE 2.1.**

rotator muscles off the femur including the quadratus femoris distally. Coagulate the vessels in this area.

- The capsule of the hip is now completely exposed posteriorly, superiorly, and inferiorly. The lesser trochanter also is visible. With the hip in internal rotation, make an incision in the capsule circumferentially, leaving at least a centimeter of capsule still attached to the femoral neck. This centimeter of capsule is later used to repair the capsule back as well as to provide protection to the intraosseous vessels needed to maintain vascularity of the femoral neck.

- Make two radial incisions in the posterior capsule to create a posterior capsular flap. This is helpful for retraction and later repair (Fig. 2.4B).

- Dislocate the femoral head and perform a complete anterior capsulotomy with sharp scissors or Bovie cautery. The inferior portion of the capsule is seen by extending and internally rotating the femur. The psoas tendon is exposed at the lesser trochanter, and the capsule is isolated just in front of the psoas tendon. While maintaining the scissors just posterior to the psoas tendon, incise the capsule from inferior to superior (Fig. 2.4C). Maintain the femur in internal rotation and apply anterior traction with a bone hook on the lesser trochanter.

- Perform the proximal end of the capsulotomy by flexing the femur 90 degrees and maintaining a narrow cobra retractor under the gluteus muscles. Incise the capsule with sharp scissors while internally rotating the femur to beyond 100 degrees. If a complete capsulotomy is not performed, exposure of the femur is compromised.

- Measure the femoral neck from superior to inferior, its longest dimension (Fig. 2.4D). The measurement tool should loosely fit over the femoral neck to avoid undersizing the femoral component, which could cause notching of the femoral neck. Femoral neck notches may weaken the neck and predispose it to early postoperative fracture. If there is any doubt, choose the next larger size of the femoral head component.

- Once the size of the femoral component is known, the acetabular component size also is known because the acetabular component is matched with components either 6 or 8 mm larger than the femoral component. Therefore, if the femoral head measures 52 mm, the acetabular component will need to be either 58 or 60 mm. That means (in this case) the acetabulum will need to be reamed to 57 or 59 mm, respectively.

- The key to exposure of the acetabulum is to dislocate the femoral head out of the way anteriorly and superiorly. Create an anterosuperior pouch large enough for the femoral head under the gluteus muscles and above the ilium. This is done by sharply dissecting the soft tissues off the bone of the ilium, including the capsule and tendons of the rectus femoris from the superior acetabular lip and the anterior inferior iliac spine.

- Once the pouch has been created, dislocate the femoral head into the pouch under the gluteus muscles and retract it with a sharp, narrow Hohmann retractor driven into the ilium superior to the acetabulum and resting on the femoral neck (Fig. 2.4E). Additional pins may be driven into the ilium and ischium to help with the acetabular exposure. A retractor also is placed inferiorly to expose the transverse acetabular ligament. Sharply excise the labrum and cotyloid fossa soft tissue (Fig. 2.5).

- Ream the acetabulum medially through the cotyloid fossa of the acetabulum to the medial wall. Take care not to ream through the medial wall. Once medialized, the reamers are used to increase the bony acetabulum to the desired size. The acetabulum usually is underreamed by 1 mm from the desired component size. Use an acetabular trial to assess the potential component's stability. The trial components in the BHR system are 1 mm smaller than their stated size to provide for tighter fitting of the actual component. Impact the trial into the acetabulum with a mallet, and excise osteophytes for unobstructed cup insertion (Fig. 2.4F,G). If that size trial is tight, the acetabular implant of the same size is selected. If the trial is loose, the acetabulum may be reamed 1 or 2 mm more to the next size acetabular component that matches the appropriate size femoral head.

- It is critical for the long-term success of the hip that the acetabular component's orientation is done correctly. Implant the acetabular component in 10 to 20 degrees of anteversion and 35 to 45 degrees of abduction (Fig. 2.4H–J).If greater than 50 degrees of abduction is accepted or there is more than 25 degrees of anteversion, components may be subjected to edge wear and associated metal debris and ion production.

- To properly insert the acetabular cup, push the insertion tool down against the inferior portion of the wound (Fig. 2.4K). The cup is implanted to the same position as the trial cup. Remove periacetabular osteophytes to avoid potential femoral component impingement.

RESURFACING OF THE FEMORAL HEAD

- To resurface the femoral head, internally rotate the femur much farther than needed to perform a THA with the soft-tissue release, which was already described, this may be safely done without risk of fracture.

- Flex the femur to 80 to 90 degrees and then internally rotate it between 120 and 150 degrees to expose the femoral head and neck circumferentially. The anterior portion of the head is most difficult to expose. A retractor between the acetabular cup and the proximal femur lifting the femur out of the wound may be helpful.

- With the femoral head and neck exposed, remove periarticular osteophytes, taking care not to violate the bone of the femoral neck. A Kerrison rongeur may be helpful anteriorly. Take care not to strip soft tissue from the femoral neck that contains vessels supplying the femoral head.

- Place a guide pin down the center of the femoral head. There are two jigs designed to help with pin placement. The jig we have most experience with is a clamp design that has two legs that clamp around the femoral neck superiorly and inferiorly (Fig. 2.6). Place a long guide rod posteriorly over the femoral neck to orient the jig in a valgus position (Fig. 2.7A). The lateral tip of that guide rod should line up with the point marked on the lateral femoral cortex and its soft-tissue mark made after measuring down from the greater trochanter. This ensures the placement of the pin down the center of the femoral neck in proper valgus alignment. View the guide pin from the medial side of the neck to be certain that it is not placed

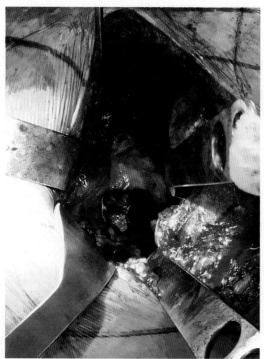

FIGURE 2.5 Acetabular exposure with femur retracted antero-superiorly. **SEE TECHNIQUE 2.1.**

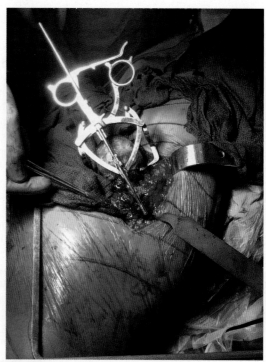

FIGURE 2.6 Femoral alignment guide in place. **SEE TECH-NIQUE 2.1.**

in retroversion (Fig. 2.7B). The guide pin position should be completely evaluated by its orientation to the femoral neck and not the femoral head. The pin usually is placed superior to the fovea, but, with wear, the head may be deformed.

- Once the guide pin is inserted down the middle of the femoral neck in anteroposterior and lateral planes, use a cannulated reamer to ream over the pin. Remove the pin and place a large reaming guide rod into the hole in the head and neck. Take circumferential measurements with a feeler-gauge to be certain the selected head size will not notch the femoral neck, especially laterally and superiorly (Fig. 2.7C). Once this has been confirmed, ream the femoral head circumferentially with the correct size reamer (Fig. 2.7D). Protect the femoral neck from notching with the measurement tool (Fig. 2.7E, F).
- Measure to see how far above the head-neck junction line the head needs to be resected (Fig. 2.7G,H) and ream the head to that line (Fig. 2.7I). Use a chamfer reamer of the correct size to finalize the shape of the femoral head to match the geometry of the interior of the femoral head component (Fig. 2.7J). Remove the reaming rod.
- Drill small to medium cement fixation holes into the femoral head around the chamfer and the tip of the head (Fig. 2.8A). Ream the hole in the femoral head and neck to a larger size with the appropriate head and neck reamer (Fig. 2.8B).
- Drill a hole into the lesser trochanter and place a metal vent in this hole to vent the proximal femur during cementing of the femoral component. This vent is attached to suction (Fig. 2.9). Mix cement in a vacuum for a short time and then inject it into the femoral component (Fig. 2.8C). While the cement is in a liquid state, cement the

component down to the femoral head (Fig. 2.10; see Fig. 2.8D). Take care not to break the femoral neck while impacting the component down onto the head. Remove excess cement and the vent tube. Carefully reduce the hip to avoid scratching the metal head against the edge of the acetabular component.

- Close the capsule with a running absorbable suture. Repair the gluteus maximus and the piriformis. Fascia is closed water-tight, and the remainder of the wound is closed in a layered fashion.

REVISION OF SURFACE REPLACEMENT ARTHROPLASTY COMPONENTS

One of the potential advantages of SRA is the ability to revise it to a more traditional THA construct. With the introduction of dual-mobility bearing surfaces, femoral SRA failures can be treated with placement of a traditional THA stem, cup retention, and conversion to a dual-mobility construct (Fig. 2.11). Recently, dual-mobility components were FDA approved for use with the BHR socket. In cases of metallosis, concerns of edge wear do exist, but modern highly cross-linked polyethylene has demonstrated reasonable resistance to edge-wear abrasion. In our experience, the BHR socket has an excellent track record of osteointegration, and increased morbidity is possible with cup revision. Osteointegration of the acetabular component should be assessed at the time of surgery, and revision of the acetabular component should be strongly considered for implants known to demonstrate poor survivorship.

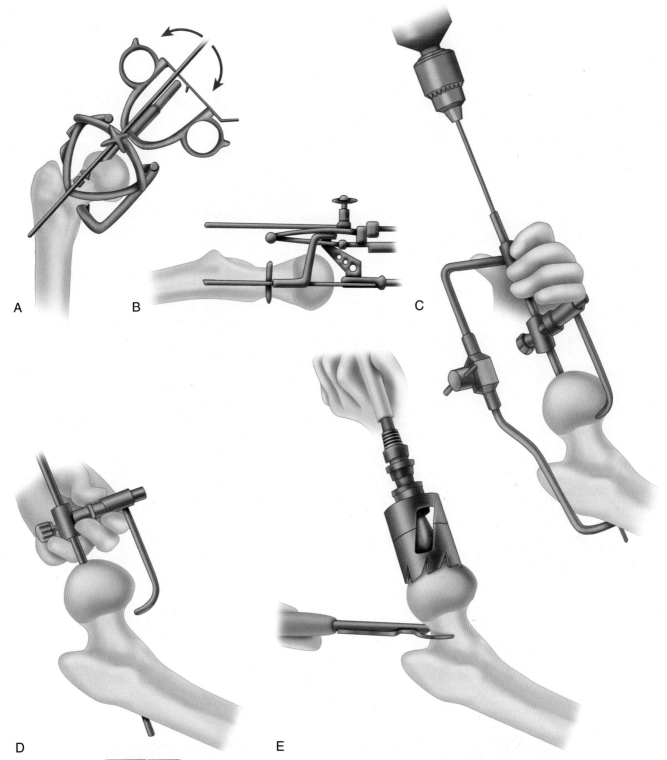

A   B   C

D   E

FIGURE 2.7 **A,** Long guide rod placed posteriorly over femoral neck to orient jig in valgus position. **B,** Guide pin viewed from medial side of neck. **C,** Guidewire inserted in desired position using alternative McMinn guide. **D,** Circumferential measurement taken to make sure head size will not notch femoral neck. **E** and **F,** Reaming of femoral head.

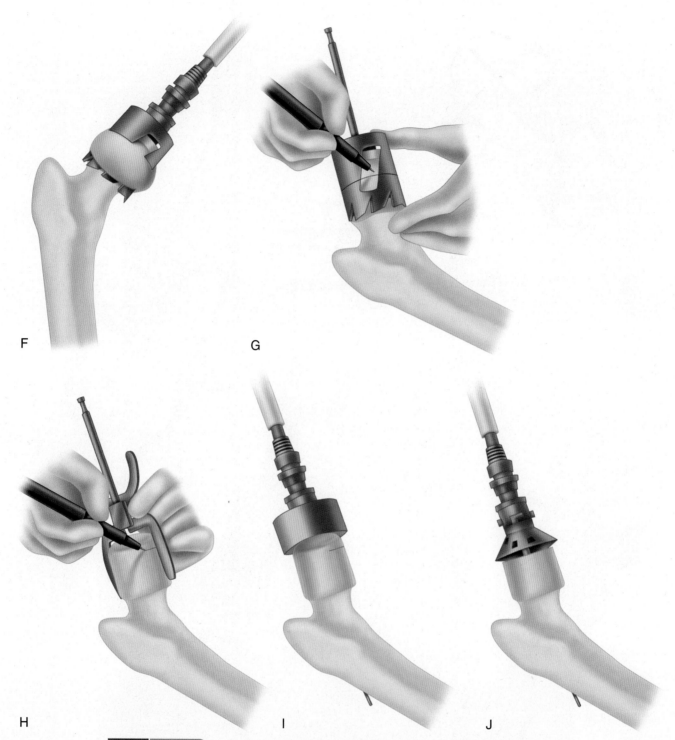

F

G

H

I

J

FIGURE 2.7, Cont'd **G-I,** Head is reamed to line after measuring how far femoral head needs to be reamed. **J,** Femoral head shaped to match geometry of femoral head component. **SEE TECHNIQUE 2.1.**

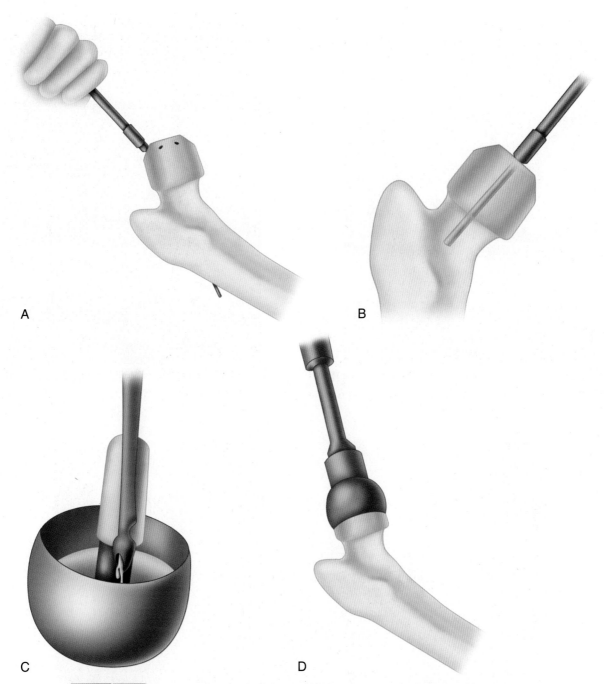

FIGURE 2.8 **A,** Cement fixation holes drilled. **B,** Reaming to accommodate component post. **C,** Cement injected into femoral component. **D,** Component cemented to femoral head. **SEE TECHNIQUE 2.1.**

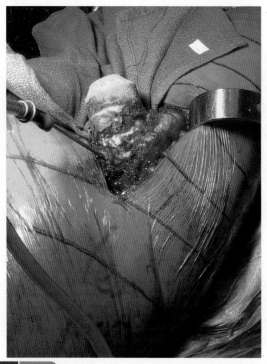

FIGURE 2.9 Femoral head prior to cementation. **SEE TECHNIQUE 2.1.**

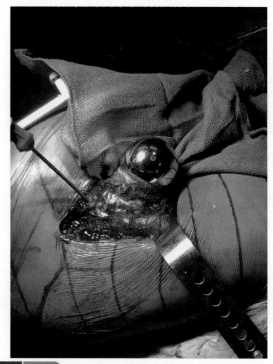

FIGURE 2.10 Final femoral component position cemented on femoral head.

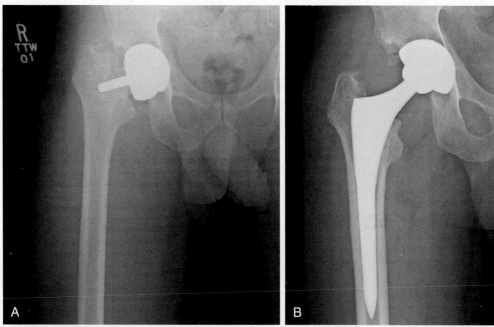

FIGURE 2.11 **A,** Failure of femoral component due to fracture. **B,** Conversion to total hip arthroplasty with retention of socket and dual mobility construct.

REFERENCES

Achten J, Parsons NR, Edlin RP, et al.: A randomised controlled trial of total hip arthroplasty versus resurfacing arthroplasty in the treatment of young patients with arthritis of the hip joint, *BMC Musculoskelet Disord* 11(8), 2010.

Amstutz HC, Le Duff MJ: Is a cementless fixation of the femoral component suitable for metal-on-metal hip resurfacing arthroplasty? *Hip Int* 1120700018815055, 2018 Nov 26. [Epub ahead of print].

Amstuta HC, Le Duff MJ: The mean ten-year results of metal-on-metal hybrid hip resurfacing arthroplasty, *Bone Joint J* 100-B:1424, 2018.

Amstutz HC, Le Duff MJ: Hip resurfacing: history, current status, and future, *Hip Int* 24:330, 2015.

Amstutz HC, Le Duff MJ, Johnson AJ: Socket position determines hip resurfacing 10-year survivorship, *Clin Orthop Relat Res* 470:3127, 2012.

Antoniou J, Bergeron SG, Ma B, et al.: The effect of the cam deformity on the insertion of the femoral component in hip resurfacing, *J Arthroplasty* 26:458, 2011.

Aulakh TS, Rao C, Kuiper JH, Richardson JB: Hip resurfacing and osteonecrosis: results from an independent hip resurfacing register, *Arch Orthop Trauma Surg* 130:841, 2010.

Azam MQ, McMahon S, Sawdon G, et al.: Survivorship and clinical outcome of Birmingham hip resurfacing: a minimum ten years' follow-up, *Int Orthop* 40(1), 2016.

Baad-Hansen T, Storgaard Jakobsen S, Soballe K: Two year migration results of the ReCap hip resurfacing system—a radiosterometric follow-up study of 23 hips, *Int Orthop* 35:497, 2011.

Bartelt RB, Yuan BJ, Trousdale RT, Sierra RJ: The prevalence of groin pain after metal-on-metal hip arthroplasty and total hip resurfacing, *Clin Orthop Relat Res* 468:2346, 2010.

Bedigrew KM, Ruh EL, Zhang Q, et al.: 2011 Marshall Urist Young Investigator Award: when to release patients to high-impact activities after hip resurfacing, *Clin Orthop Relat Res* 470:299, 2012.

Benelli G, Maritato M, Cerulli Mariani P, et al.: Revision of ASR hip arthroplasty: analysis of two hundred and ninety six recalled patients at seven years, *Int Orthop*, 2018 Sep 7, https://doi.org/10.1007/s00264-018-4128-z, [Epub ahead of print].

Bitsch RG, Loidolt T, Heisel C, Schmalzried TP: Cementing techniques for hip resurfacing arthroplasty: in vitro study of pressure and temperature, *J Arthroplasty* 26:144, 2011.

Bozic KJ, Pui CM, Ludeman MJ, et al.: Do the potential benefits of metal-on-metal hip resurfacing justify the increased cost and risk of complications? *Clin Orthop Relat Res* 468:2301, 2011.

Brooks PJ: Hip resurfacing: a large, US single-surgeon series, *Bone Joine J* 98-B(Suppl A):10, 2016.

Brown NM, Foran JR, Della Valle CJ: Hip resurfacing and conventional THA: comparison of acetabular bone stock removal, leg length, and offset, *Orthopedics* 36:e637, 2013.

Callanan MC, Jarrett B, Bragdon CR, et al.: The John Charnley Award: risk factors for cup malpositioning: quality improvement through a joint registry at a tertiary hospital, *Clin Orthop Relat Res* 469:319, 2011.

Arthroplasty Society Canadian: The Canadian Arthroplasty Society's experience with hip resurfacing arthroplasty. An analysis of 2773 hips, *Bone Joint J* 95B:1045, 2013.

Corten K, MacDonald SJ: Hip resurfacing data from national joint registries: what do they tell us? What do they not tell us? *Clin Orthop Relat Res* 468:351, 2010.

Costa ML, Achten J, Foguet P, et al: Comparison of hip function and quality of life of total hip arthroplasty and resurfacing arthroplasty in the treatment of young patients with arthritis of the hip joint at 5 years, *BMJ Open* 8(3): e018849, 18 Mar 12.

Daniel J, Pradhan C, Ziaee H, et al.: Results of Birmingham hip resurfacing at 12 to 15 years: a single-surgeon series, *Bone Joint J* 96B:1298, 2014.

Davis ET, Gallie PA, James SL, et al.: Proximity of the femoral neurovascular bundle during hip resurfacing, *J Arthroplasty* 25:471, 2010.

Della Valle CJ, Nunley RM, Raterman SJ, Barrack RL: Initial American experience with hip resurfacing following FDA approval, *Clin Orthop Relat Res* 467:72, 2009.

Delport HP, De Schepper J, Smith EJ, et al.: Resurfacing hip arthroplasty: a 3- to 5-year matched pair study of two different implant designs, *Acta Orthop Belg* 77:609, 2011.

Desloges W, Catelas I, Nishiwaki T, et al.: Do revised hip resurfacing arthroplasties lead to outcomes comparable to those of primary and revised total hip arthroplasties? *Clin Orthop Relat Res* 470:3134, 2012.

de Steiger RN, Miller LN, Prosser GH, et al.: Poor outcome of revised resurfacing hip arthroplasty, *Acta Orthop* 81:72, 2010.

Dowding C, Dobransky JS, Kim PR, et al.: Metal on metal hip resurfacing in patients 45 years of age and younger at minimum 5-year follow-up, *J Arthroplasty* 33:3196, 2018.

Eethakota VVS, Vaishnav V, Johnston L, et al.: Comparison of revision risks and complication rates between total HIP replacement and HIP resurfacing within the similar age group, *Surgeon* 16:339, 2018.

Fink Barnes LA, Johnson SH, Patrick Jr DA, Macaulay W: Metal-on-metal hip resurfacing compared with total hip arthroplasty: two to five year outcomes in men younger than sixty five years, *Int Orthop* 38:2435, 2014.

Ford MC, Hellman MD, Kazarian GS, et al.: Five to ten-year results of the Birmingham resurfacing implant in the U.S. A single institution's experience, *J Bone Joint Surg Am* 100:1879, 2018.

Frew N, Johnson G: Survival of the Birmingham hip resurfacing in young men up to 13 years post-operatively, *Acta Orthop Belg* 83:67, 2017.

Galea VP, Laaksonen I, Matuszak SJ, et al.: Mid-term changes in blood metal ion levels after articular surface replacement arthroplasty of the hip, *Bone Joint J* 99-B(Suppl B):33, 2017.

Garbuz DS, Tanzer M, Greidanus NV, et al.: The John Charnley Award: Metal-on-metal hip resurfacing versus large-diameter head metal-on-metal total hip arthroplasty: a randomized clinical trial, *Clin Orthop Relat Res* 468:318, 2010.

Garrett SJ, Bolland BJ, Yates PJ, et al.: Femoral revision in hip resurfacing compared with large-bearing metal-on-metal hip arthroplasty, *J Arthroplasty* 26:1214, 2011.

Ghomrawi HM, Dolan MM, Rutledge J, Alexiades MM: Recovery expectations of hip resurfacing compared to total hip arthroplasty: a matched pairs study, *Arthritis Care Res* 63:1753, 2011.

Girard J, Krantz N, Bocquet D, et al.: Femoral head to neck offset after hip resurfacing is critical for range of motion, *Clin Biomech* 27:165, 2012.

Girard J, Lons A, Ramdane N, et al.: Hip resurfacing before 50 years of age: a prospective study of 979 hips with a mean follow-up of 5.1 years, *Orthop Traumatol Surg Res* 104:295, 2018.

Gomes B, Olsen M, Donnelly M, et al.: Should we worry about periacetabular interference gaps in hip resurfacing? *Clin Orthop Relat Res* 471:422, 2013.

Grammatopoulos G, Pandit H, Kamali A, et al.: The correlation of wear with histological features after failed hip resurfacing arthroplasty, *J Bone Joint Surg* 95A:381, 2013.

Graves SE, Rothwell A, Tucker K, et al.: A multinational assessment of metal-on-metal bearings in hip replacement, *J Bone Joint Surg* 93A:43, 2011.

Gross TP, Liu F: Comparative study between patients with osteonecrosis and osteoarthritis after hip resurfacing arthroplasty, *Acta Orthop Belg* 78:735, 2012.

Gross TP, Liu F: Risk factor analysis for early femoral failure in metal-on-metal hip resurfacing arthroplasty: the effect of bone density and body mass index, *J Orthop Surg Res* 7(1), 2012.

Haddad FS, Konan S, Tahmassebi J: A prospective comparative study of cementless total hip arthroplasty and hip resurfacing in patients under the age of 55 years: a ten-year follow-up, *Bone Joint J* 87-B:617, 2015.

Halawi MJ, Oak SR, Brigati D, et al.: Birmingham hip resurfacing versus cementless total hip arthroplasty in patients 55 years of younger: a minimum five-year follow-up, *J Clin Orthop Trauma* 9:285, 2018.

Hart A, Matthies A, Henckel J, et al.: Understanding why metal-on-metal hip arthroplasties fail: a comparison between patients with well-functioning and revised Birmingham hip resurfacing arthroplasties. AAOS exhibit selection, *J Bone Joint Surg Am* 94:322, 2012.

Hart AJ, Muirhead-Allwood S, Porter M, et al.: Which factors determine the wear rate of large-diameter metal-on-metal hip replacements? Multivariate analysis of two hundred and seventy-six components, *J Bone Joint Surg* 95A:678, 2013.

Hart AJ, Sabah SA, Sampson B, et al.: Surveillance of patients with metal-on-metal hip resurfacing and total hip prostheses: a prospective cohort study to investigate the relationship between blood metal ion levels and implant failure, *J Bone Joint Surg* 96A:1091, 2014.

Hartmann A, Lützner J, Kirschner S, et al.: Do survival rate and serum ion concentrations 10 years after metal-on-metal hip resurfacing provide evidence for continued use? *Clin Orthop Relat Res* 470:3118, 2012.

Hawkins R, Ariamanesh AP: Hip arthrodesis in the paediatric and young adult patients; the use of hip resurfacing reamers, *Ann R Coll Surg Engl* 92:437, 2010.

Heerman KA, Highcock AJ, Moorehead JD, Scott SJ: A comparison of leg length and femoral offset discrepancies in hip resurfacing, large head metal-on-metal and conventional total hip replacement: a case series, *J Orthop Surg Res* 6:65, 2011.

Hellman MD, Ford MC, Barrack RL: Is there evidence to support an indication for surface replacement arthroplasty? A systematic review, *Bone Joint J* 1(Supple A):101, 2019.

Hunter TJA, Moores TS, Morley D, et al.: 10-year results of the Birmingham Hip Resurfacing: a non-designer case series, *Hip Int* 28:50, 2018.

Jameson SS, Baker PN, Mason J, et al.: Independent predictors of revision following metal-on-metal hip resurfacing: retrospective cohort study using national Joint Registry data, *J Bone Joint Surg* 94B:746, 2012.

Johnson AJ, LeDuff MJ, Yoon JP, et al.: Metal ion levels in total hip arthroplasty versus hip resurfacing, *J Arthroplasty* 28:2345, 2013.

Joseph J, Mullen M, McAuley A, Pillai A: Femoral neck resorption following hybrid metal-on-metal hip resurfacing arthroplasty: a radiological and biomechanical analysis, *Arch Orthop Trauma Surg* 130:1433, 2010.

Kohan L, Field C, Kerr D, Ben-Nissan B: Femoral neck remodelling after hip resurfacing surgery: a radiological study, *ANZ J Surg* 84:639, 2014.

Konan S, Rayan F, Meermans G, et al.: Preoperative digital templating of Birmingham hip resurfacing, *Hip Int* 20:14, 2010.

Krause M, Breer S, Hahn M, et al.: Cementation and interface analysis of early failure cases after hip-resurfacing, *Int Orthop* 36:1333, 2012.

Kurser TJ, Kozak KR, Cannon DM, et al.: Low rates of heterotopic ossification after resurfacing hip arthroplasty with use of prophylactic radiotherapy in select patients, *J Arthroplasty* 27:1349, 2012.

Kwon YM, Ostlere SJ, McLardy-Smith P, et al.: "Asymptomatic" pseudotumors after metal-on-metal hip resurfacing arthroplasty prevalence and metal ion study, *J Arthroplasty* 26:511, 2011.

Langton DJ, Sprowson AP, Mahdeva D, et al.: Cup anteversion in hip resurfacing: validation of EBRA and the presentation of a simple clinical grading system, *J Arthroplasty* 25:607, 2010.

Larkin B, Nyazee H, Motley J, et al.: Hip resurfacing does not improve proprioception compared with THA, *Clin Orthop Relat Res* 472:555, 2014.

Lavigne M, Therrien M, Nantel J, et al.: The John Charnley Award: the functional outcome of hip resurfacing and large-head THA is the same: a randomized, double-blind study, *Clin Orthop Relat Res* 468:326, 2010.

Lim SJ, Kim JH, Moon YW, Park YS: Femoroacetabular cup impingement after resurfacing arthroplasty of the hip, *J Arthroplasty* 27:60, 2012.

Liu F, Gross TP: A safe zone for acetabular component position in metal-on-metal hip resurfacing arthroplasty: winner of the 2012 HAP PAUL award, *J Arthroplasty* 28:1224, 2013.

Liu H, Li L, Gao W, et al.: Computer navigation vs conventional mechanical jig technique in hip resurfacing arthroplasty: a meta-analysis based on 7 studies, *J Arthroplasty* 28(98), 2013.

Madhu TS, Akula MR, Raman RN, et al.: The Birmingham Hip Resurfacing Prosthesis: an independent single surgeon's experience at 7-year follow-up, *J Arthroplasty* 26(1), 2011.

Malek IA, Hashmi M, Holland JP: Socio-economic impact of Birmingham hip resurfacing on patient employment after ten years, *Int Orthop* 35:1467, 2011.

Malhotra R, Kannan A, Kumar V, et al.: Hip resurfacing arthroplasty in inflammatory arthritis: a 3- to 5-year follow-up study, *J Arthroplasty* 27(15), 2012.

Malviya A, Lobaz S, Holland J: Mechanism of failure eleven years following a Buechel Pappas hip resurfacing, *Am J Sports Med* 38:1229, 2010.

Malviya A, Ramaskandhan JR, Bowman R, et al.: What advantage is there to be gained using large modular metal-on-metal bearing in routine primary hip replacement? A preliminary report of a prospective randomised controlled trial, *J Bone Joint Surg* 93B:1602, 2011.

Martin JW, Williams MA, Barker KL: Activity levels following hip resurfacing arthroplasty: a tool to help manage patient expectations, *J Orthop* 15:658, 2018.

Matharu GS, Berryman F, Brash L, et al.: Can blood metal ion levels be used to identify patients with bilateral Birmingham Hip Resurfacings who are at risk of adverse reaction to metal debris? *Bone Joint J* 98-B:1455, 2016.

Matharu GS, McBryde CW, Pynsent WB, et al.: The outcome of the Birmingham Hip Resurfacing in patients aged < 50 years up to 14 years post-operatively, *Bone Joint J* 95B:1172, 2013.

Matharu GS, Pandit HG, Murray DW, et al.: The future role of metal-on-metal hip resurfacing, *Int Orthop* 39:2031, 2015.

Matthies AK, Henckel J, Cro S, et al.: Predicting wear and blood metal ion levels in metal-on-metal hip resurfacing, *J Orthop Res* 32:167, 2014.

McGrory B, Barrack R, Lachiewicz PF, et al.: Modern metal-on-metal hip resurfacing, *J Am Acad Orthop Surg* 18:306, 2010.

McMinn DJ, Daniel J, Ziaee H, Pradhan C: Indications and results of hip resurfacing, *Int Orthop* 35:231, 2011.

Mehra A, Berryman F, Matharu GS, et al.: Birmingham hip resurfacing: a single surgeon series reported at a minimum of 10 years follow-up, *J Arthroplasty* 30:1160, 2015.

Miettinen SSA, Mäkinen TJ, Laaksonen I, et al.: Dislocation of large-diameter metal-on-metal total hip arthroplasty and hip resurfacing arthroplasty, *Hip Int* 11207000187983, 2018 Sep 13. [Epub ahead of print].

Morse KW, Su EP: Hip resurfacing arthroplasty for patients with inflammatory arthritis: a systematic review, *Hip Int* 28:11, 2018.

Murray DW, Grammatopoulos G, Pandit H, et al.: The ten-year survival of the Birmingham hip resurfacing: an independent series, *J Bone Joint Surg* 94(B):1180, 2012.

Nakasone S, Takao M, Sakai T, et al.: Does the extent of osteonecrosis affect the survival of hip resurfacing? *Clin Orthop Relat Res* 471:1926, 2013.

Nakasone S, Takao M, Nishii T, et al.: Incidence and natural course of initial polar gaps in Birmingham Hip Resurfacing cup, *J Arthroplasty* 27:1676, 2012.

Nall A, Robin J: Spontaneous recurrent dislocation after primary Birmingham hip resurfacing: a rare complication in a 44-year-old man, *J Arthroplasty* 25:658, 2010.

Nam D, Barrack RL, Potter HG: What are the advantages and disadvantages of imaging modalities to diagnose wear-related corrosion problems? *Clin Orthop Relat Res* 472:3665, 2014.

Nam D, Nunley RM, Ruh EL, et al.: Short-term results of Birmingham hip resurfacing in the United States, *Orthopedics* 38:e715, 2015.

Nunley RM, Zhu J, Clohisy JC, Barrack RL: Aspirin decreases heterotopic ossification after hip resurfacing, *Clin Orthop Relat Res* 469:1614, 2011.

Ollivere B, Duckett S, August A, Porteous M: The Birmingham Hip Resurfacing: 5-year clinical and radiographic results from a District General Hospital, *Int Orthop* 34:631, 2010.

Olsen M, Gamble P, Chiu M, et al.: Assessment of accuracy and reliability in preoperative templating for hip resurfacing arthroplasty, *J Arthroplasty* 25:445, 2010.

Petersen MK, Andersen NT, Mogensen P, et al.: Gait analysis after total hip replacement with hip resurfacing implant or Mallory-head Exeter prosthesis: a randomised controlled trial, *Int Orthop* 35:667, 2011.

Pritchett JW: Polyethylene hip resurfacing to treat arthritis and severe acetabular insufficiency, *J Arthroplasty* 33:3508, 2018.

Prosser GH, Yates PJ, Wood DJ, et al.: Outcome of primary resurfacing hip replacement: evaluation of risk factors for early revision, *Acta Orthop* 81:66, 2010.

Reito A, Puolakka T, Pajamäki J: Birmingham hip resurfacing: five to eight year results, *Int Orthop* 35:1119, 2011.

Rhaman L, Muirhead-Allwood SK, Alkinj M: What is the midterm survivorship and function after hip resurfacing? *Clin Orthop Relat Res* 468:3221, 2010.

Ritter MA, Galley M: Heterotopic bone formation following resurfacing total hip arthroplasty, *HSS J* 7:41, 2011.

Simpson JM, Villar RN: Hip resurfacing, *BMJ* 7:341, 2010.

Stogiannidis I, Puolakka T, Pajamäki J, et al.: Whole-mount specimens in the analysis of en block samples obtained from revisions of resurfacing hip implants: a report of 4 early failures, *Acta Orthop* 81:324, 2010.

Su EP, Su SL: Surface replacement conversion: results depend upon reason for revision, *Bone Joint J* 95B(11 Suppl A):88, 2013.

Tai SM, Millard N, Munir S, et al.: Two-year serum metal ion levels in minimally invasive total conservative hip resurfacing: preliminary results of a prospective study, *ANZ J Surg* 85:164, 2015.

Takamura KM, Amstutz HC, Lu Z, et al.: Wear analysis of 39 Conserve plus metal-on-metal hip resurfacing retrievals, *J Arthroplasty* 29:410, 2014.

Tanzer M, Tanzer D, Smith K: Surface replacement of the hip can result in decreased acetabular bone stock, *Clin Orthop Relat Res* 470:541, 2012.

Vail TP: Hip resurfacing, *J Am Acad Orthop Surg* 19:236, 2011.

Van Der Bracht H, Eecken SV, Vyncke D, et al.: Clinical and functional outcome of the hip resurfacing, *Acta Orthop Belg* 77:771, 2011.

Van Der Straeten C, Grammatopoulos G, Gill HS, et al.: The 2012 Otto Aufranc Award: the interpretation of metal ion levels in unilateral and bilateral hip resurfacing, *Clin Orthop Relat Res* 471:377, 2013.

Vendittoli PA, Ganapathy M, Roy AG, et al.: A comparison of clinical results of hip resurfacing arthroplasty and 28 mm metal on metal total hip arthroplasty: a randomised trial with 3-6 years follow-up, *Hip Int* 20:1, 2010.

Whittingham-Jones P, Charnley G, Francis J, Annapureddy S: Internal fixation after subtrochanteric femoral fracture after hip resurfacing arthroplasty, *J Arthroplasty* 25:334, 2010.

Williams DH, Greidanus NV, Masri BA, et al.: Predictors of participation in sports after hip and knee arthroplasty, *Clin Orthop Relat Res* 470:555, 2012.

Williams DH, Greidanus NV, Masri BA, et al.: Prevalence of pseudotumor in asymptomatic patients after metal-on-metal hip arthroplasty, *J Bone Joint Surg* 93A:2164, 2011.

Woon RP, Johnson AJ, Amstutz HC: The results of metal-on-metal resurfacing in patients under 30 years of age, *J Arthroplasty* 28:1010, 2013.

Yoo MC, Cho YJ, Chun UYS, Rhyu KH: Impingement between the acetabular cup and the femoral neck after hip resurfacing arthroplasty, *J Bone Joint Surg Am* 93(Suppl 2):99, 2011.

Zylberberg AD, Nishiwaki T, Kim PR, et al.: Clinical results of the Conserve plus metal-on-metal hip resurfacing: an independent series, *J Arthroplasty* 30:68, 2015.

The complete list of references is available online at Expert Consult.com.

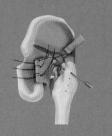

CHAPTER **3**

ARTHRODESIS OF THE HIP

Gregory D. Dabov

Arthrodesis of the hip is an infrequently performed procedure with few indications. Advances in total hip arthroplasty, which have greatly improved functional scores and patient satisfaction, have made hip fusion a much less desirable option for most patients. Good intermediate outcomes have been reported after total hip arthroplasty in patients as young as adolescence. Nevertheless, a number of recent literature reviews agree that hip arthrodesis still has a role in the treatment of carefully selected patients. In the past, a good candidate for hip fusion was a young, healthy laborer with a stiff and painful arthritic hip. In developing countries, where resources are limited or unavailable, fusion still represents a major treatment option for patients with painful hip arthritis. Internal fixation to achieve hip fusion was introduced by Watson-Jones and others in the 1930s and improved by Charnley; however, these early methods of internal fixation were associated with high rates of incomplete union and prolonged external immobilization. To gain more stability of the arthrodesis, Müller described a double compression plating technique that did not require postoperative casting. Schneider later developed a cobra-head plate that also does not require postoperative immobilization. Other internal fixation modalities, such as hip compression screws or cancellous screws alone, have been described for certain situations and can be useful alternatives as the clinical situation and available resources dictate.

INDICATIONS AND RESULTS

Arthrodesis of the hip still may be considered an alternative in patients younger than 40 years of age with severe, usually posttraumatic, arthritis and normal function of the lumbar spine, contralateral hip, and ipsilateral knee. Fusion could also be considered as primary treatment for severe trauma of the acetabulum or femoral head in select patients. Hip arthrodesis has been shown to be successful in treating painful spastic subluxed or dislocated hips in ambulatory adolescents with cerebral palsy. Before arthrodesis is considered, nonoperative treatment of arthritis, such as the use of walking aids and antiinflammatory medication, should be tried, as should less invasive and potentially less debilitating operative procedures. Hip arthrodesis can provide a functional and durable alternative to total hip replacement in properly selected younger patients. This has been confirmed by several reviews, including those by Stover et al. and Schafroth et al. Both noted that a properly performed arthrodesis can lead to years of pain relief and reasonable function.

An absolute contraindication to arthrodesis is active sepsis of the hip; the infection should be eradicated and inactive

for 3 to 6 months before arthrodesis is undertaken. Relative contraindications include severe degenerative changes in the lumbosacral spine, contralateral hip, or ipsilateral knee. Poor bone stock from osteoporosis or iatrogenic causes, such as proximal femoral resection for tumor, also is associated with lower success rates and increased disability.

Good or excellent functional results have been reported with hip arthrodesis, but low back pain, limited ambulation, and sexual dysfunction have been noted. The importance of careful patient selection cannot be overemphasized. Hip fusion increases stress in the lumbar spine, contralateral hip, and ipsilateral knee and requires greater energy expenditure for ambulation; hip fusion probably should be done only in young, otherwise healthy patients. Properly selected patients generally are satisfied with the results of hip fusion; several long-term follow-up studies have documented patient satisfaction of approximately 70% at 30 years, despite evidence of degenerative changes in the lumbar spine and adjacent joints of the lower extremities.

Degenerative changes in nearby joints typically begin to become symptomatic in 15 to 25 years after arthrodesis. A review of such patients confirmed that the average time from fusion to onset of back and joint pain was 24 years. Pain most commonly affected the back (75%), then the ipsilateral knee (54%), with fewer complaining about the contralateral knee or hip. It appears such pain symptoms are ultimately quite common but usually quite delayed in onset, especially with an optimally positioned fusion. Although ipsilateral knee pain and contralateral hip pain occur less frequently than back pain, they more often require operative intervention, such as total knee or hip arthroplasty.

Late onset of pain in patients previously asymptomatic for many years after hip arthrodesis has been reported by Wong et al. The pain in their two patients was found to be caused by implant protrusion and was resolved by implant removal.

Other less common complications can occur after hip fusion. Proximal femoral fractures, perhaps made more likely by the increased stresses in the vicinity of an immobile joint, have been reported as long as 53 years after arthrodesis. Wong et al. reported femoral shaft fractures, distal to plate hardware, treated successfully by retrograde nailing.

TECHNIQUES

Successful arthrodesis of the hip can be achieved through a variety of methods. All techniques require removal of articular cartilage for preparation of the fusion site. Acetabular reamers and hip resurfacing (reverse) reamers have been shown to be helpful in the preparation of the acetabulum and femoral head. General principles of fracture fixation, such as rigid fixation and optimal biologic environment, are applicable. Regardless of the technique selected, the ideal fusion position is 20 to 30 degrees of flexion, 0 to 5 degrees of adduction, and 0 to 15 degrees of external rotation.

ARTHRODESIS WITH CANCELLOUS SCREW FIXATION

Benaroch et al. described a simple method of hip arthrodesis for adolescent patients. Fusion was obtained in 11 of 13 patients (average age 15.6 years); two had mildly symptomatic nonunions. At an average 6.6-year follow-up, nine patients had no pain or slight pain, three had mild pain, and one had marked pain. According to a modified Harris hip scoring system, functional results were excellent in five patients, good in two, fair in five, and poor in one. The investigators noted a progressive drift into adduction averaging 7 degrees, most of which occurred within 2 years of surgery; because of this, they recommended fusion with the hip in 20 to 25 degrees of flexion and neutral or 1 to 2 degrees of abduction.

TECHNIQUE 3.1

(BENAROCH ET AL.)
- With the patient in the lateral position, make an anterolateral approach and perform an anterior capsulotomy.
- Dislocate the femoral head and denude both sides of the joint of the articular cartilage and necrotic bone.
- Place the leg in the desired position, and insert one or two cancellous screws through the femoral head into the inner surface of the ilium.

- Before tightening the screws to compress the femoral head into the acetabulum, perform an intertrochanteric osteotomy to decompress the long lever arm of the femur.

POSTOPERATIVE CARE A spica cast is worn for 8 to 12 weeks.

ARTHRODESIS WITH ANTERIOR FIXATION

Anterior plating through a modified Smith-Petersen approach is useful when there is loss of acetabular or proximal femoral bone stock. The plate is placed along the pelvic brim immediately lateral to the sacroiliac joint and posterior-superior iliac spine (Fig. 3.1A). A lag screw inserted from the trochanteric area through the center of the femoral head into the supra-acetabular bone provides additional compression because of a lateral tension-band effect (Fig. 3.1B). Matta et al. reported successful fusion in 10 of 12 patients with anterior plating.

TECHNIQUE 3.2

(MATTA ET AL.)
- With the patient supine on a fracture table, expose the hip through a combined ilioinguinal/Smith-Peterson approach.
- Proximally expose the inner table of the ilium to the sacroiliac joint using the lateral window of the ilioinguinal approach.
- Distally expose the anterior hip capsule between the tensor fascia lata and the rectus femoris as per the Smith-Peterson approach.

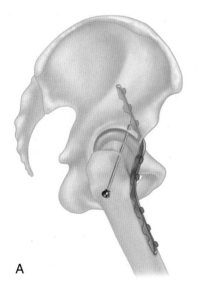
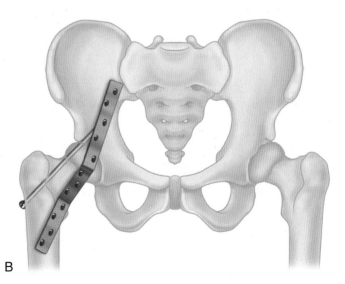

A   B

FIGURE 3.1 Anterior plate fixation for hip arthrodesis. **A,** Lateral lag screw through femoral head. **B,** Optimal position of plate. (Redrawn from Beaulé PE, Matta JM, Mast JW: Hip arthrodesis: current indications and techniques, *J Am Acad Orthop Surg* 10:249, 2002.) **SEE TECHNIQUE 3.2.**

- Expose the proximal femur by retracting the vastus lateralis medially.
- Excise the anterior hip capsule and dislocate the hip with traction and external rotation of the femur; a Steinmann pin in the proximal femur can assist with this maneuver.
- Denude the hip of articular cartilage.
- Relocate the hip and, using the fracture table, place the leg in the desired position of fusion.
- Through a percutaneous incision, place a 6.5- to 7.4-mm lag screw through the greater trochanter and femoral neck into the iliac bone superior to the acetabular dome.
- Contour a 12- to 14-hole, wide, 4.5-mm dynamic compression plate over the internal ilium, pelvic brim, femoral neck, and proximal femoral shaft. Place the proximal part of the plate just lateral to the sacroiliac joint (Fig. 3.1).
- Secure the plate to the pelvis first. Use a tensioning device distally on the femur, and fill the distal screw holes.
- Pack bone graft from reaming or from the iliac crest over the fusion site as needed.
- Irrigate and close the wound in layers.

No postoperative immobilization is required; weight bearing is protected for 10 to 12 weeks.

ARTHRODESIS WITH DOUBLE-PLATE FIXATION

Double-plating may be useful in difficult situations such as an unreduced hip dislocation, avascularity of bony surfaces, multiply operated hips, and poor patient compliance. A significant (more than 4 cm) limb-length discrepancy may require correction before the fusion. Six to 8 weeks after intertrochanteric osteotomy, a broad lateral plate is contoured over the trochanteric bed and placed anterior to the greater sciatic notch and along the lateral aspect of the femur. After removal of the anterior inferior iliac spine, a narrow anterior plate is applied along the femoral shaft (Fig. 3.2).

TECHNIQUE 3.3

(MÜLLER ET AL.)
- With the patient in the lateral position, expose the hip through a Watson-Jones approach.
- Develop the interval between the gluteus medius and tensor fascia lata, and perform a trochanteric osteotomy.
- Externally rotate the leg and develop the interval between the anterior hip capsule and the rectus femoris.
- Perform an osteotomy of the anterior-inferior iliac spine, and retract the rectus medially. Excise the anterior hip capsule.
- Dislocate the hip and remove the articular cartilage from the femoral head and acetabulum.
- Relocate the hip and place in the desired position of fusion. Use bumps and bolsters to provisionally secure the leg in this position.
- Contour the lateral plate (wide, 4.5 mm) from the ilium just anterior to the sciatic notch over the trochanteric osteotomy site and extending over the lateral femoral shaft (Fig. 3.2A). Recheck the position of the hip.
- Secure the proximal portion of the plate to the pelvis and apply a traction device distally.
- Contour the anterior plate (narrow, 4.5 mm) from just below the anterior-superior iliac spine over the inferior spine osteotomy, anterior femoral neck, and anterior femoral shaft (Fig. 3.2B). Ensure that the femur is abutting the lateral plate while contouring the anterior plate.
- Secure the proximal portion of the plate to the pelvis and apply a traction device distally.

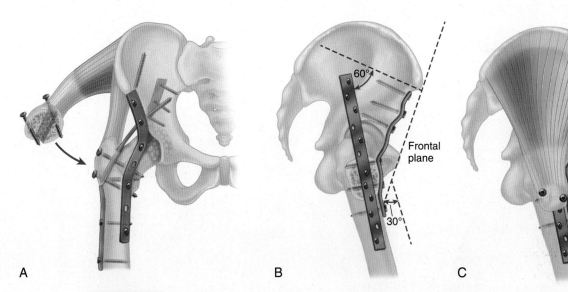

A

B

C

FIGURE 3.2 Double-plate fixation for hip arthrodesis. Optimal position of the plates. **A,** Anteroposterior view. **B,** Lateral view and after reattachment of the greater trochanter **(C).** (Redrawn from Beaulé PE, Matta JM, Mast JW: Hip arthrodesis: current indications and techniques, *J Am Acad Orthop Surg* 10:249, 2002.) **SEE TECHNIQUE 3.3.**

- Tighten both tension devices and insert the distal screws of both plates into the femur. Remove the tension devices and fill the remaining screw holes.
- Replace the greater trochanter to the osteotomy site. Some bone will need to be removed from the trochanter to accommodate the plate. Secure the greater trochanter with screws anterior and posterior to the plate (Fig. 3.2C).
- Place bone graft from reaming or the iliac crest at the fusion site as needed.
- Irrigate and close the wound in layers.

No postoperative immobilization is required; weight bearing is restricted for 10 to 12 weeks.

ARTHRODESIS WITH COBRA PLATE FIXATION

Since Schneider's development of the cobra-head plate for hip arthrodesis, the technique has been modified to allow restoration of abductor function if the fusion is later converted to a total hip arthroplasty. The technique includes a medial displacement osteotomy of the acetabulum and rigid internal fixation with the cobra plate. Murrell and Fitch reported successful fusion in eight young patients (average age 17 years) with this technique. All eight patients had diminished pain and significant improvements in function. A disadvantage of the technique is that it creates a stress riser distally that may result in femoral fracture with relatively minor trauma. Pseudarthrosis has been reported in adolescent patients at or above the 90th percentile for their age-determined weights after this technique. Alternative or supplementary stabilization methods in adolescents at or above the 90th percentile weight for age are recommended.

TECHNIQUE 3.4

(MURRELL AND FITCH)
- Place the patient supine with a sandbag under the ipsilateral buttock. Prepare and drape both lower extremities and anterior superior iliac spines to allow access to both iliac crests and both ankles.
- Make a linear longitudinal midlateral incision along the femoral diaphysis to a point 8 cm distal to the tip of the greater trochanter (Fig. 3.3A).
- Open the fascia lata in line with its fibers for the length of the wound; identify and protect the sciatic nerve throughout the procedure.
- Maintain exposure with a self-retaining retractor. Incise the origin of the vastus lateralis, and reflect it off the greater trochanteric flare and the linea aspera for a distance of 6 cm.
- Identify the anterior and posterior margins of the gluteus medius.
- Use an oscillating saw to make a greater trochanteric osteotomy so that the proximal fragment includes the insertion of the gluteus medius and minimus (Fig. 3.3B).

- Elevate the hip abductors with the greater trochanteric fragment, and hold them superiorly with two large Steinmann pins hammered into the iliac wing (Fig. 3.3C).
- Perform a superior hip capsulotomy.
- Dislocate the hip and denude the acetabulum and femoral head of the articular cartilage and necrotic bone. Reduce the hip joint.
- Elevate the periosteum of the outer table of the iliac wing superiorly to the retracting Steinmann pins, anteriorly to the anterior superior iliac spine and the anterior inferior iliac spine, and posteriorly to the sciatic notch.
- Place one blunt Hohmann retractor in the sciatic notch subperiosteally to protect the sciatic nerve and the superior gluteal artery and one anterior to the iliopectineal eminence.
- Make a transverse innominate osteotomy between the iliopectineal eminence and the sciatic notch at the superior pole of the acetabulum.
- Make the iliac cut with an oscillating saw, and complete it with an osteotome. Use osteotomes and curettes to remove any remaining cartilage and sclerotic cortical bone from the superior weight-bearing surface of the femoral head and from the acetabulum.
- Displace the distal hemipelvic fragment and the proximal femur medially 100% of the thickness of the innominate bone by placing a curved, blunt instrument in the osteotomy and levering the distal hemipelvis 1 cm.
- Remove the sandbag and place a Steinmann pin into both of the anterior-superior iliac spines; use the pins and a long-limbed protractor to determine adduction and abduction of the limb.
- Evaluate internal and external rotation by observing the patella and the malleoli relative to the two vertical Steinmann pins.
- Position the hip in 25 degrees of flexion, neutral internal and external rotation, and neutral adduction and abduction.
- Contour a nine-hole cobra plate, and secure the proximal portion to the ilium with a 4.5-mm cortical screw.
- Distal to the plate, attach an AO tensioner to the lateral femoral cortex with a single unicortical 4.5-mm cortical screw (Fig. 3.3D).
- Insert a screw in the most distal hole of the plate, hook the tensioner to the plate, and apply compression force across the hip joint to ensure good bony apposition.
- Secure the plate to the lateral femur with 4.5-mm bicortical screws in eight of the nine holes, and remove the tensioner.
- Insert 4.5-mm cortical screws in the proximal plate, taking care to protect the neurovascular structures on the inner table of the pelvis.
- Remove the retractors and the Steinmann pins holding the greater trochanter, and drill a 4.5-mm hole in the center of the proximal greater trochanteric fragment.
- Drill and tap a 3.2-mm bicortical screw in the proximal femur through the third or fourth hole of the cobra plate.
- Reattach the greater trochanter with a 4.5-mm cortical screw and washer (Fig. 3.3E, F). A trochanteric grip plate with wires may provide superior fixation if necessary.
- Pack any remaining corticocancellous bone around the hip joint, and obtain an anteroposterior pelvic radiograph to check the position of the plate, screws, and hip joint (Fig. 3.3G).

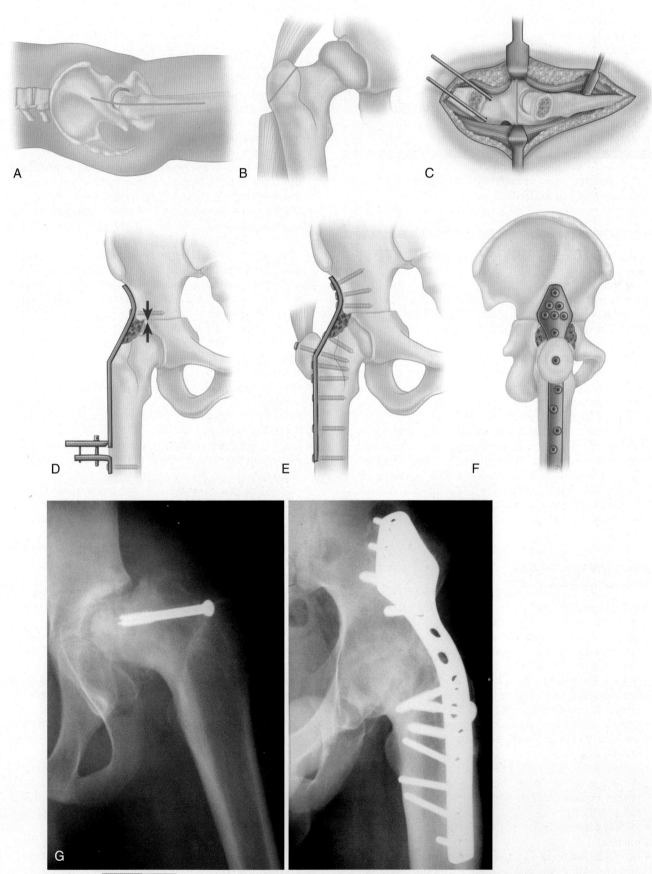

FIGURE 3.3 Hip arthrodesis with cobra plate fixation (see text). **A,** Longitudinal midlateral incision. **B,** Osteotomy of greater trochanter. **C,** Transverse innominate osteotomy. **D,** Cobra plate contoured and attached with two screws for application of compression force. **E,** Final fixation of plate. **F,** Lateral view of plate and reattachment of greater trochanter. **G,** Hip fusion with cobra plate. **SEE TECHNIQUE 3.4.**

- Thoroughly irrigate the wound, and close the soft tissue in layers over drains.
- No postoperative immobilization is applied.

POSTOPERATIVE CARE Ambulation with partial weight bearing is encouraged on day 2 or 3 after surgery. Partial weight bearing with two crutches is continued for 8 to 12 weeks.

ARTHRODESIS WITH HIP COMPRESSION SCREW FIXATION

Pagnano and Cabanela described hip arthrodesis with a sliding hip compression screw, supplemented by two or three cancellous screws placed proximal to the hip screw. They thought that this technique best met their criteria because it (1) minimizes or delays the appearance and severity of low back pain by ensuring that the hip is fused in the proper position, (2) minimizes postoperative immobilization to speed recovery, (3) allows later conversion to total hip arthroplasty if necessary, (4) preserves the abductor musculature without significantly altering the anatomy of the hip, and (5) avoids the use of bulky internal fixation devices that might damage the abductor muscles.

TECHNIQUE 3.5

(PAGNANO AND CABANELA)

- Position the patient supine on the fracture table and make a Watson-Jones approach to the hip.
- After the fascia is incised, develop the interval between the gluteus medius and the tensor fascia femoris.
- Obtain proper hemostasis, and detach the anterior third of the gluteus medius from the greater trochanter to improve access to the hip joint.
- Externally rotate the leg, and detach the reflected head of the rectus femoris from the joint capsule.
- Make an anterior capsulectomy, and take the leg off the foot holder on the fracture table.
- Dislocate the hip, and place the leg in a figure-four position. A complete capsulectomy usually is necessary at this point to gain access to the acetabulum.
- After the femoral head is retracted out of the way, use curets and reamers to remove all remaining cartilage and soft tissue and obtain a bleeding articular cancellous surface.
- Clean the femoral head in the same manner, using femoral head female reamers such as those used for surface replacement procedures.
- After both articular surfaces are reamed, reduce the femoral head into the acetabulum, replace the foot in the foot holder, and place the hip in the proper position for arthrodesis (30 degrees of flexion, neutral abduction and adduction, and slight external rotation to match the opposite limb).
- If needed, pack cancellous chips from the reamings or from the iliac crest into the interstices between the femoral head and the acetabulum.

- Expose the lateral aspect of the proximal femur.
- Drill a hole in the lateral femoral cortex 2.5 to 3 cm below the abductor ridge and, using radiographic control, insert a guide pin through the center of the femoral head and into the thick supraacetabular area of the ilium. Usually an angle of 150 degrees is required.
- Choose an appropriate compression screw and implant as described for treatment of hip fractures. Place two or three cancellous screws proximal to the hip screw for added stability.
- Close the wound in the usual manner, and apply a single hip spica cast.

POSTOPERATIVE CARE Touch-down weight bearing is continued for 8 to 10 weeks. If radiographs show evidence of bony healing, a mini-spica cast (with the knee free) is applied and partial weight bearing is progressed to full weight bearing over the next 4 to 6 weeks. The fusion is reevaluated at 12 to 14 weeks, and if stable union is questionable, another mini-spica cast is applied or a removable polypropylene orthosis is used for another 4 to 6 weeks. Full recovery often takes 6 months, and patients may require 12 months before returning to labor-intensive occupations. Routine removal of the implants is advisable after 18 months to promote bone remodeling and make later conversion to total hip arthroplasty easier.

ARTHRODESIS IN THE ABSENCE OF THE FEMORAL HEAD

Abbott and Fischer designed a method for arthrodesis of the hip after infection with complete destruction of the femoral head and neck. The procedure also has been used after nonunion of the femoral neck, in patients with osteonecrosis of the femoral head, after failed femoral head prostheses, and in patients with infected trochanteric mold arthroplasties. The operation is carried out in two or three stages: (1) correction of the deformity (rarely necessary as a separate stage), (2) arthrodesis of the hip in wide abduction, and (3) final positioning by subtrochanteric osteotomy.

TECHNIQUE 3.6

(ABBOTT, FISCHER, AND LUCAS)

CORRECTION OF DEFORMITY

- To correct severe deformity, first free the greater trochanter from the wing of the ilium, then apply heavy traction to the femur through a Steinmann pin that is inserted through the distal femoral metaphysis.
- Gradually bring the extremity into a position of wide abduction, which brings the greater trochanter near the acetabulum and permits apposition at the time of arthrodesis.

ARTHRODESIS OF THE HIP IN WIDE ABDUCTION

- Expose the acetabulum and proximal femur using an anterior iliofemoral approach.

- Excise the capsule anteriorly and superiorly.
- Debride the joint, removing all acetabular articular cartilage down to healthy cancellous bone.
- Deepen the roof of the acetabulum to permit better seating of the greater trochanter.
- Resect the remaining portion of the femoral neck at its base, and strip the abductor tendons from the greater trochanter and adjacent femoral shaft.
- Denude the greater trochanter down to bleeding cancellous bone.
- Bring the extremity into wide abduction, forcing the greater trochanter well into the prepared acetabular cavity.
- Pack any remaining space with autogenous iliac grafts.

The degree of abduction varies with the individual: In some patients 45 degrees may be sufficient, whereas 70 to 90 degrees may be required in others for accurate fitting and good apposition of the bony surfaces. The degree of abduction must be sufficient, however, to place the apposed surfaces under firm compression.

- Apply a spica cast from the nipple line to the toes on the affected side and to the knee on the opposite side.

FINAL POSITIONING BY SUBTROCHANTERIC OSTEOTOMY

- When the arthrodesis is solid, as affirmed by clinical and radiographic examination, open the distal limb of the iliofemoral approach, retract the rectus femoris medially, and incise the periosteum of the femur in the interval between this muscle and the vastus lateralis.
- Ligate branches of the lateral femoral circumflex artery as required.
- Using a transverse osteotomy 5 cm distal to the lesser trochanter, cut the shaft three-fourths through and carefully fracture the medial cortex.

Adduct and displace the shaft of the femur slightly medially so that the medial cortex of the proximal fragment fits into the medullary cavity of the distal fragment. Usually no internal fixation is necessary. Abbott and Lucas recommended a position of 5 to 10 degrees of abduction, 35 degrees of flexion, and 10 degrees of external rotation.

POSTOPERATIVE CARE Apply a bilateral spica cast; if radiographs through the cast are satisfactory, the patient is immobilized until the osteotomy is solid.

ARTHRODESIS OF THE PROXIMAL FEMUR TO THE ISCHIUM

When the femoral head is extremely diseased or absent, arthrodesis of the proximal femur to the ischium, as described by Bosworth, can be done (see earlier editions of this text for technique description).

TOTAL HIP ARTHROPLASTY AFTER HIP ARTHRODESIS

Conversion of a hip arthrodesis to total hip arthroplasty most often is indicated for pain or generalized loss of function from immobility or malposition. This is a technically demanding procedure, complications and failures are frequent, and improvement of function is uncertain. Best results have been noted in patients who are young and who have had a hip fusion for a relatively short time. Most patients are satisfied, however, with their improved mobility, maneuverability, and sitting ability. A 10% infection rate, a 10% revision rate, and a 5% resection arthroplasty rate because of infection have been reported in replacements done after hip fusions. Less than optimal results for takedown to total hip replacement have been confirmed by other studies. Richards et al. found a 54% complication rate, 74% 10-year survival, and lower outcome scores than either primary or revision total hip replacement comparison cohorts. Peterson et al. also found only 75% 10-year survival, and although 90% had minimal pain, 87% had a limp and 61% required a gait aid. Somewhat more promising results were reported by Sirikonda et al., with much improved hip scores (8.8 to 13.6), although seven of 67 patients required further revision surgery. Flecher et al. reported a 96% 15-year survival of 23 patients who had hip arthrodesis converted to total hip arthroplasty using a custom cementless stem. In a systematic review, however, Jain and Giannoudis found inconsistent reports of pain relief, and complications were reported in up to 54% of patients. Jauregui et al. recently reported a comprehensive review of 27 studies (1104 hips) on conversion of hip fusion to total hip arthroplasty and showed a 12% revision rate.

Those willing to perform this procedure may find interest in the report by Akiyama et al., who used CT-based navigation to more accurately determine the site and direction of the femoral neck osteotomy and the positioning of the acetabular socket, hoping to maximize results in this difficult procedure.

Long-standing hip arthrodeses (average 33 years) have been studied in patients who have had total knee arthroplasty, total hip arthroplasty, or both. Findings suggest that total knee arthroplasty alone is unlikely to provide satisfactory results in patients with hip fusions. Total hip arthroplasty followed by total knee arthroplasty is recommended even if severe osteoarthritis of the knee is the main complaint. Total hip arthroplasty after arthrodesis is discussed in detail in chapter 1.

REFERENCES

Aderinto J, Lulu OB, Backstein DJ, et al.: Functional results and complications following conversion of hip fusion to total hip replacement, *J Bone Joint Surg Br* 94(11 Suppl A):36, 2012.

Bittersohl B, Zaps D, Bomar JD, Hosalkar HS: Hip arthrodesis in the pediatric population: where do we stand? *Orthop Rev (Pavia)* 3:e13, 2011.

Fernandez-Fairen M, Murcia-Mazón A, Torres A, et al.: Is total hip arthroplasty after hip arthrodesis as good as primary arthroplasty? *Clin Orthop Relat Res* 469:1971, 2011.

Flecher X, Ollivier M, Maman P, et al.: Long-term results of custom cementless-stem total hip arthroplasty performed in hip fusion, *Int Orthop* 42(6):1259, 2018.

Fucs PM, Svartman C, Assumpcao RM, et al.: Is arthrodesis the end in spastic hip disease? *J Pediatr Rehabil Med* 4:163, 2011.

Fucs PM, Yamada HH: Hip fusion as hip salvage procedure in cerebral palsy, *J Pediatr Orthop* 34(Suppl 1):S32, 2014.

Gordon AB, McMulkin ML, Thompkins B, et al.: Gait findings in the adolescent subject with a stiff hip, *J Pediatr Orthop* 33:139, 2013.

Hawkins R, Ariamanesh A, Hashemi-Nejed A: Hip arthrodesis in the paediatric and young adult patients: the use of hip resurfacing reamers, *Ann R Coll Surg Engl* 92:437, 2010.

Hoekman P, Idé G, Kassoumou AS, Hayatou MM: Hip arthrodesis with the anterolateral plate: an innovating technique for an orphaned procedure, *PLoS ONE* 9:e85868, 2014.

Jain S, Giannoudis PV: Arthrodesis of the hip and conversion to total hip arthroplasty: a systematic review, *J Arthroplasty* 28:1596, 2013.

Jauregui JJ, Kim JK, Shield 3rd WP, et al.: Hip fusion takedown to a total hip arthroplasty – is it worth it? A systematic review, *Int Orthop* 41(8):1535, 2017.

Patel NK, Luff T, Whittingham-Jones P, et al.: Total hip arthroplasty in teenagers: an alternative to hip arthrodesis, *Hip Int* 22:621, 2012.

Richards CJ, Duncan CP: Conversion of hip arthrodesis to total hip arthroplasty: survivorship and clinical outcome, *J Arthroplasty* 26:409, 2011.

Schafroth MU, Blokzijl RJ, Haverkamp D, et al.: The long-term fate of the hip arthrodesis: does it remain a valid procedure for selected cases in the 21st century? *Int Orthop* 34:805, 2010.

Villaneuva M, Sobrón FB, Parra J, et al.: Conversion of arthrodesis to total hip arthroplasty: clinical outcome, complications, and prognostic factors of 21 consecutive cases, *HSS J* 9:138, 2013.

The complete list of references is available online at Expert Consult.com.

CHAPTER 4

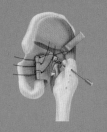

HIP PAIN IN THE YOUNG ADULT AND HIP PRESERVATION SURGERY

James L. Guyton

It has long been known that significant hip deformity resulting from childhood conditions such as developmental dysplasia of the hip and Legg-Calvé-Perthes disease can lead to secondary hip osteoarthritis in adult life. Over the past two decades, more subtle deformity of the hip has been implicated in the development of osteoarthritis in patients who previously were thought to have "primary osteoarthritis" of the hip. Primary or idiopathic osteoarthritis of the hip attributes arthritic progression to the effect of age-related chemical and mechanical deterioration of hip articular cartilage present in a subset of individuals for unknown reasons. Many patients who would formerly have been thought to fall within this primary group are now believed to have had hip impingement leading to osteoarthritis over time.

As early as 1965, Murray described the subtle "tilt deformity" of the proximal femur that he believed would lead to osteoarthritis. This theory that small deformities of the hip from childhood would inevitably lead to osteoarthritis was again stated in 1975 by Stulberg et al., who coined the term "pistol grip" deformity of the proximal femur (Fig. 4.1). In the mid-1990s, Ganz et al. refined the description of hip impingement caused by femoral and acetabular deformity and ushered in a new era of hip-preserving surgery in symptomatic young adult patients by describing techniques to correct these deformities.

Periacetabular osteotomy (PAO), with or without femoral osteotomy, for treatment of painful hip dysplasia in young adults appears to be effective in delaying prosthetic hip reconstruction when the surgical intervention occurs while the arthritic progression is fairly mild. The results of PAO in patients with more advanced arthritis have been less favorable. More recently, the disease patterns of hip impingement have been elucidated, and surgical procedures aimed at hip preservation for this condition have been applied. Similar to hip dysplasia, it appears that the articular damage resulting from hip impingement can occur while symptoms remain relatively mild and intermittent. These facts argue for early intervention in both hip dysplasia and hip impingement before the onset of irreversible arthritis. The goal of hip preservation surgery in both dysplasia and impingement is to alter the hip joint morphology to allow more unhindered physiologic range of motion while optimizing hip joint mechanics to delay or halt the progression of hip osteoarthritis.

Other sources of hip pain in young adults, including osteonecrosis of the femoral head and transient osteoporosis of the hip, are discussed in this chapter. Extraarticular sources of groin, buttock, and lateral hip pain must be differentiated from articular sources. Some of these are discussed, including sports hernias, peritrochanteric pain, and osteitis pubis.

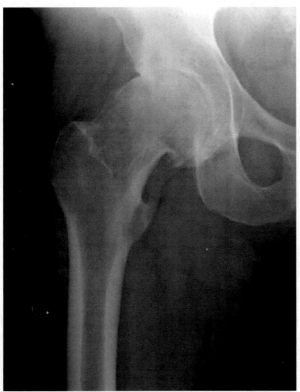

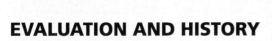

FIGURE 4.1 Pistol-grip deformity of proximal femur leading to secondary osteoarthritis.

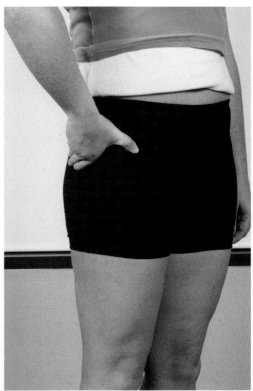

FIGURE 4.2 The "C sign" is suggestive of intraarticular hip pathology.

EVALUATION AND HISTORY

PATIENT HISTORY

The patient history can focus the physician on probable sources of hip pain, thus directing further evaluation. The onset and duration of pain can be helpful, with conditions such as osteonecrosis and stress fracture having fairly acute onsets, whereas dysplasia and hip impingement tend to have insidious onsets often described as a recurrent groin pull that occurs with certain activities. Stress fractures are common in runners, particularly amenorrheic women with lowered bone densities. Pain onset after a twisting injury is common in sports such as soccer, ice hockey, and tennis and suggests a labral injury and may also be associated with bony morphologies that predispose a patient to labral injury. Patients with labral pathology frequently describe a catching, sharp pain when twisting on a weight-bearing hip or when simultaneously flexing and internally rotating their hip, as when entering a car. Psoas tendonitis usually is described as groin pain that is made worse with active hip flexion and frequently is associated with an audible snapping of the hip.

The localization of pain also is helpful. Posterior pain along the posterosuperior iliac spine and buttock frequently is referred pain from the lumbar spine and possibly the sacroiliac joint. The radiation of this pain down the posterior thigh and past the knee is highly suggestive of a radicular origin, particularly when associated with other neurologic symptoms. Lateral hip pain is frequently peritrochanteric in origin and can radiate down the lateral thigh as in iliotibial band tendinitis. Intraarticular pathology usually presents as some amount of groin or deep, more ill-defined pain. Byrd described the frequent "C sign" suggestive of intraarticular pathology in

which the patient places his hand about the affected hip with the thumb in the groin crease and the fingers on the buttock surrounding the hip with the hand in the shape of a C (Fig. 4.2). However, intraarticular pathology can present as primarily lateral or posterior pain that must be differentiated from extraarticular sources by physical examination combined with imaging studies and occasionally diagnostic injections.

Pain that occurs with sitting for prolonged times but is minimal with standing and walking suggests hip impingement, although it also can be spine related. Weight-bearing pain that is relieved by sitting or lying is more nonspecific, with possibilities including osteoarthritis, osteonecrosis, stress fracture, dysplasia, and inflammatory arthritis. Pain associated with a popping or a snapping sensation can be caused by a labral tear or snapping psoas tendon or iliotibial band.

PHYSICAL EXAMINATION

Physical examination of the hip begins with observation of the patient's gait. An antalgic gait is described as having a decreased stance phase on the affected limb. A painful hip, however, often causes the patient to walk with an abductor lurch, in which he or she lurches toward the affected side during the stance phase of gait in an effort to reduce the joint reactive forces on the hip. This same type of gait is seen with weakness of the hip abductor. Weakness of the hip abductor is tested with the Trendelenburg test. The Trendelenburg test is positive for hip abductor weakness when the pelvis sags more than 2 cm during single-leg stance on the limb tested (Fig. 4.3).

With a fixed or painful hip flexion contracture, a patient will stand with compensatory hyperextension of the lumbar spine. During gait, extension of the hip is accomplished by

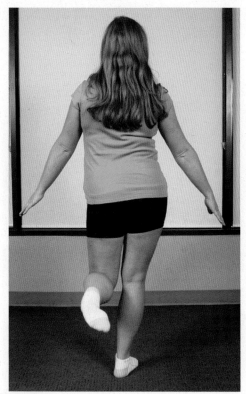

FIGURE 4.3 Trendelenburg sign is positive when affected hemipelvis sags during one-legged stance.

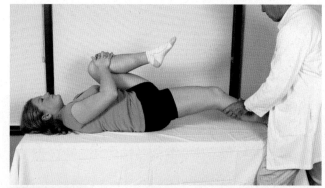

FIGURE 4.4 Thomas test detects hip flexion contracture by extending affected hip while contralateral hip is held flexed, flattening and immobilizing lumbar spine.

further extension of the lumbar spine. With a flexion contracture the pelvis also may rotate toward the affected side during extension of the hip because of the inability of the patient to extend the hip adequately. This asymmetric external rotation of the pelvis during extension of a hip with a flexion contracture is known as a pelvic wink.

Some patients experience a snapping sensation during gait or with specific standing maneuvers. The examiner may have the patient reproduce the snapping while palpating the lateral side of the hip. A snapping iliotibial band frequently can be palpated or visualized as it catches while sliding over the lateral border of the greater trochanter during gait. Many patients with a snapping iliotibial band, also known as an external snapping hip, can reproduce the snapping by bearing weight on the leg while flexing and extending the hip.

Palpation of the pelvis may identify tenderness at the pubic symphysis typical of osteitis pubis. Tenderness along the inguinal canal may represent a classic inguinal hernia or deficiency of the abdominal wall known as a sports hernia. The muscular origins of the rectus femoris and adductor longus can be tender with strains or avulsion injuries. Tenderness over the greater trochanter and abductor tendon will be present with trochanteric bursitis and partial tears of the gluteus medius or minimus.

The examination continues with the patient supine with both hips examined for symmetry of motion. Flexion, extension, abduction, and adduction, as well as internal and external rotation, are noted. Rotation is tested in both extension and 90 degrees of flexion. Rotation of the hip in extension can most reliably be tested with the patient prone on the examination table. The presence of a flexion contracture is determined by the Thomas test. With the patient supine, both hips

are flexed maximally, thus flattening any lumbar lordosis. The legs are then alternatively brought into extension with any residual flexion contracture noted while the pelvis and lumbar spine are held stationary by keeping the contralateral hip flexed (Fig. 4.4). The presence of reproducible popping or clicking during hip range of motion testing should be noted because it may be suggestive of a labral tear.

A hip with synovitis from any cause can be painful when the hip is rotated passively to the extremes of motion allowable. The range of motion in all planes may be decreased, with internal rotation and abduction tending to be most affected. When the hip is quite irritable, even log-rolling the patient's hip on the examination table can be painful. A hip that is irritable with log-rolling should make the examiner consider diagnoses such as inflammatory arthritis, sepsis, stress fracture, acute onset of osteonecrosis, or advanced degenerative arthritis.

An active straight leg raise performed by the patient produces a force of approximately two times body weight because of the joint reactive force produced by the hip flexors. Pain with an active straight-leg raise can be helpful because this force is reproducible in a given patient and can be used as a gauge of disease severity. Pain with resisted hip flexion past 30 to 45 degrees is known as a positive Stinchfield test and can detect even more subtle degrees of intraarticular hip pathology than is detected by straight leg raise alone.

The anterior impingement test or FADIR (flexion adduction internal rotation) test is performed by flexing the hip to 90 degrees, adducting across the midline, and maximally internally rotating the hip (Fig. 4.5). Hips with symptomatic anterior impingement are limited in internal rotation and are painful with this maneuver. Contralateral comparison of internal rotation is particularly helpful because this value will vary greatly between individuals. With anterior impingement, patients have distinctly more pain with the FADIR test than with other extremes of rotation. With lateral or posterior impingement, however, as in patients with a protrusio deformity, pain may be produced by pure abduction or with the FABER (flexion abduction external rotation) test (Fig. 4.6). The FABER test also may elicit posterior pelvic pain with disorders of the sacroiliac joint or lumbosacral junction.

The anterior apprehension test is performed with the patient supine on the edge of the examination table. The hip is extended and externally rotated (Fig. 4.7). Patients with hip dysplasia, including deficient anterior coverage, will experience groin discomfort or a sense of apprehension with this

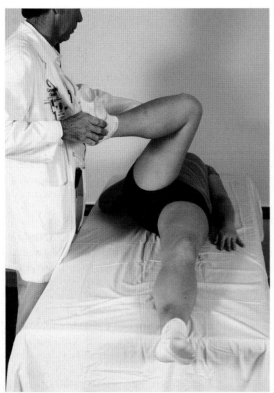

FIGURE 4.5 FADIR test: flexion, adduction, and internal rotation of hip.

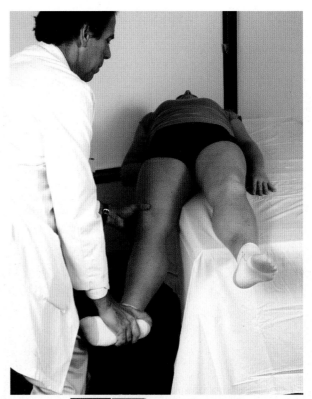

FIGURE 4.7 Apprehension test.

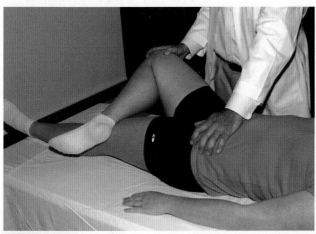

FIGURE 4.6 FABER test: flexion, abduction, and external rotation of hip.

maneuver. This maneuver also may elicit posterior or lateral pain in a patient with posterior impingement.

The test for internal snapping of the hip or a snapping iliopsoas tendon is performed by passively flexing the hip to 90 degrees in a slightly abducted and externally rotated position, and then asking the patient to extend the hip to the examination table while keeping the foot suspended. A snapping psoas tendon frequently is audible as a distinctive, low-pitched "thunk" as it crosses from lateral to medial over the iliopectineal eminence during extension of the hip. This finding is common as a normal variant in individuals with no hip pain.

The area about the greater trochanter and gluteal muscles is more easily assessed with the patient in a lateral position. Pain with resisted abduction or against gravity may be present in patients with gluteus medius or minimus tendinitis or partial tears. The Ober test is performed with the patient in the lateral position by abducting the patient's hip with the knee flexed and then letting the hip fall into adduction. A delay in adduction caused by gravity is a positive Ober test. With the hip extended past neutral, a positive Ober test signifies tightness of the iliotibial band, whereas a positive Ober test with the hip in neutral flexion/extension is indicative of a gluteus medius contracture or tendinopathy. In the lateral position, snapping of the iliotibial band over the greater trochanter can be reproduced in patients with external snapping hip syndrome by flexing and extending the hip while tensioning the iliotibial band similar to the Ober test. In thin patients, a thickened portion of the iliotibial band may produce visible snapping with this maneuver.

The use of a diagnostic intraarticular hip injection with local anesthetic can be used as a means of identifying patients with an intraarticular pathologic process when physical examination and radiographic studies are equivocal. This test can be particularly helpful when encountering a patient with an atypical pain pattern or when trying to differentiate pain from intraarticular pathology from referred pain generated from another source. Examining the patient within a couple of hours of the injection can be helpful, with the patient asked to reproduce the activities that previously elicited hip pain. Definite improvement in the patient's symptoms has been noted by Byrd to predict the presence of an intraarticular pathologic process with 90% accuracy.

RADIOGRAPHIC ASSESSMENT

Assessment of the painful hip begins with plain radiography and a standing anteroposterior pelvic view. The radiographic signs on an anteroposterior pelvic radiograph are highly sensitive to rotation and tilt of the pelvis. A satisfactory anteroposterior pelvic view displays symmetry of the iliac wings and obturator foramina with the tip of the coccyx 1 to 3 cm above the pubic symphysis (Fig. 4.8). A true anteroposterior view of the pelvis is particularly necessary when evaluating acetabular version and coverage.

The lateral center edge (LCE) angle of Wiberg (Fig. 4.9) is measured on the anteroposterior pelvic radiograph by first drawing a horizontal reference line by connecting the centers of the femoral heads or the base of the radiographic teardrops.

A line perpendicular to this horizontal reference line is drawn through the center of the femoral head and dome of the acetabulum. Another line is drawn from the center of the femoral head to the lateral edge of the sourcil or dense subchondral bone forming the dome of the acetabulum. Bone that extends lateral to the sourcil is not included in the measurement because it does not contribute to the weight-bearing support of the femoral head. The angle between these lines is the LCE angle. An LCE angle of less than 20 degrees is indicative of hip dysplasia with inadequate coverage of the femoral head by the lateral dome of the acetabulum. Hips with LCE angles in the range of 20 to 24 degrees have borderline dysplasia, and hips with an LCE angle of more than 40 degrees display overcoverage.

The version of the acetabulum is evaluated on the anteroposterior pelvic radiograph by tracing the rim of the anterior and posterior walls. In a normal hip, the anterior and posterior walls converge at the superior lateral margin of the acetabulum. The crossover sign is present when the anterior wall outline crosses over the posterior wall below the superior lateral margin of the acetabulum (Fig. 4.10). The crossover sign is indicative of either isolated anterior overcoverage of the hip or retroversion of the entire acetabulum with deficient posterior coverage. The position of the posterior wall relative to the center of the femoral head is noted. A positive posterior wall sign exists when the posterior wall lies medial to the femoral head center and indicates deficient posterior wall coverage (Fig. 4.11). When combined with a crossover sign, a positive posterior wall sign indicates relative retroversion of the acetabulum. Another sign of acetabular retroversion is ipsilateral prominence of the ischial spine in an otherwise properly rotated and positioned anteroposterior pelvic radiograph. The distinction between isolated anterior overcoverage and retroversion of the entire acetabulum is crucial because the surgical treatment is different for these two conditions. Of note, a crossover sign also may be caused by variations in the

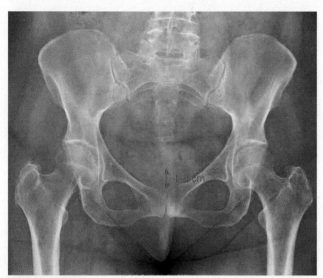

FIGURE 4.8 Satisfactory anteroposterior pelvic radiograph shows coccyx centered 1 to 3 cm above the symphysis with symmetric obturator foramina.

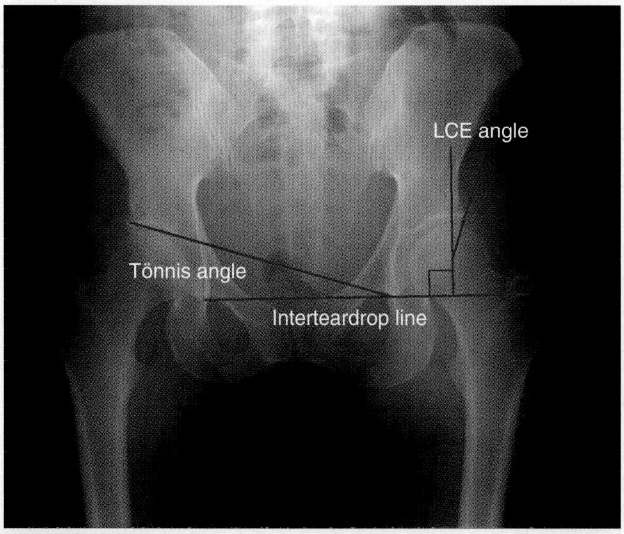

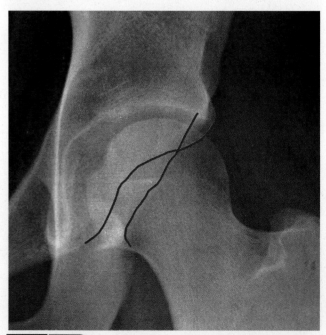

FIGURE 4.10 Crossover sign is indicative of acetabular retroversion with anterior overcoverage of femoral head.

FIGURE 4.9 Lateral center edge *(LCE)* angle of Wiberg measures arc of superolateral acetabular coverage beyond vertical line drawn through center of femoral head. Tönnis angle measures inclination of radiographic sourcil compared with interteardrop line.

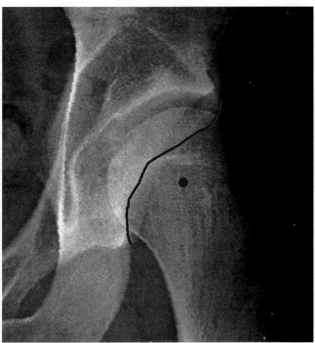

FIGURE 4.11 Posterior wall sign is present when center of femoral head lies lateral to lateral margin of posterior wall on anteroposterior pelvic radiograph.

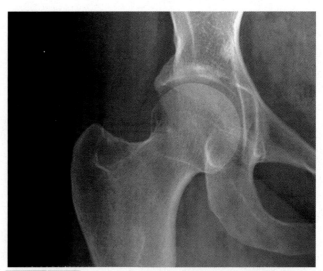

FIGURE 4.12 Coxa profunda is present when the acetabular fossa extends medial to the ilioischial line and indicates excessive acetabular depth sometimes associated with pincer type impingement.

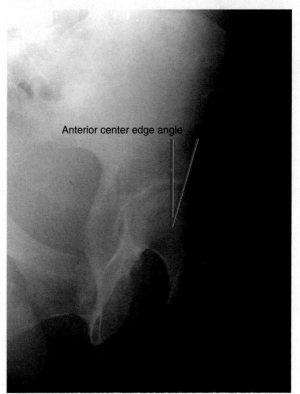

Anterior center edge angle

FIGURE 4.13 Anterior center edge angle of Lequesne is measured on false profile view and is indicative of anterior coverage of hip.

morphology of the AIIS in the presence of normal acetabular version.

The inclination of the acetabulum is measured on the anteroposterior pelvic view with the Tönnis angle, which is determined by first drawing a line from the most medial aspect of the radiographic sourcil to its most lateral aspect. A second line is drawn parallel to the interteardrop line with the apex of the angle at the medial sourcil (see Fig. 4.9). This angle normally is between 0 and 10 degrees. Angles of more than 10 degrees are present with hip dysplasia, whereas an angle of less than 0 degrees can indicate overcoverage.

The presence of coxa profunda is seen on the anteroposterior pelvic radiograph when the medial aspect of the acetabular fossa extends medial to the ilioischial line (Fig. 4.12). Coxa profunda may be present in patients with acetabular overcoverage, though it can also be a normal variant, particularly in women. Protrusio acetabuli exists when the medial aspect of the femoral head is projected crossing the ilioischial line and usually indicates excessive acetabular depth and possible acetabular overcoverage with pincer impingement morphology. Protrusio acetabuli frequently is associated with inflammatory arthropathy or Marfan syndrome, but can be isolated and idiopathic.

The anterior center edge (ACE) angle of Lequesne is generated on the false profile view of the pelvis to assess the anterior coverage of the hip. The false profile view is made with the patient standing with the affected side of the pelvis externally rotated 65 degrees from the anteroposterior projection (Fig. 4.13). The ACE angle is determined by first drawing a vertical line from the center of the femoral head through the dome of the acetabulum. A second line is drawn from the center of the femoral head to the anterior edge of the subchondral bone of the acetabulum, ignoring bone anterior to the sclerotic subchondral edge because this bone does not provide

anterior support for the femoral head. The normal ACE angle is approximately 20 degrees, with lesser values indicative of undercoverage.

Other views typically obtained in younger patients with hip pain include a frog-leg lateral, a cross-table lateral, and a 45-degree modified Dunn view of the hip. The modified Dunn view is obtained with the patient supine with the hip in 45 degrees of flexion, 20 degrees of abduction, and neutral

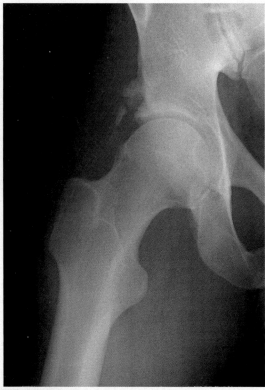

FIGURE 4.14 Modified Dunn view displays anterosuperior head-neck junction, which frequently is involved with cam impingement.

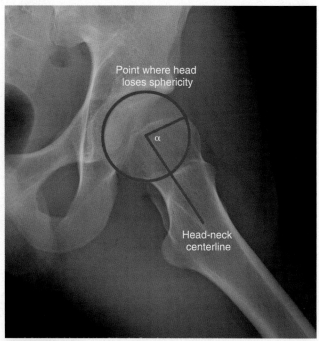

FIGURE 4.15 Alpha angle measures angle between axis of femoral neck and junction of spherical portion of femoral head with more prominent head-neck junction.

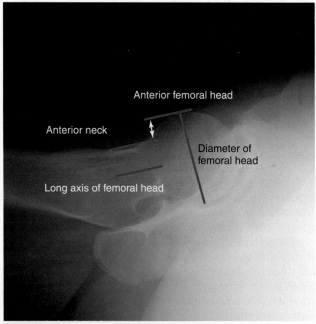

FIGURE 4.16 Anterior head-neck offset ratio (see text for description).

rotation (Fig. 4.14). With the use of these three views in addition to the anteroposterior pelvic view, the femoral head-neck junction is evaluated at different degrees of femoral rotation for the presence of head-neck offset abnormality and anterolateral prominence of the femoral neck that can cause cam impingement. The cam deformity was described by Murray as a "tilt" deformity of the femoral head and later by Stulberg et al. as a "pistol grip" deformity with flattening of the lateral head-neck junction seen on an anteroposterior view of the hip. The cam deformity appears to predispose individuals to secondary osteoarthritis. This anterolateral cam deformity is better seen on the lateral and modified Dunn views and is quantitated by the alpha angle and head-neck offset ratio.

The alpha angle is used to assess the femoral head-neck junction on AP, lateral, and modified Dunn views. The angle is formed by a line drawn from the center of the femoral neck to the center of the femoral head and a second line drawn from the center of the femoral head to the point on the anterior head-neck junction where the contour of the femoral head diverges from the spherical contour determined more medially on the head (Fig. 4.15). Nötzli et al. described the normal value for the alpha angle to be 42 degrees in asymptomatic hips. An alpha angle of more than 50 to 55 degrees is generally considered consistent with a cam deformity of the femoral head-neck junction.

The anterior head-neck offset ratio is determined from the cross-table lateral view with the hip in 10 degrees of internal rotation (Fig. 4.16). The offset of the femoral head is determined by measuring the distance between two lines drawn parallel to the axis of the femoral neck. The first line is drawn through the most anterior portion of the femoral neck, and

the second line is drawn through the most anterior portion of the femoral head. The ratio is determined by dividing this distance by the diameter of the femoral head. According to Beaulé et al., a value of less than 0.15 has a 95% positive predictive value of diagnosing femoroacetabular impingement.

The beta angle, originally described by Wyss et al. using an open MRI, determines the angle between the pathologic head-neck junction, the center of the femoral head, and the

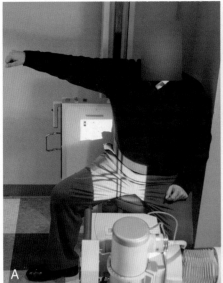
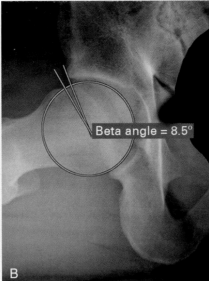
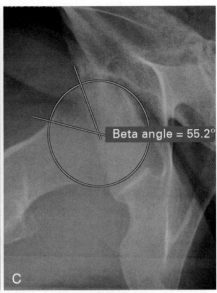

FIGURE 4.17   **A,** "Beta view" for measurement of the beta angle with the hip in 90 degrees of flexion, 20 degrees of abduction, and 0 degrees of rotation. X-ray beam is angled 15 degrees to the anteroposterior direction so that it is tangential to the acetabular plane. Beta-view radiographs showing **(B)** cam-type femoroacetabular impingement with a reduced beta angle of 8.5 degrees and **(C)** a healthy control subject with a more normal beta angle of 55.2 degrees. (From Brunner A, Hamers AT, Fitze M, Herzog RF: The plain β-angle measured on radiographs in the assessment of femoroacetabular impingement, *J Bone Joint Surg B* 92:1203, 2010. Copyright British Editorial Society of Bone and Joint Surgery.)

acetabular rim with the hip in 90 degrees of flexion. Brünner et al. described the measurement of the beta angle on plain radiographs. The radiograph is obtained with the patient seated and the hip held in 90 degrees of flexion, 20 degrees of abduction, and neutral rotation. The beam is angled 15 degrees from the anteroposterior projection to be tangential to the acetabular plane and centered on the femoral shaft approximately 6 cm lateral to the anterior-superior iliac spine. The beta angle is measured from the point where the contour of the femoral head-neck junction departs from the spherical contour of the femoral head to the center of the femoral head and then to the superior lateral bony margin of the acetabulum (Fig. 4.17). According to Brünner et al., a beta angle of less than 30 degrees is indicative of impingement morphology, including cam, pincer, and mixed types.

The Tönnis grading system is commonly used to describe the presence of osteoarthritis in hips being considered for hip preservation surgery:

Grade 0: no signs of osteoarthritis

Grade 1: sclerosis of the joint with minimal joint space narrowing and osteophyte formation

Grade 2: small cysts in the femoral head or acetabulum with moderate joint space narrowing

Grade 3: advanced arthritis with large cysts in the femoral head or acetabulum, joint space obliteration, and severe deformity of the femoral head.

The prognosis of any hip preservation surgery is improved when it is done in patients with lower Tönnis grades.

Small impingement cysts or sclerosis at the anterolateral femoral head-neck junction are radiographic evidence of femoroacetabular impingement and are present in approximately one third of symptomatic patients (Figs. 4.18 and 4.19). A calcified labrum may worsen pincer-type impingement

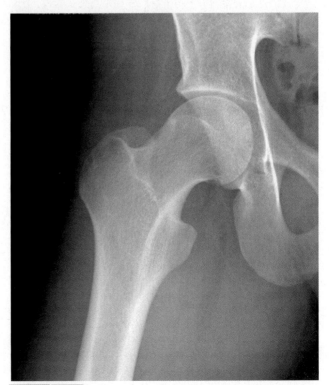

FIGURE 4.18   Sclerosis seen at femoral head-neck junction is indicative of impingement.

by producing secondary overcoverage. The sphericity of the femoral head and the congruence of the femoral head with the acetabulum are evaluated on all views. Posterior cartilage space narrowing occasionally can be discerned on the false profile view, whereas the other views remain relatively normal.

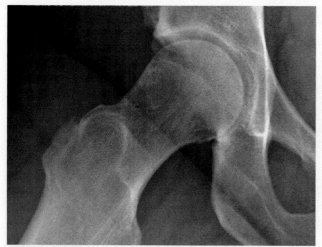

FIGURE **4.19** Impingement cyst is seen at anterolateral head-neck junction in patient with combined cam and pincer impingement.

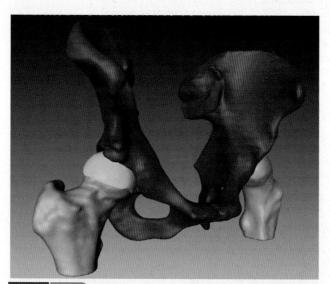

FIGURE **4.20** Computed tomography scan of pelvis with three-dimensional reconstruction shows acetabular overcoverage and direct surgical correction. (Courtesy Christopher Peters, MD.)

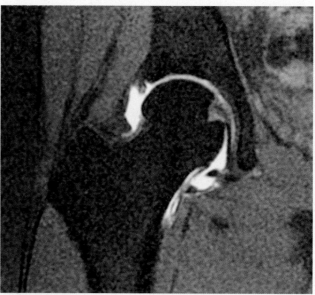

FIGURE **4.21** Magnetic resonance arthrogram shows gadolinium tracking into labral chondral junction, indicating a labral tear.

acetabulum also can be seen with impingement. Small cysts within the anterior femoral neck have been described as anatomical variants or "herniation pits." These cysts, as well as sclerosis of the femoral head-neck junction, are thought to be caused by the repetitive trauma of hip impingement. Thinning of the articular cartilage on MRA is indicative of more advanced disease, as is the presence of acetabular subchondral cysts. The alpha angle described earlier used with plain radiographs also has been applied to radial MRA and CT images of the hip for planning bony resection of both cam and pincer deformities.

Labral tears seen on MRA may occur secondary to injury alone, although they are uncommon without underlying bony deformity. Labral tears are more likely to be the result of abnormal hip mechanics with secondary injury of the labrum and adjacent acetabular rim. These abnormal mechanics may be exacerbated by physical activity as is seen in certain sports such as hockey, soccer, and tennis.

CT of the pelvis with three-dimensional reconstruction is frequently used to offer guidance with bony resection in cam- and pincer-type deformities (Fig. 4.20).

MR arthrography (MRA) of the hip has been the gold standard in detection of labral pathology, improving the sensitivity of demonstrating labral tears from around 60% to more than 90% when compared with traditional MRI of the hip performed without administration of a contrast agent (Fig. 4.21). The status of the articular cartilage is more difficult to ascertain on MRA. Occasionally, contrast medium can be seen tracking beneath the articular cartilage adjacent to the labrum because of delamination in cam-type impingement. With the evolution of MRI technology, higher resolution 3Tesla scans with various sequencing have been shown to reliably demonstrate labral and articular cartilage pathology. These scans may eventually obviate the benefit of injecting intraarticular contrast at the time of the study. Edema in the anterior femoral neck and the anterosuperior

FEMOROACETABULAR IMPINGEMENT

Femoroacetabular impingement (FAI) occurs when anatomic variation of the hip causes impingement between the femoral head-neck junction and the acetabular rim during functional range of motion. The presence of symptomatic hip impingement in adolescence and young adulthood is believed to be one of the primary causes of osteoarthritis in patients younger than the age of 50 years. In a study of patients under 50 years of age undergoing total hip replacement, Clohisy et al. found that in patients with osteoarthritis, after excluding those with developmental dysplasia of the hip, slipped capital femoral epiphysis, and Perthes disease, 97% had radiographic signs of cam, pincer, or mixed type impingement. Early recognition of hip impingement and intervention to correct the underlying pathology has been championed in an attempt to modify the

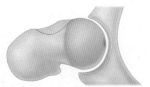

FIGURE 4.22 Cam impingement occurs when prominent head-neck junction contacts acetabular rim during hip flexion.

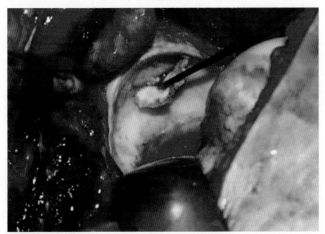

FIGURE 4.23 Delamination of articular cartilage secondary to impingement injury. (Courtesy Robert Trousdale, MD.)

natural history of the condition. Multiple approaches to hip-preserving surgery have evolved based in part on the varied pathologic processes involved as well as varied surgical philosophies and skills.

Two basic types of impingement have been described. Cam impingement occurs when the anterosuperior femoral head-neck junction is prominent or the femoral neck has a diminished offset from the adjacent femoral head (Fig. 4.22). With flexion and particularly flexion combined with internal rotation, the nonspherical portion of the femoral head-neck junction rotates into the acetabulum. A typical injury pattern with cam impingement is a tear at the base of the labrum at the labral-chondral junction. The adjacent articular cartilage then becomes injured because of compression from the femoral head with its relatively larger radius of curvature rotating into the acetabulum. Frequently, the articular cartilage delaminates from the underlying subchondral bone, progressing from the acetabular rim (Fig. 4.23). In this process, the acetabular labrum is relatively spared, with more injury incurred within the adjacent articular cartilage. Cam morphology is more common in young athletic males. Kapron et al. found 72% of collegiate football players to have an alpha angle of more than 50 degrees. The etiology of the deformity is unknown, although some authors have postulated that it may be a mild variant of slipped capital femoral epiphysis, whereas more commonly others have postulated a developmental abnormality of the lateral femoral physis, possibly related to activity level. In a cross-sectional MRI study of adolescents, abnormal alpha angles were not found in any hips with open physes, but 14% of hips with closed physes had cam deformities. The daily activity levels for patients with cam deformities were significantly higher than for those with no deformity.

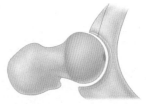

FIGURE 4.24 Pincer impingement occurs when acetabulum has localized or global overcoverage leading to contact of acetabular rim with femoral head-neck junction during normal hip motion.

There is an increasing body of evidence that cam impingement can predispose a hip to osteoarthritis. A large, prospective, cross-sectional, population-based study found 6% of men and 2% of women to have cam deformities, whereas 42% of those who had hip replacements had evidence of a cam deformity. In a longitudinal, prospective study, a cam deformity with an alpha angle of more than 60 degrees had an adjusted odds ratio of 3.67 for development of end-stage osteoarthritis, whereas an alpha angle of more than 83 degrees had an adjusted odds ratio of 9.66. In a 20-year longitudinal study of 1003 women, each degree increase in the alpha angle over 65 degrees was associated with a 5% increase in the risk of developing osteoarthritis.

Pincer impingement occurs when the acetabular rim has an area of overcoverage causing impingement against the femoral neck with functional motion (Fig. 4.24). The area of overcoverage can be global, as with protrusio acetabuli, or can be localized to the anterior acetabulum as with acetabular retroversion. Acetabular retroversion can also be global or isolated. In true global retroversion of the acetabulum, the posterior coverage of the acetabulum is deficient, with the entire acetabulum rotated or retroverted about the longitudinal axis. In isolated retroversion of the acetabulum the anterosuperior rim of the acetabulum extends farther around the femoral head whereas the remainder of the acetabulum has more normal morphology.

The injury pattern with pincer impingement is created by the femoral neck abutting the acetabular rim and labrum during the extremes of motion. The labrum is pinched between the bony surfaces and subsequently suffers more damage than the adjacent articular cartilage, which is relatively spared. Pincer impingement may worsen with time as the result of reactive bone growth at the acetabular rim or calcification of the labrum, effectively increasing the arc of overcoverage of the acetabulum (Fig. 4.25). A "contrecoup" injury frequently is seen on the posterior femoral head and posteroinferior acetabulum owing to levering of the femoral neck on the acetabular rim with subsequent increased pressure on the posterior hip cartilage. Pincer morphology is more commonly encountered in women.

Pincer impingement morphology also has been implicated in the development of osteoarthritis, though not as strongly as cam impingement morphology. In a comparison of radiographs of hips that had total hip arthroplasty (THA) for osteoarthritis to radiographs of nonarthritic hips, 20% of the arthritic hips had evidence of acetabular retroversion, although only 5% of the asymptomatic hips showed signs of retroversion. In the Copenhagen Osteoarthritis Study, deep acetabular sockets had an adjusted risk ratio of 2.4 for the development of osteoarthritis.

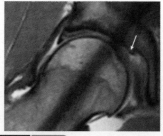
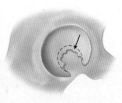

FIGURE 4.27 A "sabertooth" osteophyte seen on MRA and depicted in drawing. (From Hanke MS, Steppacher SD, Anwander H, et al: What MRI findings predict failure 10 years after surgery for femoroacetabular impingement? *Clin Orthop Relat Res* 475:1192, 2017.)

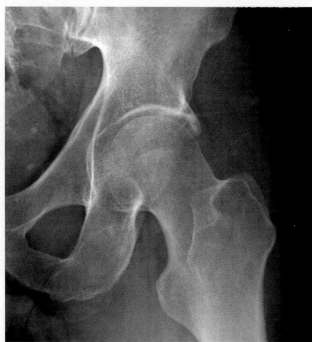

FIGURE 4.25 Calcified labrum contributing to pincer-type impingement.

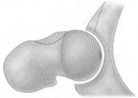

FIGURE 4.26 Combined cam and pincer femoroacetabular impingement.

Combined mechanism hip impingement occurs when cam and pincer morphology coexist in the same hip (Fig. 4.26). Associated pincer deformities have been reported in variable percentages of patients being operated on for cam-type impingement, though according to some authors, most hips treated for FAI have combined morphology. Interestingly, Bardakos and Villar described a positive posterior wall sign as a risk factor for arthritis progression when observing patients with cam deformities and Tönnis grade 1 or 2 arthritic staging over a 10-year time interval. Some of these patients are likely to have had associated acetabular retroversion, whereas others may have had a dysplastic variant.

SURGICAL INDICATIONS

As FAI has become better defined, the number of surgical procedures performed for FAI has increased dramatically, particularly hip arthroscopic procedures. Surgical indications are being refined as the short-term and midterm outcomes of open, arthroscopic, and combined procedures are reported.

Accurate diagnosis of the source of pain in young adults or adolescents is crucial in obtaining optimal surgical outcomes with FAI surgery. The diagnosis of FAI is primarily made clinically from the patient's history and physical examination and then correlated with the radiographic findings. Occasionally, a diagnostic hip injection is done at the time of MRA. A study by Hack et al. corroborates the need for a compelling clinical picture of FAI as an indication for surgery. Of 200 asymptomatic volunteers who had MRI of the hips, 14% had cam morphology of at least one proximal femur (alpha angle of more than 50.5 degrees), including 25% of the men and 5% of the women. With symptomatic individuals excluded from the study and with an estimated lifetime radiographic incidence of osteoarthritis of the hip of 8%, the radiographic appearance of a cam deformity as currently defined does not appear to always lead to osteoarthritis. The authors stated that concurrent pincer-type deformity and other environmental factors may have a role in the development of osteoarthritis.

Hanke et al. identified MRA findings that correlated with failure of FAI surgery within 10 years of surgery, including the presence of an acetabular rim cyst, involvement of 60 degrees of the articular cartilage, and the presence of a sabertooth (central acetabular) osteophyte (Fig. 4.27). They recommended routine MRA with radial cuts to search specifically for these signs of early osteoarthritis that portend a poorer outcome with FAI surgery.

The exclusion criteria for arthroscopic intervention have tended to focus on the residual hip cartilage thickness. A residual joint space of over 2 mm frequently is cited as being associated with a good result after FAI surgery. Skendzel et al. found that, at 5 years after arthroscopic FAI surgery, of those with a preoperative cartilage space measuring 2 mm or less 86% had been converted to THA, while only 16% of those with preserved cartilage spaces had been converted to THA. Byrd et al. stated that with 2-year follow-up even Tönnis grade 2 hips had meaningful improvement of patient-reported outcomes (mHHS). Outcomes with longer follow-up of Tönnis grade 2 hips have been less favorable.

Osteochondroplasty of the femoral head-neck junction is the surgical treatment for symptomatic cam impingement. This is usually accomplished arthroscopically, though it can be done through a limited open anterior approach or open surgical dislocation. The technique is determined by the extent of the pathologic process, associated pathology, and the surgeon's familiarity with a given approach.

The radiographic parameters defining pincer morphology are studied to determine the extent and regions of overcoverage or deficiency. An LCE angle of more than 40 degrees is indicative of lateral overcoverage and may be associated with a coxa profunda or protrusio acetabuli deformity with global overcoverage. Three-dimensional CT images may be helpful in determining the location and extent of acetabular overcoverage. In patients with pincer impingement caused by isolated retroversion of the anterosuperior rim of the acetabulum, the crossover sign may be the only plain radiographic finding. This type of pincer impingement can be treated arthroscopically with labral reflection, rim trimming, and labral reattachment. Limited anterior approaches have been used to treat this lesion, as well as open surgical dislocation. Larger deformities on the acetabular side of the joint involving the posterior-superior and posterior acetabular rim usually are treated with open surgical dislocation with acetabular rim trimming and labral reattachment when possible.

A crossover sign associated with a posterior wall sign and a prominent ischial spine indicates retroversion of the entire acetabulum with deficient posterior coverage. These patients have true retroversion of their entire acetabulum and are candidates for PAO. Some of these patients have a component of dysplasia with deficient lateral coverage. Some surgeons advocate arthroscopy alone for treating global acetabular retroversion, with anterior rim trimming reported to improve patient-reported outcomes 2 years postoperatively while avoiding the greater surgical intervention of a PAO. However, predominant thought is that treating these patients with acetabular rim trimming may predispose them to symptoms of instability. Performing a PAO allows the surgeon to antevert the acetabulum, with or without changing lateral coverage, as needed to optimize the position of the acetabulum from the predetermined radiographic parameters.

There is a subset of patients with borderline hip dysplasia (LCE angle of 20 to 25 degrees) with coexistent cam deformity. This is a difficult patient group because the pain may be primarily from impingement or dysplasia. Careful history and physical examination must be relied upon to determine the appropriate treatment of these patients because purely positional pain not associated with weight-bearing activity may be primarily due to impingement. Some of these patients experience pain because of instability and are appropriately treated with a PAO to correct the borderline dysplasia with combined osteochondroplasty of the femoral cam deformity and open labral repair through an anterior capsulotomy at the time of PAO or with arthroscopy.

SURGICAL DISLOCATION OF THE HIP

Surgical dislocation of the hip was described by Ganz et al. for the treatment of FAI. The surgery is designed to allow full access to the acetabulum and the femoral head-neck junction while preserving the blood supply to the femoral head. The approach protects the deep branch of the medial circumflex artery as it supplies the posterolateral retinacular vessels to the femoral head. The major advantage of the approach is its extensile nature with full access to the acetabular rim, the labrum, and the femoral head-neck junction without the limitations of arthroscopy and limited anterior approaches. Surgical dislocation of the hip also has been used for open treatment of slipped capital femoral epiphysis, the deformities of residual Perthes disease and Pipkin fractures of the femoral head. The shortcoming of the approach also relates to its extensile nature, which requires trochanteric osteotomy with a more prolonged recovery compared with more limited exposures.

SURGICAL DISLOCATION OF THE HIP

TECHNIQUE 4.1

(GANZ ET AL.)

- With the patient in the lateral decubitus position, make a Kocher-Langenbeck incision and split the fascia lata accordingly. Alternatively, make a Gibson approach and retract the gluteus maximus posteriorly.
- Internally rotate the leg and identify the posterior border of the gluteus medius. Do not mobilize the gluteus medius or attempt to expose the piriformis tendon.
- Make an incision from the posterosuperior edge of the greater trochanter extending distally to the posterior border of the ridge of the vastus lateralis.
- Use an oscillating saw to make a trochanteric osteotomy with a maximal thickness of 1.5 cm along this line. At its proximal limit, the osteotomy should exit just anterior to the most posterior insertion of the gluteus medius (Fig. 4.28A). This preserves and protects the profundus branch of the medial femoral circumflex artery.
- Release the greater trochanteric fragment along its posterior border to about the middle of the tendon of the gluteus maximus and mobilize it anteriorly with its attached vastus lateralis.
- Release the most posterior fibers of the gluteus medius from the remaining trochanteric base. The osteotomy is correct when only part of the fibers of the tendon of the piriformis have to be released from the trochanteric fragment for further mobilization.
- With the patient's leg flexed and slightly rotated externally, elevate the vastus lateralis and intermedius from the lateral and anterior aspects of the proximal femur.
- Carefully retract the posterior border of the gluteus medius anterosuperiorly to expose the piriformis tendon.
- Separate the inferior border of the gluteus minimus from the relaxed piriformis and the underlying capsule. Take care to avoid injury to the sciatic nerve, which passes inferior to the piriformis muscle into the pelvis.
- Retract the entire flap, including the gluteus minimus, anteriorly and superiorly to expose the superior capsule (Fig. 4.28B). Further flexion and external rotation of the hip makes this step easier.
- Incise the capsule anterolaterally along the long axis of the femoral neck; this avoids injury to the deep branch of the medial femoral circumflex artery (Fig. 4.28C).
- Make an anteroinferior capsular incision, taking care to keep the capsulotomy anterior to the lesser trochanter to avoid damage to the main branch of the medial femoral circumflex artery, which lies just superior and posterior to the lesser trochanter.
- Elevate the anteroinferior flap to expose the labrum.
- Extend the first capsular incision toward the acetabular rim and then turn it sharply posteriorly parallel to the labrum, reaching the retracted piriformis tendon. Take care not to damage the labrum.
- Dislocate the hip by flexing and externally rotating the leg; bring the leg over the front of the operating table and

place it in a sterile bag (Fig. 4.28D). Most of the acetabulum can now be inspected.

- Manipulation of the leg allows a 360-degree access to the acetabulum and nearly 360-degree access to the femoral head.
- After exposure of the acetabulum, reflect the labrum from the portion of the acetabular rim that displays overcoverage (Fig. 4.28E) and trim excessive bone with an osteotome or burr (Fig. 4.28F).
- If possible, reattach the labrum at the margin of the articular surface with suture anchors, recreating the seal effect of the labrum (Fig. 4.28G).
- For osteochondroplasty, outline the femoral head-neck junction with a surgical marker and then cut the articular cartilage at the proximal edge of the resection with a scalpel to avoid inadvertent extension into the normal femoral head.
- Carefully perform the resection with small osteotomes, using a burr to complete the recontouring of the head-neck junction (Fig. 4.28H). Cadaver studies have shown

that up to 30% of the diameter of the femoral neck can be removed from the anterolateral quadrant of the head-neck junction without substantially altering the strength of the femoral neck to axial load. A typical resection, however, is much less than 30% and is tailored to the specific anatomy encountered.

- Check the contour of the femoral head with a plastic template or spherometer to gauge the proximal extent of the osteochondroplasty where the femoral head becomes aspherical (Fig. 4.28I).
- Coat the exposed cancellous bone with bone wax. Reduce the hip and reproduce the position of impingement, evaluating range of motion directly and with fluoroscopy.
- Repair the capsule anatomically with nonabsorbable sutures.
- Reattach the greater trochanter with two 4.5-mm cortical screws aimed medially and distally in the region of the lesser trochanter.

POSTOPERATIVE CARE Postoperatively, the patient is mobilized with touch-down weight bearing for 6 weeks

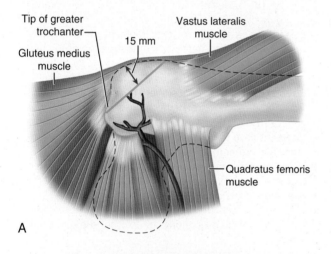

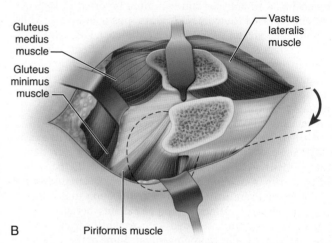

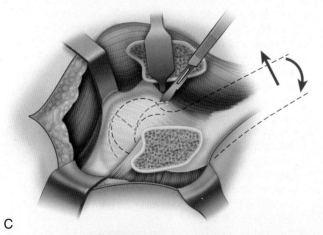

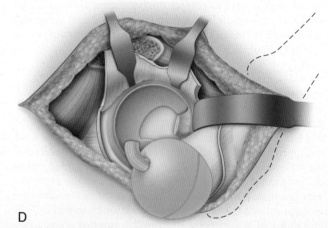

FIGURE **4.28** **A,** Trochanteric osteotomy exits proximally just anterior to most posterior attachment of gluteus medius, preserving capsular branch of medial femoral circumflex artery. **B,** Hip capsule is exposed above level of piriformis by dissecting gluteus minimus off capsule while displacing trochanteric fragment anteriorly. **C,** Z-shaped capsulotomy is performed. **D,** Hip is dislocated anteriorly while placing leg in sterile drape pouch over anterior side of operating table and cutting ligamentum teres.

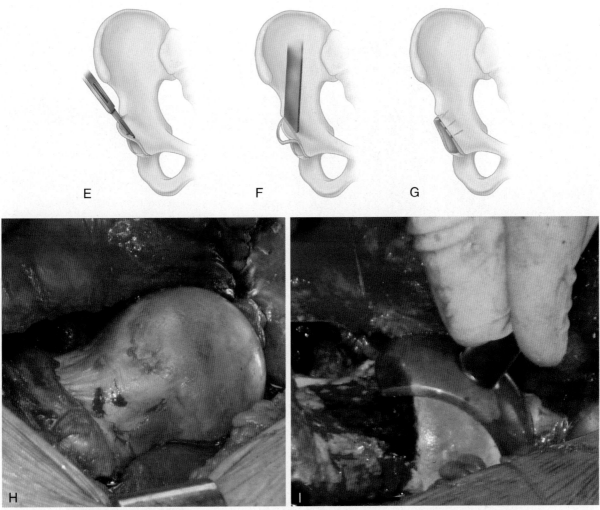

FIGURE 4.28, Cont'd **E,** Labrum is reflected off overhanging acetabulum. **F,** Excessive bone is trimmed with osteotome or burr, and intact labrum is reattached with suture anchors if possible. **G,** Labrum is reattached with suture anchors. **H,** Burr is used to recontour head-neck junction. **I,** Clear plastic spherometer can be used to judge point where femoral head becomes aspherical and to guide extent of osteochondroplasty. **SEE TECHNIQUE 4.1.**

with avoidance of active abduction and extreme flexion or rotation of the hip. After 3 weeks, pool exercises are begun, and at 6 weeks weight bearing is allowed with progressive abductor strengthening. Low-molecular-weight heparin is used for deep venous thrombosis prophylaxis for 2 weeks, followed by aspirin 325 mg per day for another 4 weeks.

■ RESULTS

In follow-up studies ranging from 2 to 10 years, the rate of good to excellent results has ranged from 68% to 94%. Hip scores improved an average 2 to 5 points as measured by the Merle d'Aubigné Score and in one study by 30 points as measured by the modified Harris Hip Score (Fig. 4.29). Conversion to total hip replacement occurred in 0% to 30% of patients. Factors that negatively impacted results included preoperative evidence of arthritis (Tönnis grade 2), intraoperative evidence of cartilage delamination, and increasing age. In a study by Anwander et al., refixation of the labrum

improved the good to excellent percentage from 48% to 83% at 10 years when compared with labral debridement, although radiographic progression of osteoarthritis and conversion to THA was not significantly affected. In a separate report from the same group, Steppacher et al. reported a 10-year survivorship free of arthritic progression for 80% of FAI patients treated with surgical dislocation including labral reattachment. Heterotopic ossification and painful trochanteric hardware requiring removal were rarely reported complications.

COMBINED HIP ARTHROSCOPY AND LIMITED OPEN OSTEOCHONDROPLASTY

This approach described by Clohisy et al., Laude et al., and others has been used for patients with cam impingement. After hip arthroscopy for intraarticular or central compartment labral debridement or repair, the anterior aspect of the hip is approached through a limited Smith-Petersen approach or Hueter approach (through the sheath of the tensor fascia lata). The osteochondroplasty of the femoral head-neck junction is performed under direct vision. With traction, the anterior rim

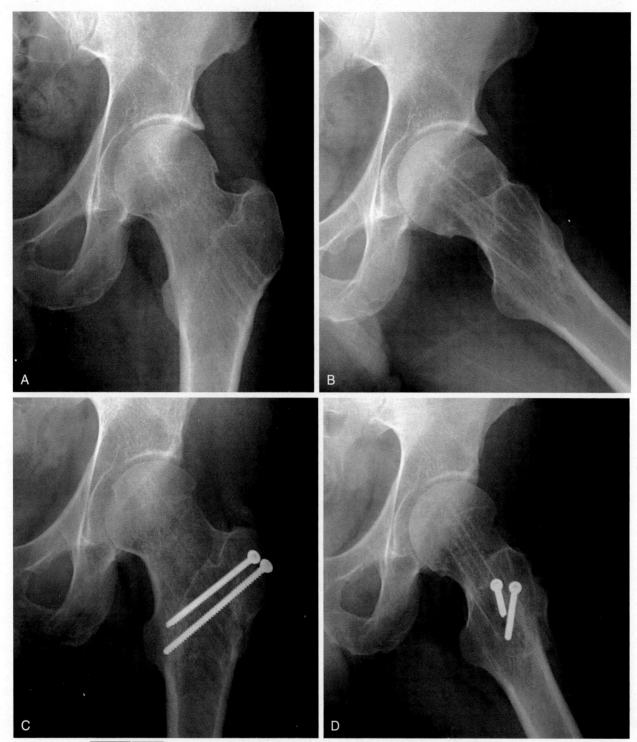

FIGURE 4.29   **A** and **B,** Preoperative anteroposterior and lateral pelvic radiographs of 32-year-old woman with combined cam and pincer impingement after treatment of femoral neck fracture. **C** and **D,** After surgical dislocation with acetabular rim trimming and femoral osteochondroplasty.

of the acetabulum can be resected with reflection of the labrum and reattachment with suture anchors although the extent of rim exposure and resection is limited. The advantage of this approach is primarily avoiding the morbidity of surgical dislocation with a larger exposure including trochanteric osteotomy. This approach allows direct vision of a typical cam deformity on the femoral head-neck junction. The limitation of this approach is that only the anterior aspect of the femoral head and neck and acetabular rim can be accessed. The lateral femoral cutaneous nerve may be injured in this approach as well. Placing the incision several centimeters lateral to the antero-superior iliac spine and approaching the anterior hip through the fascial sheath of the tensor fascia lata may lessen the risk of injury to the nerve.

COMBINED HIP ARTHROSCOPY AND LIMITED OPEN OSTEOCHONDROPLASTY

TECHNIQUE 4.2

(CLOHISY AND MCCLURE)
- With the patient supine, perform a standard arthroscopic examination of the hip for inspection of the articular cartilage of the femoral head, acetabulum, and acetabular labrum. Debride any unstable flaps of acetabular labrum and associated articular cartilage flaps.
- After arthroscopic debridement is completed, irrigate the joint, remove the arthroscopic instruments, and release the traction.
- Obtain a cross-table lateral or frog-leg lateral fluoroscopy view (Fig. 4.30A) to ensure excellent visualization of the proximal femur, specifically the femoral head-neck junction.

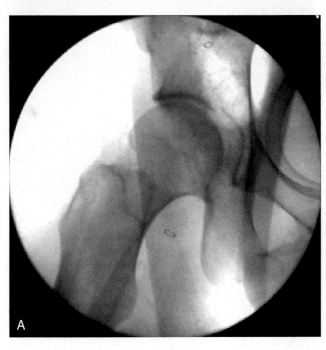

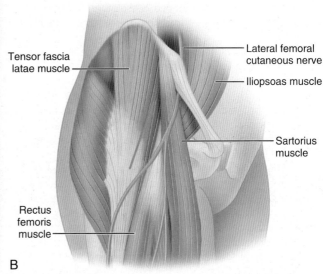

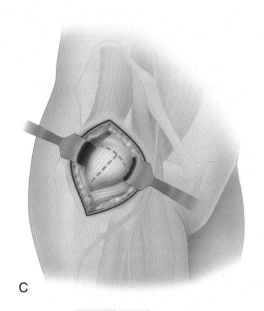

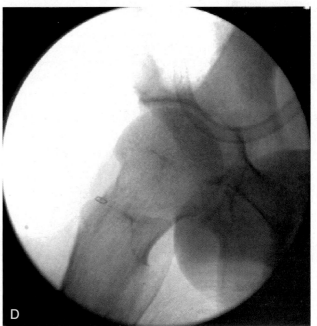

FIGURE 4.30 **A,** Frog-leg lateral fluoroscopic view shows femoral head-neck junction. **B,** Incision incorporates anterior arthroscopy portal slightly lateral to anterosuperior iliac spine to avoid lateral femoral cutaneous nerve. **C,** Tensor fascia lata muscle is retracted laterally, and rectus and iliocapsularis are reflected to access anterior hip capsule. **D,** Frog-leg lateral fluoroscopic view verifying adequate resection. **SEE TECHNIQUE 4.2.**

- Make an 8- to 10-cm incision, starting just inferior to the anterosuperior iliac spine and incorporating the anterior arthroscopy portal incision (Fig. 4.30B).
- Carry the dissection through the subcutaneous tissue laterally directly onto the fascia of the tensor fascia lata muscle.
- Incise the fascia and retract the muscle belly laterally and the fascia medially. Protect the femoral cutaneous nerve by placing the fascial incision lateral to the tensor-sartorius interval.
- Develop the interval between the tensor and sartorius, identify the rectus origin, and release the direct and reflected heads.
- Reflect the rectus distally, and dissect the adipose tissue and iliocapsularis muscle fibers off the anterior hip capsule (Fig. 4.30C).
- Make an I-shaped or T-shaped capsulotomy to provide adequate exposure of the anterolateral femoral head-neck junction.
- Using the normal head-neck offset anteromedially as a reference point for resection of the abnormal osteochondral lesion along the anterolateral head-neck junction, use a 0.5-inch curved osteotome to perform an osteoplasty at the head-neck junction.
- Direct the osteotome distally and posteriorly to make a beveled resection to prevent delamination of the retained femoral head articular head cartilage.
- After the anterolateral head-neck offset has been established, confirm accuracy of the resection with fluoroscopy using frog-leg lateral or cross-table lateral views in neutral and varying degrees of internal rotation (Fig. 4.30D).
- Examine the hip for impingement in flexion and for combined flexion and internal rotation, while palpating the anterior hip to test for residual impingement.
- If the anterior acetabular rim is overgrown secondary to labral calcification or osteophyte formation, carefully debride until adequate clearance is obtained.
- Hip motion should improve at least 5 to 15 degrees in flexion and 5 to 20 degrees in internal rotation.
- The goal of osteoplasty is to remove all prominent anterolateral osteochondral tissue that contributes to an aspherical shape of the femoral head (Fig. 4.31). If sphericity has not been achieved, perform additional resection of the femoral head-neck junction.
- Control bleeding with bone wax, irrigate the joint, and close the longitudinal and superior transverse arms of the arthrotomy with nonabsorbable suture. Close the remainder of the wound in standard fashion.

POSTOPERATIVE CARE Physical therapy is instituted for toe-touch weight bearing with crutches to minimize the risk of femoral neck stress fracture. A pillow is used under the thigh to protect the rectus repair, and active flexion is avoided for 6 weeks. Abductor strengthening is begun immediately and is continued with a home exercise program. Crutches are discontinued at 6 weeks, and activities are resumed gradually as tolerated. Impact activities, such as running, are not encouraged for at least 6 months. Aspirin, 325 mg, is taken as a thromboembolic prophylaxis, and indomethacin, 75 mg sustained release, is used for heterotopic ossification prophylaxis; therapy with both is continued for 6 weeks.

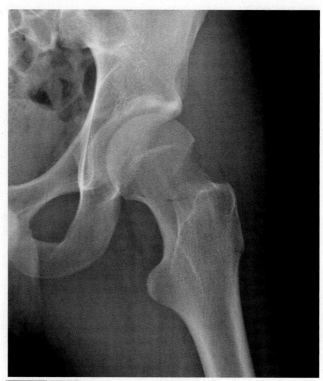

FIGURE 4.31 After limited open osteochondroplasty of femoral head-neck junction. **SEE TECHNIQUE 4.2.**

■ RESULTS

Clohisy et al. reported an average improvement in the modified Harris hip score from 64 to 87 with normalization of the alpha angle at 2-year follow-up after arthroscopic labral debridement and limited open osteochondroplasty. Two of 36 patients showed radiographic progression of arthritis from Tönnis grade 0 to grade 1. Laude et al. showed at average 58-month follow-up an increase in the nonarthritic hip score of 29 points. There was an 11% failure rate with conversion to total hip replacement, with better results obtained in patients younger than 40 years of age and patients having Tönnis grade 0 arthritis preoperatively.

MINI-OPEN DIRECT ANTERIOR APPROACH

Similar to the limited open osteochondroplasty described above, the mini-open direct anterior approach described by Ribas et al. uses the Smith-Petersen interval to access the anterior hip, but the procedure is done on a standard operating table with distraction of the hip accomplished by extension of the hip and a T-shaped anterior hip capsulotomy. No muscle is detached from the pelvis. Specialized retractors with attached fiber-optic illumination are recommended. A 70-degree arthroscope can be used through the capsulotomy to inspect the articular surface of the acetabulum. The acetabular rim can be treated in the region of the most common pathology, and cam lesions of the head-neck junction can be directly visualized and corrected. The labrum can be repaired with suture anchors. Cohen et al. reported the use of this approach in athletes and found similar activity score improvements and return to sport compared with arthroscopic and surgical dislocation techniques.

TECHNIQUE 4.3

(RIBAS ET AL.)

POSITIONING AND APPROACH

- With the patient supine on an extension table, make an incision beginning 1 cm below and 1 cm lateral to the anterosuperior iliac spine and continuing 4 to 8 cm distally toward the fibular head.
- Open the crural fascia and the tensor fascia latae approximately 1 cm posterior to the first fibers of the tensor fascia latae and identify the interval between the sartorius and the tensor fascia latae muscles. This maneuver protects the posterior branches of the lateral femorocutaneous nerve by making a "double fascial pocket" (Fig. 4.32A).
- Detach the reflected portion of the rectus femoris muscle.
- Place a curved blunt Hohmann retractor over the upper part of the capsule and a straight Hohmann retractor between the iliocapsularis muscle and the capsule with the

hip in at least 30 degrees of flexion to avoid damage to the femoral nerve.
- Make a T-shaped capsulotomy from distal to proximal through the interval between the iliofemoral ligaments, taking care to identify the labrum by lifting the capsule as the dissection reaches the acetabulum.
- Place reference sutures in both sides of the capsule and place two blunt curved Hohmann retractors intraarticularly around the femoral neck.

INSPECTION OF THE HIP JOINT

- Perform the impingement (FADIR) maneuver to observe the area of impingement.
- Apply an extension force for hip distraction. Once the hip is distracted about 10 mm, use an additional light source attached to the Hohmann retractor or a 70-degree arthroscope to inspect the joint for acetabular chondral and labral lesions in the six zones described by Ilizaliturri: zone 1, anterior inferior; zone 2, anterior superior; zone

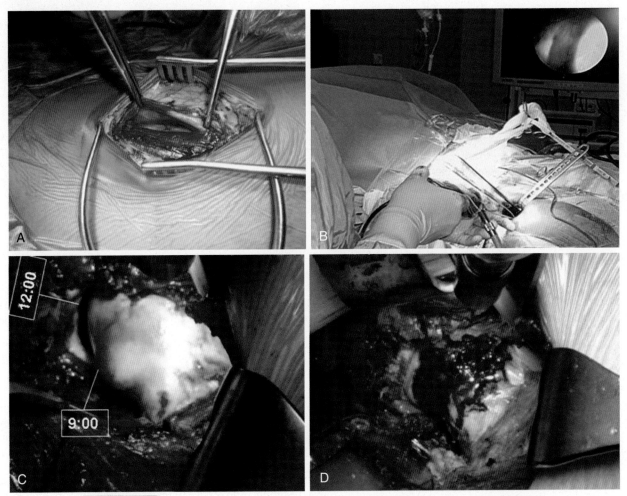

FIGURE 4.32   Mini-open direct anterior approach for osteochondroplasty. **A,** Development of "double fascial pocket" to protect lateral femoral cutaneous nerve and its posterior branches. **B,** Inspection and treatment of the internal compartment using a 70-degree arthroscope. **C,** Appearance of the cam deformity after labral suture. **D,** After completion of the femoral osteoplasty. (From Ribas M, Cardenas-Nylander C, Bellotti V, et al: Mini-open technique for femoroacetabular impingement. www.boneandjoint.org.uk/content/focus/mini-open-technique-femoroacetabular-impingement.)
SEE TECHNIQUE 4.3.

3, middle superior; zone 4, posterior superior; zone 5, posterior inferior; and zone 6, middle inferior (cotyloid fossa) (Fig. 4.32B).

ACETABULAR OSTEOPLASTY AND LABRAL REPAIR

- Repair chondrolabral delamination by detachment of the labrum and trimming of the acetabular rim with 5-mm diamond burrs.
- Reattach the labrum with 3.1-mm resorbable transosseous anchors, and release extension of the hip (Fig. 4.32C).

FEMORAL OSTEOPLASTY

- Use fluoroscopy to identify intraoperative landmarks according to preoperative planning.
- For cam-type impingement, excise the bony prominence with ultra-sharp curved osteotome and round burrs manipulated counter-clockwise to avoid excessive bone penetration.
- Start the bump resection at the posterosuperior head-neck junction with hyperextension, adduction, and internal rotation of the hip. Then flex, abduct, and externally rotate the hip to reach the posteroinferior head-neck junction and the acetabular rim (Fig. 4.32D). Use pulsed lavage throughout the procedure to prevent heterotopic ossification.
- When bone resection is complete, obtain a final fluoroscopic image and test the femoroacetabular clearance and range of motion, especially flexion and internal rotation.

CLOSURE

- Close the wound in routine fashion. Close the hip capsule with the hip in full extension to avoid capsular overtightening.
- Take care to avoid injury to the branches of the lateral femoral cutaneous nerve during superficial closure.

POSTOPERATIVE CARE Indomethacin protocol is used to prevent heterotopic ossification. Gastroprotective drugs and low-molecular-weight heparin also are administered.

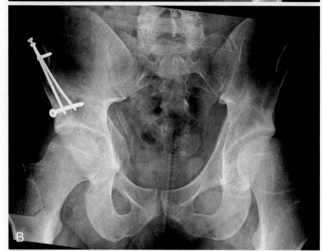

FIGURE 4.33 **A,** Preoperative radiograph of patient with both crossover and posterior wall signs indicative of acetabular retroversion with deficient posterior coverage. **B,** After "reverse" periacetabular osteotomy to increase patient's acetabular anteversion. (Courtesy Christopher Peters, MD.)

PERIACETABULAR OSTEOTOMY

Periacetabular osteotomy developed primarily for the treatment of dysplasia also has been used for the treatment of pincer-type impingement caused by global acetabular retroversion (Fig. 4.33) identified radiographically by a crossover sign with a corresponding posterior wall sign on the anteroposterior radiograph of the pelvis. Some of these patients also have deficient lateral coverage with a center edge angle of less than 20 degrees. According to the algorithm described by Peters et al., the articular cartilage of the anterior acetabulum should be judged to be intact by MR arthrogram before proceeding with a PAO because that cartilage is rotated into a more weight-bearing position with correction of the bony deformity.

■ SURGICAL TECHNIQUE

The technique of PAO is described in the section on hip dysplasia (Technique 4.4). The direction of rotation of the acetabular segment is individualized for each patient. Care must be taken not to overantevert the acetabular segment because posterior impingement can be created. In combined type

deformity, an osteochondroplasty of the femoral head-neck junction can be done through the Smith-Petersen approach used for the PAO.

■ RESULTS

Siebenrock et al. reported the use of PAO for impingement caused by acetabular retroversion in 29 hips, 24 of which had concurrent reshaping of the femoral head-neck junction. They strove for 30 degrees of internal rotation in 90 degrees of hip flexion. Seventy-one percent had good to excellent results with no evidence of osteoarthritis at an average 11-year follow-up. Predictors for poor outcome were the lack of femoral offset creation and overcorrection of the acetabular version resulting in excessive anteversion. The authors emphasized the intraoperative assessment of acetabular correction with anteroposterior pelvic images and assessment of range of motion. Peters et al. reported an improvement in the average Harris hip score from 72 to 91 in 30 hips at 4-year follow-up after PAO for acetabular retroversion with a positive posterior wall sign.

HIP ARTHROSCOPY

Management of FAI with arthroscopic osteochondroplasty of the femoral head-neck junction and/or acetabular rim trimming with labral debridement or refixation has evolved quickly, with almost all FAI surgery in the United States now performed arthroscopically. Early results of hip arthroscopy reflected primarily labral debridement without correction of underlying bony pathology. Studies by McCarthy et al. and Byrd and Jones demonstrated subsequent conversion to THA in 44.1% and 22.6%, respectively, at 13- and 10-year follow-up. Studies representing more contemporary treatment that includes correction of underlying impingement morphology as well as labral refixation appear to obtain better outcomes. Menge et al., however, in their study of 10-year results of FAI surgery with labral debridement and labral repair, found that 34% of patients underwent THA within 10 years, regardless of the technique of labral treatment. Older patients, patients treated with microfracture, and those with a preoperative joint space of less than 2 mm were most at risk for subsequent THA.

Currently, almost all FAI surgery is being done arthroscopically. More rapid recovery following arthroscopy has been reported by multiple authors, while radiographic and clinical parameters of impingement are treated effectively. Although advanced techniques of arthroscopy have been developed, there do appear to be some general limitations to the arthroscopic technique and situations in which open techniques may be preferable. A cam deformity extending into the posterior-superior head-neck junction, behind the retinacular vessels, is more difficult to access arthroscopically. Similarly, a symptomatic pincer deformity that involves the posterior-superior and posterior wall may be better treated through open surgery. Significant deformity of the proximal femur, including excessive anteversion, coxa valga, or a residual deformity from childhood from slipped capital femoral epiphysis, Perthes disease, or previous open reduction for developmental dysplasia of the hip (DDH) are reasons for possible femoral osteotomy and open assessment with correction.

Care also should be taken with a cam deformity combined with a borderline dysplastic acetabulum because arthroscopic capsulotomy with rim trimming can lead to hip instability. Some authors cite reasonable 2-year outcomes with arthroscopic FAI treatment in patients with borderline dysplasia compared to those with normal LCE angles as long as capsular plication is done. Others state that this deformity is better treated with PAO combined with an open reshaping of the femoral head-neck junction and functional assessment of impingement.

The treatment of FAI with arthroscopic techniques is discussed in other chapter.

EXTRAARTICULAR HIP IMPINGEMENT

There is a subgroup of patients who appear to have extraarticular bony impingement. The demographics, physical examination findings, and bony morphologies of these patients were characterized by Ricciardi et al. They tended to be younger women, 40% of whom had previously had a hip procedure for another diagnosis. Factors that increased clinical suspicion of extraarticular FAI included a history of lateral or posterior pain, decreased external rotation, decreased internal rotation with no evidence of a cam lesion, absence of major pelvic or acetabular deformity, a positive posterior impingement sign, incomplete response to intraarticular injection of a local anesthetic or corticosteroid, and continued impingement-type symptoms after arthroscopic treatment without a residual cam lesion.

The types of extraarticular impingement are characterized as anterior, posterior, and complex (Fig. 4.34). In the anterior type, also known as subspinal impingement, the anterior greater trochanter or intertrochanteric line impinges on prominent bone just below the anterior inferior iliac spine or on the AIIS itself. On axial imaging, this type frequently is associated with femoral retrotorsion, defined as less than 5 to 10 degrees of femoral anteversion. On examination, these patients have diminished internal rotation in 90 degrees of hip flexion with increased hip external rotation in both flexion and extension. Failure to recognize subspinal FAI is thought to be a common cause of continued pain following adequate correction of intraarticular FAI. It can be difficult to diagnose significant extraarticular impingement when obvious coexistent intraarticular FAI is present. This underscores the value of examination on the operating table after intraarticular FAI has been corrected to search for restriction of internal rotation in flexion as evidence of extraarticular impingement.

Similar to cam impingement, subspinal impingement can be iatrogenically created during PAO when the acetabular fragment is rotated forward to create more anterior coverage, bringing the AIIS caudad into an impinging position. This can be demonstrated with intraoperative fluoroscopic examination and allow correction before concluding the operation (Fig. 4.35).

Posterior type of extraarticular impingement occurs when the posterior greater trochanter and extraarticular femoral neck impinge against the ischium when the hip is flexed and externally rotated. These hips tend to have excessive femoral anteversion with limited external rotation clinically. Their internal rotation in flexion tends to be increased. If symptoms warrant, these patients can be treated with derotational osteotomy of the femur.

The complex type of extraarticular impingement occurs both anteriorly and posteriorly in femurs with diminished femoral offset and proximal femoral deformity secondary to Perthes disease with an enlarged greater trochanter and femoral head deformity. Rotation tends to be limited in both directions in flexion and limited in external rotation in extension. The surgical treatment of these patients is aimed at relieving the impinging areas by anterior or posterior trochanteric osteoplasty, relative lengthening of the femoral neck, osteochondroplasty of the femoral neck, and treatment of coexisting FAI deformities. Relative femoral neck lengthening (Fig. 4.36) is done during open surgical dislocation with careful mobilization of the retinacular vessels and osteotomy and distalization of the greater trochanter. This correction not only relieves extraarticular impingement but also improves the hip abductor function by increasing the abductor moment arm. It also provides better access to the femoral canal for subsequent THA if later required.

Ischiofemoral extraarticular impingement in extension has been described in active patients with a diminished distance between the lesser trochanter and the ischium. Pain typically is described in the lower buttock, groin, and medial thigh, with worsening pain during pronounced extension of the hip. MRI may show edema within the quadratus femoris muscle (Fig. 4.37). Small series have reported improvement with open or arthroscopic partial resection or distalization of the lesser trochanter.

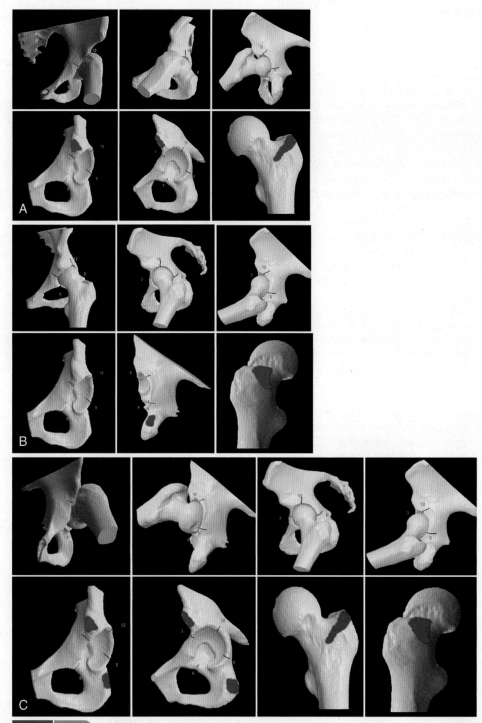

FIGURE 4.34　Classification of extraarticular FAI described by Ricciardi et al. **A,** Anterior. **B,** Posterior. **C,** Complex. (See text). (From Ricciardi BF, Fabricant PD, Fields KG, et al: What are the demographic and radiographic characteristics of patients with symptomatic extraarticular femoroacetabular impingement? *Clin Orthop Relat Res* 473:1299, 2015.)

HIP DYSPLASIA

Hip dysplasia in young adults results from residual childhood developmental dysplasia of the hip or, less frequently, Perthes disease (Fig. 4.38). The treatment of these disorders in skeletally immature patients is discussed in other chapter.

Radiographically, dysplasia of the hip is characterized by an LCE angle of less than 20 degrees, with hips in the 20- to 25-degree range having borderline dysplasia. Typically, the Tönnis angle is increased above 10 degrees. Dysplastic hips also display a lateralized hip center with a broadened radiographic teardrop. The femoral neck-shaft angle usually is increased, and the proximal femur is usually excessively anteverted. The femoral head may be small and have a flattened lateral contour. Many patients with hip dysplasia display an increased alpha angle and thus have a cam morphology.

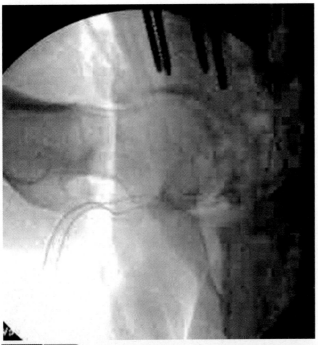

FIGURE 4.35 Iatrogenic subspinal impingement created during periacetabular osteotomy was seen on fluoroscopy, prompting decompression.

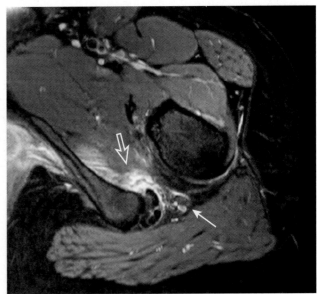

FIGURE 4.37 MRI T2 sequence of a patient with ischiofemoral impingement of the left hip. *Outlined arrow*, quadratus femoris muscle belly edema; *solid arrow*, sciatic nerve. (From Gollwitzer H, Banke IJ, Schauwecker J, et al: How to address ischiofemoral impingement? Treatment algorithm and review of the literature, *J Hip Preserv Surg* 4289, 2017.)

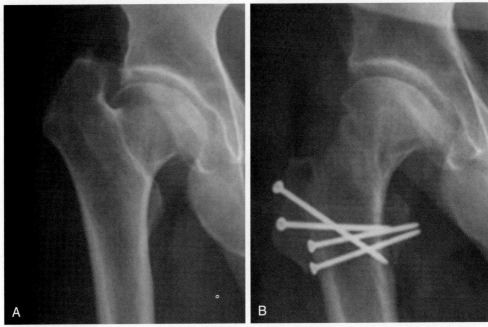

FIGURE 4.36 A, Patient with a short femoral neck and high-riding greater trochanter from Perthes disease. B, After relative femoral neck lengthening. (From Steppacher SD, Anwander H, Schwab JM, et al: Femoral dysplasia, https://musculoskeletalkey.com/femoral-dysplasia.)

Studies of patients with symptomatic acetabular dysplasia have found cam morphology in 10% to 40%. Cam morphology may lead to symptomatic FAI after acetabular reorientation. Disruption of the Shenton line is present with superior and lateral positioning of the hip center and with true hip subluxation from the hip center (Fig. 4.39).

The natural history of untreated dysplasia has been studied by a number of investigators. Murphy et al. longitudinally observed hips in patients who had undergone total hip replacement for osteoarthritis. They found that the contralateral hips having a LCE angle less than 16 degrees routinely developed significant osteoarthritis by the age of 65. Jessel et al. used dGEMRIC (delayed gadolinium-enhanced magnetic resonance imaging of cartilage) indexing to quantitate the osteoarthritic state in a cohort of dysplastic hips and found that increasing age, severity of dysplasia as defined by both the lateral and

ACE angles, and the presence of a labral tear on MRA all correlated with increasing osteoarthritis. Interestingly, a 20-year longitudinal study of women by Thomas et al. found that for each degree of reduction in the LCE angle below 28 degrees there was a 14% increase in the risk of developing secondary osteoarthritis, implying that our definition of dysplasia based on a LCE angle of 20 degrees may be too restrictive. Wyles et al. followed the contralateral hip in patients younger than 55 years of age who had a THA and found at 10-year follow-up that 1 of 33 Tönnis 1 dysplastic hips progressed to THA compared to 1 of 5 Tönnis 1 FAI morphology hips and Tönnis 1 normal morphology hips.

Typically, patients with hip dysplasia become symptomatic between their second and fifth decades of life. Initially, pain may occur only with high-stress activities or prolonged standing. Impingement or FADIR testing may become positive with injury to the labrum. Apprehension testing can be positive with insufficient anterior coverage and anterior cartilage injury.

The radiographic workup of these patients as outlined earlier includes an assessment of the acetabular coverage, depth, version, and lateralization. Sphericity of the femoral head is noted because rotational correction of the acetabulum may worsen congruence of the hip when the femoral head is aspherical. An anteroposterior view with the hip slightly flexed and abducted can be performed to simulate the congruence that would be attained with a PAO (Fig. 4.40). Any evidence of arthritic change is noted and graded by the Tönnis scale. The false profile is evaluated for evidence of subluxation or posterior cartilage wear. Evaluation

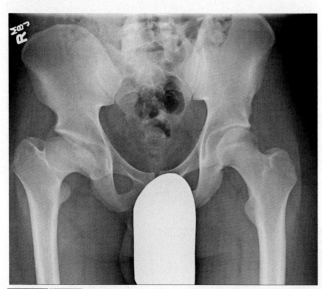

FIGURE 4.38 Twenty-year-old male with residual right hip deformity from Legg-Calvé-Perthes disease with an enlarged femoral head and shortened femoral neck. The acetabulum has secondary signs of dysplasia including an increased Tönnis angle and extrusion of the lateral portion of the head and undercoverage.

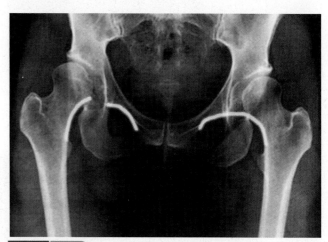

FIGURE 4.39 In more severe dysplasia, the Shenton line is disrupted, indicating superior subluxation of the femoral head and hip center.

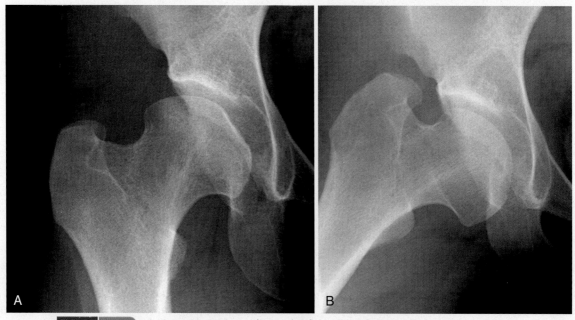

FIGURE 4.40 **A,** Anteroposterior radiograph of dysplastic hip with questionable articular congruence. **B,** Same hip held in abduction and slight flexion to mimic congruence that would be attained with periacetabular osteotomy.

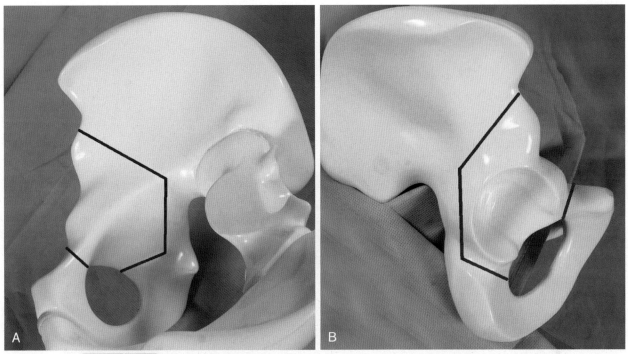

FIGURE 4.41 Bernese periacetabular osteotomy. **A,** Internal view of bony pelvis. **B,** External view of bony pelvis.

of the contour of the femoral head-neck junction is important, because rotating the acetabulum with a PAO may create anterior cam impingement requiring femoral osteochondroplasty. An MR arthrogram is performed to evaluate the status of the articular cartilage and labrum. A low-dose CT scan of the pelvis with a few slices through the epicondyles of the knee is useful to determine the pattern of acetabular dysplasia, the version of the acetabulum, and the version of the femoral neck.

PERIACETABULAR OSTEOTOMY

PAO was described by Ganz and others in the 1980s as a method of stabilizing symptomatic dysplastic hips in skeletally mature patients and preventing arthritic deterioration. The osteotomy is done through a Smith-Petersen approach with reproducible bony cuts and extensive rotational freedom for acetabular repositioning with little risk of osteonecrosis of the acetabular segment (Fig. 4.41). The labrum and anterior femoral head-neck junction can be accessed through the distal end of the Smith-Petersen approach with a capsular arthrotomy. The rotated fragment can be stabilized with screw fixation, and the patient can be mobilized relatively quickly because the posterior column is left in continuity, leaving the ischium attached to the axial skeleton.

■ SURGICAL INDICATIONS

PAO is clearly indicated for symptomatic younger patients with spherically congruent dysplasia of the hip, an LCE angle of less than 20 degrees, and minimal or no secondary arthritic changes (Tönnis grade 0 or 1). Symptomatic patients with weight bearing, activity-related pain with center edge angles between 20 and 25 degrees, particularly women with coxa valga and excessive anteversion, may be reasonable surgical candidates. Adolescent patients with hip dysplasia who have fair congruity also may be considered because they tend to

fare better than older patients and may be able to delay hip replacement for one to two decades.

Preoperative age older than 35 and fair or poor joint congruence have been reported to be independent factors predictive of failure of PAO; when both factors occurred in a given patient, the chance of resultant severe pain or conversion to total hip replacement reached 95%. Others, however, have found that patients older than 50 years of age had radiographic and clinical 2-year results similar to those in patients younger than 50 years of age. In our practice, PAO can be indicated for patients older than the age of 40 with a spherical femoral head and minimal arthritic change as evaluated on the standard radiographic views and MRA. This decision, however, is always weighed against the option of symptomatic treatment with probable future THA. Pincer-type FAI with global acetabular retroversion is another indication for PAO discussed earlier.

Intertrochanteric osteotomy of the proximal femur occasionally is done as a simultaneous procedure. Varus derotational osteotomy is done to correct excessive valgus and anteversion of the proximal femur, although guidelines for this indication are not uniform (Fig. 4.42). Valgus osteotomy can be done for coxa vara and aspherical Perthes type femoral head deformity to maintain articular congruence and to avoid impingement of the greater trochanter with the rotated acetabular rim (Fig. 4.43). A relative neck lengthening with osteochondroplasty of the femoral neck through an open surgical dislocation in combination with a PAO has been reported to have good short-term benefits in patients with typical Perthes deformity.

■ SURGICAL TECHNIQUE

The original technique described by Ganz et al. involved exposure of both inner and outer tables of the ilium through the Smith-Petersen approach with stripping of the abductors to expose the posterior column of the acetabulum on the lateral surface of the pelvis. Murphy and Millis described a modified

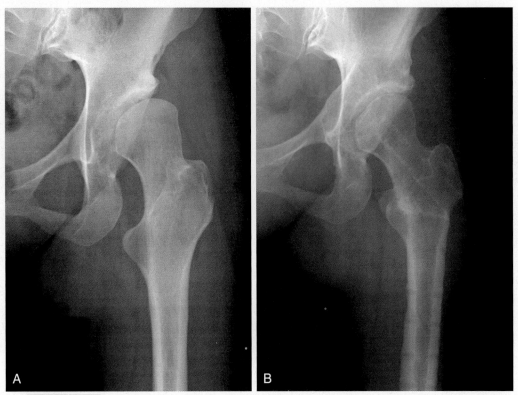

FIGURE 4.42   Preoperative **(A)** and postoperative **(B)** radiographs of a patient with hip dysplasia associated with high femoral neck-shaft angle treated with periacetabular osteotomy and intertrochanteric varus osteotomy.

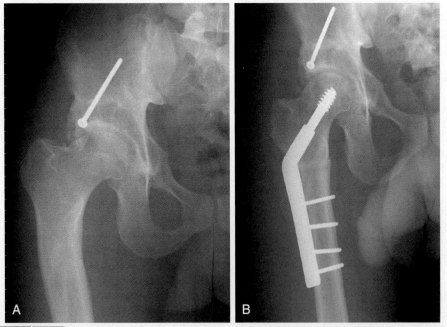

FIGURE 4.43   **A**, After periacetabular osteotomy for dysplasia, a patient with varus deformity of the proximal femur developed impingement symptoms relieved by valgus osteotomy of the proximal femur **(B)**.

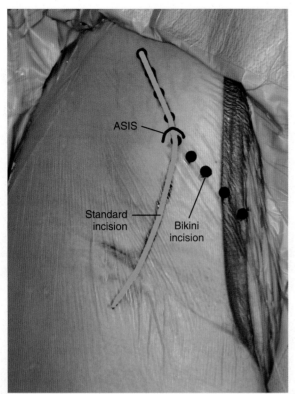

FIGURE 4.44 Smith-Petersen incision is preferred for most patients, with occasional use of more cosmetic bikini incision in thin patients. *ASIS,* Anterior superior iliac spine.

abductor-sparing variant of the Smith-Petersen approach for PAO, making the osteotomy from the internal surface of the pelvis with minimal lateral stripping. They also described a bikini-type skin incision that follows the inguinal crease medially (Fig. 4.44). Although we use this bikini-type incision in thin females, access to the hip joint for labral repair and femoral osteochondroplasty is better through a standard Smith-Petersen incision, and we prefer to use it in most patients. We currently use an abductor-sparing approach as described by Matheney et al. However, in patients with no cam deformity of the proximal femur, no labral tear or articular defect on MRA, and no mechanical symptoms suggestive of labral pathology, we use a rectus-sparing approach as described by Novais et al. With this approach, an anterior arthrotomy of hip is not made, and the direct and indirect heads of the rectus femoris are not detached from the anterior-inferior iliac spine and acetabular rim. This is done in an attempt to minimize postoperative pain and possibly improve postoperative hip flexion strength.

BERNESE PERIACETABULAR OSTEOTOMY

TECHNIQUE 4.4

(MATHENEY ET AL.)
- With the patient supine, prepare and drape the involved extremity free to the costal margin, medially to the umbilicus, and posteriorly to the posterior third of the ilium.

SUPERFICIAL DISSECTION
- Make a direct anterior longitudinal Smith-Petersen incision or an anterior bikini-type incision just below the iliac crest extending a few centimeters medial to the anterior superior iliac spine.
- Identify the fascia over the external oblique and gluteus medius and incise it posterior to the anterior superior iliac spine.
- Develop the plane between the two muscles to expose the periosteum over the iliac crest. Divide this periosteum and subperiosteally dissect the inner table of the ilium.
- Enter the compartment of the tensor fasciae latae and bluntly dissect the muscle off the septum with the sartorius muscle; this is done to protect the lateral femoral cutaneous nerve.
- Identify the floor of this compartment and follow it proximally until the anterior aspect of the ilium is palpated.
- Predrill the anterosuperior iliac spine with a 2.5-mm drill and osteotomize the anterior portion (1 × 1 × 1 cm) to make dissection and later repair easier.
- Alternatively, detach the sartorius with a thin wafer of bone that will be repaired with suture at the end of the procedure.
- Continue subperiosteal dissection to the anteroinferior iliac spine.

DEEP DISSECTION
- Flex and adduct the hip to take tension off the anterior musculature.
- Divide the reflected head of the rectus femoris at its junction with the direct head.
- Elevate the direct head of the rectus femoris and the underlying capsular portion of the iliacus as a unit and reflect them distally and medially from the underlying joint capsule.
- Reflect the iliacus, sartorius, and abdominal contents medially.
- Open the sheath of the psoas and retract its muscle and tendon medially. Alternatively, retract the psoas by subperiosteal release of its sheath from the pubic ramus and separate the sheath from the capsule. This allows exposure of the anterior portion of the superior pubic ramus medial to the iliopectineal eminence, an important landmark denoting the most medial extent of the osseous acetabulum.
- Create an interval between the medial joint capsule and the iliopsoas tendon and sequentially dilate with the tip of a long Mayo scissor and/or Lane retractor.
- Use the tips of the scissors and Lane retractors to palpate the anterior portion of the ischium at the infracotyloid groove; confirm proper placement of these instruments with fluoroscopy. The goal is to place them superior to the obturator externus tendon. If the joint capsule is accidentally entered, a second pass can be made by entering the floor of the psoas tendon sheath to develop a second, extraarticular path to reach the anterior portion of the ischium.

OSTEOTOMY OF THE ANTERIOR PORTION OF THE ISCHIUM

- Place the hip in 45 degrees of flexion and slight adduction.
- Insert a 30-degree forked, angled bone chisel (15- or 20-mm blade width) (Fig. 4.45A) through the previously created interval between the medial capsule and the psoas tendon to place its tip in contact with the superior portion of the infracotyloid groove of the anterior portion of the ischium, just superior to the obturator externus tendon. Staying proximal to the obturator externus helps prevent injury to the nearby medial femoral circumflex artery.
- Gently palpate the medial and lateral aspects of the ischium with the chisel, confirming the position of the chisel with fluoroscopy in both the anteroposterior and iliac oblique projections. The chisel should be positioned approximately 1 cm below the inferior lip of the acetabulum with its tip aimed at the ischial spine or a point slightly above the ischial spine (Fig. 4.45B).
- Impact the chisel to a depth of 15 to 20 mm through both medial and lateral cortices of the ischium. Take care not to drive the chisel too deeply through the lateral cortex because of the proximity of the sciatic nerve, especially with the hip flexed and adducted.

OSTEOTOMY OF THSE SUPERIOR PUBLIC RAMUS

- With the hip still flexed and adducted, gently retract the psoas tendon and medial structures medially. Retraction can be aided by impacting either the tip of a spiked Hohmann retractor or a large-gauge Kirschner wire into the superior pubic ramus just beyond the most medial extent of the dissection.
- Incise the periosteum over the superior pubic ramus along its axis and perform careful circumferential subperiosteal dissection. This can be aided by making a transverse periosteal incision 1 to 2 cm medial to the iliopectineal eminence and working to continue the previous subperiosteal dissection of the inner iliac table into the lateral obturator foramen.
- Place Hohmann retractors, Rang retractors, or Lane bone retractors anteriorly and posteriorly around the superior pubic ramus into the obturator foramen to protect the obturator nerve and artery. Watch for spontaneous adduction of the limb, which is indicative of stretching or irritation of the obturator nerve.
- Osteotomize the superior pubic ramus perpendicular to its long axis when viewed from above and oblique from proximolateral to distomedial when viewed from the front. The osteotomy can be made by using a Satinsky vascular clamp to pass a Gigli saw around the ramus and sawing upward, away from the retractors, or by impacting a straight osteotome just medial to the iliopectineal eminence. The key to this osteotomy is to stay medial to the iliopectineal eminence to avoid creating an intraarticular osteotomy (Fig. 4.45C).

ARTHROTOMY AND INTRACAPSULAR INSPECTION

- If there is concern about an intraarticular pathologic process, such as a torn labrum, cam lesion, or loose bodies, make a T-shaped arthrotomy centered on the anterior and lateral aspects of the femoral neck to avoid injury to the retinacular vessels that run along the posterior and superior aspects of the femoral neck.
- Make the vertical portion of the arthrotomy along the long axis of the femoral neck and the horizontal portion along the acetabular rim.
- Make the vertical portion of the arthrotomy first; this will allow observation of the labrum while making the horizontal portion (the "top" of the T).
- Repair or debride any labral tears and resect cam lesions of the femoral neck with curved or straight osteotomes or a high-speed burr. Check the adequacy of resection by moving the hip through a range of motion or with a lateral fluoroscopy view.
- Close the arthrotomy loosely with simple interrupted absorbable sutures.

SUPRA-ACETABULAR ILIAC OSTEOTOMY

- Create a 1.5- to 2.0-cm subperiosteal window beneath the anterior abductors just distal to the anterosuperior iliac spine without disturbing the abductor origin.
- Slightly abduct and extend the limb to allow an atraumatic subperiosteal dissection with a narrow elevator that is directed posteriorly toward, but not into, the apex of the greater sciatic notch.
- Place a narrow, long, spiked Hohmann retractor in this window and confirm proper placement with fluoroscopy. In the lateral projection, the spike of the retractor should point toward the apex of the sciatic notch.
- Retract the iliacus medially with a reverse Hohmann retractor, the tip of which is placed on the quadrilateral surface.
- Under direct vision, make the iliac osteotomy with an oscillating saw and cooling irrigation in line with the Hohmann retractor until reaching a point approximately 1 cm above the iliopectineal line (well anterior to the notch) (Fig. 4.45D).
- Confirm that both the lateral and medial cortices are cut before proceeding.
- The end point of the iliac saw cut represents the posterosuperior corner of the periacetabular osteotomy and is the starting point of the posterior-column osteotomy, which will be midway between the sciatic notch and posterior portion of the acetabulum.
- At this point, use a 3.2-mm drill to create a passage for a single Schanz screw on a T-handled chuck.
- Insert the Schanz screw into the acetabular fragment distal and parallel to the iliac saw cut, well above the dome of the acetabulum.

OSTEOTOMY OF THE POSTERIOR COLUMN

- Flex and adduct the hip to relax the medial soft tissues.
- Place a reverse blunt Hohmann retractor medially with the tip on the ischial spine. Dissection into the sciatic notch is not necessary.
- Make the osteotomy through the medial cortex with a long, straight 1.5-cm osteotome. The osteotomy extends from the posterior end of the iliac saw cut, passes over the iliopectineal line, through the medial quadrilateral plate, and parallel to the anterior edge of the sciatic notch as seen on iliac oblique fluoroscopy, and then is directed toward the ischial spine.

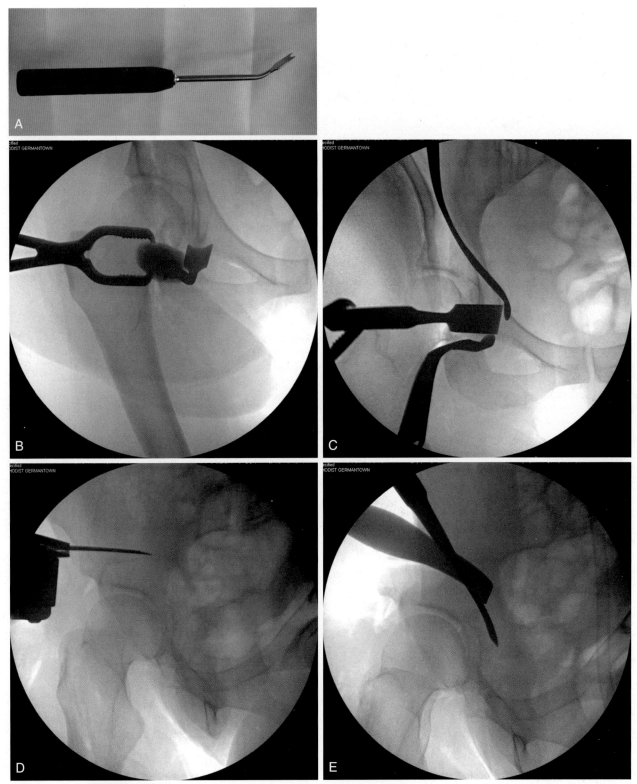

FIGURE 4.45 **A,** 30-degree Ganz osteotome. **B,** Ischial osteotomy is performed through interval between psoas tendon and hip capsule with 30-degree osteotome. **C,** Osteotomy of pubis is performed just medial to iliopectineal eminence and radiographic teardrop. **D,** Initial iliac osteotomy is made with oscillating saw aiming toward top of sciatic notch. **E,** Posterior column osteotomy proceeds from tip of iliac osteotomy through pelvic brim then through medial cortex of quadrilateral plate.

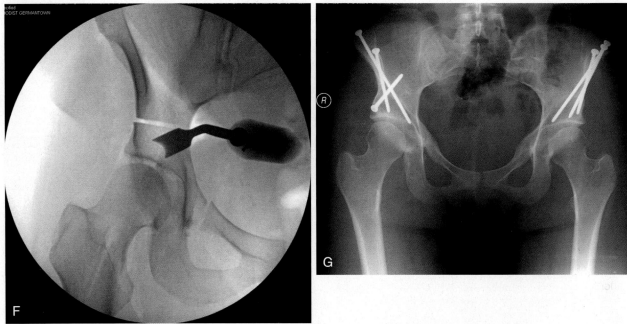

FIGURE 4.45, Cont'd **F,** 30-degree Ganz osteotome is used carefully to complete posterior column osteotomy from medial to lateral under fluoroscopic control and to connect posterior column osteotomy to ischial osteotomy. **G,** Fixation of osteotomy can be solely through screws through iliac wing into rotated fragment or include a "home run" screw that goes from antero-inferior iliac spine directed into sciatic buttress. **SEE TECHNIQUE 4.4.**

- Make the posterior cut first through the medial and then the lateral wall of the ischium. Do not set the osteotome perpendicular to the medial quadrilateral plate; instead, tip the free medial edge of the osteotome 10 to 15 degrees away from the sciatic notch to create a more true coronal plate osteotomy, perpendicular to the lateral cortex of the posterior column (Fig. 4.45E).
- Confirm correct angulation and positioning with fluoroscopy.
- Make certain the medial and lateral cortices of the posterior column are completely cut. A Ganz osteotome can be used to connect the medial and lateral cortices, beginning at the proximal posterior column, but this must be done very carefully to avoid injury to the sciatic nerve and other structures that exit the sciatic notch (Fig. 4.45F).
- Use a 30-degree angled, long-handled chisel to connect the anterior and posterior ischial cuts to complete the osteotomy of the posteroinferomedial corner of the quadrilateral plate.

ACETABULAR DISPLACEMENT

- Place a straight 1-in (2.54-cm) Lambotte chisel into the supra-acetabular iliac saw cut to both confirm completion of the lateral cortex osteotomy and protect the cancellous bone above the acetabulum during displacement.
- Place the tines of a Weber bone clamp into the superior pubic ramus portion of the acetabular fragment in such a way as to place its handle anterior and in contact with the Schanz screw.
- While gently opening the lamina spreader, use the Schanz screw and/or Weber clamp to mobilize the acetabular fragment. Be sure the posterior and anterior osteotomies are complete or the fragment will not freely rotate and

distal and lateral displacement may occur as the fragment hinges on the lateral, intact cortices. If necessary, palpate these cuts with a narrow or broad 30-degree chisel and complete the osteotomies if needed.
- Once the fragment is completely free, position it to obtain the desired correction. The most common deficiency is anterior and lateral, so the most common maneuver is to lift the acetabular fragment slightly toward the ceiling, creating an initial displacement, followed by a three-step movement of lateral, distal, and internal rotation. Internally rotate the fragment to antevert it, extend the fragment to achieve anterior coverage, and adduct the fragment to obtain lateral coverage.
- When positioning is properly done, the posterosuperior corner of the acetabular fragment should be impacted slightly into the superior intact iliac cut and the prominent superior tip of the acetabular fragment should be roughly in line with the superior aspect of the intact iliac crest. The radiographic teardrop and its relation to the femoral head should be elevated and tilted laterally, or adducted, commensurate with the amount of lateral correction that is made.
- If needed to recreate the proper position of the femoral head in relation to the medial aspect of the pelvis, medialize the acetabular fragment slightly once the desired anterior and/or lateral coverage has been obtained. This will maintain the proper biomechanical position of the femur in relation to the pelvis.

ACETABULAR FIXATION

- Once the desired acetabular position has been obtained, place smooth Kirschner wires (of the approximate diameter of the planned drill bit to be used for later fixation) from proximal to distal through the ilium and into the fragment in a divergent pattern.

■ Check the position of the fragment fluoroscopically in the anteroposterior and false-profile projections. In the false-profile view, check the anterior femoral head coverage in full extension and at 100 degrees of flexion and confirm that the femoral head is not overcovered and that impingement has not been created from a femoral-sided deformity. On the anteroposterior view, check the proper position of the sacrococcygeal junction in relation to the pubic symphysis; the sourcil should be roughly horizontal, the femoral head should be well covered, the posterior acetabular wall should overlap the center of the femoral head, the anterior wall shadow should not overlap the posterior wall, and the Shenton line should be intact.

■ Measure the Kirschner wires for depth and length and replace them with either 3.5- or 4.5-mm cortical screws. Confirm extraarticular placement of the screws with fluoroscopy.

■ If required for stability (as in patients who have ligamentous laxity, a neuromuscular condition, or poor bone quality), an additional "home run" screw can be placed anterior to posterior from the anteroinferior iliac spine posteriorly into the inferior portion of the ilium (Fig. 4.45G). We prefer not to use this screw unless necessary because the screws are removed once osseous healing is confirmed to prevent screw-head irritation or because MRI may be needed later.

■ Trim the anterior iliac prominence of the acetabular fragment and use it as bone graft.

■ Remove all sponges and copiously irrigate the wounds.

■ Repair the direct head of the rectus femoris with heavy nonabsorbable suture.

■ Place suction drains under the iliacus.

■ Reattach the anterosuperior iliac spine osteotomy fragment with a 3.5-mm partially threaded cancellous screw or with heavy absorbable sutures, depending on the thickness of the fragment.

■ Pay careful attention to proper, tight closure over the iliac crest. Pass heavy absorbable suture through the predrilled holes in the iliac crest to reattach the abductor, iliacus, and external oblique musculature.

■ Close the remainder of the wound in layers in standard fashion.

RECTUS-SPARING MODIFICATION OF BERNESE OSTEOTOMY

TECHNIQUE 4.5

(NOVAIS ET AL.)
■ Identify the iliacus muscle proximally at the pelvic brim.
■ Dissect the iliopsoas musculotendinous unit free from the periosteum of the inner table of the ilium and superior pubic ramus to expose the anatomic plane between the

rectus femoris tendon and the iliacus muscle at the level of the anteroinferior iliac spine.

■ Open the muscle fascia of the rectus femoris medially and retract the rectus femoris muscle belly laterally, exposing the underlying iliocapsularis muscle.

■ Elevate the iliocapsularis muscle from the joint capsule from lateral to medial, leaving the rectus tendon intact. It is important to release the iliocapsularis muscle insertion from the anteroinferior iliac spine and to retract it along with the iliopsoas muscle medially to allow complete exposure of the interval between the iliopsoas and the joint capsule.

■ From this point on, follow the steps described in Technique 4.4.

POSTOPERATIVE CARE Partial weight bearing is supervised by a physical therapist on the first postoperative day. Weight bearing is progressed from partial to full weight bearing, typically by 6 to 8 weeks, when there is radiographic evidence of healing and abductor strength has returned. Range of motion is limited to 90 degrees of flexion, 10 degrees from full extension, and 10 degrees of adduction, abduction, and rotation for the first 6 weeks. Resistive exercises are avoided for 6 weeks. Patients older than 16 years are given low-molecular-weight heparin for 10 to 14 days followed by 81 mg of aspirin twice a day for 4 weeks for thromboprophylaxis. Nonsteroidal antiinflammatory medications are avoided.

■ RESULTS

Preservation of the hip after PAO has been achieved in 73% to 76% of patients in two mid-term studies with longer than 9-year average follow-up (Fig. 4.46). Twenty-year results from the originating surgical center in Berne showed hip preservation in 60% of hips at 20-year follow-up. The 30-year survivorship of the first 75 PAOs done at the originating center has recently been reported as 29%. This patient population included 24% of patients with Tönnis grade 2 or greater disease that would not be considered for surgery with current indications. Since the original surgeries, technical aspects of the surgery and the indications have become clearer, with the possibility of preservation of an even higher percentage of hips in the future. The procedure has evolved to place greater emphasis on identifying and treating labral pathologic processes and avoiding or correcting postoperative impingement. Patients having more advanced arthritis are more likely to await arthroplasty rather than undergo hip preservation surgery. Factors identified as likely to negatively impact the result of PAO for dysplasia include advancing age, moderate preoperative arthritis, labral pathologic processes, postoperative impingement, and fair or poor congruence of the joint.

■ COMPLICATIONS FOLLOWING PERIACETABULAR OSTEOTOMY

In a multicenter study of 1760 periacetabular osteotomies, Sierra et al. reported a 2.1% incidence of sciatic or femoral nerve partial or complete palsy, half of which recovered fully. Recovery was more likely when the femoral nerve was involved. Other complications reported include superficial and deep infection, heterotopic ossification (though rarely

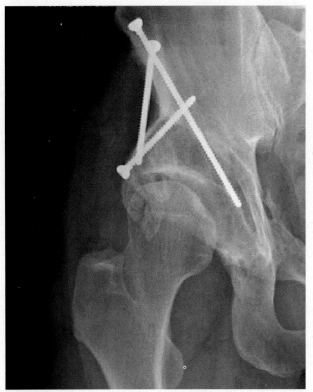

FIGURE 4.46   Fourteen years after periacetabular osteotomy for hip dysplasia, this 37-year-old man was pain free and had a well-preserved cartilage space with some posterior heterotopic ossification.

symptomatic), acetabular fragment migration requiring reoperation, and symptomatic hardware requiring removal. The rate of symptomatic thromboembolic events following PAO is approximately 1% using a variety of thromboprophylactic measures. Obesity has been cited as raising the risk of complications by a factor of 10. Larger blood loss, longer surgery, and associated femoral osteotomy have all been associated with a higher rate of perioperative complications.

Arthroscopy of the central compartment to treat labrochondral pathology at the same time as PAO has been reported, with short follow-up not demonstrating complication rates over that of PAO alone. Longer follow-up will determine the potential benefits of more routine arthroscopy combined with PAO.

■ HIP ARTHROSCOPY WITH BORDERLINE HIP DYSPLASIA

The use of arthroscopy for labral and chondral disorders due to dysplasia has been controversial, with some reports of increased instability created by the surgical procedure. Patients with borderline dysplasia with impingement (LCE angle 20 to 24 degrees) are difficult, falling between the clear indications for PAO and arthroscopic FAI surgery. A number of studies have described the use of arthroscopy in the treatment of FAI in the presence of borderline dysplasia. At 26 months, Larson et al. found good to excellent results in 61% of patients with borderline dysplasia after labral repair or debridement with associated femoral osteochondroplasty in 72% and capsular plication in 82% compared to 81% good

to excellent results in other FAI patients. The factors they found predictive of better outcome included labral repair rather than debridement and capsular plication. Domb et al. reported 2-year results for arthroscopic labral repair with capsular plication with inferior shift for patients with borderline dysplasia (LCA ≥18 degrees and ≤25 degrees) with good to excellent results in 77%. According to Bolia et al., however, these patients are more likely to have higher grades of chondral damage on both the femoral head and acetabulum at the time of FAI arthroscopic surgery compared to patients without borderline dysplasia. Predictors of poorer outcomes have included greater degrees of acetabular chondral damage, greater labral damage, and even lesser degrees of femoral head cartilage damage. Longer follow-up is needed in this patient population treated with arthroscopy alone. Further discussion of arthroscopic intervention is contained in other chapter.

TOTAL HIP REPLACEMENT FOLLOWING PERIACETABULAR OSTEOTOMY

Amanatullah et al. reported a multicenter study of total hip replacement following PAO with an abductor-sparing technique (Fig. 4.47) compared with THA performed on similar patients for hip dysplasia with no prior history of PAO. They found no difference in complications, revision rates, or modified Harris hip scores between the two groups. They did find that in hips with previous PAO, the acetabular component of the total hip was placed in an average of 17 degrees more retroversion than in hips in which THA was done for DDH without previous PAO. Baqué, Brown, and Matta described using the same Smith-Petersen interval for direct anterior THA after PAO. They claim that by using this approach for both procedures, the patient's immediate and ultimate functional recovery and hip stability are optimized. They contend that instead of compromising subsequent THA, PAO may improve THA results in dysplastic hips.

EXTRAARTICULAR SOURCES OF HIP PAIN
GREATER TROCHANTERIC PAIN SYNDROME

Lateral hip pain in the region of the greater trochanter can be caused by a number of sources including an inflamed trochanteric bursa, a snapping iliotibial band, tendinosis or tears of the gluteus medius and minimus, extraarticular impingement, referred pain from an intraarticular pathologic process, and referred pain from a pathologic process of the lumbar spine. Differentiation of referred pain from local sources of pain usually can be determined by seeking tenderness to direct palpation over the hip abductors, trochanteric bursa, and iliotibial band, noting that tenderness can also be present with radicular type pain. Pain with resisted hip abduction can suggest abductor tendinitis or a partial tear of the gluteus minimus or medius similar to a rotator cuff tear in the shoulder. Frequently, a steroid combined with a local anesthetic can be injected into the trochanteric bursa as a therapeutic intervention for trochanteric bursitis or abductor tendinitis and can aid in confirming the diagnosis by attaining pain relief and ruling out referred pain as the primary cause. Hip abductor stretching exercises and antiinflammatory medications are the mainstays of treatment for most patients with greater

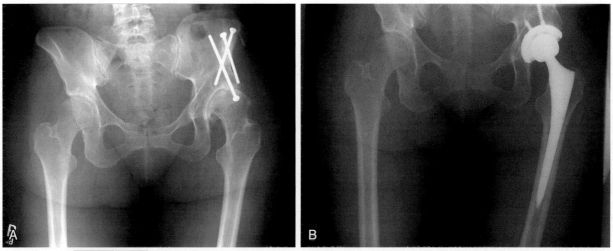

FIGURE 4.47 **A,** Twelve years after periacetabular osteotomy in a 22-year-old patient with Tönnis grade 2 arthritis now with end-stage arthritis. **B,** Subsequent total hip replacement with good superior acetabular coverage.

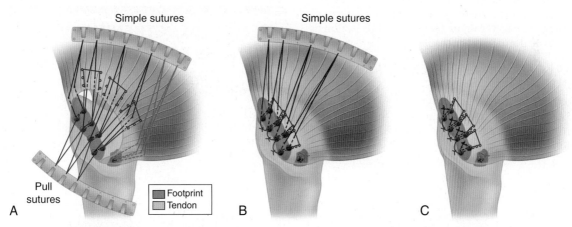

FIGURE 4.48 Open repair of gluteus medius tear. **A,** Three pull sutures *(red)* and four simple sutures *(purple)* are placed in the gluteus medius tendon; one 6.5-mm suture anchor with two sutures *(blue)* is placed in the gluteus minimus tendon. **B,** Sutures from the anchor *(blue)* are tied first to secure gluteus minimus to its facet; then pull sutures *(red)* are tied down under maximal tension to approximate the gluteus medius tendon to its footprint. **C,** Simple sutures *(purple)* are tied to secure the tendinous flap down to the greater trochanter. (From Davies JF, Stiehl JB, Davies JA, Geiger PB: Surgical treatment of hip abductor tendon tears, *J Bone Joint Surg* 95:1420, 2013.)

trochanteric pain, with one or two selective steroid injections into the area of maximal tenderness. One study reported maintenance of pain relief in 61% of hips 6 months after steroid injection. Refractory cases may warrant further investigation with MRI or diagnostic intraarticular hip injection.

GLUTEUS MEDIUS AND MINIMUS TEARS

In patients with chronic greater trochanteric bursitis, edema may be seen within the trochanteric bursa on MRI; however, this finding was reported in one study to occur in only 8% of patients with chronic lateral hip pain whereas gluteus medius tendinitis was apparent in 63%. The recognition of partial and complete gluteal tears on MRI, as well as the development of arthroscopic techniques about the hip, has led to an increase in surgical intervention for these tears.

Kagan first described atraumatic tearing of the anterior fibers of the gluteus medius as a "rotator cuff tear of the hip." Open repair with osseous tunnels has been reported to obtain pain relief and improvement in abductor strength in most patients. Davies et al. reported the results of 23 tears treated with open repair (Fig. 4.48). The tears were suspected in patients with lateral hip pain with weakness that persisted after a trochanteric injection of 1% lidocaine. Smaller tears were suspected when the patients exhibited a positive Trendelenburg fatigue test with a Trendelenburg sign that became positive after standing on the ipsilateral leg for 15 to 20 seconds. The tears were confirmed by MRI. Typical MRI findings included tendon discontinuity, elongation of the gluteus medius tendon, atrophy of the gluteus muscles, and high signal intensity superior to the greater trochanter. They reported average improvement in Harris hip scores from 53 to 87 at 1 year and 88 at 5 years after surgery with an average improvement in hip abduction strength testing from 3.1 to 4.7 out of 5. They had four poor results in patients with large tears.

ENDOSCOPIC REPAIR OF THE HIP ABDUCTORS

Endoscopic repair of the gluteus medius was reposted by Voos et al. and by McCormick et al. to have good pain relief and excellent abductor function. Alpaugh et al. performed a review of studies including patients undergoing surgical repair for partial-thickness and full-thickness abductor tears. They found that most patients are women and that the gluteus medius is almost always torn, with concomitant tearing of the gluteus minimus one-third of the time. They found that both open and endoscopic techniques are viable surgical approaches to repairing abductor tendon tears in the hip that produce good to excellent functional results and reduce pain; however, endoscopic repair appears to result in fewer postoperative complications including tendon retear.

It has been recognized that the gluteus medius will usually first tear on the undersurface creating a partial tear inaccessible to direct lateral visualization. Though partial thickness tears have traditionally been treated nonoperatively, a transtendinous endoscopic technique of repair has been described by Domb, Nasser, and Botser for patients with pain unresponsive to stretching and nonsteroidal antiinflammatory drugs (NSAIDs). Endoscopic repair of the abductor insertion is described in more detail in other chapter.

EXTERNAL SNAPPING HIP (EXTERNAL COXA SALTANS)

Snapping of a thickened posterior edge of the iliotibial band or anterior edge of the gluteus maximus over the greater trochanter during flexion and extension of the hip can lead to inflammation of the underlying bursa and is known as external coxa saltans or an external snapping hip. This condition is common in ballet dancers, runners, and soccer players. The condition is easily appreciated on physical examination with the patient in the lateral position while the patient actively flexes and extends the hip, causing this thickened band to snap across the posterior edge of the greater trochanter. The patient can frequently demonstrate the snapping while standing on the leg and flexing and extending the hip. Iliotibial band stretching and injection of steroid into the thickened area can lessen the severity of the snapping and secondary pain.

If conservative management is not successful, operative intervention may be indicated. Z-plasty lengthening of the iliotibial band has been reported to obtain resolution of snapping and relief of pain in a high percentage of patients. White et al. described a relatively minimally invasive step-cut lengthening of the iliotibial band through a 10-cm longitudinal incision; 14 of 16 patients remained asymptomatic after final surgical release and two patients had marked decreases in the severity and frequency of snapping. An endoscopic technique also has been described for release of the iliotibial band with relief of snapping in 10 of 11 hips at 2-year follow-up.

STEP-CUT LENGTHENING OF THE ILIOTIBIAL BAND

TECHNIQUE 4.6

(WHITE ET AL.)

- With the patient in the lateral decubitus position, make a 10-cm incision directly over the greater trochanter (Fig. 4.49A).

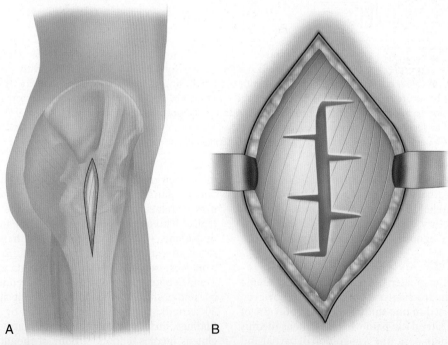

A   B

FIGURE 4.49   Step-cut lengthening of the iliotibial band for snapping hip. **A,** Lateral approach directly over the greater trochanter; incision is approximately 10 cm long. **B,** Typical 10-cm longitudinal incision through the iliotibial band with the associated 1.5-cm step-cuts.   (Redrawn from White RA, Hughes MS, Burd T, et al: A new operative approach in the correction of external coxa saltans: the snapping hip, *Am J Sports Med* 32:1504, 2004.) **SEE TECHNIQUE 4.6.**

- Carry dissection down to the iliotibial tract and make a 10-cm incision longitudinally in line with the fibers overlying the trochanter.
- Identify and excise any inflamed bursa.
- Make six transverse step-cuts, each 1.5 cm, evenly spaced along the longitudinal incision, with three anterior and three posterior in an offsetting fashion (Fig. 4.49B).
- Move the hip through provocative maneuvers, including adduction and internal and external rotation to determine if snapping is still present.
- If the release is deemed satisfactory, irrigate the wound and close only the skin.

POSTOPERATIVE MANAGEMENT The patient is allowed to go home the day of surgery, with no weight-bearing restrictions. Crutches are used for comfort and to aid in ambulation, usually for 3 to 5 days.

INTERNAL SNAPPING HIP

The internal snapping hip is a result of the iliopsoas tendon snapping over the iliopectineal eminence or the anterior hip capsule. In flexion, the psoas tendon is lateral to the iliopectineal eminence. As the hip is extended, the tendon slides across the iliopectineal eminence and anterior hip capsule, producing a snapping sensation in up to 10% of the normal population (Fig. 4.50). When symptomatic, the snapping sensation is accompanied by groin pain and usually an audible low-pitched characteristic "thunk." The patient usually is able to reproduce the snapping while lying supine and actively ranging the hip from a position of flexion, abduction, and external rotation to a position of extension, adduction, and internal rotation. In thinner patients, the snapping can be palpated in the inguinal crease.

Although the snapping phenomenon cannot be documented by MRA, there is a high incidence of associated intraarticular pathology, and an MRA usually is obtained to look for other sources of pain. The snapping can be demonstrated by bursography of the iliopsoas bursa with a dynamic examination under fluoroscopy. Ultrasound also has been used to demonstrate the snapping psoas tendon, although this technique is highly dependent on the experience of the ultrasonographer.

Activity restriction, extension stretching of the hip, the use of NSAIDs, and occasional psoas tendon sheath steroid injections are the mainstays of treatment for the hip with internal snapping. The use of an injection of a local anesthetic with a steroid into the psoas tendon sheath can help confirm the source of hip pain, although the psoas bursa does connect to the hip joint in a large number of patients, and an intraarticular pathologic process cannot be ruled out.

Open and endoscopic techniques of psoas tendon release have been described for the treatment of recalcitrant cases of internal snapping hip syndrome. The open techniques describe a limited exposure through the Smith-Petersen interval with release or lengthening of the psoas tendon. Persistent or recurrent snapping has been reported in 20% to 25% of patients after open inguinal approach with fractional lengthening of the psoas tendon, and iliopsoas release through a medial approach provided relief of snapping in 63% of hips and pain resolution in 94%.

Endoscopic techniques of psoas tendon release have been described with good success. The release can be done either at the level of the lesser trochanter or by a transcapsular technique. In a systemic review of open and endoscopic release of snapping psoas tendons by Khan et al., resolution of snapping was achieved in 100% of hips treated endoscopically compared with 77% treated through an open approach, with a lower complication rate for the endoscopically treated hips. Bitar et al. reported 82% relief of painful internal snapping with arthroscopic release at 2-year follow-up.

OSTEITIS PUBIS

Disorders of the pubic symphysis and the adjoining musculotendinous structures can occur in athletic adults and must be distinguished from the other musculoskeletal sources of groin and pubic pain covered in this chapter. Genitourinary and gynecologic origins of pain should be considered as well. Osteitis pubis is seen in athletes involved in running and cutting sports such as soccer and hockey, as well as with trauma or pregnancy and vaginal delivery. The typical radiographic appearance is that of widening of the symphysis with blurring of the cortical margins and occasionally a cyst within the pubic body adjacent to the fibrocartilaginous disc of the symphysis (Fig. 4.51). This probably represents a stress reaction to overuse or excessive mobility. On a bone scan, the symphysis demonstrates increased uptake, whereas MRI can show bone marrow edema. Notably, some asymptomatic athletes demonstrate bone marrow edema in the pubis as well. A cleft sign can be seen on MRI when there is a tear of the ligamentous capsule that envelops the fibrocartilaginous disc of the symphysis. Other related MRI findings include tendinosis of the rectus abdominis and adductor longus insertions into the pubis; chronic strains of these tendons frequently are confused with true osteitis pubis.

Treatment of osteitis pubis is primarily conservative because the condition tends to be self-limiting when the inciting stress of overuse is withdrawn. Rehabilitation aimed

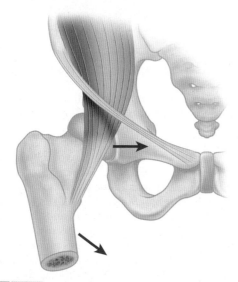

FIGURE 4.50 Internal snapping of hip occurs when psoas tendon snaps over iliopectineal eminence from lateral to medial as hip goes from flexion to extension.

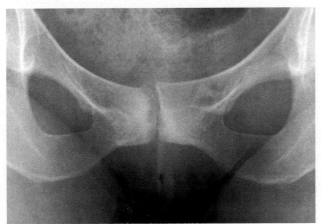

FIGURE 4.51 Osteitis pubis with blurring of cortical margins of pubis.

at strengthening of the patient's abdomen and hip adductors should be done in a graded fashion. Operative intervention has been described for recalcitrant cases, including open or endoscopic symphysis curettage, resection of the symphysis, and symphysis fusion. Our experience with these surgical techniques is limited, and we favor nonoperative treatment.

SPORTS HERNIA (ATHLETIC PUBALGIA)

Sports hernia as a cause of chronic groin pain in running, twisting athletes is a diagnosis made with increasing frequency and represents a deficiency in the abdominal wall in the region of the inguinal canal. Many anatomic variations have been described, although the most common is incompetence of the posterior wall of the inguinal canal, with or without involvement of the internal inguinal ring. Frequently, tendinosis of the adductor longus origin is present and may be the primary source of pain, and an association between athletic pubalgia and FAI has been identified.

Sports hernia is a condition that is very difficult to appreciate on physical examination, because the classic signs of an inguinal hernia are not typically present. Referral to a general surgeon familiar with subtle inguinal abnormalities can be helpful when sports hernia is clinically suspected. Dynamic ultrasound has been reported to have diagnostic utility in this condition. Surgical repair of the deficient abdominal wall has been reported to be successful when the correct diagnosis is made. Messaoudi et al. found that, in soccer players, adding adductor longus release to abdominal wall repair led to more reliable pain relief and return to sport.

OSTEONECROSIS OF THE FEMORAL HEAD

Osteonecrosis of the femoral head is a progressive disease that generally affects patients in the third through fifth decades of life. Formerly referred to as *avascular necrosis,* the term *osteonecrosis* is now preferred. Simply defined, *osteonecrosis* means "dead bone." The "avascular" state of the necrotic bone is the result of a loss of circulation from numerous potential causes. When symptomatic, it typically leads to collapse of the femoral head and eventual deterioration of the hip joint. It is estimated that 20,000 new cases of osteonecrosis are diagnosed

---

BOX 4.1

Pathogenic Mechanisms for Osteonecrosis

Ischemia
- Vascular disruption
  - Femoral head fracture
  - Hip dislocation
  - Surgery
- Vascular compression or constriction
  - Increased intraosseous pressure caused by marrow fatty infiltration
  - Corticosteroids, alcohol
- Vasoconstriction of arteries perfusing femoral head
  - Corticosteroids, eNOS, polymorphisms
- Intravascular occlusion
  - Thrombosis
    - Thrombophilia
      - Low protein C and S
      - Activated protein
        - C resistance, factor V mutation
    - High homocysteine
    - eNOS polymorphisms
  - Hypofibrinolysis
    - High PAI activity, PAI-1 polymorphisms
    - High lipoprotein(a)
  - Embolization
    - Fat, air
  - Sickle cell occlusion

Direct Cellular Toxicity
- Pharmacologic agents
- Irradiation
- Oxidative stress

Altered Differentiation of Mesenchymal Stem Cells
- Altered differentiation of mesenchymal stem cells
- Corticosteroids, alcohol

eNOS, Endothelial nitric oxide synthase; *PAI,* plasminogen activator inhibitor. Modified from Zalavras CG, Lieberman JR: Osteonecrosis of the femoral head: evaluation and treatment, *J Am Acad Orthop Surg* 22:455, 2014.

---

each year in the United States. Currently, up to 12% of all total hip arthroplasties performed in the United States are done for osteonecrosis.

Osteonecrosis describes an end condition that is the result of many possible pathogenic pathways. The list of risk factors for osteonecrosis is long and includes trauma, corticosteroid use, alcohol abuse, smoking, hemoglobinopathies (e.g., sickle cell anemia), coagulation disorders, myeloproliferative disorders (Gaucher disease, leukemia), hyperbaric decompression, hyperlipidemias, chronic kidney disease, autoimmune diseases, and human immunodeficiency virus infection. In many cases a cause cannot be identified, and these patients are designated as having idiopathic osteonecrosis.

Several theories on the pathogenesis of osteonecrosis have been proposed (Box 4.1). Hypotheses include ischemia from a variety of mechanisms, direct cellular toxicity, and alteration of differentiation of mesenchymal stem cells. None of these theories can fully account for the variety of causes. Most patients with the risk factors just mentioned never

TABLE 4.1

Ficat and Arlet Classification of Osteonecrosis of the Femoral Head

STAGE	SYMPTOMS	RADIOGRAPHY	BONE SCAN	PATHOLOGIC FINDINGS	BIOPSY
0	None	Normal	Decreased uptake?		
1	None/mild	Normal	Cold spot on femoral head	Infarction of weight-bearing portion of femoral head	Abundant dead marrow cells, osteoblasts, osteogenic cells
2	Mild	Density change in femoral head Sclerosis or cysts, normal joint line, normal head contour	Increased uptake	Spontaneous repair of infarcted area	New bone deposited between necrotic trabeculae
3	Mild to moderate	Flattening (crescent sign) Loss of sphericity, collapse	Increased uptake	Subchondral fracture, collapse, compaction, and fragmentation of necrotic segment	Dead bone trabeculae and marrow cells on both sides of fracture line
4	Moderate to severe	Joint space narrowing, acetabular changes	Increased uptake	Osteoarthritic changes	Degenerative changes in acetabular cartilage

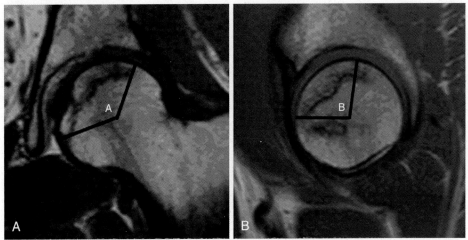

FIGURE 4.52 Calculation of the combined necrotic angle from magnetic resonance imaging scans. **A,** Angle of necrotic area in the midcoronal image. **B,** Angle of necrotic area in the midsagittal image. The combined necrotic angle = A + B. (From Ha, YC, Jung WH, Kim JR, et al: Prediction of collapse in femoral head osteonecrosis: a modified Kerboul method with use of magnetic resonance images, *J Bone Joint Surg* 88 (suppl 3):35, 2006.)

develop osteonecrosis, suggesting possible individual susceptibility, and many patients without identifiable risk factors do acquire the disease. The process is most likely multifactorial.

The most commonly used classification schemes for osteonecrosis of the femoral head are the Ficat and Arlet system (Table 4.1) and the Steinberg system (Table 4.2). Both are based on the evaluation of plain radiographs with the addition of MRI to the Steinberg system. The Steinberg classification adds modifiers A to C for percentage of involvement of the femoral head or articular surface involvement for stages I through IV. The Association Research Circulation Osseous (ARCO) system is used occasionally and is similar in concept to the Steinberg system (see Table 4.2). The combined angle of articular involvement of the head measured from midsagittal and midcoronal MRI cuts (Fig. 4.52) has been shown to be predictive of collapse in hips with precollapse osteonecrosis.

DIAGNOSIS

Patients are typically asymptomatic early in the course of osteonecrosis and eventually have groin pain on ambulation. A thorough history and physical examination should be done to discover potential risk factors and to determine the clinical status of the patient. Plain radiographs should be obtained, including anteroposterior and frog-leg lateral views. Radiographic changes seen in osteonecrosis depend on the stage of the disease. Plain films may appear normal in the early stages, but changes are noted as the disease progresses, such as increased density or lucency in the femoral head. With further progression, the pathognomonic crescent sign is visible on plain films (best seen on frog-leg lateral views) (Fig. 4.53). The crescent sign is a subchondral fracture overlying the necrotic segment of the femoral head. In the end stages of the disease, femoral head collapse occurs, and severe arthritic changes may be seen on both sides of the joint.

TABLE 4.2

Additional Classifications for Osteonecrosis

STAGE	STEINBERG ET AL.	ARCOS
0	Normal or nondiagnostic radiographic, bone scan, and MRI findings	Bone biopsy results consistent with osteonecrosis; other test results normal
I	Normal radiographic findings, abnormal bone scan and/or MRI findings	Positive findings on bone scan, MRI, or both
	A: Mild: <15% of head affected	IA: <15% head involvement (MRI)
	B: Moderate: 15%–30% affected	IB: 15%–30% involvement
	C: Severe: >30% affected	IC: >30% involvement
II	Lucent and sclerotic changes in the femoral head	Mottled appearance of femoral head, osteosclerosis, cyst formation, and osteopenia on radiographs; no signs of collapse of femoral head on radiograph or CT; positive findings on bone scan and MRI; no changes in acetabulum
	A: Mild: <15%	A: Mild: <15%
	B: Moderate: 15%–30%	B: Moderate: 15%–30%
	C: Severe: >30%	C: Severe: >30%
III	Subchondral collapse (crescent sign) without flattening	Presence of crescent sign lesions classified on basis of appearance on anteroposterior and lateral radiographs
	A: Mild: <15% of articular surface	A: <15% crescent or <2-mm depression
	B: Moderate: 15%–30%	B: 15%–30% crescent sign or 2- to 4-mm depression
	C: Severe: >30%	C: >30% crescent sign or >4-mm depression
IV	Flattening of the femoral head	Articular surface flattened; joint space narrowing; change in acetabulum with evidence of osteosclerosis, cyst formation, and marginal osteophytes
	A: Mild: <15% of surface or <2-mm depression	
	B: Moderate: 15%–30% of surface or 2- to 4-mm depression	
	C: Severe: >30% of surface or >4-mm depression	
V	Joint narrowing and/or acetabular changes A: Mild: Average of femoral head involvement as in stage IV and estimated acetabular involvement B: Moderate involvement C: Severe involvement	
VI	Advanced degenerative changes	

CT, Computed tomography; *MRI,* magnetic resonance imaging.

MRI is the imaging modality of choice for earlier stages of osteonecrosis of the femoral head, allowing determination of the exact stage and extent of the pathologic process without use of invasive methods. When both hips demonstrate typical femoral head collapse, MRI is not necessary because it does not alter clinical decision-making. However, when plain radiographs show changes in only one joint, MRI of the pelvis is indicated, not only to define clearly the extent of the disease in the symptomatic hip but also to evaluate the asymptomatic hip. This can allow detection of the disease in the early stages when most treatments are potentially more effective. Differentiation between transient osteoporosis and osteonecrosis usually is possible, with the bone marrow edema of transient osteoporosis extending into the intertrochanteric region of the femur with no demarcation of a proximal necrotic segment. MRI also is useful in following the progression of the asymptomatic disease and in evaluating the efficacy of treatment.

Bone scanning can occasionally be useful, when the patient has a contraindication to MR imaging or when assessing the status of multiple other joints. The uptake of technetium-99m usually is decreased in the very early stage of disease and is variable or increased at a stage when symptoms occur. When symptoms appear, however, there is no relationship between the scintigraphic appearance of the femoral head and the pain and function of the hip.

TREATMENT

The natural history of osteonecrosis in its early stage, before subchondral collapse, is still unclear, but evidence suggests that the rate of progression is high, especially in symptomatic patients. Asymptomatic osteonecrosis in which the lesion was less than 30% of the area of the femoral head was shown to remain asymptomatic in most patients (95%) for more than 5 years; as lesion size increased, however, the percentage of painful osteonecrosis increased, up to 83% in hips with large lesions (>50% of the area of the femoral head). Using the modified Kerboul method in a 5-year longitudinal study of precollapsed femoral heads with osteonecrosis, Ha et al. found that no femoral heads with a combined necrotic angle of less than 190 degrees went on to collapse, whereas all the femoral heads with a combined necrotic angle of more than 240 degrees collapsed. When subchondral collapse occurs and joint space is lost, progressive osteoarthritis

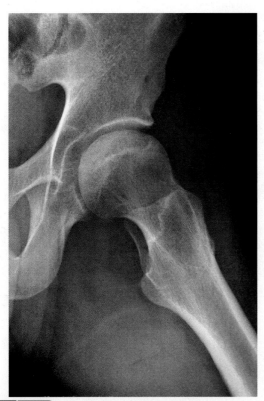

FIGURE 4.53   Crescent sign in stage III osteonecrosis of the hip.

generally is considered inevitable. Many studies have reported an extremely poor prognosis, with a rate of femoral head collapse of greater than 85% at 2 years in symptomatic patients (Ficat stage I or II disease).

No treatment method has proved to be completely effective in arresting the disease process before subchondral collapse or in slowing the progression of femoral head destruction and osteoarthritis after subchondral collapse. The rate and course of progression of the disease are unpredictable, and the radiographic picture may not correlate with the clinical symptoms; some patients maintain tolerable function for an extended period after femoral head collapse. Spontaneous remission of even Ficat stage II osteonecrosis has been reported, but this is rare. Conservative treatment, such as crutch ambulation or bed rest, generally is ineffective. Symptomatic patients who may benefit from a femoral head preserving technique can be placed on crutches, however, until surgical treatment is performed with hope to prevent collapse in the interim.

■ NONOPERATIVE TREATMENT

The use of bisphosphonates in osteonecrosis has been studied in animal models, with demonstrated inhibition of osteoclast function of bone resorption and subsequent reduction of bone turnover. However, a multicenter level 1 study comparing alendronate to placebo failed to show any differences in the rate of THA, disease progression, and quality of life at 2-year follow-up.

Statins have been proposed to potentially be beneficial in the early stages of osteonecrosis in renal failure patients as they reduce intraosseous adipose deposition and may decrease vascular congestion. Hyperbaric oxygen has been suggested in limited studies to benefit patients with early disease, and extracorporeal shock wave therapy used for the breakdown

of renal stones has been shown to incidentally increase pelvic bone density. Its use has been reported as beneficial in some studies though its use has not been widely accepted.

■ CORE DECOMPRESSION

The theoretical advantage of core decompression is based on the belief that the procedure relieves intraosseous pressure caused by venous congestion, allowing improved vascularity and possibly slowing the progression of the disease. The initial promising results of core decompression have not been matched by more recent investigations. Several authors noted, however, that the results of core decompression are better than the results of nonoperative treatment. Several reports noted that the earlier the stage of the disease, the better the results with core decompression, with the best results reported in Ficat stage I hips. Others have found core decompression to be less effective even in early stages, with reported failure rates of 60% in hips treated in precollapse stages and in 100% of hips treated after collapse.

Some authors have suggested the placement of nonstructural, nonvascularized bone grafts or bone graft substitutes in the void left after core decompression. There also has been interest in the use of growth factors to enhance osteogenesis (bone morphogenetic protein) or angiogenesis (fibroblast growth factor or vascular endothelial growth factor). Favorable outcomes have been reported with the use of autologous bone grafts that include bone marrow cells, with or without growth factors. The insertion of porous tantalum rods has been advocated by some after core decompression to provide structural support. Although early reported outcomes of tantalum rod use were encouraging (92% survival at 48 months), subsequent studies have reported less favorable outcomes. A retrieval analysis of failed tantalum implants found little bone ingrowth and insufficient mechanical support of subchondral bone. The effect of high-density metal particles seen on radiographs also is a concern.

Review of the literature currently supports the use of core decompression for the treatment of Ficat stages I and IIA small central lesions in young, nonobese patients who are not taking steroids. This surgery is relatively simple to perform and has a very low complication rate. The surgical field for subsequent THA, if needed, is not substantially altered. For more advanced disease (Ficat stage III), the results of core decompression are much less predictable, so alternative treatment methods should be explored. Patients should be advised that more than 30% of patients, even with early-stage disease, will likely require THA within 4 to 5 years of core decompression surgery.

CORE DECOMPRESSION

TECHNIQUE 4.7

(HUNGERFORD)

■ With the patient supine on a hip fracture table, approach the hip through a 2- to 3-cm midlateral longitudinal incision centered over the subtrochanteric region using image intensification as a guide.

■ As an alternative, with the patient in the lateral decubitus position and the operative limb draped free, position the C-arm to obtain an anteroposterior view; the limb can be

moved to a frog-leg position for a lateral view. This avoids the need to move the fluoroscopy unit during surgery.
- Split the fascia lata in the direction of its fibers.
- Using image intensification, place a 3.2-mm threaded guide pin between the lateral cortex of the inferior portion of the greater trochanter and the distal portion of the lesser trochanter. Cortical windows made below the lesser trochanter increase the possibility of postoperative fracture.
- Direct the tip of the guide pin to the center of the diseased portion of the bone. MRI and plain films should be reviewed to help locate the optimal position for the guide pin.
- Overream the guide pin with an 8-mm reamer. If histologic examination is necessary, a coring reamer can be used.
- Close the wound in layers.

POSTOPERATIVE CARE Partial weight bearing (50%) on crutches is continued for at least 6 weeks to protect the cortical window. In patients with advanced disease, protected weight bearing is prolonged.

CORE DECOMPRESSION— PERCUTANEOUS TECHNIQUE

A percutaneous technique has been described for core decompression using multiple small drillings with a 3.2-mm Steinmann pin. The technique is reported to have a lower rate of femoral head collapse than traditional core decompression, with low morbidity and few or no surgical complications.

TECHNIQUE 4.8

(MONT ET AL.)
- With the patient supine on a hip fracture table, mark the position of the femoral head and prepare and drape the hip in standard fashion.
- Insert a 3.2-mm Steinmann pin laterally and percutaneously under fluoroscopic guidance (Fig. 4.54).

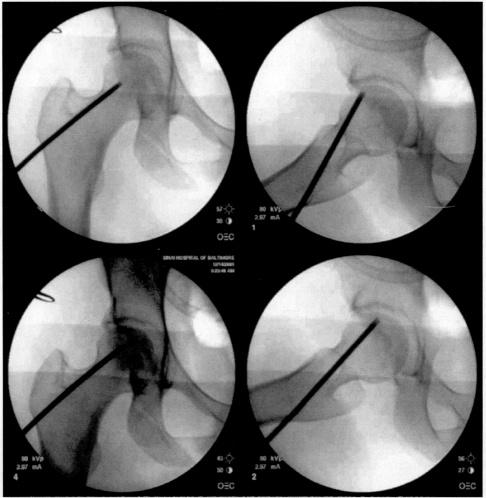

FIGURE 4.54 Percutaneous technique for core decompression (see text). Fluoroscopic images show entry into femoral neck and head. Lateral views are obtained to avoid penetration of cortical bone. (From Mont MA, Ragland PS, Etienne, G: Core decompression of the femoral head for osteonecrosis using percutaneous multiple small-diameter drilling, *Clin Orthop Rel Res* 429:131–138, 2004.) **SEE TECHNIQUE 4.8**.

- Advance the pin until it reaches the lateral cortex in the metaphyseal region opposite the superior portion of the lesser trochanter.
- Penetrate the femur and advance the pin through the femoral neck into the femoral head and the site of the lesion (as determined on preoperative radiographs or MR images). Use anteroposterior and lateral fluoroscopic views while advancing the pin to ensure the correct track in the medullary canal of the femoral neck.
- Using the one skin entry point, make two passes with the pin through small lesions and three through large lesions. Try to avoid penetration of the femoral head cartilage when advancing the pin.
- Remove the pin and close the wound with a simple bandage or a single nylon suture.

POSTOPERATIVE CARE Physical therapy, including gait reconditioning with a cane or crutches, is encouraged. Protected weight bearing (approximately 50%) is maintained for 5 to 6 weeks and then advanced to full weight bearing as tolerated. High-impact loading such as jogging or jumping is not permitted for 12 months. If there is no radiographic evidence of collapse and the patient is asymptomatic at 12 months after surgery, return to usual activities, including higher-impact loading activities such as running, is allowed.

BONE GRAFTING

Successful results after core decompression with structural bone grafting for the treatment of osteonecrosis of the femoral head have been reported in 50% to 80% of patients. Structural bone grafting techniques after core decompression have been described using cortical bone, cancellous bone, vascularized bone graft, and debridement of necrotic bone from the femoral head, each with promising results. One small study of core decompression combined with cortical press-fit structural bone grafting for stage I or II osteonecrosis found no difference in results between hips in which tibial or fibular autogenous grafts were used and hips in which fibular allografts were used. A prospective case-controlled study comparing vascularized and nonvascularized fibular grafts for large lesions (involvement of more than 30% of the femoral head) found better clinical results and more effective prevention of femoral head collapse with vascularized grafting.

Accurate placement of the graft within the lesion and under subchondral bone is essential (Fig. 4.55). The bone grafts can be introduced with a standard core track technique, "trapdoor" technique, or a "light bulb" technique. Advantages of the standard core track technique include a wide debridement of necrotic bone, simple technique, avoidance of surgical dislocation of the hip, and a low complication rate. In the trapdoor technique, the hip is surgically dislocated, a portion of the chondral surface of the femoral head is lifted to expose the lesion, the necrotic bone is removed, the cavity is filled with bone graft, and the cartilage flap is replaced and secured (Fig. 4.56A). Advantages of this approach include direct evaluation of the cartilage surface and necrotic femoral head segment and precise placement of the bone graft; disadvantages include technical difficulty, iatrogenic cartilage damage, and risk of iatrogenic osteonecrosis from the surgical dislocation. In the

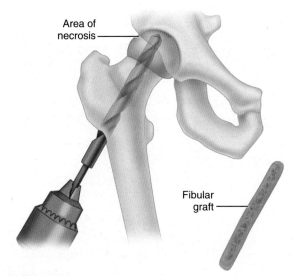

FIGURE 4.55 Core decompression and cortical press-fit structural bone grafting for osteonecrosis of femoral head (stage I or II).

light bulb technique, a bone window measuring approximately 2 cm × 2 cm is removed at the femoral head-neck junction with a micro-oscillating saw and osteotomes (Fig. 4.56B); the bone plug is saved in normal saline–wrapped gauze for later use. Through the entry, a mushroom-tipped burr is used to curet a cavity in the femoral head, removing all the necrotic bone (the shape of the cavity resembles a light bulb). Allograft is packed into the cavity, and the bone plug is replaced and fixed with three 2-mm absorbable pins. Advantages of this technique are similar to those for the trapdoor technique, but the creation of a cortical defect in the femoral neck raises the risk of fracture.

VASCULARIZED FIBULAR GRAFTING

After advances in microsurgical techniques made it possible to preserve the intrinsic vascularity of bone graft, several authors independently proposed implanting a vascularized bone graft into the core of the femoral head. The rationale for vascularized bone grafting is based on four aspects of the operation and postoperative care: (1) decompression of the femoral head, which may interrupt the cycle of ischemia and intraosseous hypertension that is believed to contribute to the disease; (2) excision of the sequestrum, which might inhibit revascularization of the femoral head; (3) filling of the defect that is created with osteoinductive cancellous graft and a viable cortical strut to support the subchondral surface and to enhance the revascularization process; and (4) protection of the healing construct by a period of limited weight bearing. Proposed advantages of free vascularized fibular grafting compared with THA are the presence of a healed femoral head, which may allow more activity, and, if performed before the development of a subchondral fracture, the procedure offers the possibility of survival of a viable femoral head for the life of the patient. Disadvantages include a longer recovery period, less reliable relief of pain, donor site morbidity, and less predictable survivorship in terms of subsequent surgery when compared with THA.

Most reports have shown good results in 80% to 91% of patients after vascularized fibular grafting, and it may be a reasonable option for patients younger than 50 years without collapse of the femoral head; for patients older than 50, THA is indicated

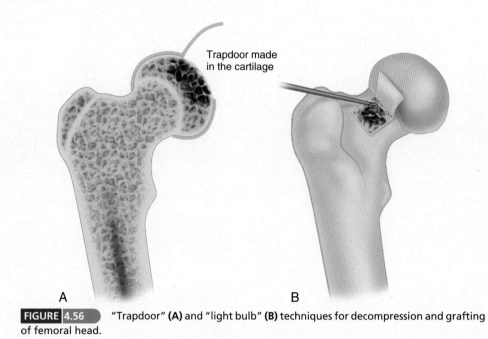

Trapdoor made in the cartilage

A   B

FIGURE 4.56 "Trapdoor" **(A)** and "light bulb" **(B)** techniques for decompression and grafting of femoral head.

if symptoms warrant surgical intervention. Concurrent steroid use is not a contraindication for this procedure. Vascularized fibular grafting remains controversial for patients with asymptomatic early-stage osteonecrosis because the donor site morbidity can be significant and the results of core decompression are debatably equally effective for this group of patients.

■ PROXIMAL FEMORAL OSTEOTOMY

If osteonecrosis of the femoral head develops, the involved segment tends to be in the weight-bearing portion. Various proximal femoral osteotomies have been developed for the treatment of osteonecrosis with the intent to move the involved necrotic segment of the femoral head from the principal weight-bearing area. These procedures have achieved best results for small-sized or medium-sized lesions (<30% femoral head involvement) in young patients in whom it is optimal to delay a THA. Patients younger than 55 years did better than older patients, and patients with idiopathic or posttraumatic osteonecrosis did better than patients with alcohol-induced or steroid-induced necrosis. A valgus-extension intertrochanteric osteotomy combined with curettage of the avascular segment and autogenous bone grafting was reported to have an 87% success rate at 65 months.

A transtrochanteric rotational osteotomy of the femoral head for idiopathic osteonecrosis was developed to reposition the necrotic anterosuperior part of the femoral head to a non–weight-bearing locale. The femoral head and neck segment is rotated anteriorly around its longitudinal axis so that the weight-bearing force is transmitted to what was previously the posterior articular surface of the femoral head, which is not involved in the ischemic process (Fig. 4.57). This technically challenging procedure has reports of success in the Japanese literature that have not been reproduced elsewhere. We have no experience with this procedure; for a description of the technique, see earlier editions of this text.

■ ARTHROPLASTY

If osteonecrosis involves more than 30% of the head, the success rates of the aforementioned techniques tend to diminish.

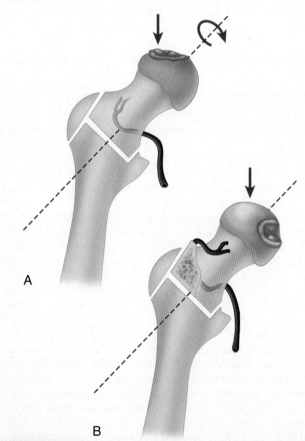

A

B

FIGURE 4.57 Sugioka transtrochanteric anterior rotational osteotomy (see text). Transposition of the necrotic portion of the femoral head anteroinferiorly away from the weight-bearing area is accomplished by anterior rotation of the femoral head. **A,** Before rotation. **B,** After rotation.

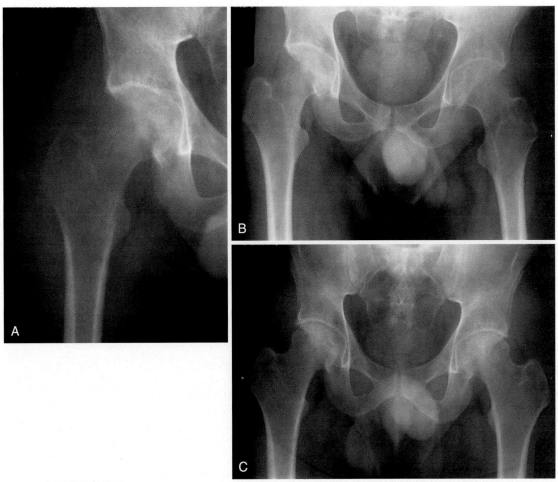

FIGURE 4.58 Idiopathic transient osteoporosis of hip. **A,** Onset and early radiographic changes; note diffuse haziness of right hip. **B,** At 6 months, radiographic changes are still evident. **C,** At 36-month follow-up, complete resolution of radiographic changes.

Once collapse has begun, the hip inevitably progresses to end-stage arthritis. Options for large lesions and advanced disease include resurfacing arthroplasty and total hip replacement. The acetabular articular cartilage in hips with Ficat stage 3 disease has routinely been shown to have significant damage, arguing for avoidance of hemiarthroplasty. Additionally, similar to the treatment of femoral neck fractures, longer follow-up has favored the use of total hip replacement over hemiarthroplasty. There have been proponents of resurfacing arthroplasty in this patient population; however, the results are inferior to the outcomes of total hip replacement. When adding the concerns of resurfacing arthroplasty as a metal-on-metal bearing, we favor the use of total hip replacement for patients once collapse has occurred and symptoms warrant surgical intervention.

THA in patients with femoral head osteonecrosis is discussed in chapter 1.

IDIOPATHIC TRANSIENT OSTEOPOROSIS

Idiopathic transient osteoporosis of the hip occurs most often in middle-aged men, but it sometimes occurs in women, usually in late pregnancy (Fig. 4.58). Increasing pain and limp with local muscle wasting are typical, and the symptoms are bilateral in approximately one third of patients. Demineralization may not be apparent on plain radiographs for 6 weeks after onset of symptoms. An abnormal bone scan may precede radiographically visible osteoporosis of the femoral head and neck. MRI is highly sensitive in the detection of this condition, but other entities, such as osteonecrosis, osteomyelitis, and neoplasms, can mimic idiopathic transient osteoporosis on MRI. These entities should be ruled out by evaluation of the patient's clinical history, physical examination, and laboratory values. The MRI appearance of transient osteoporosis includes edema in the femoral head and neck that extends into the intertrochanteric region, usually with a joint effusion. The lack of involvement of the subchondral bone can differentiate its appearance from early osteonecrosis.

Because transient osteoporosis resolves with conservative measures over several months as evidenced clinically, radiographically, and on MRI, surgical intervention for this condition is rarely, if ever, indicated. We recommend conservative treatment for transient osteoporosis. Physical therapy to maintain range of motion and protected weight bearing to avoid secondary fracture are mainstays of treatment. Bisphosphonates and calcitonin have both been advocated to limit the duration of recovery. It is important to identify this

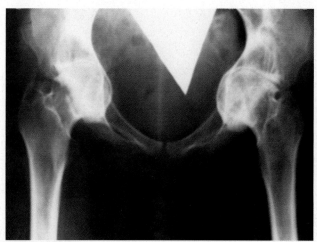

FIGURE 4.59 Intrapelvic protrusio acetabuli. Severe bilateral progressive protrusion of acetabulum with severe pain and decreased motion in both hips.

process and differentiate it from osteonecrosis so that early core decompression is not mistakenly done for osteoporosis.

PROTRUSIO ACETABULI

Protrusio acetabuli is characterized by a chronic progressive protrusion of the femoral head into the acetabulum and pelvis (Fig. 4.59). About two thirds of these lesions are unilateral and occur most often in patients of middle age but may develop during adolescence or childhood. The cause of primary protrusio acetabuli, also known as Otto pelvis, is undefined and the diagnosis is one of exclusion. It typically is bilateral and is most common in young and middle-aged women. Osteomalacia may play a role in its development. Infectious, neoplastic, inflammatory, metabolic, traumatic, and genetic factors have been implicated in the development of secondary protrusio acetabuli (Box 4.2). Pain and limitation of motion usually are the indications for surgery. THA (see chapter 1) is the preferred treatment at this clinic. For a young adult, valgus intertrochanteric proximal femoral osteotomy may be successful.

ADULT-ONSET RHEUMATOID ARTHRITIS

Rheumatoid arthritis generally affects adults aged 35 to 50 years, but it can occur in children and adolescents. The hip is less frequently involved with rheumatoid arthritis than the knee; most often rheumatoid arthritis involves the small joints of the hands and feet. Treatment for the early stages of rheumatoid arthritis of the hip is primarily medical, although physical and occupational therapy often can be helpful. The availability of newer and more effective medications has made surgery less frequently needed in patients with rheumatoid arthritis. If surgery is required, THA (see chapter 1) is indicated for most patients (Fig. 4.60).

JUVENILE IDIOPATHIC ARTHRITIS

Because approximately 97% of children with polyarticular juvenile arthritis are rheumatoid factor (RF) negative, the

---

BOX 4.2

Causes of Secondary Protrusio Acetabuli

Infectious
Gonococcus
  Echinococcus
  Staphylococcus
  Streptococcus
  Mycobacterium tuberculosis

Neoplastic
Hemangioma
  Metastatic carcinoma (breast, prostate most common)
  Neurofibromatosis
  Radiation-induced osteonecrosis

Inflammatory
Rheumatoid arthritis
  Ankylosing spondylitis
  Juvenile rheumatoid arthritis
  Psoriatic arthritis
  Acute idiopathic chondrolysis
  Reiter syndrome
  Osteolysis following hip replacement

Metabolic
Paget disease
  Osteogenesis imperfecta
  Ochronosis
  Acrodysostosis
  Osteomalacia
  Hyperparathyroidism

Traumatic
Sequelae of acetabular fracture
  Surgical error during hip replacement

Genetic
Trichorhinophalangeal syndrome
  Stickler syndrome
  Trisomy 18
  Ehlers-Danlos syndrome
  Marfan syndrome
  Sickle cell disease

Modified from McBride MT, Muldoon MP, Santore RF, et al: Protrusio acetabuli: diagnosis and treatment, *J Am Acad Orthop Surg* 9:79, 2001.

---

term *juvenile idiopathic arthritis* has become more commonly used than *juvenile rheumatoid arthritis* to describe this group of diseases. Juvenile idiopathic arthritis is a heterogeneous group of diseases characterized by the onset of chronic arthritis in childhood. The diagnostic criteria for and types of juvenile rheumatoid arthritis are outlined in chapter 7.

Involvement of the hip in juvenile idiopathic arthritis can cause significant difficulties with walking and can severely limit activity in young patients (Fig. 4.61). Clinically, hip joint involvement is marked by pain, limitation of range of motion, and rapid-onset cartilage destruction, which can affect other lower extremity joints and the spine.

Four categories of involvement of the hip have been described in patients with juvenile idiopathic arthritis. In the first group, only mild disability and slight radiographic

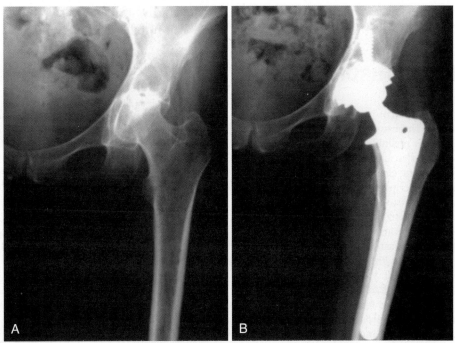

FIGURE 4.60   Total hip arthroplasty for rheumatoid arthritis. **A,** Advanced disease with articular cartilage destruction. **B,** After total hip arthroplasty.

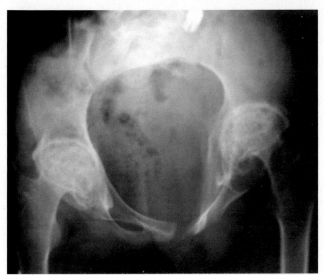

FIGURE 4.61   Polyarticular juvenile idiopathic arthritis in 16-year-old girl with severe bilateral hip involvement; note deformity of femoral head and acetabulum (protrusio acetabuli).

changes are present. In the second group, episodic disability is correlated with the activity of the disease. In the third group, progressive disability is associated with radiographic changes; this group of patients requires surgery most frequently. In the fourth group, clinical and radiographic findings are marked but functional disability is minimal.

Because of the success of medical therapy in the treatment of juvenile idiopathic arthritis, surgical treatment is infrequently needed. Reconstructive procedures that may be required in patients with juvenile idiopathic arthritis include soft-tissue procedures for correction of contractures, osteotomy, arthrodesis, joint excision, and arthroplasty. Combinations of these procedures may be necessary to relieve pain and correct deformity. Osteotomies are most commonly required to correct severe angular deformities. THA is the procedure of choice for severe pain and limitation of motion in the hip in adolescent patients with juvenile idiopathic arthritis.

OSTEOARTHRITIS

The lifetime risk of hip osteoarthritis has been estimated to be 8%. Osteoarthritis of the hip is most often brought on by an anatomic deformity that may be subtle and asymptomatic for decades. The mechanisms by which FAI and dysplasia lead to cartilage injury and subsequent osteoarthritis have been discussed earlier in this chapter, as has intervention with hip-preserving surgery before the development of significant osteoarthritis. Once the hip displays Tönnis grade 2 changes of osteoarthritis, hip preservation surgery provides little benefit, and other nonsurgical and surgical approaches are more appropriate.

Several randomized controlled trials support the use of corticosteroid injections to provide transient (approximately 1 month) relief of pain and improve function; steroid injections have been reported to be effective in up to 90% of patients with mild arthritis compared with only 9% to 20% of those with severe arthritis. Intraarticular corticosteroid injection also can be helpful in excluding extraarticular causes of hip pain. Viscosupplementation, although not approved for hip arthritis by the U.S. Food and Drug Administration, has had long-term use in Europe, with varying outcomes. However, two randomized controlled trials reported that a single intraarticular injection of hyaluronic acid was no more effective than placebo in relieving symptoms of hip arthritis, and it currently cannot be recommended for treatment of hip osteoarthritis.

The primary treatment for significant osteoarthritis of the hip is THA (see chapter 1). Although uncommon, there still remains the occasional indication for hip arthrodesis in young patients with hip abductor deficiency or chronic infection.

NEUROPATHIC ARTHROPATHY (CHARCOT JOINT)

Neuropathic arthropathy (Charcot joint) develops most often in weight-bearing joints. The causes are manifold. The predominant cause is diabetes mellitus, but it also is associated with leprosy, yaws, congenital insensitivity to pain, spina bifida, myelomeningocele, syringomyelia, aerodystrophic neuropathy, amyloid neuropathy, peripheral neuropathy secondary to alcoholism and avitaminosis, spinal cord injury, peripheral nerve injury, postrenal transplant arthropathy, and intraarticular steroid injections. Syphilis is an infrequent but increasingly common cause of neuropathic arthropathy. According to the Centers for Disease Control and Prevention, the rate of syphilis has increased dramatically each year over the past 10 years. Because of inadequate treatment of primary or secondary syphilis, or exposure to antibiotics for treatment of unrelated infections, many patients with neurosyphilis do not have the classic signs or symptoms. A high index of clinical suspicion and the appropriate serologic testing are necessary for correct diagnosis and appropriate treatment. The cause of neuropathic arthropathy should be sought, and, if indicated, specific treatment is rendered in addition to treatment of the joint itself. On histologic examination of the synovium from trophic joints, osteochondral fragments can be seen embedded within the synovium, which is diagnostic of neuropathic arthropathy.

Radiographically, Charcot arthropathy of the hip is characterized by rapid joint destruction with fragmentation of the femoral head and adjacent subchondral bone of the acetabulum with subsequent subluxation (Fig. 4.62).

Surgery of any kind is not indicated except for severe disability. The few reports of THA in neuropathic joints indicate that recurrent dislocation and loosening are frequent

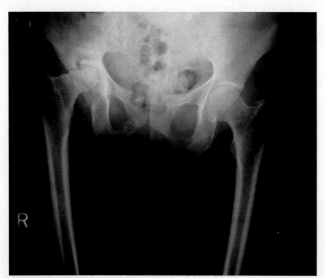

FIGURE 4.62 Charcot neuropathic hip disease in a patient who had a normal appearing radiograph 3 months earlier. Fragmentation of the femoral head and acetabular dome is seen as well as a fracture of the inferior pubic ramus.

sequelae; in our opinion, total joint arthroplasty is rarely indicated for a neuropathic hip joint.

REFERENCES

RADIOGRAPHIC ASSESSMENT

Clohisy JC, Dobson MA, Robison JF, et al.: Radiographic structural abnormalities associated with premature, natural hip-joint failure, *J Bone Joint Surg* 93A(Suppl 2):3, 2011.

Linda DD, Naraghi A, Murnaghan L, et al.: Accuracy of non-arthrographic 3T MR imaging in evaluation of intra-articular pathology of the hip in femoroacetabular impingement, *Skeletal Radiol* 46:299, 2017.

Zaltz I, Beaulé P, Clohisy J, et al.: Incidence of deep vein thrombosis and pulmonary embolus following periacetabular osteotomy, *J Bone Joint Surg* 93(Suppl 2):62, 2011.

Zaltz MD, Kelly BT, Hetsroni I, et al.: The crossover sign overestimates acetabular retroversion, *Clin Orthop Relat Res* 471:2463, 2013.

FEMOROACETABULAR IMPINGEMENT

Alradwan H, Khan M, Hamel-Smith Grassby M, et al.: Gait and lower extremity kinematic analysis as on outcome measure after femoroacetabular impingement surgery, *Arthroscopy* 31:339, 2015.

Anwander H, Siebenrock KA, Tannast M, et al.: Labral reattachment in femoroacetabular impingement surgery results in increased 10-year survivorship compared with resection, *Clin Orthop Relat Res* 475:1178, 2017.

Audenaert EA, Peeters I, Van Onsem S, Pattyn C: Can we predict the natural course of femoroacetabular impingement? *Acta Orthop Belg* 77:188, 2011.

Belzile EL, Beaulé PE, Ryu JJ, et al.: Outcomes of joint preservation surgery: comparison of patients with developmental dysplasia of the hip and femoroacetabular impingement, *J Hip Preserv Surg* 3:270, 2016.

Bernstein J: The myths of femoroacetabular impingement, *Clin Orthop Relat Res* 472:3623, 2014.

Bolia IK, Briggs KK, Locks R, et al.: Prevalence of high-grade cartilage defects in patients with borderline dysplasia with femoroacetabular impingement: a comparative cohort study, *Arthroscopy* 34:2347, 2018.

Botser IB, Smith Jr TW, Nasser R, Domb BG: Open surgical dislocation versus arthroscopy for femoroacetabular impingement: a comparison of clinical outcomes, *Arthroscopy* 27:270, 2011.

Brünner A, Hamers AT, Fitze M, Herzog RF: The plain ß-angle measured on radiographs in the assessment of femoroacetabular impingement, *J Bone Joint Surg Br* 92:1203, 2010.

Byrd JWT, Bardowski EA, Jones KS: Influence of Tönnis grade on outcomes of arthroscopic management of symptomatic femoroacetabular impingement, *Arthroscopy* 34:2353, 2018.

Carton P, Filan D: Anterior inferior iliac spine (AIIS) and subspine hip impingement, *Muscles Ligaments Tendons J* 6:324, 2016.

Chandrasekaran S, Darwish N, Martin TJ, et al.: Arthroscopic capsular plication and labral seal restoration in borderline hip dysplasia: 2-year clinical outcomes in 55 cases, *Arthroscopy* 33:1332, 2017.

Cohen SB, Huang R, Ciccotti MG, et al.: Treatment of femoroacetabular impingement in athletes using a mini-direct anterior approach, *Am J Sports Med* 40(7):1620, 2012.

Cvetanovich GL, Levy DM, Weber AE, et al.: Do patients with borderline dysplasia have inferior outcomes after hip arthroscopic surgery for femoroacetabular impingement compared with patients with normal acetabular coverage? *Am J Sports Med* 45:2116, 2017.

Degen RM, Nawabi DH, Bedi A, et al.: Radiographic predictors of femoroacetabular impingement treatment outcomes, *Knee Surg Sports Traumatol Arthrosc* 25:36, 2017.

Ejnisman L, Philippon MJ, Lertwanich P: Femoroacetabular impingement: the femoral side, *Clin Sports Med* 30:369, 2011.

Evans PT, Redmond JM, Hammarstedt JE, et al.: Arthroscopic treatment of hip pain in adolescent patients with borderline dysplasia of the hip: minimum 2-year follow-up, *Arthroscopy* 33:1530, 2017.

Fabricant PD, Fields KG, Taylor SA, et al.: The effect of femoral and acetabular version on clinical outcomes after arthroscopic femoroacetabular impingement surgery, *J Bone Joint Surg Am* 87:537, 2015.

Flores SE, Chambers CC, Borak KR, et al.: Arthroscopic treatment of acetabular retroversion with acetabuloplasty and subspine decompression: a matched comparison with patients undergoing arthroscopic treatment for focal pincer-type femoroacetabular impingement, *Orthop J Sports Med* 6: 2325967118783741, 2018.

Freeman CR, Azzam MG, Leunig M: Hip preservation surgery: surgical care for femoroacetabular impingement and the possibility of preventing hip osteoarthritis, *J Hip Preserv Surg* 1:46, 2014.

Fukui K, Briggs KK, Trindade CA, et al.: Outcomes after labral repair in patients with femoroacetabular impingement and borderline dysplasia, *Arthroscopy* 31:2371, 2015.

Gebhart JJ, Streit JJ, Bedi A, et al.: Correlation of pelvic incidence with cam and pincer lesions, *Am J Sports Med* 42:2649, 2014.

Gollwitzer H, Banke IJ, Schauwecker J, et al.: How to address ischiofemoral impingement? Treatment algorithm and review of the literature, *J Hip Preserv Surg* 4:289, 2017.

Hack K, Di Primio G, Rakhra K, Beaule P: Prevalence of cam-type femoroacetabular impingement morphology in asymptomatic volunteers, *J Bone Joint Surg* 92A:2436, 2010.

Haefeli PC, Tannast M, Beck M, et al.: Subchondral drilling for chondral flaps reduces the risk of total hip arthroplasty in femoroacetabular impingement surgery at minimum five years follow-up, *Hip Int*, 2018 Jun 1: 1120700018781807. [Epub ahead of print].

Hanke MS, Steppacher SD, Anwander H, et al.: What MRI findings predict failure 10 years after surgery for femoroacetabular impingement? *Clin Orthop Relat Res* 475:1192, 2017.

Hartofilakidis G, Bardakos NV, Babis GC, Georgiades G: An examination of the association between different morphotypes of femoroacetabular impingement in asymptomatic subjects and the development of osteoarthritis of the hip, *J Bone Joint Surg* 93B:580, 2011.

Haviv B, Burg A, Velkes S, et al.: Trends in femoroacetabular impingement research over 11 years, *Orthopedics* 34:353, 2011.

Hetsroni I, Larson CM, Dela Torre K, et al.: Anterior inferior iliac spine deformity as an extra-articular source for hip impingement: a series of 10 patients treated with arthroscopic decompression, *Arthroscopy* 28:1644, 2012.

Ida T, Nakamura Y, Jagio T, Naito M: Prevalence and characteristics of cam-type femoroacetabular deformity in 100 hips with symptomatic acetabular dysplasia: a case control study, *J Orthop Surg Res* 9:93, 2014.

Jäger M, Bittersohl B, Zilkens C, et al.: Surgical hip dislocation in symptomatic cam femoroacetabular impingement: what matters in early good results? *Eur J Med Res* 16:217, 2011.

Kaldau NC, Brorson S, Hölmich P, et al.: Good midterm results of hip arthroscopy for femoroacetabular impingement, *Dan Med J* 65:pii A5483, 2018.

Kapron AL, Aoki SK, Peters CL, Anderson AE: Subject-specific patterns of femur-labrum contact are complex and vary in asymptomatic hips and hips with femoroacetabular impingements, *Clin Orthop Relat Res* 472:3912, 2014.

Khan O, Witt J: Evaluation of the magnitude and location of cam deformity using three dimensional CT analysis, *Bone Joint J* 96-B:1167, 2014.

Klit J, Gosvig K, Magnussen E, et al.: Cam deformity and hip degeneration are common after fixation of a slipped capital femoral epiphysis, *Acta Orthop* 85:585, 2014.

Leunig M, Ganz R: The evolution and concepts of joint-preserving surgery of the hip, *Bone Joint J* 96-B:5, 2014.

Leunig M, Ganz R: Relative neck lengthening and intracapital osteotomy for severe Perthes and Perthes-like deformities, *Bull NYU Hosp Jt Dis* 69(Suppl 1):62, 2011.

Litrenta J, Mu B, Chen AW, et al.: Radiographic and clinical outcomes of adolescents with acetabular retroversion treated arthroscopically, *J Pediatr Orthop*, 2018 Apr 30, https://doi.org/10.1097/BPO.0000000000001063, [Epub ahead of print].

Locks R, Utsunomiya H, Bolia I, et al.: Arthroscopic focal subspinal decompression and management of pincer-type femoroacetabular impingement, *Arthrosc Tech* 6:e1029, 2017.

Mamisch TC, Kain MS, Bittersohl B, et al.: Delayed gadolinium-enhanced magnetic resonance imaging of cartilage (dGEMRIC) in femoroacetabular impingement, *J Orthop Res* 29:1305, 2011.

Matsuda DK, Carlisle JC, Arthurs SC, et al.: Comparative systematic review of the open dislocation, mini-open, and arthroscopic surgeries for femoroacetabular impingement, *Arthroscopy* 27:252, 2011.

Matsuda DK, Gupta N, Khatod M, et al.: Poorer arthroscopic outcomes of mild dysplasia with cam femoroacetabular impingement versus mixed femoroacetabular impingement in absence of capsular repair, *Am J Orthop (Belle Mead NJ)* 46:E47, 2017.

McCarthy B, Ackermann IN, de Steiger R: Progression to total hip arthroplasty following hip arthroscopy, *ANZ J Surg* 88:702, 2018.

Menge TJ, Briggs KK, Dornan GJ, et al.: Survivorship and outcomes 10 years following hip arthroscopy for femoroacetabular impingement: labral debridement compared with labral repair, *J Bone Joint Surg Am* 99:997, 2017.

Naal FD, Miozzari HH, Wyss TF, Nötzli HP: Surgical hip dislocation for the treatment of femoroacetabular impingement in high-level athletes, *Am J Sports Med* 39:544, 2011.

Nassif NA, Schoenecker PL, Thorsness R, Clohisy JC: Periacetabular osteotomy and combined femoral head-neck junction osteochondroplasty: a minimum two-year follow-up cohort study, *J Bone Joint Surg* 94:2012, 1959.

Nawabi DH, Degen RM, Fields KG, et al.: Outcomes after arthroscopic treatment of femoroacetabular impingement for patients with borderline hip dysplasia, *Am J Sports Med* 44:1017, 2016.

Nepple JJ, Clohisy JC: ANCHOR Study Group Members: Evolution of femoroacetabular impingement treatment: the ANCHOR experience, *Am J Orthop (Belle Mead NJ)* 46:28, 2017.

Nepple JJ, Clohisy JC: The dysplastic and unstable hip: a responsible balance of arthroscopic and open approaches, *Sports Med Arthrosc Rev* 23:180, 2015.

Nepple JJ, Vigdorchik JM, Clohisy JC: What is the association between sports participation and the development of proximal femoral cam deformity? A systematic review and meta-analysis, *Am J Sports Med* 43:2833, 2015.

Nepple JJ, Riggs CN, Ross JR, Clohisy JC: Clinical presentation and disease characteristics of femoroacetabular impingement are sex-dependent, *J Bone Joint Surg* 96:1683, 2014.

Nwachukwu BU, Rebolledo BJ, McCormick F, et al.: Arthroscopic versus open treatment of femoroacetabular impingement: a systematic review of medium- to long-term outcomes, *Am J Sports Med* 44:1062, 2016.

Packer JD, Safran MR: The etiology of primary femoroacetabular impingement: genetics or acquired deformity? *J Hip Preserv Surg* 2:249, 2015.

Parry JA, Swann RP, Erickson JA, et al.: Midterm outcomes of reverse (anteverting) periacetabular osteotomy in patients with hip impingement secondary to acetabular retroversion, *Am J Sports Med* 44:672, 2016.

Peters CL, Anderson LA, Erickson JA, et al.: An algorithmic approach to surgical decision in acetabular retroversion, *Orthopedics* 34:10, 2011.

Peters CL, Schabel K, Anderson L, Erickson J: Open treatment of femoroacetabular impingement is associated with clinical improvement and low complication rate at short-term followup, *Clin Orthop Relat Res* 468:504, 2010.

Pollard TC: A perspective on femoroacetabular impingement, *Skeletal Radiol* 40:815, 2011.

Pollard TC, McNally EG, Wilson DC, et al.: Localized cartilage assessment with three-dimensional dGEMRIC in asymptomatic hips with normal morphology and cam deformity, *J Bone Joint Surg* 92A:2557, 2010.

Ribas M, Cardenas-Nylander C, Bellotti V, et al.: Mini-open approach for femoroacetabular impingement: 10 years experience and evolved indications, *Hip Int* 26(Suppl 1):38, 2016.

Ricciardi BF, Sink EL: Surgical hip dislocation: techniques for success, *J Pediatr Orthop* 34(Suppl 1):S25, 2014.

Riley GM, McWalter EJ, Stevens KJ, et al.: MRI of the hip for the evaluation of femoroacetabular impingement: past, present, and future, *J Magn Reson Imaging* 41:558, 2015.

Ross JR, Nepple JJ, Philippon MJ, et al.: Effect of changes in pelvic tilt on range of motion to impingement and radiographic parameters of acetabular morphologic characteristics, *Am J Sports Med* 42:2401, 2014.

Ross JR, Schoenecker PL, Clohisy JC: Surgical dislocation of the hip: evolving indications, *HSS J* 9:60, 2013.

Schilders E, Dimitrakopoulou A, Bismil Q, et al.: Arthroscopic treatment of labral tears in femoroacetabular impingement: a comparative study of refixation and resection with a minimum two-year follow-up, *J Bone Joint Surg* 93B:1027, 2011.

Schoenecker PL, Clohisy JC, Millis MB, Wenger DR: Surgical management of the problematic hip in adolescent and young adult patients, *J Am Acad Orthop Surg* 19:275, 2011.

Siebenrock KA, Steppacher SD, Haefeli PC, et al.: Valgus hip with high antetorsion causes pain through posterior extraarticular FAI, *Clin Orthop Relat Res* 471:3774, 2013.

Skendzel JG, Philippon MJ, Briggs KK, et al.: The effect of joint space on midterm outcomes after arthroscopic hip surgery for femoroacetabular impingement, *Am J Sports Med* 42:1127, 2014.

Steppacher SD(1), Anwander H, Zurmühle CA, et al.: Eighty percent of patients with surgical hip dislocation for femoroacetabular impingement have a good clinical result without osteoarthritis progression at 10 years, *Clin Orthop Relat Res* 473:1333, 2015.

Wall PD, Brown JS, Parsons N, et al.: Surgery for treating hip impingement (femoroacetabular impingement), *Cochrane Database Syst Rev* (9):CD010796, 2014.

Wyles CC, Heidenreich MJ, Jeng J, et al.: The John Charnley Award: Redefining the natural history of osteoarthritis in patients with hip dysplasia and impingement, *Clin Orthop Relat Res* 475:336, 2017.

Zaltz I, Kelly BT, Larson CM, et al.: Surgical treatment of femoroacetabular impingement: what are the limits of hip arthroscopy? *Arthroscopy* 30:99, 2014.

ACETABULAR DYSPLASIA

Albers CE, Steppacher SD, Ganz R, et al.: Impingement adversely affects 10-year survivorship after periacetabular osteotomy for DDH, *Clin Orthop Relat Res* 47:1602, 2013.

Amanatullah DF, Stryker L, Schoenecker P, et al.: Similar clinical outcomes for THAs with and without prior periacetabular osteotomy, *Clin Orthop Relat Res* 473:685, 2015.

Anderson LA, Erickson JA, Swann RP, et al.: Femoral morphology in patients undergoing periacetabular osteotomy for classic or borderline acetabular dysplasia: are cam deformities common? *J Arthroplasty* 31(9 Suppl):259, 2016.

Anderson LA, Gililland J, Pelt C, et al.: Center edge angle measurement for hip preservation surgery: technique and caveats, *Orthopedics* 34:86, 2011.

Clohisy JC, Nepple JJ, Ross JR, et al.: Does surgical hip dislocation and periacetabular osteotomy improve pain in patients with Perthes-like deformities and acetabular dysplasia? *Clin Orthop Relat Res* 473:1370, 2015.

Domb BG, Lareau JM, Baydoun H, et al.: Is intraarticular pathology common in patients with hip dysplasia undergoing periacetabular osteotomy? *Clin Orthop Relat Res* 472:674, 2014.

Domb BG, LaReau JM, Hammarstedt JE, et al.: Concomitant hip arthroscopy and periacetabular osteotomy, *Arthroscopy* 31:2199, 2015.

Domb BG, Stake CE, Lindner D, et al.: Arthroscopic capsular plication and labral preservation in borderline hip dysplasia: two-year clinical outcomes of a surgical approach to a challenging problem, *Am J Sports Med* 41:2591, 2013.

Fukui K, Trindale CA, Briggs KK, et al.: Arthroscopy of the hip for patients with mild to moderate developmental dysplasia of the hip and femoroacetabular impingement: outcomes following hip arthroscopy for treatment of chondrolabral damage, *Bone Joint J* 97-B:1316, 2015.

Ganz R, Horowitz K, Leunig M: Algorithm for femoral and periacetabular osteotomies in complex hip deformities, *Clin Orthop Relat Res* 268:3168, 2010.

Gray BL, Stambough JB, Baca GR, et al.: Comparison of contemporary periacetabular osteotomy for hip dysplasia with total hip arthroplasty for hip osteoarthritis, *Bone Joint J* 97-B:1322, 2015.

Ida T, Nakamura Y, Hagio T, et al.: Prevalence and characteristics of camtype femoroacetabular deformity in 100 hips with symptomatic acetabular dysplasia: a case control study, *J Orthop Surg Res* 9:93, 2014.

to II H, Tanino H, Yamanaka Y, et al.: Intermediate to long-term results of periacetabular osteotomy in patients younger and older than forty years of age, *J Bone Joint Surg* 93A:1347, 2011.

Kain MS, Novais EN, Vallim C, et al.: Periacetabular osteotomy after failed hip arthroscopy for labral tears in patients with acetabular dysplasia, *J Bone Joint Surg* 93A(Suppl 2):57, 2011.

Larson CM, Ross JR, Stone RM, et al.: Arthroscopic management of dysplastic hip deformities: predictors of success and failures with comparison to an arthroscopic FAI cohort, *Am J Sports Med* 44:447, 2016.

Lehmann CL, Nepple JJ, Baca G, et al.: Do fluoroscopy and postoperative radiographs correlate for periacetabular osteotomy corrections? *Clin Orthop Relat Res* 470:3508, 2012.

Lerch TD, Steppacher SD, Liechti EF, et al.: One-third of hips after periacetabular osteotomy survive 30 years with good clinical results, no progression of arthritis, or conversion to THA, *Clin Orthop Relat Res* 475:1154, 2017.

Nepple JJ, Wells J, Ross JR, et al.: Three patterns of acetabular deficiency are common in young adult patients with acetabular dysplasia, *Clin Orthop Relat Res* 475:1037, 2017.

Novais EN, Kim YJ, Carry PM, Millis MB: The Bernese periacetabular osteotomy: is transection of the rectus femoris tendon essential? *Clin Orthop Relat Res* 472:3142, 2014.

Novais EN, Potter GD, Sierra RJ, et al.: Surgical treatment of adolescent acetabular dysplasia with a periacetabular osteotomy: does obesity increase the risk of complications, *J Pediatr Orthop* 35:561, 2015.

Peters CL, Erickson JA, Anderson MB, Anderson LA: Preservation of the rectus femoris during periacetabular osteotomy does not compromise acetabular reorientation, *Clin Orthop Relat Res* 473:608, 2015.

Ricciardi BF, Mayer SW, Fields KG, et al.: Patient characteristics and early functional outcomes of combined arthroscopic labral refixation and periacetabular osteotomy for symptomatic acetabular dysplasia, *Am J Sports Med* 44:2518, 2016.

Sankar WN, Beaulé PE, Clohisty JC, et al.: Labral morphologic characteristics in patients with symptomatic acetabular dysplasia, *Am J Sports Med* 43:2152, 2015.

Sierra RJ, Beaule P, Zaltz I, et al.: Prevention of nerve injury after periacetabular osteotomy, *Clin Orthop Relat Res* 470:2209, 2012.

Steppacher SD, Anwander H, Schwab JM, et al.: Femoral dysplasia. https://musculoskeletalkey.com/femoral-dysplasia.

Thawrani DP, Feldman DS, Sala DA: Not all hip dysplasias are the same: preoperative CT version study and the need for reverse Bernese periacetabular osteotomy, *J Pediatr Orthop* 37:47, 2017.

Wassilew GI, Perka C, Janz V, et al.: Tranexamic acid reduces the blood loss and blood transfusion requirements following peri-acetabular osteotomy, *Bone Joint J* 97-B:1604, 2015.

Wells J, Millis M, Kim YJ, et al.: Survivorship of the Bernese periacetabular osteotomy: what factors are associated with long-term failure? *Clin Orthop Relat Res* 475:396, 2017.

Wells J, Nepple JJ, Crook K, et al.: Femoral morphology in the dysplastic hip: three-dimensional characterizations with CT, *Clin Orthop Relat Res* 475:1045, 2017.

Wingerter SA, Keith AD, Schoenecker PL, et al.: Does tranexamic acid reduce blood loss and transfusion requirements associated with the periacetabular osteotomy? *Clin Orthop Relat Res* 473:2639, 2015.

Zaltz I, Baca G, Kim YJ, et al.: Complications associated with the periacetabular osteotomy: a prospective multicenter study, *J Bone Joint Surg Am* 96:2014, 1967.

GREATER TROCHANTERIC PAIN SYNDROME/GLUTEUS TENDINOPATHY

Alpaugh K, Chilelli BJ, Xu S, Martin SD: Outcomes after primary open or endoscopic abductor tendon repair in the hip: a systematic review of the literature, *Arthroscopy* 31:530, 2014.

Davies JF, Stiehl JB, Davies JA, Geiger PB: Surgical treatment of hip abductor tendon tears, *J Bone Joint Surg* 95:1420, 2013.

Domb BG, Nasser RM, Botser IB: Partial-thickness tears of the gluteus medius: rationale and technique for transtendinous endoscopic repair, *Arthroscopy* 26(12):1697, 2010.

McCormick F, Alpaugh K, Nwachukwu BU, et al.: Endoscopic repair of full-thickness abductor tendon tears: surgical technique and outcome at minimum of 1-year follow-up, *Arthroscopy* 29:1941, 2013.

Redmond JM, Chen AW, Domb BG: Greater trochanteric pain syndrome, *J Am Acad Orthop Surg* 24:231, 2016.

Ricciardi BF, Fabricant PD, Fields KG, et al.: What are the demographic and radiographic characteristics of patients with symptomatic extraarticular femoroacetabular impingement? *Clin Orthop Relat Res* 473:1299, 2015.

Strauss EJ, Nho SJ, Kelly BT: Greater trochanteric pain syndrome, *Sports Med Arthrosc* 18:113, 2010.

Walsh N, Walsh M, Walton J, Millar N: Surgical repair of the abductor mechanism of the hip, *J Bone Joint Surg* 93B(Suppl 1):25, 2011.

Yen YM, Lewis CL, Kim YJ: Understanding and treating the snapping hip, *Sports Med Arthrosc Rev* 23:194, 2015.

ILIOPSOAS TENDINOPATHY

Brandenburg JB, Kapron AL, Wylie JD, et al.: The functional and structural outcomes of arthroscopic iliopsoas release, *Am J Sports Med* 44:1286, 2016.

Chandrasekaran S, Close MR, Walsh JP, et al.: Arthroscopic technique for iliopsoas fractional lengthening for symptomatic internal snapping of the hip, iliopsoas impingement lesion, or both, *Arthrosc Tech* 7:e915, 2018.

El Bitar YF, Stake CE, Dunne KF, et al.: Arthroscopic iliopsoas fractional lengthening for internal snapping of the hip: clinical outcomes with a minimum 2-year follow-up, *Am J Sports Med* 42:1696, 2014.

Gupta A, Redmond JM, Hammarstedt JE, et al.: Endoscopic pubic symphysectomy for recalcitrant osteitis pubis, *Arthrosc Tech* 4:e115, 2015.

Ilizaliturri Jr VM, Buganza-Tepole M, Olivos-Meza A, et al.: Central compartment release versus lesser trochanter release of the iliopsoas tendon for the treatment of internal snapping hip: a comparative study, *Arthroscopy* 30:790, 2014.

Khan M, Adamich J, Simunovic N, et al.: Surgical management of internal snapping hip syndrome: a systematic review evaluating open and arthroscopic approaches, *Arthroscopy* 29:942, 2013.

Strosberg DS, Ellis TJ, Renton DB: The role of femoroacetabular impingement in core muscle injury/athletic pubalgia: diagnosis and management, *Front Surg* 3:6, 2016.

SPORTS HERNIA

Hopkins JN, Brown W, Lee CA: Sports hernia: definition, evaluation, and treatment, *JBJS Rev* 5:e6, 2017.

Litwin DE, Sneidre EB, McEnaney PM, Busconi BD: Athletic pubalgia (sports hernia), *Clin Sports Med* 30:417, 2011.

Messaoudi N, Jans C, Pauli S, et al.: Surgical management of sportsman's hernia in professional soccer players, *Orthopedics* 35(9):e1371, 2012.

Minnich JM, Hanks JB, Muschaweck U, et al.: Sports hernia: diagnosis and treatment highlighting a minimal repair surgical technique, *Am J Sports Med* 39:1341, 2011.

Ostrom E, Joseph A: The use of musculoskeletal ultrasound for the diagnosis of groin and hip pain in athletes, *Curr Sports Med Rep* 15:86, 2016.

Vasileff WK, Nekhline M, Kolowich PA, et al.: Inguinal hernia in athletes: role of dynamic ultrasound, *Sports Health* 9:414, 2017.

OSTEONECROSIS OF THE FEMORAL HEAD

Ali SA, Christy JM, Griesser MJ, et al.: Treatment of avascular necrosis of the femoral head utilizing free vascularized fibular graft: a systematic review, *Hip Int* 24:5, 2014.

Amstutz HC, Le Duff MJ: Hip resurfacing results for osteonecrosis are as good as for other etiologies at 2 to 12 years, *Clin Orthop Relat Res* 468:375, 2010.

Babis GC, Sakellariou V, Parvizi J, Soucacos P: Osteonecrosis of the femoral head, *Orthopedics* 34:39, 2011.

Bertrand T, Urbaniak JR, Lark RK: Vascularized fibular grafts for avascular necrosis after slipped capital femoral epiphysis: is hip preservation possible? *Clin Orthop Relat Res* 471:2206, 2013.

Bose VC, Baruah BD: Resurfacing arthroplasty of the hip for avascular necrosis of the femoral head: a minimum follow-up of four years, *J Bone Joint Surg* 92B:922, 2010.

Carli A, Albers A, Séguin C, et al.: The medical and surgical treatment of ARCO stage I and II osteonecrosis of the femoral head: a critical analysis review, *JBJS Rev* 2:pii: 01874474-201402000-00001, 2014.

Chen CH, Chang JK, Lai KA, et al.: Alendronate in the prevention of collapse of the femoral head in nontraumatic osteonecrosis: a two-year multicenter, prospective, randomized, double-blind, placebo-controlled study, *Arthritis Rheum* 64:1572, 2012.

Cui Q, Botchwey EA: Emerging ideas: treatment of precollapse osteonecrosis using stem cells and growth factors, *Clin Orthop Relat Res* 469:2665, 2011.

Eward WC, Rineer CA, Urbaniak JR, et al.: The vascularized fibular graft in precollapse osteonecrosis: is long-term hip preservation possible? *Clin Orthop Relat Res* 470:2819, 2012.

Fang T, Zhang EW, Sailes FC, et al.: Vascularized fibular grafts in patients with avascular necrosis of femoral head: a systematic review and meta-analysis, *Arch Orthop Trauma Surg* 133:1, 2013.

Gagala J, Tarczynska M, Gaweda K: A seven- to 14-year follow-up study of bipolar hip arthroplasty in the treatment of osteonecrosis of the femoral head, *Hip Int* 24:14, 2014.

Gupta AK, Frank RM, Harris JD, et al.: Arthroscopic-assisted core decompression for osteonecrosis of the femoral head, *Arthrosc Tech* 3:e7, 2013.

Ha YC, Kim HJ, Kim SY, et al.: Effects of age and body mass index on the results of transtrochanteric rotational osteotomy for femoral head osteonecrosis: surgical technique, *J Bone Joint Surg* 93A(Suppl 1):75, 2011.

Hwang KT, Kim YH, Kim YS, Choi IY: Is bipolar hemiarthroplasty a reliable option for Ficat stage III osteonecrosis of the femoral head? 15- to 24-year follow-up study, *Arch Orthop Trauma Surg* 132:1789, 2012.

Issa K, Pivec R, Kapadia BH, et al.: Osteonecrosis of the femoral head: the total hip replacement solution, *Bone Joint J* 95B(11 Suppl A):46, 2013.

Johannson HR, Zywiel MG, Marker DR, et al.: Osteonecrosis is not a predictor of poor outcomes in primary total hip arthroplasty: a systematic literature review, *Int Orthop* 35:465, 2011.

Johnson AJ, Mont MA, Tsao AK, Jones LC: Treatment of femoral head osteonecrosis in the United States: 16-year analysis of the Nationwide Inpatient Sample, *Clin Orthop Relat Res* 472:617, 2014.

Kang JS, Moon KH, Kwon DG, et al.: The natural history of asymptomatic osteonecrosis of the femoral head, *Int Orthop* 37:379, 2013.

Karantanas AH, Drakonaki EE: The role of MR imaging in avascular necrosis of the femoral head, *Semin Musculoskelet Radiol* 15:281, 2011.

Kim YH, Kim JS, Park JW, Joo JH: Contemporary total hip arthroplasty with and without cement in patients with osteonecrosis of the femoral head: a concise follow-up, at an average of seventeen years, of a previous report, *J Bone Joint Surg* 93A:1806, 2011.

Korompilias AV, Beris AE, Lykissas MG, et al.: Femoral head osteonecrosis: why choose free vascularized fibula grafting, *Microsurgery* 31:223, 2011.

Leiberman JR, Engstrom SM, Meneghini RM, SooHoo NF: Which factors influence preservation of the osteonecrotic femoral head? *Clin Orthop Relat Res* 470:525, 2012.

Liu ZH, Guo WS, Li ZR, et al.: Porous tantalum rods for treating osteonecrosis of the femoral head, *Genet Mol Res* 13:8342, 2014.

Mont MA, Zywiel MG, Marker DR, et al.: The natural history of untreated symptomatic osteonecrosis of the femoral head: a systematic literature review, *J Bone Joint Surg* 92A:21265, 2010.

Nakasone S, Takao M, Sakar T, et al.: Does the extent of osteonecrosis affect the survival of hip resurfacing? *Clin Orthop Relat Res* 471:2013, 1926.

Park KS, Tumin M, Peni I, Yoon TR: Conversion total hip arthroplasty after previous transtrochanteric rotational osteotomy for osteonecrosis of the femoral head, *J Arthroplasty* 29:813, 2014.

Pyda M, Koczy B, Widuchowski W, et al.: Hip resurfacing arthroplasty in treatment of avascular necrosis of the femoral head, *Med Sci Monit* 21:304, 2015.

Rajagopal M, Balch Samora J: Ellis TJ: Efficacy of core decompression as treatment for osteonecrosis of the hip: a systematic review, *Hip Int* 22:489, 2012.

Sabesan BJ, Pedrotty DM, Urbaniak JR, et al.: Free vascularized fibular grafting preserves athletic activity level in patients with osteonecrosis, *J Surg Orthop Adv* 21:242, 2012.

Sayeed SA, Johnson AJ, Stroh DA, et al.: Hip resurfacing in patients who have osteonecrosis and are 25 years or under, *Clin Orthop Relat Res* 469:1582, 2011.

Sun W, Li ZR, Wang BL, et al.: Relationship between preservation of the lateral pillar and collapse of the femoral head in patients with osteonecrosis, *Orthopedics* 37:e24, 2014.

van der Jagt D, Mokete L, Pietrzak J, et al.: Osteonecrosis of the femoral head: evaluation and treatment, *J Am Acad Orthop Surg* 23:69, 2015.

Wang BL, Sun W, Shi ZC, et al.: Treatment of nontraumatic osteonecrosis of the femoral head using bone impaction grafting through a femoral neck window, *Int Orthop* 34:635, 2010.

Zalavras CG, Lieberman JR: Osteonecrosis of the femoral head: evaluation and treatment, *J Am Acad Orthop Surg* 22:455, 2014.

Zhang Y, Li L, Shi ZJ, et al.: Porous tantalum rod implant is an effective and safe choice for early-stage femoral head necrosis: a meta-analysis of clinical trials, *Eur J Orthop Surg Traumatol* 23:211, 2013.

Zhao D, Zhang Y, Wang W, et al.: Tantalum rod implantation and vascularized iliac grafting for osteonecrosis of the femoral head, *Orthopedics* 36:789, 2013.

IDIOPATHIC TRANSIENT OSTEOPOROSIS

Lidder S, Lang KJ, Lee HJ, et al.: Bilateral hip fractures associated with transient osteoporosis of pregnancy, *J R Army Med Corps* 157:176, 2011.

Rochietti March M, Tovaglia V, Meo A, et al.: Transient osteoporosis of the hip, *Hip Int* 20:297, 2010.

PROTRUSIO ACETABULI

Asadipooya K, Graves L, Greene LW: Transient osteoporosis of the hip: review of the literature, *Osteoporosis Int* 28:2016, 1805.

Baghadi YM, Larson AN, Sierra RJ: Restoration of the hip center during THA performed for protrusion acetabuli is associated with better implant survival, *Clin Orthop Relat Res* 471:3251, 2013.

Shah K, Shah H: Primary protrusio acetabuli in childhood, *Pediatr Radiol* 40(Suppl 1):S55, 2010.

ADULT-ONSET RHEUMATOID ARTHRITIS

Aulah TS, Kuiper JH, Dixey J, Richardson JB: Hip resurfacing for rheumatoid arthritis: independent assessment of 11-year results from an international register, *Int Orthop* 35:803, 2011.

Yun HH, Song SY, Park S, Lee JW: Rapidly destructive arthropathy of the hip joint in patients with rheumatoid arthritis, *Orthopedics* 35:e958, 2012.

JUVENILE IDIOPATHIC ARTHRITIS

Bertamino M, Rossi F, Pistorio A, et al.: Development and validation of a radiographic scoring system for the hip in juvenile idiopathic arthritis, *J Rheumatol* 37:432, 2010.

Cruz-Pardos A, Garcia-Rey E, Garcia-Cimbrelo E, Ortega-Chamarro J: Alumina-on-alumina THA in patients with juvenile idiopathic arthritis: a 5-year followup study, *Clin Orthop Relat Res* 470:1421, 2012.

de Oliveira Sato J, Corrente JE: Saad Magalhaes C: Progression of articular and extraarticular damage in oligoarticular juvenile idiopathic arthritis, *Clin Exp Rheumatol* 29:871, 2011.

Malviya A, Walker LC, Avery P, et al.: The long-term outcome of hip replacement in adults with juvenile idiopathic arthritis: the influence of steroids and methotrexate, *J Bone Joint Surg* 93B:443, 2011.

OSTEOARTHRITIS

Barros HJ, Camanho GL, Bernabé AC, et al.: Femoral head-neck junction deformity is related to osteoarthritis of the hip, *Clin Orthop Relat Res* 468:2010, 1920.

Browne JA: The mature athlete with hip arthritis, *Clin Sports Med* 30:453, 2011.

Chee YH, Teoh KH, Sabnis BM, et al.: Total hip replacement in morbidly obese patients with osteoarthritis: results of a prospectively matched study, *J Bone Joint Surg* 92B:1066, 2010.

Davis AM, Wood AM, Kennan AC, et al.: Does body mass index affect clinical outcome post-operatively and at five years after primary unilateral hip replacement performed for osteoarthritis? A multivariate analysis of prospective data, *J Bone Joint Surg* 93B:1178, 2011.

Deshmukh AJ, Panagopoulos G, Alizadeh A, et al.: Intra-articular hip injection: does pain relief correlate with radiographic severity of osteoarthritis? *Skeletal Radiol* 40:1449, 2011.

Franklin J, Ingvarsson T, Englund M, et al.: Natural history of radiographic hip osteoarthritis: a retrospective cohort study with 11-28 years of followup, *Arthritis Care Res (Hoboken)* 63:689, 2011.

Gosvig KK, Jacobsen S, Sonne-Holm S, et al.: Prevalence of malformations of the hip joint and their relationship to sex, groin pain, and risk of osteoarthritis: a population-based survey, *J Bone Joint Surg* 92A:1162, 2010.

Jiang L, Rong J, Wang Y, et al.: The relationship between body mass index and hip osteoarthritis: a systematic review and meta-analysis, *Joint Bone Spine* 78:150, 2011.

Klit J, Gosvig K, Jacobsen S, et al.: The prevalence of predisposing deformity in osteoarthritic hip joints, *Hip Int* 21:537, 2011.

Murphy LB, Helmick CG, Schwartz TA, et al.: One in four people may develop symptomatic hip osteoarthritis in his or her lifetime, *Osteoarthritis Cartilage* 18:1372, 2010.

Sayeed SA, Johnson AJ, Jaffe DE, Mont MA: Incidence of contralateral THA after index THA for osteoarthritis, *Clin Orthop Relat Res* 470:535, 2012.

Skytta ET, Jarkko L, Antti E, et al.: Increasing incidence of hip arthroplasty for primary osteoarthritis in 30- to 59-year-old patients, *Acta Orthop* 82:1, 2011.

Thomas GER, Palmer AJR, Batra EN, et al.: Subclinical deformities of the hip are significant predictors of radiographic osteoarthritis and joint replacement in women. A 20 year longitudinal cohort study, *Osteoarthritis Cartilage* 22:1504, 2014.

NEUROPATHIC ARTHROPATHY (CHARCOT JOINT)

Drago L, De Vecchi E, Pasqualini M, et al.: Rapid, progressive neuropathic arthropathy of the hip in a patient co-infected with human immunodeficiency virus, hepatitis C virus and tertiary syphilis: case report, *BMC Infect Dis* 11:159, 2011.

Viens NA, Watters TS, Vinson EN, Brigman BE: Case report: Neuropathic arthropathy of the hip as a sequela of undiagnosed tertiary syphilis, *Clin Orthop Relat Res* 468:3126, 2010.

The complete list of references is available online at Expert Consult.com.

PART II

RECONSTRUCTIVE PROCEDURES OF THE KNEE IN ADULTS

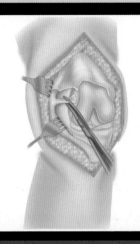

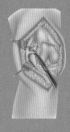

MODERN PROSTHESIS EVOLUTION AND DESIGN

Although many total knee designs predate the total condylar prosthesis designed by Insall and others, its introduction in 1973 marked the beginning of the total knee arthroplasty (TKA) era (Fig. 5.1). This prosthesis design allowed mechanical considerations to outweigh the desire to reproduce anatomically the kinematics of normal knee motion. Influenced largely by the previous Imperial College/London Hospital design, both cruciate ligaments were sacrificed, with sagittal plane stability maintained by the articular surface geometry. The original cemented total condylar prosthesis not only set the standard for survivorship of TKA but also formed the basis of designs for decades to follow. Newer knee replacement designs have now evolved to the point where several have reported long-term survivorships of over 90% at 15- to 20-year follow-up.

Since the concept of the total condylar design was introduced, total knee replacement design has yet to see another major leap in advancement. One of the original designs was the Insall-Burstein total condylar knee. This design had symmetric medial and lateral condyles with a decreasing sagittal radius of curvature posteriorly. The symmetric condyles were individually convex in the coronal plane. The double-dished articular surface of the tibial polyethylene component was perfectly congruent with the femoral component in extension and congruent in the coronal plane in flexion. Translation and dislocation of the components were resisted by the anterior and posterior lips of the tibial component and the median eminence. The tibial component has a metaphyseal stem to resist tilting of the prosthesis during asymmetric loading. The tibial component originally was all polyethylene (see Fig. 5.1), but metal backing was added later to allow more uniform stress transfer to the underlying cancellous metaphyseal bone and to prevent polyethylene deformation at the implant-cement interface. The patella was resurfaced with a dome-shaped, all-polyethylene patellar component with a central fixation lug. Many of these design characteristics are retained in modern designs.

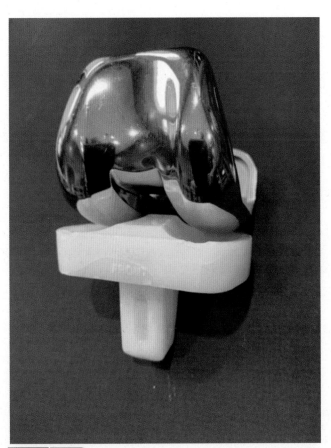

FIGURE 5.1 Total condylar prosthesis introduced by Insall in 1973. After almost five decades there has not been another large technologic advancement.

Concurrent with the development of the cruciate-sacrificing total condylar prosthesis, the duopatellar prosthesis was developed with the sagittal plane contour of the femoral component being anatomically shaped. This prosthesis included retention of the posterior cruciate ligament (PCL). Originally, the medial and lateral tibial plateau components were separate, but this was soon revised to a one-piece tibial component with a cutout for retention of the PCL. The patellar component of the duopatellar prosthesis was an all-polyethylene dome similar to that used in the total condylar knee. The duopatellar prosthesis evolved into the kinematic condylar prosthesis, which was widely used in the 1980s (Fig. 5.2).

Two early criticisms of the total condylar prosthesis were its tendency to subluxate posteriorly in flexion if the flexion gap was larger than the extension gap and its lack of femoral rollback and smaller range of flexion if the PCL was not functioning. By not "rolling back," the posterior femoral metaphysis in a total condylar knee impinged against the tibial articular surface at approximately 95 degrees of flexion (Fig. 5.3). The early clinical reviews of the total condylar prosthesis documented average flexion of only 90 to 100 degrees. To correct these problems, the Insall-Burstein posterior cruciate-substituting or posterior-stabilized (PS) design was developed in 1978 by adding a central cam mechanism to the articular surface geometry of the total condylar prosthesis (Fig. 5.4). The cam on the femoral component engaged a central post on the tibial articular surface at approximately 70 degrees of flexion and caused the contact point of the femoral-tibial articulation to be posteriorly displaced, effecting femoral rollback and allowing further flexion.

Most current total knee designs are derivatives of the Insall-Burstein and kinematic designs. During the late 1980s

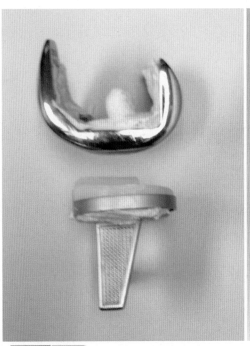
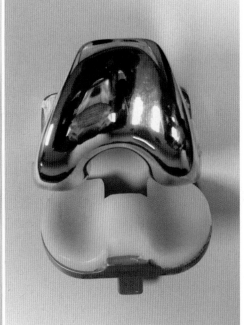

FIGURE 5.2 Kinematic condylar prosthesis obtained during revision procedure.

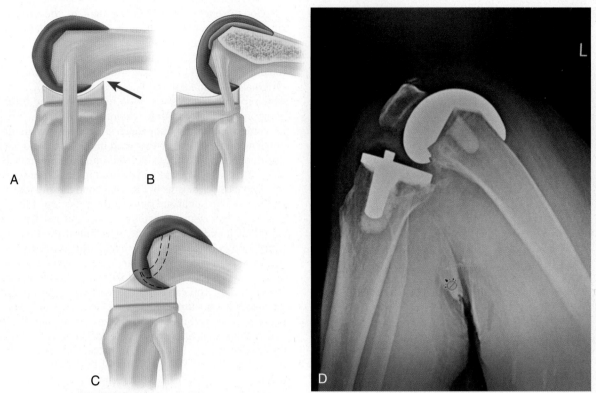

FIGURE 5.3 **A,** With loss of posterior condylar offset and roll forward of femoral component on tibial tray, there can be limited flexion from abutment of posterior femur against polyethylene insert. **B,** With proper posterior femoral offset and functioning posterior cruciate ligament (PCL), flexion can be optimized without impingement of posterior aspect of femur against tibial insert. **C,** A posterior stabilized implant with post and cam drives rollback of femoral condyles on tibial tray, optimizing flexion. **D,** In this radiograph an example of posterior-stabilized TKA shows optimal flexion with complete support of posterior condyles and no edge loading on posterior lip of polyethylene.

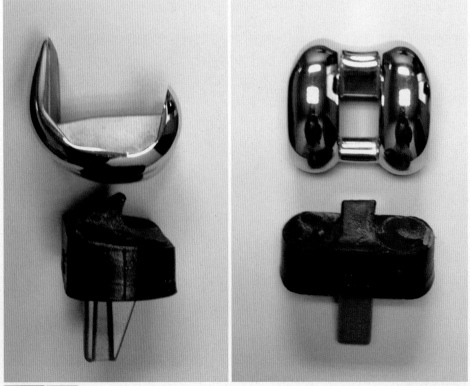

FIGURE 5.4 Insall-Burstein posterior-stabilized knee went through multiple design iterations and enhancements. One iteration included monoblock tibia available with carbon-reinforced polyethylene.

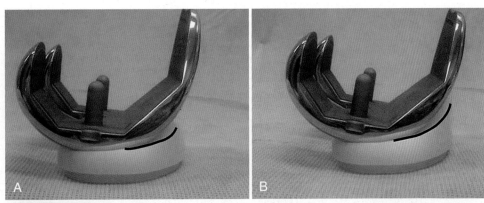

FIGURE 5.5   Posterior cruciate–retaining total knee designs. Deep-dish polyethylene option **(A)** adds stability by building up anterior aspect and preventing significant roll forward of femoral condyles on tibial polyethylene **(B)**.

and 1990s, patellofemoral complications became one of the primary causes for reoperation in TKA. Consequently, improved reconstruction of the patellofemoral joint has received attention in more recent designs. Newer designs incorporate greater areas of patellofemoral contact by elongating the length of the trochlear groove through a larger range of motion and with the addition of more asymmetric anterior flanges designed to resist patellar subluxation and soft-tissue reaction from articulating on a short trochlear groove. Many newer designs now deepen the trochlear groove by adding a sulcus cut to the anterior chamfer of the femur.

Cruciate-retaining (CR) designs have evolved over the past 3 decades. These designs attempt to recreate femoral roll-back by retaining the PCL. Without a post-cam mechanism, advocates point to less constraint and lower forces imparted to the tibial tray. Their resulting kinematics, however, have shown roll-forward contact on the medial side of the joint. Some total knee systems have incorporated a deep polyethylene insert or tray option to their CR designs to combat this and for use when the PCL is not supportive. This design is similar to the original total condylar design that uses sagittal plane concavity or dishing alone to control anterior and posterior translational stability (Fig. 5.5). A comparison of deep-dish components with PS post-cam devices using the same femoral components found no difference at follow-up in range of motion, ability to climb or descend stairs, or pain scores. There have been reports of sagittal-plane laxity in some designs that are not as stable as PS designs. This deep-dish design incorporated many of the previously mentioned advantages of cruciate sacrifice without the obligatory bone sacrifice in the intercondylar region of the femur, which may predispose to fracture. With proper flexion-extension gap balancing, posterior impingement in flexion was reportedly avoided, yielding flexion in many reported series similar to the PS design.

Many designs, however, have still shown a tendency for the femoral articulation to roll forward with increasing flexion (Fig. 5.6). Range of motion after posterior cruciate–retaining TKA has been reported to be improved when the posterior condylar offset is re-established. If the posterior condyles are over resected, the posterior aspect of the tibia may butt up against the posterior aspect of the femur and result in suboptimal flexion. Later reports have shown that measuring this variable radiographically is difficult and that a combination of

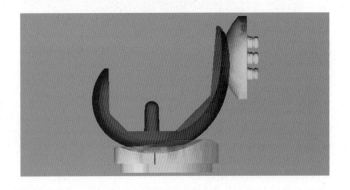

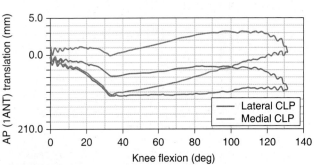

FIGURE 5.6   Computer model depicts roll forward of medial femoral condyle *(red area)* starting just after 30 degrees of flexion.

variables including implant design and tibial slope also play a role in the amount of flexion obtained (Fig. 5.7).

Some newer PS total knee designs have incorporated more complex post-cam interactions and even a dual-cam mechanism in which the anterior aspect of the post drives a screw-home mechanism as the knee is moved into full extension. The transverse plane rotation pattern in this type of design has been shown to be closer to normal knee kinematics than with older PS designs. Many manufacturers now change the positioning of the post and the cam, as well as their geometry, to guide a more normal tibiofemoral articulation pattern throughout the range of motion (Fig. 5.8).

More modern efforts to normalize knee kinematics have been made by either substituting both the anterior cruciate ligament (ACL) and PCL or by retaining them. Although the

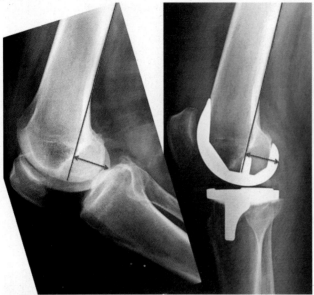

FIGURE 5.7 Important surgical technique points for a cruciate-retaining knee replacement include posterior tibial slope and maintaining posterior condylar offset as measured from posterior aspect of femoral diaphysis.

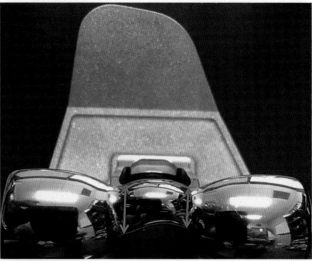

FIGURE 5.8 Newer designs now guide medial pivot through varying diameter of cam. This allows more rollback on lateral side with larger diameter while guiding medial side to stay more centered. (This is implant seen in Fig. 5.3D.)

bicruciate-substituting design has shown more consistent motion in fluorokinematic studies, it still does not normalize motion. The bicruciate-retaining implant designs have shown kinematic patterns that are most comparable to the native knee, but because their application is technically demanding and there is lack of long-term outcomes, their popularity has not increased substantially.

VARUS-VALGUS CONSTRAINED PROSTHESES

The original constrained condylar knee (CCK) was developed from the posterior-substituting design by enlarging the central post of the tibial polyethylene insert, constraining it against the medial and lateral walls of a deepened central box of the femoral component (Fig. 5.9). Varus-valgus stability is controlled by this mechanism with a small amount of varus-valgus toggle allowed. This type of prosthesis otherwise functions as a PS design and is used in patients with instability that might otherwise require a hinged prosthesis. It cannot be used for recurvatum deformity because it does not control hyperextension. Originally designed with cemented intramedullary stems on femoral and tibial components, the design evolved to include modular press-fit or cemented intramedullary stems on the tibial and femoral components.

The CCK design has been used extensively for revision arthroplasty when instability is present and for difficult primary arthroplasties in patients with extreme valgus deformity and medial collateral ligament insufficiency. Although no loosening was reported at 8 years in a group of 28 CCK knees implanted for severe valgus deformities in an older patient group (average age 73), the added constraint of the CCK design raises the concern of whether it might incur increased rates of loosening, particularly when used in younger patients. Progressive bone-cement radiolucencies have been reported in 16% of patients at an average of 44 months after arthroplasty with the total

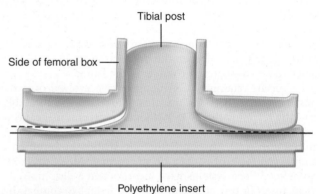

Tibial post

Side of femoral box

Polyethylene insert

FIGURE 5.9 Original constrained condylar knee enlarged central post of tibial polyethylene insert to constrain it against medial and lateral walls of deepened central box of femoral component. Most designs allow small tolerance within the box against post as shown.

condylar prosthesis III, the precursor of the CCK, and nonprogressive radiolucent lines were found in 16% of 148 knees with CCK implants without stem extensions used for correction of significant deformities. Reported failure rates are low, ranging from no failures to 2.5% failures at 4-year follow-up. Most total knee systems include a variation of a varus-valgus constrained design. More recent reports have also shown similar results after primary TKA using a CCK type of implant. Maynard et al. reported 127 primary TKAs using a CCK type of implant and found that at an average 110-month follow-up the revision rate was 0.8%, with a 10-year survivorship of 97.6%. These reports seem to indicate that for complicated primary TKAs with balancing issues that cannot be resolved with standard implants, a CCK implant can be a valid option for consideration. To combat higher forces from being imparted to the tibial implant, a mobile-bearing option can be added to the tibial side of the implant (see next section).

MOBILE-BEARING PROSTHESES

Mobile-bearing knee designs have seen an increase in popularity, and requests have been made to the United States Food and Drug Association (FDA) to down-classify these devices for clearance purposes. The meniscal-bearing version of the low contact stress (LCS) prosthesis developed by Buechel and others incorporated many of the features of the earlier Oxford knee. Individual polyethylene menisci articulate with the femoral component above and with a polished tibial baseplate below. The LCS design has additional dovetailed arcuate grooves on the tibial baseplate that control the anteroposterior course of the menisci. The femoral component has a decreasing radius of curvature posteriorly. This modification of the Oxford design decreases the posterior excursion of the menisci in flexion, helping to decrease the incidence of posterior extrusion of the menisci.

The LCS total knee system also includes a rotating platform design with congruent tibiofemoral geometry in extension similar to other current deep-dish designs; however, the tibial polyethylene is additionally free to rotate within the stem of the tibial baseplate. This design has had rare rotational dislocations of the tibial inserts because of inadequate flexion-extension gap balancing, but it has exhibited excellent longevity. Callaghan et al. reported a 100% prosthesis survival rate in 82 patients at a minimum of 9-year follow-up of the cemented rotating platform LCS design. In a later follow-up study, Callaghan et al. reported the status of 53 knees in 37 of these patients who were still living at a minimum follow-up of 15 years. None of the knees had required revision because of loosening, osteolysis, or wear; three knees had required reoperation (two for periprosthetic fractures and one for infection), but none of the components was revised as part of the reoperations. Buechel, one of the developers of the LCS design, reported a 98% 20-year survivorship with this design and a similar survivorship at 18 years with the cementless rotating platform design. A recent meta-analysis comparing outcomes with fixed-bearing and mobile-bearing TKA found no clinically significant differences in patient-specific or clinical outcome parameters. One reason these implant designs are not offered by many manufacturers is their designation as a class III device by the FDA. In vivo fluorokinematic studies have shown that the bearing rotation in the transverse plane may be nonphysiologic in some patients. A meta-analysis found that there was moderate to low-quality evidence that CR mobile-bearing TKA was as good as fixed-bearing TKA.

Potential advantages of mobile-bearing knees include lower contact stresses at the articulating surfaces, rotational motion of the tibial polyethylene during gait, and self-alignment of the tibial polyethylene compensating for small rotational malalignment of the tibial baseplate during implantation. Recent studies have found a higher revision rate in both the short-term and mid-term follow-up period with a mobile-bearing insert compared with fixed-bearing TKA. Whether mobile-bearing designs will outperform fixed-bearing designs has yet to be determined and may be specific to individual manufacturer design as well as proper surgical technique.

UNICOMPARTMENTAL PROSTHESES

There are some reported results of unicompartmental knee arthroplasty (UKA) that are as good as those of TKA, but controversy remains about indications and the use of unicompartmental prostheses in patients with high body mass indices (BMIs); some reports show higher revision rates at 2-year follow-up in these patients. Many surgeons advocate the use of UKA for arthritis limited to only one knee compartment (Fig. 5.10). These prostheses replace the articular surface of either the medial or the lateral femoral condyle and the adjacent tibial plateau surface. The current trend toward minimally invasive surgery has rekindled enthusiasm for these devices despite the fact that most studies, with some notable exceptions, have shown a slightly worse survivorship for UKA compared with TKA but is better than the revision rates for a revision TKA.

Marmor introduced a unicompartmental replacement in the early 1970s, obtaining better results with replacement of the lateral compartment than of the medial compartment. The Marmor prosthesis was anatomically shaped with a flat, all-polyethylene tibial component. Squire et al. observed 87.5% 15-year survivorship using this prosthesis. Subsequent unicompartmental prostheses with metal-backed tibial components and thin polyethylene occasionally exhibited rapid polyethylene wear.

Meniscal-bearing unicompartmental knee replacements allow translational motion at the polyethylene tibial baseplate interface similar to meniscal-bearing TKA and are enthusiastically supported by some authors, with reports of a 96% 10-year survivorship of the unicompartmental Oxford meniscal knee arthroplasty. In the Swedish National Registry, the Oxford unicompartmental knee fared worse, having a 7% revision rate by 6 years.

Sparing of the cruciate ligaments, the opposite tibiofemoral compartment, and the patellofemoral joint in UKA is purported to result in more normal knee kinematics and to allow easy revision to a tricompartmental prosthesis at a later time. A more normal knee possibly can be obtained with UKA with quicker rehabilitation time and greater range of motion than with TKA. The second purported advantage, bone stock preservation, is more controversial. Revision of UKA to tricompartmental prostheses, requiring special components, bone grafting, or cement with screw augmentation to fill osseous defects, was necessary in 76% of patients reported by Padgett, Stern, and Insall and in 45% reported by Barrett and Scott. McAuley, Engh, and Ammeen reported a 26% use of local autograft, whereas 21% required wedge augmentation. They commented that the UKA revisions to TKA were simpler than typical revision TKA. An emphasis on more limited tibial resection with many newer designs may lessen the incidence of significant bony defects at the time of revision.

Mobile-bearing medial compartment UKA designs have the advantage of a congruent femoral polyethylene articular surface that allows the medial compartment to roll back and maintain more physiologic motion. Indications typically include a functioning ACL and limited flexion contracture with a flexion arc of greater than 100 degrees. To ensure bearing stability, a gap-balancing approach typically is used. The results have been good, and recent reports other than those of the design surgeons have been good to excellent.

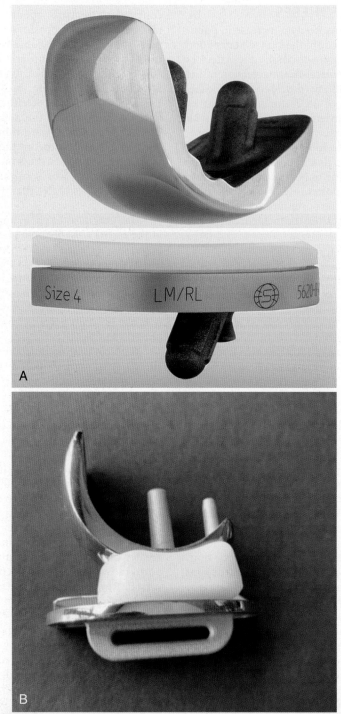

FIGURE 5.10 Fixed-bearing unicompartmental knee arthroplasty system (Stryker Triathlon) **(A)**, and mobile-bearing unicompartmental systems (Oxford Unicompartmental Zimmer/Biomet) **(B)** are current options, with pros and cons for each.

HINGED IMPLANTS

The Kinematic Rotating Hinge (Howmedica, Rutherford, NJ) (Fig. 5.11) has been a widely used linked, hinged knee replacement. Two polyethylene and cobalt chrome bearings allow flexion-extension and axial rotation. The rotating hinge type of implant offers constraint in the sagittal and coronal planes while allowing free rotation in the transverse plane to limit the transfer of forces to the implant-bone interfaces and allow substitution of soft-tissue constraint in the coronal

plane because of insufficient collateral support. The implant provides a block to extension as well, which prevents recurvatum. This implant often is necessary in salvage revision TKA but can be used in a primary TKA when significant deformity and loss of soft-tissue support does not allow a stable knee to be obtained or a flexion gap is created that might "jump" a constrained condylar type of implant. An early report found outcomes with the Kinematic Rotating Hinge no better than those with the earlier GUEPAR prosthesis with respect to

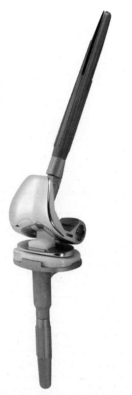

FIGURE 5.11 Kinematic II Rotating Hinge (Stryker) total knee implant.

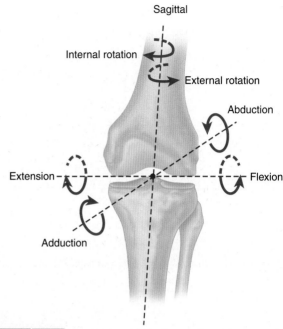

FIGURE 5.12 Motion in knee occurs in three separate planes during course of normal gait cycle and is referred to as "triaxial motion."

infection, loosening, and patellar complications. A more recent study of hinged prostheses found a much lower complication rate at 4-year follow-up of the S-ROM hinged prosthesis (Joint Medical Products/Johnson & Johnson, Stamford, CT). This type of prosthesis is used in patients with severe ligamentous insufficiency, severe flexion or extension gap mismatch, recurvatum deformity, neuromuscular disease, and limb salvage procedures. Use of a hinged implant for primary TKA should be reserved for patients with these problems because of the tendency for worse outcomes and more complications than with other types of implants.

KNEE REPLACEMENT SYSTEMS

Different types of prostheses are necessary for varying amounts of arthritic involvement, deformity, laxity, and bone loss. Prostheses used range from unicompartmental designs for single-compartment disease with minimal deformity to hinged prostheses for severe deformity and or ligamentous deficiencies and for salvage procedures. Many surgeons advocate the use of PCL-retaining prostheses for mild deformity and PCL-substituting designs for more severe deformity while for many surgeons the choice is based on training and experience. Knee prosthesis manufacturers have developed newer systems that offer either PCL retention or PCL substitution through modular tibial polyethylene inserts and PCL-substituting and PCL-retaining femoral components that require similar bone cuts. These prostheses typically use shared operative instrumentation and allow an intraoperative change from PCL retention to PCL substitution or even a constrained condylar design. If balancing of the PCL is difficult, the arthroplasty can be converted to a PCL-substituting design with relative ease in most cases. Many prosthesis designs also include a tibial polyethylene component with

significant dishing (or increased AP congruency or constraint) in the sagittal plane for optional use instead of the PS design when the PCL is incompetent. Modular stems and metal augments and constrained condylar components are typically available in most systems.

Many other factors are important in prosthesis design and selection, including prosthesis fixation, the handling of the patellofemoral articulation, modularity, and polyethylene issues. These are discussed in subsequent sections of this chapter. It is the surgeon's responsibility to understand the indications, contraindications, expected functional outcome, and longevity for each prosthesis type and for specific prostheses. Every surgeon should be familiar with the options and instrumentation of his or her choice to ensure that all bases are covered in the operating room. Long-term follow-up studies will continue to improve our understanding of appropriate indications for the variety of available knee prostheses.

KNEE AND IMPLANT BIOMECHANICS
FUNCTIONAL ANATOMY AND KINEMATICS

Knee motion during normal gait has been studied by many investigators, who have found it to be much more complex than simple flexion and extension. Knee motion during gait occurs in all three anatomic planes around the long axis of the limb (Fig. 5.12). Knee flexion, which occurs around a varying transverse axis (Fig. 5.13), is a function of the articular geometry of the knee and the ligamentous restraints. Dennis et al. described the flexion axis as varying in a helical fashion in a normal knee, with an average of 2 mm of posterior translation of the medial femoral condyle on the tibia during flexion compared with 21 mm of translation of the lateral femoral condyle. This observation was acquired by dynamic fluoroscopy

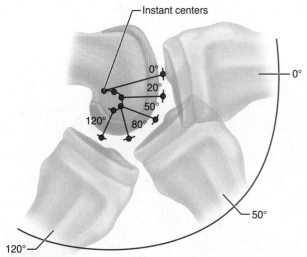

FIGURE 5.13 Transverse axis of flexion and extension of knee constantly changes and describes J-shaped curve around femoral condyles.

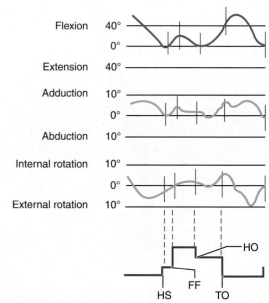

FIGURE 5.14 Triaxial motion of normal knee during walking, as measured by electrogoniometer. Flexion and extension are about 70 degrees during swing phase and 20 degrees during stance phase. About 10 degrees of abduction and adduction and 10 to 15 degrees of internal and external rotation occur during each gait cycle. *FF*, Flatfoot; *HO*, heel-off; *HS*, heel-strike; *TO*, toe-off.

coupled with three-dimensional CT scans of the studied knees. The axis became more variable after sectioning of the anterior cruciate ligament, with an average 5 mm of medial condylar translation and 17 mm of lateral condylar posterior translation in flexion. This pattern of medially based pivoting of the knee explains the observed external rotation of the tibia on the femur during extension, known as the "screw-home mechanism," and internal rotation of the tibia during knee flexion. The inability of many early knee prosthesis designs to accommodate these complex knee motions and their attendant stresses was an unforeseen shortcoming. Many current prosthesis designs attempt to reproduce normal knee kinematics closely, whereas others settle for an approximation of normal motion, placing other concerns, such as polyethylene contact stresses, ahead of accurate reproduction of knee kinematics.

The use of gait laboratories, biomechanical models, and fluoroscopic analyses to study normal subjects and patients before and after knee arthroplasty has become an important tool in prosthesis design and functional evaluation of TKA patients (Fig. 5.14). In kinematic studies of the knee during selected activities of daily living (ADLs), normal gait required 67 degrees of flexion during the swing phase, 83 degrees for stair climbing, 90 degrees for descending stairs, and 93 degrees to rise from a chair. Computer modeling now can be used to predict the effects of prosthetic designs on motion and how they respond to malpositioning during surgery, aiding in the development of designs that are more forgiving and provide more physiologic motion and kinematics. Variation in implant positioning in the transverse plane has been investigated by Milhalko and Williams using a dynamic kinematic model, and significant variations in internal and external rotation during a simulated deep-knee bend have been described. This enforces the need for forgiveness in implant designs so that the knee is not constrained in any one way that may increase the implant-bone interface stresses.

■ ROLE OF THE POSTERIOR CRUCIATE LIGAMENT IN TOTAL KNEE ARTHROPLASTY

Since the concurrent development of PCL-retaining and PCL-substituting prostheses, the relative merits of each design

have been debated. Each design boasts multiple series with comparable excellent 10- to 15-year results. Studies of bilateral TKA with a PCL-retaining prosthesis on one side and a PCL-substituting prosthesis on the other side have failed to show significant subjective performance or patient satisfaction differences. A closer look at the differences in these designs illustrates, however, many of the factors involved in successful arthroplasty.

PCL retention achieves an increased potential range of motion by effective femoral rollback. In vivo kinematic analysis has shown that with a CR design there may be a "roll forward" positioning of the medial femoral condyle on the polyethylene insert with flexion, which may limit flexion. The designs now compensate for this and have evolved from a relatively flat articulation to a higher constrained anterior aspect in most CR designs to prevent the medial femoral condyle from sliding forward in an excessive manner. PCL substitution achieves femoral rollback by a tibial post and femoral cam mechanism. Compared with the original total condylar design, both of the modern designs of PCL retaining and substituting attain greater flexion (see Fig. 5.3). In multiple studies comparing PCL-retaining and PCL-substituting prostheses, the average flexion attained at long-term follow-up has been similar. When the PCL is retained, it frequently needs to be partially released or recessed to allow adequate flexion, especially in the varus-deformed knee because it is a more medial anatomic structure and may be involved in the coronal plane deformity. More recently, deep-dish designs with increased sagittal plane conformity have been studied (with PCL recession and with PCL sacrifice). The flexion with these more conforming devices is similar to that with the PCL-retaining and PCL-substituting devices with which they have been compared.

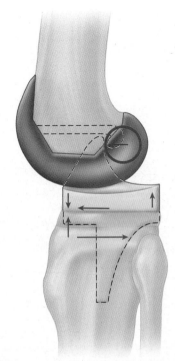

FIGURE 5.15 One argument against posterior cruciate ligament substitution is that added prosthetic constraint may ultimately transfer more stress to prosthesis-bone interface.

In PCL-substituting designs, posterior displacement in flexion is produced by the tibial post contacting the femoral cam, with the resultant stress borne by the prosthetic construct and ultimately transferred to the bone-cement interface (Fig. 5.15). Originally, this situation led many authors to suggest that PCL-substituting designs would have higher failure rates than PCL-retaining devices because of loosening. The loosening rates in most reported studies show equal survivorships of PS and CR TKA. A recent study from the Mayo Clinic, however, compared 5389 CR TKAs to 2728 PS TKAs and found 15-year survivorships of 90% and 77%, respectively, a statistically significant difference. Higher mid-term and late-term revision rates in PS TKA have also been reported in other studies. This finding appears to support the theory that higher transfer of stress to the implant interface of some PS designs may decrease their longevity.

Early gait analysis studies have found that individuals with PCL-retaining prostheses have a more symmetric gait, especially during stair climbing, than do individuals with either PCL-sacrificing or PCL-substituting designs. They showed decreased knee flexion during stair climbing and a tendency to lean forward in a quadriceps-sparing posture in patients with PCL-sacrificing and PCL-substituting designs. They postulated that these observations may indicate inadequate rollback of these designs or possibly the loss of a proprioceptive role of the PCL. These observations have been cited as reasons to retain the PCL. Later gait analysis contradicts the conclusions of these earlier studies, however, after comparing PCL-substituting knees with normal controls. These earlier observations are refuted further by in vivo studies using fluoroscopy during single-stance deep knee bends to show a paradoxic forward translation of the femorotibial contact point during weight-bearing flexion in some PCL-retaining knees, whereas PCL-substituting knees studied showed more uniform femoral rollback.

The patellofemoral joint functions with a larger extensor lever arm when femoral rollback, as a function of PCL retention or PCL substitution, moves the tibial tubercle more anteriorly. The patellofemoral joint also is affected by joint line elevation, the extent to which the new prosthetic joint line is raised relative to the native joint line. PCL-retaining designs do not tolerate much alteration in the level of the preoperative joint line while balancing the flexion and extension gaps, whereas PCL-substituting designs frequently balance with some mild elevation of the joint line in extension to aid in the balancing of the increased flexion gap that occurs when the PCL is sacrificed. The PCL functions as a secondary stabilizer in the coronal plane, and its release often necessitates less collateral ligament balancing to obtain a symmetric flexion and extension gap during surgery (Videos 5.1 and 5.2). In a cadaver study, Mihalko and Krackow showed that release of the PCL may increase the flexion gap 4 to 6 mm while increasing the extension gap less than 2 mm, but it should be pointed out that this was in a cadaver study with nonarthritic specimens. Figgie et al. suggested that joint line elevation may alter patellofemoral mechanics and result in postoperative pain and subluxation.

PCL-substituting femoral components have a cutout for a cam mechanism that begins just below the trochlea of the patellofemoral joint. Additional bone is removed from the femur when PCL-substituting designs are used to accommodate this box-and-cam mechanism. Additionally, the degree of flexion at which the patella contacts this "box" varies among different PS designs. The patella and hypertrophic synovium on the undersurface of the quadriceps tendon can bind in this mechanism. This clinical entity, termed *patellar clunk syndrome,* is a potential complication of PCL-substituting designs. Many posterior stabilized implant designs now offer a longer trochlear groove to combat the build-up of synovium from a shorter trochlear-groove-to-box length, but this continues to be reported in the literature, albeit less frequently, despite this design change.

Many authors argue that it is difficult to balance a diseased or contracted PCL in the presence of a significant varus deformity in a reproducible fashion. Although intraoperative tests of PCL balance have been devised by advocates of PCL retention, other investigators have stated that it is difficult, even in a laboratory setting, to reproduce near-normal PCL strain and function in a PCL-retaining knee arthroplasty. To have near-normal strain, the PCL needs to be balanced to an accuracy of approximately 1 to 2 mm. A PCL that is too tight in flexion can limit the extent of flexion attained postoperatively and lead to excessive femoral rollback, which multiple retrieval studies have shown to accelerate posterior tibial polyethylene wear. Some authors have suggested that attaining reliable balance of the PCL requires experience and that surgeons who perform fewer than 20 TKAs a year should use PCL-substituting prostheses. Late rupture of the PCL is also thought to be a cause of late instability in PCL-retaining designs. It should be pointed out, however, that a posterior stabilized implant does not recreate the normal kinematics of the knee either, and there are proponents for both designs, which have had similar 15- to 20-year survivorships reported in the literature. The argument that the PCL in an osteoarthritic knee is involved in the osteoarthritic process is one

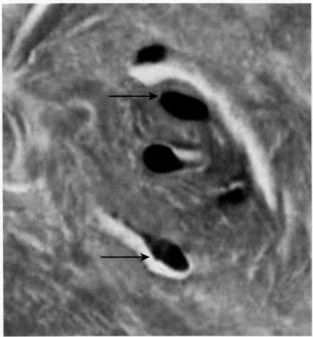

FIGURE 5.16 After a posterior cruciate–retaining total knee arthroplasty (TKA), posterior cruciate ligament (PCL) has been shown to retain its mechanoreceptors, as determined at time of necropsy. Arrows show positive S-100 protein staining in mechanoreceptors in PCL after it functioned for 10 years in a PCL-retaining TKA.

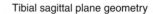

Tibial sagittal plane geometry

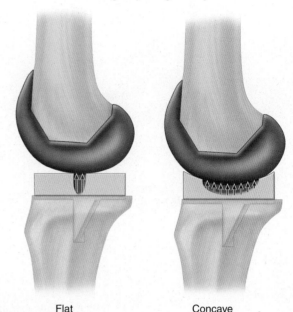

Flat   Concave

FIGURE 5.17 Earlier posterior cruciate–retaining prostheses had flatter sagittal plane geometry that increased the contact forces (*longer arrows* over a smaller area of the polyethylene). This, along with poor polyethylene, created delamination and higher wear. Most current designs of posterior cruciate ligament-retaining knee implants have more conforming surfaces to decrease the forces on the polyethylene (*smaller arrows* over a larger area).

used by proponents of PCL-sacrificing and PCL-substituting techniques. The mechanoreceptors in knees with osteoarthritis (OA) have been shown to be decreased but still present. PCLs retrieved at necropsy from CR TKAs (Fig. 5.16) have been shown to be similar to those from osteoarthritic knees with PCL-sacrificing TKAs, suggesting that the mechanoreceptors are functioning and may contribute to proprioception after TKA.

Another argument in favor of PCL substitution is that significant deformity can be more reliably corrected with its use. Extensive collateral ligament release on the concave side of a fixed knee deformity may not be effective without release of the contracted PCL, which acts as a tether. Similarly, if the collateral ligament on the convex side of a deformity is significantly stretched or attenuated, opposite collateral ligament release is effective only in achieving varus-valgus balance to the extent that is allowed by the intact PCL. The tethering effect of the PCL on soft-tissue balancing of the varus or valgus knee also has been shown in cadaver studies. In a series of patients with preoperative fixed varus or valgus deformities of 15 degrees or more associated with flexion contractures, knees treated with PCL retention had less postoperative flexion, more severe residual flexion contractures, and less correction of the mechanical axis than knees with PCL substitution. In another large series of knees treated with PCL retention, however, no correlation was found between preoperative deformity and postoperative outcome.

Polyethylene wear is affected by prosthesis design and by its in vivo kinematics. The tibial articular surface of PCL-retaining prostheses is typically less conforming to the femoral component in the sagittal plane to allow femoral

rollback. This less-conforming geometry in the sagittal plane is responsible for higher tibial polyethylene contact stresses in PCL-retaining prostheses (Fig. 5.17). Several authors have suggested that these greater contact stresses are responsible in part for accelerated polyethylene wear. This wear can be compounded by an excessively tight PCL that may increase the polyethylene contact stress as it becomes tight in flexion. In the extreme, a PCL that is tight in flexion can cause the femoral condyles to override the posterior edge of the tibial polyethylene, causing extremely high polyethylene contact stresses. This mechanism of accelerated posterior wear has been proposed after study of retrieved polyethylene specimens by various authors, who expressed concern that paradoxic anterior tibial translation in flexion in a poorly functioning PCL-retaining knee may lead to early polyethylene wear. Conversely, the tibial post on many PCL-substituting designs has been shown to be a site of wear and occasional breakage, particularly when the femoral component can impinge on the post anteriorly in hyperextension. This condition is accentuated when the femoral component is implanted in a flexed position, when the tibial component is implanted with a greater posterior slope, and when the knee hyperextends. Other design features where the cam climbs the post in flexion and transfers load at the upper aspect of the post may also contribute to post wear and breakage (see Fig. 5.26D).

■ AXIAL AND ROTATIONAL ALIGNMENT OF THE KNEE

Numerous studies have shown a correlation between long-term success of TKA and restoration of near-normal limb alignment. Suboptimal alignment of total knee prostheses

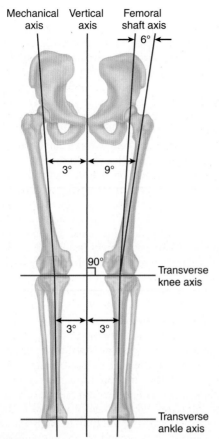

Mechanical
axis

Vertical
axis

Femoral
shaft axis

6°

3°   9°

90°

Transverse
knee axis

3°   3°

Transverse
ankle axis

FIGURE 5.18   Mechanical axis of lower limb extends from center of femoral head to center of ankle joint and passes near or through center of knee. It is in 3 degrees of valgus from vertical axis of body. Anatomic axis of femur is in 6 degrees of valgus from mechanical axis of lower limb and 9 degrees of valgus from true vertical axis of body. Anatomic axis of tibia lies in 2 to 3 degrees of varus from vertical axis of body.

has been implicated in long-term difficulties, including tibiofemoral instability, patellofemoral instability, patellar fracture, stiffness, accelerated polyethylene wear, and implant loosening. The use of accurate instrumentation and an understanding of the basic principles inherent to the instruments are necessary to implant reproducibly well-aligned prostheses. Computer-assisted navigation and robotic techniques are now being used by some surgeons to try to improve the reproducibility of component alignment and to improve functional outcomes.

Normally, the anatomic axes of the femur and the tibia form a valgus angle of 6 ± 2 degrees. The mechanical axis of the lower limb is defined as the line drawn on a standing long-leg anteroposterior radiograph from the center of the femoral head to the center of the talar dome (Fig. 5.18). This mechanical axis typically should project through the center of the knee joint, described as a "neutral" mechanical axis. When the mechanical axis lies to the lateral side of the knee center, the knee is in mechanical valgus alignment. In mechanical varus alignment, the mechanical axis of the limb lies to the medial side of the knee center. The amount of varus or valgus deformity can be determined on an anteroposterior long-standing radiograph by first drawing the mechanical axis of the femur, a line from the center of the femoral head to the center of

the intercondylar notch, and extending this line distally. The mechanical axis of the tibia runs from the center of the tibial plateau to the center of the tibial plafond, discounting any bowing of the tibia. The angle formed between these separate mechanical axes of the femur and tibia determines the varus or valgus deviation from the neutral mechanical axis. By determining the tibial mechanical axis using the center of the tibial plateau and the femoral mechanical axis using the center of the intercondylar notch, any medial or lateral subluxation through the knee joint is disregarded. Insall argued that rotation affects the mechanical axis of the femur apparent on an anteroposterior radiograph, lessening the value of these preoperative and postoperative measurements.

In a normal knee, the tibial articular surface is in approximately 3 degrees of varus with respect to the mechanical axis and the femoral articular surface is in a corresponding 9 degrees of valgus. Multiple studies have shown that tibial components placed in more than 5 degrees of varus tend to fail by subsiding into more varus. Consequently, tibial components generally are implanted perpendicular to the mechanical axis of the tibia in the coronal plane, with varying amounts of posterior tilt in the sagittal plane, depending on the articular design of the component to be implanted. The femoral component usually is implanted in 5 to 7 degrees of valgus, the amount necessary to reestablish a neutral mechanical axis of the femur (Fig. 5.19). Most implant systems offer various options, usually from 5 to 7 degrees of valgus for the distal femoral resection, but the proper angle can be calculated from the standing hip-to-knee radiograph by measuring the angle between the mechanical axis of the femur (line from the center of the femoral head to the center of the distal femur) and a line drawn from the entry point of the intramedullary rod to the diaphyseal line that the rod travels. Once the distal femoral cut is made, the use of an intramedullary goniometer to measure the actual cut distal femoral surface to the intramedullary femoral angle has been shown to be more accurate.

Recently, kinematic alignment of the lower extremity for TKA surgery has been described and advocated by many surgeons. Although this method has been used in the past, advocates point out that today we face less severe deformity correction than we did 20 years ago and that a kinematic alignment with a 3-degree varus joint line at the tibia and an increased distal valgus cut on the femur may improve functional results after TKA. Proponents also point to the ease of balancing the varus knee when using kinematic alignment. Opponents of the kinematic alignment method point to the fact that if outliers on the tibia reach 4 or more degrees varus, the rate of short-term and mid-term failures is much higher. We continue to recommend that the normal mechanical axis of the femur and the tibia be established and the joint line maintained parallel to the ground.

Rotational alignment of total knee components is difficult to discern radiographically, making the assessment of rotation primarily an intraoperative determination. The rotation of the femoral component has effects not only on balancing of the flexion space but also on patellofemoral tracking. Because the proximal tibial cut is made perpendicular to the mechanical axis of the limb instead of in the anatomically correct 3 degrees of varus, rotation of the femoral component also must be altered from its anatomic position to create a symmetric flexion space (Fig. 5.20). To create this rectangular flexion space, with equal tension on the medial and lateral collateral

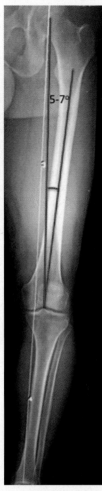

FIGURE 5.19 Implantation of femoral component in 5 to 7 degrees of valgus usually restores neutral mechanical axis of the femur.

ligaments, the femoral component is externally rotated an average of 3 degrees relative to the posterior condylar axis or perpendicular to the anteroposterior axis. In an average male femur, this technique rotationally places the femoral component with the posterior condylar surfaces parallel to the epicondylar axis. This technique fails when the posterior aspect of the native femoral condyle has significant wear, or when the lateral femoral condyle is hypoplastic, as is frequently seen in knees with valgus deformity. In these instances, the surgeon can use the epicondylar axis or the anteroposterior axis popularized by Whiteside (see Technique 5.1 for details). The epicondylar axis has been shown in multiple studies to be difficult to determine in vivo when comparing different observers and when comparing the measured axis with one determined by CT. Each of these techniques of determining femoral component rotation is based on the geometry of the femur primarily, with subsequent ligamentous releases to create symmetric flexion and extension gaps.

Knowledge of each of these techniques is necessary because arthritic deformity or previous surgery may obscure one or more of these landmarks. In revision TKA, the epicondylar axis usually is the only native landmark left to ensure proper femoral component rotation.

Two primary techniques are used to align the tibial component rotationally. The first technique aligns the center of the tibial tray with the junction of the medial third of the tibial tubercle with the lateral two thirds. The second technique places the knee through a range of motion with trial components in place, allowing the tibia to align with the flexion axis of the femur. This second technique tends to align the tibial component rotationally with the rotation of the femoral component, lowering the chance of a rotation mismatch that could lead to accelerated polyethylene wear, although combined internal rotation of both components may lead to patellofemoral maltracking, as shown by Berger et al., and a higher incidence of patellofemoral pain.

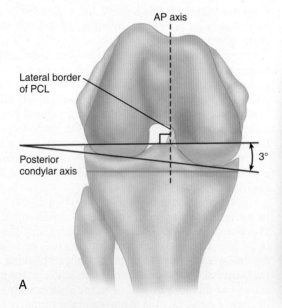

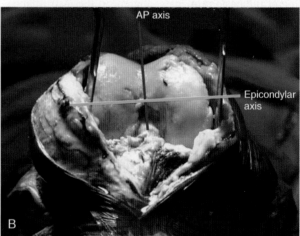

FIGURE 5.20 **A,** To form rectangular flexion space, after tibia has been cut perpendicular to its axis, plane of posterior femoral condylar cuts must be externally rotated approximately 3 degrees from posterior condylar axis. **B,** Location of epicondylar axis and anteroposterior axis of the knee.

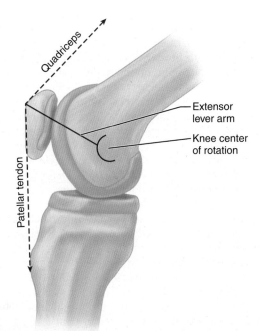

FIGURE 5.21   Patella acts to lengthen extensor lever arm by displacing force vectors of quadriceps and patellar tendons away from center of rotation (COR) of knee. Length of extensor lever arm changes with varying amounts of knee flexion.

Proponents of rotating platform designs claim that the rotational freedom of the tibial polyethylene allows self-correction of minor malrotation of the tibial tray. Although this factor may improve the congruency of the tibiofemoral articulation, tracking of the patella may not be improved and may be related to the existing and proposed femoral rotational alignment.

■ PATELLOFEMORAL JOINT BIOMECHANICS AND FUNCTIONAL ANATOMY

The primary function of the patella is to optimize the lever arm of the extensor mechanism around the knee, improving the efficiency of quadriceps contraction. The quadriceps and patellar tendons insert anteriorly on the patella, with the thickness of the patella displacing their respective force vectors away from the center of rotation of the knee (Fig. 5.21). This displacement or lengthening of the extensor lever arm changes throughout the arc of knee motion. The length of the lever arm varies as a function of the geometry of the trochlea, the varying patellofemoral contact areas, and the varying center of rotation of the knee. The extensor lever arm is greatest at 20 to 30 degrees of flexion, and the quadriceps force required for knee extension increases significantly in the last 20 degrees of extension as less of the patella is in contact with the trochlear groove.

Patellofemoral stability is maintained by a combination of the articular surface geometry and soft-tissue restraints. The Q angle is the angle between the extended anatomic axis of the femur and the line between the center of the patella and the tibial tubercle (Fig. 5.22). The quadriceps acts primarily in line with the anatomic axis of the femur, with the exception of the vastus medialis obliquus, which acts to medialize the patella in terminal extension. Limbs with larger Q angles have a greater tendency for lateral patellar subluxation. Because the patella does not contact the trochlea until early flexion, lateral subluxation of the patella in this range is resisted primarily by the vastus medialis obliquus fibers. As the angle of flexion increases, the bony and subsequent prosthetic constraints play a dominant

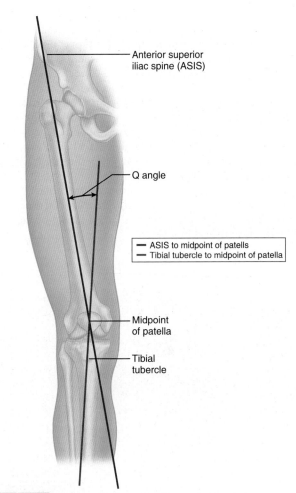

FIGURE 5.22   Q angle, as described by Hvid, is angle between extended anatomic axis of femur and line between center of patella and tibial tubercle.

role in preventing subluxation. In most current femoral component designs, the lateral flange of the trochlea has been made more prominent, producing a more anatomic reconstruction. Many designs add a built-in trochlear groove angle of up to 7 degrees to enhance patellar mechanics and tracking (Fig. 5.23). Trochlear enhancements and attention to femoral component rotation, reproduction of preoperative patellar thickness, and maintenance of joint line height have improved patellofemoral stability and have decreased the rate of lateral patellar retinacular release significantly. The application of these principles is discussed further in the section on surgical technique.

As a consequence of its role in transmitting the force of contraction of the quadriceps muscle to the patellar tendon around a variably flexed knee, the patella experiences a joint reaction force as the trochlea opposes its posterior displacement. This joint reaction force depends on the angle of knee flexion and the magnitude of the forces transmitted to the patella from the quadriceps and patellar tendons. During standing, the joint reaction force increases with increasing knee flexion as the force vectors of the quadriceps and patellar tendons become more parallel to the joint reaction force. Multiple investigators have calculated patellofemoral joint reaction forces of two to five times body weight during activities of daily living. However, during squatting with knee flexion up to 120 degrees, the joint reaction force may be seven to eight times body weight. These forces in a normal knee are resisted by thick articular cartilage, but they may exceed the yield strength of polyethylene, especially in the case of edge loading, which may lead to deformation of polyethylene patellar components over time.

Many authors have described variations in the area of contact between the patella and the trochlea during knee flexion (Fig. 5.24). The inferior articular surface of the patella first contacts the trochlea in approximately 20 degrees of knee flexion. The midportion of the patella articulates with the trochlea in approximately 60 degrees of flexion, and the superior portion of the patella articulates at 90 degrees of flexion. In extreme flexion, beyond 120 degrees, the patella articulates only medially and laterally with the femoral condyles, and the quadriceps tendon articulates with the trochlea. A third articulating facet often is present on the medial aspect of the patella that articulates with the lateral aspect of the medial femoral condyle at more than 90 degrees of flexion.

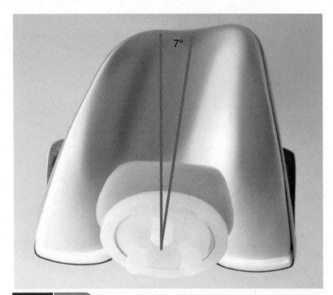

FIGURE 5.23 Built-in trochlear groove angle up to 7 degrees enhances patellar mechanics and patellar tracking.

As discussed in the earlier section on knee kinematics, the normal tibia internally rotates with respect to the femur during flexion with greater posterior translation of the lateral femoral contact point on the tibia relative to the medial femoral contact point. The net effect of this internal rotation of the tibia during flexion is to centralize the tibial tubercle in flexion or diminish the Q angle. These relationships may be altered in TKA with nonanatomic patellofemoral geometry, malrotation of the femoral and tibial components, elevation of the joint line relative to the tibial tubercle, and patella infera from patellar tendon contracture. Dennis et al. and Harman et al. noted that with multiple designs of TKA tested during fluorokinematic analyses, at least 19% had a reverse rotational pattern with deep knee bend. This indicates a need for less constraint during deep flexion to ensure that excessive implant-bone interface stresses are avoided and that the femoral component is supported in the deep flexed state without edge loading of the polyethylene insert (see Fig. 5.3D).

Changes in the patellar area of contact with flexion have a significant effect on the prosthetic patellofemoral joint. Eccentric loading of the patellofemoral joint leads to shear forces within the patellar component and at the prosthesis-bone interface (Fig. 5.25). Even if the mediolateral geometry of the patellofemoral articulation is perfectly conforming, the inferior-to-superior migration of the area of contact on the patella with increasing knee flexion leads to eccentric forces on the polyethylene patellar component. These forces may lead to failure of metal-backed patellar components, localized polyethylene wear, or component loosening.

POLYETHYLENE AND BEARING CHOICES

Ultrahigh-molecular-weight polyethylene articular surfaces have been an integral part of TKA from its conception. Catastrophic wear leading to early failure and osteolysis, although seen less frequently than in total hip arthroplasty, historically has occurred more frequently in some TKA designs. Studies of polyethylene have provided information on its varying wear characteristics after different fabrication and sterilization processes and its limitations in TKA applications. Several manufacturers have converted to utilizing

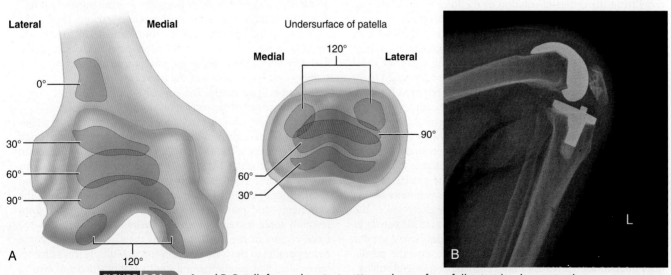

FIGURE 5.24 **A** and **B**, Patellofemoral contact patterns change from full extension (no contact) to initiating contact around 10 degrees on inferior aspect of patella and then moving superior with flexion. Past 90 degrees contact moves periphery of the patella in two different contact areas. As the knee flexes and passes 120 degrees, patella eventually may lose contact altogether.

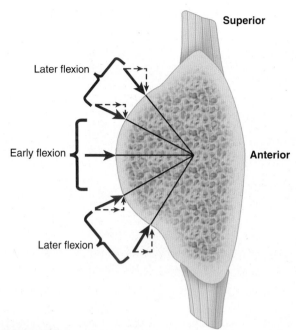

Superior

Later flexion

Early flexion

Anterior

Later flexion

Resultant forces on patellofemoral joint change with knee flexion. Eccentric loading increases shear component of resultant force (shear component is tangential or, in drawing, in vertical direction). Patellar tilt and subluxation magnify shear force.

either highly crosslinked polyethylene or polyethylene with vitamin E to improve long-term wear. Early results do seem to show a resistance to fatigue-related damage and wear.

Compared with the perfectly conforming articulations of total hip arthroplasties, the tibiofemoral articulations in modern TKA are typically less conforming, with the femoral condyles having a decreasing radius of curvature posteriorly. PCL-retaining prostheses tend to have an even greater degree of sagittal plane nonconformity because the tibial surface remains relatively flat to allow femoral rollback without excessive PCL tension. This nonconformity creates areas of high contact stress within the polyethylene that is design specific (see Fig. 5.17). Retrieval studies by various authors document polyethylene wear in areas of high contact stress. Wear is pronounced in areas of unusual stress caused by prosthesis malalignment or ligamentous imbalance. Several authors have emphasized "double dishing" as a tibial polyethylene geometry that appears to avoid areas of high contact stress. Conformity in the coronal and sagittal planes should be enough to allow stability without constraining the transverse plane or without causing edge loading (Fig. 5.26). This type of geometry also aids in condylar lift-off with designs that do not include coronal plane dishing of the individual tibial plateaus and corresponding femoral condyles.

A thinner tibial polyethylene also has been correlated with accelerated wear. Several studies have recommended a minimal polyethylene thickness of 8 mm to avoid the higher contact stresses that occur with thinner polyethylene. Retrieval studies showing accelerated wear in knees implanted with thin polyethylene have supported this recommendation. An average 10-year follow-up study showed no difference, however, in radiographic loosening, wear, or osteolysis in patients with a thin, one-piece, compression-molded, metal-backed polyethylene component (polyethylene thickness 4.4 mm) in

one knee compared with a similar, although thicker (minimal thickness 6.4 mm), tibial component in the contralateral knee. Other reports have shown that survivorship decreases with less polyethylene thickness in some designs.

Retrieval data suggest that variations in polyethylene quality are partly responsible for reports of accelerated wear in the past. Landy and Walker found delamination only in areas of polyethylene that contained granular fusion defects. Whether ram extrusion with subsequent machining or direct compression molding of the components is the optimal polyethylene manufacturing process is debatable. Various manufacturers are attempting to improve the wear characteristics of polyethylene either by reprocessing bar stock purchased commercially to achieve a higher degree of uniformity within the polymer or by compression molding their own implants in an inert gas environment. Newer indications for TKA revision surgery have now been reported by Sharkey et al., and wear and osteolysis as reported more than a decade ago have fallen from the top of the list.

Polyethylene "enhancements" do not always improve the survivorship of their associated total knee components. In the mid-1980s, carbon fiber–reinforced polyethylene was introduced with the hope of improving wear characteristics of standard ultrahigh-molecular-weight polyethylene (Fig. 5.27). This polyethylene was available for a brief period before it was withdrawn from the market because of accelerated and catastrophic wear. A dark carbon staining of the synovium can be seen at revision arthroplasty in knees with carbon fiber–reinforced polyethylene. Another unsuccessful polyethylene modification was the process of heat-pressing the prosthetic articular surface after the insert had been milled in an attempt to create a very smooth articular surface. This process led to a physical transition zone 1 mm beneath the articular surface of the polyethylene, which is in a region of high subsurface stress concentration. This coincidence in some early porous-coated anatomic knees, along with an articular geometry that was characterized by high contact stresses, led to a high rate of failure because of polyethylene delamination (Fig. 5.28), particularly with thin polyethylene.

The method of polyethylene implant sterilization can affect polyethylene properties, with evidence that gamma radiation in an oxygen environment causes detrimental effects that can hasten polyethylene wear. Over a period of years, a subsurface white band appears in polyethylene sterilized in this manner (Fig. 5.29). This occurs even in prostheses that have not been implanted and represents an area of high oxidation and chain scission within the polyethylene. McGovern et al. reported a failure rate of 49% at 18 months after surgery in a series of UKAs sterilized by gamma radiation in an air environment and stored preoperatively for 4.4 years or more before implantation. They found an inverse relationship between the shelf life of the tibial components (after sterilization but before implantation) and the time to revision surgery. Removed components showed high degrees of oxidation, wear, and fragmentation. Alternative approaches to prevent accelerated oxidation include radiation sterilization and packaging in an inert gas environment and sterilization by ethylene oxide or gas plasma.

The introduction of highly crosslinked polyethylene produced by high-dose gamma irradiation with subsequent annealing has produced dramatic decreases in wear in simulated hip and knee studies. Many authors caution, however, that the wear mechanisms in the knee are different from the mechanisms in the hip, and that highly crosslinked

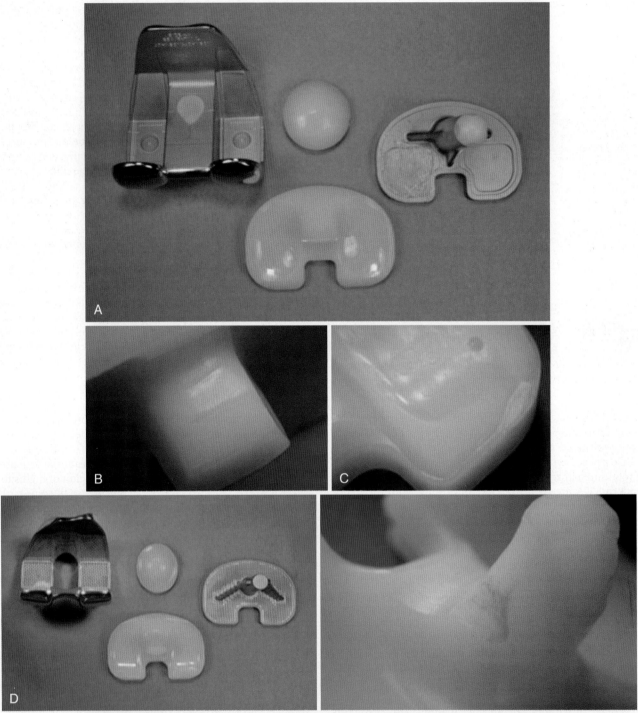

FIGURE 5.26 Retrieved implants. **A,** Posterior-stabilized total knee system at time of necropsy. **B,** Posterior wear scars are evident on post from articulation with cam. **C,** There is evidence of posterior edge-loading from posterior femoral condyles or possibly retained osteophytes. **D,** Anterior post wear can occur from anterior box impinging on anterior post in full extension as seen in this example of retrieval study.

polyethylene may not be beneficial in TKA applications, especially when a PS implant is used with a post-cam bearing surface that is under higher shear than the tibiofemoral articulation. Some manufacturers have introduced the use of vitamin E–stabilized polyethylene in their knee replacement lines to correct the possible issue related to highly crosslinked polyethylene. Although mechanical studies have shown the benefits of vitamin E polyethylene with decreased wear properties in vitro, it remains to be seen whether this will translate into improved wear in vivo in the long term. The fact that an updated publication has indicated that wear and osteolysis have dropped from the top of the list may mean that we are on the right track with updated polyethylene formulas and sterilization techniques.

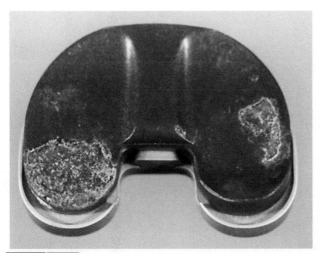

FIGURE 5.27 Reinforcement of tibial polyethylene with carbon fiber often led to rapid wear and failure.

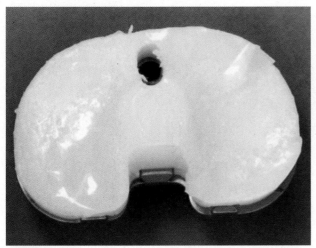

FIGURE 5.28 Process of heat pressing of early porous-coated anatomic tibial polyethylene led to early delamination from subsurface oxidation.

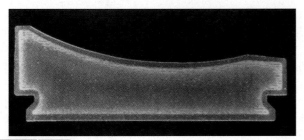

FIGURE 5.29 Subsurface white band appears over time in polyethylene sterilized by gamma radiation in oxygen environment.

Some surgeons advocate alternative bearing surfaces in primary TKA. One type of bearing surface available is oxidized zirconium on the femoral components as a means to reduce polyethylene wear. This technology incorporates a zirconium oxide ceramic coating on a zirconium metal alloy femoral component. Developers claim that this surface is more scratch resistant than cobalt chrome, lessening wear debris from the polyethylene tibial articular surface.

Ezzet et al. showed a 42% wear volume reduction in a knee simulator at 5 million cycles using this device. Other alternative bearing surfaces on the femoral side of the knee are now being introduced to decrease polyethylene wear. These include solid ceramic femoral components (still under FDA investigational trials) and zirconium or titanium nitride types of coatings; however, not all zirconium or titanium nitride coatings are the same since monolayer types of coating can be susceptible to mechanical ablation, and the surface can peel off the substrate metal layer through an eggshell effect wherein the underlying substrate is much softer than the thin coating. Using a multilayer coating as one implant manufacturer does with a top layer of zirconium nitride can combat this eggshell effect (Aesculap Inc.). Other manufacturers utilize a transformed layer of the surface alloy as with some titanium nitride or oxidized zirconium options.

The use of a modular metal-alloy baseplate backing for tibial polyethylene inserts became standard in the early 1980s. Multiple studies stated theoretical advantages of metal backing, including more even distribution of weight-bearing stresses to the underlying fixation interface and cancellous bone and a reduction in the potential polyethylene deformity caused by creep. A multisurgeon, multiprosthesis study of 9200 knee arthroplasties showed a 98% 5-year survivorship of knees with metal backing of the tibial polyethylene compared with 94% survivorship of knees with all-polyethylene tibial components. A Hospital for Special Surgery study reported a 97% 7-year survival of all-polyethylene, PS tibial components and a 99% 7-year survival of metal-backed components. In a more recent review of the literature concerning cruciate condylar TKAs, there were no significant differences, however, in prosthesis survival or periprosthetic lucencies between metal-backed tibial polyethylene and all-polyethylene tibial components. Similar survival rates of 98% have been reported for all-polyethylene and metal-backed tibial components in patients older than 80 years old at the time of surgery, suggesting that one-piece, all-polyethylene, cemented tibial components of sufficient thickness may be appropriate for use in low-demand, elderly patients.

COMPONENT FIXATION

Prosthetic fixation in TKA with polymethyl methacrylate (PMMA) has consistently shown long-term durability. Cementless fixation with bone ingrowth has been less reliable in long-term studies, however, with a few notable exceptions. The more successful cementless TKA designs typically have multiple attributes to attain baseplate stability while ingrowth occurs (Figs. 5.30 and 5.31).

Retrieval analysis of some failed cementless implants has shown little, if any, bony ingrowth into tibial trays removed at the time of component revision. The bony ingrowth that did occur tended to be centered around fixation screws. Other reports of bony ingrowth have been more favorable. In 13 Miller-Galante prostheses removed for reasons other than loosening or infection, the average area of bone ingrowth was 27% of the available porous surface. They found a propensity for bone ingrowth in the region of fixation screws and pegs and in the anterior half of the tray. They postulated that the area of bony ingrowth necessary for stable fixation may be significantly less than 100%.

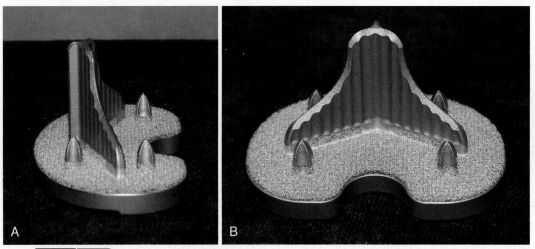

FIGURE 5.30 The press-fit Triathlon total knee implant (Stryker, Mahwah, NJ) tibial baseplate has a 3-D printed porous ingrowth surface to allow bony ingrowth and spiked press-fit pegs for added stability.

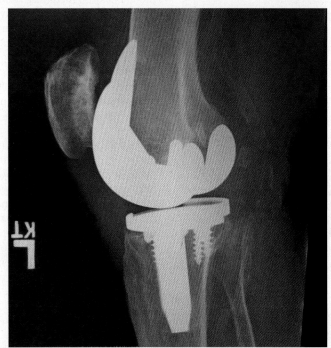

FIGURE 5.31 Cementless Profix knee (Smith & Nephew, Memphis, TN) uses metaphyseal stem and keel with multiple screws to provide necessary initial fixation for bone ingrowth.

Clinically, many of the early cementless TKA systems had poor survival rates because of associated failure of metal-backed patellar components. Even discounting this factor, however, a 72% 10-year survivorship was reported with a cementless press-fit condylar design (Johnson & Johnson, Raynham, MA) compared with a 94% 10-year survivorship with similar cemented TKA. These results are being improved on as newer designs are now showing similar survivorship in the short term. A recent study on a medial pivot CR-designed implant in 54 patients showed 100% survival at 9 years in both cemented and cementless baseplates. A recent review of the literature also concluded that newer designs have had excellent results but cautioned that longer follow-up studies were necessary.

There are some notable exceptions in earlier press-fit designs with excellent long-term success. The Ortholoc (Wright Medical, Arlington, TN) prosthesis was reported to have one loosening in 184 knees followed for a minimum of 15 years, and the cementless LCS rotating platform knee was reported to have a survivorship of 98% at 18 years. Because of the importance of adequate initial fixation of cementless implants, stems with keels and multiple screws have been incorporated into the design of modern cementless tibial baseplates (see Figs. 5.30 and 5.31). A purported advantage of a biologic interface over cemented fixation is its durability, reported to result in better long-term pain relief; however, excellent long-term durability of cement fixation has been reported. Despite claims that cementless fixation may be more durable over time, most authors believe cemented fixation has produced more uniformly reliable long-term fixation with less osteolysis in multiple prosthesis designs. This belief is supported by the Swedish National Registry data, which showed that cementless designs had a 1.4 times higher rate of revision than did cemented designs.

Modular stems that engage the diaphyseal bone on the femur and the tibia are used for revision when there is bone loss and when components with varus-valgus constraint are used. These stems typically are press-fit in cementless reconstructions and either cemented or press-fit when the articular portion of the prosthesis is cemented. Because of deformity and anatomic variations, the stems occasionally need to be offset to achieve alignment.

Newer three-dimensional printed ingrowth surfaces are being used, and there has been a resurgence in popularity of cementless fixation for primary knee replacement. With the success of newer designs and ingrowth surfaces noted in primary total hip replacement, adopting these into modern knee implants is a logical next step as biologic interface should become more robust over a longer time period.

INDICATIONS AND CONTRAINDICATIONS
TOTAL KNEE ARTHROPLASTY

The primary indication for TKA is to relieve pain caused by severe arthritis, with or without significant deformity. Other sources of knee and leg pain must be sought and systematically excluded. These include radicular pain from spinal disease, referred pain from the ipsilateral hip pathology, peripheral vascular disease, meniscal pathology, and bursitis of the knee. Radiographic findings must correlate with a clear clinical impression of knee arthritis. Before surgery is considered, conservative treatment measures should be exhausted, including physical therapy, antiinflammatory medications, intraarticular injections, activity modifications, and the use of a cane for ambulation. Patients who do not have complete cartilage space loss before surgery tend to be less satisfied with their clinical result after TKA.

Because knee replacement has a finite expected survival that is adversely affected by activity level, it generally is indicated in older patients with more sedentary lifestyles. It also is clearly indicated in younger patients who have a significant functional impairment from OA or from other pathologic causes such as systemic arthritis with multiple joint involvement or osteonecrosis with subchondral collapse of a femoral condyle. Severe pain from chondrocalcinosis and pseudogout in an elderly patient is an occasional indication for arthroplasty in the absence of complete cartilage space loss. Occasionally, severe patellofemoral arthritis in an elderly patient may justify TKA because the expected outcome of arthroplasty is better than that of patellectomy or patellofemoral replacement in these patients.

Deformity can become the principal indication for arthroplasty in patients with moderate or severe arthritis and variable levels of pain when the progression of deformity begins to threaten the expected outcome of an anticipated arthroplasty. As a flexion contracture progresses beyond 20 degrees, gait is significantly hampered and difficulty with regaining extension may warrant surgical intervention. Similarly, as

varus or valgus laxity becomes severe, a constrained condylar type of prosthesis may become necessary to prevent subsequent coronal plane instability. Intervening before this degree of laxity is present allows the use of a prosthesis that lacks coronal plane constraint and has a more favorable expected survivorship.

Absolute contraindications to TKA include recent or current knee sepsis; a remote source of ongoing infection; extensor mechanism discontinuity or severe dysfunction; recurvatum deformity secondary to neuromuscular weakness; and the presence of a painless, well-functioning knee arthrodesis. Relative contraindications are numerous and debatable and include medical conditions that compromise the patient's ability to withstand anesthesia, the metabolic demands of surgery and wound healing, immunodeficiency, and the significant rehabilitation necessary to ensure a favorable functional outcome. A severely osteoarthritic ipsilateral hip joint also should be considered for arthroplasty before the symptomatic osteoarthritic knee, because rehabilitation is easier with a total hip arthroplasty and an osteoarthritic knee than with a TKA and an osteoarthritic hip joint. Other relative contraindications include significant atherosclerotic disease of the operative leg, skin conditions such as psoriasis within the operative field, venous stasis disease with recurrent cellulitis, neuropathic arthropathy, superobesity (BMI ≥ 45), recurrent urinary tract infections, and a history of osteomyelitis in the proximity of the knee. This list is not all inclusive, and any preoperative condition that can adversely affect the patient's outcome can be considered a relative contraindication.

Outcome studies have now shown that patient optimization is key to ensuring the best chance of a good long-term outcome. Certain modifiable risk factors should be considered before elective TKA, including low vitamin D levels, metabolic syndrome (MetS), low albumin, neutropenia, superobesity, and a BMI less than 20. The current AAOS Clinical Practice Guidelines on Knee Osteoarthritis Treatment states that delaying primary TKA for up to 8 months while a patient works to improve a modifiable risk factor does not appear to worsen the outcome. A recent review noted an increasing rise in infection and other complications as obesity classification increased from severe to super-obese. Although these issues need to be weighted by the surgeon, quality of life in superobese individuals can be attained cost effectively and without a higher incidence of early aseptic loosening.

UNICONDYLAR KNEE ARTHROPLASTY

UKA is being selected for increasing numbers of patients, particularly with minimally invasive techniques that allow overnight hospital stays or outpatient procedures. Ten-year follow-up studies of two designs of UKA, the Oxford mobile bearing knee (Biomet Orthopaedics, Warsaw, IN) and the Miller-Galante knee (Zimmer, Warsaw, IN), have shown survivorship approaching that of TKA. Newer techniques are now available, including robotic-arm–assisted surgical procedures. These procedures involve preoperative computed tomographic studies for determining appropriate component sizing and accurate positioning of the implants. Many of the studies of UKA were conducted in older patients, and many authors doubted that the survivorship of UKA into the second decade would parallel the survivorship of TKA. A long-term survivorship analysis of over 500 medial compartment

Oxford meniscal-bearing unicompartmental arthroplasties, however, found a 10-year survivorship of 94% and a 20-year survivorship of 91%, indicating that the implant remains durable into the second decade.

UKA currently is advocated for different reasons in two patient populations. The first patient group for whom UKA has been advocated comprises elderly, thin individuals with unicompartmental disease who would otherwise undergo TKA. The suggested benefits of UKA over TKA are a shorter rehabilitation time; a greater average postoperative range of motion; and preservation of the proprioceptive function of the cruciate ligaments, which give a more natural-feeling knee. The procedure can be done with a shorter hospital stay and with less blood loss. The argument in this patient group is that a UKA is a less invasive procedure that has a good likelihood of lasting the patient's lifetime. Berger et al. reported a 10-year survivorship of 98% with a cemented UKA design in older patients using stringent selection criteria. UKA should not be considered in an elderly patient who has evidence of arthritis in more than one compartment of the knee unless there are medical contraindications to TKA.

The second group currently considered for UKA comprises younger individuals with unicompartmental disease in whom UKA is used as a "first" arthroplasty, usually instead of high tibial osteotomy (HTO) in patients with isolated medial compartment arthritis. This indication is becoming more prevalent with the increasing popularity of minimally invasive surgery and the increasing demands of patients and higher BMIs of the general population. Although this is a frequently stated indication for UKA, few studies that have been published to date have reported results in this patient group. One study described an 11-year survivorship of 92% in patients younger than 60 years old, with another 22% showing progression of the unresurfaced compartment, although not requiring revision at the time of follow-up.

There has been continued discussion concerning whether the patellofemoral compartment should be a determining factor in the decision to perform a UKA. One recent study pointed out that patellofemoral congruence is improved after UKA and that this may be the reason for reports of good outcomes after UKA done for patellofemoral osteoarthritis (OA). The type of bearing used in medial compartment arthroplasty also has been debated, with many advocating the use of a mobile-bearing UKA. A recent study found that the difficulty of revision surgery is comparable, regardless of the bearing used. In this series mobile-bearing UKA required more medial augments for conversion to primary TKA.

It has been suggested that UKA is a bone-sparing operation that would allow an uncomplicated revision later, but earlier studies of failed UKA did not show this anticipated benefit, with significant bone grafting, tibial wedges, or long-stem components necessary in nearly half of revisions and major osseous defects in 76% of knees. With more contemporary UKAs, the need for structural grafts is rare and results of revision approach those of primary TKA. In a matched retrospective review, the results of revision of a failed UKA to TKA were slightly worse than conversion of a previous HTO to TKA. The selection of UKA or HTO in this patient population remains unclear because many studies have cited difficulties with exposure and slightly less satisfactory clinical outcomes with TKA after previous HTO compared with primary TKA.

Another argument favoring TKA over UKA is the unfamiliarity of many surgeons with UKA. According to Stern, Becker, and Insall, only 6% of patients needing arthroplasty have none of the contraindications to UKA. Because the success of the procedure is dictated by the technical performance of the operation, surgeons who rarely perform UKA may have difficulty reproducing the reported results from large reconstructive centers. Gioe and Bowman described an 89% 10-year survivorship for UKA performed in a community hospital setting compared with a 95% survivorship of TKA done in the same time period. A recent review of patient-reported outcomes after both UKA and TKA from a large European registry found no significant differences between the two groups; however, some registries have reported higher short-term and mid-term revision rates with UKA. Another report pointed out that superior outcomes typically have been reported by high-volume centers and surgeons, which raises concerns about poorer outcomes with low-volume surgeons and centers. A recent systematic review also pointed out slightly better results in patients with UKA but confirmed higher revision rates. Another review reported no detrimental effects of preexisting patellofemoral disease on 10-year outcomes.

Although the certain indications for UKA are debatable, the contraindications are fairly well defined: inflammatory arthritis, a flexion contracture of 15 degrees or more, a preoperative arc of motion of less than 90 degrees, angular deformity of more than 10 degrees from the mechanical axis for varus knees or 5 degrees for valgus knees, significant cartilaginous erosion in the weight-bearing areas of the opposite compartment, and anterior cruciate ligament deficiency. Obesity also has been cited as a relative contraindication to UKA.

PATELLOFEMORAL ARTHROPLASTY

Although historically controversial, new interest in patellofemoral arthroplasty over the past few years has been fueled by contemporary implant designs that have produced improved clinical outcomes. First-generation designs failed because of narrow trochlear grooves and high constraint, which often produced maltracking, patellar catching, or persistent anterior knee pain. Despite improvements in the current designs, the most common reason for failure of the second-generation implants is progression of tibiofemoral arthritis, making careful patient selection the key to a successful outcome. The use of custom-designed implants to allow the least amount of bone loss has been reported. These implants, although more expensive than the off-the-shelf sizing that most manufacturers offer, are being reported to have excellent outcomes and short-term to mid-term survivorship.

The ideal candidate for patellofemoral arthroplasty is a patient who is younger than 65 years of age and has debilitating, isolated patellofemoral arthritis with minimal coronal deformity; pain during daily activities is localized to the patellofemoral joint and has not responded to nonsteroidal antiinflammatory medications or injection. Patellofemoral arthroplasty is recommended for isolated patellofemoral OA to provide a conservative, bone-sparing alternative to TKA, which may not have as good patient satisfaction in young, active patients. A recent report indicated that conversion of a patellofemoral arthroplasty is comparable to performing a primary TKA. Parratte et al. compared 21 patellofemoral arthroplasty conversions to TKA with 21 primary and revision TKAs. Although there were more complications in the patellofemoral arthroplasty conversion group, this was not comparable to the revision cohort. To date there are no published studies showing that outcomes of patellofemoral arthroplasty are age dependent. All of these considerations should be taken into account before offering a patellofemoral arthroplasty over a TKA.

Good results have been reported after patellofemoral arthroplasty in patients with posttraumatic arthritis, primary patellofemoral OA, and patellofemoral dysplasia without malalignment. In patients with posttraumatic arthritis, patellofemoral arthroplasty may be considered as an alternative to patellectomy. Primary patellofemoral arthritis includes Outerbridge type IV chondromalacia of the patella or trochlea or both. Note that progression of tibiofemoral arthritis is more frequent with primary OA than with posttraumatic arthritis or patellofemoral dysplasia. Malalignment is most often determined using the quadriceps angle (Q angle). Angles of more than 15 degrees in men and 20 degrees in women are considered abnormal. Any condition that increases the Q angle increases the lateral displacement forces on the patella and may lead to subluxation or dislocation. Patellofemoral arthroplasty alone cannot correct patellar malalignment and/or instability. Malalignment and/or instability of the patellofemoral joint is not an indication for the procedure. Mild patellar tilt or subluxation can be corrected at the time of patellofemoral arthroplasty with lateral retinacular release, medialization of the patellar component, and possibly partial lateral facetectomy. Malalignment should be corrected before or during patellofemoral arthroplasty. No particular patellar or trochlear wear pattern has been determined to be a contraindication to patellofemoral arthroplasty, unlike various tubercle osteotomy procedures. Lateral and inferior patellar facet lesions in younger patients can be treated with anterior medialization of the tibial tubercle. A recent analysis showed that patients with trochlear dysplasia tend to have an internally rotated placement of the trochlear groove and that patellofemoral arthroplasty can compensate for this pathologic alignment.

Progression of tibiofemoral arthritis is the most common reason for revision to TKA, emphasizing that tibiofemoral arthrosis is a principal contraindication to patellofemoral arthroplasty. Inflammatory arthropathies involve the entire joint and currently are a contraindication to patellofemoral arthroplasty because of progressive tibiofemoral arthritis and painful synovitis. This includes chondrocalcinosis, which can be indicative of an inflammatory arthropathy and can lead to altered joint mechanics because of abnormal menisci.

Patellofemoral arthroplasty also is not indicated in patients with severe coronal deformity of the knee (valgus of more than 8 degrees or varus of more than 5 degrees) unless the deformity is corrected by osteotomy before arthroplasty. Flexion of 120 degrees in the sagittal plane, with less than 10 degrees of flexion contracture, is recommended as long as the flexion contracture is not caused by OA in the medial or lateral compartment of the knee. Knee joint stiffness should be carefully assessed because this patient population has a high rate of previous surgery that increases the frequency of arthrofibrosis and patellar height abnormalities. Patients with patella baja from quadriceps muscle atrophy or patellar tendon scarring are not good candidates for patellofemoral

arthroplasty. Although few data exist correlating the outcome of patellofemoral arthroplasty with BMI, currently it is not recommended in obese patients because of concerns about overloading of the implant. A recent study showed a higher rate of revision to TKA in obese patients (BMI > 30) than in nonobese patients, whereas primary diagnosis, age, or sex did not significantly affect the revision rate.

Reported results of patellofemoral arthroplasty indicate that it provides excellent pain relief and functional improvement and is a reliable alternative to TKA for the treatment of patellofemoral arthritis in carefully selected patients (Fig. 5.32). Good-to-excellent 3- to 17-year results have been reported in 66% to 100% of patients (Table 5.1); less mean blood loss, shorter hospital stays, and better functional outcomes have been reported in patients with patellofemoral arthroplasty compared to those in patients with TKA. Recent studies, however, have found that revision rates after conversion of a patellofemoral arthroplasty to a TKA are higher than revision rates for a primary TKA. These findings should be considered when making decisions concerning the possible effectiveness of patellofemoral replacement (see Table 5.1).

INDICATIONS AND CONSIDERATIONS FOR PATELLAR RESURFACING IN PRIMARY TOTAL KNEE ARTHROPLASTY

The role of universal patellar resurfacing in TKA is somewhat controversial, with some advocating it because of clinical series indicating that knee scores after patellar resurfacing are slightly better because of less residual peripatellar pain and improved quadriceps strength. In a large retrospective study, patellofemoral complications occurred in 4% of patients with patellar resurfacing compared with 12% of patients in whom the patella was unresurfaced. Significant residual anterior knee pain was the most common complication in the unresurfaced group. A 5-year prospective, randomized study of a single knee design found that 25% of patients with unresurfaced patellas complained of anterior knee pain, whereas only 5% of patients with patellar resurfacing complained of anterior knee pain. Secondary resurfacing of the patella for residual anterior knee pain after TKA has been studied by various authors who found that pain relief after secondary resurfacing was inferior to what would be expected with primary resurfacing and found a higher rate of complications, including patellar fracture and postoperative stiffness.

Other authors have advocated selective resurfacing of the patella. The major argument in favor of selective resurfacing of the patella is that complications of resurfaced patellae account for most of the reoperations after TKA in many series. Also, with selective resurfacing of the patella, using a femoral component that incorporates an anatomically shaped femoral trochlea, essentially equal knee scores have been reported for resurfaced and unresurfaced groups. Prospective studies comparing TKA with and without patellar resurfacing have found no significant differences in patient preferences, functional scores, anterior knee pain, or revision rates. However, these reports have found that those with an unresurfaced patella who have secondary procedures for resurfacing are not always satisfied after secondary resurfacing. This has led some to suggest that anterior knee pain after TKA is related more to component design and proper alignment in the transverse plane than to patellar retention or resurfacing. A recent report from the Australian registry on selective

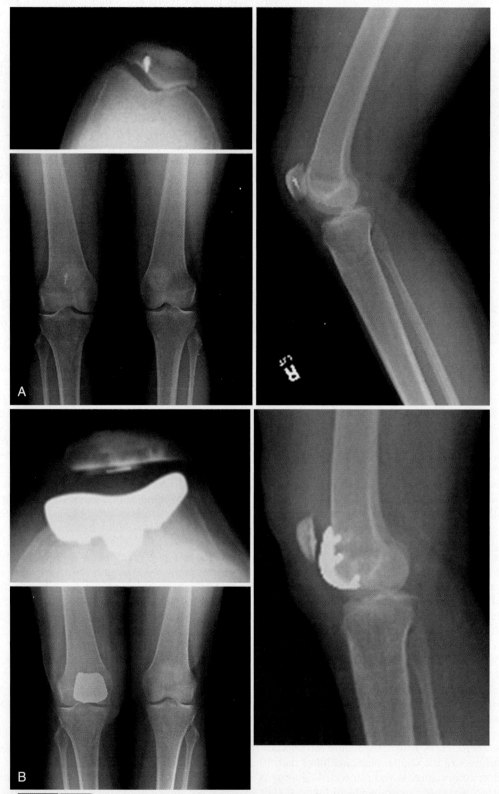

FIGURE 5.32 **A,** Preoperative radiograph of patient who had medial patellofemoral ligament repair for patellar maltracking after dislocation; overtightening caused medial facet arthropathy. **B,** Results of patellofemoral arthroplasty were excellent at 6 weeks, with pain-free range of motion and no pain with full squat maneuver.

TABLE 5.1

Reported Results of Patellofemoral Arthroplasty

AUTHOR(S), YEAR	NO. PATIENTS (KNEES)	IMPLANT	FOLLOW-UP	OUTCOME
de Winter et al., 2001	24 (26)	Richards II (Smith & Nephew, Memphis, TN)	11 years	76% excellent/good results
Tauro et al., 2001	48 (62)	Lubinus (Waldemar Link, Hamburg, Germany)	7.5 years	65% survivorship
Smith et al., 2002	34 (45)	Lubinus	4 years	64% excellent/good results
Kooijman et al., 2003	51 (56)	Richards	17 years	86% excellent/good results
Board et al., 2004	17	Lubinus	19 months	53% satisfactory results
Merchant, 2004	15	LCS (DePuy, Warsaw, IN)	3.75 years	93% excellent/good results
Cartier et al., 2005	70 (79)	Richards II and III	10 years	75% survivorship Main cause of failure: osteoarthritic degeneration of tibiofemoral joint (8 TKAs)
Ackroyd and Chir, 2005	240 (306)	Avon (Stryker Howmedica Osteonics, Mahwah, NJ)	2-5 years	Revision to TKA required in 3.5% of patients because of progression of tibiofemoral arthritis
Argenson et al., 2005	66	Autocentric (DePuy, Warsaw, IN)	16 years	58% survivorship Revision to TKA in 29: tibiofemoral arthritis in 14, loosening in 11, and stiffness in 4
Sisto and Sarin, 2006	22 (25)	Kinematch (Kinamed, Camarillo, CA)	6 years	100% excellent/good results
Ackroyd et al., 2007	85 (109)	Avon	5 years	96% 5-year survivorship Main complication—radiographic progression of arthritis (28%)
Mohammed et al., 2008	91 (101)	Avon Lubinus FPV (Wright Medical, UK)	4 years	72% "did very well"—did not require subsequent surgery Conversion to TKA—3 patients with progressive arthritis, 1 with infection
Leadbetter et al., 2009	70 (79)	Avon (second generation)	3 years	90% without pain in daily activity and stair climbing 84% with Knee Society Scores of more than 80 points 7.5% revision to TKA
van Wagenberg et al., 2009	20 (24)	Autocentric II (DePuy, Warsaw, IN)	4 years	Additional surgery needed in 21 knees (87.5%) Conversion to TKA in 7 (29%), primarily for progressive tibiofemoral osteoarthritis and patellar maltracking
van Jonbergen et al., 2010	161 (185)	Richards II	13 years	84% survivorship at 10 years, 69% at 20 years Tibiofemoral arthritis in 45%, conversion to TKA in 13% Revision more frequent in obese patients
Dahm et al., 2010	23 PFA 22 TKA	Avon	28 months	Knee Society Scores: 89 PFA, 90 TKA UCLA Scores: 6.6 PFA, 4.2 TKA Mean blood loss and hospital stay significantly lower in PFA
Odumenya et al., 2010	32 (50)	Avon	5.3 years	100% survivorship at 5 years Main complication—progression of disease (22%)
Charalambous et al., 2011	35 (51)	LCS	2 years	Estimated 3-year survival rate 63%

Continued

TABLE 5.1

Reported Results of Patellofemoral Arthroplasty—cont'd

AUTHOR(S), YEAR	NO. PATIENTS (KNEES)	IMPLANT	FOLLOW-UP	OUTCOME
Mont et al., 2012	37 (43)	Avon	7 years	5-year survivorship 95%, 7-year survivorship 82% Conversion to TKA in 5 knees
Yadav et al., 2012	49 (51)	LCS	4 years	High revision rate (20%) 7-point improvement in Oxford Knee Score Estimated survival rate 73% at 4.5 years, 48% at 5.5 years
Morris et al., 2013	30 (37)	Vanguard (26) Gender Solutions (15) Kinematch (4) Other? (2)	31 months	All Knee Society Pain, Functional, and Clinical scores improved. Two complications (arthrofibrosis, painful crepitus) Overall revision rate at short-term 97%
Davies, 2013	52	Femoro-Patella Vialla (FPV)	1 year	Oxford Knee Scores improved 30 points, American Knee Society Scores 51 points, and function scores 28 points. 21% had little improvement (knees similar to or worse than before surgery). Early revision rate high: 7 (13%) revisions to TKA
Hernigou, Caton, 2014	70	Hermes	10 years	No late complications Disease progression in 5 patients; 3 required revision Persistent anterior knee pain in 4
Al-Hadithy et al., 2014	41 (53)	Femoro-Patella Vialla	3 years	Progression of OA in 12% Oxford Knee Scores improved 18 points; good pain relief 2 revisions to TKA at 7 months
Goh et al., 2015	51 (51)	SIGMA HP Partial Knee	4 years	All functional scores improved significantly; 76% satisfied 2 wound infections (4%) Survivorship 92%; 4 revisions
Akhbari et al., 2015	57 (61)	Avon	5 years	Significant improvements in functional scores 2 revisions
Kazarian et al., 2016	53 (70)	Gender Solutions	5 years	ROM and functional scores improved significantly. <4% revision rate Less than 2/3 of patients satisfied; dissatisfied patients had lower Mental Health Scores on SF-36

LCS, Low-contact stress; *OA,* osteoarthritis; *PFA,* patellofemoral arthroplasty; *ROM,* range of motion; *SF-36,* Medical Outcomes Study Questionnaire Short Form 36; *SIGMA HP,* SIGMA High Performance; *TKA,* total knee arthroplasty.

resurfacing found a higher rate of revision compared to those who routinely resurface the patella.

The desirability of resurfacing continues to be debated, and the results of selective patellar resurfacing seem to be dependent on the design of the trochlear groove, with a native patella articulating within an anatomic trochlear groove giving results similar to those of TKA with resurfacing of the patella. Suggested indications for leaving the patella unresurfaced are a primary diagnosis of OA, satisfactory patellar cartilage with no eburnated bone, congruent patellofemoral tracking, a normal anatomic patellar shape, and no evidence of crystalline or inflammatory arthropathy. A report using a similar implant with a resurfaced patella on one knee and

an unresurfaced patella on the contralateral side found that patients could not discern a difference.

Patient weight also seems to be a factor, with lighter patients tending to do well with unresurfaced patellae. This may be one factor in the trend to routinely leave the native patella seen in the European literature. Some have suggested that resurfacing the patella in "super-obese" patients (BMI ≥ 50) may overload the sesamoid bone and be a generator of pain, but no clinical series has been published showing a difference in pain scores in this patient population and lighter-weight patients. A report of the Australian registry indicated that PS TKA designs with unresurfaced patellae had higher revision rates after surgery than those with resurfaced patellae.

They found that the minimally constrained (CR) designs with resurfaced patellae had the lowest rate of revision followed by PS designs with resurfaced patellae. In addition, onlay resurfacing fared better than inlay patellar designed buttons. Another report determined that resurfacing was cost effective based on the number of revisions reported after unresurfaced TKA.

INDICATIONS AND CONSIDERATIONS FOR SIMULTANEOUS BILATERAL TOTAL KNEE ARTHROPLASTY

Numerous studies in the literature have documented the safety and cost effectiveness of simultaneous bilateral TKA compared with separate staged procedures. With respect to cost, simultaneous bilateral procedures can reduce hospital charges by 58% compared with staged procedures because of overall decreases in operative time and total length of hospital stay. Lane et al. questioned, however, if this is a true savings because 89% of their patients with bilateral TKA required an additional rehabilitation hospital stay, whereas only 45% of their patients with unilateral TKA required rehabilitation hospital stays. Other outcomes, as measured by infection rate, knee scores, and radiographic criteria, have been similar between the two groups.

Controversy continues regarding the relative incidences of complications in simultaneous and staged procedures. Various studies have shown total blood loss to be equal in the two groups, whereas others have shown significantly more blood loss with simultaneous procedures. A greater degree of postoperative thrombocytopenia the second day after surgery and more frequent deep vein thrombosis (DVT) and pulmonary embolism (PE) also have been reported after simultaneous procedures, but many other authors reported similar or lower rates of DVT and PE after simultaneous bilateral TKA than after staged procedures.

Fat embolism is a risk of TKA when intramedullary stems or alignment devices are used, and the risk of clinically significant fat embolism syndrome probably is increased with simultaneous bilateral TKA. Dorr et al. found a 12% prevalence of fat embolism syndrome with simultaneous bilateral TKA, as documented by neurologic changes with hypoxemia. Other authors found no differences in the occurrence of clinically significant fat embolism between the two groups. Venting of the intramedullary canal with fluted intramedullary alignment rods and a slightly enlarged entrance hole for intramedullary alignment rod insertion have been recommended to decrease the risk of fat embolism syndrome.

In considering patients for simultaneous bilateral TKA, comorbidities and physiologic age should be considered because significant cardiopulmonary disease may sway the surgeon toward unilateral procedures. An increased risk of cardiovascular and neurologic complications has been noted in patients older than 70 years undergoing simultaneous bilateral TKA. No increased risks of complications with bilateral TKA have been identified in patients with a BMI of 30 or more compared with those with a lower BMI. An analysis of over 4 million hospital discharges over a 14-year period compared unilateral, bilateral, and revision TKA procedures and found that bilateral TKA had higher complication and mortality rates than either unilateral or revision TKA. Before choosing staged or simultaneous TKA procedures, each patient should be carefully evaluated, considering his or her age, cardiac risk factors, and other comorbidities. The risks associated with both approaches should be thoroughly discussed with the patient before a choice is made (Video 5.3). Newer reports have been mixed concerning whether bilateral versus staged TKA is cost effective, and it appears that this should not currently have a bearing on the decision-making process. Other reports have shown that bilateral primary TKA surgery is as safe as simultaneous TKA in the right patient population.

CONSIDERATIONS FOR OUTPATIENT KNEE JOINT ARTHROPLASTY

Many centers have now begun to offer outpatient surgery for both TKA and UKA. To safely accomplish this, a complete team setup is required, including office staff, operating room personnel, anesthesia, physical therapy, and ancillary providers. The use of tranexamic acid to reduce the need for blood transfusion also has helped provide a safer path to ambulatory surgery joint replacement. Pain modalities, including intraarticular injections with liposomal encased or plain bupivacaine with or without the addition of Toradol, morphine, and dexamethasone also have helped provide adequate pain relief in the immediate postoperative period to allow centers to successfully and safely perform knee joint arthroplasty procedures in the ambulatory or 23-hour setting (see section on pain management modalities). A visit to a center that has a successful program is helpful before implementing a short-stay/ambulatory arthroplasty program. Having a program that educates patients on the process so that they and their immediate family or caregivers understand what to expect can be beneficial. Using a family member as a "joint coach" has also been shown to be beneficial, with education being a key to success and patient satisfaction.

RESULTS OF PRIMARY TOTAL KNEE ARTHROPLASTY
FUNCTIONAL AND RADIOGRAPHIC OUTCOME MEASURES

Over the past 3 decades the most popular knee rating systems have been those of the Hospital for Special Surgery and the Knee Society. The Knee Society released a knee rating system in 1989 and updated it in 2011 (Box 5.1). Because of increased patient demands and expectations over the past 2 decades, this latest update has been tailored to incorporate patient-specific activities and patient-perceived expectations. The updated system now consists of preoperative and postoperative objective measurements recorded by the surgeon and patient-driven measures evaluated by patients concerning their perceptions of the most important and deleterious aspects of their knee arthritis and replacement surgery.

The first parts of the score include patient demographics and the patient's Charnley functional score. The objective measures and knee score (out of 100 points depending on range of motion measures) include alignment and instability, which account for up to 50 points. The patient's range of motion is considered by giving one point for each 5 degrees of total measured arc of motion, with deductions taken for flexion contracture and extension lag. The next part of the score takes into account patient-perceived measures including symptoms, satisfaction concerning pain and function during daily activities (40 points), and expectations after

BOX 5.1

Knee Society Scoring System (2011)

Objective Knee Score (7 Items, 100 Points)
Anteroposterior alignment (25 points)
    Stability (25 points)
    Medial/lateral (15 points)
    Anterior/posterior (10 points)
Range of motion (25 points)
Symptoms (25 points)
Deductions
    Malalignment (–10 points)
    Flexion contracture (–2/–5/–10/–15 points)
    Extensor lag (–5/–10/–15 points)

Satisfaction Score (5 Items, 40 Points)
Pain level while sitting (8 points)
Pain level while lying in bed (8 points)
Knee function while getting out of bed (8 points)
Knee function while performing light household duties (8 points)
Knee function while performing leisure recreational activities (8 points)

Expectation Score (3 Items, 15 Points)
Pain relief (5 points)
Ability to carry out activities of daily living (5 points)
Ability to perform leisure, recreational, or sports activities (5 points)

Functional Activity Score (19 Items, 100 Points)
Walking and standing (5 items, 30 points)
Standard activities (6 items, 30 points)
Advanced activities (5 items, 25 points)
Discretionary activities (3 items, 15 points)

TKA concerning pain and daily and recreational activities (15 points). Functional activities (100 points) are assessed by the patient and include walking and standing (30 points), standard everyday activities (30 points), and advanced activities (25 points). The section on discretionary activities (15 points) allows the patient to pick three of his or her most important activities from a list and rate the level of difficulty he or she perceives in performing these activities. In this newest version of the rating system, the Knee Society has placed more importance on patient perceptions, possibly because patient- and surgeon-perceived outcomes have been reported to be significantly different. The preoperative and postoperative questionnaires are the same to allow direct comparison. Any surgeon can apply for a license through the Knee Society to use the Knee Society Scoring System.

Other activity-related scoring systems have been developed and validated. The Lower Extremity Activity Score (LEAS) was developed as a simple way to allow patients to report their highest level of possible activity before and after surgery, choosing from a list of activities that progress in the level of functional capacity. The LEAS was validated using the Western Ontario and McMasters Universities Osteoarthritis Index (WOMAC) and comparison to responses to pedometer readings from patients. The scale also has been shown to be accurate when filled out by next of kin, making it a unique measure of functional activity.

In 1989, the Knee Society introduced the Total Knee Arthroplasty Radiographic Evaluation and Scoring System (Fig. 5.33) to standardize the radiographic parameters to be measured when reporting radiographic outcomes of TKA: component alignment, tibial surface coverage, radiolucencies, and a patellar problem list that includes angle of the prosthesis, eccentric component placement, subluxation, and dislocation. A score is tabulated for each component based on the width and extent of its associated radiolucencies. For a seven-zone tibial component, a nonprogressive score of 4 or less probably is insignificant, a score of 5 to 9 indicates a need for close follow-up for progression, and a score of 10 or more signifies possible or impending failure regardless of symptoms. Developers of total knee prostheses are requested to superimpose silhouettes of their designs on the Knee Society form and assign radiographic zones to be used by all authors in subsequent reports.

The Knee Injury and Osteoarthritis Outcome Score for Joint Replacement (KOOS JR) has gained popularity. It is a one-page questionnaire, with a seven-item instrument, that is easily administered. Since the questions represent "knee health" in patients, it can be used to determine pain, symptom severity, and activities of daily living (ADL). Movements or activities that are difficult for patients with advanced knee osteoarthritis before surgery are then compared to after TKA.

PROSTHESIS SURVIVAL

Modern knee arthroplasty began in the early 1970s with the development of the total condylar knee prosthesis. Survivorship studies with this prosthesis are the standard with which modern knee replacement is compared. Long-term series have documented the longevity of the original total condylar prosthesis to be 95% at 15 years and 91% at 21 and 23 years. More recently, the reported 15- to 18-year survivorship of a cementless CR TKA was 98.6%, with 79% of patients reporting no pain.

Multiple studies of PCL-retaining and PCL-substituting designs have documented 10-year survivorship of 95% or greater, and most registry data agree with this figure. As discussed in the earlier section on component fixation, cementless fixation has had mixed results with respect to prosthesis survivorship in the past, but more modern, next-generation ingrowth surface technologies are now demonstrating similar mid-term results to cemented TKA. An update on why TKA fails was recently given by Sharkey et al. Of the 781 revisions performed at their institution over a 10-year period, the most common failure mechanisms were loosening (39.9%), infection (27.4%), instability (7.5%), periprosthetic fracture (4.7%), and arthrofibrosis (4.5%). Infection was the most common reason for failure in early revision (<2 years from primary surgery), and aseptic loosening was the most common reason in late revision. They reported that polyethylene wear was no longer the major cause of failure, which can be attributed to better forms of polyethylene and better designs. When they compared these results to their previous report, the percentage of revisions performed for polyethylene wear, instability, arthrofibrosis, malalignment, and extensor mechanism deficiency had all decreased.

TKA Scoring System

Evaluator name _____ Date _____

Patient
name/number _____ Preop ☐ Postop ☐

Surgeon name _____ Hospital number _____

X-ray date _____ Prior implants _____

Joint: Left knee ☐   Right knee ☐

Alignment: Recumbent ☐   Standing ☐

Anteroposterior	Angle in degrees
Femoral flexion (α)	_____
Tibial angle (β)	_____
Total valgus angle (Ω)	_____
18" Film	_____
3' Film	_____

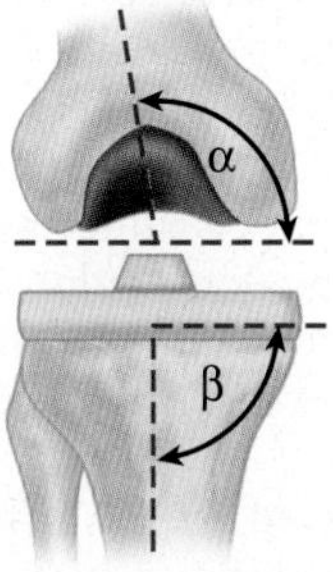

Lateral	Angle in degrees
Femoral flexion (γ) ±	_____
Tibial angle (σ)	_____

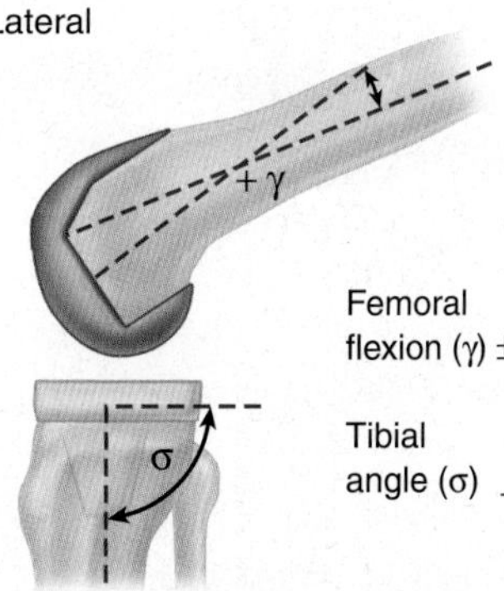

Implant/bone surface area
Percent area of tibial surface covered by implant

Radiolucencies: Indicate depth in millimeters in each zone

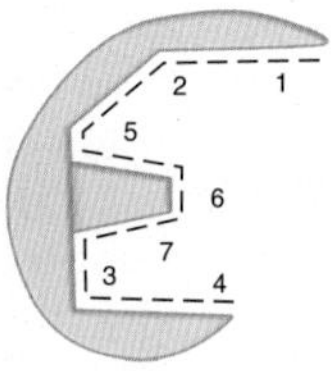

	RLL
	1 ____
	2 ____
	3 ____
	4 ____
	5 ____
	6 ____
	7 ____
Total	____

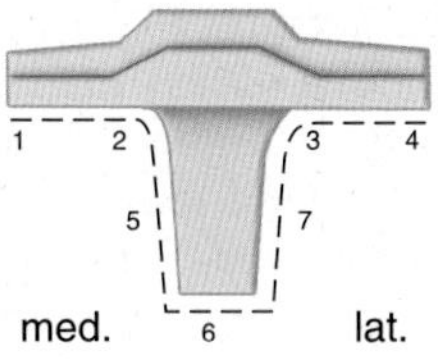

	RLL
	1 ____
	2 ____
	3 ____
	4 ____
	5 ____
	6 ____
	7 ____
Total	____

anterior posterior

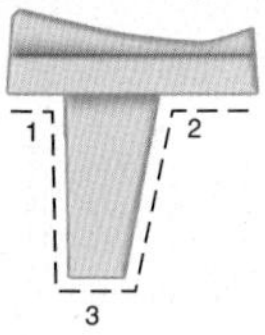

	RLL
	1 ____
	2 ____
	3 ____
Total	____

medial lateral

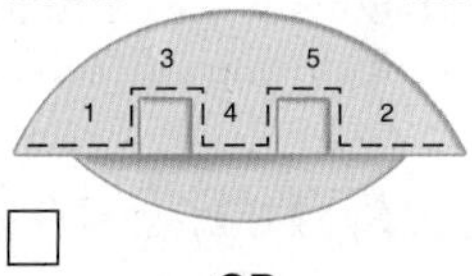

OR

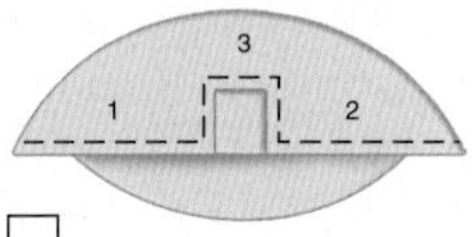

	RLL
	1 ____
	2 ____
	3 ____
	4 ____
	5 ____
Total	____

Patellar problem list
Angle of prosthesis _____   Subluxation _____
Placement Med-Lat _____
Sup-Inf _____   Dislocation _____

FIGURE 5.33 Knee Society radiographic evaluation and TKA scoring system.

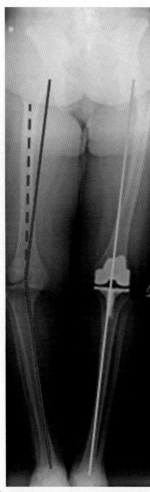

FIGURE 5.34 Anatomic and mechanical axes of femur and tibia are determined independently on preoperative long leg radiographs, with the goal of centering postoperative mechanical axis of limb within center of prosthetic knee. *1,* Angle between anatomic *(2)* and mechanical *(3)* axes of femur. *4,* Mechanical axis of tibia (see text).

PREOPERATIVE EVALUATION

The most important part of preoperative evaluation is determining that TKA is clearly indicated (see earlier section on indications and contraindications for TKA). Preoperative knee radiographs should include a standing anteroposterior view, a lateral view, and a skyline view of the patella. A long leg standing anteroposterior radiograph can be beneficial in determining the mechanical axis of the limb, particularly when deformity secondary to trauma or previous surgical procedure is present (Fig. 5.34).

The long leg film also is useful to determine if significant bowing of the tibia precludes the use of an intramedullary tibial alignment guide. Templates can be used to anticipate approximate component size and bone defects that would need to be treated intraoperatively. The mechanical axis of the femur can be measured to determine the proper distal femoral valgus angle to properly make the resection and obtain neutral mechanical axis during the procedure.

The preoperative medical evaluation of candidates for TKA must be detailed and thorough to prevent potential complications that can threaten life or limb. Because most patients who undergo TKA are elderly, comorbid diseases must be considered. Patients with multiple medical risk factors have

been shown to require longer hospital stays. Smokers, in particular, tend to have longer operative times and increased hospital charges after undergoing joint replacement.

Patients must have adequate cardiopulmonary reserve to withstand general or epidural anesthesia and to withstand a blood loss of 1000 to 1500 mL over the perioperative period. A routine preoperative electrocardiogram should be obtained. Patients who have a history of coronary artery disease, mild congestive heart failure, chronic obstructive pulmonary disease, or restrictive pulmonary disease should be evaluated by appropriate medical consultants. Vascular supply to the operative leg also should be evaluated. If adequate vascularity is questionable, noninvasive arterial studies should be obtained and a vascular surgery consultation may be necessary.

Routine preoperative laboratory evaluation should include complete blood cell count, electrolytes, and urinalysis. Preferably, these tests are performed a few days before surgery so that measures can be undertaken for any correctable abnormalities. The routine use of a chest radiograph usually is not cost effective as a screening tool, but it is indicated in patients with a history of cardiopulmonary disease. Similarly, routine preoperative evaluation of coagulation studies is unnecessary except in patients with a history of bleeding or coagulopathy. Patients receiving anticoagulant medications must be managed appropriately to limit blood loss while ensuring medical stability in the perioperative period.

Medical clearance usually is requested by the orthopaedic surgeon when any medical comorbidity exists, but the orthopaedic surgeon should carefully evaluate certain medical conditions that the primary care physician may not think important but which have been shown to increase postoperative morbidity after total joint arthroplasty. Smoking cessation should be encouraged to decrease the risk of morbidity after total joint arthroplasty. Poor nutrition, frequently present in elderly patients and severely obese individuals, often can be detected by a low albumin level in the serum (<3.5 mg/dL). Patients with total lymphocyte counts of less than 1200 cells/mL also have been shown to have higher hospital charges, longer hospital stays, and longer anesthesia and surgery times than those with higher counts. Patients with type II diabetes should have a hemoglobin A1c test preoperatively, and their blood glucose level should be well controlled (A1c < 7.5). In one study fructosamine was shown to be a better indicator of glycemic control and more responsive to changes in glucose homeostasis. A subset of patients with an A1c under 7 but high fructosamine went on to have a primary joint infection. In this Knee Society award-winning paper, patients with high fructosamine (>293 µmol/L) were 11.2 times more likely to develop a prosthetic joint infection compared with patients with low fructosamine. Obesity with the addition of two other comorbidities (hypertension, hypercholesterolemia, or blood glucose intolerance) is referred to as metabolic syndrome (MetS) and is associated with a higher risk of complications after total joint arthroplasty. A preoperative conversation with obese patients with MetS should explain that this modifiable risk factor can be associated with a poor outcome. Patient involvement is necessary to ensure that he or she will do whatever possible to improve the risk profile. Outcome studies of morbidly obese patients show a high patient satisfaction rate but also a higher risk of revision surgery. In super-obese patients (BMI ≥ 50) the reported rate of any complication after surgery is over 50%, and elective surgery should be carefully considered in this patient population. No clear BMI cutoff for proceeding with TKA has been established, but clearly as the number of comorbidities increases in an obese patient the more likely that he or she will have a poor outcome or a complication.

AMBULATORY AND SHORT-STAY CONSIDERATIONS

Many centers have now turned to outpatient surgery for both UKA and TKA. To safely accomplish this endeavor, one must have a complete team setup, including office staff, operating room personnel, anesthesiology, physical therapy, and ancillary providers. The use of tranexamic acid to reduce the need for blood transfusion also has helped to provide a safer path to ambulatory surgery for joint replacement. Pain modalities, including intraarticular injections with liposomal-encased or plain bupivacaine, with or without the addition of ketorolac, morphine, or dexamethasone, help to provide adequate pain relief in the immediate postoperative period (see section on Pain Management Strategies below). These measures allow centers to successfully and safely perform knee joint arthroplasty procedures in an ambulatory or a 23-hour setting. We established a 24/7 total joint hotline for patients with issues to call so that they feel more at ease and have access to a provider. Having a program that educates patients on the process so that they and their immediate families or caregivers understand what to expect can be beneficial. Before implementing an outpatient TKA it is helpful to first visit a center that has a successful program in place.

ANESTHETIC OPTIONS

The selection of regional or general anesthesia for TKA is a complicated issue that is affected by comorbid medical conditions. The anesthesiologist has the ultimate responsibility for this selection, with input from the surgeon. Cardiovascular outcomes of regional and general anesthesia have not been proved to be significantly different, and perioperative mortality in patients with hip fractures is the same with both techniques. Cognitive function after surgery has been shown to be similar with regional and general anesthesia after the initial postoperative period. Most studies, as well as the AAOS Clinical Practice Guidelines, now advocate regional over general anesthesia for primary TKA because of better pain control and outcomes. A spinal anesthetic is preferred because it affords better pain control and has lower complications after primary TKA.

The effect of general versus epidural anesthesia on thromboembolic complications is controversial. A slight, but not statistically significant, decrease in overall DVT and PE rates has been reported in patients who have had epidural anesthesia compared with general anesthesia, whereas another randomized trial showed no difference in overall thromboembolic disease but did show a decrease in proximal thrombus formation with epidural anesthesia. Possible benefits of epidural anesthesia include vasodilation of the lower extremity, resulting in increased blood flow, hemodilution, and decreased blood viscosity. A fibrinolytic effect also has been postulated for epidural anesthesia; however, in a study comparing epidural and general anesthesia there was no difference in intraoperatively obtained blood markers for fibrinolysis or thrombogenesis.

PAIN MANAGEMENT STRATEGIES AFTER PARTIAL AND TOTAL KNEE ARTHROPLASTY

Many different pain management modalities have been used to alleviate pain after total or partial knee arthroplasty. Most surgeons advocate a multimodal approach that includes a preoperative dose of a COX-2 antiinflammatory and gabapentin, which has been shown to be beneficial in patients with chronic pain who have TKA. The use of femoral nerve catheters is now under scrutiny because they can inhibit postoperative mobilization, especially on and after the day of surgery. Intraarticular injections that infiltrate the surrounding soft tissues with either a bupivacaine or ropivacaine (lower cardiotoxicity) product or that are placed in the intraarticular space have been studied, as has the use of liposomal-encased bupivacaine. Use of one nonnarcotic oral preoperative medication with either a femoral nerve block or intraarticular injection can give excellent pain relief. These modalities have been compared in prospective studies, with several studies finding no significant difference in visual analog scale (VAS) scores or narcotic usage after surgery. The use of liposomal-encased bupivacaine has come under some scrutiny because of its expense and lack of improvement in some reports over plain bupivacaine injections combined with epinephrine, with or without addition of ketorolac and dexamethasone. The PILLAR study, however, did show an advantage in postoperative pain control after primary TKA using 20 mL of liposomal bupivacaine with 20 mL of 0.5% plain bupivacaine and 80 mL of normal saline in a targeted infiltration technique.

A recent publication has reported that up to 40% of patients remain chronic users of narcotics after primary TKA; therefore, surgeons should make all efforts to wean patients off narcotics after surgery. Cryoneurolysis of the anterior femoral cutaneous and infrapatellar branch of the saphenous nerve before TKA surgery has been shown to decrease the amount of daily morphine equivalents needed after TKA, and this may be a beneficial treatment in high-risk patients or those who are under chronic pain management.

BLOOD PRESERVATION MANAGEMENT IN PARTIAL AND TOTAL KNEE ARTHROPLASTY

The use of tranexamic acid either intravenously, topically before closure, or orally has been shown to significantly decrease postoperative hemoglobin drop and the need for postoperative transfusions after primary TKA. All of the delivery modes have been shown to be safe with no increased risk of thromboembolic events after surgery in the proper patient population. Advocates for intravenous administration argue that there is no wait to close the operative approach, whereas advocates of topical administration believe it may be a safer route of administration. For intravenous administration, the dose should be 10 to 15 mg/kg or 1 g, with consideration of a preoperative dose given 20 minutes before tourniquet inflation and a repeat dose given about 15 minutes before tourniquet deflation. For topically administered dosing, 1.5 to 3 g diluted in 100 mL normal saline should be placed in the wound and intracapsular space for 5 minutes before tourniquet deflation. Some surgeons who still use drains administer the dose through the drain and then activate the closed suction after 5 minutes. Contraindications to intravenous tranexamic acid use include a history of a clotting disorder, bleeding disorder, subarachnoid hemorrhage, pulmonary embolus, DVT, cardiovascular accident, or myocardial infarction, as well as the presence of a coronary stent. Oral tranexamic acid and has been shown to be effective. Doses of 2000 mg given 2 hours before surgery and then two doses after surgery (4 to 6 hours and 12 hours postoperatively) have been reported to be effective and equivalent to intravenous or topical dosing. It is also more cost effective.

SURGICAL TECHNIQUE FOR PRIMARY TOTAL KNEE ARTHROPLASTY

The following description of surgical technique includes principles that are applicable to knee replacement in general; it is not intended to replace the individual technique manuals that are available or the implant-specific instrumentation guides that are unique to each available implant system. An understanding of the principles involved allows the surgeon to use sound judgment in any knee reconstruction, regardless of the particular type of implant being used.

SURGICAL APPROACH FOR PRIMARY TOTAL KNEE ARTHROPLASTY

The most commonly used skin incision for primary TKA is an anterior midline incision. Variations may be considered, but in general most incisions will compromise the infrapatellar branch of the saphenous nerve and result in an area of numbness on the outer aspect of the knee; this should be discussed with the patient before surgery. There are many variations to the approach to the knee deep to the subcutaneous level of dissection.

TECHNIQUE 5.1

- Make the incision with the knee in flexion to allow the subcutaneous tissue to fall medially and laterally, which improves exposure.
- If a preexisting anterior scar on the knee is in a usable position, incorporate it into the skin incision. If multiple previous incisions are present, choose the most lateral usable incision because the blood supply to the skin of the anterior knee tends to come predominantly from the medial side. Generally, previous direct medial and lateral incisions and transverse incisions can be ignored.
- Make the skin incision long enough to avoid excessive skin tension during retraction, which can lead to areas of skin necrosis or use the mobile window technique to expose all aspects of the knee as needed.
- The standard retinacular incision in TKA is a medial parapatellar retinacular approach (Fig. 5.35).
- Keep the medial skin flap as thick as possible by keeping the dissection just superficial to the extensor mechanism.

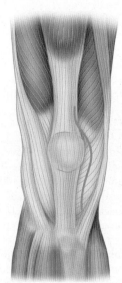

FIGURE **5.35**   Medial parapatellar retinacular approach. **SEE TECHNIQUE 5.1.**

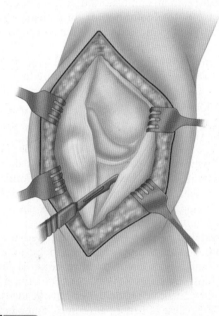

FIGURE **5.36**   Medial capsule and deep portion of medial collateral ligament are elevated subperiosteally. **SEE TECHNIQUE 5.1.**

- Extend the retinacular incision proximally the length of the quadriceps tendon, leaving a 3- to 4-mm cuff of tendon on the vastus medialis for later closure.
- Continue the incision around the medial side of the patella, extending 3 to 4 cm onto the anteromedial surface of the tibia along the medial border of the patellar tendon.
- Expose the medial side of the knee by subperiosteally elevating the anteromedial capsule and deep medial collateral ligament off the tibia to the posteromedial corner of the knee (Fig. 5.36).
- Extend the knee and evert the patella to allow a routine release of lateral patellofemoral plicae (Fig. 5.37). In obese patients, if eversion of the patella is difficult, develop the

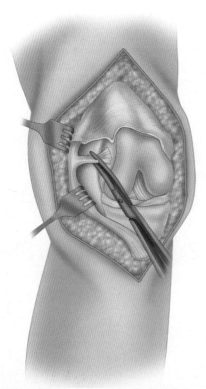

FIGURE 5.37 Lateral patellofemoral plicae are cut to allow mobilization of extensor mechanism. **SEE TECHNIQUE 5.1.**

lateral subcutaneous flap further so that the patella can be everted underneath this tissue. Alternatively, the patella can be subluxated laterally if this provides adequate exposure.

- Flex the knee and remove the anterior cruciate ligament and the anterior horns of the medial and lateral menisci, along with any osteophytes that may lead to component malposition or soft-tissue imbalance. The posterior horns of the menisci can be excised after the femoral and tibial cuts have been made. If a PCL-substituting prosthesis is to be used, the PCL can be resected at this time or can be removed later in the procedure along with the box cut made in the distal femur for the PCL-substituting femoral component.

- With PCL substitution and PCL retention, subluxate and externally rotate the tibia. External rotation relaxes the extensor mechanism, decreases the chance of patellar tendon avulsion, and improves exposure.

- Expose the lateral tibial plateau by a partial or complete excision of the infrapatellar fat pad and retraction of the everted extensor mechanism with a levering-type retractor placed carefully adjacent to the lateral tibial plateau.

- During all maneuvers that place tension on the extensor mechanism, especially knee flexion and patellar retraction, pay careful attention to the patellar tendon attachment to the tibial tubercle. Avulsion of the patellar tendon is difficult to repair and can be a devastating complication.

See also Video 5.4.

In an effort to reduce patellofemoral complications and expedite the return of quadriceps function postoperatively, alternative methods of exposure have been described. The subvastus ("Southern") approach differs from Technique 5.1 in the method of subluxating the extensor mechanism laterally for knee exposure (Fig. 5.38). The same anterior midline knee incision is used, but the proximal retinacular incision is performed by incising the superficial fascia overlying the vastus medialis and bluntly mobilizing the distal medial border of the vastus medialis posteriorly to the medial intermuscular septum. The origin of the vastus medialis is lifted off the medial intermuscular septum to approximately 10 cm proximal to the adductor tubercle, staying distal to the aperture for the femoral vessels. The synovium is incised, and the entire extensor mechanism is dislocated laterally. Advocates of this approach claim that leaving the extensor mechanism intact results in a more rapid return of quadriceps strength, preserves more of the vascularity to the patella, improves patient satisfaction while decreasing postoperative pain, and decreases the need for lateral release. Compared with the medial parapatellar approach, the exposure may be limited, especially in obese patients and patients with previous knee surgeries.

Engh and Parks described the midvastus approach, which differs from the subvastus approach in that the vastus medialis muscle is split in line with its fibers, rather than subluxated laterally in its entirety. The split in the vastus medialis starts at the superomedial border of the patella and extends proximally and medially toward the intermuscular septum (Fig. 5.39).

A safe zone of 4.5 cm of the vastus medialis can be sharply split from the margin of the patella and can be bluntly dissected further if desired. This approach preserves the supreme genicular artery to the patella and the quadriceps tendon. Relative contraindications to the midvastus approach include obesity, previous upper tibial osteotomy, and preoperative flexion of less than 80 degrees. Careful attention to hemostasis is mandatory because postoperative hematomas have been described with the subvastus and midvastus approaches. Extensile exposures are described in the section on revision TKA.

INTRAMEDULLARY AND EXTRAMEDULLARY ALIGNMENT INSTRUMENTATION

Intramedullary alignment instrumentation is crucial on the femoral side of a TKA because femoral landmarks are not easily palpable. The entry portal for the femoral alignment rod typically is placed a few millimeters medial to the midline, at a point anterior to the origin of the PCL. Preoperative radiographs should be scrutinized for a wide canal or excessive femoral bowing because these conditions may result in alignment errors. Cadaver studies have shown that positioning of the entry point of the femoral intramedullary alignment rod significantly affects the resulting alignment of the distal femoral cut by as much as 5 degrees in the sagittal plane.

Extramedullary femoral alignment is useful only in limbs with severe lateral femoral bowing, femoral malunion, or stenosis from a previous fracture, or when an ipsilateral total hip arthroplasty or other hardware fills the isthmus of the intramedullary canal. A palpable marker can be placed over the center of the femoral head based on preoperative hip radiographs

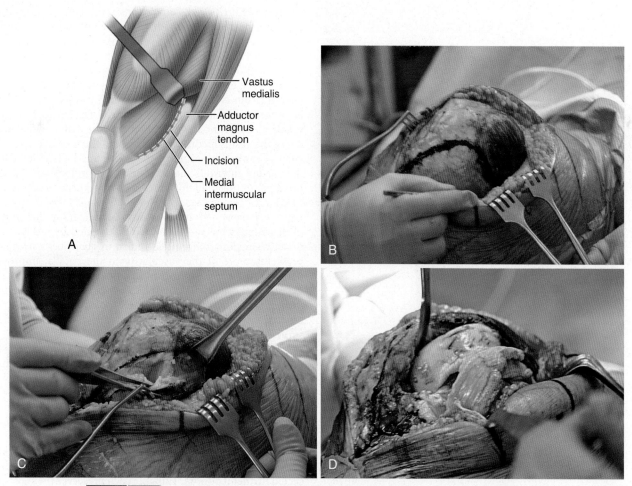

FIGURE 5.38 **A** and **B,** Subvastus approach involves lifting entire extensor mechanism off medial intermuscular septum and subluxing it laterally for exposure. **C,** Tine retractor placed over top of femur and secured on lateral surface places vastus medialis under tension while muscle attachment to intermuscular septum is sharply detached with scissors. **D,** Complete release of quadriceps to medial intermuscular septum. Exposure obtained after full eversion of patella. (From Miller MD: Knee and lower leg. In Miller MD, Chhabra AB, Hurwitz S, et al, editors: *Orthopaedic surgical approaches*, Philadelphia, 2008, Elsevier.)

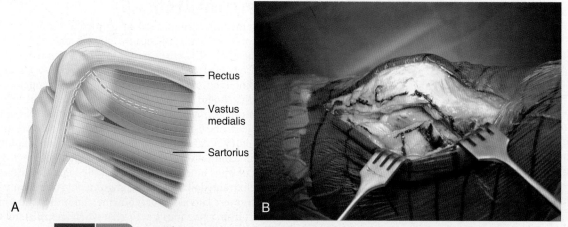

FIGURE 5.39 **A,** Midvastus approach shown as *green dashed line* with right knee in 90 degrees flexion. **B,** Operative photograph. (From Miller MD: Knee and lower leg. In Miller MD, Chhabra AB, Hurwitz S, et al, editors: *Orthopaedic surgical approaches*, Philadelphia, 2008, Elsevier.)

or by fluoroscopic imaging with the patient on the operating table. The anterior superior iliac spine has been shown to be unreliable for determining the hip center and should not be used as the primary landmark when extramedullary femoral alignment is chosen. Currently, when preexisting deformity or hardware is present, more modern techniques such as computer navigation or custom cutting blocks are used (see Computer-Assisted Alignment Technique).

The use of tibial intramedullary alignment guides is slightly more controversial. One concern about the use of these guides is the risk of fat embolism. A greater elevation of pulmonary arterial pressures and slightly diminished cardiac indices were found in patients undergoing bilateral TKAs using intramedullary tibial alignment guides compared with extramedullary tibial alignment guides and venting of the femoral intramedullary canals; however, these slight changes were not believed to constitute any contraindication to the use of intramedullary alignment devices. Because of a 12% prevalence of postoperative neurologic changes believed to be consistent with fat embolism after bilateral TKA, the use of pulmonary arterial pressure monitoring has been recommended by some surgeons. Drilling an oversized 12.7-mm hole in the distal femur and using an 8-mm fluted rod were shown to eliminate the negative cardiopulmonary effects of intramedullary femoral alignment rods.

The relative accuracy of intramedullary and extramedullary tibial alignment also has been debated. In one study, 94% of tibial components were within 2 degrees of 90 degrees with intramedullary alignment compared with 85% with extramedullary alignment. Another study found extramedullary alignment to be more accurate, with 88% of tibial components within 2 degrees of the 90-degree goal, whereas only 72% of the components placed using intramedullary alignment met this criterion. Neutral tibial component alignment was reported to be obtained with intramedullary devices in 83% of varus knees, but in only 37% of valgus knees; tibial bowing was more common in valgus knees (Fig. 5.40A), and the use of long leg films for templating and intraoperatively double checking the alignment of the tibial cut with an extramedullary device were recommended (Fig. 5.40B). In a cadaver study comparing intramedullary and extramedullary devices to computer navigation for tibial alignment, intramedullary alignment was not as accurate as extramedullary alignment in determining posterior slope. The anterior tibial crest also has been used by some surgeons during extramedullary alignment of the tibia. This technique has been shown in a cadaver study to be variable, resulting in a range from 3.2 degrees varus to 2.1 degrees valgus with a consistent anterior slope in the sagittal plane. Currently, most surgeons at our institution use intramedullary femoral alignment with extramedullary tibial alignment; one uses computer navigation techniques as well. When determining where the center of the ankle lies between the malleoli, some now advocate a slightly medial-based position from the center of the malleolar axis in the coronal plane. This has been reported to be approximately 2 mm medial to this center point, so many surgeons aim the tip of the tibial extramedullary alignment rod slightly medial to the center of the ankle, and the amount of tibial torsion and subcutaneous tissue present can affect where the radiographic center of the ankle lies. Assessment of a long-standing radiograph can help determine where the radiographic center of the tibia lies on an individual basis and should be reviewed before every case.

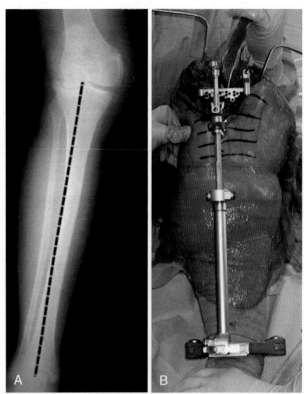

FIGURE 5.40 **A,** Bowed tibia may preclude use of intramedullary alignment guide for making tibial cut. **B,** Extramedullary alignment guide is recommended in this situation.

BONE PREPARATION FOR PRIMARY TOTAL KNEE ARTHROPLASTY

Bone surface preparation is based on the following principles: appropriate sizing of the individual components, alignment of the components to restore the mechanical axis, recreation of equally balanced soft tissues and gaps in flexion and extension, and optimal patellar tracking.

TECHNIQUE 5.2

- Make the distal femoral cut at a valgus angle (usually 5 to 7 degrees), and for more accuracy this angle can be measured off of a long-standing radiograph by measuring the angle between the mechanical and anatomic axes of the femur (see Fig. 5.19) perpendicular to the predetermined mechanical axis of the femur. The amount of bone removed generally is the same as that to be replaced by the femoral component. If a significant preoperative flexion contracture is present, additional resection can be done to aid in correction of the contracture, but elevation of the joint line over 4 mm should be avoided. If a posterior cruciate–substituting prosthesis is used, an additional 2 mm of distal femoral resection can be performed to equal the increase in the flexion gap that occurs when the PCL is sacrificed.
- The anterior and posterior femoral cuts determine the rotation of the femoral component and the shape of the

flexion gap. Excessive external rotation widens the flexion gap medially and may result in flexion instability. Internal rotation of the femoral component can cause lateral patellar tilt or patellofemoral instability.

- Femoral component rotation can be determined by one of several methods. The transepicondylar axis, anteroposterior axis, posterior femoral condyles, and cut surface of the proximal tibia all can serve as reference points (Fig. 5.41).
- If the transepicondylar axis is used, make the posterior femoral cut parallel to a line drawn between the medial and lateral femoral epicondyles. Determine the anteroposterior axis by drawing a line between the bottom of the sulcus of the femur and the top of the intercondylar notch, and make the posterior femoral cut perpendicular to this axis.
- When the posterior condyles are referenced, make the cut in 3 degrees of external rotation off a line between them. A valgus knee with a hypoplastic lateral femoral condyle may lead to an internally rotated femoral component if the posterior condyles alone are referenced (Fig. 5.42).
- Using the cut surface of the proximal tibia or the "gap" technique, make the posterior femoral cut parallel to the proximal tibial cut after the soft tissues have been balanced in extension (Fig. 5.43). This technique often is used for mobile-bearing TKA because precise gap balancing in flexion is necessary to ensure that "spinout" of the polyethylene bearing does not occur.

- Caution should be exercised when using the gap technique because reliance on ligaments of nonanatomic length can lead to suboptimal femoral component rotation in the transverse plane. It is important for the surgeon to be familiar with each of these reference points because reliance on a single reference could result in suboptimal femoral component rotation in the transverse plane.

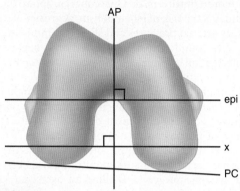

FIGURE 5.41 Alignment axes in knee with normal condylar shape. Resection perpendicular to anteroposterior (*AP*) axis or parallel to epicondylar (*epi*) axis results in resection line (*x*) that is slightly externally rotated relative to posterior condylar (*PC*) axis by 3 degrees on average. This results in correct positioning of femoral component. **SEE TECHNIQUE 5.2.**

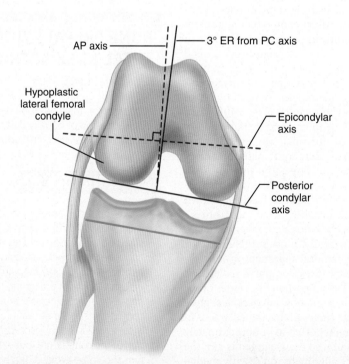

FIGURE 5.42 Hypoplastic lateral condyle causes relative internal rotation of the femoral component if the posterior condylar axis is utilized while the anteroposterior axis places it in the proper position. **SEE TECHNIQUE 5.2.**

- Regardless of the method used for rotational alignment, the thickness of bone removed from the posterior aspect of the femoral condyles should equal the thickness of the posterior condyles of the femoral component. This is determined directly by measuring the thickness of the posterior condylar resection with "posterior referencing" instrumentation. "Anterior referencing" instruments measure the anteroposterior dimension of the femoral condyles from an anterior cut based off the anterior femoral cortex to the articular surface of the posterior femoral

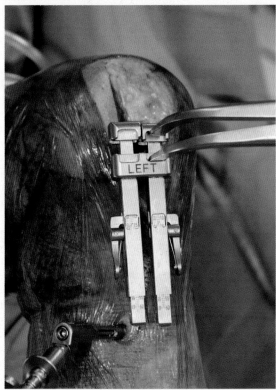

FIGURE 5.43 Rectangular flexion gap is obtained by externally rotating cutting jig of femur parallel to cut surface of tibia while collateral ligaments are under equal tension, obtained with tensioning device as shown or with spacer blocks. **SEE TECHNIQUE 5.2.**

condyles. The femoral component chosen must be equal to or slightly less than the measured anteroposterior dimension to avoid tightness in flexion.

- Posterior referencing instruments are theoretically more accurate in recreating the original dimensions of the distal femur; however, anterior referencing instruments have less risk of notching the anterior femoral cortex and place the anterior flange of the femoral component more reliably against the anterior surface of the distal femur. It is absolutely necessary that the surgeon knows whether the implant system being used is an anterior- or posterior-based reference system because this will be important when balancing flexion-to-extension gap inequalities.
- Complete the distal femoral preparation for a PCL-retaining prosthesis by making anterior and posterior chamfer cuts for the implant. If a PCL-substituting design is chosen, remove the bone for the intercondylar box to accommodate the housing for the post and cam mechanism (Fig. 5.44).
- Cut the tibia perpendicular to its mechanical axis with the cutting block oriented by an intramedullary or extramedullary cutting guide. The amount of posterior slope depends on the individual implant system being used. Many systems incorporate 3 degrees of posterior slope into the polyethylene insert, which allows more accurate slope to be aligned by the implant rather than with the cutting block. The amount of tibial resection depends on which side of the joint (more or less arthritic) is used for reference. When measured off the unaffected side of the joint, the resection should be close to the size of the implant being used, typically 8 to 10 mm. If the more arthritic side of the joint is used for reference, the amount of resection usually is 2 mm or less. Protect the patellar tendon and collateral ligaments during this portion of the procedure.
- Alternatively, the proximal tibia can be cut before completion of the distal femoral cuts.

GAP BALANCING TECHNIQUE

- If the distal femoral resection has not been completed, balance the flexion and extension gaps at this time by placing spacer blocks or a tensioner within the gaps with the knee in flexion and extension. Varus-valgus balance

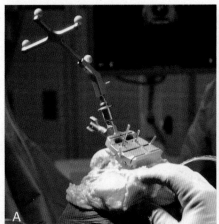
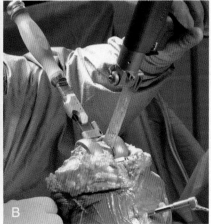

FIGURE 5.44 **A,** Chamfer cuts complete distal femoral resection in cruciate-retaining arthroplasty. **B,** Intercondylar notch cut to accommodate post and cam mechanism in cruciate-substituting arthroplasty. **SEE TECHNIQUE 5.2.**

can be fine-tuned with further medial or lateral releases (see "Soft-Tissue Balancing").

- Before any soft-tissue release, remove any medial or lateral osteophytes about the tibia and femur. Remove posterior condylar osteophytes because they can block flexion and tent posterior soft-tissue structures in extension, causing a flexion contracture.
- The flexion and extension gaps must be roughly equal. If the extension gap is too small or tight, extension is limited. Similarly, if the flexion gap is too tight, flexion is limited. Laxity of either gap can lead to instability.
- If the extension gap is smaller than the flexion gap, remove more bone from the distal femoral cut surface, or release the posterior capsule from the distal femur, but first make certain that all posterior condylar osteophytes have been removed before raising the joint line.
- If the flexion gap is smaller than the extension gap, remove more bone from the posterior femoral condyles by making appropriate cuts for the next smaller available femoral component; make sure this is done with anterior referencing so that the posterior condyles are shortened and the anterior cortex is not notched.
- If the flexion and extension gaps are equal, but there is not enough space for the desired prosthesis, remove more bone from the proximal tibia because bone removed from the tibia affects the flexion and extension gaps equally.
- When the flexion and extension gaps are equal but lax, a larger spacer block and a thicker tibial polyethylene insert are required to obtain stability.

COMPUTER-ASSISTED ALIGNMENT TECHNIQUE

Computer navigation has not seen a significant adoption for use during primary TKA. The most popular technique uses imageless computer navigation with the surgeon determining the anatomic landmarks by direct or indirect measures during the procedure. Despite multiple studies in the literature confirming that imageless computer navigation decreases the number of outliers in coronal mechanical axis alignment after TKA, the technique has not been universally adopted in the United States.

The technique typically involves the attachment of active or passive trackers on the femur and the tibia, which are then tracked by a computer-assisted infrared camera, which must have a clear line of sight during the procedure (Fig. 5.45). The markers are removable from a reference base that is anchored to the bone to ensure they are not damaged or loosened during the procedure. Once the trackers are attached to the reference bases, the surgeon typically performs a registration of the anatomic landmarks so that the computer can determine and track the femoral and tibial anatomy during the procedure to guide the surgeon in alignment of the bony cuts and implants. The anatomy within the surgical field typically is registered using a pointing device that the computer can track, and the center of the femoral head is determined by indirect means of a center-of-rotation mathematic algorithm. Palpated landmarks of a combination of center-of-rotation and external landmarks can be used to determine the center of the ankle. In a cadaver study, using the most medial and most lateral aspects of the medial and lateral malleoli and using a percentage of the distance between the two points was the most accurate method for determining the center of the ankle. Once the registration is complete, the computer can give real-time feedback about the alignment of the bony cuts of the femur and tibia in all three anatomic planes, which allows the surgeon to make changes and to measure the accuracy of the bony cuts rather than relying solely on the alignment of the cutting jig, which may not translate into an accurate bony cut because of sclerotic or osteopenic bone.

Computer navigation systems also can aid in determining the proper implant size and alignment. Soft-tissue balancing and measurement of flexion and extension gaps during the procedure are other significant advantages to computer-assisted TKA. Objective measurement of the gaps ensures proper soft-tissue balancing and gaps that will provide a stable joint throughout a range of motion. A gap balancing and equalization technique was found to produce better flexion at 1- to 4-year follow-up, but no patient-derived outcome measures were different than those with conventional techniques. In a meta-analysis of 22 studies of computer-assisted TKA, better overall alignment and implant positioning were

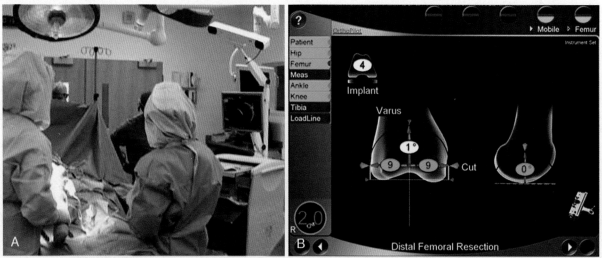

FIGURE 5.45   **A,** Computer-assisted alignment uses trackers placed on the femur and tibia, which are tracked by a computer-assisted camera. **B,** Computer allows real-time planning during case.

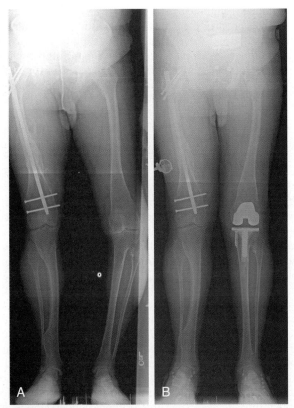

FIGURE 5.46 **A,** Malunion of the femur. **B,** Computer navigation was used to perform TKA.

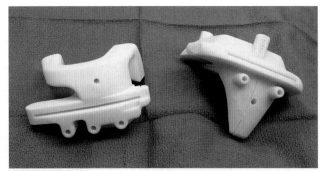

FIGURE 5.47 Custom cutting-block produced from preoperative magnetic resonance images.

ROBOTIC-ASSISTED SURGERY CONSIDERATIONS

As technology advances, companies have turned to active and/or semi-active robotic systems to improve accuracy of primary TKA procedures. It is important to point out that these systems utilize the image-free tracking technology that computer navigation techniques have been using for years. The advancement has been in the haptics and casting systems and in real-time operative planning routines that allow surgeons to change or "tweak" component placement during surgery. To date no improvements or cost-effective results have been reported, however. Most opponents to this technology point out the large up-front costs, the need for preoperative imaging with some platforms, and the lack of improvement in outcomes. Proponents of these systems point to better accuracy and less soft-tissue damage during the procedure, which seems to show some benefit in preliminary studies and outcomes.

CUSTOM CUTTING BLOCKS

After the introduction of custom cutting blocks, there were reports that they offered a more accurate, less invasive technique for achieving proper implant alignment during TKA. This technique uses preoperative MRI or CT scans of the lower extremity that include the hip and ankle to produce custom cutting blocks for the distal femur (Fig. 5.47) and the proximal tibia. With this technique, the "computer alignment" is done outside the operating room using three-dimensional imaging to determine the position of the distal femoral cut and the rotational position of the femoral component in the transverse plane. Rapid prototyping technology and image shape-fitting software typically are used to manufacture these custom cutting blocks. Although initial reports showed alignment after TKA with a custom cutting block to be comparable to that using computer navigation, there are monetary concerns associated with the cost of imaging and production of the cutting jigs. Advocates of the custom cutting blocks report shorter operating room times and less cost to sterilize instrument sets. However, the technique cannot tell the surgeon if the cutting block is secured in the proper position or if the resulting bony cut is in the proper position, and there is no way to determine this until postoperative radiographs are obtained. A retrospective study compared 120 patients who had TKA with standard instrumentation with 124 who had TKA with a custom cutting guide and found no difference at 2-year follow-up in UCLA activity scores, the Oxford Knee Scores, or SF-36 reported outcome measures, nor were

found, but no improvement in functional outcome was noted. A recent prospective study randomized 195 patients to TKA with conventional instrumentation (97 knees) or computer-assisted navigation (98 knees). At 5-year follow-up Knee Society Scores were significantly higher in the navigated group, possibly suggesting that the effects of computer assistance may not be apparent until further along in the survivorship curves of TKA patients.

Another advantage of computer navigation is that it avoids violation of the femoral intramedullary canal. This may reduce blood loss and cardiac-related complications because fewer emboli are placed into the venous system than with placement of an intramedullary alignment rod. These imageless navigation systems are helpful when existing hardware is present or extraarticular deformity precludes the use of conventional instruments because they avoid the morbidity of an additional procedure to remove existing hardware or correct a deformity (Fig. 5.46).

Disadvantages of computer navigation systems include the cost of the system, increased operating times, and the lack of current clinical outcome studies showing improved survivorship. Periprosthetic fractures through the reference-base anchoring holes in the femur and tibia have been reported. Currently, there are only limited reports showing improved functional results with computer navigation assisted TKA. In a prospective study of 115 primary TKA procedures, patients in whom computer navigation was used had significantly higher SF-12 and Knee Society Scores up to 1 year postoperatively, but other studies reproducing these outcomes have not been prominent.

there any differences in coronal alignment on CT scan measurements. Another study comparing the two procedures in 97 patients also found no differences in alignment using the UCLA and Oxford knee scores.

SOFT-TISSUE BALANCING

Soft-tissue balancing is essential to providing a stable joint after TKA. If a matched resection surgical technique is being used, the bone preparation is completed first, and then the flexion and extension gaps should be evaluated for symmetry for equal height in flexion and extension. This can be done with laminar spreaders, spacer blocks, or computer navigation techniques. Before release of any anatomic soft-tissue supporting structure about the knee, all peripheral osteophytes should be removed from the femur and tibia. The removal of osteophytes alone may be enough to balance existing coronal plane deformities. If a tibial resection first (gap balancing) surgical technique is being used, the osteophytes should be removed before determining any bony cuts on the femur. Eventual knee range of motion can be restricted by excessive collateral or PCL tension, and excessive laxity may lead to clinically unacceptable instability. As a general guideline, 1 to 2 mm of balanced varus-valgus opening in the medial and lateral compartments of the prosthetic knee is a reasonable goal. Regardless of the type of deformity being corrected, stability should be checked after each stage of soft-tissue release because overrelease can lead to excessive coronal plane instability and require conversion to an implant with a constrained post.

■ SOFT-TISSUE BALANCING TECHNIQUES (PIE-CRUSTING OR STANDARD RELEASE)

The traditional way of releasing tight structures is by subperiosteal release. In a varus deformity, the tight medial structures are released subperiosteally from the proximal tibia, while in a valgus deformity the tight structures are released off the femoral side of the joint. On the tibial side the releases can be performed with an elevator or an osteotome. On the femoral side these are typically performed by sharp dissection.

For a varus deformity, when the flexion or extension gap is tight medially, one can direct the portion of the medial soft-tissue sleeve to release. In general, the anterior half of the superficial medial collateral ligament affects the flexion gap more, while the posterior half and the posterior oblique ligament portions affect the extension gap more than the flexion gap. For a valgus deformity, when the lateral aspect of the flexion and/or extension gap is tight, one can direct the releases as determined by previous anatomical or biomechanical studies. The iliotibial band (ITB) can be released to affect the extension gap. The lateral collateral ligament tends to affect both the extension and flexion gaps, while the posterolateral corner affects the extension space more than the flexion gap.

The popliteus tendon release tends to affect the flexion gap more than the extension gap. In severe deformities it may be necessary to assess the lateral head of the gastrocnemius to see if it is involved in the extension gap deformity and consider releasing it as well. In either a varus or valgus knee deformity, if after complete release of structures there continues to be a trapezoidal extension gap, advancing the opposite collateral ligament may be considered to balance the gap, but this mostly is needed in extreme deformities.

Another technique used for soft-tissue balancing in knees with valgus or varus deformity is pie-crusting of the lateral or medial soft-tissue sleeve. This technique allows the surgeon to direct the lengthening of soft-tissue supporting structures according to which areas are taut under tension or under varus and valgus stress of the joint space in the operating room. During balancing, whether using a matched-resection or gap-balancing surgical technique, the contracted side of the soft-tissue sleeve is assessed for tight structures. Multiple stab incisions are made with a scalpel blade or large needle parallel to the joint line to effectively elongate the areas of the soft-tissue sleeve that are under undue tension (see Fig. 5.49C). Multiple studies have reported good outcomes in both valgus and varus deformities with this technique. The advantage of pie-crusting, especially on the lateral soft-tissue sleeve, is that it leaves a supporting tether that does not allow a larger gap opening on the lateral side of the knee in flexion. Cadaver studies have shown that larger releases are not possible with this technique until the lateral collateral ligament is resected. Care is needed when pie-crusting is done in the posterolateral corner because the peroneal nerve is within 1.5 cm of this area. Because the nerve is farther away when the knee is flexed, flexing the knee can help protect the nerve during pie-crusting of the posterolateral corner. In a varus knee, if pie-crusting cannot obtain enough elongation of the medial soft-tissue sleeve, then moving to more traditional releases off of the proximal tibia can be utilized for balancing. Regardless of the technique used, the surgeon should understand which anatomic structures will affect the extension and flexion gaps so that each individual type of gap asymmetry can be properly corrected. Multiple cadaver biomechanical studies have delineated which anatomic structures affect the flexion and extension gaps of the knee. In general, remember that release of the posterior structures from the posterior oblique ligament to the posterior capsule and semimembranosus insertion on the tibia affects the extension space more than the flexion space, and release of the anterior half of the superficial medial collateral and the pes anserinus insertion affects the flexion space more. Targeting these structures by pie-crusting has been shown to be safe and effective, and by feeling the tight bands, selective soft tissues can be targeted.

PIE-CRUSTING

TECHNIQUE 5.3

- After the distal femur is prepared using the anteroposterior and epicondylar axes as a rotational guide, cut the proximal tibia perpendicular to the mechanical axis and remove osteophytes.
- Place the knee in full extension and evaluate the medial and lateral soft-tissue balance with either a spacer block or trial components under varus and valgus stress or place tensioners medially and laterally between the posterior femoral condyles and proximal tibial cut surfaces. Careful placement of the tensioners is crucial to avoid crushing and deforming osteoporotic bone.

- Remove any retractors that are causing tension on the affected side and replace them with rake retractors.
- Palpate the soft tissues on the affected side and release them by pie-crusting until a rectangular flexion gap is achieved.
- Move the knee into 90 degrees of flexion and repeat the balancing assessment.
- If the knee is still tight medially or laterally in flexion, remove the trial components and reinsert the tensioning devices with the knee in flexion.
- Repeat pie-crusting with the knee in 90 degrees flexion until a rectangular flexion gap is achieved (Fig. 5.49).
- Replace the trial components and confirm coronal plane stability in flexion and extension.
- Correct any residual discrepancies in the flexion and extension gaps with pie-crusting or, if necessary, standard gap balancing techniques (see Technique 5.2).

POSTERIOR STABILIZED TOTAL KNEE ARTHROPLASTY IN A VARUS KNEE

TECHNIQUE 5.4

- Make the initial exposure to include release of the deep medial collateral ligament off the tibia to the posteromedial corner of the knee.
- Make the bone cuts using the preferred technique (intramedullary or extramedullary guide, computer navigation, custom cutting blocks).
- Remove all osteophytes on the femur and the tibia because they can tent the medial soft-tissue sleeve and effectively shorten the medial collateral ligament.
- Make sure the PCL is resected before balancing. Because the PCL is a secondary medial stabilizer, take care not to release the entire soft-tissue sleeve off the tibia because it may overshoot the gap. In general, less soft-tissue release is needed to balance a varus knee once the PCL is resected.
- Assess the flexion and extension gaps. If the gaps are tight medially, release the appropriate tight portion of the medial soft-tissue sleeve with your preferred method. Recheck the gaps in flexion and extension.
- If the extension gap is tight only medially in extension, the posterior oblique ligament portion can be targeted for release now or later in the soft-tissue balancing procedure. If the extension gap remains tight medially, the semimembranosus and posteromedial capsule can be targeted for release.
- If the flexion gap is tight, the anterior aspect of the superficial medial collateral ligament and tight bands within the structure can be targeted for release.
- If the entire soft-tissue sleeve is released and the medial gap is still tight (as is usually the case with severe varus deformity), consider advancing the lateral collateral ligament or use of a more constrained implant.

POSTERIOR CRUCIATE–RETAINING TOTAL KNEE ARTHROPLASTY OF A VARUS KNEE

TECHNIQUE 5.5

- Make the initial exposure to include release of the deep medial collateral ligament off the tibia to the posteromedial corner of the knee.
- Make the bone cuts using the preferred technique (intramedullary or extramedullary guide, computer navigation, custom cutting blocks). Care needs to be taken to protect the bony insertion on the tibia of the PCL.
- Remove all osteophytes on the femur and the tibia because they can tent the medial soft-tissue sleeve and effectively shorten the medial collateral ligament.
- Assess the flexion and extension gaps and target the appropriate soft-tissue structures with your preferred balancing technique. With a CR TKA with the PCL intact, the release may need to be more significant to effectively balance the gap since the PCL is a secondary coronal stabilizing structure.
- If the extension gap is tight only medially, the posterior oblique ligament portion can be targeted now or later in the soft-tissue balancing procedure. If the extension gap remains tight medially, the semimembranosus and posteromedial capsule can be targeted for release (Fig. 5.48).
- If the flexion gap is tight, the anterior aspect of the superficial medial collateral ligament and the pes anserinus insertion can be targeted for release (see Fig. 5.48).
- If the entire soft-tissue sleeve is released and the medial gap is still tight, consider balancing the posterior cruciate ligament if it is tight (see section on Balancing of the Posterior Cruciate Ligament and Fig. 5.48). If after recession of the PCL it no longer functions in the sagittal plane, consider conversion to an anterior-lipped, deep-dish insert if available with the implant system being used or consider conversion to a posterior stabilized implant.
- If after complete release of the medial soft-tissue sleeve and PCL recession (see Fig. 5.48) there is still a tight medial gap, make certain the posterior capsule is not tight. If it is, release the capsule. If a tight medial gap still persists, consider advancing the lateral collateral ligament and/or using a constrained condylar implant (this usually is needed for severe varus deformity cases)

VALGUS DEFORMITY CORRECTION

Valgus deformity is common in patients with rheumatoid and inflammatory arthropathies and also can occur in those with hypoplastic lateral femoral condyle or previous trauma or reconstructive procedures that change the weight-bearing axis of the lower extremity or tighten the lateral side of the joint. The three-layer anatomy of the lateral side of

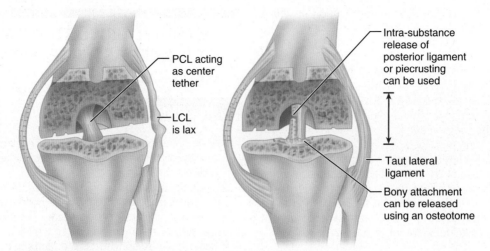

Intra-substance
release of
posterior ligament
or piecrusting
can be used

Taut lateral
ligament

Bony attachment
can be released
using an osteotome

PCL acting
as center
tether

LCL
is lax

FIGURE 5.48   The posterior cruciate ligament (PCL) is a more medial structure and may be involved in coronal plane deformity in osteoarthritic varus knee. After release of medial structures, PCL may still be affecting medial gap, especially in flexion, and may need to be released to equalize gaps. This can be done intrasubstance or off tibial insertion with or without piece of bone to effectively elongate ligament. PCL less likely acts as central tether in valgus deformity because of its more medial location. If it is involved in more severe valgus deformities, it may need to be released. **SEE TECHNIQUE 5.5.**

the knee joint makes its soft-tissue balancing more complex than with varus deformity. The surgeon should have detailed knowledge of the three soft-tissue layers to understand the release and balancing techniques used to correct tight lateral gaps in valgus deformity.

TECHNIQUE 5.6

- During exposure of a knee with a valgus deformity, take care not to compromise the medial soft-tissue sleeve, which may already be attenuated.
- Make the bone cuts using the preferred technique (intramedullary or extramedullary guide, computer navigation, custom cutting blocks).
- Remove osteophytes to the level of the native articular margins to avoid tenting of the soft tissues.
- The order of soft-tissue release on the lateral side of the knee varies, depending on the extent of fixed contracture and associated deformity.
- The structure released first depends on whether both the extension and flexion gaps are tight on the lateral side. If both are tight, then feel for the tight structures in both flexion and extension and target the appropriate structure with your preferred balancing technique to achieve a balanced gap. Try and leave the insertion of the popliteus tendon intact as long as it is not tight (see Fig. 5.49). Check for tight structures in both extension and flexion.
- If at any point during the balancing of the valgus knee only the extension gap is tight, release the tight portions of the iliotibial band by your preferred technique. For the ITB we recommend pie-crusting as opposed to complete release. Make certain all fibers are released and evaluate the biceps aponeurosis to make sure it is not involved in the contracture.
- Release of the posterolateral corner has been shown to effectively increase the extension space more than the flexion space and should be considered before release of the lateral collateral ligament if only a small amount of correction is needed.

- Release of the popliteus tendon will tend to increase the flexion gap laterally more than the extension gap.
- If the knee is still not balanced in full extension after release of all of these structures, release the posterior capsule off the lateral femoral condyle; then release of the lateral head of gastrocnemius may be considered if further correction is needed.
- Because it is a medial structure, the PCL often is attenuated in a knee with a valgus deformity. If complete release did not balance the gaps, inspect the PCL to determine whether it is involved in the deformity.
- If complete release of all of the above structures does not balance the flexion and extension gaps on the lateral side, consider advancement of the medial collateral ligament (Fig. 5.50).
- If the lateral flexion gap opens more than the extension gap, make certain that the "jump height" of a posterior stabilized peg is not exceeded; if this is a possibility, consider using a constrained condylar type of implant.

When a combined severe valgus and flexion contracture deformity is present, acute correction can cause stretching of the peroneal nerve and subsequent palsy. Close attention to the neurologic examination after surgery is recommended in these patients and, if a palsy presents itself after surgery, the knee should be flexed to alleviate traction on the nerve. Another, more commonly used approach is to immobilize the knee postoperatively in some degree of flexion to allow gradual stretching of the nerve as the knee is moved into extension.

Occasionally, because of attenuation of the medial collateral ligament, adequate ligament balance cannot be obtained. In elderly patients, a constrained condylar type of prosthesis may be a reasonable option. The other option in this circumstance is medial collateral ligament advancement, which includes elevation of the femoral origin of the medial collateral ligament and proximal advancement using

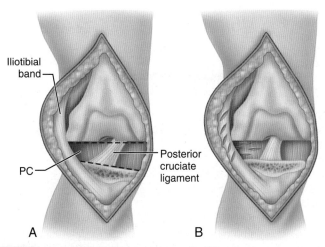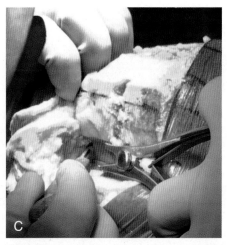

FIGURE 5.49 Pie-crusting technique. **A,** Knee with valgus deformity before intraarticular release of posterolateral aspect of capsule (PC). Note trapezoidal extension gap. **B,** Correction of deformity after release of posterolateral aspect of capsule and pie-crusting of iliotibial band. Note resulting rectangular extension gap. **C,** Surgical photo (**C,** From Mihalko WM, Woodard EL, Hebert CT, et al: Biomechanical validation of medial pie-crusting for soft tissue balancing in knee arthroplasty, *J Arthroplasty* 30:296, 2015.) **SEE TECHNIQUE 5.3.**

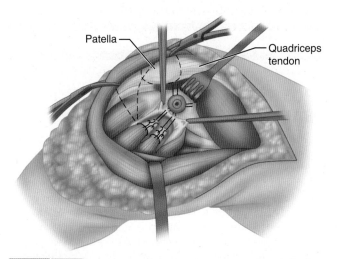

FIGURE 5.50 Advancement of femoral origin of medial collateral ligament and fixation in medial epicondyle with screw and washer.

a locking-loop type of suture within the substance of the ligament. This suture is secured around a screw and washer with a staple placed in its desired attachment in the medial epicondyle (Fig. 5.50).

FLEXION CONTRACTURE CORRECTION

Most preoperative flexion deformities improve with appropriate soft-tissue balancing for coronal plane deformity. If a flexion contracture persists despite balanced medial and lateral soft tissues, the shortened posterior structures must be effectively lengthened. If the contracture persists, the joint line may need to be elevated by increasing the

amount of distal femoral bone resection. With severe flexion contracture, elevation of the joint line more than 4 mm should be avoided because it can create midflexion instability, and an increase in implant constraint may be necessary.

TECHNIQUE 5.7

- Perform the bone cuts and ligament balancing using the surgeon's preferred techniques.
- To recreate the normal posterior capsular recesses of the knee joint, strip the adherent posterior capsule proximally off the femur a short distance above the femoral condyles. This usually is done after the posterior condylar cuts are made, allowing access to this space. Stripping farther proximally should be carried out carefully because of the risk of avulsing the superior geniculate artery at this level; bleeding can be difficult to control in this area.
- Make sure that all posterior condylar osteophytes have been removed off the femoral condyles and that no loose bodies are tenting the posterior capsule in this area. Remove posterior condylar osteophytes with a curved osteotome. Large osteophytes on the posterior aspect of the femur can be difficult to remove if they are adherent to the posterior capsule within the posterior capsular recess. Using a curet to peel these osteophytes off the posterior capsule makes removal easier.
- If necessary, release the posterior capsule further by stripping more proximally up the posterior aspect of the femur and releasing the tendinous origins of the gastrocnemius muscles if necessary. Alternatively, posterior capsular release off the proximal tibia can be considered, but extreme caution is required to protect neurovascular structures.
- If the flexion contracture persists, increase the distal femoral bone cut by 2 mm and recheck to see if the knee

will move into full extension with the trial components in place. This can be increased by another 2 mm (total of 4 mm over a matched resection) but make certain that midflexion instability does not exist. If it does, consider a constrained condylar type of implant.

When excessive distal femoral resection is performed in an effort to obtain extension, the knee may be stable in full extension because of a posterior tension band effect, but with slight flexion the knee may lack enough varus-valgus stability. In this situation, the collateral ligaments are relatively longer than the posterior soft-tissue restraints. A constrained condylar type of prosthesis may be necessary to resolve this "midflexion" instability, or in some severe cases, a hinge-type of implant.

We prefer to obtain full knee extension intraoperatively, using the steps outlined in Technique 5.7. No correlation has been found between patients who require increased distal femoral bone resection and the amount of coronal plane deformity. In a PCL-retaining TKA the PCL does not contribute to the flexion contracture deformity. Although it may be part of the coronal plane contracture and need to be released or balanced to correct the extension and flexion gap, releasing the PCL for a flexion deformity only further increases the flexion gap, making the disparity with the extension gap greater.

RECURVATUM CORRECTION

Recurvatum deformity is rare in patients who have TKA, reported to be present in less than 1% of patients. Regardless of the diagnosis for which TKA is indicated (OA, posttraumatic arthritis, or inflammatory arthritis), the presence of a recurvatum deformity presents a unique situation. Recurvatum often occurs in conjunction with a valgus knee deformity caused by a hypoplastic lateral femoral condyle that allows a larger extension space. A careful medical history and physical examination are necessary to identify any neuromuscular disease or any quadriceps weakness that may be the cause of the recurvatum deformity. Because recurvatum deformity tends to recur in patients with these conditions, a hinged implant with an extension stop may be needed to compensate for the loss of quadriceps power.

In a patient who has a recurvatum deformity but no neuromuscular weakness, the operative procedure must be planned so that the flexion and extension gaps are equal to prevent recurrent deformity after TKA. Simply adding height to the tibia will also tighten the flexion space and possibly decrease the amount of flexion after surgery; moving the joint line distally and/or using a smaller femoral component with anterior referencing is a preferable technique. Although possibly counterintuitive, using a smaller femoral component referenced from the anterior aspect of the femur requires removal of more posterior femoral condylar bone, which will increase the flexion gap. This will allow the height of the tibial polyethylene component to be used to fill the gap and create a joint space that is stable in extension and flexion. Whiteside and Mihalko found that moving the joint line 3 to 5 mm distally and using a smaller femoral component with anterior referencing corrected recurvatum deformities in 10 patients, with no recurrence at 1-year follow-up. In a report of 53 patients with recurvatum deformi-

ties not related to neuromuscular disease, only two of the 57 knees treated with a PCL-retaining implant had postoperative recurvatum of 10 degrees.

TECHNIQUE 5.8

- If the distal femoral cut is being made first, decrease the amount of bone to be removed by 2 to 3 mm depending on the severity of the recurvatum deformity.
- Place the sizing jig, and with anterior referencing determine the appropriate component size. If in between sizes, or if a significant recurvatum deformity exists, choose the smaller size to increase the amount of posterior condylar bone removed.
- If the tibial resection is done first, measure the extension gap with a spacer block to determine the amount of distal femoral resection necessary to fill the extension gap and decrease the distal femoral resection by that amount.
- Regardless of which resection is done first, make certain during trial component reduction that the knee is no longer in recurvatum and that the flexion space is not tight once the appropriate height polyethylene component is chosen to correct the recurvatum deformity.

POSTERIOR CRUCIATE LIGAMENT BALANCING

With retention of the PCL, femoral rollback is accomplished by tension developed within the PCL during knee flexion (see Fig. 5.3). A PCL that is too tight in flexion can lead to poor postoperative knee flexion or excessive femoral rollback, which is thought to be a factor in accelerated polyethylene wear. Conversely, if the PCL does not develop adequate tension in flexion, femoral rollback does not occur. Accurate balancing of the PCL is necessary for optimal functioning and longevity of a PCL-retaining prosthesis.

TECHNIQUE 5.9

- Correct excessive PCL tension by partial release or recession of the PCL, which is accomplished in a stepwise fashion with frequent retesting of the PCL tension.
- Release the PCL from the superior surface of the bone island on the tibia (see Figs. 5.48 and 5.51).
- Release it subperiosteally in 1- to 2-mm intervals along the posterior surface of the tibia. The PCL bone island can be partially or completely removed. The PCL has a broad insertion over approximately 2 cm on the posterior surface of the proximal tibia.
- If partial release is unsuccessful in balancing the PCL, make certain that the appropriate amount of posterior slope for the implant being used was obtained in the proximal tibial cut.
- More commonly, a smaller femoral component, with anterior referencing for sizing, can be used to enlarge the flexion gap relative to the extension gap if necessary.

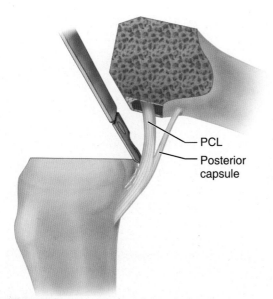

FIGURE 5.51 Posterior cruciate ligament can be "recessed" by releasing it from superior surface of tibia and proximal portion of its posterior tibial attachment. **SEE TECHNIQUE 5.9.**

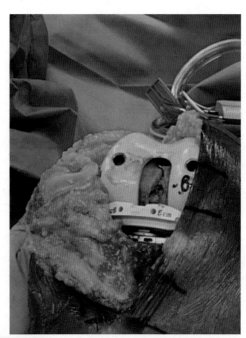

FIGURE 5.52 One sign of tight flexion space in cruciate-retaining TKA is seen in this intraoperative photo showing lift-off of trial poly insert in flexion. In this case osteophytes in intracondylar notch were removed to balance PCL.

■ Alternatively, with difficulty balancing the PCL or with PCL incompetence because of complete release, sacrifice it completely and convert to a PCL-substituting design or use a high anterior wall or deep-dish tibial polyethylene component if the implant system provides that option to prevent anterior translation of the femoral condyles with knee flexion.

A trial tibial component that lacks a stem can be used to evaluate PCL balancing. If the tibial tray lifts off anteriorly with knee flexion, PCL tension is excessive (Fig. 5.52). The patella should be located within the trochlear groove during this and other tests of PCL tension because the everted patella externally rotates the tibia in flexion and can lead to a false-positive result. Direct observation of femoral rollback during flexion also can be used: the tibiofemoral contact point should not move onto the posterior third of the tibial articular surface. With the knee in 90 degrees of flexion, firm digital pressure should cause the PCL to deflect 1 to 2 mm. If more than 75% of the PCL is released, a prosthesis with greater posterior constraint should be chosen to avoid late posterior instability. Cadaver studies have shown that the posterior slope has more of an effect than partial release of the PCL. Because complete release of the PCL affects the flexion space more than the extension space, balancing or release of the PCL does not correct a flexion contracture nor create a recurvatum deformity during TKA.

MANAGEMENT OF BONE DEFICIENCY

Bone deficiencies encountered during TKA can have multiple causes, including arthritic angular deformity, condylar hypoplasia, osteonecrosis, trauma, and previous surgery such as HTO and previous TKA. The method used to compensate for a given bone defect depends on the size and the location of the defect. Contained or cavitary defects have an intact rim of cortical bone surrounding the deficient area, whereas noncontained or segmental defects are more peripheral and lack a bony cortical rim (Fig. 5.53).

Rand classified these defects into three types:

Type I: focal metaphyseal defect, intact cortical rim
Type II: extensive metaphyseal defect, intact cortical rim
Type III: combined metaphyseal and cortical defect

Small defects (<5 mm) typically are filled with cement. Contained defects can be filled with impacted cancellous bone graft. Larger noncontained defects can be treated by a variety of methods, including the use of structural bone grafts, metal wedges attached to the prosthesis, or screws within cement that fills the defect. The Anderson Orthopaedic Research Institute (AORI) further delineated bone loss into either femoral (F1, F2, and F3) or tibial (T1, T2, and T3) descriptions. Type 2 defects were further classified into A (bone loss in one condyle) or B (bone loss in both condyles).

Before contemporary augments were released, larger contained defects in primary TKA were reported with use of PMMA and screw fixation. In 145 TKAs (20 all-polyethylene tibial components and 125 metal-backed trays) with medial tibial defects treated with screws and cement, medial collapse occurred in two and lateral collapse in one, all in metal-backed tibial components; no revisions were required.

No progression of tibial radiolucencies was seen over 7 years in 25 knees in which screw-augmented cement was used to fill large tibial defects (Fig. 5.54).

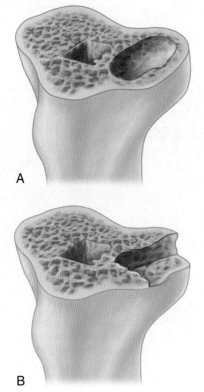

FIGURE 5.53   **A,** Contained defects have intact rim of cortical bone surrounding area. **B,** Noncontained defects are more peripheral and lack bony cortical rim.

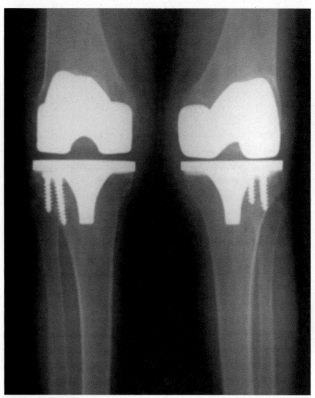

FIGURE 5.54   Screws used to augment polymethyl methacrylate for filling tibial defect.

BONE GRAFTING OF PERIPHERAL TIBIAL DEFECTS

TECHNIQUE 5.10

(WINDSOR, INSALL, AND SCULCO)

- Convert the concave, irregular defect to a flat one by minimal bone removal with a saw (Fig. 5.55).
- Attach bone removed from the distal femur or proximal tibia to the flattened defect and secure it with threaded Steinmann pins or screws (Fig. 5.56).
- Carefully recut the upper tibial surface to create a flat upper tibial surface.
- During cementing, premix a small batch of cement and use it to seal the junction of the bone graft with the tibia to prevent extrusion of cement into this interface during final component cement fixation.
- If the defect cannot be corrected with this type of reconstruction because too much bone must be removed from the tibia or femur to allow apposition of flat bone surfaces, level the irregular bone surfaces with a burr to allow maximal graft-host bone apposition.
- Fashion the graft to fit the defect.

Restoration of neutral alignment is essential because this has been shown to affect bone graft survival and prosthesis loosening. Intramedullary stems on the femoral and tibial

components commonly are used to protect peripheral bone grafts from stress.

Brand et al. first reported the use of modular metal wedges attached to the tibial tray to compensate for tibial bone deficiencies (Fig. 5.57). They reported no tibial loosening in 22 knees observed an average of 3 years. Most modern total knee systems employ modular wedges and blocks that can be attached to femoral and tibial components to compensate for multiple bone deficiencies. With these structural additions, a surgeon can literally build a custom prosthesis in the operating room for a given defect or combination of defects.

Although not often necessary in primary TKA, porous metal augments and cones also are now available, and good results have been reported with their use (Fig. 5.58A). Some of these cones are press fit into the distal femoral or proximal tibial cavitary defect and then the implant is cemented into these types of augments to create a composite type of construct. Sleeves also are available that are attached to the implant to create a single implant construct when the defects are contained (see Fig. 5.58B and C). Most of these devices are used for revision cases involving significant defects. These cone-types of augments have shown successful integration even when the implant construct has failed.

PATELLOFEMORAL TRACKING

Patellofemoral tracking is affected by multiple factors, each of which must be inspected during trial reduction and before final component implantation. Any factor that increases the Q angle of the extensor mechanism can cause lateral maltracking of the patella. Internal rotation of the tibial component lateralizes the tibial tubercle, increasing the Q angle and

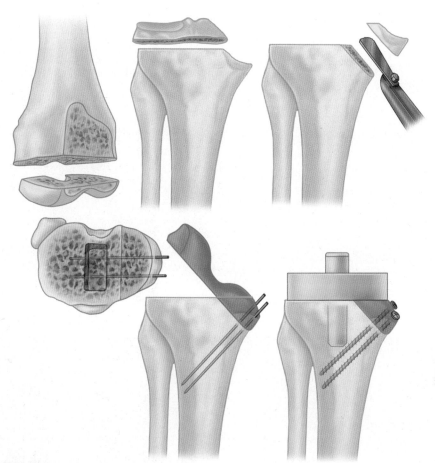

FIGURE 5.55 Technique of Windsor et al. for grafting of peripheral tibial defects. **SEE TECHNIQUE 5.10.**

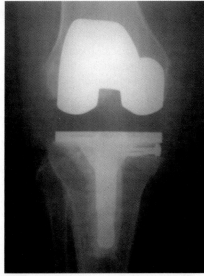

FIGURE 5.56 Medial segmental tibial defect filled with autogenous bone block from distal femoral resection fixed with cancellous screws. **SEE TECHNIQUE 5.10.**

the tendency to lateral patellar subluxation. Similarly, internal rotation or medial translation of the femoral component can increase lateral patellar subluxation by moving the trochlea medially. If the patella is to be resurfaced, the prosthetic patella should be medialized to approximate the median

eminence of the normal patella, rather than simply centering the prosthetic button on the available bone (Fig. 5.59). Centralization of the patellar component requires the bony patella to track medially, which forces it to function with a higher Q angle. Increasing the anterior displacement of the patella during knee motion also can lead to patellar instability or limited flexion. Anterior displacement can be caused by placing the trochlea too far anterior with an oversized femoral component or by underresection of the patella, which results in an overall increase in patellar thickness (Fig. 5.60).

The "no thumb" test of patellar tracking should be used as a guide of adequate patellar stability. The reduced patella is observed within the femoral trochlea throughout the range of knee motion before retinacular closure. If the patellar button tracks congruently with minimal or no pressure applied to the lateral side of the patella, patellofemoral tracking is adequate. If the patella tends to subluxate, the knee should be inspected for the previously discussed causes of patellar subluxation. If none of these factors is identified, a lateral patellar retinacular release may be necessary. Lateral retinacular release is accomplished by cutting the synovium and retinaculum longitudinally, to a variable extent, from Gerdy's tubercle distally to the muscle fibers of the vastus lateralis proximally (Fig. 5.61). Frequently, release of only small transverse bands is sufficient, but occasionally the entire release is necessary. Most commonly, this release is performed from inside the knee joint with anterior and lateral retraction of the patella, although some surgeons prefer

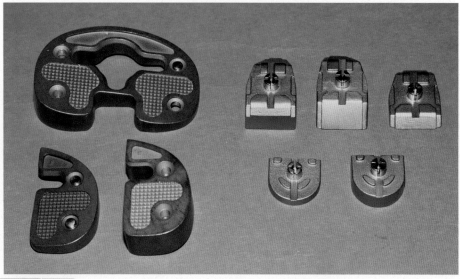

FIGURE 5.57 Modular wedges for femoral and tibial augmentation.

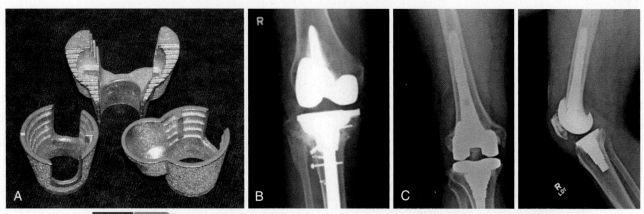

FIGURE 5.58 **A,** Porous metal cones are placed into metaphyseal defects for enhanced fixation. **B,** Radiograph of bi-lobed tibial cone used to augment defect from tibial plateau fracture nonunion. **C,** Sleeves that are attached to implant stem construct can enhance metaphyseal-contained or uncontained defects as seen in this anteroposterior and lateral radiograph of revision TKA in rheumatoid patient with poor bone.

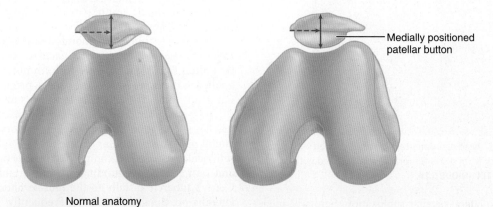

FIGURE 5.59 The patellar button should be positioned medially to recreate location of apex of the native patella and improve tracking. Care should be taken not to "overreplace" patella, which will increase the height and possibility of tilt and/or lateral subluxation and patellar maltracking.

to release the retinaculum from the exterior surface, leaving the lateral synovium intact. The latter approach requires creation of a large lateral subcutaneous flap superficial to the retinaculum but can provide exposure of the superior lateral geniculate vessels and allow their preservation.

Lowering the tourniquet and reassessing patellar tracking before lateral retinacular release have been shown to avoid an unnecessary lateral retinacular release. One study found that 48% of knees showed initial maltracking, which reverted to normal after tourniquet release, and another reported that tourniquet deflation improved patellar tracking in 31% of patients who otherwise would have required lateral release.

The greatest risk in lateral release is devascularization of the patella caused by interruption of the superior lateral geniculate artery. This artery is located at the musculotendinous junction of the vastus lateralis and usually can be preserved. An increased prevalence of patellar fracture also has been correlated with lateral release. Other potential problems associated with lateral release include increased postoperative pain and swelling, slower rehabilitation, and increased wound complications. Nevertheless, the potential complications of lateral release are far outweighed by the detrimental effect of patellar subluxation.

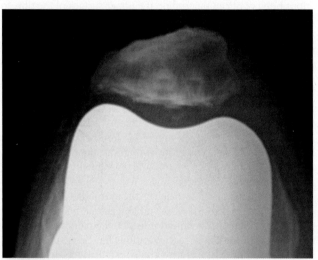

FIGURE 5.60   Radiograph depicting improper resection of the patella and button placement.

COMPONENT IMPLANTATION

TECHNIQUE 5.11

- After bone deficiencies have been treated, ligamentous balancing is satisfactory, and the extensor mechanism is tracking properly, remove the trial components. Do not hyperextend the knee because the joint is unstable with the trial components removed and the posterior neurovascular structures can be injured.
- If an intramedullary guide has been used on the tibia, occlude the tibial intramedullary canal with a plug of previously resected bone distal to the level of the tibial stem. Occlude the femoral canal in a similar fashion.
- If sclerotic bone surfaces are present, use a small drill to make multiple perforations into the underlying cancellous bone to allow cement intrusion.

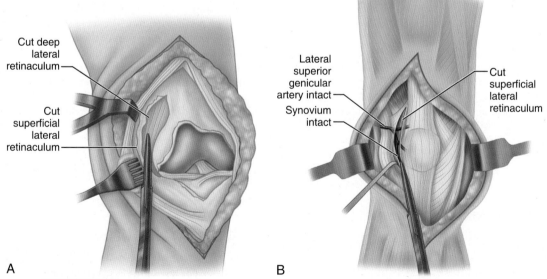

FIGURE 5.61   **A,** Lateral retinacular release can be done from inside out, which releases synovial layer and lateral retinaculum but can expose joint to subcutaneous tissue. Release is made from vastus lateralis muscle fibers proximally and distally to Gerdy's tubercle if necessary. **B,** Outside-in technique also can be used, which allows synovial membrane to remain intact, leaving layer between subcutaneous tissue and intraarticular space. This also allows identification of lateral geniculate artery, which can be preserved.

- Clean the cut bone surfaces with a pulsatile lavage irrigator using saline containing an added antibiotic solution such as cefazolin or genitourinary irrigant.
- Dry surfaces with clean sponges.
- Generally, the tibial tray is implanted first. Apply PMMA cement in its initial setting phase right after mixing when it is "sticky" onto the cemented surfaces of the tibial baseplate, including the keel and the femoral component. Then pressurize the tibial keel and cancellous bone surface. Add a suction drain to one of the tibial cutting block pin sites to keep blood and fat from mixing with the cement and to keep it out of the cement-prosthesis interface.
- Impaction of the tibial prosthesis generally results in intrusion of early dough-phase cement to a depth of 2 to 5 mm in cancellous bone, which is sufficient for long-term fixation.
- Remove excess cement from the periphery of the component.
- Cement the femoral and patellar components in a similar fashion. Usually, all components can be cemented simultaneously, but this requires an efficient and experienced surgical team.
- Cementing of the tibia and femur also can be done by preparing two batches of cement. Using a two-batch cementation technique by starting the mixture of the second batch at the time of cement application to the tibial baseplate may be better in settings in which the operating room staff are not familiar with cementation procedures.
- The patella can be cemented with the femur or the tibia, but use cement in an early dough phase to allow adequate cement intrusion.
- Access to the posterior femoral recesses is limited after the femoral and tibial components have been implanted. To minimize the amount of cement that may have to be removed from the posterior femoral recesses, apply a small amount of cement to the posterior femoral bone surface and a limited amount on the posterior condyles of the femoral implant when applying the cement to the femoral implant.
- After the femoral component has been seated, carefully extend the knee with a trial tibial spacer in place to ensure complete seating of the femoral prosthesis.
- Ensure that the tibial spacer is of adequate thickness to hold the knee in full extension. If a thinner tibial trial is substituted, hyperextension of the knee and posterior lift-off of the tibial component posteriorly could result.
- Carefully searching for any bone or cement debris before implantation of the final tibial polyethylene articular surface is paramount to keep any remaining debris from causing third body wear of the polyethylene.

All surgeons should be familiar with the manufacturer's recommendations for implantation and fixation techniques of the system being used. It is extremely important that surgeons follow the directions specific to the bone cement used because small variations in technique could be detrimental to the long-term survivorship of the primary TKA implants. We also recommend cementation of the keel because it has been shown in biomechanical studies to be comparable to using an extended press-fit stem.

For cementless fixation of total knee components, the technique of implantation is less demanding, but the preparation of the cut bone surfaces requires more accuracy than with cement fixation. Cementless fixation relies on intimate apposition of the fixation surface to the cut bone surfaces and rigid immediate fixation to minimize micromotion. To evaluate apposition, the trial tibial tray without a keel/stem extension can be placed in the center of the tibial cut surface and held with an index finger. The periphery of the tray can then be stressed to observe any movement of the tray on the bony surface. If any movement is detected, the surface should be revised to allow complete support of the tibial tray with no visual movement when peripheral load is manually applied. In experimental models, bone-prosthesis gaps of more than 0.5 mm tend to fill with fibrous tissue. A fine autogenous bone graft can be used on the upper surface of the tibia to level small irregularities. Retrieval studies have repeatedly shown maximal bone ingrowth around fixation screws and pegs, and the use of such adjunctive fixation is crucial to obtain the stability necessary for bone ingrowth and long-term prosthesis fixation.

WOUND CLOSURE

Conventionally, after the final prosthesis has been implanted, the tourniquet is released, the knee is packed with moist sponges, and pressure is applied. Hemostasis is obtained by sequentially removing the sponges from the lateral and medial sides of the knee, looking specifically for bleeding from the geniculate arteries.

Although we continue to deflate the tourniquet before wound closure to obtain hemostasis, we no longer routinely use suction drains. No difference in wound infection, hematoma formation, or reoperation for wound complications has been substantiated with or without postoperative drain use. Patients with drains were found to be more likely to receive transfusions, whereas undrained wounds required more frequent dressing reinforcement. The use of a femoral intramedullary plug has been shown to decrease blood loss associated with TKA by 20% to 25%.

After hemostasis is obtained, the retinacular incision is closed, taking care to approximate the elevated periosteal tissues to the patellar tendon. The knee should be flexed past 90 degrees to ensure that no part of the closure limits flexion, that the patella tracks normally, and that none of the repair sutures are compromised and fail. The use of double-barbed running suture for closure can improve water tightness and capsular closure and has been reported to be cost effective. The subcutaneous tissue and skin are closed with the knee in approximately 40 degrees of flexion to aid in skin flap alignment.

ARTHROPLASTY TECHNIQUES (UNICONDYLAR AND PATELLOFEMORAL KNEE ARTHROPLASTIES)

UNICONDYLAR KNEE ARTHROPLASTY

If the strict indications outlined in 1989 by Kozinn and Scott were followed, few patients would be candidates for UKA. In most reports, long-term prosthesis survival in UKA to date has been less than that in TKA. A few current UKA prostheses have performed better than their predecessors, however, with survivorship at 10 years ranging from 82% to 98%. Important selection criteria include an intact anterior cruciate ligament, unicompartmental arthritis, passively correctable deformity, and reasonable body weight. Multiple techniques for UKA now exist, including fixed bearing (inset or onlay designs), mobile bearing, and computer or robotically assisted methods (MAKOplasty, Mako Surgical Corp., Ft. Lauderdale, FL). Just as in primary TKA, the differences between fixed and mobile-bearing techniques involve strict adherence to equalization of flexion and extension gaps to avoid bearing "spit-out." The MAKOplasty technique uses preoperative CT studies to register anatomic landmarks in the operating room. The computer-assisted system then aids preparation of the bone on the femoral and tibial sides for proper implant positioning to match the preoperative plan.

TECHNIQUE 5.12

- Make a longitudinal skin incision along the medial or lateral aspect of the patellar tendon depending on the compartment being replaced. A medial approach can be used for a lateral unicondylar replacement, but the exposure must be more extensive to allow adequate patellar eversion or subluxation; a minimally invasive technique requires a lateral approach.
- Make sure the capsular incision does not go above the vastus medialis or lateralis. A Hohmann-type retractor can be used to lever the patella medially or laterally with the knee in flexion to expose the entire femoral condyle.
- To expose the medial compartment, incise the coronary ligament, remove the anterior horn of the medial meniscus, and raise the periosteal sleeve from the anteromedial aspect of the tibia.
- To expose the lateral compartment, raise the anterolateral periosteal sleeve to the medial aspect of Gerdy's tubercle.
- Carefully inspect the two compartments being preserved to be sure the patient is a candidate for UKA.
- Remove all peripheral osteophytes before the bone cuts are made to allow better exposure, especially when a minimally invasive approach is used (Fig. 5.62). Removal of the tibial peripheral osteophytes should be enough to adequately balance the arthritic compartment (Fig. 5.63). Make certain intercondylar osteophytes also are removed because they can impinge on the cruciate ligaments and damage them.
- A need for more extensive soft-tissue balancing may indicate inadequate bony resection or a varus deformity that is too severe for UKA.
- With most fixed bearing systems, the matched resection begins with the tibial resection. Use an extramedullary guide to align the proximal tibial cut with the center of the ankle distally and recreate the posterior tibial slope with a 2-mm deep resection or as indicated by the implant system. For onlay tibial implants, use a reciprocating saw to complete the tibial bone cut just medial to the medial tibial eminence.
- With the knee flexed, use a spacer block to make sure the gap is large enough for the smallest tibial resection (this varies according to the implant system used but usually is about 8 mm).
- Move the knee into full extension and use another spacer block to determine the distal femoral resection needed to balance the flexion and extension gaps. Use the implant-specific cutting jig to make the distal femoral cut.

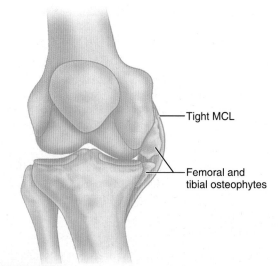

FIGURE 5.62 Osteophytes on medial side of femur and tibia prevent correction of varus deformity. **SEE TECHNIQUE 5.12**

Tight MCL

Femoral and tibial osteophytes

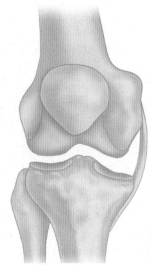

FIGURE 5.63 After osteophyte resection, knee passively corrects to normal alignment. **SEE TECHNIQUE 5.12.**

- Once the distal femoral cut is made, insert the femoral sizing guide and determine the appropriate sized cutting block. Make the posterior condylar bone resection and chamfer cut as indicated.
- Take care to resect the medial meniscus and remove any loose bodies from the posterior recess of the knee.
- Insert the tibial trial implant and perform a trial reduction to ensure that the joint is stable in extension and flexion and that a full range of motion is possible without overstuffing or excessive laxity.
- Complete bone preparation specific to implant design and cementation of the implants as described in Technique 5.11. Take care to ensure that no loose or excessive amount of bone cement remains in the posterior aspect of the tibia or posterior femoral condyle.
- Close the wound as described in the earlier section, Wound Closure.

PATELLOFEMORAL ARTHROPLASTY

A successful patellofemoral arthroplasty relies on strict adherence to operative indications. Most implant systems now offer second- or third-generation, minimally constrained patellofemoral components that have reported long-term survivorship of 70% or more at 8 to 10 years after surgery. Custom implants are available, with the suggested advantage of conserving more bone. Conversion rates to TKA are higher after patellofemoral arthroplasty than after UKA, and progression of arthritis in the tibiofemoral articulation is the most common reason for reoperation.

TECHNIQUE 5.13

- Use the same midline approach as described in Technique 5.1, taking care not to incise the coronary meniscal ligament.
- Carefully inspect the tibiofemoral articulations to ensure that the patient is a candidate for patellofemoral arthroplasty.
- Femoral trochlear preparation uses an intramedullary starting point similar to that for TKA, and a cutting block for the anterior femoral resection is pinned in place perpendicular to the anteroposterior axis of Whiteside.
- If the trochlear groove is hypoplastic, as is the case in many candidates for patellofemoral arthroplasty, slightly flex the anterior femoral trochlear cutting block to allow more bone removal without notching or overstuffing the patellofemoral mechanism.
- Prepare the trochlear intercondylar bone using the appropriate size femoral component and removing bone with a burr or curet, or by using a template with a routing tool. Final component preparation is implant specific, most commonly using pegs for cementation support.
- Prepare the patella as described in Technique 5.11, making certain that no overstuffing of the patella results.
- Cementation is as described in Technique 5.11 and wound closure as described in an earlier section.

POSTOPERATIVE MANAGEMENT

Postoperative physical therapy and rehabilitation greatly influence the outcome of TKA. Initially, a compressive dressing is worn to decrease postoperative bleeding, and a knee immobilizer may be used until quadriceps strength is adequate to ensure stability during ambulation.

Range-of-motion exercises are performed postoperatively, with or without the assistance of a continuous passive motion machine. Continuous passive motion has been shown in multiple studies to assist in obtaining knee flexion more quickly, which may decrease the length of stay in the hospital. Continuous passive motion has not been proved to affect the prevalence of DVT, long-term knee range of motion, or knee functional scores.

Passive knee extension is encouraged by placing the patient's foot on a pillow while in bed. Dangling the legs over the side of the bed is used to promote flexion. Patients are instructed in a home exercise program. Many surgeons have their patients instructed by a physical therapist preoperatively because postoperative pain and analgesics may hinder the patient's understanding of the necessary rehabilitation. In addition to range-of-motion exercises, the postoperative rehabilitation protocol includes lower extremity muscle strengthening, concentrating on the quadriceps; gait training, with weight bearing as allowed by the particular knee reconstruction; and instruction in performing basic ADLs.

Retention of the cruciate ligaments and limited surgical dissection typically allows patients with unicondylar or patellofemoral arthroplasty to have shorter hospital stays and faster rehabilitation.

SURGICAL PROBLEMS RELATIVE TO SPECIFIC DISORDERS
PREVIOUS HIGH TIBIAL OSTEOTOMY

HTO frequently is used to treat unicompartmental OA of the knee (see chapter 7), usually as a time-buying procedure to delay eventual TKA. Although HTO previously was thought to have no effect on the outcome of eventual TKA, multiple studies have shown less successful outcomes after HTO, along with predictable surgical challenges. Factors cited as contributing to poor results include the presence of patella infera, difficulties in exposure, and poor lateral skin flap vascularity. A review of 166 TKAs after HTO found an 8% revision rate at 6 years' follow-up and identified several risk factors for failure, including male gender, obesity, young age, varus-valgus laxity, and preexisting limb malalignment. Other studies have found no difference in postoperative knee function or complications compared with primary TKA without previous osteotomy.

Several technical problems unique to patients with previous HTO must be expected and accounted for to improve results with conversion to TKA. Although transverse skin incisions may be ignored, lateral longitudinal skin incisions must be respected, and an adequate intervening skin bridge of at least 8 cm must be left between new midline and old lateral incisions. Scarring over the lateral compartment and infrapatellar region may be encountered, making patellar eversion and lateral compartment exposure more difficult. Lateral retinacular release, V-Y quadricepsplasty, or a tibial tubercle osteotomy may be necessary for exposure. Medial subperiosteal exposure also must be done carefully to maintain the continuous soft-tissue sleeve necessary for closure and medial soft-tissue stability. Because ligamentous balancing may be difficult, many authors recommend routine PCL substitution.

After failed valgus closing wedge osteotomy of the proximal tibia, only minimal bone resection from the lateral tibial plateau usually is necessary. The tibial cut should be referenced off the intact medial compartment, which may leave a defect on the lateral side of the tibia that requires bone grafting or placement of a metal augmentation wedge or block (Fig. 5.64). Another common problem after previous HTO is medial offset of the intramedullary canal of the tibia relative to the center of the tibial tray. Extramedullary alignment usually is advocated in this situation, and medialization of the tibial tray or an offset tibial stem may be needed to accommodate the deformity. Rotational deformity also may be

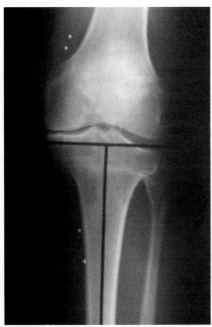

FIGURE 5.64 Frequently after high tibial osteotomy, lateral tibial bone is deficient after proximal tibial resection.

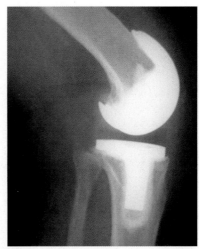

FIGURE 5.65 Posterior cruciate ligament–substituting arthroplasty performed for previous patellectomy and osteoarthritis.

encountered with previous HTO because the proximal fragment may be rotated relative to the tibial shaft. The tibial tray must be inserted carefully to avoid internal rotation and subsequent patellar tracking problems.

Over the past decade, opening-wedge proximal tibial osteotomy techniques have become popular for correction of varus deformity in the arthritic knee. Opening-wedge osteotomies are purported to cause less anatomic change to the proximal tibia than do closing lateral wedge techniques, making conversion to TKA easier; however, there is currently little information in the literature regarding this technique. In a series of 76 valgus opening wedge osteotomies using external fixation, 9 knees (12%) had required conversion to TKA at 7-year follow-up; only one knee had patella infera, and the authors reported no technical difficulties caused by altered proximal tibial anatomy. More recently, the outcomes of TKA after opening wedge tibial osteotomy in 36 patients were compared with a cohort of over 1300 primary TKA patients. Although the authors found TKA technically straightforward in most patients, clinical results were inferior in those with previous osteotomy, who had lower knee scores and more pain. Another study compared results of TKA after UKA and HTO and found both procedures resulted in a higher risk of revision.

PREVIOUS PATELLECTOMY

Early clinical studies of TKA after patellectomy reported varied results, with most reporting persistent pain and functional disability because of quadriceps weakness. More recent studies are more encouraging, although the type of prosthesis that is optimal in this setting is debated. Comparison of the results of TKA after patellectomy in patients treated with PCL-retaining and PCL-substituting prostheses with a control group of TKA patients without previous patellectomy found that Knee Society Scores were greater for PCL-substituting designs, whereas PCL-retaining knees showed

greater anteroposterior instability (Fig. 5.65). Presumably, the four-bar linkage of the quadriceps tendon, patellar tendon, and cruciate ligaments is disrupted by patellectomy, and the PCL and posterior capsule are incapable of maintaining long-term sagittal plane stability (Fig. 5.66). The resultant vector of the force exerted on the tibial tubercle by the patellar tendon changes after patellectomy, and not only is there less of a moment arm imparted by the extensor mechanism but also a more posterior force on the tibia results from the loss of the patella (see Fig. 5.66). Although these patients have less of a mechanical advantage to their extensor mechanism, treatment of tibiofemoral arthritis results in good pain relief and function, although not as good as in knees with an intact patella. A highly porous tantalum-based patellar implant has been used in an attempt to recreate the patella and improve the extensor mechanism moment arm; however, high failure rates because of loosening, wound complications, or continued anterior knee pain have been reported in several studies. Results appear to be better when there is remaining patellar bone stock to allow ingrowth into the trabecular metal.

NEUROPATHIC ARTHROPATHY

Although neuropathic arthropathy generally is considered a relative contraindication to TKA, fair results have been reported after arthroplasty for Charcot arthropathy. Keys to improving results include proper surgical technique, with attention to limb alignment, ligamentous balancing, bone grafting or prosthetic augmentation for bony defects, and use of revision-type components when necessary. In the longest follow-up study to date (12 years), Bae et al. reported one infection and two dislocations in 11 arthroplasties in nine patients with neuropathic arthropathy. Because of the propensity of Charcot knees to develop early postoperative dislocation and progress to symptomatic instability, they recommended the use of a rotating hinge prosthesis and postoperative protection with a knee brace or immobilizer to prevent early dislocation. Although TKA in this patient population is technically demanding and has a relatively high complication rate, patients with Charcot neuropathy can have relatively good outcomes with TKA.

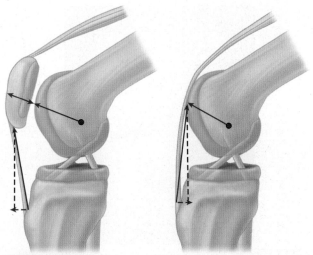

FIGURE 5.66 Four-bar linkage system of cruciate ligaments reveals that patellar tendon is roughly parallel to posterior cruciate ligament and quadriceps tendon is roughly parallel to anterior cruciate ligament at 30 degrees of flexion when patella is engaged with trochlear groove. Loss of patella results in alteration of extensor mechanism moment arm and loss of contraction strength of quadriceps.

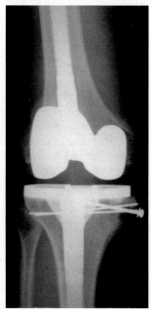

FIGURE 5.67 Total knee arthroplasty performed for hemophilic arthropathy with medial tibial structural autograft and press-fit stems.

OTHER MEDICAL CONDITIONS

Knee arthroplasty can relieve pain in patients with hemophilic arthropathy, but restoration of motion is suboptimal and the risk of perioperative complications is considerable (Fig. 5.67). Significant postoperative complications after TKA in hemophilic patients include hemorrhage, superficial skin necrosis, nerve palsies, and deep infection. Because a perioperative factor VIII level of less than 80% has been associated with a greater probability of complications, the perioperative factor VIII level should be maintained at 100%. In a report of 60 primary TKAs in patients with hemophilia, 95% had good or excellent results at 9-year follow-up and only one deep infection was noted. Use of newer techniques of continuous infusion of clotting factor was cited as the primary reason for the low complication rate.

Many patients with hemophilic arthropathy have been infected with human immunodeficiency virus (HIV) contracted from contaminated transfusions of coagulation factors. The most common complication after TKA in these patients is infection, with reported rates of 30%. In patients with HIV, it should be noted that a clearance note from their infectious disease specialist should state a lowered viral load and adequate CD4 counts before considering surgery. TKA in patients who are HIV positive, with or without hemophilia, has a high complication rate. Surgeons should have a frank discussion with patients who are HIV positive concerning the high rates of infection and other complications before TKA is considered. A recent review of the literature pointed out an infection rate of 7.7% in patients with HIV compared to 3.3% in patients without HIV but with comparable survivorship.

TKA in patients with diabetes is associated with an increased wound complication rate, increased infection, and more frequent revisions, with no significant differences noted between insulin-dependent and non–insulin-dependent diabetics. When the presence of metabolic syndrome was added, these complication rates were up to 10 times that of healthy patients, and optimization of the patient should be considered prior to surgery.

An inflammatory arthritis similar to rheumatoid arthritis develops in approximately 7% of patients with psoriasis. The exfoliating plaques seen on extensor surfaces harbor bacterial pathogens, which increases the risk of deep infection after TKA. Optimal control of psoriatic lesions in the vicinity of proposed skin incisions should be obtained before TKA.

COMPLICATIONS
THROMBOEMBOLISM

One of the most significant complications after TKA is the development of DVT, possibly resulting in life-threatening PE. Factors that have been correlated with an increased risk of DVT include age older than 40 years, estrogen use, stroke, nephrotic syndrome, cancer, prolonged immobility, previous thromboembolism, congestive heart failure, indwelling femoral vein catheter, inflammatory bowel disease, obesity, varicose veins, smoking, hypertension, diabetes mellitus, and myocardial infarction. The overall prevalence of DVT after TKA without any form of mechanical or pharmaceutical prophylaxis has been reported to range from 1% to 84%. Proximal thrombi in the popliteal vein and above have been reported in 0% to 16% of patients. These pose a greater risk of PE than thrombi in calf veins, which have been reported in 1% to 67% of patients. Thrombi in the calf veins, however, do have a propensity to propagate proximally. The risk of asymptomatic PE may be 0% to 12%, with symptomatic PE reported in 0% to 1% of patients and a fatal PE in 0% to 1.5%. In 2017 Dua et al. reported national trends in DVT after TKA and THA. They noted a significant decrease in incidence from 2001 to 2011, with DVT after TKA decreasing by almost half even though TKA procedures almost doubled during that same time. They concluded that the significant increase in DVT prophylaxis administration may be responsible for the decreased rates of DVT in patients after total joint replacement.

Clinical examination is unreliable in detecting DVT because most clots occur without signs or symptoms. Venography is the classic radiographic method of detection of DVT and is still considered the gold standard, especially for research purposes. Venography carries the risk of anaphylactic reaction to the contrast media and a small risk of inducing DVT. Duplex ultrasound has been reported as an alternative method of diagnosis of DVT after total joint arthroplasty, with documented sensitivities of 67% to 86% using venography for comparison. In a multicenter study, however, only a 52% overall sensitivity, with a range of 20% to 90%, was found, raising the question of whether reliable detection rates can be reproduced in all institutions. Duplex ultrasound seems to be useful, especially as a screening test, because of its minimal morbidity, low cost, and repeatability with minimal patient discomfort, but its accuracy depends on the experience of the ultrasound technologist.

Many methods of DVT prophylaxis are available, including mechanical devices such as compression stockings or foot pumps and pharmaceutical agents such as low-dose warfarin, low-molecular-weight heparin (LMWH), factor Xa inhibitor, and low- and high-dose aspirin. Mechanical compression boots and foot pumps are advantageous because they are without significant risk to the patient, but they are limited by patient compliance and short duration of hospitalization with same-day or 24-hour stays.

Low-molecular-weight heparin and fondaparinux have been shown to be effective in DVT prophylaxis after TKA. The benefits of these medications include a standard dose regimen and the absence of routine laboratory monitoring. The disadvantages include greater medication cost, subcutaneous administration, and increased incidence of bleeding. Low-molecular-weight heparin with epidural or spinal anesthesia must be used with extreme caution because epidural hematomas with disastrous neurologic complications have been reported. The time of utmost risk apparently occurs on postoperative day 3 when the indwelling catheter is removed from a patient being treated with low-molecular-weight heparin for DVT prophylaxis. Guidelines from the American College of Chest Physicians in 2008 recommend that low-molecular-weight heparin, fondaparinux, or a vitamin K antagonist (e.g., warfarin) be used for DVT prophylaxis in TKA patients for a minimum of 10 days.

Oral factor Xa inhibitor (rivaroxaban, apixaban, and edoxaban) for DVT prophylaxis after TKA has been reported to be effective. In a multicenter prospective study (Regulation of Coagulation in Orthopedic Surgery to Prevent Deep Venous Thrombosis and Pulmonary Embolism [RECORD] trials), 3148 patients were randomized to receive enoxaparin (30 mg subcutaneously twice a day, beginning 12 to 14 hours after surgery) or rivaroxaban (10 mg orally one a day, beginning 6 to 8 hours after surgery). Venography at 11 and 15 days after surgery found a significantly higher rate of DVT in those taking enoxaparin; a nonsignificant increase in the number of wound complications was found in those taking rivaroxaban. A retrospective study of 1048 patients who had TKA or total hip arthroplasty and received either low-molecular-weight heparin or rivaroxaban had similar results: a return to the operating room because of wound complications was required in approximately twice as many patients taking rivaroxaban as in those taking low-molecular-weight heparin. The lower cost of rivaroxaban is an advantage, as is the lower rate of documented DVT, but the frequency of wound complications may require further investigation. Bawa et al., using a Medicare dataset review from 2004 to 2013, found a higher rate of DVT in patients using warfarin and LMWH than those using aspirin, fondaparinux, and rivaroxaban.

INFECTION

Infection is one of the most dreaded complications affecting TKA patients, with reported frequencies of 2% to 3% in several large series. According to current Medicare data, 1.5% of patients develop a periprosthetic infection in the first 2 years after TKA. Preoperative factors associated with a higher rate of infection after TKA include rheumatoid arthritis (especially in seropositive men), skin ulceration, previous knee surgery, use of a hinged-knee prosthesis, obesity, concomitant urinary tract infection, steroid use, renal failure, diabetes mellitus, poor nutrition, malignancy, and psoriasis.

Efforts to reduce bacterial contamination, optimize the status of the wound, and maximize the available host response should be employed to minimize postoperative sepsis. Prevention of infection in TKA begins in the operating room, with strict adherence to aseptic technique. The number and ingress and egress of operating room personnel should be minimized as much as possible. Operating room surveillance with adherence to such policies has been shown to decrease the incidence of postoperative infection in total joint arthroplasty.

The use of filtered vertical laminar flow operating rooms, body exhaust suits, and prophylactic antibiotics has greatly reduced postoperative infection rates in total joint arthroplasty. In one clinical series, however, the use of horizontal laminar flow was shown to increase the postoperative infection rate in TKA, probably because of positioning of operating room personnel between the source of the airflow and the open wound. Ultraviolet light is preferred by some centers to create an ultraclean air environment, with bacterial counts equal to or better than those of standard laminar flow systems.

Because the most common organisms causing postoperative infection are *Staphylococcus aureus, Staphylococcus epidermidis,* and *Streptococcus* species, the usual choice of prophylactic antibiotic is a first-generation cephalosporin, such as cefazolin. In patients with significant penicillin allergy, vancomycin or clindamycin may be used. Infecting organisms should be monitored by individual hospitals, with the choice of prophylactic antibiotic determined by such routine surveillance.

The diagnosis of infection after TKA should begin with a careful history and physical examination. The timing of an infection can have a profound effect on the outcome of its treatment and should be used in guiding treatment decisions. Infection should be considered in any patient with a consistently painful TKA or an acute onset of pain in the setting of a previously pain-free, well-functioning arthroplasty. A history of subjective swelling, erythema, or prolonged wound drainage suggests TKA sepsis, but these signs are not uniformly present. Swelling, tenderness, painful range of motion, erythema, and increased warmth of the affected limb may accompany a TKA infection.

Although the white blood cell count and erythrocyte sedimentation rate may be elevated in the presence of deep

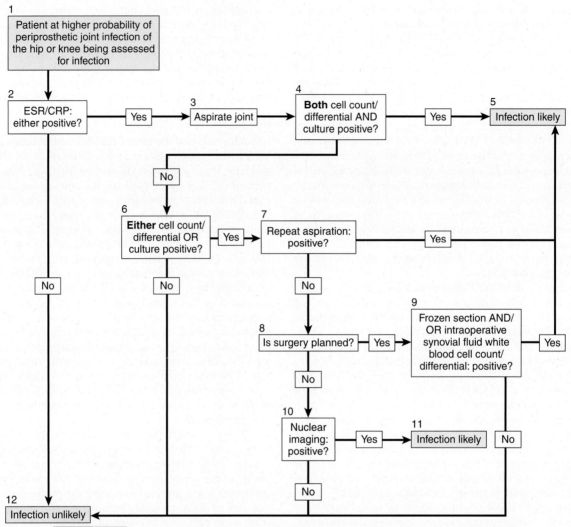

FIGURE 5.68 Algorithm for patients with higher probability of having periprosthetic joint infection. (Modified from The diagnosis of periprosthetic joint infections of the hip and knee. Guideline and evidence report. Adopted by the American Academy of Orthopaedic Surgeons Board of Directors June 18, 2010. www.aaos.org/Research/guidelines/PJIguideline.pdf. Copyright American Academy of Orthopaedic Surgeons, Rosemont, IL.)

infection, this does not occur consistently. The C-reactive protein level is a more reliable marker for infection because it typically returns to normal in a reliable manner.

Radiographic changes of bone resorption at the bone-cement interface, cyst formation, and occasionally periosteal new bone formation may be present but usually are seen only in advanced infections. Nuclear medicine scans can be helpful in the evaluation of a painful TKA when the diagnosis is not clear. Comparing the differential periprosthetic uptake on a technetium scan with the uptake on an indium-labeled white blood cell scan is a technique for differentiating infection from aseptic loosening, with reported sensitivities of 64% to 77% and specificities ranging from 78% to 86%. Although these scans cannot be advocated for routine use, they may be indicated when results of the clinical examination, radiography, and laboratory information are equivocal in diagnosing infection.

Aspiration remains the standard for diagnosing infection in TKA, although the reported sensitivity ranges from 45%

to 100%. This sensitivity can be improved by repeated aspiration and by deferring aspiration for 2 weeks in patients taking systemic antibiotics. The fluid cell count obtained at aspiration can be helpful, with a white blood cell count of more than 2500 cells/mm^3 and 60% or higher polymorphonuclear cells indicative of probable infection. In 2011, the American Academy of Orthopaedic Surgeons published a clinical practice guideline on the diagnosis of periprosthetic joint infections of the hip and knee, which provides recommendations as to testing studies and procedures that are supported by high levels of evidence or expert consensus. Testing strategies are determined based on whether a patient has a high or low probability of periprosthetic infection (Figs. 5.68 and 5.69). Because of the lack of a standard definition of periprosthetic joint infection, an international consensus group and a work group by the Musculoskeletal Infection Society (MSIS) convened to develop a list of diagnostic criteria. Although the consensus group voted on questions and criteria for diagnosis and treatment, the MSIS group gave a diagnosis criteria

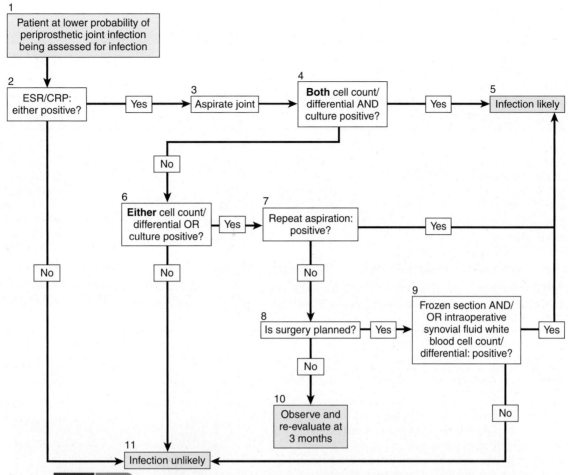

FIGURE 5.69 Algorithm for patients with a lower probability of having a periprosthetic joint infection. (Modified from The diagnosis of periprosthetic joint infections of the hip and knee. Guideline and evidence report. Adopted by the American Academy of Orthopaedic Surgeons Board of Directors June 18, 2010. www.aaos.org/Research/guidelines/PJIguideline.pdf. Copyright American Academy of Orthopaedic Surgeons, Rosemont, IL.)

for hip and knee periprosthetic infections. These criteria use a system of points, with six points or more resulting in a likely diagnosis of a periprosthetic joint infection. Newer markers such as alpha defensin, C-reactive protein, and leucocyte esterase have all been reported to have some degree of reliability.

The MSIS has now published the new set of criteria (Table 5.2) that most have adopted for diagnosing prosthetic joint infection. These are divided into major and minor criteria. Any one of two major criteria, with two positive same-organism aspiration cultures or a draining sinus track, meets the definition of prosthetic joint infection. The minor criteria are scored by points: two points are given for serum C-reactive protein or D-dimer threshold levels of 100 mg/L in the acute and 10 mg/L in the chronic setting for C-reactive protein, and 860 mg/L for D-dimer; an elevated percentage of polymorphonuclear leukocytes (PMNs; 70% in acute or 90% in chronic setting); and a single positive culture. Three points are given for elevated white blood cell counts in acute (10,000 cells/μL) and chronic (3000 cells/μL) infections, and positive intraoperative histology or presence of purulence.

When the diagnosis of infection is established, treatment options include antibiotic suppression, debridement with prosthesis retention, resection arthroplasty, knee arthrodesis, one-stage or two-stage reimplantation, and amputation. The choice between the various options depends on the general medical condition of the patient, the infecting organism, timing and extent of infection, the residual usable bone stock, status of the soft-tissue envelope, and extensor mechanism continuity.

Suppression with antibiotics rarely is indicated. Antibiotic suppression generally is indicated only when prosthesis removal is not feasible (usually because of medical comorbidities) and the infecting microorganism is of low virulence and susceptible to an oral antibiotic of low toxicity. Antibiotic suppression should not be considered in patients with multiple joint arthroplasties who run the risk of hematogenously seeding their unaffected joints should antibiotic suppression fail. Suppression must be lifelong and should be limited to patients in whom no other more successful treatment options are available. Risks of antibiotic suppression include the development of resistant strains of bacteria, progressive loosening, extensive infection, and possible septicemia.

Joint debridement with prosthesis retention is similarly limited to a small subset of patients: those with an early (<4 weeks) postoperative infection or an acute hematogenous

TABLE 5.2

Musculoskeletal Infection Society Criteria for Prosthetic Joint Infection

MAJOR CRITERIA (AT LEAST ONE OF THE FOLLOWING)	DECISION
Two positive growth of the same organism using standard culture methods	Infected
Sinus track with evidence of communication to the joint or visualization of the prosthesis	

MINOR CRITERIA	THRESHOLD		SCORE	DECISION
	ACUTE*	CHRONIC		
Serum C-reactive protein (mg/L)	100	10	2	**Combined preop-**
Or D-dimer (μg/L)	Unknown	860		**erative and post-**
Elevated serum ESR (μL/hr)	No role	30	1	**operative score:**
Elevated synovial WBC (cells/μL)	10,000	3,000	3	**≥6 Infected**
Or Leukocyte esterase	++	++		**3-5 Inconclusive‡**
Or Positive alpha-defensin (signal/cutoff)	1.0	1.0		**<3 Not infected**
Elevated synovial polymorphonuclear PMN (%)	90	70	2	
Single positive culture			2	
Positive histology			3	
Positive intraoperative purulence†			3	

*These criteria were never validated on acute infections.
†No role in suspected adverse local tissue reaction.
‡Consider further molecular diagnostics such as next-generation sequencing.

infection (>4 weeks postoperatively, acute onset of symptoms) with a well-fixed prosthesis. Debridement and prosthesis retention in the setting of late chronic infection (>4 weeks postoperatively, insidious onset of symptoms) have been universally unsuccessful and should not be attempted. Infection with *S. aureus* is another relative contraindication to debridement and component retention.

Several points have been recommended that could lead to higher success rates for debridement:
1. Infectious disease consultation and antibiotic monitoring
2. Diagnosis and treatment of hematogenous sources of infection
3. Newer antibiotics
4. Six-week duration of postoperative intravenous antibiotics
5. Repeat cultures within 2 weeks of the initial debridement and repeat debridement if these cultures were positive
6. Polyethylene exchange at the time of debridement; exchange of gown, gloves, and instruments; and redraping at the time of wound closure

Resection arthroplasty consists of removal of the infected prosthesis and cement and debridement of the synovium (Fig. 5.70). The bone ends can be temporarily apposed with heavy sutures or pins. To maximize stability, the leg is maintained in a cast for 6 months. Resection arthroplasty is ideal for a patient with an infected TKA and severe polyarticular rheumatoid arthritis with limited ambulation. Such treatment is preferable to fusion in these patients because it allows some knee flexion for sitting. Although infection can be controlled in most patients, function is poor because of instability and mild-to-moderate residual pain with standing.

Knee arthrodesis as treatment of an infected TKA can provide a stable, generally painless limb with some expected shortening. Indications for knee arthrodesis after failed TKA

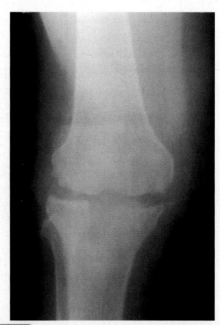

FIGURE 5.70 Resection arthroplasty of knee.

include high functional demands, disease involving a single joint, young age, deficient extensor mechanism, poor soft-tissue coverage, immunocompromised patient, and infection with a highly virulent microorganism that necessitates highly toxic antimicrobial therapy. Relative contraindications include ipsilateral hip or ankle arthritis, contralateral knee arthritis or limb amputation, and severe segmental bone loss. Various techniques of arthrodesis have been used, including external fixation, plating, and intramedullary nailing. Regardless of the method of fixation, the conversion of

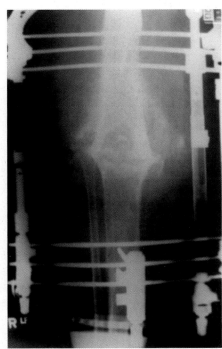

FIGURE 5.71 Knee arthrodesis with biplanar external fixation may be indicated for persistent infection.

resurfacing-type arthroplasties to arthrodesis has been more successful than attempts at fusion of hinged, constrained prostheses. A meta-analysis of the literature showed a 64% fusion rate with external fixation compared with a 95% rate for intramedullary nailing. Gram-positive organisms carried a favorable prognosis with a 100% union rate compared with 73% for mixed and gram-negative infections.

Advantages of external fixation include minimal soft-tissue stripping, adequate wound access, and compression at the arthrodesis site (Fig. 5.71). Disadvantages include pin track infection, possible neurovascular damage with pin insertion, limited stability, and the stress riser effect after pin removal. An anterior midline incision generally is used. The prosthesis, all of the cement, hypertrophic synovium, and as much scar tissue as possible are removed. Extramedullary total knee guides can be used to make bone cuts that maximize apposition. The amount of bone removed should be the least amount necessary to allow apposition of viable cancellous bone surfaces with approximately 10 degrees of knee flexion. The knee should be in neutral to 5 degrees of valgus. The biplanar fixator is assembled with crossed pins placed medial to lateral in the femur and lateral to medial in the tibia, avoiding the neurovascular structures. Anterior half-pins are placed in the tibia and the femur and attached to the assembled frame. Partial weight bearing is encouraged, and the fixator is removed when clinical union is present, usually after 3 months. A cylinder cast, long leg cast, or knee brace is worn, with weight bearing to tolerance until radiographic union is apparent.

Arthrodesis with an intramedullary nail has the advantage of immediate partial weight bearing without external immobilization and a reliable fusion rate. Most authors recommend a two-stage technique with complete debridement and component removal followed by an intervening period of 4 to 6 weeks of intravenous antibiotics. The initial procedure

is performed with or without the use of antibiotic-impregnated beads. We prefer to do a repeat aspiration of the knee joint 2 weeks after completion of a 4- to 6-week course of appropriate intravenous antibiotics. With a sterile culture, the intramedullary arthrodesis can be undertaken. Templating is performed from full-length anteroposterior and lateral views of the limb, with magnification markers to determine the appropriate length and diameter of the nail. The length should account for the expected shortening through the knee joint and should extend from the tip of the greater trochanter into the distal metaphysis of the tibia. The diameter of the nail is limited by the size of the medullary canal of the tibia.

ARTHRODESIS WITH AN INTRAMEDULLARY NAIL FOR AN INFECTED TOTAL KNEE ARTHROPLASTY

TECHNIQUE 5.14

- Position the patient supine on a radiolucent table with a bean bag under the affected buttock to allow access to the piriformis fossa.
- Reopen the old knee incision and make an incision in the buttock for the proximal entry portal.
- Remove scar tissue from the knee joint to allow apposition of the bone surfaces.
- Ream the tibia antegrade from the knee joint to 1 mm larger than the diameter of the nail, allowing for some mismatch between the bow of the nail and the medullary canal of the tibia.
- Ream the femur retrograde or antegrade 1 to 1.5 mm larger than the diameter of the nail to allow for mismatch of the bow of the nail and the bow of the femur.
- Drive the nail from the piriformis fossa across the knee to the level of the distal tibial metaphysis. We prefer to use a locked nail with a cylindrical cross section with the locking holes rotated 45 degrees from their standard position. This allows the bow of the nail to be positioned anteromedially, creating slight flexion and valgus alignment (Fig. 5.72).
- Make final corrections in the distal femoral and proximal tibial surfaces before final driving of the nail and impaction of the arthrodesis site.
- Compression at the fusion site can be done with a femoral distractor in the compression mode before distal interlocking.
- Do not notch the surface of the nail with any power instruments.
- Lock the nail proximally and distally and apply bone graft in areas of suboptimal apposition.
- Closure of the tissue can be difficult because of the excess of knee soft-tissue sleeve, which causes a redundant overfolding of soft tissue. Take care to obtain a sealed closure of the knee, which may require excision of some redundant tissue.

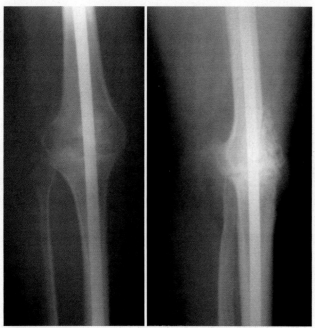

FIGURE 5.72 Knee arthrodesis with intramedullary nail fixation after failed total knee arthroplasty. **SEE TECHNIQUE 5.14.**

POSTOPERATIVE CARE Postoperatively, partial weight bearing is allowed immediately and increases to full weight bearing with radiographic progression of bony union.

Exchange arthroplasty in one or two stages offers the greatest chance of functional knee recovery after an infected TKA. One-stage exchange arthroplasty is performed essentially as a revision arthroplasty with an emphasis on debridement and surgically rendering the wound as close to sterile as possible. The reported success rate of one-stage exchange is approximately 89%.

More commonly, exchange arthroplasty is done in two stages: initial prosthesis removal and debridement followed by a period of intravenous antibiotics and later reimplantation. The most commonly accepted protocol calls for 6 weeks of intravenous antibiotics, maintaining a minimal bactericidal titer of 1:8, followed by reimplantation of another prosthesis. Success rates reported with this protocol range from 89% to 100% and may depend on the bacterial species.

Antibiotic-impregnated PMMA spacers are used by many surgeons to maintain soft-tissue tension of the knee during the interval between debridement and reimplantation in two-stage procedures (Fig. 5.73). Other suggested benefits of this technique include high levels of local antibiotic delivery, improved exposure at the time of reimplantation, and the ability to maintain weight bearing during the interval period. Some authors have expressed concern about leaving a foreign body within the wound, along with potential bone loss from weight bearing on the spacer block. Some suggestions to improve the effectiveness of antibiotic-containing cement spacers have included mixing 3.6 g of tobramycin with 3 g of vancomycin per pack of Palacos cement (Zimmer, Warsaw, IN) to improve elution rates, holding the knee distracted in full extension to allow maximal soft-tissue tension while the spacer hardens, maximal coverage of the femoral

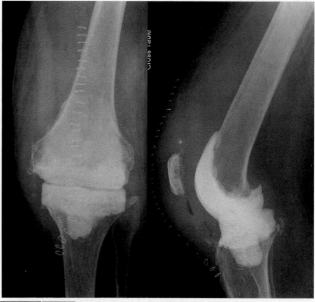

FIGURE 5.73 Antibiotic-impregnated polymethyl methacrylate spacers are useful to maintain joint space and ligamentous relationships, as well as motion of knee, during interval between debridement and reimplantation.

and tibial bone surfaces by the spacer to avoid bone loss, and fabrication of intramedullary portions of the spacer to avoid displacement.

Articulating spacers with temporary prosthetic components have been advocated for two-stage exchange to improve range of motion, maintain functional status of the limb during treatment, and minimize bone loss between stages (see Fig. 5.73). Success rates of 88% to 96% and flexion arcs of 100 to 104 degrees have been reported.

Whiteside et al. described a one-stage debridement and revision with a cementless prosthesis and intraarticular infusion of vancomycin for methicillin-resistant *Staphylococcus aureus* (MRSA) infections. After debridement and implantation of the prosthesis, patients received two 1-g doses of vancomycin intravenously over 24 hours, and then only intraarticular infusion of vancomycin, keeping blood levels between 3 and 10 µg/mL. Seventeen of 18 documented MRSA infections were successfully treated using this technique, as was one recurrent infection. The technique relies on the use of a cementless revision, which can be technically demanding.

Recently Parvizi et al. reviewed the Rothman results for treating patients with prosthetic joint infection. They found that of the 570 patients with prosthetic joint infection, 458 had reimplantation at a mean of 4.1 months. The bigger issues, however, were that the mortality was 13.9%, with 6.7% occurring before reimplantation, and that treatment success was highly variable depending on the definition utilized (54.2% to 88.9%). There have been other reports with sobering results, such as those by Gomez et al. in which success rates were 82%. It has been pointed out that these results are lower than many treatment successes for certain cancer diagnoses.

The last option for the treatment of the infected TKA is above-knee amputation. Amputation is indicated only for life-threatening infection or persistent local infection with massive bone loss not suitable for arthrodesis or resection arthroplasty.

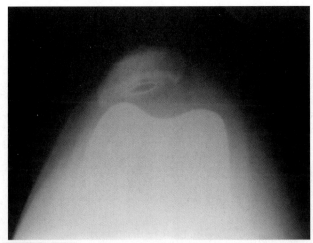

FIGURE 5.74　Lateral patellar subluxation shown on skyline view.

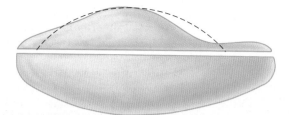

FIGURE 5.75　Often, lateral facet resection must be much shallower than medial facet resection because of normal asymmetry of patellar facets.

PATELLOFEMORAL COMPLICATIONS

Patellofemoral complications include patellofemoral instability, patellar fracture, patellar component failure, patellar component loosening, patellar clunk syndrome, and extensor mechanism rupture. Improvements in design and surgical technique have decreased their frequency; nonetheless, they remain as difficult problems that are best avoided by careful attention to detail.

Patellofemoral instability can be caused by many factors, including extensor mechanism imbalance in which the lateral retinaculum is too tight or the medial soft tissues are too loose (Fig. 5.74). If the lateral retinaculum is tight, lateral release is indicated, sparing the superior lateral geniculate artery if possible (see Fig. 5.61). Medial retinacular laxity may occur with postoperative rupture of the medial capsular repair, which can be caused by a closure that is too tight or by a traumatic event in the early postoperative period. Some authors have advised closing the retinacular-capsular layer with the knee in 90 degrees of flexion to ensure proper medial tensioning. The knee should be placed through a full range of motion after the medial capsular closure to evaluate patellar tracking and the adequacy of the repair.

Suboptimally positioned patellar, femoral, or tibial components also may lead to patellofemoral instability. Excessive lateral patellar facet resection is possible because of the normal asymmetry of the medial and lateral patellar facets. Often, the level of the lateral facet resection must be much shallower than the medial facet resection to avoid tilting of the patellar component (Fig. 5.75). Lateral placement of the patellar component on the cut surface of the patella fails to reproduce the normal median eminence of the patella and can lead to lateral subluxation of the patella in extension.

Suboptimal position of the tibial component in an internally rotated position increases the Q angle by moving the tibial tubercle laterally (see Fig. 5.22). The increased Q angle leads to lateral subluxation. The tibial component should be centered on the medial border of the tibial tubercle, with any deviation into slight external rotation. Similarly, internal rotation and medial translation of the femoral component move the trochlea more medial relative to the extensor mechanism, leading to lateral subluxation.

The intraoperative evaluation of femoral component rotational alignment is based on anatomic landmarks. The posterior femoral condyles, epicondylar axis, and anteroposterior axis all are useful in the primary knee arthroplasty setting. In revision arthroplasty, the position of the previous component and the epicondylar axis are usually the only landmarks available for this assessment.

Surgical treatment of patellar subluxation should be aimed at the cause. The components should be inspected for malposition as outlined in the previous paragraphs and revised if necessary. If the components are positioned appropriately, surgical efforts to improve patellar tracking should proceed in a step-wise fashion. Lateral retinacular release should be performed first, although this rarely has been sufficient as an isolated procedure. If patellar subluxation persists, a proximal realignment procedure should be done. Distal realignment procedures, such as tibial tubercle osteotomy, should be undertaken only with extreme caution because serious functional loss would result if nonunion of the transferred tibial tubercle occurred.

Patellar fracture after TKA is uncommon, occurring in less than 1% of patients (Fig. 5.76). Patellar fracture has been correlated with multiple factors, including excessive patellar resection, vascular compromise secondary to lateral release, patellar maltracking secondary to component malposition, excessive joint line elevation, knee flexion of more than 115 degrees, trauma, thermal necrosis from PMMA polymerization, and revision TKA. The relationship of patellar fracture to lateral release has been carefully studied. In a series of 1146 TKAs, a statistically significant association was found between lateral release and patellar fracture. Patellar thickness and sacrifice of the superior lateral geniculate artery were not associated with fracture. In some patellar fractures after lateral release, pathologic evidence of osteonecrosis has been apparent; however, patellar fracture remains relatively infrequent compared with the number of lateral releases performed.

The results of operative treatment of patellar fractures after TKA vary significantly from the results of treatment of patellar fractures in normal knees. Nonunion and hardware failure are frequent after internal fixation, leading some authors to recommend nonoperative treatment of displaced and nondisplaced fractures with no extensor lag and no loosening of the patellar component from a large fracture fragment.

Periprosthetic patellar fractures have been classified according to the integrity of the extensor mechanism and stability of the implant. Fractures associated with an intact extensor mechanism and stable implant (type I) should be treated nonoperatively with a knee immobilizer or cylinder cast for 6 weeks. Displaced fractures with extensor mechanism discontinuity (type II) should be treated operatively. Transverse middle-third fractures are treated with tension band wiring and retinacular repair. Loose patellar components (type III) should be excised and not replaced because this may impair fracture healing. Stable patellar components that impair fracture fixation also should be removed. Proximal or distal pole fractures should be treated with partial patellectomy and suture repair. Postoperative rehabilitation and range of motion are based on the stability of the fixation achieved at the time of surgery. Patellectomy and extensor mechanism repair are indicated when extreme comminution or poor bone stock preclude stable bony fixation. Patients should be cautioned when operative intervention is recommended because complication rates are high.

Failure of metal-backed patellar components has been attributed to various mechanisms, including fatigue fracture of the metal baseplate from the fixation lugs, delamination of the polyethylene from the baseplate, failure of the ingrowth interface, and wear in areas of thin polyethylene exposing the underlying metal baseplate and leading to metal-on-metal wear between the baseplate and the femoral component (Fig. 5.77). Patients with metal-backed patellar implants require close follow-up to watch for signs of failure. Radiographically, skyline and lateral views of the knee show polyethylene wear, interface failure, and patellar subluxation. Clinically, the onset of a knee effusion, patellofemoral crepitus, or audible squeaking and scraping all suggest component failure. Early revision of the failed components

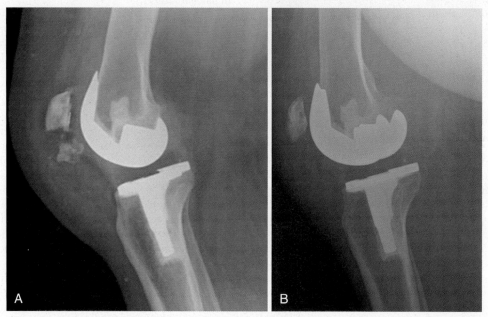

FIGURE 5.76　**A,** Patella is intact in postoperative lateral radiograph. **B,** Six weeks later, patellar fracture with displacement is clearly visible.

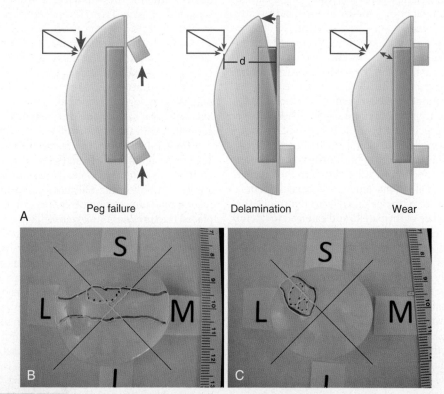

FIGURE 5.77　**A,** Inadequate patellar resection can add undue forces and wear on the patellar polyethylene button. **B,** If proper resection and patellar tracking are obtained, a more symmetric wear pattern results. **C,** Maltracking patella leaves an asymmetric wear pattern.

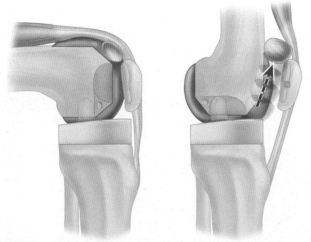

FIGURE 5.78 Patellar clunk syndrome. Synovium just superior to patella can form hypertrophic nodule that catches in box cutout of posterior stabilized total knee design.

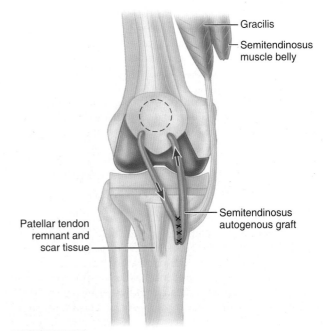

FIGURE 5.79 Reconstruction of patellar ligament with use of semitendinosus tendon.

is recommended to prevent extensive metallosis of the knee. Usually, revision consists of exchange of the tibial polyethylene insert, synovectomy, and revision or removal of the patellar component. Occasionally, metal-on-metal wear damages the femoral component to the extent that revision of the femoral component also is necessary. Techniques for removal of well-fixed metal-backed patellar components have been described using diamond-tipped saws and high-speed burrs to separate the fixation pegs from the baseplate. Berry and Rand, in a series of 42 isolated patellar revisions, found a significant complication rate (33%), including five late patellar fractures and three instances of patellar instability.

Patellar component loosening occurs in 0.6% to 2.4% of arthroplasties. Predisposing factors include deficient bone stock, component malposition and subluxation, patellar fracture, osteonecrosis of the patella, and loosening of other knee components. Some patients tolerate radiographic loosening with only mild anterior knee pain, whereas more symptomatic patients require revision, component removal, or patellectomy, depending on the status of the remaining patellar bone.

Patellar clunk syndrome was described by Hozack et al. in association with PS knee arthroplasties. A fibrous nodule forms on the posterior surface of the quadriceps tendon just above the superior pole of the patella (Fig. 5.78). This nodule can become entrapped in the intercondylar notch of the femoral prosthesis and cause the knee to pop or "clunk" at 30 to 45 degrees of knee flexion as the knee is actively extended. Two causes for this condition have been proposed. Proximal placement of the patellar button so that it overhangs the cut surface of the patella is one possible cause, as the prominent button could impinge on the quadriceps tendon, with resultant fibrous tissue proliferation. Femoral component design is another possible cause. Early PS components with a relatively high, sharp femoral sulcus also could impinge on the quadriceps tendon because they allow the patellar component to fall into the notch with lesser degrees of flexion.

The recommended treatment for this condition is arthroscopic debridement of the nodule. Arthrotomy and nodule excision are reserved for patients with recurrence after arthroscopic treatment or in the setting of loose or malpositioned patellar components that may require revision. Insall recommended a limited synovectomy of the posterior surface

of the quadriceps tendon as a prophylactic measure for this condition when performing a PS arthroplasty.

Rupture of the quadriceps or the patellar tendon is an infrequent but severe complication of TKA, occurring in 0.1% to 0.55% of patients. Quadriceps rupture may be related to lateral release in part because of vascular compromise of the tendon and possibly extension of the release anteriorly that weakens the tendon. Nonoperative treatment is recommended for partial tears. Surgical repair is advocated for complete tears, although the results are suboptimal, with frequent diminished range of motion, weakness, extensor lag, and rerupture.

Patellar tendon rupture is associated with previous knee surgery, knee manipulation, and distal realignment procedures of the extensor mechanism. Multiple procedures have been described to treat patellar tendon rupture after TKA, including direct repair; augmentation with hamstring tendons or synthetic ligament substitutes; gastrocnemius muscle flap; and use of an extensor mechanism allograft consisting of the quadriceps tendon, patella, patellar tendon, and tibial tubercle (Fig. 5.79). None of these procedures has been routinely successful.

The largest series of extensor allografts reported by Nazarian and Booth showed reasonable results in an extremely challenging group of patients, one third of whom had previous infections. Of the 36 patients analyzed, eight had rerupture, with six occurring at the quadriceps tendon level and two at the tibial tubercle. All eight patients with failed procedures underwent repeat allograft reconstruction, with two patients in this group having recurrent ruptures. Burnett et al. stressed the importance of tensioning the allograft with the knee in full extension to avoid extensor lag and clinical failure. Browne and Hanssen described a salvage technique using a knitted monofilament polypropylene graft for repair of the patellar tendon after TKA. The technique involves cementation of the graft into the tibial bone-implant interface of immediate fixation and suture of the graft into surrounding tissue for incorporation, with the graft serving as a scaffold for tissue ingrowth. Of 13 patients in whom this technique was used, three had failure of the graft and one had recurrence of infection; the nine patients treated successfully had less than a 10-degree extensor lag and no loss of flexion compared with preoperative values. Suggested advantages of this technique are the lack of risk of disease transmission from an allograft and lower cost than allografts, which also can be difficult to obtain.

If patellar bone stock allows, distal primary repair seems warranted with the addition of a tension band wire from the proximal patella to the tibial tubercle or hamstring augmentation or both. When the patella is absent or insufficient for distal repair, extensor mechanism allograft reconstruction or gastrocnemius muscle flap should be considered in centers that have experience with these techniques.

NEUROVASCULAR COMPLICATIONS

Arterial compromise after TKA is a rare but devastating complication that occurs in 0.03% to 0.2% of patients, with 25% resulting in amputation. The circulatory status of the limb should be examined carefully in all patients before operation. Noninvasive vascular studies are indicated in patients with questionable vascular supply, and vascular surgical consultation should be obtained if these studies are abnormal. Several authors have recommended performing TKA without the use of a tourniquet in patients with significant vascular disease.

Peroneal nerve palsy is the only commonly reported nerve palsy after TKA, with a reported prevalence of less than 1% to nearly 2%. The true incidence may be higher because mild palsies may recover spontaneously and not be reported. A recent review of over 383,000 primary TKA in the New York State database found an incidence of 0.12%; valgus deformity and previous spine surgery were common risk factors. Peroneal nerve palsy occurs primarily with correction of long-standing combined fixed valgus and flexion deformities, as are common in patients with rheumatoid arthritis. Suggested risk factors for peroneal palsy after TKA include postoperative epidural anesthesia, previous laminectomy, tourniquet time of more than 90 minutes, high body mass index, and valgus deformity. When a peroneal nerve palsy is discovered postoperatively, the dressing should be released completely and the knee should be flexed. Recent studies have suggested that many of these peroneal nerve palsies resolve within a year. The value of intraoperative exposure and possible decompression of the peroneal nerve is questionable.

PERIPROSTHETIC FRACTURES

Supracondylar fractures of the femur occur infrequently after TKA (0.3% to 2%) (Fig. 5.80). Reported risk factors include anterior femoral notching, osteoporosis, rheumatoid arthritis, steroid use, female gender, revision arthroplasty, and neurologic disorders. The anterior femoral flange of condylar-type prostheses creates a stress riser at its proximal junction with the relatively weak supracondylar bone.

In a biomechanical study and review of the literature, Lesh et al. reported that 30.5% of periprosthetic supracondylar femoral fractures were associated with a notched femur. Their biomechanical study found a decrease in load to failure in bending and torsion for cadaver femurs notched experimentally. Also, short oblique fractures occurred with a bending load in specimens that were notched. These authors recommended avoiding manipulation if the femur has been inadvertently notched and considering the use of a stemmed femoral component if the notch is discovered intraoperatively. In a later study, however, the relationship between

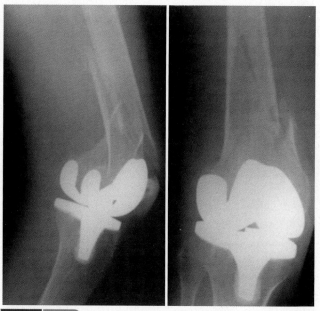

FIGURE **5.80** Supracondylar fracture of femur above total knee arthroplasty.

femoral notching and periprosthetic fracture was disputed. In a series of 1089 TKAs, 30% of patients had a notched distal femur. Only two fractures occurred in this consecutive series, both in femurs without notching.

Treatment of femoral fracture after TKA has varied, with early studies generally recommending nonoperative management. More recent studies have favored operative treatment by a variety of techniques: open reduction and internal fixation using blade plates, condylar screw plates, and buttress plates with bone grafting; Rush pins inserted under image intensification with minimal surgical dissection; or fixation with a locked supracondylar intramedullary nail (Fig. 5.81). Our personal experience with intramedullary nailing of periprosthetic femoral fractures has been good. In 12 patients with 13 fractures, 11 (85%) healed primarily within an average of 16 weeks. In osteoporotic or noncompliant patients, external immobilization with a hinged knee brace and limited weight bearing are recommended in the early postoperative period.

Some TKA designs and sizes do not allow passage of the supracondylar nail through the intercondylar region because of a closed intercondylar box, an intercondylar dimension that is too narrow, or a stemmed implant. If intramedullary fixation is chosen in these circumstances, the intercondylar box can be opened with a high-speed burr if retrograde nailing is desired, or antegrade nailing can be used in these circumstances. Information on which prosthesis types and sizes can be treated with this device is available from the manufacturer of the supracondylar nail.

Indirect reduction and locked distal plating of these fractures have been reported with good results (Fig. 5.82). Reported advantages include minimal soft-tissue stripping, and fixed-angle fixation with the screws, which are locked into the plate. Early range of motion and mobilization have been reported with plating techniques in patients with satisfactory results. Several reports have shown age at the time of the fracture to be predictive of outcome, with older age patients having a high mortality rate 1 year after surgery. In older individuals with comminuted and/or osteoporotic bone, revision to a distal femoral replacement should be considered.

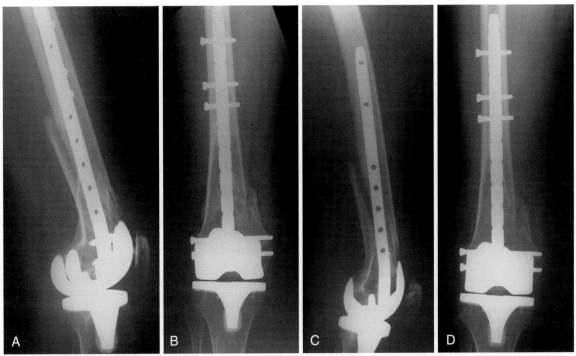

FIGURE 5.81 **A** and **B,** Supracondylar intramedullary nail used for fixation of fracture shown in Figure 5.80. **C** and **D,** Healed fracture.

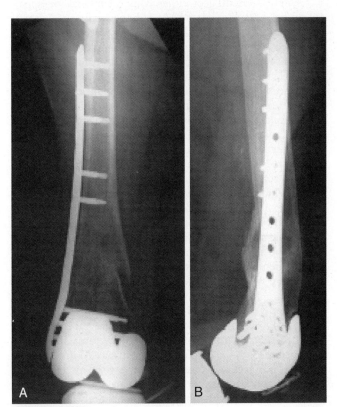

FIGURE 5.82 **A** and **B,** Less invasive surgical stabilization (LISS) plate fixation of periprosthetic femoral fracture. (From Althausen PL, Lee MA, Finkemeier CG, et al: Operative stabilization of supracondylar femur fractures above total knee arthroplasty: a comparison of four treatment methods, *J Arthroplasty* 18:834, 2003.)

Rorabeck, Angliss, and Lewis classified supracondylar periprosthetic femoral fractures on the basis of fracture displacement and implant stability and proposed a corresponding treatment algorithm (Fig. 5.83):

Type I: undisplaced fracture, prosthesis stable

Type II: displaced fracture, prosthesis stable

Type III: unstable prosthesis with or without fracture displacement

When the fracture extends to the fixation surface or if the femoral component is loose, revision arthroplasty with a long intramedullary stem extending into the femoral diaphysis may be necessary. Strut femoral allografts have been used in conjunction with this technique. Kassab et al. reported the use of a distal femoral allograft-prosthetic composite for primary treatment of these fractures when severe osteoporosis led to extensive comminution and precluded adequate fixation with standard fracture management techniques. In nine of 10 patients, the graft-host junction united and the patients achieved full weight bearing. Despite three complications requiring reoperation, the authors concluded that this was a useful technique for treatment of fractures in patients with extremely compromised bone stock.

Tibial fractures below TKAs are uncommon. Felix, Stuart, and Hanssen classified these fractures on the basis of their location, implant stability, and timing (intraoperative versus postoperative) (Fig. 5.84). Fractures associated with loose implants are treated with revision, bone grafting, and stemmed implants as needed. Nondisplaced, stable fractures with well-fixed implants are treated nonoperatively; displaced fractures with well-fixed implants are treated with internal fixation.

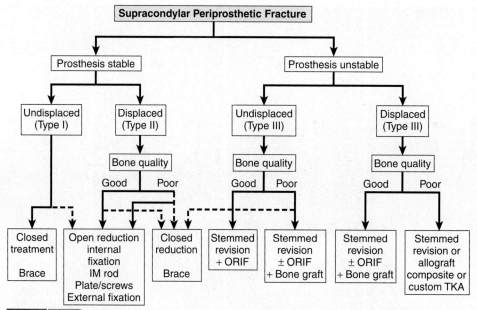

FIGURE 5.83   Treatment algorithm for supracondylar periprosthetic fractures. *IM*, Intramedullary rod; *ORIF*, open reduction and internal fixation; *TKA*, total knee arthroplasty.

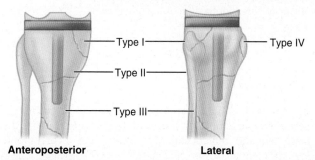

FIGURE 5.84   Anatomic locations of tibial fractures associated with total knee arthroplasty.

Treatment of periprosthetic fractures around TKAs requires a variety of techniques depending on the characteristics of the individual fracture. Ultimate function of the TKA after fracture healing depends on restoration of alignment, adequate patellofemoral function, maintenance of prosthesis fixation, and early range of motion.

REVISION TOTAL KNEE ARTHROPLASTY

The rate of revision of primary TKA remains relatively low. Most registry data list primary TKA survivorship at 10 years to be around 95%. The reasons for revision have shifted over the past decade as reported by Sharkey et al. Osteolysis and aseptic loosening are now not as common. Infection and instability are the more common reasons for revision surgery.

ASEPTIC FAILURE OF PRIMARY TOTAL KNEE ARTHROPLASTY

Aseptic failure of TKA can be caused by several factors, including component loosening, polyethylene wear with osteolysis, ligamentous laxity, periprosthetic fracture, arthrofibrosis, and patellofemoral complications. To date, tibial

component loosening has been more common than femoral component loosening. It has been associated with malalignment of the limb, ligamentous laxity, duration of implantation, patients with high activity demands, polyethylene wear, and excessive component constraint.

Aseptic loosening of either component may be apparent on radiograph as a complete radiolucent line of 2 mm or more around the prosthesis at the bone-cement interface in cemented arthroplasty (Fig. 5.85). Incomplete radiolucencies of less than 2 mm are common and have not been shown to correlate with poor clinical outcomes in cemented TKA. Radiolucent lines around uncemented total knee implants indicate areas where bone ingrowth has not occurred. If these lines are extensive, progressive, or associated with symptoms, aseptic loosening must be considered as well. A radiolucent line under a metal-backed tibial component can be obliterated by 4 degrees of knee flexion. For the evaluation of progressive lucency, comparable views must be obtained at each examination. Fluoroscopic examination may be helpful in patients with unexplained pain after TKA and normal radiographs. Such studies allow careful positioning of the x-ray beam parallel to the surfaces of the implant so that subtle radiolucencies can be detected and correlated with clinical evaluation of these patients. Component loosening also can be manifested by implant migration shown on sequential radiographs (Fig. 5.86).

Polyethylene wear can cause failure of TKA by contributing to loosening and osteolysis or more rarely by catastrophic failure through polyethylene fracture. The factors responsible for polyethylene wear are discussed in the earlier section on polyethylene issues. Rarely, worn modular polyethylene inserts may be exchanged as an isolated procedure, provided that the remaining components are well fixed and well aligned.

Instability is an increasingly frequent cause of TKA failure that requires revision (Fig. 5.87). The main causes of instability are ligamentous imbalance and incompetence, malalignment and late ligamentous incompetence, deficient extensor

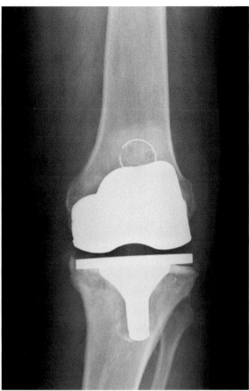

FIGURE 5.85   Lucency at entire bone-cement interface of tibial component, with deformity and subsidence of component.

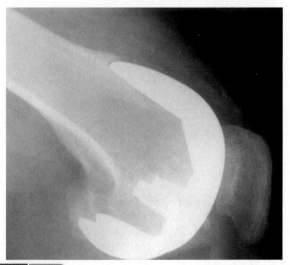

FIGURE 5.86   Loose uncemented femoral component with subsidence into extended position relative to distal femur.

mechanism, inadequate prosthetic design, and surgical error. Besides physical examination, stress radiographs can be used to document less severe instabilities.

Implant selection is based on the ligamentous instability that requires correction, using the lowest level of constraint possible to treat the problem adequately. McAuley, Engh, and Ammeen made recommendations for treating unstable TKAs, dividing them into (1) anteroposterior or flexion space instability, (2) varus-valgus or extension space instability, and (3) multiplanar or global instability. Anteroposterior instability is treated with conversion to a PS implant. CR insert

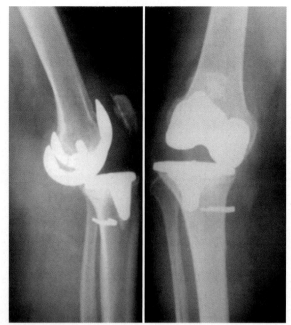

FIGURE 5.87   Instability from polyethylene wear or loss of ligamentous support may be indication for revision knee arthroplasty.

exchange is recommended only with an intact PCL and balanced flexion space with a thicker insert. For varus-valgus instability, which can be corrected with soft-tissue balancing, a constrained condylar design may be used. If the native soft tissues are inadequate or cannot be reconstructed, a linked implant is required. Global instability also requires linked implants if the host soft tissues cannot be balanced or reconstructed adequately. Implant systems with variable levels of constraint are extremely helpful in the revision setting but must be combined with careful attention to implant alignment, ligamentous balancing in flexion and extension, joint line restoration, and patellar tracking.

SURGICAL EXPOSURES

Operative exposure in revision TKA should use the previous TKA skin incision if possible. Parallel longitudinal anterior knee incisions place the intervening skin at risk for necrosis. When two previous incisions already exist, the more lateral of the two should be selected if possible because of the more favorable superficial blood supply from the medial side of the knee.

A standard medial parapatellar arthrotomy can be used in most revisions; however, the scarred capsule may need to be thinned, especially in reimplantation for infection. Scarring of the peripatellar fat pad and adjacent retinaculum may make patellar eversion difficult. Recreation of the medial and lateral gutters, subperiosteal release of the medial soft tissues from the proximal tibia, external rotation of the tibia, and lateral retinacular release often are required to allow eversion without placing excessive stress on the insertion of the patellar tendon. Avulsion of the patellar tendon from the tibial tubercle can compromise knee function drastically and must be avoided. During eversion of the patella and flexion of the knee, the tibial insertion of the patellar tendon should be directly observed. If the medial fibers of the insertion begin to peel away from the tibial tubercle, tension should be released

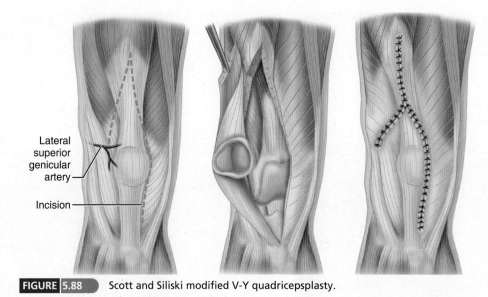

FIGURE 5.88 Scott and Siliski modified V-Y quadricepsplasty.

and a more extensive, quadriceps-relaxing exposure should be considered.

The quadriceps turndown procedure consists of a standard medial parapatellar retinacular incision with an additional limb extending as an inverted V across the quadriceps tendon through the lateral patellar retinaculum (Fig. 5.88). The superior lateral geniculate artery, which runs at the inferior border of the vastus lateralis, is identified and preserved if possible. Excessive thinning of the scarred peripatellar fat pad should be avoided to prevent further devascularization of the patella. During closure of the quadriceps turndown, the inverted V can be converted to a Y by allowing the patella and attached quadriceps tendon to be advanced distally. This is useful in obtaining flexion in knees with quadriceps contractures from long-standing lack of flexion. The closure must be secured with nonabsorbable sutures to allow early passive motion within a "safe" range determined at the time of surgery to avoid excessive stress on the repair. Intraoperatively, a useful guide is to perform the repair so that gravity alone produces 90 degrees of knee flexion. Postoperatively, ambulation should be allowed only in a hinged-knee brace, locked in extension, for 2 to 3 months. The brace is unlocked for active flexion within the "safe" range and passive extension with quadriceps-setting exercises is begun 3 weeks postoperatively. At 6 weeks, active knee extension against gravity alone is allowed along with progression of active and passive flexion.

A V-Y quadriceps turndown results in a postoperative extension lag that tends to resolve over several months. Studies have shown that long-term quadriceps strength can return to near-normal levels. Radiographic changes consistent with osteonecrosis of the patella were documented in eight of 29 revision total knee exposures using a quadriceps turndown, although clinical symptoms were absent.

Insall described the rectus "snip" as a modification of the quadriceps turndown procedure (Fig. 5.89). The proximal extent of a medial parapatellar arthrotomy is extended laterally across the quadriceps tendon to incise the rectus tendon and the underlying tendinous insertion of the vastus muscles. The lateral attachment from the vastus lateralis is left intact along with the superior lateral geniculate vessels; a lateral release can be added distally.

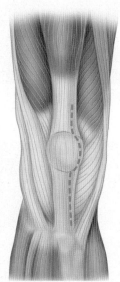

FIGURE 5.89 Insall rectus snip modification of quadriceps turndown procedure (see text).

Tibial tubercle osteotomy was originally described for quadriceps relaxation during primary or revision TKA (Fig. 5.90). Whiteside and Ohl recommended elevation of an 8- to 10-cm segment of the bone that includes the tibial tubercle and a portion of the anterior crest of the tibia, leaving the anterior compartment musculature attached to the fragment laterally for vascularity. The tubercle can be advanced proximally for patella baja or if the joint line is elevated significantly (Fig. 5.91). They described reattaching the tubercle with multiple wires; other authors have advocated using screws. With secure fixation, passive range of motion can be begun early, but active extension still must be delayed. Complications, including nonunion or proximal migration of the osteotomized fragment, tibial shaft fracture, wound infection, wound necrosis, and prominent hardware, have been reported with this technique.

In a comparison of the standard medial arthrotomy, rectus snip, V-Y quadricepsplasty, and tibial tubercle osteotomy in revision TKA, the outcomes with the standard approach and rectus snip were identical in all clinical parameters. V-Y quadricepsplasty resulted in greater extensor lag but increased patient satisfaction compared with tibial tubercle osteotomy, which resulted in more difficulty with kneeling and stooping. The quadricepsplasty and osteotomy groups had significantly lower outcome ratings compared with the standard arthrotomy and rectus snip.

COMPONENT REMOVAL

After exposure, the prosthesis-bone interface should be examined on the tibial and femoral components. We prefer to

femoral component. When the arthroplasty is cemented, the osteotome should be directed at the prosthesis-cement interface rather than at the cement-bone interface. Cement can be removed more easily from the surface of the bone after component extraction with less risk of further bone loss. A thin flexible osteotome blade often is useful; the flat portion of the blade should be placed against the implant so that the bevel of the blade is forced against the implant and not into the bone. Offset osteotomes are useful to reach the posterior condylar interfaces of the femoral component, as well as the intercondylar interfaces. A Gigli saw can be used on some of

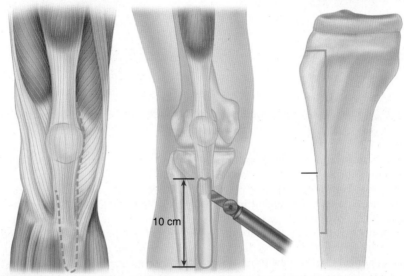

FIGURE 5.90 Tibial tubercle osteotomy can relax extensor mechanism and improve exposure, with benefit of bony healing rather than scar formation as with V-Y turndown procedure. Making step-cut proximally will help prevent escape of tubercle postoperatively.

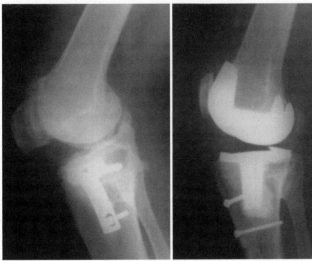

FIGURE 5.91 Proximal advancement of tibial tubercle osteotomy for treatment of patella baja.

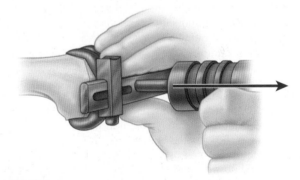

FIGURE 5.92 Slap hammer delivers longitudinal force during femoral component extraction, minimizing chance of fracturing femoral condyle.

remove the femoral component first because this allows better clearance for the tibial component during its extraction. Even with components that appear grossly loose on radiographs, the interface should be carefully disrupted with a variety of osteotomes before component extraction. It is extremely easy to fracture a femoral condyle in the process of removing the

the interfaces when exposure is adequate. After all the fixation surfaces have been disrupted, including the posterior condylar surfaces, the component should be removed with an extraction device that uses a slap hammer that delivers only a longitudinal force to the component (Fig. 5.92). Tilting of the component by peripheral blows may result in a fracture of one of the condyles. If the prosthesis does not extract easily, an osteotome should be used again to disrupt the fixation surface.

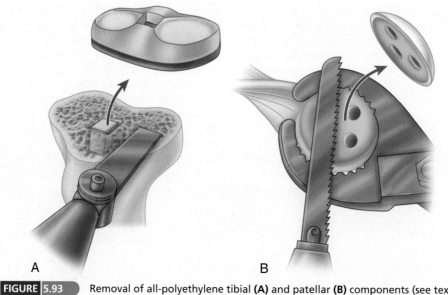

A   B

FIGURE 5.93 Removal of all-polyethylene tibial **(A)** and patellar **(B)** components (see text).

The tibial component is removed in a similar fashion. With all-polyethylene tibial components, the interface can be disrupted with an oscillating saw, cutting through the polyethylene stem and allowing access to its bone-cement interface before extraction (Fig. 5.93A). With metal-backed tibial components, the interface cannot be easily disrupted around a cemented stem or keel. Usually, freeing the undersurface of the tibial baseplate allows component extraction without significant bone loss. If a long stem is present and has extensive cement fixation or a porous ingrowth surface, however, access can be gained by performing a long tibial tubercle osteotomy, as previously described. The tibial baseplate also can be cut with a diamond-tipped saw to gain access to this interface.

The patellar component should be removed if there is evidence of patellar component wear, loosening, or associated osteolysis. If a well-bonded patellar button shows no significant wear, however, the component can be retained because removal may significantly compromise the residual bone stock, leading to fracture or component loosening. The bone-cement interface of an all-polyethylene patellar component is easily disrupted with an oscillating saw (Fig. 5.93B). The remaining fixation pegs can be removed with a small curet or burr. Metal-backed patellar components are more difficult to remove, requiring small osteotomes to fit between the fixation lugs and possibly cutting the metal fixation pegs off the baseplate with a diamond-tipped saw.

KNEE REVISION AND RECONSTRUCTION PRINCIPLES

The steps necessary in revision knee arthroplasty vary greatly among patients, although some general principles should be followed:

1. The joint line should be reconstructed as close as possible to its anatomic position. When significant bone loss is present, it may take some detective work to track down original radiographic studies, especially if the patient did not have the index procedure at the same facility.
2. Bone defects must be treated appropriately, with an emphasis on bone preservation and reconstitution. Metal augments and/or porous augments or cones should be

used to maintain as much bone stock as possible for future reconstructions if needed.
3. Knee stability must be restored by appropriate soft-tissue balancing; when soft-tissue support is inadequate, increasing the prosthetic constraint to a constrained condylar or if necessary a hinge type of prosthesis may need to be considered.
4. Appropriate limb alignment must be ensured, often using the medullary canals of the femur and tibia as reference points. The option of distal femoral alignment from extended stems should be considered. Determination of the proper distal femoral alignment can be aided by preoperative planning and long-standing radiographs.
5. Solid stem fixation with either diaphyseal-engaged press-fit stems or shorter cemented stems should be considered.
6. Rigid fixation is necessary for prolonged implant survival.
7. Patellofemoral mechanics must be optimized.
8. Revision components should have a comprehensive variety of metal augmentations, stem extensions, and constraints (Fig. 5.94).
9. Flexion and extension gaps should be filled using components, augments, and offset stems to give a stable joint throughout a range of motion.

First, the soft-tissue envelope should be reconstructed by debridement of hypertrophic synovium that may contain particulate debris and by thinning of any present scarred capsular tissue. The suprapatellar pouch, medial and lateral gutters, and posterior femoral recesses must be reconstituted. Because the PCL usually is scarred or incompetent, most surgeons prefer PCL-substituting prostheses for revision arthroplasty. When there is gross incompetence of the medial collateral ligament or the combined lateral supporting structures, the decision to use a more constrained type of prosthesis can be made early in the revision procedure.

The tibia usually is prepared first with minimal additional bone resection. Defects of less than 5 mm can be filled with cement. Larger contained defects may be filled with cancellous graft, and noncontained defects are treated with modular wedges and blocks or structural bone grafts. Circumferential contact should be maintained between the augmented trial

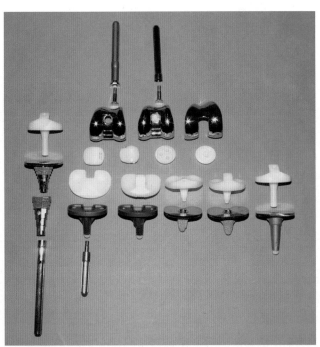

FIGURE 5.94 Modular total knee system with available augmentations and levels of constraint.

tibial baseplate and the tibial cortex. With more severe bone loss, the addition of cones or sleeves should be considered to ensure optimal implant fixation. Modular stem extensions should be used to provide additional component stability to compromised metaphyseal bone stock and to protect bone grafts and oblique fixation interfaces beneath metal augmentation wedges from stress. Care must be taken that a long press-fit stem does not cause angulation or offset of the tibial component; using a stem of smaller diameter or length or an offset stem extension is preferable (Fig. 5.95). The level of the joint line, determined by the depth of the tibial resection and the thickness of the tibial polyethylene, should be established roughly one fingerbreadth above the proximal tip of the fibula and one fingerbreadth distal to the inferior pole of the patella if patella baja does not exist (Fig. 5.96). Rarely, a custom tibial component or a proximal tibial allograft may be necessary because of extensive bone loss (Fig. 5.97). This should be anticipated by preoperative templating in patients with significant bone loss.

The femur is prepared, adhering to the principles of the flexion-extension gap technique (see Technique 5.2). The main difference between primary and revision arthroplasty is the frequent need for augmentation of the femoral condyles distally or posteriorly or both to balance the flexion and extension gaps without significant joint line elevation. In revision TKA, increasing the tibial implant height either with augments or polyethylene thickness will fill both the extension and flexion gaps; distal femoral augments fill only the extension gap, and increasing the femoral component size fills the flexion gap. A gap that is trapezoidal rather than rectangular must be corrected with soft-tissue balancing techniques, as discussed in the section on primary TKA, or with femoral component rotation in the transverse plane when appropriate. Laxity with the knee in flexion and extension frequently is caused by an undersized prosthesis placed too proximally

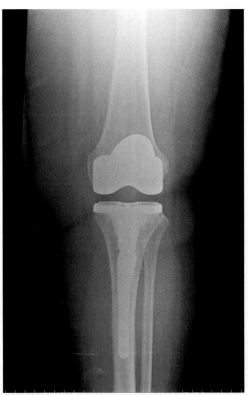

FIGURE 5.95 Tibial component revised with medially offset, press-fit tibial stem.

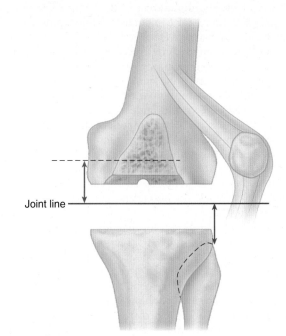

FIGURE 5.96 Joint line in revision total knee arthroplasty can be measured from tip of fibular head (average 14 mm) or from epicondylar axis (average 23 mm from lateral epicondyle and 28 mm from medial epicondyle).

on the femur. It is better to use a larger femoral component in the anteroposterior dimension, with distal and posterior metal augmentation, than to elevate the joint line by using a thicker tibial polyethylene spacer. Knowledge of the anteroposterior dimension of the previous femoral component or a

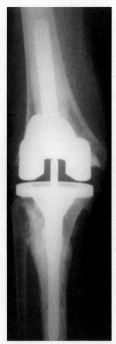

FIGURE 5.97 Revision total knee arthroplasty with proximal tibial allograft, cemented stems, and constrained condylar articulation for massive bone loss.

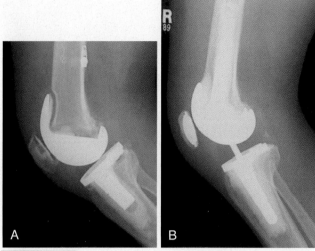

FIGURE 5.98 **A,** Lateral radiograph shows femoral and patellar osteolysis before revision total knee arthroplasty. **B,** After revision with trabecular metal patellar shell. (From Nelson CL, Lonner JH, Lahiji A, et al: Use of a trabecular metal patella for marked patella bone loss during revision total knee arthroplasty, *J Arthroplasty* 18(7 Suppl 1):37, 2003.)

lateral radiograph of the contralateral knee can be helpful in determining the appropriate size of the femoral component. Rotation of the femoral component should be determined using the epicondylar axis (see Fig. 5.41).

Bone defects on the femur generally are managed with metal augmentation including wedges, cones, or sleeves, although cancellous bone graft is useful in contained defects, which are common with some earlier prosthetic designs. Small defects and larger defects under the anterior flange of the revision component can be filled with cement or if large enough a cone augment can be considered. Structural allografts or custom femoral components can be used for extensive bone loss, and the need for these must be anticipated. Stem extensions should be used when condylar bone stock is tenuous and with constrained condylar prostheses.

Multiple options exist for handling the patellofemoral joint during revision TKA surgery, including retention, replacement, or excision of the original patellar prosthesis. Retention may be done when a securely fixed component shows minimal wear. Replacement is possible when the residual bone stock allows preparation of an adequate bony bed with fixation holes and the possibility for cement intrusion. Inadequate bone stock can be treated with component excision, with trimming of the residual patellar bone to allow tracking within the trochlea of the femoral component. A trabecular metal-backed patellar implant and grafting can be used to aid in the reconstruction of the patella, but varying results have been reported using this technique (Fig. 5.98). Advancement of the vastus medialis may improve tracking of the extensor mechanism in the absence of a patellar component.

Most revision knee arthroplasties are cemented at the interfaces between the prostheses and the bone, with stem extensions used in a press-fit fashion or in a fully cemented technique. When press-fit stems are used, applying cement only to the fixation surfaces of the prosthesis makes it easier to keep cement out of the diaphysis. Staggering the cementing of the tibial and femoral components by 5 to 7 minutes is helpful when the bone stock is tenuous or small defects are filled with cement. The patella can be cemented concurrently with the femur or the tibia. When cement is used to fill a defect beneath the anterior flange of the femoral component or with other peripheral defects, it is useful to allow the cement to polymerize partially and use a knife to trim excess cement sharply from the edge of the prosthesis. A curet can be used to extract cement from beneath the edge of the prosthesis. We agree with the routine use of antibiotic-impregnated cement in TKA revision because of the increased risk of postoperative infection.

RESULTS

The clinical results of revision TKA also are not as good as the results of primary TKA. Short-term follow-up studies have shown lower clinical scores and higher complication rates. Long-term studies are limited to early revision prostheses with minimal modularity. Series with at least 5 years of follow-up reported good-to-excellent results in 46% to 74% of patients.

Complications after revision TKA, especially extensor mechanism complications and deep infection, are significantly more frequent than after primary TKA, and patients requiring repeat revision surgery fare worse. In a series of 60 patients, reoperation after revision TKA was required because of infection in 20% and for complications of the extensor mechanism in 41%. Other causes for repeat surgery included aseptic loosening, wound problems, and tibiofemoral instability. In a prospective multicenter study, the North American Knee Arthroplasty Revision Study Group followed 221 patients from 17 centers for 2 years and found that surgical technique factors did not necessarily correlate with patient-specific outcome measures. Worsening pain and knee-specific function scores were evident in the second year after revision TKA, and the study group emphasized the need to follow patients past the 1-year recovery point after TKA. An analysis of 42 patients who had polyethylene exchange because of instability, stiffness, or aseptic effusions after TKA determined that those who had exchange less than 3 years after their primary TKA were nearly four times as likely to require re-revision than those who had exchange longer than 4 years after primary TKA. Recent studies have reported good mid-term results of revision TKA using cones and sleeves for AORI IIb and III defect reconstruction to ensure optimal implant fixation in poor bone stock.

REFERENCES

COMPONENT DESIGN, SELECTION, AND BIOMECHANICS

Abdel MP, Morrey ME, Jensen MR, Morrey BF: Increased long-term survival of posterior cruciate–retaining versus posterior cruciate–stabilizing total knee replacements, *J Bone Joint Surg* 93A:2072, 2011.

Abdelgaied A, Brockett CL, Liu F, et al.: Quantification of the effect of cross-shear and applied nominal contact pressure on the wear of moderately cross-linked polyethylene, *Proc Inst Mech Eng H* 227:18, 2013.

Alnachoukati OK, Barrington JW, Berend KR, et al.: Eight hundred twenty-five medial mobile-bearing unicompartmental knee arthroplasties: the first 10-year US multi-center survival analysis, *J Arthroplasty* 33(3):677, 2018.

Appy Fedida B, Krief E, Havet E, Massin P, Mertl P: Cruciate-sacrificing total knee arthroplasty and insert design: a radiologic study of sagittal laxity, *Orthop Traumatol Surg Res*, 2015 Nov 19.

Baker P, Critchley R, Gray A, et al.: Mid-term survival following primary hinged total knee replacement is good irrespective of the indication for surgery, *Knee Surg Sports Traumatol Arthrosc* 22(3):599, 2014.

Blakeney W, Clément J, Desmeules F, et al.: Kinematic alignment in total knee arthroplasty better reproduces normal gait than mechanical alignment, *Knee Surg Sports Traumatol Arthrosc* 27(5):1401, 2019.

Bonutti PM, Goddard MS, Zywiel MG, et al.: Outcomes of unicompartmental knee arthroplasty stratified by body mass index, *J Arthroplasty* 26:1149, 2011.

Chakravarty R, Elmallah RD, Cherian JJ, et al.: Polyethylene wear in knee arthroplasty, *J Knee Surg* 28:370, 2015.

Cohen RG, Sherman NC, James SL: Early clinical outcomes of a new cementless total knee arthroplasty design, *Orthopedics* 41(6):e765, 2018.

Dayan I, Moses MJ, Rathod P, et al.: No difference in failure rates or clinical outcomes between non-stemmed constrained condylar prostheses and posterior-stabilized prostheses for primary total knee arthroplasty, *Knee Surg Sports Traumatol Arthrsc*, 2019 Aug 27.

Dolan MM, Kelly NH, Nguyen JT, et al.: Implant design influences tibial post wear damage in posterior-stabilized knees, *Clin Orthop Relat Res* 469:160, 2011.

Flament EM, Berend KR, Hurst JM, et al.: Early experience with vitamin E antioxidant-infused highly cross-linked polyethylene inserts in primary total knee arthroplasty, *Surg Technol Int* 29:334, 2016.

Fransen B, Hoozemans MJ, Keijser LC, et al.: Does insert type affect clinical and functional outcome in total knee arthroplasty? A randomised controlled clinical trial with 5-year follow-up, *J Arthroplasty* 30:1931, 2015.

Gascoyne TC, Teeter MG, Guenther LE, et al.: In vivo wear performance of cobalt-chromium versus oxidized zirconium femoral total knee replacements, *J Arthroplasty* 31:137, 2016.

Grazette AJ, Wylde V, Dixon S, et al.: A 15 to 17-year follow-up of the Kinemax total knee replacement, *Knee* 25(6):1292, 2018.

Haider H, Weisenburger JN, Kurtz SM, et al.: Does vitamin E-stabilized ultra-high-molecular-weight polyethylene address concerns of cross-linked polyethylene in total knee arthroplasty? *J Arthroplasty* 27:461, 2012.

Hernández-Vaquero D, Sandoval-Garcia MA: Hinged total knee arthroplasty in the presence of ligamentous deficiency, *Clin Orthop Relat Res* 468:1248, 2010.

Heyse TJ, Khefacha A, Peersman G, Cartier P: Survivorship of UKA in the middle-aged, *Knee* 19:585, 2011.

Hofer JK, Ezzet KA: A minimum 5-year follow-up of an oxidized zirconium femoral prosthesis used for total knee arthroplasty, *Knee* 21:168, 2014.

Hoffart HE, Langenstein E, Vasak N: A prospective study comparing the functional outcome of computer-assisted and conventional total knee replacement, *J Bone Joint Surg* 94B:194, 2012.

Hofstede SN, Nouta KA, Jacobs W, et al.: Mobile bearing vs fixed bearing prostheses for posterior cruciate retaining total knee arthroplasty for postoperative functional status in patients with osteoarthritis and rheumatoid arthritis, *Cochrane Database Syst Rev* (2)CD003130, 2015.

Hutt JRB, Sur A, Sur H, Ringrose A, Rickman MS: Outcomes and early revision rate after medial unicompartmental knee arthroplasty: prospective results from a non-designer single surgeon, *BMC Musculoskelet Disord* 19(1):172, 2018.

Innocenti M, Matassi F, Carulli C, et al.: Oxidized zirconium femoral component for TKA: a follow-up note of a previous report at a minimum of 10 years, *Knee* 21:858, 2014.

Ishii Y, Noguchi H, Takeda M, et al.: Posterior condylar offset does not correlate with knee flexion after TKA, *Clin Orthop Relat Res* 471:2995, 2013.

Järvenpää J, Ketunen J, Miettinen H, Kröger H: The clinical outcome of revision knee replacement after unicompartmental knee arthroplasty versus primary total knee arthroplasty: 8-17 years follow-up study of 49 patients, *Int Orthop* 34:649, 2010.

Karachalios T, Komnos G, Amprazis V, et al.: A 9-year outcome study comparing cancellous titanium-coated cementless to cemented tibial components of a single knee arthroplasty design, *J Arthroplasty* 33(12):3672, 2018.

Kim YH, Park JW, Kim JS: The long-term results of simultaneous high-flexion mobile-bearing and fixed-bearing total knee arthroplasties performed in the same patients, *J Arthroplasty* 34(3):501, 2019.

Kowalczewski J, Marczak D, Synder M, Sibinski M: Primary rotating-hinge total knee arthroplasty: good outcomes at mid-term follow-up, *J Arthroplasty* 29(6):1202, 2014.

Makaram N, Clement ND, Hoo T, et al.: Survival of the low contact stress rotating platform total knee replacement is influenced by age: 1058 implants with a minimum follow-up of 10 years, *Knee* 25(6):1283, 2018.

McMahon SE, Doran E, O'Brien S, et al.: Seventeen to twenty years of follow-up of the low contact stress rotating-platform total knee arthroplasty with a cementless tibial in all cases, *J Arthroplasty* 34(3):508, 2019.

Mihalko WM, Conner DJ, Benner R, Williams JL: How does TKA kinematics vary with transverse plane alignment changes in a contemporary implant? *Clin Orthop Relat Res* 470:186, 2012.

Mihalko WM, Krackow KA: Posterior cruciate ligament effects on the flexion space in total knee arthroplasty, *Clin Orthop Relat Res* 360:243, 1999.

Mihalko WM, Williams JL: Computer modeling to predict effects of implant malpositioning during TKA, *Orthopedics* 33(Suppl 10):71, 2010.

Mihalko WM, Williams JL: Total knee arthroplasty kinematics may be assessed using computer modeling: feasibility study, *Orthopedics* 35(Suppl 10):40, 2012.

Minoda Y, Hata K, Iwaki H, et al.: No difference in in vivo polyethylene wear particles between oxidized zirconium and cobalt-chromium femoral component in total knee arthroplasty, *Knee Surg Sports Traumatol Arthrosc* 22:680, 2014.

Molloy J, Kennedy J, Jenkins C, et al.: Obesity should not be considered a contraindication to medial Oxford UKA: long-term patient-reported outcomes and implant survival in 1000 knees, *Knee Surg Sports Traumatol Arthrosc* 27(7):2250, 2019.

Namba R, Graves S, Robertsson O, et al.: International comparative evaluation of knee replacement with fixed or mobile non-posterior-stabilized implants, *J Bone Joint Surg* 96(Suppl 1):52, 2014.

Newman JM, Sodhi N, Khlopas A, et al.: Cementless total knee arthroplasty: a comprehensive review of the literature, *Orthopedics* 41(5):263, 2018.

Normand X, Pinçon JL, Ragot JM, et al.: Prospective study of the cementless "New Wave" total knee mobile-bearing arthroplasty: 8-year follow-up, *Eur J Orthop Surg Traumatol* 25:349, 2015.

Onodera T, Majima T, Nishiike O, et al.: Posterior femoral condylar offset after total knee replacement in the risk of knee flexion contracture, *J Arthroplasty* 28:1112, 2013.

Pang HN, Jamieson P, Teeter MG, et al.: Retrieval analysis of posterior stabilized polyethylene tibial inserts and its clinical relevance, *J Arthroplasty* 29:365, 2014.

Papasoulis E, Karachalios T: A 13- to 16-year clinical and radiological outcome study of the Genesis II cruciate retaining total knee arthroplasty with an oxidised zirconium femoral component, *Knee* 26(2):492, 2019.

Pearse AJ, Hooper GJ, Rothwell A, Frampton C: Survival and functional outcome after revision of a unicompartmental to a total knee replacement: the New Zealand National Joint Registry, *J Bone Joint Surg* 92:508, 2010.

Pfitzner T, Abdel MP, von Roth P, et al.: Small improvements in mechanical axis alignment achieved with MRI versus CT-based patient-specific instruments in TKA: a randomized clinical trial, *Clin Orthop Relat Res* 472:2913, 2014.

Pijls BG, Van der Linden-Van der Zwaag HM, Nelissen RG: Polyethylene thickness is a risk factor for wear necessitating insert exchange, *Int Orthop* 36:1175, 2012.

Puah KL, Chong HC, Foo LSS, Lo NN, Yeo SJ: Clinical and functional outcomes: primary constrained condylar knee arthroplasty compared with posterior stabilized knee arthroplasty, *J Am Acad Orthop Surg Glob Res Rev* 2(2):e084, 2018.

Rai S, Liu X, Feng X, et al.: Primary total knee arthroplasty using constrained condylar knee design for severe deformity and stiffness of knee secondary to post-traumatic arthritis, *J Orthop Surg Res* 13(1):67, 2018.

Reinitz SD, Currier BH, Levine RA, Van Citters DW: Crosslink density, oxidation and chain scission in retrieved, highly cross-linked UHMWPE tibial bearings, *Biomaterials* 35:4436, 2014.

Ritter MA, Davis KE, Meding JB, et al.: The effect of alignment and BMI on failure of total knee replacement, *J Bone Joint Surg* 93A:1588, 2011.

Ritter MA, Meneghini RM: Twenty-year survivorship of cementless anatomic graduated component total knee arthroplasty, *J Arthroplasty* 25:507, 2010.

Riviere C, Dhaif F, Shah H, et al.: Kinematic alignment of current TKA implants does not restore the native trochlear anatomy, *Orthop Traumatol Surg Res* 104(7):983, 2018.

Sartawi M, Zurakowski D, Rosenberg A: Implant survivorship and complication rates after total knee arthroplasty with a third-generation cemented system: a 15-year follow-up, *Am J Orthop (Bell Mead NJ)* 47(3), 2018.

Schüttler KF, Efe T, Heyse TJ, Haas SB: Oxidized zirconium bearing surfaces in total knee arthroplasty: lessons learned, *J Knee Surg* 28:376, 2015.

Spece H, Schachtner JT, MacDonald DW: Reasons for revision, oxidation, and damage mechanisms of retrieved vitamin E-stabilized highly cross-linked polyethylene in total knee arthroplasty, *J Arthroplasty*, 2019 Jul 18.

Spekenbrink-Spooren A, Van Steenbergen LN, Denissen GAW, et al.: Higher mid-term revision rates of posterior stabilized compared with cruciate retaining total knee arthroplasties: 133,841 cemented arthroplasties for osteoarthritis in the Netherlands in 2007-2016, *Acta Orthop* 89(6):640, 2018.

Sykes J, Snearly C, Benner R, et al.: Comparison of mobile bearing and fixed bearing total knee arthroplasty outcomes: a review of the literature, *J ASTM International* 8:1, 2011.

Takahashi T, Ansari J, Pandit HG: Kinematically aligned total knee arthroplasty or mechanically aligned total knee arthroplasty, *J Knee Surg* 31(10):999, 2018.

Takemura S, Minoda Y, Sugama R, et al.: Comparison of a vitamin E-infused highly crosslinked polyethylene insert for primary total knee arthroplasty at two years postoperatively, *Bone Joint J* 101-B(5):559, 2019.

Teeter MG, Parikh A, Taylor M, et al.: Wear and creep behavior of total knee implants undergoing wear testing, *J Arthroplasty* 30:130, 2015.

Vaidya C, Alvarez E, Vinciguerra J, et al.: Reduction of total knee replacement wear with vitamin E blended highly cross-linked ultra-high molecular weight polyethylene, *Proc Inst Mech Eng H* 225:1, 2011.

van IJsseldijk EA, Harman MK, Luetzner J, et al.: Validation of a model-based measurement of the minimum insert thickness of knee prostheses: a retrieval study, *Bone Joint Res* 3:289, 2014.

Victor J, Mueller JK, Komistek RD, et al.: In vivo kinematics after a cruciate-substituting TKA, *Clin Orthop Relat Res* 468:807, 2010.

Wernle JD, Mimnaugh KD, Rufner AS, et al.: Grafted vitamin-E UHMWPE may increase the durability of posterior stabilized and constrained condylar total knee replacements, *J Biomed Mater Res B Appl Biomater* 105(7):1789, 2017.

Zhang K, Mihalko WM: Posterior cruciate mechanoreceptors in osteoarthritic and cruciate-retaining TKA retrievals: a pilot study, *Clin Orthop Relat Res* 470:1855, 2011.

INDICATIONS AND CONTRAINDICATIONS

Chaudhry H, Ponnusamy K, Somerville L, et al.: Revision rates and functional outcomes among severely, morbidly, and super-obese patients following primary total knee arthroplasty: a systematic review and meta-analysis, *J Bone Joint Surg Rev* 7(7):e9, 2019.

Godshaw BM, Ojard CA, Adams TM, et al.: Preoperative glycemic control predicts perioperative serum glucose levels in patients undergoing total joint arthroplasty, *J Arthroplasty* 33(7S):S76, 2018.

Hadley S, Day M, Schwarzkopf R, et al.: Is simultaneous bilateral total knee arthroplasty (BTKA) as safe as staged BTKA? *Am J Orthop (Belle Mead NJ)* 46(4):E224, 2017.

Naziri Q, Issa K, Malkani AL, et al.: Bariatric orthopaedics: total knee arthroplasty in super-obese patients (BMI > 50 kg/m2). Survivorship and complications, *Clin Orthop Relat Res* 471(11):3523, 2013.

Phillips JLH, Rondon AJ, Gorica Z, et al.: No difference in total episode-of-care cot between staged and simultaneous bilateral total joint arthroplasty, *J Arthroplasty* 33(12):3607, 2018.

Ponnusamy KE, Vasarhelyi EM, Somerville L, et al.: Cost-effectiveness of total knee arthroplasty vs nonoperative management in normal, overweight, obese, severe obese, morbidly obese, and super-obese patients: a Markov model, *J Arthroplasty* 33(7S):S32, 2018.

Ponnusamy KE, Marsh JD, Somerville LE, et al.: Ninety-day costs, reoperations, and readmissions for primary total knee arthroplasty patients with varying body mass index levels, *J Arthroplasty* 33(7S):S157, 2018.

Raja A, Williamson T, Horst PK: Extrapolation of normative KOOS, JR data for the young patient population undergoing knee arthroplasty procedures, *J Arthroplasty* 33(12):3655, 2018.

Richardson SS, Kahlenberg CA, Blevins JL, et al.: Complications associated with staged versus simultaneous bilateral total knee arthroplasty: an analysis of 7747 patients, *Knee* (19), 2019, Pii:S0968-0160(19)30124-3.

Schroer WC, Diesfeld PJ, LeMarr AR, et al.: Modifiable risk factors in primary joint arthroplasty increase 90-day cost of care, *J Arthroplasty* 33(9):2740, 2018.

Sharkey PF, Hozack WJ, Rothman RH, et al.: Insall Award paper. Why are total knee arthroplasties failing today?, *Clin Orthop Relat Res* 404, 2002, 7.

Shohat N, Tarabichi M, Tischler EH, et al.: Serum fructosamine: a simple and inexpensive test for assessing preoperative glycemic control, *J Bone Joint Surg Am* 99(22):1900, 2017.

Wyles CC, Robinson WA, Maradit-Kremers H, et al.: Cost and patient outcomes associated with bilateral total knee arthroplasty performed by 2-surgeon teams vs a single surgeon, *J Arthroplasty* 34(4):671, 2019.

Yong TM, Young EC, Molloy IB, et al.: Long-term implant survivorship and modes of failure in simultaneous concurrent bilateral total knee arthroplasty, *J Arthroplasty* 2019. Pii:S0883-5403(19)30742-9.

CONSIDERATIONS FOR OUTPATIENT KNEE JOINT REPLACEMENT

Adelani MA, Barrack RL: Patient perceptions of the safety of outpatient total knee arthroplasty, *J Arthroplasty* 34(3):462, 2019.

Darrith B, Frisch NB, Tetreault MW, et al.: Inpatient versus outpatient arthroplasty: a single-surgeon, matched cohort analysis of 90-day complications, *J Arthroplasty* 34(2):221, 2019.

Edwards PK, Milles JL, Stambough JB, et al.: Inpatient versus outpatient total knee arthroplasty, *J Knee Surg* 32(8):730, 2019.

Kelly MP, Calkins TE, Culvern C, et al.: Inpatient versus outpatient hip and knee arthroplasty: which has higher patient satisfaction? *J Arthroplasty* 33(11):3402, 2018.

Li J, Rubin LE, Mariano ER: Essential elements of an outpatient total joint replacement programme, *Curr Opin Anaesthesiol* 32(5):643, 2019.

Meneghini RM: Outpatient joint replacement: practical guidelines for your program based on evidence, success, and failures, a moderator introduction, *J Arthroplasty* 34(7S):S38, 2019.

Menehini R, Gibson W, Halsey D, et al.: The American Association of Hip and Knee Surgeons, Hip Society, Knee Society, and American Academy of Orthopaedic Surgeons Position Statement on Outpatient Joint Replacement, *J Arthroplasty* 33(12):3599, 2018.

Sah A: Considerations for office and staff protocols for outpatient joint replacement, *J Arthroplasty* 34(7S):S44, 2019.

PATELLOFEMORAL ARTHROPLASTY

Akhbari P, Malak T, Dawson-Bowling S, et al.: The Avon patellofemoral joint replacement: mid-term prospective results from an independent centre, *Clin Orthop Surg* 7:171, 2015.

Al-Hadithy N, Patel R, Navadgi B, et al.: Mid-term results of the FPV patellofemoral joint replacement, *Knee* 21:138, 2014.

Bohu Y, Klouche S, Seer HB, et al.: Hermes patellofemoral arthroplasty: annual revision rate and clinical results after two to 20 years of follow-up, *Knee* 26(2):484, 2019.

Charalambous CP, Abiddin Z, Mills SP, et al.: The low contact stress patellofemoral replacement: high early failure rate, *J Bone Joint Surg* 93B(4):484, 2011.

Clement ND, Howard TA, Immelman RJ, et al.: Patellofemoral arthroplasty versus total knee arthroplasty for patients with patellofemoral osteoarthritis: equal function and satisfaction but higher revision rate for partial arthroplasty at a minimum eight years' follow-up, *Bone Joint J* 101-B(1):41, 2019.

Coory JA, Tan KG, Whitehouse SL, et al.: The outcome of total knee arthroplasty with and without patellar resurfacing up to 17 years: a report from the Australian Orthopaedic Association National Joint Replacement Registry, *J Arthroplasty* 2019. Pii: S0883-5403(19)30738-7.

Dahm DL, Al Rayashi W, Dajani K, et al.: Patellofemoral arthroplasty versus total knee arthroplasty in patients with isolated patellofemoral osteoarthritis, *Am J Orthop* 39:487, 2010.

Davies AP: High early revision rate with the FPV patello-femoral unicompartmental arthroplasty, *Knee* 20:482, 2013.

Fabi DW, Mohan V, Goldstein WM, et al.: Unilateral vs bilateral total knee arthroplasty risk factors increasing morbidity, *J Arthroplasty* 26:668, 2011.

Goh GS, Liow MH, Tay DK, et al.: Four-year follow up outcome study of patellofemoral arthroplasty at a single institution, *J Arthroplasty* 30:959, 2015.

Hernigou P, Caton J: Design, operative technique and ten-year results of the Hermes patellofemoral arthroplasty, *Int Orthop* 38:437, 2014.

Hoogervorst P, de Jong RJ, Hannink G, van Kampen A: A 21% conversion rate to total knee arthroplasty of a first-generation patellofemoral prosthesis at a mean follow-up of 9.7 years, *Int Orthop* 39:1857, 2015.

Kazarian GS, Tarity TD, Hansen EN, et al.: Significant functional improvement at 2 years after isolated patellofemoral arthroplasty with an onlay trochlear implant, but low mental health scores predispose to dissatisfaction, *J Arthroplasty* 31:389, 2016.

King AH, Engasser WM, Sousa PL, et al.: Patellar fracture following patellofemoral arthroplasty, *J Arthroplasty* 30:1203, 2015.

Koh IJ, Kim MS, Sohn S, et al.: Patients undergoing total knee arthroplasty using a contemporary patella-friendly implant are unaware of any differences due to patellar resurfacing, *Knee Surg Sports Traumatol Arthrosc* 27(4):1156, 2019.

Lewis PL, Graves SE, Cuthbert A, et al.: What is the risk of repeat revision when patellofemoral replacement is revised to TKA? An analysis of 482 cases from a large National Arthroplasty Registry, *Clin Orthop Relat Res* 477(6):1402, 2019.

Lonner JH, Bloomfield MR: The clinical outcome of patellofemoral arthroplasty, *Orthop Clin North Am* 44:271, 2013.

Lyman S, Lee YY, Franklin PD, et al.: Validation of the KOOS JR: a Short-Form knee arthroplasty outcomes surgery, *Clin Orthop Relat Res* 47496:1461, 2016.

Lyman S, Lee YY, McLawhorn AS, et al.: What are the minimal and substantial improvements in the HOOS and KOOS and JR versions after total joint replacement? *Clin Orthop Relat Res* 476(12):2432, 2018.

Middleton SWF, Toms AD, Schranz PJ, Mandalia VI: Mid-term survivorship and clinical outcomes of the Avon patellofemoral joint replacement, *Knee* 25(2):323, 2018.

Mofidi A, Veravalli K, Jinnah RH, Poehling GG: Association and impact of patellofemoral dysplasia on patellofemoral arthropathy and arthroplasty, *Knee* 21:509, 2014.

Mont MA, Johnson AJ, Naziri Q, et al.: Patellofemoral arthroplasty: 7-year mean follow-up, *J Arthroplasty* 27:358, 2012.

Morris MJ, Lombardi Jr AV, Berend KR, et al.: Clinical results of patellofemoral arthroplasty, *J Arthroplasty* 28(Suppl 9):199, 2013.

Odumenya M, Costa ML, Parsons N, et al.: The Avon patellofemoral joint replacement: five-year results from an independent centre, *J Bone Joint Surg* 92:56, 2010.

Parratte S, Lunebourg A, Ollivier M, et al.: Are revisions of patellofemoral arthroplasties more like primary or revision TKAs? *Clin Orthop Relat Res* 473:213, 2015.

Pilling RW, Moulder E, Allgar V, et al.: Patellar resurfacing in primary total knee replacement: a meta-analysis, *J Bone Joint Surg* 94:2270, 2012.

Price AJ, Svard U: A second-decade lifetable survival analysis of the Oxford unicompartmental knee arthroplasty, *Clin Orthop Relat Res* 469:174, 2011.

Taylor BC, Simitris C, Mowbray JG, et al.: Perioperative safety of two-team simultaneous bilateral total knee arthroplasty in the obese patient, *J Orthop Surg Res* 5:38, 2010.

van Jonbergen HP, Werkman DM, Barnaart LF, van Kampen A: Long-term outcomes of patellofemoral arthroplasty, *J Arthroplasty* 25:166, 2010.

Vertullo CJ, Graves SE, Cuthbert AR, Lewis PL: The effect of surgeon preference for selective patellar resurfacing on revision risk in total knee replacement: an instrumental variable analysis of 136,116 Procedures from the Australian Orthopaedic Association National Joint Replacement Registry, *J Bone Joint Surg Am* 101(1):1261, 2019.

Walker T, Perkinson B, Mihalko WM: Patellofemoral arthroplasty: the other unicompartmental knee replacement, *J Bone Joint Surg* 94:1712, 2012.

Weeks CA, Marsh JD, MacDonald SJ, et al.: Patellar resurfacing in total knee arthroplasty: a cost-effectiveness analysis, *J Arthroplasty* 33(11):3412, 2018.

Woon CYL, Christ AB, Goto R, et al.: Return to the operating room after patellofemoral arthroplasty versus total knee arthroplasty for isolated patellofemoral arthritis – a systematic review, *Int Orthop* 43(7):1611, 2019.

Yadav B, Shaw D, Radcliffe G, et al.: Mobile-bearing, congruent patellofemoral prosthesis: short-term results, *J Orthop Surg (Hong Kong)* 20:348, 2012.

RESULTS OF TOTAL KNEE ARTHROPLASTY

Australian Orthopaedic Association National Joint Replacement Registry: *Annual Report*, 2015. https://aoanjrr.sahmri.com/en/annual-reports-2015.

Camera A, Biggi S, Cattaneo G, Brusaferri G: Ten-year results of primary and revision condylar-constrained total knee arthroplasty in patients with severe coronal plane instability, *Open Orthop J* 9:379, 2015.

Cholewinski P, Putman S, Vasseur L, et al.: Long-term outcomes of primary constrained condylar knee arthroplasty, *Orthop Traumatol Surg Res* 101(4):449, 2015.

Hart A, Antoniou J, Brin YS, et al.: Simultaneous bilateral versus unilateral total knee arthroplasty: a comparison of 30-day readmission rates and major complications, *J Arthroplasty* 31:31, 2016.

Kowalczewski J, Marczak D, Synder M, Sibiński M: Primary rotating-hinge total knee arthroplasty: good outcomes at mid-term follow-up, *J Arthroplasty* 29:1202, 2014.

Maempel JF, Riddoch F, Calleja N, Brenkel IJ: Longer hospital stay, more complications, and increased mortality but substantially improved function after knee replacement in older patients, *Acta Orthop* 86:451, 2015.

Maynard LM, Sauber TJ, Kostopoulos VK, et al.: Survival of primary condylar-constrained total knee arthroplasty at a minimum of 7 years, *J Arthroplasty* 29:1197, 2014.

National Joint Registry for England: Wales and Northern Ireland 10th Annual Report 2013. , www.njrcentre.org.uk/njrcentre/Reports,Publicationsand Minutes/Annualreports/tabid/86/Default.aspx.

New Zealand Joint Registry Fourteen year report 1999 to 2012. www.nzoa.org.nz/nz-joint-registry.

Norwegian Arthroplasty Register 2010 Publication, ISBN: 978-82-91847-15-3. http://nrlweb.ihelse.net/eng/#Publications.

SURGICAL TECHNIQUE

Abdel MP, Parratte S, Blanc G, et al.: No benefit of patient-specific instrumentation in TKA on functional and gait outcomes: a randomized clinical trial, *Clin Orthop Relat Res* 472:2468, 2014.

Babazadeh SM, Dowsey MM, Swan JD, et al.: Joint line position correlated with function after primary total knee replacement: a randomised controlled trial comparing conventional and computer-assisted surgery, *J Bone Joint Surg* 93B:1223, 2011.

Beldame J, Boisrenoult P, Beaufils P: Pin track induced fractures around computer-assisted TKA, *Orthop Traumatol Surg Res* 96:249, 2010.

Bellemans J: Multiple needle puncturing: balancing the varus knee, *Orthopedics* 34:e510, 2011.

Blakeney WG, Kahn RJ, Wall SJ: Computer-assisted techniques versus conventional guides for component alignment in total knee arthroplasty: a randomized controlled trial, *J Bone Joint Surg* 93A:1377, 2011.

Browne JA, Cook C, Hoffmann AA, Bolognesi MP: Postoperative morbidity and mortality following total knee arthroplasty with computer navigation, *Knee* 17:152, 2010.

Bruzzone M, Ranawat A, Castoldi F, et al.: The risk of direct peroneal nerve injury using the Ranawat "inside-out" lateral release technique in valgus total knee arthroplasty, *J Arthroplasty* 25:161, 2010.

Chotanaphuti T, Wangwittayakul V, Khuangsirikul S, Foojareonyos T: The accuracy of component alignment in custom cutting blocks compared with conventional total knee arthroplasty instrumentation: prospective control trial, *Knee* 21:185, 2014.

Choy WS, Yang DS, Lee KW, et al.: Cemented versus cementless fixation of a tibial component in LCS mobile-bearing total knee arthroplasty performed by a single surgeon, *J Arthroplasty* 29:2397, 2014.

Cinotti G, Sessa P, Rocca AD, et al.: Effects of tibial torsion on distal alignment of extramedullary instrumentation in total knee arthroplasty, *Acta Orthop* 84:275, 2013.

Davis JJ, Bono JV, Lindeque BG: Surgical strategies to achieve a custom-fit TKA with standard implant technique, *Orthopedics* 33:569, 2010.

Dossett HG, Estrada NA, Swartz GJ, et al.: A randomised controlled trial of kinematically and mechanically aligned total knee replacements: two-year clinical results, *Bone Joint J* 96:907, 2014.

Elkassabany NM, Abraham D, Huang S, et al.: Patient education and anesthesia choice for total knee arthroplasty, *Patient Educ Couns* 100(9):1709, 2017.

Fricka KB, Sritulanondha S, McAsey CJ: To cement or not? Two-year results of a prospective, randomized study comparing cemented vs. cementless total knee arthroplasty (TKA), *J Arthroplasty* 30(Suppl 9):55, 2015.

Fukagawa S, Matsuda S, Mitsuyasu H, et al.: Anterior border of the tibia as a landmark for extramedullary alignment guide in total knee arthroplasty for varus knees, *J Orthop Res* 29:919, 2011.

Harman MK, Banks SA, Kirschner S, Lützner J: Prosthesis alignment affects axial rotation motion after total knee replacement: a prospective in vivo study combining computed tomography and fluoroscopic evaluations, *BMC Musculoskelet Disord* 13:206, 2012.

Hoke D, Jafari SM, Orozco F, Ong A: Tibial shaft stress fractures resulting from placement of navigation tracker pins, *J Arthroplasty* 26:504.e5, 2011.

Howell SM, Papadopoulos S, Kuznik KT, Hull ML: Accurate alignment and high function after kinematically aligned TKA performed with generic instruments, *Knee Surg Sports Traumatol Arthrosc* 21:2271, 2013.

Jiang Y, Yao JF, Xiong YM, et al.: No superiority of high-flexion vs standard total knee arthroplasty: an update meta-analysis of randomized controlled trials, *J Arthroplasty* 30:980, 2015.

Jung KA, Lee SC, Ahn NK, et al.: Delayed femoral fracture through a tracker pin site after navigated total knee arthroplasty, *J Arthroplasty* 26:505.e9–505.e11, 2011.

Khakha RS, Chowdhry M, Norris M, et al.: Low incidence of complications in computer assisted total knee arthroplasty-a retrospective review of 1596 cases, *Knee* 22:416, 2015.

Kim K, Kim YH, Park WM, Rhyu KH: Stress concentration near pin holes associated with fracture risk after computer navigated total knee arthroplasty, *Comput Aided Surg* 15:98, 2010.

Kwong LM, Nielsen ES, Ruiz DR, et al.: Cementless total knee replacement fixation: a contemporary durable solution—affirms, *Bone Joint J* 96B(11 Suppl A):87, 2014.

Meneghini RM, Daluga AT, Sturgis LA, Lieberman JR: Is the pie-crusting technique safe for MCL release in varus deformity correction in total knee arthroplasty? *J Arthroplasty* 28:1306, 2013.

Mihalko WM, Conner DJ, Benner R, Williams JL: How does TKA kinematics vary with transverse plane alignment changes in a contemporary implant? *Clin Orthop Relat Res* 470:186, 2012.

Mihalko WM, Williams JL: Total knee arthroplasty kinematics may be assessed using computer modeling: a feasibility study, *Orthopedics* 35(Suppl 10):40, 2012.

Mihalko WM, Woodard EL, Hebert CT, et al.: Biomechanical validation of medial pie-crusting for soft-tissue balancing in knee arthroplasty, *J Arthroplasty* 30:296, 2015.

Nam D, Park A, Stambough JB, et al.: The Mark Coventry Award: Custom cutting guides do not improve total knee arthroplasty clinical outcomes at 2 years followup, *Clin Orthop Relat Res* 474:40, 2016.

Novicoff WM, Saleh KJ, Mihalko WM, et al.: Primary total knee arthroplasty: a comparison of computer-assisted and manual techniques, *Instr Course Lect* 59:109, 2010.

Raynauld JP, Martel-Pelletier J, Haraoui B, et al.: Risk factors predictive of joint replacement in a 2-year multicentre clinical trial in knee osteoarthritis using MRI: results from over 6 years of observation, *Ann Rheum Dis* 70:1382, 2011.

Sando T, McCalden RW, Bourne RB, et al.: Ten-year results comparing posterior cruciate-retaining versus posterior cruciate-substituting total knee arthroplasty, *J Arthroplasty* 30:210, 2015.

Seon JK, Song EK, Park SJ, Lee DS: The use of navigation to obtain rectangular flexion and extension gaps during primary total knee arthroplasty and midterm clinical results, *J Arthroplasty* 26:582, 2011.

Siddiqui MM, Yeo SJ, Sivaiah P, et al.: Function and quality of life in patients with recurvatum deformity after primary total knee arthroplasty: a review of our joint registry, *J Arthroplasty* 27:1106, 2011.

Thein R, Zuiderbaan HA, Khamaisy S, et al.: Medial unicondylar knee arthroplasty improves patellofemoral congruence: a possible mechanistic explanation for poor association between patellofemoral degeneration and clinical outcome, *J Arthroplasty* 30:1917, 2015.

Tsukeoka T, Lee TH, Tsuneizumi Y, Suzuki M: The tibial crest as a practical useful landmark in total knee arthroplasty, *Knee* 21:283, 2014.

Watters TS, Mather 3rd RC, Browne JA, et al.: Analysis of procedure-related costs and proposed benefits of using patient-specific approach in total knee arthroplasty, *J Surg Orthop Adv* 20:112, 2011.

Weinstein SM, Baaklini LR, Liu J, et al.: Neuraxial anaesthesia techniques and postoperative outcomes among joint arthroplasty patients: is spinal anaesthesia the best option? *Br J Anaesth* 121(4):842, 2018.

Woolson ST, Harris AH, Wagner DW, Giori NJ: Component alignment during total knee arthroplasty with use of standard or custom instrumentation: a randomized clinical trial using computed tomography for postoperative alignment measurement, *J Bone Joint Surg* 96:366, 2014.

Wyles CC, Jacobson SR, Houdek MT, et al.: The Chitranjan Ranawat Award: Running subcuticular closure enables the most robust perfusion after TKA: a randomized clinical trial, *Clin Orthop Relat Res* 474:47, 2016.

PARTIAL AND TOTAL KNEE ARTHROPLASTY

Bagsby DT, Ireland PH, Meneghini RM: Liposomal bupivacaine versus traditional periarticular injection for pain control after total knee arthroplasty, *J Arthroplasty* 29(8):1687, 2014.

Billi F, Kavanaugh A, Schmalzried H, Schmalzried TP: Techniques for improving the initial strength of tibial tray-cement interface bond, *Bone Joint J* 101-B(1 Suppl A): 53, 2019.

Cancienne JM, Patel KJ, Browne JA, Werner BC: Narcotic use and total knee arthroplasty, *J Arthroplasty* 33(1):113, 2018.

Cao G, Xie J, Huang Z, et al.: Efficacy and safety of multiple boluses of oral versus intravenous tranexamic acid at reducing blood loss after primary total knee arthroplasty without a tourniquet: a prospective randomized clinical trial, *Thromb Res* 171:68, 2018.

Chan VWK, Chan PK, Chiu KY, et al.: Does barbed suture lower cost and improve outcome in total knee arthroplasty? A randomized controlled trial, *J Arthroplasty* 32(5):1474, 2017.

Dasa V, Lensing G, Parsons M, et al.: Percutaneous freezing of sensory nerves prior to total knee arthroplasty, *Knee* 23(3):523, 2016.

Deep K, Shankar S, Mahendra A: Computer assisted navigation in total knee and hip arthroplasty, *SICOT J* 3:50, 2017.

De Martino I, De Santis V, Sculco PK, et al.: Tantalum cones provide durable midterm fixation in revision TKA, *Clin Orthop Relat Res* 473(10):3176, 2015.

Derome P, Sternheim A, Backstein D, Malo M: Treatment of large bone defects with trabecular metal cones in revision total knee arthroplasty: short-term clinical and radiographic outcomes, *J Arthroplasty* 29(1):122, 2014.

Elmallah RK, Chugtai M, Khlopas A, et al.: Pain control in total knee arthroplasty, *J Knee Surg* 31(6):504, 2018.

Gong L, Dong JY, Li ZR: Effects of combined application of muscle relaxants and celecoxib administration after total knee arthroplasty (TKA) on early recovery: randomized, double-blind, controlled study, *J Arthroplasty* 28(8):1301, 2013.

Grupp TM, Saleh KJ, Holderied M, et al.: Primary stability of tibial plateaus under dynamic compression-shear loading in human tibiae – influence of keel length, cementation area and tibial stem, *J Biomech* 59(9), 2017.

Kayani B, Konan S, Tahmassebi J, et al.: Robotic-arm assisted total knee arthroplasty is associated with improved early functional recovery and reduced time to hospital discharge compared with conventional jig-based total knee arthroplasty: prospective cohort study, *Bone Joint J* 100-B(7):930, 2018.

Kazerooni R, Tran MH: Evaluation of celecoxib addition to pain protocol after total hip and knee arthroplasty stratified by opioid tolerance, *Clin J Pain* 31(10):903, 2015.

Khlopas A, Chughtai M, Hampp EL, et al.: Robotic-arm assisted total knee arthroplasty demonstrated soft tissue protection, *Surg Technol Int* 30:441, 2017.

Kim HJ, Lee OS, Lee SH, Lee YS: Comparative analysis between cone and sleeve in managing severe bone defect during revision total knee arthroplasty: a systematic review and meta-analysis, *J Knee Surg* 31(7):677, 2018.

Kobayashi S, Niki Y, Harato K, et al.: The effects of barbed suture on watertightness after knee arthrotomy closure: a cadaveric study, *J Orthop Surg Res* 13(1):323, 2018.

Kovalak E, Dogan AT, Üzümcügil O, et al.: A comparison of continuous femoral nerve block and periarticular local infiltration analgesia in the management of early period pain developing after total knee arthroplasty, *Acta Orthop Traumatol Turc* 49(3):260, 2015.

Lonner JH, Fillingham YA: Pros and cons: a balanced view of robotics in knee arthroplasty, *J Arthroplasty* 33(7):207, 2018.

Morales-Avolos R, Ramos-Morales T, Espinoza-Galindo AM, et al.: First comparative study of the effectiveness of the use of tranexamic acid against ε-Aminocapróic acid via the oral route for the reduction of postoperative bleeding in TKA: a clinical trial, *J Knee Surg*, 2019.

Nam D, Park A, Stambough JB, et al.: The Mark Coventry Award: Custom cutting guides do not improve total knee arthroplasty clinical outcomes at 2 years followup, *Clin Orthop Relat Res* 474(1):40, 2016.

Ponzio DY, Austin MS: Metaphyseal bone loss in revision knee arthroplasty, *Curr Rev Musculoskelet Med* 8(4):361, 2015.

Potter 3rd GD, Abdel MP, Lewallen DG, Hanssen AD: Midterm results of porous tantalum femoral cones in revision total knee arthroplasty, *J Bone Joint Surg Am* 98(15):1286, 2016.

Radnovich R, Scott D, Patel AT, et al.: Cryoneurolysis to treat the pain and symptoms of knee osteoarthritis: a multicenter, randomized, double-blind, sham-controlled trial, *Osteoarthritis Cartilage* 25(8):1247, 2017.

Reinhardt KR, Duggal S, Umunna BP, et al.: Intraarticular analgesia versus epidural plus femoral nerve block after TKA: a randomized, double-blind trial, *Clin Orthop Relat Res* 472(5):1400, 2014.

Saleh KJ, El Othmani MM, Tzeng TH, et al.: Acrylic bone cement in total joint arthroplasty: a review, *J Orthop Res* 34(5):737, 2016.

Sawan H, Chen AF, Viscusi ER, et al.: Pregabalin reduces opioid consumption and improves outcome in chronic pain patients undergoing total knee arthroplasty, *Phys Sportsmed* 42(2)::10 2014.

Schmitz HC, Klauser W, Citak M, et al.: Three-year followup utilizing tantal cones in revision total knee arthroplasty, *J Arthroplasty* 28(9):1556, 2013.

Schroer WC, Diesfeld PG, LeMarr AR, et al.: Does extended-release liposomal bupivacaine better control pain than bupivacaine after total knee arthroplasty (TKA)? A prospective, randomized clinical trial, *J Arthroplasty* 30(9 Suppl):64, 2015.

Tsukada S, Wakui M, Hoshino A: Pain control after simultaneous bilateral total knee arthroplasty: a randomized controlled trial comparing periarticular injection and epidural analgesia, *J Bone Joint Surg Am* 97(5):367, 2015.

Wang D, Wang HY, Luo ZY, et al.: Blood-conserving efficacy of multiple doses of oral tranexamic acid associated with an enhanced-recovery programme in primary total knee arthroplasty: a randomized controlled trial, *Bone Joint J* 100-B(8):1025, 2018.

Wang D, Zhu H, Meng WK, et al.: Comparison of oral versus intra-articular tranexamic acid in enhanced-recovery primary total knee arthroplasty without tourniquet application: a randomized controlled trial, *BMC Musculoskelet Disord* 19(1):85, 2018.

Yang HY, Seon JK, Shin YJ, et al.: Robotic total knee arthroplasty with a cruciate-retaining implant: a 10-year follow-up study, *Clin Orthop Surg* 9(2):169, 2017.

Zhang LK, Ma JX, Kuang MJ, et al.: The efficacy of tranexamic acid using oral administration in total knee arthroplasty: a systematic review and meta-analysis, *J Orthop Surg Res* 12(1):159, 2017.

INTRAOPERATIVE AND POSTOPERATIVE MANAGEMENT

Aguilera X, Martínez-Zapata MJ, Hinarejos P, et al.: Topical and intravenous tranexamic acid reduce blood loss compared to routine hemostasis in total knee arthroplasty: a multicenter, randomized, controlled trial, *Arch Orthop Trauma Surg* 135:1017, 2015.

Bagsby DT, Ireland PH, Meneghini RM: Liposomal bupivacaine versus traditional periarticular injection for pain control after total knee arthroplasty, *J Arthroplasty* 29:1687, 2014.

Bagsby DT, Samujh CA, Vissing JL, et al.: Tranexamic acid decreases incidence of blood transfusion in simultaneous bilateral total knee arthroplasty, *J Arthroplasty* 30:2106, 2015.

Chahal GS, Saithna A, Brewster M, et al.: A comparison of complications requiring return to theatre in hip and knee arthroplasty patients taking enoxaparin versus rivaroxaban for thromboprophylaxis, *Ortop Traumatol Rehabil* 15:125, 2013.

Duggal S, Flics S, Cornell CN: Intra-articular analgesia and discharge to home enhance recovery following total knee replacement, *HSS J* 11:56, 2015.

Elmallah RK, Cherian JJ, Pierce TP, et al.: New and common perioperative pain management techniques in total knee arthroplasty, *J Knee Surg* 29:169, 2015.

Feng W, Wu K, Liu Z, et al.: Oral direct factor Xa inhibitor versus enoxaparin for thromboprophylaxis after hip or knee arthroplasty: Systemic review, traditional meta-analysis, dose-response meta-analysis and network meta-analysis, *Thromb Res* 136:1133, 2015.

Fuji T, Wang CJ, Fujita S, et al.: Safety and efficacy of edoxaban, an oral factor Xa inhibitor, versus enoxaparin for thromboprophylaxis after total knee arthroplasty: the STARS E-3 trial, *Thromb Res* 134:1198, 2014.

Gao F, Sun W, Guo W, et al.: Topical administration of tranexamic acid plus diluted-epinephrine in primary total knee arthroplasty: a randomized double-blinded controlled trial, *J Arthroplasty* 30:1354, 2015.

Gomez-Barrena E, Ortega-Andreu M, Padilla-Eguiluz NG, et al.: Topical intra-articular compared with intravenous tranexamic acid to reduce blood loss in primary total knee replacement: a double-blind, randomized, controlled, noninferiority clinical trial, *J Bone Joint Surg* 96:1937, 2014.

Gong L, Dong JY, Li ZR: Effects of combined application of muscle relaxants and celecoxib administration after total knee arthroplasty (TKA) on early recovery: a randomized, double-blind, controlled study, *J Arthroplasty* 28:1301, 2013.

Kazerooni R, Tran MH: Evaluation of celecoxib addition to pain protocol after total hip and knee arthroplasty stratified by opioid tolerance, *Clin J Pain* 31:903, 2015.

Kovalak E, Doğan AT, Üzümcügil O, et al.: A comparison of continuous femoral nerve block and periarticular local infiltration analgesia in the management of early period pain developing after total knee arthroplasty, *Acta Orthop Traumatol Turc* 49:260, 2015.

Lassen MR, Gent M, Kakkar AK, et al.: The effects of rivaroxaban on the complications of surgery after total hip or knee replacement: results from the RECORD programme, *J Bone Joint Surg* 94:1573, 2012.

Mahmoudi M, Sobieraj DM: The cost-effectiveness of oral direct factor Xa inhibitors compared with low-molecular-weight heparin for the prevention of venous thromboembolism prophylaxis in total hip or knee replacement surgery, *Pharmacotherapy* 33:1333, 2013.

Melvin JS, Stryker LS, Sierra RJ: Tranexamic acid in hip and knee arthroplasty, *J Am Acad Orthop Surg* 23:732, 2015.

Nawabi DH: Topical tranexamic acid was noninferior to intravenous tranexamic acid in controlling blood loss during total knee arthroplasty, *J Bone Joint Surg* 97:343, 2015.

Reinhardt KR, Duggal S, Umunna BP, et al.: Intraarticular analgesia versus epidural plus femoral nerve block after TKA: a randomized, double-blind trial, *Clin Orthop Relat Res* 472:1400, 2014.

Sawan H, Chen AF, Viscusi ER, et al.: Pregabalin reduces opioid consumption and improves outcome in chronic pain patients undergoing total knee arthroplasty, *Phys Sportsmed* 42:10 2014.

Schroer WC, Diesfeld PG, LeMarr AR, et al.: Does extended-release liposomal bupivacaine better control pain than bupivacaine after total knee arthroplasty (TKA)? A prospective, randomized clinical trial, *J Arthroplasty* 30(Suppl 9):64, 2015.

Shemshaki H, Nourian SM, Nourian N, et al.: One step closer to sparing total blood loss and transfusion rate in total knee arthroplasty: a meta-analysis of different methods of tranexamic acid administration, *Arch Orthop Trauma Surg* 135:573, 2015.

Springer BD, Odum SM, Fehring TK: What is the benefit of tranexamic acid vs reinfusion drains in total joint arthroplasty? *J Arthroplasty* 31:76, 2016.

Tsukada S, Wakui M, Hoshino A: Pain control after simultaneous bilateral total knee arthroplasty: a randomized controlled trial comparing periarticular injection and epidural analgesia, *J Bone Joint Surg* 97:367, 2015.

Wang C, Cai XZ, Yan SG: Comparison of periarticular multimodal drug injection and femoral nerve block for postoperative pain management in total knee arthroplasty: a systematic review and meta-analysis, *J Arthroplasty* 30:1281, 2015.

Whiting DR, Duncan CM, Sierra RJ, Smith HM: Tranexamic acid benefits total joint arthroplasty patients regardless of preoperative hemoglobin value, *J Arthroplasty* 30:2098, 2015.

UNICOMPARTMENTAL KNEE ARTHROPLASTY

Arirachakaran A, Choowit P, Putananon C, et al.: Is unicompartmental knee arthroplasty (UKA) superior to total knee arthroplasty (TKA)? A systematic review and meta-analysis of randomized controlled trial, *Eur J Orthop Surg Traumatol* 25:799, 2015.

Baker P, Jameson S, Critchley R, et al.: Center and surgeon volume influence the revision rate following unicondylar knee replacement: an analysis of 23,400 medial cemented unicondylar knee replacements, *J Bone Joint Surg* 95:702, 2013.

Baker PN, Petheram T, Jameson SS, et al.: Comparison of patient-reported outcome measures following total and unicondylar knee replacement, *J Bone Joint Surg* 94:919–927, 2012.

Cross MB, Berger R: Feasibility and safety of performing outpatient unicompartmental knee arthroplasty, *Int Orthop* 38:443, 2014.

Drager J, Hart A, Khalil JA, et al.: Shorter hospital stay and lower 30-day readmission after unicondylar knee arthroplasty compared to total knee arthroplasty, *J Arthroplasty* 31:356, 2016.

Dunbar NJ, Roche MW, Park BH, et al.: Accuracy of dynamic tactile-guided unicompartmental knee arthroplasty, *J Arthroplasty* 27:803, 2011.

Ghomrawi HM, Eggman AA, Pearle AD: Effect of age on cost-effectiveness of unicompartmental knee arthroplasty compared with total knee arthroplasty in the U.S, *J Bone Joint Surg* 97:396, 2015.

Gondusky JS, Choi L, Khalaf N, et al.: Day of surgery discharge after unicompartmental knee arthroplasty: an effective perioperative pathway, *J Arthroplasty* 29:516, 2014.

Hang JR, Stanford TE, Graves SE, et al.: Outcome of revision of unicompartmental knee replacement, *Acta Orthop* 81:95, 2010.

Kang SN, Smith TO, Sprenger De Rover WB, Walton NP: Pre-operative patellofemoral degenerative changes do not affect outcome after medial Oxford unicompartmental knee replacement: a report from an independent centre, *J Bone Joint Surg* 93B:476, 2011.

Labek G, Sekyra K, Pawelka W, et al.: Outcome and reproducibility of data concerning the Oxford unicompartmental knee arthroplasty: a structured literature review including arthroplasty registry data, *Acta Orthop* 82:131, 2011.

Liddle AD, Pandit H, Judge A, Murray DW: Patient-reported outcomes after total and unicompartmental knee arthroplasty: a study of 14,076 matched patients from the National Joint Registry for England and Wales, *Bone Joint J* 97B:793, 2015.

Lim JW, Chen JY, Chong HC, et al.: Pre-existing patellofemoral disease does not affect 10-year survivorship in fixed bearing unicompartmental knee arthroplasty, *Knee Surg Sports Traumatol Arthrosc* 27(6):2030, 2019.

Lonner JH, John TK, Conditt MA: Robotic arm-assisted UKA improves tibial component alignment: a pilot study, *Clin Orthop Relat Res* 468:141, 2010.

Lygre SH, Espehug B, Havelin LI, et al.: Pain and function in patients after primary unicompartmental and total knee arthroplasty, *J Bone Joint Surg* 92A:2890, 2010.

Niinimäki T, Eskelinen A, Mäkelä K, et al.: Unicompartmental knee arthroplasty survivorship is lower than TKA survivorship: a 27-year Finnish registry study, *Clin Orthop Relat Res* 472:1496, 2014.

O'Donnell T, Neil MJ: The Repicci Ii(r) unicondylar knee arthroplasty: 9-year survivorship and function, *Clin Orthop Relat Res* 468:3094, 2010.

Pandit H, Jenkins C, Gill HS, et al.: Minimally invasive Oxford phase 3 unicompartmental knee replacement: results of 1000 cases, *J Bone Joint Surg* 93B:198, 2011.

Pearle AD, O'Loughlin PF, Kendoff DO: Robot-assisted unicompartmental knee arthroplasty, *J Arthroplasty* 25:230, 2010.

Scott RD: Mobile- versus fixed-bearing unicompartmental knee arthroplasty, *Instr Course Lect* 59:57, 2010.

Vasso M, Del Regno C, Perisano C, et al.: Unicompartmental knee arthroplasty is effective: ten year results, *Int Orthop* 39:2341, 2015.

W-Dahl A, Robertsson O, Lidgren L, et al.: Unicompartmental knee arthroplasty in patients aged less than 65, *Acta Orthop* 81:90, 2010.

Wilson HA, Middleton R, Abram SFG, et al.: Patient relevant outcomes of unicompartmental versus total knee replacement: systematic review and meta-analysis, *BMJ* 364:1352, 2019.

SURGICAL PROBLEMS IN SPECIFIC DISORDERS

Badway M, Fenstad AM, Indrekam K, et al.: The risk of revision in total knee arthroplasty is not affected by previous high tibial osteotomy, *Acta Orthop* 86:734, 2015.

Cancienne JM, Werner BC, Browne JA: Complications after TKA in patients with hemophilia or Von Willebrand's disease, *J Arthroplasty* 30:2285, 2015.

Chen JY, Lo NN, Chong HC, et al.: Cruciate retaining versus posterior stabilized total knee arthroplasty after previous high tibial osteotomy, *Knee Surg Sports Traumatol Arthrosc* 23:3607, 2015.

Dimitriou D, Ramokgopa M, Pietrzak JRT, et al.: Human immunodeficiency virus infection and hip and knee arthroplasty, *JBJS Rev* 5(9):e8, 2017.

Erak S, Naudie D, MacDonald SJ, et al.: Total knee arthroplasty following medial opening wedge tibial osteotomy: technical issues early clinical results, *Knee* 18:499, 2011.

Goddard NJ, Mann HA, Lee CA: Total knee replacement in patients with end-stage haemophilic arthropathy: 25-year results, *J Bone Joint Surg* 92B:1085, 2010.

Han JH, Yang JH, Bhandare NN, et al.: Total knee arthroplasty after failed high tibial osteotomy: a systematic review of open versus closed wedge osteotomy, *Knee Surg Sports Traumatol Arthrosc* 2015, [Epub ahead of print].

Kamath AF, Horneff JG, Forsyth A, et al.: Total knee arthroplasty in hemophiliacs: gains in range of motion realized beyond twelve months postoperatively, *Clin Orthop Surg* 4:121, 2012.

KarimA, Andrawis J, Bengoa F, et al.: Hip and knee section, diagnosis, algorithm: proceedings of international consensus on orthopedic infections, *J Arthroplasty* 34(2S):S339, 2019.

Lin CA, Takemoto S, Kandermi U, Kuo AC: Mid-term outcomes in HIV-positive patients after primary total hip or knee arthroplasty, *J Arthroplasty* 29:177, 2014.

Maslow J, Zuckerman JD, Immerman I: Total knee arthroplasty in patients with a previous patellectomy, *Bull Hosp Jt Dis* 71:227, 2013.

Panotopoulos J, Ay C, Trieb K, et al.: Outcome of total knee arthroplasty in hemophilic arthropathy, *J Arthroplasty* 29:749, 2014.

Reinhardt KR, Huffaker SJ, Thornhill TS, Scott RD: Cruciate-retaining TKA is a option in patients with prior patellectomy, *Clin Orthop Relat Res* 473:111, 2015.

Rodriguez-Merchan EC: Total knee arthroplasty in haemophilic arthropathy, *Am J Orthop* 44:E503, 2015.

Rodriguez-Merchan EC: Unicompartmental knee osteoarthritis (UKOA): unicompartmental knee arthroplasty (UKA) or high tibial osteotomy (HTO)? *Arch Bone Jt Surg* 4(4):307, 2016.

Warth LC, Pugely AJ, Martin CT, et al.: Total joint arthroplasty in patients with chronic renal disease: is it worth the risk? *J Arthroplasty* 30(Suppl 9):51, 2015.

Westberg M, Paus AC, Holme PA, Tjønnfjord GE: Haemophilic arthropathy: long-term outcomes in 107 primary total knee arthroplasties, *Knee* 29:749, 2014.

Xuedong S, Zheng S: A meta-analysis of unicompartmental knee arthroplasty revised to total knee arthroplasty versus primary total knee arthroplasty, *J Orthop Surg Res* 13:158, 2018.

Yao R, Lyons MC, Howard JL, McAuley JP: Does patellectomy jeopardize function after TKA? *Clin Orthop Relat Res* 471:544, 2013.

Zingg PO, Fucentese SF, Lutz W, et al.: Haemophilic knee arthropathy: long-term outcome after total knee replacement, *Knee Surg Sports Traumatol Arthrosc* 20:2465, 2012.

COMPLICATIONS

Bala A, Huddleston 3rd JI, Goodman SB, et al.: Venous thromboembolism prophylaxis after TKA: aspirin, warfarin, enoxaparin, or factor Xa inhibitors? *Clin Orthop Relat Res* 475(9):2205, 2017.

Bawa H, Weick JW, Dirschl DR, Luu HH: Trends in deep vein thrombosis prophylaxis and deep vein thrombosis rates after total hip and knee arthroplasty, *J Am Acad Orthop Surg* 26(19):698, 2018.

Bokshan SL, Ruttiman RJ, DePasse JM, et al.: Reported litigation associated with primary hip and knee arthroplasty, *J Arthroplasty* 32(12):3573, 2017.

Browne JA, Hanssen AD: Reconstruction of patellar tendon disruption after total knee arthroplasty: results of a new technique utilizing synthetic mesh, *J Bone Joint Surg* 93A:1137, 2011.

Chang MJ, Song MK, Kyung MG, et al.: incidence of deep vein thrombosis before and after total knee arthroplasty without pharmacologic prophylaxis: a 128-row multidetector CT indirect venography study, *BMC Musculoskelet Disord* 19(1):274, 2018.

Christ AB, Chiu YF, Joseph A, et al.: Incidence and risk factors for peripheral nerve injury after 383,000 total knee arthroplasties using a New York State Database (SPARCS), *J Arthroplasty* 34(10):2473, 2019.

Courtney PM, Rozell JC, Melnic CM, Lee GC: Who should not undergo short stay hip and knee arthroplasty? Risk factors associated with major

medical complications following primary total joint arthroplasty, *J Arthroplasty* 30(9 Suppl):1, 2015.

Daines BK, Dennis DA, Amann S: Infection prevention in total knee arthroplasty, *J Am Acad Orthop Surg* 23:356, 2015.

D'Apuzzo MR, Novicoff WM, Browne JA: The John Insall Award: Morbid obesity independently impacts complications, mortality, and resource use after TKA, *Clin Orthop Relat Res* 473:57, 2015.

Deirmengian C, Kardos K, Kilmartin P, et al.: The alpha-defensin test for periprosthetic joint infection outperforms the leukocyte esterase test strip, *Clin Orthop Relat Res* 473(1):198, 2015.

Della Valle C, Parvizi J, Bauer TW, et al.: American Academy of Orthopaedic Surgeons clinical practice guideline on the diagnosis of periprosthetic joint infections of the hip and knee, *J Bone Joint Surg* 93A:1355, 2011.

Drew JM, Griffin WL, Odum SM, et al.: Survivorship after periprosthetic femur fracture: factors affecting outcome, *J Arthroplasty* 31(6):1283, 2019.

Dua A, Desai SS, Lee CL, Heller JA: National trends in deep vein thrombosis following total knee and total hip replacement in the United States, *Ann Vasc Surg* 38:310, 2017.

Faour M, Piuzzi NS, Brigati DP: Low-dose aspirin is safe and effective for venous thromboembolism prophylaxis following total knee arthroplasty, *J Arthroplasty* 33(7S):S131, 2018.

Garvin KL, Konigsberg BS: Infection following total knee arthroplasty, *J Bone Joint Surg* 93A:1167, 2011.

Goel R, Fleischman AN, Tan T, et al.: Venous thromboembolic prophylaxis after simultaneous bilateral total knee arthroplasty: aspirin versus warfarin, *Bone Joint J* 100-B(1 Supple A):68, 2018.

Gomez MM, Tan TL, Manrique J, et al.: The fate of spacers in the treatment of periprosthetic joint infection, *J Bone Joint Surg Am* 97:1495e502, 2015.

Huang R, Greenky M, Kerr GJ, et al.: The effect of malnutrition on patients undergoing elective joint arthroplasty, *J Arthroplasty* 28(Suppl 8):21, 2013.

Jensen CD, Steval A, et al.: Return to theatre following total hip and knee replacement before and after the introduction of rivaroxaban: a retrospective cohort study, *J Bone Joint Surg* 93B:91, 2011.

Jacobs JJ, Mont MA, Bozic KJ, et al.: American Academy of Orthopaedic Surgeons clinical practice guideline on preventing venous thromboembolic disease in patients undergoing elective hip and knee arthroplasty, *J Bone Joint Surg Am* 94(8):746, 2012.

Jergesen HE, Yi PH: Early complications in hip and knee arthroplasties in a safety net hospital vs a university center, *J Arthroplasty* 31(4):754–758, 2016.

Khan S, Schmidt AH: Distal femoral replacement for periprosthetic fractures around total knee arthroplasty: when and how? *J Knee Surg* 32(5):388, 2019.

Kheir MM, Ackerman CT, Tan TL, et al.: Leukocyte esterase strip test can predict subsequent failure following reimplantation in patients with periprosthetic joint infection, *J Arthroplasty* 32(6):1976, 2017.

Koh IJ, Cho WS, Choi NY, et al.: How accurate are orthopedic surgeons in diagnosing periprosthetic joint infection after total knee arthroplasty? A multicenter study, *Knee* 22(3):180, 2015.

Ledford CK, Ruberte Thiele RA, et al.: Percent body fat more associated with perioperative risks after total joint arthroplasty than body mass index, *J Arthroplasty* 29(Suppl 9):150, 2014.

Leung KH, Chiu KY, Yan CH, et al.: Review Article: venous thromboembolism after total joint replacement, *J Orthop Surg* 21(3):351, 2013.

Lewis S, Kink S, Rahl M, et al.: Aspirin: are patients actually taking it? A quality assessment study, *Arthroplast Today* 4(4):475, 2018.

Lotzien S, Hoberg C, Hoffmann MF, Schildhauer TA: Clinical outcome and quality of life of patients with periprosthetic distal femur fractures and retained total knee arthroplasty treated with polyaxial locking plates: a single-center experience, *Eur J Orthop Surg Traumatol* 29(1):189, 2019.

Mackie A, Muthumayandi K, Shirley M, et al.: Association between body mass index change and outcome in the first year after total knee arthroplasty, *J Arthroplasty* 30:206, 2015.

Manning DW, Edelstein AI, Alvi HM: Risk prediction tools for hip and knee arthroplasty, *J Am Acad Orthop Surg* 24:19, 2016.

Mason JB, Callaghan JJ, Hozack WJ, et al.: Obesity in total joint arthroplasty: an issue with gravity, *J Arthroplasty* 29:1879, 2014.

Mihalko WM, Bergin PF, Kelly FB, Canale ST: Obesity, orthopaedics, and outcomes, *J Am Acad Orthop Surg* 22:683, 2014.

Minarro JC, Urbano-Luque MT, Quevedo-Reinoso R, et al.: Is obesity related with periprosthetic fractures around the knee?, *Int Orthop* 2015, [Epub ahead of print].

Mont MA, Jacobs JJ, et al.: AAOS clinical practice guideline: preventing venous thromboembolic disease in patients undergoing elective hip and knee arthroplasty, *JAAOS* 19(12):777, 2011.

Nagwadia H, Joshi P: Outcome of osteosynthesis for periprosthetic fractures after total knee arthroplasty: a retrospective study, *Eur J Orthop Surg Traumatol* 28(4):683, 2018.

Naziri Q, Issa K, Malkani AL, et al.: Bariatric orthopaedics: total knee arthroplasty in super-obese patients (BMI > 50 kg/m2). Survivorship and complications, *Clin Orthop Relat Res* 471:3523, 2013.

Park JH, Restrepo C, Norton R, et al.: Common peroneal nerve palsy following total knee arthroplasty: prognostic factors and course of recovery, *J Arthroplasty* 28(9):1538, 2013.

Parvizi J, Della Valle CJ: AAOS clinical practice guideline: diagnosis and treatment of periprosthetic joint infections of the hip and knee, *JAAOS* 18(12):771, 2010.

Parvizi J, Tan TL, Goswami K, et al.: The 2018 definition of periprosthetic hip and knee infection: an evidence-based and validated criteria, *J Arthroplasty* 33(5):1309, 2018.

Parvizi J, Zmistowski B, Berbari EF, et al.: New definition for periprosthetic joint infection: from the Workgroup of the Musculoskeletal Infection Society, *Clin Orthop Relat Res* 469:2992, 2011.

Ponce B, Raines BT, Reed RD, et al.: Surgical site infection after arthroplasty: comparative effectiveness of prophylactic antibiotics: do surgical care improvement project guidelines need to be updated? *J Bone Joint Surg* 96:970, 2014.

Ruder JA, Hart GP, Kneisl JS, et al.: Predictors of functional recovery following periprosthetic distal femur fractures, *J Arthroplasty* 32(5):1571, 2017.

Scolaro JA, Schwarzkopf R: Management of interprosthetic femur fractures, *J Am Acad Orthop Surg* 25(4):e63, 2017.

Shohat N, Goswami K, Tan TL, et al.: Increased failure after irrigation and debridement for acute hematogenous periprosthetic joint infection, *J Bone Joint Surg Am* 101(8):696, 2019.

Speelziek SJA, Staff NP, Johnson RL, et al.: Clinical spectrum of neuropathy after primary total knee arthroplasty: a series of 54 cases, *Muscle Nerve* 59(6):679, 2019.

Sun G, Wu J, Wang Q, et al.: Factor Xa Inhibitors and direct thrombin inhibitors versus low-molecular-weight heparin for thromboprophylaxis after total hip or total knee arthroplasty: a systematic review and meta-analysis, *J Arthroplasty* 34(4):789, 2019.

Teeter MG, McAuley JP, Naudie DD: Fracture of two moderately cross-linked polyethylene tibial inserts in a TKR patient, *Case Rep Orthop* 2014:491384, 2014.

Wallace SS, Bechtold D, Sassoon A: Periprosthetic fractures of the distal femur after total knee arthroplasty: plate versus nail fixation, *Orthop Traumatol Surg Res* 103(2):257, 2017.

Werner BC, Burrus MT, Novicoff WM, Browne JA: Total knee arthroplasty within six months after knee arthroscopy is associated with increased postoperative complications, *J Arthroplasty* 30:1313, 2015.

Whiteside LA, Nayfeh TA, Lazear R, Roy ME: Reinfected revised TKA resolves with an aggressive protocol and antibiotic infusion, *Clin Orthop Relat Res* 470:236, 2012.

Whiteside LA, Peppers M, Nayfeh TA, Roy ME: Methicillin-resistant *Staphylococcus aureus* in TKA treated with revision and direct intra-articular antibiotic infusion, *Clin Orthop Relat Res* 469:26, 2011.

REVISION TOTAL KNEE ARTHROPLASTY

Agarwal S, Kabariti R, Kakar R, et al.: Why are revision knee replacements failing? *Knee* 26(3):774, 2019.

Belmont Jr PJ, Goodman GP, Rodriguez M, et al.: Predictors of hospital readmission following revision total knee arthroplasty, *Knee Surg Sports Traumatol Arthrosc*, 2015, [Epub ahead of print].

Bloom KJ, Gupta RR, Caravella JW, et al.: The effects of primary implant bearing design on the complexity of revision unicondylar knee arthroplasty, *J Arthroplasty* 29:106, 2014.

Bugler KE, Maheshwari R, Ahmed I, et al.: Metaphyseal sleeves for revision total knee arthroplasty: good short-term outcomes, *J Arthroplasty* 30:1990, 2015.

Burastero G, Cavagnaro L, Chiarlone F, et al.: The use of tantalum metaphyseal cones for the management of severe bone defects in septic knee revision, *J Arthroplasty* 33(12):3739, 2018.

Cross MB, Yi PY, Moric M, et al.: Revising an HTO or UKA to TKA: is it more like a primary TKA or a revision TKA? *J Arthroplasty* 29(Suppl 9):229, 2014.

De Martino I, De Santis V, Sculco PK, et al.: Tantalum cones provide durable mid-term fixation in revision TKA, *Clin Orthop Relat Res* 473:3176, 2015.

Derome P, Sternheim A, Backstein D, Malo M: Treatment of large bone defects with trabecular metal cones in revision total knee arthroplasty: short term clinical and radiographic outcomes, *J Arthroplasty* 29:122, 2014.

Keswani A, Lovy AJ, Robinson J, et al.: Risk factors predict increased length of stay and readmission rates in revision joint arthroplasty, *J Arthroplasty* 31:603, 2016.

Kim YH, Park JW, Kim JS, Oh HK: Long-term clinical outcomes and survivorship of revision total knee arthroplasty with use of a constrained condylar knee prosthesis, *J Arthroplasty* 30:1804, 2015.

Kurtz S, Ong K, Lau E, et al.: Projections of primary and revision hip and knee arthroplasty in the United States from 2005 to 2030, *J Bone Joint Surg* 89A:780, 2007.

Robertsson O, W-Dahl A: The risk of revision after TKA is affected by previous HTO or UKA, *Clin Orthop Relat Res* 473:90, 2015.

Schmitz HC, Klauser W, Citak M, et al.: Three-year follow up utilizing tantal cones in revision total knee arthroplasty, *J Arthroplasty* 28:1556, 2013.

Stevens J, Clement ND, MacDonald D, et al.: Survival and functional outcome of revision total knee arthroplasty with a total stabilizer knee system: minimum 5 years of follow-up, *Eur J Orthop Surg Traumatol*, 2019.

Zanirato A, Cavagnaro L, Basso M, et al.: Metaphyseal sleeves in total knee arthroplasty revision: complications, clinical and radiological results. A systematic review of the literature, *Arch Orthop Trauma Surg* 138(7):993, 2018.

Zanirato A, Formica M, Cavagnaro L, et al.: Metaphyseal cones and sleeves in revision total knee arthroplasty: two sides of the same coin? Complications, clinical and radiological results – a systematic review of the literature, *Musculoskelet Surg* 2019.

The complete list of references is available online at Expert Consult.com.

CHAPTER 6

ARTHRODESIS OF THE KNEE

Anthony A. Mascioli

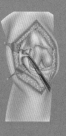

INDICATIONS AND RESULTS

With the success of total knee arthroplasty, knee arthrodesis seldom is performed as a primary operation and usually is reserved for those few patients who are not candidates for total knee replacement. Occasionally, arthrodesis may be more appropriate than arthroplasty in a young patient with severe arthrosis because of the patient's weight, occupation, or activity level. Other possible indications for primary arthrodesis include painful ankylosis after infection, loss of the extensor mechanism, tuberculosis, trauma, severe deformity in paralytic conditions, neuropathic arthropathy, and malignant or potentially malignant lesions around the knee. The most frequent indication for knee arthrodesis is currently salvage of a failed total knee arthroplasty, most often secondary to infection.

Most current series of knee arthrodesis report successful fusion in most patients, up to 100% in some series. Most properly selected patients are satisfied with a fused knee, especially with the decrease in pain postoperatively; however, some patients report functional difficulty and continued pain. Arthrodesis as a salvage procedure after failed total knee arthroplasty can be expected to have some inferior results compared with primary knee arthrodesis, including lower fusion rates, higher infection rates, and shortening (often 2 to 5 cm in this setting).

Frequent concerns expressed by patients after knee fusion include the attention they attract in public, difficulty riding public transportation, difficulty sitting in theaters and stadiums, and difficulty getting up after a fall. Patients should be counseled about these difficulties preoperatively. Some patients may benefit psychologically from a preoperative trial of long-leg immobilization (cast or brace) to decide if they can manage with a fused knee. Harris et al. found that walking speeds and efficiency are similar after amputation, arthrodesis, and arthroplasty for tumors around the knee. Although patients with arthrodeses had the most stable limbs and could perform the most demanding physical work and recreational activities, they had difficulty sitting and were more self-conscious about the limb than were patients with arthroplasty.

Above-knee amputation is another procedure for treating chronic prosthetic joint infections. Arthrodesis should still be considered first because it allows better function and ambulation compared with amputation.

TECHNIQUES

Numerous techniques have been described for knee arthrodesis, and these can be categorized by the type of fixation used. The amount and quality of bone present are important in determining appropriate fixation and the need for bone grafting. The selection of arthrodesis technique also is based on the individual patient and the surgeon's experience.

Arthrodesis can be performed as a one- or two-stage procedure, depending on the circumstances. Arthrodesis has been found to be more predictable with a two-stage method.

Published arthrodesis techniques for the knee include compression with external fixation, intramedullary nailing, plate, screws, or various combinations of the above.

COMPRESSION ARTHRODESIS WITH EXTERNAL FIXATION

Compression arthrodesis is generally indicated for knees with minimal bone loss and broad cancellous surfaces with adequate cortical bone to allow good bony apposition and compression. Advantages of compression arthrodesis include the application of good, stable compression across the fusion site and the placement of fixation at a site remote from the infected or neuropathic joint. Some series suggest that the recurrent infection rates may be lower when using external fixation compared with intramedullary nailing (e.g., 4.9% compared with 8.3% reported by Mabry et al.) for arthrodesis after infected total knee replacement.

Disadvantages of external fixation include external pin track problems, poor patient compliance, and the frequent need for early removal and cast immobilization. Several studies have demonstrated reduced fusion rates after external fixation compared with intramedullary nailing (29% to 67% vs. 91% to 95%, respectively) in arthrodesis for failed total knee replacement. These patients differ from those with primary arthrodesis in whom fusion has been reported in up to 100% with the use of external fixation. A variety of monolateral, bilateral, and ring multiple-pin fixators are now used, with fusion rates ranging from 31% to 100%. Stability, limited tissue damage, and high patient comfort are the cited advantages of using anterior unilateral external fixation.

Single-plane and biplane external fixators have similar fusion rates, although complications are numerous with both devices. Despite biomechanical advances in external fixator design, knee arthrodesis remains difficult to achieve in patients who have had multiple previous procedures, a failed total knee arthroplasty, or an infected total knee arthroplasty with significant bone loss. One series reported successful arthrodesis for treatment of sepsis using augmented external fixation with crossed Steinmann pins. No recurrences of infection were noted over a mean follow-up of 8.2 years. Other authors have used fine wire external fixation, Ilizarov external fixation, or a similar device for treatment of septic failure of total knee arthroplasty, persistent knee sepsis, or septic sequelae after knee trauma. Fusion was obtained in 77%, 96%, and 100%, respectively. Achieving fusion in the face of major bone loss can be particularly challenging and may be facilitated by using the Ilizarov device and bone transport. Ilizarov-type devices do have the advantage of bone lengthening.

COMPRESSION ARTHRODESIS USING EXTERNAL FIXATION

TECHNIQUE 6.1

- When extensive exposure is necessary, use an anterior longitudinal incision; otherwise, a transverse incision can be used. For arthrodesis after total knee arthroplasty, approach the knee through a midline incision or through previous scars when appropriate.
- Split the quadriceps and patellar tendons and excise the patella.
- Detach the joint capsule from the tibia anteriorly and divide the collateral ligaments.
- Flex the knee so that the capsule and quadriceps mechanism fall posteriorly on each side.
- Remove the synovium and excise the menisci, cruciate ligaments, and infrapatellar fat pad.

- With a power saw, cut the superior surface of the tibia exactly transverse to the long axis of the bone, and remove a wafer of cartilage and bone 1 cm thick.
- Remove an appropriately sized segment of bone from the distal femur so that raw bony surfaces are apposed with the knee in the desired position. We have found total knee instruments useful in making these bone cuts.
- If arthrodesis is performed after failed total knee arthroplasty, do not remove more bone from the femur and tibia but thoroughly clean the surfaces and attempt to interdigitate irregular surfaces to give the best possible contact.
- Charnley recommended a position of almost complete extension for cosmetic reasons; we prefer arthrodesis with the knee in 0 to15 degrees of flexion, 5 to 8 degrees of valgus, and 10 degrees of external rotation.
- Insert the appropriate pins for the compression device. Tighten the clamps so that a compression load of 45 kg is attained.
- Close and dress the wound. If a compression clamp is used, a long leg cast incorporating the clamp is applied; if a more rigid external fixator is used, the cast can be omitted.
- The compression device is removed after 6 to 8 weeks, and either a long leg or a cylinder cast is applied; graduated weight bearing is initiated. The cast is worn until fusion is solid, usually another 6 to 8 weeks.
- If a multiple-pin, biplanar fixator is used, place three parallel transfixation pins through the distal femur and three through the upper tibia (Fig. 6.1A); if bony surfaces are adequate, fixation usually is sufficient. If anteroposterior instability is present, insert additional half-pins above and below the knee at angles different from the initial pins (Fig. 6.1B). Connect all pins to the frame and apply compression.
- A triangular frame configuration also can be used, with 6.5-mm half-pins placed at a 45-degree angle to the anteroposterior and mediolateral planes (Fig. 6.1C). This configuration provides rigid stability and is tolerated by the patient.

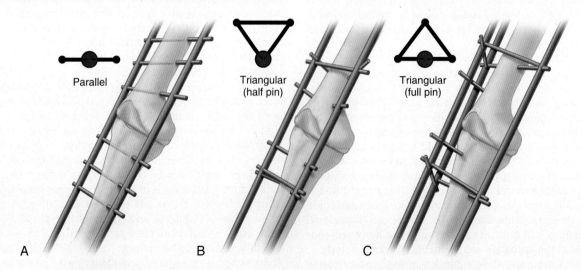

Parallel

Triangular (half pin)

Triangular (full pin)

A　　　　　B　　　　　C

FIGURE 6.1 External fixator configurations for knee arthrodesis. **A,** Parallel; standard Hoffmann-Vidal configuration. **B,** Triangular half-pin configuration. **C,** Triangular full-pin configuration provides rigid multiplanar stability. **SEE TECHNIQUE 6.1.**

POSTOPERATIVE CARE The triangular frame configuration usually is rigid enough to allow early weight bearing and should be left in place for 3 months. After removal of the triangular frame, the patient is allowed protected weight bearing with crutches until clinical and radiographic union is noted.

ARTHRODESIS WITH INTRAMEDULLARY ROD FIXATION

Intramedullary nailing techniques may be more appropriate when extensive bone loss does not allow compression to be exerted across broad areas of cancellous bone, such as after tumor resection or failed total knee arthroplasty.

The advantages of intramedullary nailing include immediate weight bearing, easier rehabilitation, absence of pin track complications, and a high fusion rate. Higher union rates have been frequently noted with intramedullary nail fixation compared with external fixation. Disadvantages of intramedullary nails include increased risk of fat embolism, potential intramedullary dissemination of infection, increased rates of infection and blood loss, and potential impediment to obtaining correct alignment.

Despite excellent fusion rates with intramedullary nailing, it is a technically demanding procedure that requires lengthy operative time (often up to 6 hours) and has significant blood loss and frequent complications. Nevertheless, the high percentage of fusion and the ability of most patients to bear full weight soon after surgery make this technique attractive in selected patients. Donley et al. used a two-stage procedure for all patients with an infected total knee arthroplasty. They also used stainless steel wire loops passed through the eye of the nail and through a hole drilled into the greater trochanter to prevent proximal migration of the nail.

Similar high rates of fusion have been reported when attempting salvage after infected total knee replacement using various one- and two-stage intramedullary nailing techniques (80% to 95%). Although residual functional difficulties have been noted, it appears that arthrodesis using intramedullary nail fixation can be considered a reasonably reliable and successful technique overall.

Nonunion is a known complication of any arthrodesis. One study showed that obtaining large surfaces of bleeding contact bone enhances union of the arthrodesis.

The intramedullary nailing technique has also been extended to other, more challenging arthrodesis situations. Mack et al. reported successfully treating a patient with a blast injury using intercalary femoral cortical autograft to fuse the remaining knee over a long intramedullary device. It has also been used successfully after resection of aggressive bone tumors. Intercalary autograft or allografts have been used as fusion material with similar results.

For large skeletal defects caused by the resection of tumors around the knee, intramedullary nailing and vascularized fibular bone grafting have been successful. However, this should be considered only when a massive loss of bone has occurred after a failed constrained total knee arthroplasty, failed arthrodesis, or tumor resection. The use of massive segmental autogenous grafts from the femur, tibia, and fibula for resection arthrodesis in 40 patients with tumors around the knee has been reported. Despite a high complication rate

(52%), most patients obtained support-free ambulation and 25 (78%) of 32 evaluated an average of 17 years after surgery had satisfactory function.

Short, locked intramedullary nails designed specifically for knee fusions have the advantages of avoiding a second incision required for insertion of long nails, the bulkiness of double-plating techniques in the relatively subcutaneous anterior knee area, and the difficulties of prolonged external fixation.

Intramedullary nail fixation for knee arthrodesis is especially useful when bone loss is extensive, as in infected total knee arthroplasty; in this situation, it is best to stage the arthrodesis, first removing the implant and polymethyl methacrylate, allowing the infection to clear, and then performing the arthrodesis. Techniques are described for primary arthrodesis using intramedullary nail fixation and for "salvage arthrodesis" after removal of total knee arthroplasty, the latter using an intramedullary nail that can be locked proximally and distally for added stability and rotational control.

ARTHRODESIS USING INTRAMEDULLARY NAIL FIXATION

TECHNIQUE 6.2

- Place a sandbag under the affected hip and extremity so that the greater trochanter can be palpated. Prepare and drape the entire limb, including the hemipelvis, so that the iliac crest, greater trochanter, and knee are visible. A fluoroscopic table-top study and image intensification are helpful.
- Approach the knee through a previous incision, if present, or through a straight anterior incision 10 to 12 cm proximal and distal to the joint line.
- Carry the dissection down to the quadriceps tendon and the medial patellar retinaculum.
- Elevate the soft tissue medially and laterally in flaps containing skin, subcutaneous tissue, capsule, and periosteum.
- Debride the joint in the standard fashion.
- Total knee alignment guides are helpful in resection of the tibial and femoral surfaces. Minimal bone should be resected.
- Excise the patella; set it aside for use later as a bone graft, if necessary.
- Make an incision 3 to 5 cm long proximal to the tip of the greater trochanter.
- Incise the gluteus maximus fascia and split the muscle fibers longitudinally.
- Identify the device-specific entry point and insert a tip-threaded guidewire at that site.
- Use a reamer to open the proximal femoral canal and pass a ball-tipped guide down the canal to the knee. Also use the reamer to open the tibial medullary canal and insert the ball-tipped guide into the canal and advance it to the metaphyseal area of the distal tibia.

- Ream the tibial medullary canal progressively; the amount of reaming required usually is determined by preoperative measurements of the tibia and femur in the anteroposterior and lateral planes. In most situations, a 12- to 14-mm nail is used.
- Ream the femur and tibia over the femoral guide pin in 1-mm increments in an antegrade fashion until cortical bone is encountered and then ream in 0.5-mm increments. Ream the canals to accommodate at least a 12-mm nail.
- If a Küntscher nail is used, overream the bones at least 0.5 mm. For a solid type nail, overreaming by 1 to 2 mm is recommended.
- The length of the nail should be determined before surgery from standing anteroposterior and lateral full-length radiographs of the lower extremity or with the aid of image intensification.
- Insert the nail antegrade from the greater trochanter over the guidewire.
- Maintain compression at the arthrodesis site to prevent distraction as the nail enters the tibia.
- The nail should be bowed concave laterally to reconstitute the normal valgus of the tibiofemoral angle and nearly approximate the normal axis of the lower extremity.
- Drive the nail until it reaches the metaphysis of the distal tibia. Its tip should not end in the diaphyseal area because this might cause stress concentration and pain or fracture of the tibia.
- Sink the nail beneath the tip of the greater trochanter to prevent irritation of the abductor muscles.
- Pack the patella or other bone grafts obtained in the standard fashion around the arthrodesis.
- Consider using suction drainage tubes and close both incisions.
- Apply a compressive dressing and a posterior plaster splint from the groin to the toes.

POSTOPERATIVE CARE Drains, if used, are removed in 2 or 3 days, and walking with crutches with touchdown weight bearing on the operated side is allowed. If adequate healing appears to be occurring after 6 weeks, progressive weight bearing is allowed. Crutches are used until union is achieved clinically and radiographically (Figs. 6.2 and 6.3).

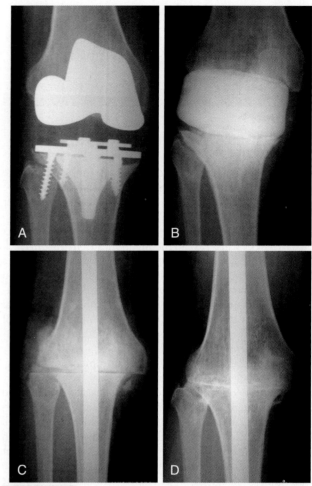

FIGURE 6.2 **A,** Infected total knee arthroplasty. **B,** After debridement with antibiotic spacer. **C,** Early postoperative radiograph. **D,** Solid arthrodesis of the knee. **SEE TECHNIQUE 6.2.**

Arthrodesis with a locked, long intramedullary nail is especially appropriate after failed total knee arthroplasty (Fig. 6.4). These nails are available in multiple lengths and diameters. Smaller diameter and stepped nails are available to match each individual patient's femoral and tibial anatomy. The nail should extend from the greater trochanter to within 2 to 6 cm from the plafond of the ankle. During preoperative planning, the thickness of the femoral and tibial components and any bone defects that will be resected should be subtracted from the length measured on the preoperative long-leg radiographs of the hip, knee, and ankle.

The next technique described is specific for knee arthrodesis after failed total knee arthroplasty. Modifications are necessary for arthrodesis for other reasons. For example, when done for infection, modification to a two-stage procedure may be indicated because it often yields superior results.

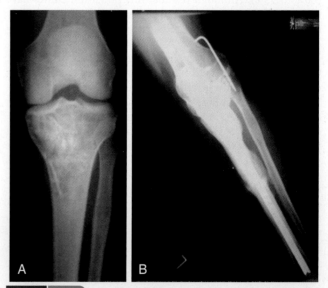

FIGURE 6.3 Resection arthrodesis of knee for hemangioendothelioma. **A,** Before surgery. **B,** After resection and arthrodesis using intramedullary nail and Kirschner wire for internal fixation. Fusion is solid. **SEE TECHNIQUE 6.2.**

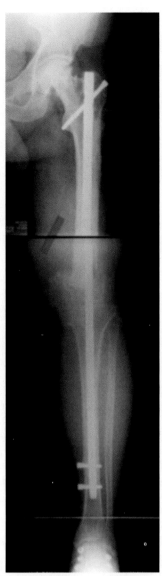

FIGURE 6.4 Knee arthrodesis with intramedullary nail fixation after infected total knee arthroplasty.

KNEE ARTHRODESIS WITH LOCKED INTRAMEDULLARY NAIL AFTER FAILED TOTAL KNEE ARTHROPLASTY

TECHNIQUE 6.3

- With the patient supine on a fluoroscopic operating table and a sandbag under the ipsilateral pelvis, prepare and drape the lower extremity to allow access from the greater trochanter to the foot; the foot should be visible to help with rotational alignment.
- Begin an incision at the tip of the greater trochanter and carry it proximally about 5 cm.
- Adduct and internally rotate the limb and identify the greater trochanter and piriformis fossa on fluoroscopy.

- Determine the correct entry portal for the nail, specific for the nail device used, and insert a tip-threaded guide pin at that site.
- Using a skin protector, ream over the guide pin with a 9-mm cannulated reamer down to the level of the lesser trochanter.
- Remove the guide pin and the reamer and insert a ball-tip guidewire down the medullary canal to just above the knee; insert the smooth end of the guidewire, rather than the ball-tip end. Leave this wire in place while the knee is being exposed.
- Apply and inflate a sterile tourniquet.
- Make an incision over the knee at approximately the same location as the incision used for the total knee arthroplasty. Use a medial parapatellar incision to enter the knee joint.
- Before removing the total knee components, place a long ruler anteriorly over the distal femur and proximal tibia. Use an osteotome or electrocautery to draw vertical lines superficially on the anterior tibial and femoral shafts along the line of the ruler (Fig. 6.5). These lines are used to determine rotational alignment when inserting the nail; ensure that the lines are not removed with bone cuts or resection of tibial implants.
- Using osteotomes and appropriate total knee instrumentation, remove all total knee components. Curet and clean out all debris and bone erosion, preserving as much bone as possible. If the patella is in good condition, preserve it to be used as a bone graft; otherwise, remove it.
- If the distal femur and proximal tibia need to be recut to allow good bony apposition, use standard intramedullary knee resection guides for total knee prostheses, resecting a minimal amount of bone.
- When the total knee components, cement, and debris have been removed and any necessary proximal tibial and distal femoral resection has been done, remove the tourniquet, insert a ball-tip guidewire into the tibial canal down past the tibial isthmus, and ream the femoral and tibial medullary canals.
- Ream both canals 1 to 2 mm larger than the nail diameter selected; ream the intertrochanteric region to 13 mm.
- Use fluoroscopy to confirm proper nail length.
- Place a marker over the greater trochanter and over the distal tibia where the tip of the nail should be driven and measure the distance with the tibia and femur apposed.
- Remove the guidewires and insert a nail of the appropriate length and diameter. Insert the nail so that the normal anterior bow is internally rotated about 45 degrees; this position provides some flexion and valgus to the limb.
- Carefully drive the nail down the femoral shaft without using excessive force. Watch for signs of impending incarceration or fracture.
- As the tip of the nail exits the femur, reduce the tibia on the femur using the previously placed "marker lines" to determine correct rotational alignment; carefully drive the nail across the knee into the proximal tibia. Sink the nail so that the proximal tip of the nail is flush with the greater trochanter. The distal end of the nail should lie distal to the tibial isthmus and proximal to the ankle joint.
- Compress or fill any defects or gaps in the knee region. If necessary, remove small segments of bone to improve

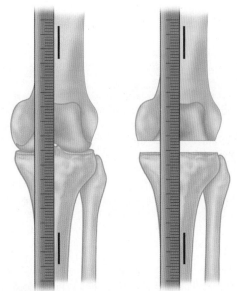

FIGURE 6.5 Knee arthrodesis with intramedullary nail fixation (see text). A long ruler is placed anteriorly over distal femur and proximal tibia, and lines are drawn on bones to be used for determining rotational alignment. **SEE TECHNIQUE 6.3.**

medial and lateral contact. If the knee is not actively infected, use bone grafts to fill any gaps.

■ Insert proximal and distal locking screws as described for subtrochanteric fractures; close the wounds in the usual manner.

POSTOPERATIVE CARE The patient is instructed in hip abduction and flexion exercises and ankle exercises. Touch-down weight bearing is allowed for 4 to 6 weeks; then weight bearing is progressed as tolerated. If significant gaps are noted at the knee at 6 to 12 weeks, the proximal or distal locking screws can be removed to dynamize the nail. Additional bone grafting may be required if significant defects are present. Nail removal is usually unnecessary.

ARTHRODESIS WITH PLATE FIXATION

Arthrodesis using dual-plate fixation was first reported by Lucas and Murray and later by Nichols et al. with good results. Lucas and Murray applied one plate medially and the other anteriorly, whereas Nichols et al. placed the plates medially and laterally to prevent the difficulties with wound closure that are sometimes encountered with an anterior plate. They suggested staggering the plates to reduce the risk of fracture at the plate margin. Compared with external fixation, the advantages of dual-plate fixation are that pin track infection and pin loosening are avoided and earlier weight bearing may be possible. Dual-plate fixation is not recommended in grossly and acutely infected knees, but if the infection seems to be low grade, a positive culture result is not considered an absolute contraindication to the use of the dual-plate method.

The use of a combined intramedullary rod and medial compression plate fixation in eight arthrodeses has been reported previously; all knees fused in that study. This technique is recommended for difficult salvage cases, especially when bone loss may require segmental allografting.

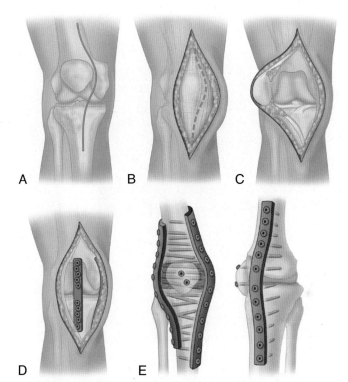

FIGURE 6.6 Lucas and Murray technique of knee arthrodesis. **A,** Skin incision. **B,** Skin and subcutaneous tissue have been reflected, exposing quadriceps tendon, patella, and patellar tendon. **C,** Stripping subperiosteally, flaps have been raised medially and laterally, exposing femur, tibia, knee joint, and deep surface of patella. **D,** Femur and tibia have been fixed by two stainless steel plates, one applied medially and one anteriorly. **E,** Dynamic compression plates placed medially and laterally in staggered fashion. **SEE TECHNIQUE 6.4.**

ARTHRODESIS USING PLATE FIXATION

TECHNIQUE 6.4

■ Make a long medial parapatellar incision extending about 12.5-cm proximal and distal to the joint (Fig. 6.6A).
■ Develop the interval between the quadriceps tendon and the vastus medialis muscle and carry the dissection through the periosteum of the femur (Fig. 6.6B).
■ Incise the periosteum of the tibia; strip subperiosteally and raise flaps of skin, subcutaneous tissue, muscle, periosteum, and joint capsule and retract them to expose the femur, tibia, knee joint, and deep surface of the patella (Fig. 6.6C).
■ Excise the patella and put it aside for use later.
■ Excise the menisci, cruciate ligaments, and any joint debris.
■ Cut the distal femur and proximal tibia with a saw to remove all the articular cartilage. We have found instruments used for total knee arthroplasty useful in making these bone cuts.
■ Place the femur and tibia in the desired position. The bones can be temporarily fixed with a transfixing Steinmann pin.

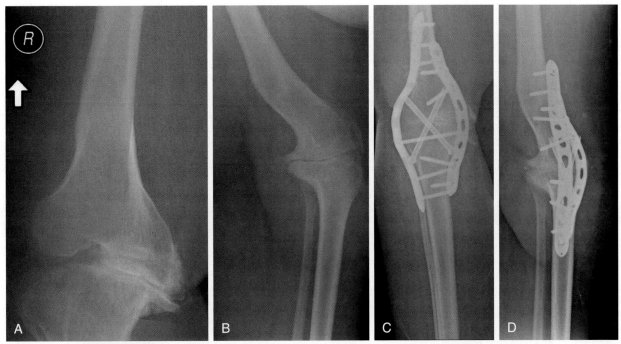

FIGURE 6.7   A 51-year-old patient with arthrogryposis. **A** and **B,** After extension osteotomy with advanced knee arthritis. **C** and **D,** Deformity would not allow for intramedullary nailing, hence plate fixation was performed.

- Use a plate bender to contour two broad, 8- to 12-hole AO plates to fit anteriorly and medially or laterally and medially. Apply the plates and fix them with screws through both cortices using standard AO plates to fit anteriorly and medially (Fig. 6.6D) or laterally and medially (Fig. 6.6E). It may be helpful to use fully threaded cancellous screws in the metaphyseal areas or to consider contourable locking plate/screws if the bone quality seems poor.
- Cut the patella into pieces and pack pieces into any defects around the joint margins or secure them to the arthrodesis site with screws.
- Close the wound in layers and apply a long leg cast.

POSTOPERATIVE CARE Partial weight bearing is begun as tolerated and is progressed over 10 to 12 weeks. The knee immobilizer is worn until fusion is solid. The plates can be removed after the fusion is mature but are typically left in (Fig. 6.7).

Lim et al. suggested an alternative method of arthrodesis, using only cannulated screws. They reported fusion in eight of eight patients; one patient required secondary grafting for delayed union. We have no experience with this method; however, the reduced hardware load may make this method attractive in selected patients.

Finally, although knee fusion effectively relieves pain and provides stability in most patients, the awkwardness in sitting and walking, along with the limited endurance and potential for development of low back pain prompts some patients who had previous arthrodesis to choose revision to total knee arthroplasty. This can be successful even in patients with long-standing fusions; however, reported complication rates have been high (up to 53%). In a comparison of total knee arthroplasty after spontaneous ankylosis and total knee arthroplasty after takedown of surgical arthrodesis, improvements in knee scores (Hospital for Special Knee Surgery) and ambulatory status were similar in both groups; all patients were satisfied with their results. Total knee arthroplasty after knee fusion is further discussed in chapter 5.

REFERENCES

Anderson DR, Anderson LA, Haller JM, Feyissa AC: The SIGN nail for knee fusion: technique and clinical results, *SICOT J* 2(6), 2016.

Balato G, Rizzo M, Ascione T, Smeraglia F, Mariconda M: Re-infection rates and clinical outcomes following arthrodesis with intramedullary nail and external fixator for infected knee prosthesis: a systematic review and meta-analysis, *BMC Musculoskelet Disord* 19(1):361, 2018.

Bruno AA, Kirienko A, Peccati A, et al.: Knee arthrodesis by the Ilizarov method in the treatment of total knee arthroplasty failure, *Knee* 24(1):91, 2017.

Carr 2nd JB, Werner BC, Browne JA: Trends and outcomes in the treatment of failed septic total knee arthroplasty: comparing arthrodesis and above-knee amputation, *J Arthroplasty* 31(7):1574, 2016.

Chen AF, Kinback NC, Heyl AE, et al.: Better function for fusions versus above-the-knee amputations for recurrent periprosthetic knee infection, *Clin Orthop Relat Res* 470:2737, 2012.

De Amesti M, Ortiz-Muñoz, Irarrázaval S: What are the benefits and risks of total arthroplasty in arthrodesed knees? *Medwave* 18(5):37258, 2018.

Friedrich M, Schmolders J, Wimmer MD, et al.: Two-stage knee arthrodesis with a modular intramedullary nail due to septic failure of revision total knee arthroplasty with extensor mechanism deficiency, *Knee* 33(4):1288, 2018.

Gallusser N, Goetti P, Luyet A, Borens O: Knee arthrodesis with modular nail after failed TKA due to infection, *Eur J Orthop Surg Traumatol* 25(8):1307, 2015.

Gathen M, Wimmer MD, Ploeger MM, et al.: Comparison of two-stage revision arthroplasty and intramedullary arthrodesis in patients with failed infected knee arthroplasty, *Arch Orthop Trauma Surg* 138(10):1443, 2018.

Gottfriedsen TB, Schrøder HM, Odgaard A: Knee arthrodesis after failure of knee arthroplasty: a nationwide register-based study, *J Bone Joint Surg Am* 98(16):1370, 2016.

Hawi N, Kendoff D, Citak M, Gehrke T, Haasper C: Septic single-stage knee arthrodesis after failed total knee arthroplasty using a cemented coupled nail, *Bone Joint J* 97-B(5):649, 2015.

Jauregui JJ, Buitrago CA, Pushilin SA, et al.: Conversion of a surgically arthrodesed knee to a total knee arthroplasty – is it worth it? A meta-analysis, *J Arthroplasty* 31(8):1736, 2016.

Kernkamp WA, Verra WC, Pijls BG, et al.: Conversion from knee arthrodesis to arthroplasty: systematic review, *Int Orthop* 40(10):2069, 2016.

Lucas EM, Marais NC, DesJardins JD: Knee arthrodesis: procedures and perspectives in the US from 1993 to 2011, *Springerplus* 5(10):1606, 2016.

Razii N, Abbas AM, Kakar R, Agarwal S, Morgan-Jones R: Knee arthrodesis with a long intramedullary nail as limb salvage for complex periprosthetic infections, *Eur J Orthop Surg Traumatol* 26(8):907, 2016.

Robinson M, Piponov HI, Ormseth A, et al.: Knee arthrodesis outcomes after infected total knee arthroplasty and failure of two-stage revision with an antibiotic cement spacer, *J am Acad Orthop Surg Glob Res Rev* 2(1):e077, 2018.

Röhner E, Windisch C, Neuetzmann K, et al.: Unsatisfactory outcome of arthrodesis performed after septic failure of revision total knee arthroplasty, *J Bone Joint Surg Am* 97(4):298, 2015.

Roy AC, Albert S, Gouse M, Inja DB: Functional outcome of knee arthrodesis with a monorail external fixator, *Strategies Trauma Limb Reconstr* 11(1):31, 2016.

Sambri A, Bianchi G, Parry M, et al.: Is arthrodesis a reliable salvage option following two-stage revision for suspected infection in proximal tibial replacements? A multi-institutional study, *J Knee Surg*, 2018 Sep 18, Epub ahead of print.

Spina M, Gualdrini G, Fosco M, Giunti A: Knee arthrodesis with the Ilizarov external fixator as treatment for septic failure of knee arthroplasty, *J Orthop Trauma* 11:81, 2010.

White CJ, Palmer AJR, Rodriguez-Merchan EC: External fixation vs intramedullary nailing for knee arthrodesis after failed infected total knee arthroplasty: a systematic review and meta-analysis, *J Arthroplasty* 33(4):1288, 2018.

Wilding CP, Cooper GA, Freeman AK, Parry MC, Jeys L: Can a silver-coated arthrodesis implant provide a viable alternative to above-knee amputation in the unsalvageable, infected total knee arthroplasty? *J Arthroplasty* 31(11):2542, 2016.

Wood JH, Conway JD: Advanced concepts in knee arthrodesis, *World J Orthop* 6(2):202, 2015.

The *complete list of references is available online at* Expert Consult.com.

CHAPTER 7

SOFT-TISSUE PROCEDURES AND OSTEOTOMIES ABOUT THE KNEE

Andrew H. Crenshaw Jr.

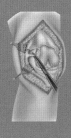

This chapter discusses the surgical treatment of nontraumatic abnormalities involving the bone, muscles, tendons, tendon sheaths, fascia, and bursae of the knee. The cause of these disorders may be degenerative, developmental, related to repetitive use, or a combination of these factors. Many of these disorders are encountered frequently in office practice, but few require surgery. Most respond favorably to treatment such as rest, application of ice or heat, elevation, and local or systemic antiinflammatory medication.

MUSCLE CONTRACTURES

Contractures can develop in almost any muscle group. The cause can be obscure, as in congenital contractures, or obvious, as in infection, ischemia, trauma, or injection myositis. Injection fibrosis most commonly occurs in the quadriceps muscle but also has been described in the gluteal, deltoid, and triceps muscles. Contractures in infants often follow intramuscular antibiotic injections. We have seen several adults with multiple areas of fibrosis and contracture after the addictive intramuscular use of the opioid pentazocine (Talwin). Oral pentazocine now comes compounded with naloxone (Talwin NX), which will cause opioid withdrawal symptoms if the pills are crushed and injected. Chronic intramuscular use of other opioid analgesics also can induce muscular fibrosis and contracture.

QUADRICEPS CONTRACTURE OF INFANCY AND CHILDHOOD

The etiology of quadriceps contracture is divided into congenital and acquired types, and in some cases there is a mixture of both types. The congenital type appears to have a familial component because it can occur in siblings, and it often occurs in patients of central and eastern Asian descent. The acquired type is seen in association with multiple injections or infusions into the thigh soon after birth. The Ad Hoc Committee of the Japanese Orthopaedic Association for Muscular Contractures classified quadriceps contractures into three types (Table 7.1). The exact mechanism causing these contractures is unclear, but suggested causes include compression of the muscle bundles and capillaries by the volume of medication injected and the toxicity of the drug. Whatever the cause, a delay between injection and contracture of several years is common.

The most common symptom is progressive, painless limitation of knee flexion. Hyperextension and subluxation of the knee may occur with continued growth. Normal skin creases over the knee may be absent, and a characteristic dimple may be present over the area of fibrosis, especially when the knee is flexed. Habitual dislocation of the patella is common.

Radiographic changes are not apparent early, but if left untreated, the muscle contracture can cause changes in the soft tissues and in the articular cartilage of the femur and tibia. Progressive displacement and hypoplasia of the patella can occur with long-standing quadriceps contracture. In older children with early onset of symptoms but delayed treatment, flattening of the femoral condyles, genu recurvatum, anterior dislocation of the tibia, and gross degenerative changes in the joint can be seen.

Early recognition and prevention of quadriceps contracture through passive exercise in children receiving intramuscular injections is crucial. When the scar contracture is well established, however, surgical treatment is indicated to prevent late changes in the femoral condyles and the patella. Surgical treatment is indicated early in patients with habitual dislocation of the patella.

TABLE 7.1

Quadriceps Contracture Classification

	KNEE FLEXION	WHEN KNEE IS FORCED TO FLEX IN PRONE POSITION
Rectus femoris type	Restricted with hip extension	Hip is forced to flex
Vastus type	Restricted with hip flexion	Hip remains the same
Mixed type	Slightly restricted with hip extension	Hip is forced to flex

From Santo S, Kokubun S: Report of the diagnosis and treatment of muscular contracture. The Ad Hoc Committee of the Japanese Orthopaedic Association for Muscular Contracture, *J Jpn Orthop Assoc* 59(2):223–253, 1985.

The following may be involved in quadriceps contracture: (1) fibrosis of the vastus intermedius muscle tying down the rectus femoris to the femur in the suprapatellar pouch and proximally, (2) adhesions between the patella and the femoral condyles, (3) fibrosis and shortening of the lateral expansions of the vasti and their adherence to the femoral condyles, and (4) actual shortening of the rectus femoris muscle. To correct the deformity, Thompson devised an operation known as "quadricepsplasty." Its success depends on (1) whether the rectus femoris muscle has escaped injury, (2) how well this muscle can be isolated from the scarred parts of the quadriceps mechanism, and (3) how well the muscle can be developed by active use.

During the early stage of contracture, when no significant joint changes have occurred, proximal release has been recommended to eliminate extensor lag and hemarthrosis of the knee. When more extensive changes are apparent, a Thompson type of quadricepsplasty is indicated. When genu recurvatum has developed, a supracondylar femoral osteotomy can restore some flexion if severe degenerative changes have occurred. Arthrodesis may be indicated if symptoms are severe.

Sasaki et al. found that best results were obtained using a longitudinal skin incision over the rectus muscle through which the fibrotic muscle was released with a transverse incision. After surgery, the leg was positioned with the knee in 90 degrees of flexion and the hip in full extension but a cast was not used. Active exercises were begun at 2 days. Results were found to deteriorate with time, and surgery was recommended at age 6 years or older. An isolated contracture of the rectus femoris can be treated in this manner.

Moderate contractures, before significant bony changes have occurred, are treated best with a proximal release of the quadriceps (Fig. 7.1).

PROXIMAL RELEASE OF QUADRICEPS

TECHNIQUE 7.1

(SENGUPTA)
- Make a curved incision along the base of the greater trochanter and vertically downward along the lateral aspect

of the thigh for a variable distance, depending on the extent of fibrosis (Fig. 7.1A).
- Through the upper part of the incision, section the iliotibial band transversely. Often the iliotibial band is thickened and fibrotic, contributing to the contracture.
- Expose the upper attachment of the vastus lateralis below the greater trochanter (Fig. 7.1B). Detach the origin of the vastus lateralis from the trochanteric line and distally along the lateral intermuscular septum (Fig. 7.1C).
- As the vastus lateralis retracts to expose the vastus intermedius, use a periosteal elevator to release the vastus intermedius from the femoral surface.
- Flex the knee, and release any remaining adhesions.
- If the rectus component also is contracted, expose its origin at the upper part of the incision and detach it, after identifying and retracting the femoral nerve (Fig. 7.1D).
- Full knee flexion should be possible; release of the joint capsule usually is unnecessary in children.
- Close the wound in routine fashion, and apply a posterior splint with the knee in maximal flexion.

POSTOPERATIVE CARE The splint is worn until all tenderness has disappeared, usually 3 to 4 weeks, and then vigorous quadriceps exercises are begun. Extension lag improves rapidly, and the child usually can walk in 4 weeks and stand up from a squatting position in 3 months. Knee stretching exercises should be continued throughout growth to prevent recurrence of the contracture.

QUADRICEPSPLASTY FOR POSTTRAUMATIC CONTRACTURE OF THE KNEE

Hahn et al. achieved 90% good to excellent results in 20 patients with a mean active flexion arc of approximately 115 degrees with this release technique. Liu et al. described successful release of extension knee contracture in 12 patients using a combination of manipulation and percutaneous pie-crusting of the distal and lateral quadriceps with an 18-gauge needle with the knee in flexion. An average of 70 degrees of increased flexion was achieved at 8 months. There was a positive correlation between the number of punctures and knee flexion achieved. Birjandinejad et al. achieved good to excellent results in 87% of 64 patients at a mean of 36 months. Preoperative range of motion, number of previous surgeries, duration of extension contracture, and body mass index influenced the final flexion achieved.

TECHNIQUE 7.2

(MODIFIED THOMPSON QUADRICEPSPLASTY AS DESCRIBED BY HAHN ET AL.)
- Perform the procedure using a tourniquet.
- Make medial and lateral parapatellar incisions for arthrolysis (Fig. 7.2A).
- Flex the knee, and if adequate flexion is not obtained, make an anterolateral or lateral incision in the distal two

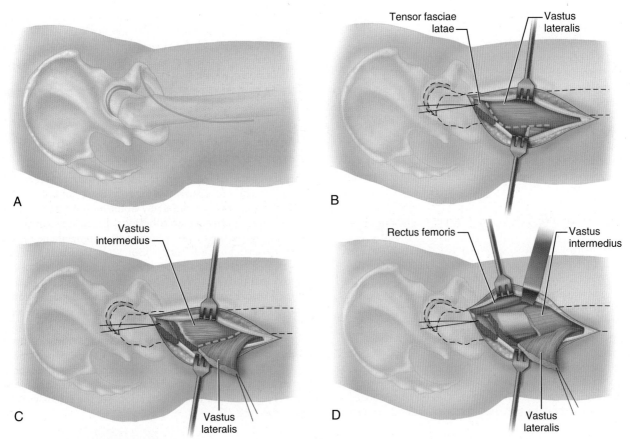

FIGURE 7.1 Sengupta proximal release of quadriceps (see text). **A,** Incision. **B,** Iliotibial band and tensor fasciae latae are cut to expose vastus lateralis, which is released along its origin. **C,** Vastus origin is detached from trochanteric line and distally along lateral intermuscular septum. **D,** If necessary, rectus femoris is released. **SEE TECHNIQUE 7.1.**

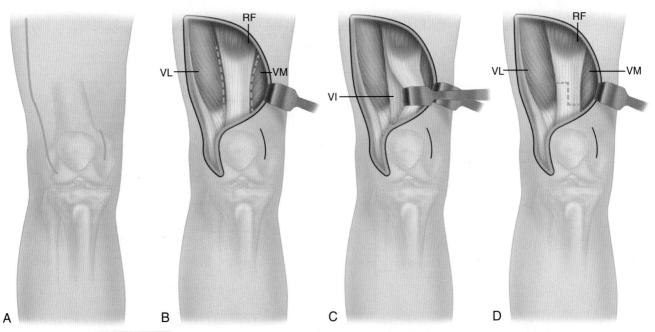

FIGURE 7.2 Modified Thompson quadricepsplasty. **A,** Parapatellar and anterolateral incisions. **B,** Release of rectus femoris *(RF)* from vastus lateralis *(VL)* and vastus medialis *(VM)* close to its patellar insertion. **C,** Vastus intermedius *(VI)* and scar adhesions dissected and released from rectus femoris, the anterior surface of the femur, and the upper pole of the patella. **D,** *RF* lengthened by Z-plasty if necessary. (From Hahn SB, Lee WS, Han DY: A modified Thompson quadricepsplasty for the stiff knee, *J Bone Joint Surg* 82B:992, 2000. Copyright British Editorial Society of Bone and Joint Surgery.) **SEE TECHNIQUE 7.2.**

thirds of the thigh and release adhesions around the quadriceps muscle.

- Divide the tensor fascia lata transversely in the distal thigh. Isolate the vastus lateralis from the rectus femoris, and release it close to its patellar insertion. Release the vastus medialis from the rectus femoris by blunt dissection (Fig. 7.2B).
- Free the rectus femoris from the vastus intermedius, the anterior surface of the femur, and the upper pole of the patella (Fig. 7.2C).
- Perform a Z-plasty lengthening of the rectus femoris tendon if satisfactory flexion has not been achieved (Fig. 7.2D).

POSTOPERATIVE CARE The extremity is immobilized in a splint in about 50 degrees less than the maximal flexion obtained during surgery; this is maintained for 2 to 3 days. The extremity is then placed in a continuous passive motion machine, range of motion is begun, and the patient remains hospitalized until 90 degrees of passive flexion is achieved. Passive and active exercises for the quadriceps and hamstrings continue and are crucial to the success of this procedure. The knee is kept in full extension during the night and is exercised during the day with active and active-assisted exercises. If 90 degrees of flexion is not obtained after 3 months, gentle manipulation with the patient under anesthesia may be required. The patient should expect slow return of active quadriceps

extension. Most patients can expect improvement in range of motion of the knee after quadricepsplasty but should expect severe quadriceps weakness for many months. If the patient is not skeletally mature, some of the improvement in flexion may be lost as growth occurs.

FLEXION, EXTENSION, AND COMBINED CONTRACTURES

Posttraumatic stiffness can be caused by intraarticular adhesions, fibrosis of the surrounding soft tissues, or both. Flexion contractures can be caused by anterior bony impingement or posterior periarticular adhesions. Extension contractures can be the result of posterior bony impingement or anterior periarticular adhesions. Bony impingements need to be treated first followed by soft-tissue releases. Pujol et al. stated that the exact cause(s) of contracture should be determined before surgery. Any complex regional pain syndrome should be controlled and surgery delayed if the patient is in the active phase. Associated fractures must be healed. A thorough workup is necessary and may include a computed tomography (CT) arthrogram, magnetic resonance imaging (MRI), bone scan, and plain radiographs. A combination of open and arthroscopic procedures may be necessary for success (Fig. 7.3). For more information, see the extensive review by Pujol et al.

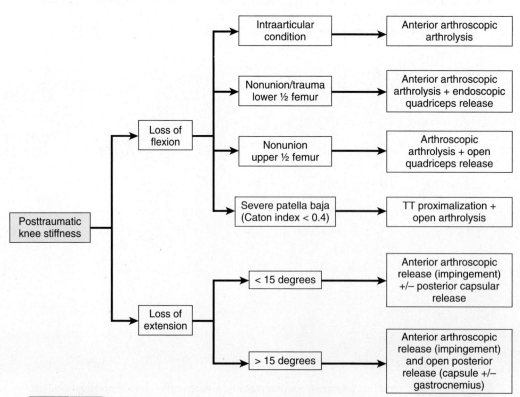

FIGURE 7.3   Algorithm used by the Versailles (France) Orthopedic and Trauma Surgery Department for posttraumatic knee stiffness without osteoarthritis or intraarticular malunion. (From Pujol N, Boisrenoult P, Beaufils P: Post-traumatic knee stiffness: surgical techniques, *Orthop Traumatol Surg Res* 101:S179, 2015.)

SNAPPING SYNDROMES

It is common for a patient to hear or feel snapping or popping of joints. Disability or pain sufficient to justify surgery for this is rare. Most patients respond favorably to reassurance and avoidance of the specific activity that produces the snapping sensation.

Snapping symptoms are rare in the knee. True snapping of the knee is extraarticular. Intraarticular catching or locking in the knee usually is caused by meniscal tears, meniscal cysts, loose bodies, patellofemoral disorders, or arthritic joint changes.

Snapping of the knee can occur in patients with an abnormal anterior insertion of the biceps femoris tendon on the fibular head. This can be treated by reinsertion of the tendon (Fig. 7.4) or resection of the fibular head with reattachment of the tendon if conservative treatment fails. Biceps femoris snapping caused by a fibular exostosis has been reported, as well as snapping from a direct injury to the tendon. Snapping caused by direct injury can be treated by rerouting the tendon insertion through a tunnel in the fibular head.

The popliteus tendon can cause snapping of the knee, which usually is palpable midway between the lateral epicondyle and lateral joint line. If conservative treatment fails, a popliteus release or tenodesis of the popliteus tendon to the fibular collateral ligament can be done.

Knee snapping also can be caused by abnormal insertion of the semitendinosus tendon, causing it to snap over a prominence on the medial tibial condyle. This can be treated by dividing the semitendinosus tendon at its insertion and transferring it to the semimembranosus tendon. A hamstring tendon sliding over an osteochondroma of the femur likewise can cause snapping, and excision of this generally benign lesion is indicated if it is severe. Shapiro et al. recommend using dynamic ultrasonography to diagnose the cause of mechanical snapping.

PAINFUL PARAARTICULAR CALCIFICATIONS

Painful paraarticular calcifications similar to those found within the rotator cuff of the shoulder also develop around the knee. These calcific deposits may be located within a tendon or the soft tissues adjacent to a tendon or ligament near its attachment to bone (Fig. 7.5). The calcification most probably is located in an area of focal necrosis or degeneration.

Although most paraarticular calcifications occur without direct trauma, calcification within tendons or ligaments may be a response to degenerative changes within the structures as a result of chronic use or subclinical injury.

The presence of calcification in the tibial collateral ligament, as in Pellegrini-Stieda disease, usually is more directly related to trauma, such as a sprain or tear of the tibial collateral ligament. The treatment is the same as that for a calcification around the shoulder.

Spontaneous recovery may occur without treatment, and the deposit may partially or completely disappear in time. Infiltration with a local anesthetic agent, supplemented, if desired, by injection of 40 mg of methylprednisolone (Depo-Medrol) or its equivalent, produces immediate relief and can be curative. Ultrasound and extracorporeal shock wave therapy also have been reported to be of benefit. The calcific deposit should be excised if response to nonoperative measures is unsatisfactory.

TENDINITIS AND BURSITIS

In the evaluation of patients with tendinitis of the lower extremity, a careful history of work conditions and exercise routines is necessary. Overuse (repetitive activity) or overload (sudden increase in activity) often accentuates tendinitis. Tendinitis from these causes usually responds to relative rest,

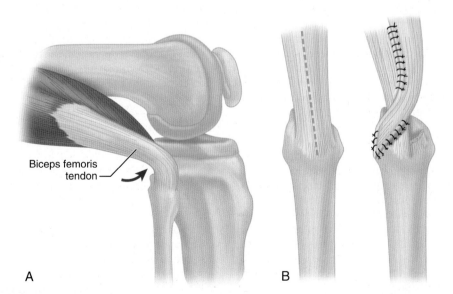

Biceps femoris tendon

A   B

FIGURE 7.4 **A,** Snapping mechanism of biceps femoris tendon over hump of fibular head *(arrow)* on flexion-extension. **B,** Anterior half of tendon is divided and sutured back over posterolateral part of fibular head covering hump. (Technique by Lokiec F, Velkes S, Schindler A, et al: The snapping biceps femoris syndrome, *Clin Orthop Relat Res* 283:205, 1992.) **SEE TECHNIQUE 7.2.**

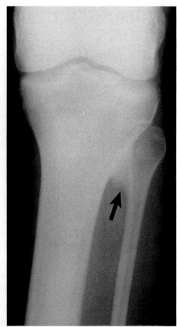

FIGURE 7.5 Calcification of proximal tibiofibular articulation resulting in peroneal nerve entrapment *(arrow)* in professional basketball player.

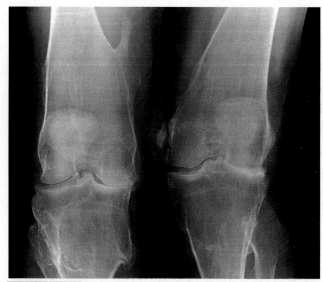

FIGURE 7.6 Multiple osteochondromas as seen in Ollier disease.

ice, the use of a Neoprene sleeve, antiinflammatory medications, and alterations in work or exercise habits. Mechanical abnormalities, leg-length inequality, and leg malalignment may respond to the use of a properly fitted shoe orthosis. Muscle imbalance should be treated with appropriate flexibility and strengthening exercise programs.

Bursae are sacs lined with a membrane similar to synovium; they usually are located around joints or where skin, tendon, or muscle moves over a bony prominence, and they may or may not communicate with a joint. Their function is to reduce friction and to protect delicate structures from pressure. Bursae are similar to tendon sheaths and the synovial membranes of joints and are subject to the same disturbances: (1) acute or chronic trauma; (2) acute or chronic pyogenic infection; and (3) low-grade inflammatory conditions such as gout, syphilis, tuberculosis, or rheumatoid arthritis. There are more than 140 bursae in the human body; bursae consist of two types: those normally present (e.g., over the patella and olecranon) and adventitious ones (e.g., develop over a bunion, an osteochondroma, or kyphosis of the spine). Adventitious bursae are produced by repeated trauma or constant friction or pressure.

Treatment is determined primarily by the cause of the bursitis and only secondarily by the pathologic change in the bursa. Surgery is not required in most instances. Systemic causes, such as gout or syphilis, and local trauma or irritants should be eliminated, and, when necessary, the patient's occupation or posture should be changed. One or more of the following local measures usually are helpful: rest, moist heat, elevation, protective padding, and, if necessary, immobilization of the affected part. Surgical procedures useful in treating bursitis are (1) aspiration and injection of an appropriate steroid preparation or antibiotic, (2) incision and drainage when an acute suppurative bursitis fails to respond to nonsurgical treatment, (3) excision of chronically infected and thickened bursae, and (4) removal of an underlying bony prominence.

The usual principles of treating general infections are employed in treating infected bursae. The responsible organisms should be identified if feasible, and the infection should be treated with appropriate systemic antibiotics. Aspiration of the bursa and injection of the appropriate antibiotic may be indicated in addition to the supportive measures just described; a compression dressing should be applied after aspiration. Surgical drainage occasionally is necessary.

Traumatic bursitis often responds favorably to nonoperative treatment, consisting of ice, rest, antiinflammatory medication, and protection with external padding. Occasionally, aspiration and injection of an appropriate steroid preparation are required if symptoms do not respond to the usual nonoperative treatment.

Adventitious bursae that develop as a result of repeated trauma usually have a much thicker fibrous wall than do normal bursae and are more susceptible to inflammatory changes. This type of bursa is treated by removing the cause (e.g., excising an osteochondroma of the distal femur; Fig. 7.6); at the time of operation, the bursal sac usually is excised. Only bursae that most often require surgical drainage or excision are described.

PREPATELLAR BURSITIS

Traumatic prepatellar bursitis (Fig. 7.7) can be caused by an acute injury, such as a fall directly onto the patella, or by recurrent minor injuries, such as those that produce "housemaid's knee." Either type usually responds to conservative treatment. If fibrosis or synovial thickening with painful nodules fails to respond to such treatment, however, excision of the bursa is indicated.

Pyogenic prepatellar bursitis is common, especially in children. If the bursa is unusually large, the swelling may be so pronounced that a diagnosis of pyogenic arthritis of the knee joint can be made by mistake. A careful physical examination should lead to the correct diagnosis. This septic prepatellar bursitis often responds to one or two daily aspirations, appropriate immobilization, and antibiotic coverage. If symptoms have not improved significantly in 36 to 48 hours, incision and drainage should be done. Smason reported a patient

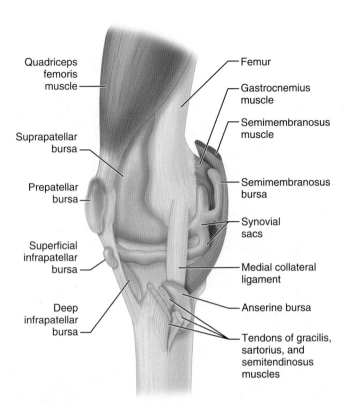

Quadriceps
femoris
muscle

Suprapatellar
bursa

Prepatellar
bursa

Superficial
infrapatellar
bursa

Deep
infrapatellar
bursa

Femur

Gastrocnemius
muscle

Semimembranosus
muscle

Semimembranosus
bursa

Synovial
sacs

Medial collateral
ligament

Anserine bursa

Tendons of gracilis,
sartorius, and
semitendinosus
muscles

FIGURE 7.7   Multiple bursae around knee that may become acutely or chronically inflamed.

in whom a posttraumatic fistula connected the prepatellar bursa with the knee joint. This could present a problem in diagnosis and treatment, especially in a pyogenic bursitis. The bursa is easily drained as follows.

DRAINAGE OF BURSA

TECHNIQUE 7.3

- Approach the bursa through two longitudinal incisions, one medial and one lateral, or through a single transverse incision.
- Open the bursa, evacuate its contents, and pack it loosely with petrolatum gauze, or close it loosely over a drain as seems appropriate.

POSTOPERATIVE CARE Because cellulitis is always present, the extremity is immobilized in a posterior splint, and appropriate antibiotics are given. If gauze has been used to pack the bursa, it is changed at least twice weekly. Despite sufficient drainage, sinuses often persist for a time on one or both sides of the knee. Immobilization is continued until the sinus has closed.

EXCISION OF BURSA

The patient should be informed when first seen that complete excision of the bursa may be necessary if healing fails

to occur after simple drainage. If the walls of the bursa are thickened from chronic inflammation, resecting the entire bursa usually is easy, but if the lesion is acute and the effusion is serous, excising the bursa completely may be impossible; however, enough can be excised to relieve symptoms.

TECHNIQUE 7.4

- Make a transverse incision of appropriate length centered over the bursa.
- Dissect the bursal sac from the overlying skin and subcutaneous tissue and from the patellar aponeurosis beneath it.
- If possible, excise the bursa without rupturing or perforating it.
- Trim away the redundant skin, obtain complete hemostasis, and close the wound primarily.
- Because the most common complication after excising a superficial bursa is a large hematoma, obliteration of the dead space by inserting one or more mattress sutures through the skin and deeper tissues on each side of the incision is recommended. After the skin edges have been apposed with interrupted sutures, the mattress sutures are tied over large buttons.

POSTOPERATIVE CARE A moderately large compression dressing is applied, and the extremity is immobilized from groin to ankle for at least 2 weeks until the wound has healed completely. Alternatively, suction drainage can be used to obliterate the dead space. Quadriceps-setting exercises are begun the day after surgery. Antibiotics are indicated if an infection is present or is possible.

Dillon et al. reported excellent results with no complications in eight patients who had endoscopic excision of septic prepatellar bursae. Huang and Yeh described endoscopic excision of posttraumatic prepatellar bursae in 60 patients in whom conservative treatment failed. The procedures were done through two or three small portals. There were no recurrences.

TIBIAL COLLATERAL LIGAMENT FIBROSITIS AND BURSITIS

Voshell and Brantigan observed bursae between the longitudinal part of the tibial collateral ligament and the capsule of the knee (Fig. 7.8); these bursae can be located in five different positions, and three have been found beneath the ligament in a single knee. These authors also reported instances of calcification in one or more of these bursae and suggested that this may be identical to Pellegrini-Stieda disease. We consider most disorders that cause pain and tenderness beneath the tibial collateral ligament (not directly opposite the knee joint) to be fibrositis of the ligament; most have responded favorably to the injection of an appropriate steroid preparation and to other nonoperative measures.

Tibial collateral ligament bursitis should be included in the differential diagnoses in patients with medial joint line pain and no history of mechanical symptoms of instability or laxity. Tenderness usually is localized to just below the joint line. This can be treated with local steroid injection followed by early exercise. If symptoms do not respond to one or two injections, MRI or arthroscopy should be considered

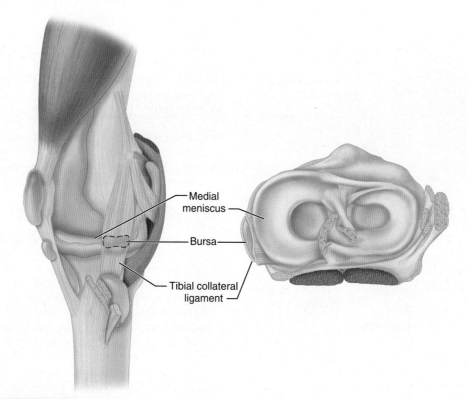

FIGURE 7.8 Voshell bursa located just below the joint line between the tibial collateral ligament and the joint capsule. (Described by Voshell and Brantigan.)

for evaluation of possible intraarticular derangement or stress fracture of the medial tibial plateau. Tibial collateral ligament bursitis has a characteristic MRI appearance of fluid deep to the tibial collateral ligament in the shape of an inverted "U." We have seen several patients who were unresponsive to one or two local steroid injections and had stress fractures visible only by MRI or bone scan.

FIBULAR COLLATERAL LIGAMENT BURSITIS

Bursitis beneath the fibular collateral ligament causes localized, tender swelling on the lateral side of the knee and often is confused with a cyst of the lateral meniscus. The distended bursa varies from 0.6 to 2.5 cm or more in diameter, is extrasynovial, and lies beneath or just anterior or posterior to the fibular collateral ligament. Varus strain of the knee is painful, but typical signs and symptoms of an internal derangement of the knee are absent. Other lesions that should be considered include biceps tendinitis, partial biceps avulsion with pain and popping at 30 to 45 degrees of flexion, and posterolateral popping caused by a previous injury to the posterolateral corner or by a bony tubercle that causes popping of the popliteus tendon.

If a mass is not evident, injections of a local anesthetic agent or a steroid preparation into the area of tenderness, together with support and rest, usually relieve the symptoms. When a mass is palpable, excision is curative.

INFRAPATELLAR BURSITIS

A small, deep, subpatellar or infrapatellar bursa is located between the tuberosity of the tibia and the patellar tendon and is separated from the synovium of the knee by a pad of fat. When distended, this bursa causes a fluctuant swelling that obliterates the depression on each side of the ligament.

Infrapatellar bursal infection should be considered when symptoms resemble septic arthritis or osteomyelitis of the proximal tibia, such as loss of full extension of the knee, resistance to full flexion, and maximal tenderness near the patellar ligament. The infrapatellar bursa should be aspirated, taking care not to enter the knee joint. If infection is found, immediate drainage is recommended in addition to evaluation of the proximal tibial metaphysis for evidence of osteomyelitis. A sterile effusion of the knee joint, which may accompany an infrapatellar bursitis, should not be confused with infection. The bursa can be drained through a small medial parapatellar incision without entering the knee joint. A knee immobilizer is used after surgery until acute symptoms have resolved, and then range-of-motion exercises are begun.

POPLITEAL CYST (BAKER CYST)

A Baker cyst, described by Baker in 1877, has since borne his name even though it had been described previously by Adams in 1840. In most instances, a Baker, or popliteal, cyst is a distended bursa. Numerous bursae are located in the popliteal space between the hamstring tendons and the collateral ligaments or condyles of the tibia; a bursa also is located deep to each head of the gastrocnemius muscle. Symptoms develop most often in the bursa beneath the medial head of the gastrocnemius or in the semimembranosus bursa; the latter is a double bursa located between the semimembranosus tendon and the medial tibial condyle and between the semimembranosus tendon and the medial head of the gastrocnemius.

A popliteal cyst can be produced by herniation of the synovial membrane through the posterior part of the capsule of the knee or by the escape of fluid through the normal communication of a bursa with the knee, that is, the semimembranosus or the medial gastrocnemius bursa. Kim et al. described the arthroscopic anatomy of the posteromedial capsule and found an association between the presence of capsular folds and holes in the capsule and the incidence of popliteal cysts in 194 knees treated arthroscopically for a variety of knee problems.

Diagnosing a popliteal cyst usually is not difficult. One third to one half of patients with these cysts are children. The cyst must be distinguished from a lipoma, xanthoma, vascular tumor, fibrosarcoma, and other tumors; occasionally, the cyst may be confused with an aneurysm. A pyogenic abscess may sometimes be located in the popliteal space, but this can be diagnosed easily. Usually, the diagnosis can be made by transilluminating the cyst. Other diagnostic techniques, such as arthrography, MRI, and ultrasound, can be helpful in establishing the diagnosis. MRI is the preferred modality because it also can show intraarticular pathology. In children, the cyst infrequently communicates with the joint, and intraarticular pathologic findings are rare. Rarely, a popliteal cyst can dissect down into the calf in an intramuscular path. Fang et al. reported three cases involving the medial head of the gastrocnemius. These were confirmed with MRI. It was hypothesized that the dissection took the path of least resistance through a weakness in the medial gastrocnemius fascia.

Giant synovial cysts of the calf often are associated with rheumatoid arthritis. They arise from and communicate with the knee in the popliteal area, as can be shown by arthrography or MRI. If a popliteal cyst is suspected, arthrography or MRI of the knee or ultrasound examination of the calf is done, and the popliteal cyst is excised. In patients with rheumatoid arthritis who have a giant synovial cyst removed, a synovectomy should be performed later to prevent recurrence of the cyst. Development of acute compartment syndrome as a result of a ruptured Baker cyst and spontaneous venous bleeding have been reported. We have seen several patients on strong anticoagulants bleed into popliteal cysts, leading to dissection into the calf. Popliteal vein thrombosis can occur, and a dissecting popliteal cyst can occur concurrently. Venous thrombosis should be excluded as part of the evaluation of suspected pseudothrombophlebitis caused by a dissecting or ruptured popliteal cyst.

The results of simple excision usually are excellent even if incomplete. In our experience with a large series of children, these cysts generally resolve with benign neglect. Occasionally, aspiration may be attempted, provided that the diagnosis is certain. In adults, intraarticular pathologic findings are common, and the cyst can recur if the intraarticular pathologic condition is not corrected. Most involve the posterior horn of the medial meniscus. Saylik and Gökkus reported 103 knees treated with posterior open cystectomy with valve and posterior capsule repair and arthroscopic treatment of intraarticular lesions. Cyst recurrence was seen in fewer than 2% of patients. Ko and Ahn recommended removal of the capsular fold of the valvular mechanism of the popliteal cyst with a motorized shaver arthroscopically. Takahashi and Nagano reported success using posterior portals to arthroscopically resect the popliteal cyst origin. Yang et al. found significantly better outcomes in patients treated with arthroscopic cystectomy compared with patients who underwent arthroscopy followed by open cystectomy or those who had open cystectomy alone. The open cystectomy alone group had a 40% recurrence rate.

Careful arthroscopic evaluation should be performed before excision of a popliteal cyst. Intraarticular pathologic conditions, such as patellofemoral chondromalacia or a degenerative tear of the posterior horn of the medial meniscus, can be identified and treated by debridement of loose cartilaginous fragments or partial meniscectomy. Significant intraarticular pathologic conditions are present in more than 50% of adults with popliteal cysts. Kp et al. recommended careful study of prearthroscopic cystectomy MR images because these cysts can be predictive of potential popliteal artery injury. When the popliteal artery is close to the cyst, the lateral wall of the cyst should not be removed. Zhou et al. performed a systematic review and meta-analysis of the surgical treatment of popliteal cysts. They concluded that arthroscopic excision of the cyst wall, enlarging the communication between the articular cavity and the cyst, and arthroscopic management of intraarticular lesions produce the best results.

Froelich and Hillard-Sembell demonstrated that loose bodies can intermittently travel between the intraarticular space and an extraarticular popliteal cyst. If a known posteromedial loose body cannot be found, a capsular opening into the cyst should be sought. The loose body can then be removed through an accessory posteromedial portal.

If the cyst does not appear to communicate with the joint or if significant changes cannot be treated arthroscopically, an open procedure is indicated. Most cysts can be approached by a posteromedial (Henderson) incision. Very large or midline lesions can be approached through a posterior incision.

POPLITEAL CYST EXCISION

For a popliteal cyst that requires excision, Hughston et al. described a posteromedial approach made through a medial hockey-stick incision. The procedure can be performed with the patient supine. If an arthroscopic evaluation is part of the procedure, the leg does not have to be rescrubbed or redraped and the patient does not need to be turned prone for open excision of the cyst.

TECHNIQUE 7.5

(HUGHSTON, BAKER, AND MELLO)

- With the patient supine, externally rotate the hip fully and flex the knee to 90 degrees. Make a medial hockey-stick incision at the joint line (Fig. 7.9A).
- Use only the posteromedial portion of the incision if an arthroscopic examination already has been performed. Otherwise, inspect the joint through an anteromedial retinacular incision (Fig. 7.9B).
- Make a posteromedial capsular incision beginning between the medial epicondyle and adductor tubercle along the posterior border of the tibial collateral ligament (Fig. 7.9B).
- Retract the posterior oblique ligament posteriorly and inspect the posteromedial compartment. Identify the popliteal cyst; it is usually in the area between the medial head of the gastrocnemius and semimembranosus tendon (Fig. 7.9B).
- Inspect the posteromedial joint and cyst lining for an intraarticular communication (Fig. 7.9C).
- Separate the adherent cyst lining from the surrounding soft tissues, and trace it to the posterior capsule.

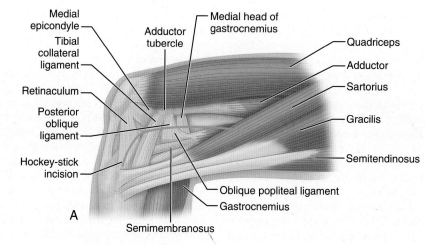

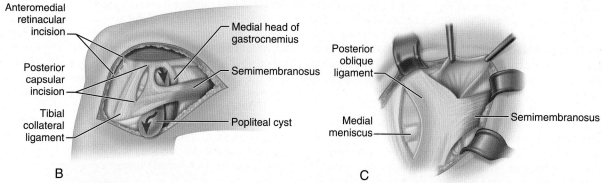

FIGURE 7.9 Posteromedial approach for excision of a popliteal (Baker) cyst. **A,** Skin incision at the level of the joint line with knee flexed to 90 degrees. **B,** Skin and subcutaneous tissue retracted. **C,** Cyst opened and retracted before excision. **SEE TECHNIQUE 7.5.**

- Excise the cyst at the base of its stalk on the capsule.
- Close the orifice if possible with one or two nonabsorbable sutures.
- At closure, the posterior oblique ligament may be lax because of pressure from the cyst beneath it. If it is lax, advance it onto the medial epicondyle and tibial collateral ligament to restore tension to the posteromedial capsular ligaments and semimembranosus capsular aponeurosis. Close the wound in layers.

POSTOPERATIVE CARE The limb is placed in a knee immobilizer, and weight bearing to tolerance is allowed. Straight leg raising and quadriceps-setting exercises are begun on the first day after surgery. The immobilizer is discontinued, and active range-of-motion exercises are begun when acute inflammation has resolved. Mild prophylactic anticoagulation is recommended for 6 weeks. If the patient develops a synovial fistula, reapply the knee immobilizer until the fistula closes.

MEDIAL GASTROCNEMIUS BURSITIS

If the medial gastrocnemius bursa is involved, a palpable mass is located in the midline of the popliteal space or extends beneath the head of the gastrocnemius and manifests between the medial head of the muscle and the semimembranosus tendon, simulating an enlarged semimembranosus bursa. In the latter instance, the bursa is excised through a posteromedial incision after arthroscopy with the patient supine, as described for semimembranosus bursitis; when in the midline of the popliteal space, it is excised as follows.

MEDIAL GASTROCNEMIUS BURSA EXCISION

TECHNIQUE 7.6

(MEYERDING AND VAN DEMARK)
- With the patient prone, make an oblique incision directly over the mass (Fig. 7.10A).
- Divide the deep fascia, expose the protruding sac, and by blunt dissection free it down to its attachment to the posterior aspect of the capsule of the knee. In some instances, relaxing the muscles and tendons on each side of the cyst by flexing the knee increases the exposure.
- Clamp the pedicle of the cyst at its attachment to the capsule of the joint and divide it, but leave enough pedicle to permit its inversion (Fig. 7.10B).
- Invert the pedicle and close it; Meyerding and Van Demark recommended permanent sutures for this closure.

POSTOPERATIVE CARE The postoperative care is the same as for Technique 7.5.

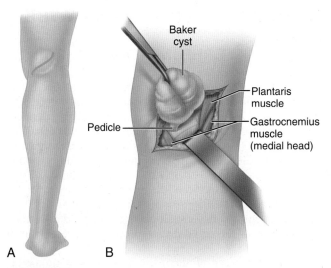

FIGURE 7.10 Meyerding and Van Demark removal of midline Baker cyst. **A,** Skin incision. **B,** After being exposed, pedicle is clamped, ligated, divided, and inverted. **SEE TECHNIQUE 7.6.**

SEMIMEMBRANOSUS BURSITIS

A distended semimembranosus bursa occurs on the medial side of the popliteal space on the medial or more usually the lateral side of the semimembranosus tendon. The bursa can be approached easily through a posteromedial incision with the patient supine or through a posterior incision as described.

SEMIMEMBRANOSUS BURSA EXCISION

TECHNIQUE 7.7

- With the patient supine, make a slightly oblique or curved longitudinal incision 7.5 cm long over the medial aspect of the popliteal space; a common error is to place this incision too far proximally. Incise the deep fascia; the proper plane for dissection is then usually evident.
- Develop the interval between the semimembranosus and the medial head of the gastrocnemius, and separate the cyst wall from these structures. No important nerves or vessels lie in this plane of cleavage.
- Continue the dissection; it becomes increasingly difficult to separate the cyst from adjacent structures. In the depths of the wound, the wall usually is adherent and requires sharp dissection that should include some of the fibrous parts of the semimembranosus or of the gastrocnemius; otherwise, the cyst is ruptured, making it difficult to outline and to determine whether it has a pedicle or communicates with the joint.
- Often the base of the cyst is intimately attached to the capsule and synovium. A small opening may be located, if desired, by injecting air or a physiologic saline solution containing a little methylene blue through the posterior part of the capsule into the joint, but closing any opening in the joint capsule probably is unnecessary.

- The technique for excising cysts on the medial side of the semimembranosus tendon is performed in a similar manner.

POSTOPERATIVE CARE Postoperative care is the same as for Technique 7.5.

SEMIMEMBRANOSUS TENDINITIS

Semimembranosus tendinitis can be diagnosed by eliciting point tenderness over the posteromedial corner of the knee just distal to the joint line. The tendon usually is easily palpated. A provocative test of resisted internal tibial rotation of a knee flexed at 90 degrees also may pinpoint the pain. A negative McMurray test in the absence of tenderness over the joint line can help rule out a torn meniscus or osteonecrosis of the tibial plateau. Ray et al. divided their 115 patients into two groups: patients with primary isolated semimembranosus tendinitis and patients with secondary tendinitis with an associated intraarticular abnormality. The group with primary tendinitis generally included younger, athletic patients with overuse injuries incurred during running or a triathlon. Secondary tendinitis was related to degenerative medial meniscal tears, degenerative changes of the medial compartment, or chondromalacia of the patella resulting in gait alterations and overuse of the tendon. Semimembranosus tendinitis generally responds to conservative therapy. If conservative treatment fails, bone scanning or MRI can be helpful to confirm the diagnosis. Occasionally, a semitendinosus tendon transfer may be necessary and is the treatment of choice. For secondary tendinitis, Ray et al. recommended evaluation and treatment of the intraarticular disorder at the time of treatment of the semimembranosus tendinitis.

SEMITENDINOSUS TENDON TRANSFER

TECHNIQUE 7.8

(RAY, CLANCY, AND LEMON)
- Make a 10-cm longitudinal posteromedial incision over the direct head insertion of the semimembranosus tendon, and free the tendon from surrounding tissue proximally and distally.
- Open the tendon sheath, and make a longitudinal incision in the tendon.
- Excise any necrotic areas. If there is no obvious necrosis, make several longitudinal incisions in the tendon to stimulate a healing reaction.
- Drill the insertion site with a small Kirschner wire.
- Pull the direct head and proximal portion of the tendon upward and parallel to the posterior edge of the tibial collateral ligament, and suture it here to redirect the tendon.

POSTOPERATIVE CARE Postoperative care is the same as for Technique 7.5.

CHRONIC SYNOVITIS

Chronic synovitis is a persistent, nonspecific, proliferative lesion of the synovium, usually monarticular, with little or no involvement of bone or cartilage and without clear evidence of any other primary pathologic process. Although joint cultures are negative, the process may seem to be related to an infection elsewhere. During World War II it was found that chronic synovitis of one or both knees often developed 3 weeks after an acute gonorrheal urethritis. Although the urethritis had already subsided after treatment with penicillin, the synovitis of the knee was believed to be of gonococcal origin. The synovitis was subacute or chronic, however, and organisms were not found in joint aspirates. Chronic synovitis also occurred after acute purulent lesions of joints had subsided with treatment with penicillin; in these cases, effusion and thickening of the synovial membrane persisted for weeks after cultures of the fluid became negative. Chronic synovitis also has been found to occur years after a traumatic injury to the joint after the joint had seemed to recover completely with no evidence of arthritis. We also have seen chronic synovitis in joints adjacent to bone infarcts where the joint space was maintained and evidence of arthritis was absent.

Because monarticular synovitis can mimic gout and pseudogout, joint fluid should be sent for evaluation for crystals to rule out these pathologic processes. Cytology also can be obtained to rule out pigmented villonodular synovitis. MRI can show areas of bone infarct not visible on plain radiographs. Lyme serologic testing also should be performed.

The initial treatment of chronic synovitis is conservative. If conservative treatment fails, synovial biopsy may be indicated. This can be performed using a standard arthroscopic technique in which the joint can be visually inspected and specific biopsy sites can be chosen. In addition, arthroscopic examination may reveal hypertrophy and hyperplasia of the synovial layer of the cells, thickening of the subsynovial layers by dermatofibrosis, and engorgement of blood vessels. These findings are nonspecific, but the more characteristic features of rheumatoid arthritis, osteoarthritis, and Charcot joints are not found. A persistent swelling of the joint with fluctuation but without edema of the surrounding soft tissues is characteristic of chronic synovitis.

SYNOVECTOMY OF THE KNEE

Although synovectomy in rheumatoid arthritis, chronic synovitis, or other arthritides (e.g., psoriatic arthritis) may temporarily decrease the pain, increase in motion is doubtful, and some loss of motion may occur. Arthroscopic synovectomy has been used successfully in adult and pediatric patients with rheumatoid arthritis, sarcoid synovitis, and hemophilic arthropathy. The advantages of arthroscopic synovectomy over open synovectomy include decreased postoperative pain and early joint mobility. Arthroscopic synovectomy is a demanding procedure, however, and should be performed by experienced arthroscopists.

In a comparative study of open and arthroscopic synovectomy, both techniques were found to be successful; however, patients who had arthroscopic synovectomy had less scarring, less pain, and faster recovery than patients who had open synovectomy.

RHEUMATOID ARTHRITIS OF THE KNEE

ADULT-ONSET RHEUMATOID ARTHRITIS

Rheumatoid arthritis is a chronic, systemic, inflammatory disease, most often involving the small joints of the hands and feet, although any synovial joint can be affected. It affects 1% to 2% of the world population, with a female-to-male ratio of 2.5:1. Adult rheumatoid arthritis usually is polyarticular; systemic involvement in the visceral organs or eyes is rare. The test for rheumatoid factor in adults is positive in 70% to 80% of patients in whom rheumatoid arthritis is diagnosed. The American Rheumatism Association developed criteria for the diagnosis of rheumatoid arthritis (Table 7.2). A patient is considered to have rheumatoid arthritis if at least four of the seven criteria have been present for at least 6 weeks.

The exact cause of rheumatoid arthritis is unknown. Knowledge of the nature and pathogenesis of the disease has increased in more recent years, however, and medical and surgical management of the disease has improved. The goal of medical and surgical management of patients with rheumatoid arthritis is to maintain or improve functional capacity.

The clinical picture of rheumatoid arthritis is characterized by synovitis and joint destruction. The synovitis tends to wax and wane and initially is treated pharmacologically. The joint destruction starts within the first or second year of the disease, however, and continues to progress. Radiographically, this destruction is shown by joint space narrowing, periarticular erosions, and subchondral osteopenia. The structural damage manifests as pain with activity and deformity. A few patients go into remission within the first year and lead fairly normal lives with few symptoms. Others have permanent disability as the disease progresses to the point of incurring joint destruction.

Treatment of the early stages of rheumatoid arthritis is primarily medical, although physical and occupational therapy often can be helpful. Pharmacologic agents used in rheumatoid arthritis include nonsteroidal antiinflammatory drugs, corticosteroids, methotrexate, and biologic agents. Biologic agents are recombinant proteins that generally target an inflammatory cytokine, such as tumor necrosis factor. These agents have shown excellent results. There is hope that they may decrease or eliminate the need for surgical intervention in many patients; however, these agents inhibit the immune system and cause an increased risk of infection in patients taking them.

Jämsen et al. reviewed the Finnish Arthroplasty Register covering the years 1995 to 2010 and found a 48% decrease in the number of primary arthroplasties performed for rheumatoid arthritis. They attributed this decrease to the effectiveness of improved medical management.

Goodman et al. published an extensive review of antirheumatologic agents and included recommendations for perioperative adjustments in medications for rheumatoid patients (Table 7.3). Patients who are on corticosteroids generally require preoperative "stress" dosages of hydrocortisone (Table 7.4). In general, agents that inhibit the immune system should be withheld at least 1 week before and 1 week after a surgical procedure. Patients with rheumatoid arthritis can

TABLE 7.2	
The 2010 American College of Rheumatology/European League Against Rheumatism Classification Criteria for Rheumatoid Arthritis	

	SCORE
Target population (Who should be tested?): Patients who 1. have at least 1 joint with definite clinical synovitis (swelling)[a] 2. with the synovitis not better explained by another disease[b] Classification criteria for RA (score-based algorithm: add score of categories A–D; A score of ≧6/10 is needed for classification of a patient as having definite RA)[c]	
A. Joint involvement[d]	
1 large joint[e]	0
2–10 large joints	1
1–3 small joints (with or without involvement of large joints)[f]	2
4–10 small joints (with or without involvement of large joints)	3
>10 joints (at least 1 small joint)[g]	5
B. Serology (at least 1 test result is needed for classification)[h]	0
Negative RF *and* negative ACPA	2
Low-positive RF *or* low-positive ACPA	3
High-positive RF *or* high-positive ACPA	0
C. Acute-phase reactants (at least 1 test result is needed for classification)[i]	1
Normal CRP *and* normal ESR	0
Abnormal CRP *or* abnormal ESR	1
D. Duration of symptoms[j]	
<6 weeks	
≧6 weeks	

[a]The criteria are aimed at classification of newly presenting patients. In addition, patients with erosive disease typical of rheumatoid arthritis (RA) with a history compatible with prior fulfillment of the 2010 criteria should be classified as having RA. Patients with long-standing disease, including those whose disease is inactive (with or without treatment) who, based on retrospectively available data, have previously fulfilled the 2010 criteria should be classified as having RA.

[b]Differential diagnoses vary among patients with different presentations but may include conditions such as systemic lupus erythematosus, psoriatic arthritis, and gout. If it is unclear about the relevant differential diagnoses to consider, an expert rheumatologist should be consulted.

[c]Although patients with a score of less than 6/10 are not classifiable as having RA, their status can be reassessed, and the criteria might be fulfilled cumulatively over time.

[d]Joint involvement refers to any *swollen* or *tender* joint on examination, which may be confirmed by imaging evidence of synovitis. Distal interphalangeal joints, first carpometacarpal joints, and first metatarsophalangeal joints are *excluded from assessment*. Categories of joint distribution are classified according to the location and number of involved joints, with placement into the highest category possible based on the pattern of joint involvement.

[e]"Large joints" refers to shoulders, elbows, hips, knees, and ankles.

[f]"Small joints" refers to the metacarpophalangeal joints, proximal interphalangeal joints, second through fifth metatarsophalangeal joints, thumb interphalangeal joints, and wrists.

[g]In this category, at least 1 of the involved joints must be a small joint; the other joints can include any combination of large and additional small joints, as well as other joints not specifically listed elsewhere (e.g., temporomandibular, acromioclavicular, sternoclavicular, etc.).

[h]Negative refers to IU values that are less than or equal to the upper limit of normal (ULN) for the laboratory and assay; low-positive refers to IU values that are higher than the ULN but ≤3 times the ULN for the laboratory and assay; high-positive refers to IU values that are greater than three times the ULN for the laboratory and assay. Where rheumatoid factor (RF) information is only available as positive or negative, a positive result should be scored as low-positive for RF. *ACPA,* Anti-citrullinated protein antibody.

[i]Normal/abnormal is determined by local laboratory standards. *CRP,* C-reactive protein; *ESR,* erythrocyte sedimentation rate.

[j]Duration of symptoms refers to patient self-report of the duration of signs or symptoms of synovitis (EG, pain, swelling, tenderness) of joints that are clinically involved at the time of assessment, regardless of treatment status.

From Aletaha D, Neogi T, Silman AJ, et al: 2010 Rheumatoid Arthritis Classification criteria: an American College of Rheumatology/European League against Rheumatism collaborative initiative, *Arthritis Rheum* 62[9]:2569, 2010.

have atlantoaxial instability secondary to bony erosion and ligamentous laxity from chronic synovitis. Cranial settling also can be present. During preoperative evaluation, consideration should be given to obtaining flexion and extension lateral radiographs to check for instability, which will be a factor during intubation if present.

Surgery for rheumatoid arthritis should accomplish one or more of the following: relieve pain; prevent destruction of cartilage or tendon; or improve function of joints by increasing or decreasing motion, correcting deformity, increasing stability, improving effective muscle forces, or any combination of these measures. Surgery in rheumatoid arthritis can be preventive and corrective; surgery can be done in some situations during spontaneous or induced remissions of the disease. Surgery may be indicated to relieve pain or to improve function or both. Currently, the activity of the disease often is disregarded, and preventive surgery is done early.

Synovectomy has played a role in the management of rheumatoid arthritis for many years. The current indications are mostly for pain in patients with minimal structural damage to the joint refractory to pharmacologic agents. Open synovectomy is being performed less frequently as arthroscopic synovectomy

TABLE 7.3

2017 American College of Rheumatology/American Association of Hip and Knee Surgeons Guideline for Perioperative Management of Antirheumatic Medication in Patients with Rheumatic Diseases Undergoing Elective Total Hip or Total Knee Arthroplasty

DMARDS: CONTINUE THESE MEDICATIONS THROUGH SURGERY	DOSING INTERVAL	CONTINUE/WITHHOLD
Methotrexate	Weekly	Continue
Sulfasalazine	Once or twice daily	Continue
Hydroxychloroquine	Once or twice daily	Continue
Leflunomide (Arava)	Daily	Continue
Doxycycline	Daily	Continue
BIOLOGIC AGENTS: STOP these medications prior to surgery and schedule surgery at the end of the dosing cycle. RESUME medications at minimum 14 days after surgery in the absence of wound healing problems, surgical site infection, or systemic infection	Dosing Interval	Schedule Surgery (relative to last biologic agent dose administered) during
Adalimumab (Humira)	Weekly or every 2 weeks	Week 2 or 3
Etanercept (Enbrel)	Weekly or twice weekly	Week 2
Golimumab (Simponi)	Every 4 weeks (SQ) or every 8 weeks (IV)	Week 5 Week 9
Infliximab (Remicade)	Every 4, 6, or 8 weeks	Week 5, 7, or 9
Abatacept (Orencia)	Monthly (IV) or weekly (SQ)	Week 5 Week 2
Certolizumab (Cimzia)	Every 2 or 4 weeks	Week 3 or 5
Rituximab (Rituxan)	2 doses 2 weeks apart every 4–6 months	Month 7
Tocilizumab (Actemra)	Every week (SQ) or every 4 weeks (IV)	Week 2 Week 5
Anakinra (Kineret)	Daily	Day 2
Secukinumab (Cosentyx)	Every 4 weeks	Week 5
Ustekinumab (Stelara)	Every 12 weeks	Week 13
Belimumab (Benlysta)	Every 4 weeks	Week 5
Tofacitinib (Xeljanz): STOP this medication 7 days prior to surgery	Daily or twice daily	7 days after last dose
SEVERE SLE-SPECIFIC MEDICATIONS: CONTINUE these medications in the perioperative period	Dosing Interval	Continue/Withhold
Mycophenolate mofetil	Twice daily	Continue
Azathioprine	Daily or twice daily	Continue
Cyclosporine	Twice daily	Continue
Tacrolimus	Twice daily (IV and PO)	Continue
NOT-SEVERE SLE: DISCONTINUE these medications 1 week prior to surgery	Dosing Interval	Continue/Withhold
Mycophenolate mofetil	Twice daily	Withhold
Azathioprine	Daily or twice daily	Withhold
Cyclosporine	Twice daily	Withhold
Tacrolimus	Twice daily (IV and PO)	Withhold

Dosing intervals were obtained from prescribing information provided online by pharmaceutical companies. *DMARDS,* Disease-modifying antirheumatic drugs; *IV,* intravenous; *PO,* oral; *SLE,* systemic lupus erythematosus; *SQ,* subcutaneous.
(Reproduced with permission from: Goodman SM, Springer B, Guyatt G, et al: 2017 American College of Rheumatology/American Association of Hip and Knee Surgeons guideline for perioperative management of antirheumatic medication in patients with rheumatic diseases undergoing elective total hip or total knee arthroplasty, *J Arthroplasty* 32:2628, 2017.)

has increased in popularity, especially for a rheumatoid knee. However, one meta-analysis of 2589 patients demonstrated that although both approaches relieved pain, arthroscopic synovectomy was associated with more recurrences of synovitis and disease progression. In addition, another study of two-stage surgical synovectomy in patients with rheumatoid arthritis demonstrated a decrease in sensory nerve fibers followed by a wound healing cell response, leading to reduced pain and better mobility. The authors did concede, however, that not all patients benefit from surgical synovectomy.

TABLE 7.4

Supplemental Hydrocortisone for Surgical Stress Levels

PROCEDURE CLASS/LEVEL OF STRESS	PROCEDURE	RECOMMENDED SUPPLEMENTAL HYDROCORTISONE
Minor/minimal	Carpal tunnel release Tenosynovectomy Knee arthroscopy Hammer toe correction First metatarsophalangeal fusion	25 mg hydrocortisone on day of procedure only (prednisone 5 mg)
Moderate/moderate	Hip arthroplasty Knee arthroplasty Ankle arthroplasty Shoulder arthroplasty Elbow arthroplasty Metacarpophalangeal arthroplasty Complex foot reconstruction with arthrodesis and tendon transfer Anterior cruciate ligament reconstruction	50–75 mg hydrocortisone on day of procedure with expeditious tapering over 1–2 days to preoperative dose (prednisone 10–15 mg)
Intensive/significant	Multiple trauma Bilateral knee arthroplasty Revision arthroplasty Multiple level spinal fusion	100–150 mg hydrocortisone on day of procedure with expeditious tapering over 1–2 days to preoperative dose (prednisone 20–40 mg)

From Howe CR, Gardner GC, Kadel NJ: Perioperative medication management for the patient with rheumatoid arthritis, *J Am Acad Orthop Surg* 14:544, 2006.

BOX 7.1

Diagnostic Criteria for Classification of Juvenile Rheumatoid Arthritis

- Age at onset younger than 16 years
- Arthritis in one or more joints defined as swelling or effusion or by the presence of two or more of the following signs: limitation of motion, tenderness or pain on motion, and increased heat
- Duration of disease 6 weeks to 3 months
- Type of onset of disease during the first 4–6 months classified as:
  - Polyarthritis: 5 joints or more
  - Monarthritis: 4 joints or fewer
  - Systemic disease: intermittent fever, rheumatoid rash, arthritis, visceral disease
- Exclusion of other rheumatic diseases

Modified from Brewer LJ Jr, Bass JC, Cassidy JT, et al: Criteria for the classification of juvenile rheumatoid arthritis, *Bull Rheum Dis* 23:712–719, 1972.

With current techniques of total joint arthroplasty, surgical options for the treatment of adult-onset rheumatoid arthritis have expanded greatly. In patients with moderate-to-severe destruction of cartilage and subchondral bone, total joint arthroplasty can relieve pain and improve function in most joints.

JUVENILE RHEUMATOID ARTHRITIS

Juvenile rheumatoid arthritis differs significantly from the adult form. The diagnosis of juvenile rheumatoid arthritis usually is made by exclusion. Other, more common types of arthritis in children and other rheumatic and connective tissue disorders must be ruled out. The diagnostic criteria for juvenile rheumatoid arthritis listed in Box 7.1 are similar to the criteria for the adult form. Rheumatoid factor is positive in less than 25% of patients with juvenile rheumatoid arthritis. After patients pass the age of 8 years, laboratory tests show an increasingly higher percentage of positive results, however. Similar to the adult form, juvenile rheumatoid arthritis is best treated by a multispecialty team approach.

Juvenile rheumatoid arthritis clinically consists of three types: polyarticular (involving five or more joints), monarticular (involving four or fewer joints), and systemic. Polyarthritis occurs in almost half of all children with juvenile rheumatoid arthritis. The knees, wrists, elbows, and ankles are most frequently affected, and the pattern of involvement usually is symmetric. Monarticular arthritis occurs in approximately one third of children with juvenile rheumatoid arthritis. In about half of these, the disease begins in only one joint, usually the knee. Systemic disease occurs in 10% to 20% of patients. Severe constitutional symptoms precede the development of overt arthritis. A high spiking fever and a "rheumatoid rash" are virtually diagnostic of systemic disease.

Psychosocial problems are common in patients with symptomatic juvenile rheumatoid arthritis. The timing of any surgical procedure in these patients should consider psychosocial factors, and counseling should be provided.

The chief cause of morbidity in systemic and polyarticular arthritis is severe joint disease, which occurs in 25% of patients. The chief cause of morbidity in monarticular disease is chronic iridocyclitis, which occurs in 25% to 30% of patients. Schaller reported that 90% of patients with juvenile rheumatoid arthritis and iridocyclitis had a positive antinuclear antibody test. Permanent blindness can occur from iridocyclitis, and patients with monarticular arthritis, especially patients with positive tests for antinuclear antibodies, should be evaluated by an ophthalmologist approximately every 3 months.

Open synovectomy for the treatment of juvenile rheumatoid arthritis has produced inconsistent results. Granberry and Brewer noted that patients with mild monarticular or polyarticular disease tend to have the best results after synovectomy. Patients with poor results after synovectomy included children with systemic disease and polyarticular involvement and children younger than 7 years old. Very young patients apparently had relief of pain but were unable to cooperate in the range-of-motion exercise programs to improve the function of the joint. Jacobsen et al. found few, if any, benefits from synovectomy in regard to relief of pain or improvement in range of motion, but the operation seemed to provide permanent relief of joint swelling. In their opinion, the one indication for synovectomy in juvenile rheumatoid arthritis is monarticular synovitis of long duration that has not responded to other treatment.

Although good results have been reported after arthroscopic synovectomy of the knee in adults with rheumatoid arthritis, the differences between adult-onset and juvenile rheumatoid arthritis prohibit application of these findings to children. In contrast to adult-onset disease, joint destruction can become extensive before pain becomes a serious problem. Juvenile rheumatoid arthritis also is more cyclical than the adult form, which tends to be relentlessly progressive. In one of the few studies of arthroscopic knee synovectomy in children, Vilkki et al. reported 22 such procedures in children 5 to 16 years old. They concluded that arthroscopic synovectomy is preferable to open synovectomy in these patients because mobilization and full weight bearing can be started soon after the procedure, morbidity is less, and rehabilitation is more rapid. Although arthroscopic synovectomy may provide a palliative treatment option for some children with juvenile rheumatoid arthritis, the procedure cannot be routinely recommended.

Ideal indications for synovectomy include involvement of one or only a few joints; hyperplastic, "wet" type of rheumatoid synovitis; failure to respond to an adequate trial of nonoperative treatment; and no radiographic evidence of articular cartilage destruction. Few patients meet all these criteria, however, and the decision to perform synovectomy requires astute clinical judgment. Contraindications to synovectomy include "dry" synovitis, involvement of multiple joints in the acute inflammatory phase, and systemic disease (Box 7.2).

Reconstructive procedures that may be required in patients with juvenile rheumatoid arthritis include soft-tissue procedures for correction of contractures, osteotomy, arthrodesis, joint excision, and arthroplasty. Combinations of these procedures often are necessary to relieve pain and correct deformity. Osteotomies are most commonly required to correct severe angular deformities. Arthrodesis usually is reserved for severely damaged joints unsuited for arthroplasty, such as the wrist, the foot, and occasionally the fingers. Excision of one of the articular surfaces occasionally is indicated at skeletal maturity for severely painful, contracted joints unsuited for arthroplasty. Arthroplasty may be indicated for destruction of the articular cartilage, especially in patients with multiple and bilateral joint destruction. The young age and lifestyles of these patients should be considered, however, before such an extensive procedure is undertaken. Generally, young adults with severe multiple joint involvement and low activity levels are best suited for arthroplasty.

Parvizi et al. (25 patients), Palmer et al. (15 patients), and Thomas et al. (17 patients) all reported excellent pain relief and improvement in functional capacity after total knee arthroplasty in patients with juvenile rheumatoid arthritis; however, repeat surgery and complications were more

---

> ### BOX 7.2
> ## Synovectomy in Juvenile Rheumatoid Arthritis
>
> **Ideal Indications**
> - Involvement of one or few joints
> - Hyperplastic, "wet" rheumatoid synovitis
> - Failure to respond to adequate trial of nonoperative treatment
> - No radiographic evidence of articular cartilage destruction
>
> **Relative Indications**
> - Severe pain
> - Significant loss of motion
> - Contractures despite several months of nonoperative treatment
>
> **Contraindications**
> - Seronegative "dry" synovitis
> - Polyarticular involvement
> - Acute inflammatory stage
> - Systemic disease

From Canale ST, Beaty JH, editors: *Operative pediatric orthopaedics*, ed 2, St Louis, 1995, Mosby.

frequent than reported after total knee arthroplasty in adults with osteoarthritis.

SURGICAL PROCEDURES

In rheumatoid arthritis, flexion contractures of both knees are common; when they exceed 30 degrees, the patient usually is confined to a wheelchair. The following surgical procedures are useful in properly selected patients with rheumatoid arthritis: (1) arthroscopic synovectomy, (2) proximal tibial osteotomy, (3) arthrodesis, and (4) arthroplasty or reconstruction.

▪ ARTHROSCOPIC SYNOVECTOMY

The basic indication for synovectomy in rheumatoid arthritis is failure of the disease to respond to appropriate medical treatment after 6 months. If the operation is to be successful, the disease should be limited almost entirely to the synovial membrane (Fig. 7.11) with little, if any, involvement of the cartilage or bone and consequently with little, if any, radiographic evidence of narrowing of the joint space. The involvement of two or more joints and the presence of acute inflammation are no longer considered contraindications for synovectomy. Although temporary symptomatic relief has been highly successful, range of motion often decreases and progression of the disease is rarely affected. Nonetheless, the palliative benefits often make the procedure worthwhile. Late synovectomy performed on knees with advanced arthritic changes has an unacceptably high failure rate and is not recommended.

The technique for arthroscopic synovectomy has evolved over the past 30 years. Consequently, arthroscopic synovectomy of the knee has become the standard because of advantages over the open procedure (Box 7.3).

Studies have shown that arthroscopic knee synovectomy in patients with rheumatoid arthritis successfully controls synovitis and improves pain. In one study, improvement was seen in all measured criteria. Although range of motion is preserved, it does not increase. Results seem to be better in patients with less cartilaginous damage. Ogawa et al. evaluated the results of 30 arthroscopic synovectomies at 6-year follow-up. All knees with

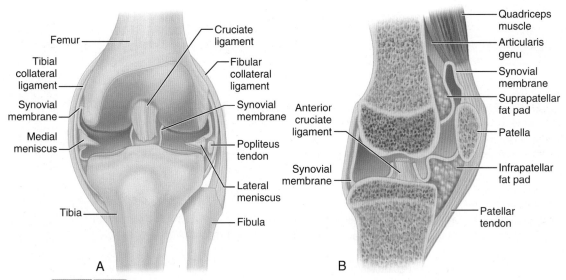

FIGURE 7.11 **A,** Location of synovium in knee joint in anteroposterior projection. **B,** Lateral projection. Only small portion of posterior synovium can be removed by anterior synovectomy.

BOX 7.3

Advantages of Arthroscopic Synovectomy

1. Synovial resection is more complete.
2. Incision is minimal.
3. Quadriceps muscle remains intact.
4. Incidence of infection is decreased.
5. Incidence of hemarthrosis is decreased.
6. Range of motion is maintained or increased.
7. It is cost-effective as an outpatient procedure.
8. Postoperative physical therapy is minimal or none.
9. Menisci are spared.
10. Patient acceptance is high.

From Salisbury RB: Synovectomy. In: Fu FH, Harner CD, Vince KG, editors: *Knee surgery*, Baltimore, 1994, Williams & Wilkins.

---

grade I changes (Larsen classification) maintained the same grade, whereas some with grade II changes and all with grade III changes required total knee arthroplasty.

For patients with adult-onset rheumatoid arthritis in whom a minimum of 6 months of conservative treatment has been ineffective and who do not have late erosive arthritic changes, arthroscopic knee synovectomy can be palliative. Although some of the erosive changes seen on radiographs may be delayed, the ultimate natural progression of the disease is unchanged. If performed by an experienced arthroscopist, arthroscopic synovectomy may decrease pain without sacrificing significant motion and decrease operative and postoperative morbidity compared with open synovectomy.

Arthroscopic synovectomy should be performed systematically after examination of the joint. Knee joint synovium is found diffusely throughout the interior lining of the joint, in the cruciate ligaments, and on the undersurface of the menisci (Fig. 7.11). For adequate and safe synovectomy in these regions, the posterior pouches of the knee joint should be examined thoroughly but cautiously. The superficial layers of the synovium are removed with a shaver, and resection is carried down to a defining plane between the synovium and subsynovial tissues.

When this plane is reached, the smooth shiny fibers of the capsule can be seen, with the superficial capillaries lying over the interior of the capsule. The surgeon should view the knee as a series of compartments, spending an equal amount of time in each compartment to remove an even distribution of the synovium. Because of the risk of serious neurovascular complications, arthroscopic synovectomy should be performed by an experienced arthroscopist. The technique for arthroscopic knee synovectomy is described in other chapter.

■ PROXIMAL TIBIAL OSTEOTOMY

Proximal tibial osteotomy (see Technique 7.9) is useful for correcting varus or valgus deformities of an arthritic knee resulting from unicompartmental arthritis. It realigns the weight-bearing axis through the knee to distribute the forces of weight to the less involved or uninvolved compartment. This operation usually is contraindicated in patients with rheumatoid arthritis because the disease process is likely to be more evenly distributed between the medial and lateral compartments and the patellofemoral articulation. In addition, the osteoporotic bone in rheumatoid patients makes the procedure more demanding than in patients with osteoarthritis, with an increased chance of fracture into the joint during the osteotomy, avulsion of the patellar tendon, or loss of fixation.

■ ARTHRODESIS

Arthrodesis (see chapter 6) offers the advantages of stability and freedom from pain. With advances in total joint arthroplasty, however, it is rarely indicated except for severe unilateral joint involvement in young, active patients. If there is any question that the contralateral hip is involved, knee arthrodesis is contraindicated.

■ ARTHROPLASTY OR RECONSTRUCTION

Improvements in total knee arthroplasty have made it the surgical treatment of choice for most patients with rheumatoid arthritis involving the knees. In advanced disease, when synovectomy is of no benefit, total joint arthroplasty can relieve pain and in certain instances increase motion. It is most appropriate for patients in class III or class IV (American

TABLE 7.5

American Academy of Orthopaedic Surgeons' Recommendations for Less Invasive Treatment of Osteoarthritis of the Knee

RECOMMENDATION	YES/NO	STRENGTH OF RECOMMENDATION
1. Participation in self-management programs, strengthening low-impact aerobic exercises, and neuromuscular education; engagement in physical activity consistent with national guidelines is recommended.	Yes	Strong
2. Weight loss in patients with a body mass index of greater than 25.	Yes	Moderate
3A. Acupuncture	No	Strong
3B. Physical agents (including electrotherapeutic modalities)	?	Inconclusive
3C. Manual therapy	?	Inconclusive
4. Valgus directing force brace (medial compartment unloader)	?	Inconclusive
5. Lateral wedge insoles for symptomatic medial compartment osteoarthritis	No	Moderate
6. Glucosamine and chondroitin	No	Strong
7A. Nonsteroidal antiinflammatory drugs or Tramadol	Yes	Strong
7B. Acetaminophen, opioids, pain patches	?	Inconclusive
8. Intraarticular corticosteroids	?	Inconclusive
9. Hyaluronic acid	No	Strong
10. Growth factor injections and/or platelet- rich plasma	?	Inconclusive
11. Needle lavage	No	Moderate

Derived from Jevsevar DS, Brown GA, Jones DL, et al: The American Academy of Orthopaedic Surgeons evidence-based guideline on treatment of osteoarthritis of the knee, 2nd Edition, *J Bone Joint Surg* 95(20):1885–1886, 2013.

Rheumatism Association classification) with involvement of multiple joints, especially the ipsilateral hip or ankle or contralateral knee or both, when involvement of other joints does not preclude adequate rehabilitation. Excellent or good results have been reported after total knee arthroplasty, and one study found a lower failure rate in patients with rheumatoid arthritis than in other diagnostic groups.

The outcomes of total knee arthroplasty are good with posterior cruciate–retaining and posterior cruciate–sacrificing designs. Although previous reports of total knee arthroplasty in patients with rheumatoid arthritis have been favorable, a 50% rate of posterior cruciate ligament instability in the sagittal plane has been reported, although others have not duplicated this finding. We use posterior cruciate ligament–substituting prostheses for total knee arthroplasty in patients with rheumatoid arthritis.

Complications may be more frequent after total knee arthroplasty in patients with rheumatoid arthritis than in patients with osteoarthritis because of (1) poor healing of tissue, (2) deep wound infections, (3) severe flexion contracture, (4) severe joint laxity, (5) severe osteopenia, and (6) involvement of multiple other joints limiting rehabilitation. To help minimize some of the problems in our patients with rheumatoid arthritis for whom total knee arthroplasty is planned, we try to optimize nutritional status preoperatively, use antibiotic-containing bone cement, and frequently use stemmed components for primary arthroplasty in patients with severe osteopenia. Rodriguez et al. reported delayed infections in 4.1% of patients an average of 7 years after primary total knee arthroplasty. It has been theorized that the role of corticosteroids, more than the disease process itself, may be responsible for wound complications and infection. Indications, contraindications, and procedures for total knee arthroplasty are described in chapter 5.

OSTEOARTHRITIS OF THE KNEE

Osteoarthritis of the knee can cause symptoms ranging from mild to disabling. Initial management of most patients should be nonoperative and may include physical therapy, bracing, orthoses, ambulatory aids, nonsteroidal antiinflammatory medications, intraarticular injections of a steroid or hyaluronic acid, and analgesics. Changes in daily, work, and recreational activities also may be necessary. Obesity is a known risk factor for osteoarthritis of the knee, and weight loss has been shown to slow the progression of the disease. Because of the progressive nature of the disease, many patients with osteoarthritis of the knee eventually require operative treatment. Table 7.5 lists recommendations made by the American Academy of Orthopaedic Surgeons on less invasive treatments.

SURGICAL PROCEDURES

A variety of procedures have been described for treatment of the osteoarthritic knee, including arthroscopic debridement, osteochondral or chondrocyte transplantation, high tibial osteotomy, distal femoral osteotomy, arthroplasty, and arthrodesis. The choice of procedure depends on the patient's age and activity expectations, the severity of the disease, and the number of knee compartments involved.

◼ DEBRIDEMENT

Surgical debridement of the osteoarthritic knee generally includes limited synovectomy, excision of osteophytes, removal of loose bodies, chondroplasty, and removal of damaged menisci. Satisfactory results have been reported after open debridement of an osteoarthritic knee. We have had limited success with this procedure; symptoms generally recur, sometimes quite rapidly. This procedure is painful and

---

TABLE 7.6

Prognostic Factors for Arthroscopic Debridement of Osteoarthritic Knee

PROGNOSIS	HISTORY	PHYSICAL EXAMINATION	RADIOGRAPHIC FINDINGS	ARTHROSCOPIC FINDINGS
Good	Short duration Associated trauma First arthroscopy Mechanical symptoms	Medial tenderness Effusion Normal alignment Ligament stable	Unicompartmental Normal alignment Minimal Fairbank lesions Loose bodies Relevant osteophytes	Outerbridge I or II Meniscal flap tear Chondral fracture/flap Loose bodies Osteophyte at symptom site

Poor	Long duration
	Insidious onset
	Multiple procedures
	Rest pain
	Litigation
	Work related
		Lateral tenderness
		No effusion
		Malalignment
		Varus >10 degrees
		Valgus >15 degrees
		Ligaments unstable
			Bicompartmental or
			  tricompartment
			Malalignment
			Significant Fairbank lesions
			Irrelevant osteophytes
				Outerbridge III or IV
				Degenerative meniscus
				Diffuse chondrosis
				Osteophyte away from
				  symptom site

From Cole BJ, Harner CD: Degenerative arthritis of the knee in active patients: evaluation and management, *J Am Acad Orthop Surg* 7:389–402, 1999.

---

often requires 6 months of postoperative rehabilitation. With the advent of arthroscopic techniques, open debridement of the knee for osteoarthritis rarely is used. The technique can be found in older editions of *Campbell's Operative Orthopaedics*.

Arthroscopic techniques result in less postoperative pain and shorter rehabilitation than open procedures. Arthroscopic treatments of osteoarthritis of the knee include simple lavage, debridement, and abrasion chondroplasty. Although good initial results have been reported after arthroscopic lavage, outcomes tend to deteriorate over time. The initial relief of symptoms after arthroscopic lavage is thought to be secondary to the removal of cartilaginous debris and inflammatory factors. Some studies have cited the benefits of arthroscopic debridement of the osteoarthritic knee, with a success rate of about 70%.

Patients with symptoms of short duration and patients with mechanical symptoms tend to do well, but those with radiographic malalignment, especially valgus deformities, tend to have poor outcomes, as do patients with pending litigation or workers' compensation claims. Only 25% of knees with severe arthritis, limb malalignment, and a joint space width of less than 2 mm have substantial relief of symptoms. Table 7.6 lists the prognostic factors for arthroscopic debridement in one study. Arthroscopic abrasion chondroplasty and microfracture techniques also have been advocated to stimulate cartilage regeneration. On average, about 60% of patients have a good result from an abrasion procedure. Abrasion chondroplasty is contraindicated in patients with inflammatory arthritis, significant knee stiffness, deformity, or instability and in patients who are unwilling or unable to comply with 2 months of non–weight bearing after surgery.

Several authors have reported a "placebo effect" after arthroscopy for osteoarthritis of the knee that occurs even when no specific procedure is performed, but most suggested that this effect was of short duration. In 2002, Moseley et al. reported a placebo-controlled, randomized study of 180 patients in which they concluded that there was no difference between arthroscopic debridement or arthroscopic lavage and sham surgery. Dervin et al. prospectively evaluated 126 arthroscopic debridement procedures done for osteoarthritis of the knee and found that 44% of patients had significant pain relief at 2 years after surgery. Three variables were significantly associated with improvements in symptoms: (1) medial joint line tenderness, (2) positive Steinmann test (forced external and internal rotation of a knee

that is flexed to 90 degrees and recording pain that is referable to either joint line), and (3) an unstable meniscal tear identified at arthroscopy. Arthroscopic debridement procedures cannot significantly alter the natural progression of osteoarthritis. Wai et al. retrospectively reviewed more than 14000 arthroscopic debridement procedures performed for osteoarthritis and found that almost 20% of the patients had total knee arthroplasty within 3 years of the surgery. This study showed that the rate of total knee arthroplasty after arthroscopic debridement increases significantly with age; patients older than age 70 years were almost five times more likely to have total knee arthroplasty within 1 year after debridement than were patients younger than 60 years. At best, arthroscopic techniques may delay the need for a more definitive procedure, especially in younger, active patients with localized degenerative arthritis that causes pain at rest without malalignment or instability. The role of arthroscopic knee debridement in the treatment of osteoarthritis remains controversial.

The American Academy of Orthopaedic Surgeons does not recommend arthroscopic debridement for osteoarthritis.

Arthroscopic techniques for debridement, drilling, and chondroplasty are described in other chapter.

■ OSTEOCHONDRAL AND AUTOLOGOUS CHONDROCYTE TRANSPLANTATION

Overall satisfactory results have been reported after osteochondral allograft transplant (78%); however, only 30% of knees with arthritis had satisfactory results. The technique has been described as a salvage procedure for young, active patients with severe articular cartilage degeneration of the patellofemoral joint.

Brittberg et al. of Sweden reported their results with autologous chondrocyte transplantation in 23 knees with deep cartilage defects. Two years after transplantation, 14 of 16 patients with femoral condylar transplants had good or excellent results; however, only two of seven patients with patellar transplants had good or excellent results. Other systematic reviews have shown autologous chondrocyte implantation to be no more effective than other methods of treatment, such as microfracture and mosaicplasty. Sharpe et al. combined autologous chondrocyte implantation with osteochondral autografts. Autologous chondrocytes were injected under a periosteal patch covering the osteochondral autograft cores. All patients had significant improvement in symptoms at 1 year, with improvement maintained at 3 years. Franceschi et al. concluded that simultaneous arthroscopic implantation of autologous chondrocytes and medial opening wedge osteotomy of the proximal tibia is a viable option for the treatment of chondral defects of the medial tibial plateau in the varus knee.

Although satisfactory short-term results have been reported, currently data are insufficient to recommend autologous chondrocyte implantation as more effective than other treatments. Indications are limited and include isolated, full-thickness, grade IV femoral defect and a tibial surface with no more than grade II chondromalacia. Patients must be willing to restrict activity for 12 months to allow the new cartilage to mature. A more detailed description of these techniques can be found in other chapter.

Improved knee scores at 2 years have been reported after arthroscopic debridement followed by stem cell injection derived from the infrapatellar fat pad.

PROXIMAL TIBIAL OSTEOTOMY

High tibial osteotomy is a well-established procedure for the treatment of unicompartmental osteoarthritis of the knee. Most reports have shown approximately 80% satisfactory results at 5 years and 60% at 10 years after high tibial osteotomy. These results also have been shown to deteriorate over time, however. The rate of proximal tibial osteotomies performed in North America has declined significantly in recent years, whereas the rate of total and unicompartmental knee arthroplasties has steadily increased. Nevertheless, high tibial osteotomy still is a useful procedure for properly selected patients.

Varus or valgus deformities are fairly common and cause an abnormal distribution of the weight-bearing stresses within the joint. The most common deformity in patients with osteoarthritis of the knee is a varus position, which causes stresses to be concentrated medially, accelerating degenerative changes in the medial part of the joint; if the deformity is one of valgus position, changes are accelerated in the lateral part. The biomechanical rationale for proximal tibial osteotomy in patients with unicompartmental osteoarthritis of the knee is "unloading" of the involved joint compartment by correcting the malalignment and redistributing the stresses on the knee joint.

Some authors have reported arthroscopic evidence of fibrocartilaginous repair in patients who have had a high tibial osteotomy. At second-look arthroscopy of 58 knees an average of 18 months after lateral closing wedge osteotomy, Kanamiya et al. found that only three of the 58 knees showed no signs of repair, and 55% of patients had partial or complete coverage of eburnated lesions with fibrocartilage. Wakabayashi et al. also noted reparative signs in 62% of completely eburnated bony lesions at arthroscopic examination 12 months after high tibial osteotomy.

The indications for proximal tibial osteotomy are (1) pain and disability resulting from osteoarthritis that significantly interfere with high-demand employment or recreation and (2) evidence on weight-bearing radiographs of degenerative arthritis that is confined to one compartment with a corresponding varus or valgus deformity. The patient must be able to use crutches or a walker and have sufficient muscle strength and motivation to carry out a rehabilitation program. Contraindications to a proximal tibial osteotomy are (1) narrowing of lateral compartment cartilage space, (2) lateral tibial subluxation of more than 1 cm, (3) medial compartment tibial bone loss of more than 2 or 3 mm, (4) flexion contracture of

more than 15 degrees, (5) knee flexion of less than 90 degrees, (6) more than 20 degrees of correction needed, (7) inflammatory arthritis, and (8) significant peripheral vascular disease.

Many techniques have been described for valgus proximal tibial osteotomy. Four basic types are most commonly used: medial opening wedge, lateral closing wedge, dome, and medial opening hemicallotasis. The technique with the longest "track record" is lateral closing wedge osteotomy first described by Coventry (see Technique 7.9). A medial opening wedge osteotomy with iliac crest bone graft and rigid fixation was described by Hernigou et al. Opening wedge hemicallotasis, described by Turi et al., uses an external fixator to distract the osteotomy site gradually. There is no distinct advantage to using an opening wedge or closing wedge osteotomy. A randomized trial between the two demonstrated no difference in clinical outcome or radiographic alignment. The opening wedge group had more complications, but the closing wedge group experienced more early conversion to total knee arthroplasty.

Maquet described a "barrel vault," or dome, osteotomy, which he believed allowed more accuracy and adjustability of correction (Fig. 7.12). Because this osteotomy is inherently stable, internal fixation usually is not required, but pins, plate-and-screw devices, or external fixation can be used if necessary. If no internal fixation is used, postoperative adjustments in alignment can be made by adjustments in the cast. Disadvantages of the technique include technical difficulty, intraarticular fracture, and scarring around the patellofemoral extensor mechanism.

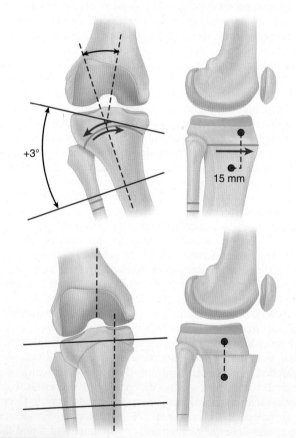

FIGURE 7.12 Barrel vault osteotomy of Maquet uses special jigs to orient dome osteotomy properly. Distal tibia can be translated if needed to change patellar tracking for patellofemoral degenerative changes.

Because isolated lateral compartment osteoarthritis is not as common as medial compartment involvement, varus osteotomies to correct valgus deformities are infrequently done in patients with osteoarthritis. Marti et al. used a lateral opening wedge osteotomy with iliac crest bone grafting and rigid fixation to treat 34 osteoarthritic patients with valgus deformities. At a mean follow up of 11 years, 88% had excellent or good results. Coventry recommended a medial closing wedge osteotomy to correct valgus deformity; however, if the valgus deformity is larger than 12 degrees, or if the joint surface tilt of the tibia after osteotomy will be more than 10 degrees, he recommended a supracondylar medial closing wedge femoral osteotomy instead (Technique 7.11).

LATERAL CLOSING WEDGE OSTEOTOMY

Coventry described a closing wedge osteotomy made proximal to the tibial tuberosity. He recommended a lateral approach to correct a varus deformity and a medial approach to correct a valgus deformity. The advantages of this osteotomy are that (1) it is made near the deformity, that is, the knee joint; (2) it is made through cancellous bone, which heals rapidly; (3) it permits the fragments to be held firmly in position by staples or a rigid fixation device, such as a plate-and-screw construct; and (4) it permits exploration of the knee through the same incision. After this operation, the danger of delayed union or nonunion is slight and prolonged immobilization in a cast is unnecessary, especially with rigid internal fixation.

Coventry found that the major complication was recurrence of deformity, which coincided with the recurrence of pain. He also found that the risk of failure was increased if alignment was not overcorrected to at least 8 degrees of valgus and if the patient was substantially overweight (30% over ideal body weight).

Longer-term follow-up (>10 years) confirmed a gradual deterioration of results over time. Most reports have shown satisfactory results in about 80% at 5 years and 60% at 10 years after high tibial osteotomy. Berman et al. identified several factors associated with favorable results, including (1) age younger than 60 years, (2) purely unicompartmental disease, (3) ligamentous stability, and (4) preoperative arc of motion of at least 90 degrees. Sprenger and Doerzbacher reported a 90% 10-year survival rate in a retrospective study of 76 lateral closing wedge osteotomies.

Normally, there is valgus alignment of 5 to 8 degrees in the tibiofemoral angle as measured on radiographs taken in the weight-bearing position. The amount of correction of the arthritic knee needed to achieve a normal angle is calculated, and an additional 3 to 5 degrees of overcorrection is added to achieve approximately 10 degrees of valgus. With a varus deformity, the only limitation in the amount of correction from a valgus osteotomy is the size of the bone wedge that can be taken proximal to the patellar tendon.

Coventry used the method of Bauer et al. for calculating the size of the wedge removed as roughly 1 degree of correction for each 1 mm of length at the base of the wedge (e.g., 20 degrees of correction = a 20-mm base of the wedge). This is true only if the tibia is 57 mm wide, however, and we prefer using exact measurements for the width of the base of the osteotomy, with a right triangle constructed from a preoperative drawing (Fig. 7.13) or the formula W = diameter × 0.02 × angle or tangent tables. Alternately, full-length, near actual size, standing anteroposterior radiographs can be used to determine the size of the wedge needed. The desired alignment, based on the

mechanical axis from the center of the femoral head through the knee to the center of the ankle, can be achieved by cutting the appropriate-sized wedge from the proximal tibia.

We also have used the technique of Slocum et al. of leaving a thin posteromedial lip of bone on the proximal tibial fragment. When the osteotomy is closed after removal of the wedge of bone, this posterior lip overrides the proximal end of the distal fragment and gives added support and stability to the osteotomy (Fig. 7.14). If the deformity is undercorrected, we also have found it helpful to curet cancellous bone just medial to the lateral edge of the proximal tibia instead of removing more cortical bone; this allows the lateral cortical edge of the inferior margin of the osteotomy to slide beneath the proximal lateral cortex and lock the osteotomy further in place before internal fixation. Sadek, Osman, and Laklok found that anterior translation of the distal osteotomy fragment of greater than 1.5 cm led to significantly better postoperative functional knee scores.

Completion of the osteotomy and realigning the extremity requires disruption of the proximal tibiofibular joint. This can be accomplished by either removing the inferomedial portion of the fibular head (Fig. 7.15) or careful disruption of the proximal tibiofibular syndesmosis to allow posterosuperior migration of the fibula when the osteotomy is closed. Care should be taken to not injure the peroneal nerve.

Steinmann pins and a drill guide can be used to determine accurate placement of the osteotomy cuts (Fig. 7.16). Hofmann et al. compared the results of tibial osteotomies performed using an osteotomy jig, rigid fixation (L-buttress plate), and early motion (immediate continuous passive motion machine and 50% weight bearing) with results of procedures in which the osteotomy cuts were determined by measuring the lateral cortex and cylinder casts were used for postoperative stabilization. They reported quicker union (3 vs. 4.5 months), fewer complications (5% vs. 42%), and less time to return of 90 degrees of flexion with the jig technique. An advantage of this technique is that postoperative cast immobilization, which has been associated with patella baja, is not required. We also have had good results with this technique and prefer the use of jigs when performing a lateral closing wedge high tibial osteotomy (Fig. 7.17). Müller and Strecker reviewed 340 osteotomy procedures with same-session arthroscopy and found it indispensable to check the indication for osteotomy, to modify the degree of correction or procedure according to the cartilage status, and to perform therapeutic procedures. Wu et al. stated after a meta-analysis that using navigation produced superior alignment accuracy and precision but no significant improvement in clinical results.

The following technique outlines the basics for use of an osteotomy jig. There are several brands available.

LATERAL CLOSING WEDGE OSTEOTOMY

TECHNIQUE 7.9

(MODIFIED COVENTRY; HOFMANN, WYATT, AND BECK)
- With the patient supine, place a sandbag under the involved hip to allow easier access to the lateral aspect of the knee.

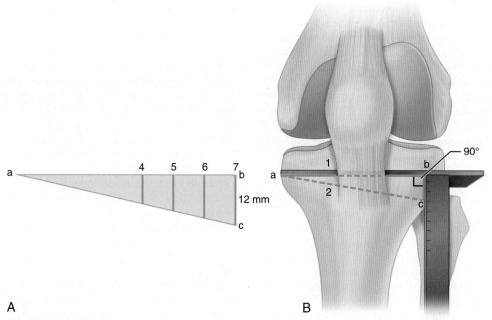

FIGURE 7.13 **A,** Calculation of size of bone wedge to be removed to accomplish desired degrees of correction with high tibial osteotomy. Apex angle *(a)* is number of degrees of correction desired for wedge osteotomy. Line *ab* corresponds to width of tibia and is marked off in 4-, 5-, 6-, and 7-cm distances from point *a.* Height of base of wedge can be measured (line *bc* for tibia, 7 cm wide). When tibia is 4 cm wide, height of base measured from diagram is 8 mm. **B,** Transferring calculations of size to wedge of osteotomy of tibia. Line *ab* represents transverse saw cut 2 cm below joint line with metal ruler inserted into cut. Angle at *a* represents correction desired and distance down second ruler. Line *bc* represents height of base of wedge to achieve this angular correction when *ab* represents width of tibia being osteotomized.

A sandbag taped to the operating table helps maintain 90 degrees of knee flexion during the operation. This position is important because it carries the popliteal vessels and peroneal nerve posteriorly and relaxes the iliotibial band.

- Drape and prepare the limb from the anterior superior iliac spine to the ankle; apply and inflate a thigh tourniquet.
- Make an inverted-L–shaped incision for a lateral approach to the proximal tibia (Fig. 7.18A). The transverse limb of the incision is at the lateral joint line and extends posteriorly to the fibular head. The vertical limb is midline to the tibia and extends 10 cm distally.
- Carefully divide the proximal tibiofibular capsule with a sharp ¾-inch curved osteotome. Use a blunt Hohmann retractor to protect the neurovascular structures throughout the procedure.
- Use Keith needles or small Kirschner wires to identify the joint line and insert the transverse osteotomy jig with the top portion touching the needles or wires (Fig. 7.18B).
- Stabilize the jig by drilling to the third mark (3 inches) on the 3.2-mm drill bit and filling the hole with a smooth pin (⅛ inch).
- Flex and extend the osteotomy guide to match the patient's posterior slope and to determine proper plate positioning.

This can be confirmed by placing the plate over the smooth pin in the jig (Fig. 7.18C).

- When proper positioning is determined, drill a second hole, and fill it with a smooth pin.
- Through the central hole in the transverse osteotomy guide, adjacent to the osteotomy slot, drill completely across the tibia, and use a depth gauge to measure the tibial width.
- Insert the calibrated saw blade, and make the transverse limb of the osteotomy, keeping a 10-mm bridge of the medial cortex intact.
- Replace the transverse osteotomy jig with the slotted oblique jig; this jig is slotted in 2-mm increments to allow the desired degree of correction (6 to 20 degrees).
- Make the oblique portion of the osteotomy (Fig. 7.18D), and remove the oblique jig, leaving the pins in place.
- Remove the wedge of bone, and carefully inspect the osteotomy site to ensure no residual bone is left.
- Apply a buttress plate over the two smooth pins. Remove one pin, and replace it with a 6.5-mm cancellous screw, using the second pin as a parallel alignment marker (Fig. 7.18E). Remove the second pin, and replace it with a cancellous screw. Screws 60 to 70 mm long usually are used in men, and screws 50 to 60 mm long usually are used in women. Shorter (50 mm) screws can be used in very young patients to make hardware removal easier

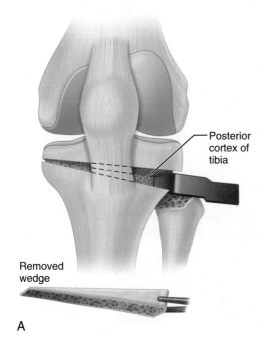

A

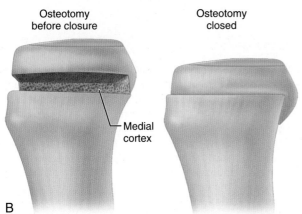

B

FIGURE 7.14 **A,** Bone wedge is cut to but not through posterior cortex of tibia before its removal. **B,** Lower saw cut is deepened through posterior cortex and osteotomy wedge closed as illustrated on right. This permits posterior lip of bone above to override cortex distal to osteotomy for stability. The distal segment of the osteotomy translates anteriorly for a short distance to improve patellofemoral tracking.

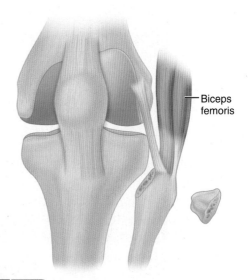

FIGURE 7.15 Partial removal of fibular head in lateral or valgus osteotomy of proximal tibia.

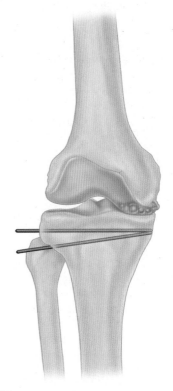

FIGURE 7.16 Steinmann pins used as an osteotomy guide. Cuts are made with a broad osteotome viewed with an image intensifier.

when healing is complete. Do not tighten these screws until the distal cortical screws have been inserted.

- Using the two distal holes in the L-plate as a reference, use the drill alignment guide to place a single-cortex, 3.2-mm hole in line with and distal to the plate (Fig. 7.18F). Slight toggling of the bit makes application of the compression clamp easier.

- Insert the curved pin at the end of the compression clamp into this hole, while placing the straight pin on the end of the clamp into the most distal hole of the L-plate, and apply slow compression (Fig. 7.18G).

- Compression often takes 5 minutes, allowing plastic deformation to occur through the incomplete osteotomy site. If compression is difficult, check that the proximal

tibiofibular joint is completely disrupted and that any residual bone wedge has been removed.

- When the osteotomy is closed, evaluate overall alignment with either a long alignment rod or an electrocautery cord. When aligned from the center of the hip to the center of the ankle, the plumb line should pass through the lateral compartment of the knee.

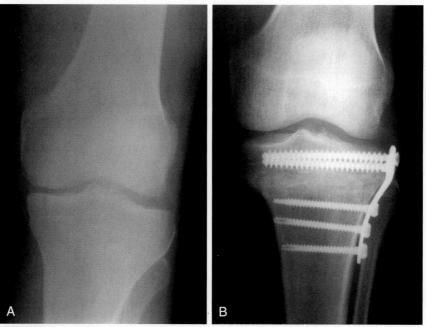

FIGURE 7.17 **A,** Medial joint collapse resulting in varus deformity and medial knee pain. **B,** After high tibial osteotomy.

- Confirm alignment and placement of the plate with anteroposterior and lateral radiographs or fluoroscopy.
- Through the central round hole in the plate, drill a hole with the 3.2-mm drill bit and insert a self-tapping cortical screw (Fig. 7.18H).
- Remove the compression device and insert a cortical screw in the most distal hole in the plate. Tighten the proximal cancellous screws. Do not apply severe torque when tightening any of the screws, especially the cortical screws. A power screwdriver is not recommended for final tightening.
- Release the tourniquet and obtain hemostasis with electrocautery. Irrigate the wound, insert a small suction drain, and loosely approximate the fascia of the anterior compartment and the iliotibial band with interrupted sutures. Close the subcutaneous tissue with interrupted absorbable sutures, and close the skin with staples and sterile strips. Apply a large compressive Jones dressing.

POSTOPERATIVE CARE Continuous passive motion is begun immediately after surgery in the recovery room, usually from 0 to 30 degrees of flexion, progressing 10 degrees each day. Ambulation is begun on the second day after surgery, and 50% weight bearing is allowed for the first 6 weeks with the use of crutches. Muscle strengthening and active range-of-motion exercises also are begun on postoperative day 2. Full weight bearing is allowed after 6 weeks.

MEDIAL OPENING WEDGE OSTEOTOMY

Hernigou et al. described a medial opening wedge tibial osteotomy (Fig. 7.19), which they thought is more precise and allows more exact correction than does a lateral closing wedge osteotomy. Use of an osteotomy jig and rigid plate fixation is recommended. Tricortical iliac crest autograft with supplemental cancellous graft material also is recommended; however, other structural graft material, such as hydroxyapatite wedges, can be successful. Opening wedge osteotomy should be done if the involved extremity is 2 cm or more shorter than the contralateral extremity. Opening wedge osteotomy also may be indicated in patients with laxity of the medial collateral ligament or combined anterior cruciate ligament deficiency. Arthur et al. performed proximal tibial opening wedge osteotomies as the initial treatment for chronic grade III posterolateral corner instability with a combined varus deformity in 21 patients. Two thirds of these patients did not require second-stage ligament reconstruction procedures. In a biomechanical study, LaPrade et al. demonstrated that opening wedge proximal tibial osteotomy decreased varus and external rotation laxity for posterolateral corner–deficient knees. They thought that this was, in part, caused by tightening of the superficial medial collateral ligament. After reviewing 117 medial opening wedge osteotomies, Stanley et al. found no significant difference in radiographic correction of alignment between navigated and fluoroscopic techniques.

A lateral hinge fracture with extension into the lateral tibial plateau is a common complication with medial opening wedge osteotomy occurring in 15% to 18% of patients. Ogawa et al. stated that a sufficient osteotomy of both anterior and posterior cortices with the endpoint at the level of the fibular head is necessary to avoid a lateral hinge fracture.

Leg-length discrepancy is a common finding after open wedge osteotomy. Careful leg-length measurements should be made before surgery. If the leg involved is of equal length or longer than the contralateral leg, consideration should be given to a lateral closing wedge osteotomy because there is minimal change in leg length with that procedure.

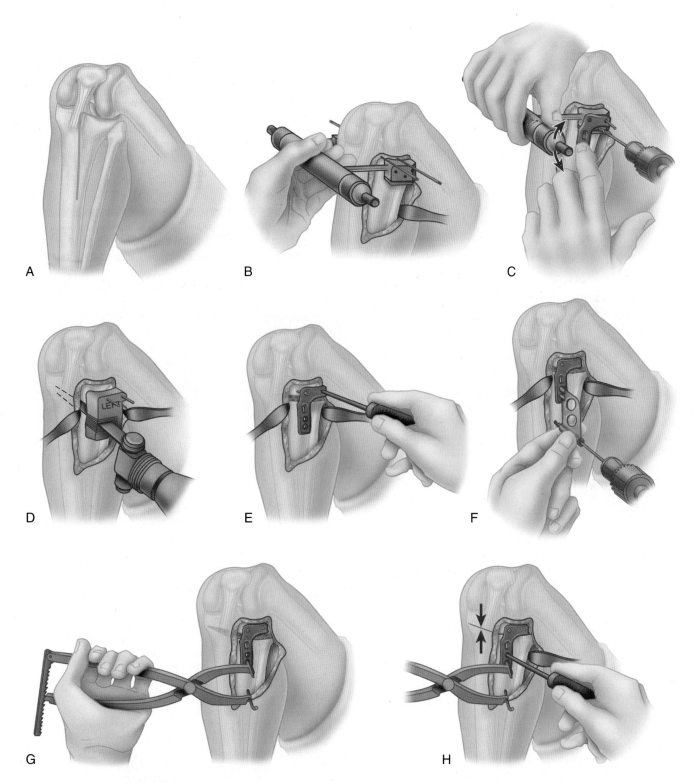

FIGURE 7.18 High tibial osteotomy with use of osteotomy jig (see text). **A,** Incision. **B,** Positioning of transverse osteotomy guide. **C,** Determination of correct position of jig. **D,** Placement of oblique osteotomy guide over 3.2-mm smooth pins and performance of osteotomy. **E,** Placement of L-shaped osteotomy plate. **F,** Application of compression clamp. **G,** Application of slow compression. **H,** Fixation of distal plate. **SEE TECHNIQUE 7.9.**

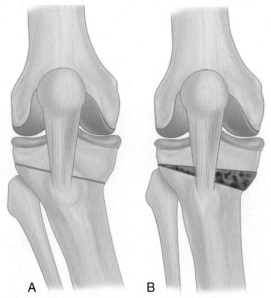

FIGURE 7.19 Hernigou et al. medial opening wedge tibial osteotomy. **A,** Osteotomy proximal to tibial tubercle begins 3.5 cm distal to medial joint line and is directed toward proximal tip of fibula, leaving lateral part of cortex intact. **B,** Osteotomy is pried open, and wedge-shaped bicortical iliac bone grafts are inserted. Osteotomy is fixed with plate and screws.

OPENING WEDGE HEMICALLOTASIS

Schwartsman advocated the use of circular external fixation after percutaneous tibial osteotomy (Ilizarov technique) distal to the tibial tuberosity so that accurate adjustments can be made postoperatively on the basis of standing, weight-bearing radiographs. He suggested that healing is more reliable after opening wedge percutaneous corticotomy than after open closing wedge osteotomy and that placement of the osteotomy below the tibial tubercle minimizes the chance of patella infera and loss of proximal tibial bone stock that may complicate later total knee arthroplasty. He also cited as advantages the ability to translate the distal fragment to restore mechanical alignment, improved stability of fixation, and immediate weight bearing and knee motion of 0 to 90 degrees in the circular frame. Disadvantages of the Ilizarov technique for proximal tibial osteotomy include poor patient acceptance of the external fixator, pin loosening, the possibility of pin track infection that may compromise later total knee arthroplasty, and the need for extremely close follow-up. This technique also requires patients to make numerous daily adjustments to the fixator, which can be overwhelming for some patients.

Turi et al. described an opening wedge osteotomy with a dynamic uniplanar external fixator using hemicallotasis techniques. In this procedure, the medial osteotomy is made below the tibial tuberosity. A dynamic external fixator is applied, and beginning 7 days postoperatively, the fixator is distracted 0.25 mm four times a day until correction is obtained. Five-year and 10-year survivorships of 89% and 63%, respectively, have been reported after this procedure, with few serious complications, although superficial pin track infections were frequent. Opening wedge hemicallotasis has been compared with dome osteotomy in patients with osteoarthritic varus deformities. Patients in the hemicallotasis group had little change in patellar tendon length or direction

angle of the tibial plateau compared with patients with dome osteotomies, who showed decreases in both. Closing wedge valgus osteotomy has been compared with opening wedge osteotomy hemicallotasis, with no clinical differences found between the two groups at 2 years.

Mizuta et al. compared distraction frequencies in patients who had opening wedge hemicallotasis. Those who had distraction of 0.25 mm eight times each day had significantly higher radiographic mineral density compared with those who had distraction 0.125 mm four times each day. Pulsed ultrasound during the consolidation phase has been shown to accelerate callus maturation. The consolidation phase begins when the mineral density of the gap is thought to be strong enough to allow fixator removal.

OPENING WEDGE HEMICALLOTASIS

Turi's opening wedge osteotomy hemicallotasis technique uses an articulated dynamic fixator, in which the patient distracts the osteotomy four times a day until correction is achieved.

TECHNIQUE 7.10

(TURI ET AL.)

- With the patient supine, tape a sandbag to the operating table to help maintain 90 degrees of flexion during the surgery. Use a tourniquet and image intensification.
- Position the fixator over the leg to check the position of the pin clamps, osteotomy site, and hinge. The proximal pins should be placed at least 15 mm below the joint line to avoid intracapsular pin placement.
- The osteotomy site is below the tibial tuberosity. Make the incision for the osteotomy before placement of the fixator so that the dissection is not encumbered. Make a longitudinal incision just medial to the tibial tuberosity extending distally 3 to 4 cm.
- Reflect the pes anserinus subperiosteally to expose the proximal tibial osteotomy site.
- Superimpose the hinge of the fixator over the lateral tibial cortex at the level of the osteotomy (Fig. 7.20A).
- When the fixator is in the proper position, secure it to the bone with temporary Kirschner wires placed through holes in the frame (Fig. 7.20B). Ensure that the fixator is at least one fingerbreadth from the skin to allow for soft-tissue swelling. Check the placement of the Kirschner wires with fluoroscopy to ensure they are perpendicular to the tibial shaft.
- Place the screw guide through the clamp for the lateral proximal pin, and push against the skin to determine the location of the incision. Make the incision, and use a 4.8-mm drill bit to make a pilot hole for the pin. Manually screw the pin into the bone through the screw guide (Fig. 7.20C).
- Repeat the procedure for the medial proximal pin. Both pins should engage the posterior cortex (Fig. 7.20D). Tighten the clamps to the pins, and remove the provisional Kirschner wires.
- Repeat the pin placement procedure for the distal pins using the fixator as a guide, and tighten the clamp to the distal pins (Fig. 7.20E).

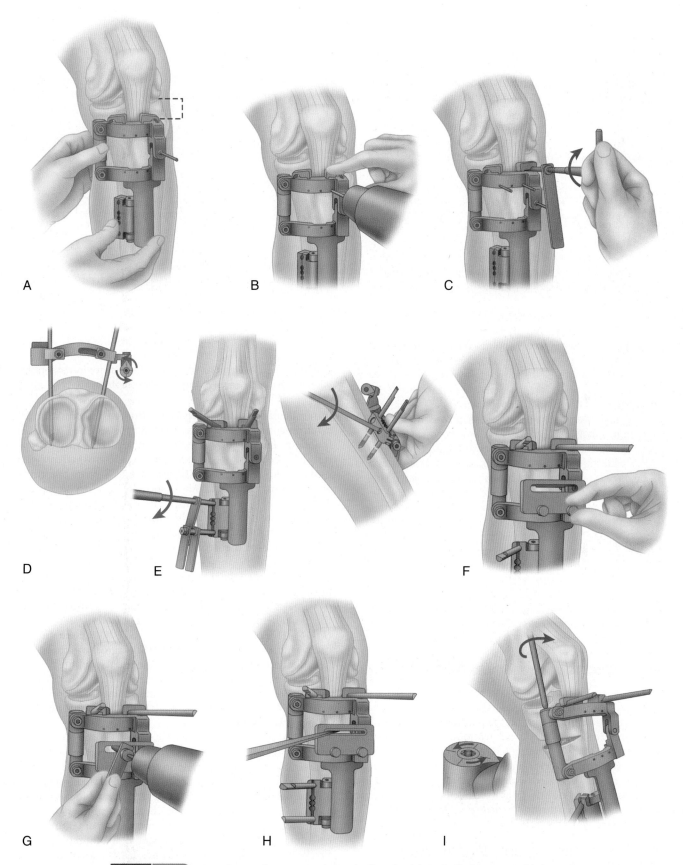

FIGURE 7.20 Opening wedge osteotomy hemicallotasis with Orthofix (Verona, Italy) dynamic external fixator. **A,** Positioning of fixator. **B,** Fixator provisionally secured with Kirschner wires. **C,** Proximal fixator pin inserted. **D,** Medial and lateral proximal fixator pins. **E,** Distal fixator pins placed. **F,** Osteotomy guide attached. **G,** Series of holes drilled at osteotomy site. **H,** Holes connected with osteotome or saw. **I,** Distraction of osteotomy. **SEE TECHNIQUE 7.10.**

- Ensure that all fixator locking and hinge screws are tightened.
- Use the plastic thumb screws to attach the osteotomy guide to the fixator (Fig. 7.20F).
- Insert a drill guide through the slot of the osteotomy guide, and make a series of holes in the medial two thirds of the proximal tibia using a drill bit (Fig. 7.20G). Complete the osteotomy by connecting the holes with a thin, straight osteotome placed through the slot of the osteotomy guide (Fig. 7.20H). Alternatively, a thin saw blade can be used.
- Remove the osteotomy guide, and open the fixator to the desired correction angle by turning the distraction mechanism (Fig. 7.20I). This ensures that the osteotomy is complete and that the desired amount of correction can be achieved. The mechanical axis of the limb can be fluoroscopically checked using a Bovie cord held from the hip joint center to the center of the ankle joint. At the knee joint, the cord should be at or just lateral to the tibial eminence.
- When the proper correction is achieved, check and record the distraction level from the markings on the fixator. At this point, close the distraction mechanism to compress the osteotomy site. Lock the fixator and carefully suture the periosteum to cover the osteotomy site.

POSTOPERATIVE CARE Continuous passive motion is begun immediately after surgery in the recovery room, usually from 0 to 45 degrees of flexion, progressing at least 20 degrees each day. Ambulation is begun the day after surgery, allowing weight bearing to tolerance with crutches. The drain is removed 1 or 2 days after surgery, depending on the output. Patients are instructed on proper pin site care and on the distraction technique. Seven days after surgery, the patient begins distracting the fixator at a rate of 1 mm/day by turning the distracter a quarter turn four times a day until the desired correction angle is achieved. Close follow-up is necessary to check weight-bearing radiographs and pin sites and to ensure that the patient is distracting the fixator properly. When the appropriate correction is achieved, the fixator is locked. If radiographs show good callus formation, the locking nut is released and dynamic loading is started. The fixator is removed after solid union is achieved, generally by 12 weeks after surgery.

Complications. Although medial opening wedge hemicallotasis avoids problems with the patellar tendon and tibial inclination, the procedure is not without complications (up to 76% in one study, including pin track infections, deep vein thrombosis, technical error, and septic arthritis). Psychosocial issues also are associated with the use of external fixation devices, and pin track infections have been reported to cause delayed septic gonarthritis. Inadequate correction also has been reported with this technique.

GENERAL COMPLICATIONS OF HIGH TIBIAL OSTEOTOMY

Other reported complications of proximal tibial osteotomy include recurrence of deformity (loss of correction), peroneal nerve palsy, nonunion, infection, knee stiffness or instability,

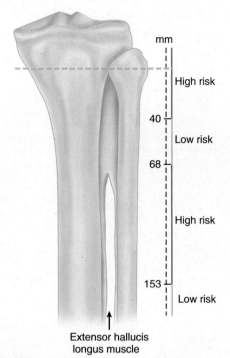

FIGURE 7.21 Regions at high and low risk for intraoperative injury of peroneal nerve during fibular osteotomy.

intraarticular fracture, deep vein thrombosis, compartment syndrome, patella infra, and osteonecrosis of the proximal fragment. Inadequate correction and recurrent varus deformity have been reported to occur in 5% to 30% of patients with proximal tibial osteotomy. Recurrence of a varus deformity was the most common complication in Coventry's report of 213 proximal tibial osteotomies. He attributed the recurrence to inadequate correction at the time of surgery and suggested that overcorrection beyond the normal 5 degrees of anatomic valgus decreased the frequency of this complication.

Peroneal nerve injury most often is related to fibular osteotomy performed in conjunction with proximal tibial osteotomy. The peroneal nerve is most at risk with osteotomy of the proximal fibula, where the nerve wraps around the neck of the fibula before dividing into deep and superficial branches (Fig. 7.21). Popliteal artery injury is rare but devastating. A cadaver study demonstrated that at 90 degrees of flexion, the distance between the osteotomy blade and the popliteal artery averaged only 10.6 mm. The authors of that study recommended keeping something substantial between the proximal tibia and the popliteal artery especially when using an oscillating power saw.

Most patients develop significant patella baja after proximal tibial osteotomy. Several factors may cause this, including shortening of the patellar tendon after prolonged immobilization, new bone formation at the site of the osteotomy in the area of the insertion of the patellar tendon, and fibrosis of the patellar tendon. The decrease in the height of the patella has no appreciable effect, however, on the success or failure of the osteotomy or the need for subsequent total joint replacement. Patella baja is likely, however, to make a subsequent total knee arthroplasty more technically demanding.

High Tibial Osteotomy or Arthroplasty. A meta-analysis by Fu et al. of clinical outcomes after high tibial osteotomy and medial compartment arthroplasty showed better knee function in the arthroplasty group but no difference in knee score. The 10-year survival rate for medial compartment arthroplasty reported by Pandit et al. was 91%. The 10-year survival rate for high tibial osteotomy was 60%. Unicompartmental arthroplasty is becoming much more popular and is less stressful for the patient than total knee arthroplasty. Of the two arthroplasty procedures, a unicompartmental arthroplasty is more likely to be "forgotten" by the patient according to Zuiderbaan et al. Becker and Hirschmann stated that patients with the varus morphotype may be better served with an osteotomy to unload the already overloaded medial compartment. Careful patient selection is necessary for the best outcome. If the underlying cause is significant malalignment, then osteotomy may be preferred. Unicompartmental arthroplasty may be best suited for true medial compartment arthritis. If the problem is an undiagnosed early inflammatory arthritis, then the best choice may be a total knee arthroplasty.

TOTAL KNEE ARTHROPLASTY AFTER PROXIMAL TIBIAL OSTEOTOMY

At 10 to 15 years after proximal tibial osteotomy, 40% of patients require conversion to total knee arthroplasty. Most series of total knee arthroplasties after proximal tibial osteotomies report slightly lower rates of good and excellent clinical results than those reported for primary total knee arthroplasty.

Studies have shown that the outcome of total knee arthroplasty in patients with previous high tibial osteotomies was not significantly different from outcomes after primary total knee arthroplasty, although total knee arthroplasty after high tibial osteotomy is technically demanding and is a longer operative procedure. Unicompartmental arthroplasty has poor results after high tibial osteotomy (28% failure at 5 years).

The operative technique of total knee arthroplasty can be complicated by several factors in patients with proximal tibial osteotomies. Obtaining adequate exposure is the most frequently encountered technical difficulty. Lateral ligamentous laxity can occur because of proximal "riding" of the fibula, and maintaining continuity of the medial soft-tissue sleeve during exposure can be difficult because scarring at the level of the osteotomy causes laxity of the medial collateral ligament. The posterior cruciate ligament usually is scarred, making posterior cruciate ligament substitution necessary. The lateral tibial plateau usually is the more deficient side and may require bone grafting or metal block augmentation. Offset of the proximal fragment laterally or posteriorly can make stem placement difficult. Patella baja may require tibial tubercle osteotomy.

Parvizi et al. reported their results of 166 total knee arthroplasties in 118 patients with previous lateral closing wedge proximal tibial osteotomies done for osteoarthritis. At the 15-year follow-up, the survival rate was 89%. Risk factors for early failure requiring revision were male gender, obesity, and age older than 60 years at the time of total knee arthroplasty. In a subgroup of patients who had bilateral total knee arthroplasties, one knee in each had not had a proximal tibial osteotomy, and the other knee had a previous proximal tibial osteotomy. In contrast to the patients reported by Meding et al., the knees with previous osteotomies did not do as well as the knees without osteotomies. The total knee arthroplasties after osteotomy had a significantly higher number of radiolucent lines than those without osteotomy. Techniques for total knee arthroplasty after proximal tibial osteotomy are described in detail in chapter 5.

DISTAL FEMORAL OSTEOTOMY

If the valgus deformity at the knee is more than 12 to 15 degrees, or the plane of the knee joint deviates from the horizontal by more than 10 degrees, Coventry recommended a distal femoral varus osteotomy rather than a proximal tibial varus osteotomy. In a comparative study, Berruto et al. found that functional results after supracondylar osteotomy did not differ significantly from those after total knee arthroplasty, and they suggested that femoral osteotomy is a valid alternative to total knee arthroplasty in active patients younger than 65 years with valgus angulation of no more than 15 degrees (Fig. 7.22). Reported success rates for distal femoral osteotomies performed for osteoarthritis range from 71% to 86% good or excellent results. Poor outcomes have been noted in patients with rheumatoid arthritis and patients with inadequate motion of the knee before distal femoral osteotomy.

Total knee arthroplasty after distal femoral osteotomy can be complicated by exposure difficulties from scarring and difficulty in hardware removal. Blade plates and supracondylar compression screw devices usually must be removed before preparation of the distal femur for total knee arthroplasty. If a supracondylar locking plate (Fig. 7.23) is used for the osteotomy, distal femoral instrumentation can be performed after percutaneous locking screw removal and the use of a short intramedullary guide rod and extramedullary alignment instrumentation. Opening wedge distal femoral varus osteotomy techniques have been described for lateral compartment osteoarthritis of the knee. One 5-year follow-up study of 18 opening wedge osteotomies demonstrated a cumulative survival of 80% comparable to that after closing wedge osteotomy. The technique is, however, technically demanding and reoperation is common.

The technique for a closing wedge distal femoral varus osteotomy is described next. The use of patient-specific, printed cutting guides can significantly reduce operative and fluoroscopy time according to Shi et al. in a 54-patient comparative study.

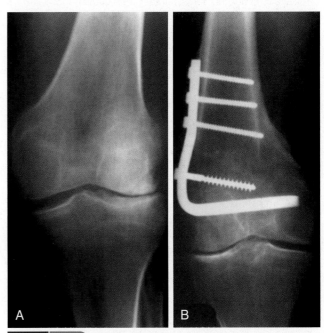

FIGURE 7.22 Varus distal femoral osteotomy. **A,** Preoperative radiograph. **B,** Radiograph 10 years postoperatively.

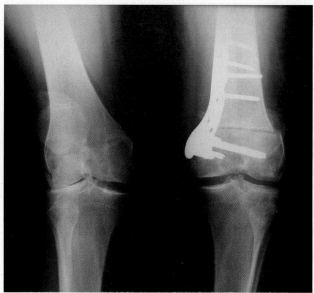

FIGURE 7.23 Distal femoral locking plate. Supracondylar osteotomy performed with a locking plate. Distal screws can be removed percutaneously to allow instrumentation of the distal femur without the need for plate removal.

VARUS DISTAL FEMORAL OSTEOTOMY

In Coventry's method, a medial approach is used. An anterior total knee incision also can be used by exposing the medial distal femur through a subvastus approach. This can avoid skin bridges if subsequent total knee arthroplasty is required.

TECHNIQUE 7.11

(COVENTRY)
- Make a medial incision separating the rectus femoris and vastus medialis at their junction, expose the lower part of the femur, and displace the suprapatellar pouch distally without opening it until the base of the medial femoral condyle is exposed.
- To achieve the desired position of the femoral condyles, construct a template (1) to indicate the proper size of the wedge of bone to be removed and (2) to establish the required angle between the plate of the blade plate used for internal fixation and the lateral surface of the cortex at the time the blade plate is inserted (Fig. 7.24). The tip of the blade should just penetrate the opposite cortex for firm fixation. Use an appropriate retractor and maintain knee flexion to protect the neurovascular structures.
- Determine the proper site and angle of insertion and the length of the blade by evaluating radiographs of a Kirschner wire inserted in the distal fragment. Use this wire, when in the desired position, as a guide for insertion of the nail.
- Use a power saw to cut the femur after insertion of the blade of the plate.
- Bring the plate into contact with the diaphysis after removing a wedge or simply cutting across the bone and countersinking the distal end of the proximal fragment into the medullary cavity of the distal portion.

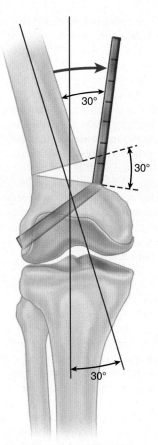

FIGURE 7.24 Coventry technique of lower femoral osteotomy. Angle to be corrected is measured on preoperative radiograph, and nail of blade plate is driven into femoral metaphysis so that plate can accomplish desired correction when attached to osteotomized femoral shaft. Wedge with apical angle equal to amount of correction is removed with osteotomy. **SEE TECHNIQUE 7.11.**

- Secure the plate to the proximal fragment with screws. Correct any flexion deformity by appropriate placement of the nail plate. Insert suction drainage tubes and close the wound.

POSTOPERATIVE CARE The extremity is treated in the same manner as after a proximal tibial osteotomy. (see also Video 7.1.)

REFERENCES

GENERAL

Liu HX, Wen H, Hu YZ, et al.: Percutaneous quadriceps tendon pie-crusting release of extension contracture of the knee, *Orthop Traumatol Surg Res* 100:333, 2014.

Pujol N, Boisrenoult P, Beaufils P: Post-traumatic knee stiffness: surgical techniques, *Orthop Traumatol Surg Res* 101:S179, 2015.

PAINFUL PARAARTICULAR CALCIFICATIONS, BURSITIS, AND TENDINITIS

Shapiro SA, Hernandez LO, Montero DP: Snapping pes anserinus and the diagnostic utility of dynamic ultrasound, *J Clin Imaging Sci* 7:39, 2017.

Painful Paraarticular Calcifications, Bursitis, and Tendinitis

Huang YC, Yeh WL: Endoscopic treatment of prepatellar bursitis, *Int Orthop* 35:355–358, 2011.

Pan X, Zhang X, Liu Z, et al.: Treatment for chronic synovitis of knee: arthroscopic or open synovectomy, *Rheumatol Int* 32:1733, 2012.

Saylik M, Gökkus K: Treatment of baker cyst, by using open posterior cystectomy and supine arthroscopy on reclacitrant cases (103 knees), *BMC Musculoskelet Disord* 17(1):435, 2016.

Yang B, Wang F, Lou Y, et al.: A comparison of clinical efficacy between different surgical approaches for popliteal cyst, *J Orthop Surg Res* 12(1):158, 2017.

RHEUMATOID ARTHRITIS

Aletaha D, Neogi T, Solman AJ, et al.: 2010 Rheumatoid Arthritis Classification criteria. An American College of Rheumatology/European League against Rheumatism collaborative initiative, *Arthritis Rheumatism* 62(9):2569, 2010.

Chalmers PN, Sherman SL, Raphael BS, Su EP: Rheumatoid synovectomy: does the surgical approach matter? *Clin Orthop Relat Res* 469:2062, 2011.

Goodman SM, Springer B, Guyatt G, et al.: 2017 American College of Rheumatology/American Association of Hip and Knee Surgeons Guideline for the perioperative management of antirheumatic medication in patients with rheumatic diseases undergoing elective total hip or total knee arthroplasty, *J Arthroplasty* 32:2628, 2017.

Jämsen E, Virta LJ, Hakala M, et al.: The decline in joint replacement surgery in rheumatoid arthritis is associated with a concomitant increase in the intensity of anti-rheumatic therapy: a nationwide register-based study form 1995 through 2010, *Acta Orthop* 84:331, 2013.

Ossyssek B, Anders S, Grifka J, Straub RH: Surgical synovectomy decreases density of sensory nerve fibers in synovial tissue of noninflamed controls and rheumatoid arthritis patients, *J Orthop Res* 29:297, 2011.

OSTEOARTHRITIS

Becker R, Hirschmann M: The pertinent question in treatment of unicompartmental osteoarthritis of the knee: high tibial osteotomy or unicondylar knee arthroplasty or total knee arthroplasty, *Knee Surg Sports Traumatol Arthrosc* 25:637, 2017.

Darnis A, Villa V, Debette C, et al.: Vascular injuries during closing-wedge high tibial osteotomy: a cadaveric angiographic study, *Orthop Traumatol Surg Res* 100:891, 2014.

Dillon JP, Freedman I, Tan JS, et al.: Endoscopic bursectomy for the treatment of septic pre-patellar bursitis: a case series, *Arch Orthop Trauma Surg* 132:921, 2012.

Duivenvoorden T, Brouwer RW, Baan A, et al.: Comparison of closing-wedge and opening-wedge high tibial osteotomy for medial compartment osteoarthritis of the knee: a randomized controlled trial with a six-year follow-up, *J Bone Joint Surg* 96A:1425, 2014.

Fu D, Li G, Chen K, et al.: Comparison of high tibial osteotomy and unicompartmental knee arthroplasty in the treatment of unicompartmental osteoarthritis: a meta-analysis, *J Arthroplasty* 28:759, 2013.

Jevsevar DS, Brown GA, Jones DL, et al.: The American Academy of Orthopaedic Surgeons evidence-based guideline on treatment of osteoarthritis of the knee, ed 2, *J Bone Joint Surg* 95(20):1885–1886, 2013.

Kim KI, Lee SH, Ahn JH, Kim JS: Arthroscopic anatomic study of posteromedial joint capsule in knee joint associated with popliteal cyst, *Arch Orthop Trauma Surg* 134:979, 2014.

Koh YG, Jo SB, Kwon OR, et al.: Mesenchymal stem cell injections improve symptoms of knee osteoarthritis, *Arthroscopy* 30:420, 2014.

Liu HX, Wen H, Hu YZ, et al.: Percutaneous quadriceps tendon pie-crusting release of extension contracture of the knee, *Orthop Traumatol Surg Res* 100:333, 2014.

Ogawa H, Matsumoto K, Akiyama H: The prevention of a lateral hinge fracture as a complication of a medial opening wedge high tibial osteotomy: a case control study, *Bone Joint J* 99-B(7):887, 2017.

Pandit H, Hamilton TW, Jenkins C, et al.: The clinical outcome of minimally invasive phase 3 Oxford unicompartmental knee arthroplasty: a 15-year follow-up of 1000 UKAs, *Bone Joint J England* 97B:1493, 2015.

Pujol N, Boisrenoult P, Beaufils P: Post-traumatic knee stiffness: surgical techniques, *Orthop Traumatol Surg Res* 101:S179, 2015.

Sadek AF, Osman MK, Laklok MA: Management of combined knee medial compartmental and patellofemoral osteoarthritis with lateral closing wedge osteotomy with anterior translation of the distal tibial fragment: Does the degree of anteriorization affect the functional outcome and posterior tibial slope? *Knee* 23(5):857, 2016.

Saithna A, Kundra R, Getgood A, Spalding T: Opening wedge distal femoral varus osteotomy for lateral compartment osteoarthritis of the valgus knee, *Knee* 21(1):172, 2014.

Shi J, Lv W, Wang Y, et al.: Three dimensional patient-specific printed cutting guides for closing-wedge distal femoral osteotomy, *Int Orthop* 2019. [Epub ahead of print].

Stanley JC, Robinson KG, Devitt BM, et al.: Computer assisted alignment of opening wedge high tibial osteotomy provides limited improvement of radiographic outcomes compared to flouroscopic alignment, *Knee* 23(2):289, 2016.

Wu ZP, Zhang P, Bai JZ, et al.: Comparison of navigated and conventional high tibial osteotomy for the treatment of osteoarthritic knees with varus deformity: a meta-analysis, *Int J Surg* 55:211, 2018.

Zhou XN, Li B, Wang JS, Bai LH: Surgical treatment of popliteal cyst: a systematic review and meta-analysis, *J Orthop Surg Res* 11:22, 2016.

Zuiderbaan HA, van der List JP, Khamaisy S, et al.: Unicompartmental knee arthroplasty versus total knee arthroplasty: which type of artificial joint do patients forget? *Knee Surg Sports Traumatol Arthrosc* 25(3):681, 2017.

The complete list of references is available online at Expert Consult.com.

PART III

RECONSTRUCTIVE PROCEDURES OF THE ANKLE IN ADULTS

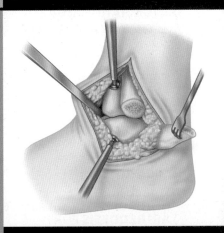

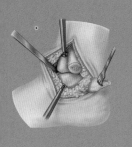

CHAPTER **8**

TOTAL ANKLE ARTHROPLASTY

G. Andrew Murphy

Although many orthopaedic surgeons abandoned ankle arthroplasty because of high failure and complication rates, the continued search for alternatives to ankle arthrodesis for ankle arthritis has led to a renewal of interest. The development of contemporary designs more biomechanically compatible with the anatomy and kinematics of the ankle, improved techniques and instrumentation, and the introduction of biologic ingrowth for component fixation have led to a profusion of studies evaluating the design, technique, and outcomes of total ankle arthroplasty (TAA). The results of these studies have spurred an increase in the use of TAA as an alternative to traditional ankle arthrodesis for a number of conditions. As surgeons become more experienced with the technique, the frequency of TAA has increased dramatically over the past decade, particularly in patients with posttraumatic arthritis and osteoarthritis.

DEVELOPMENT OF TOTAL ANKLE ARTHROPLASTY SYSTEMS

Since the first report of TAA in the 1970s, many TAA systems have been introduced. The first-generation, cemented, constrained designs were very stable but required extensive bony resection for implantation and frequently failed because of loosening, subsidence, and extensive osteolysis. Second-generation, less constrained implants required less bone resection and did not require cement fixation; because shear forces and torsion at the bone-prosthesis were reduced, loosening was less frequent.

However, increased polyethylene wear and failure compromised the stability of the components, often leading to painful impingement and subluxation or complete dislocation of the components. Contemporary, third-generation, semi-constrained total ankle systems consist of three components: a metallic baseplate that is fixed to the tibia, a domed or condylar-shaped metallic component that resurfaces the talus, and an ultrahigh-molecular-weight polyethylene bearing surface interposed between the tibial and talar components. Systems in which the polyethylene component is locked into the baseplate are often referred to as "two-piece" or "fixed-bearing" designs, whereas those with the polyethylene component not attached to the baseplate are called "three-piece" or mobile or meniscal bearing systems. Currently, there are over 50 different TAA systems in use worldwide, most of which have not been approved for use by the US Food and Drug Administration (FDA). There is no convincing evidence of the clear superiority of one design over another among the currently available systems; choice of a prosthesis depends on individual patient factors, institutional factors, and the surgeon's training and experience.

DESIGN RATIONALE

The development of an implant system that mimics the normal anatomy and biomechanics of the ankle and achieves success rates similar to those of hip and knee arthroplasty has been hampered by several anatomic features of the ankle joint: (1) the ankle has significantly less contact area between joint surfaces than the hip or knee; (2) the ankle experiences 5.5 times body weight with normal ambulation, compared with three times body weight at the knee; and (3) the articular cartilage surface of the ankle is uniformly thinner than that of the knee.

The biomechanical concepts that have resulted in the most recent generation of ankle arthroplasties are somewhat beyond the scope of a surgical-oriented textbook; however, the number and variety of implants on the market demand a familiarity of basic principles of component design.

The design of TAA systems continues to evolve as we learn more about the modes of failure from longer-term studies. First-generation implants had high rates of osteolysis, implant loosening, tibial and talar bone loss, and wound complications. Second-generation designs used porous metal-backed surfaces to improve osseous integration; replaced the tibiotalar, talofibular, and medial-malleolar-talar articulations; and/or improved stability by fusing the syndesmosis. Complications related to nonunion of the syndesmosis, polyethylene wear, and migration and impingement of the implants led to a number of modifications in third- and fourth-generation designs: less bone resection, more bony ingrowth, retention of ligamentous support, and anatomic balancing.

FIXED-BEARING VERSUS MOBILE-BEARING DESIGNS

Most modern implants fall into two basic groups: those with a mobile polyethylene component that has the ability, at least in theory, to move under the tibial component to adapt to changes in joint forces (Fig. 8.1A) and those with the polyethylene component fixed rigidly to the tibial component (Fig. 8.1B). Mobile-bearing designs are used most commonly in Europe and have a long history of outcomes from which they can be evaluated. Another theoretical advantage of these designs is the "forgiveness" of the implant, which allows small variances in alignment to be compensated for by a reorientation of the prosthesis to accommodate the joint forces. The ability of the polyethylene component to move should, in theory, keep the articulation between the talar component and the polyethylene component more congruent and less likely to lead to edge load and advanced wear. In experienced hands, however, there is a question of how much the polyethylene component actually moves under the tibia. Barg et al. found very little anteroposterior movement of the talar component under the tibia in follow-up radiographs of a three-component, mobile-bearing design. They noted that the prosthesis functioned largely like a fixed-bearing design, but with a possible advantage of allowing an individualized position of the polyethylene insert in response to individual soft-tissue loads produced by different ankle joint configurations. Aside from the STAR ankle implants (Fig. 8.2), implants approved for use in the United States are fixed-bearing designs.

Proponents of fixed-bearing designs suggest that the normal ankle joint, as opposed to the knee, has a more stable central axis of motion and less need for an additional degree of freedom of motion. Backside polyethylene wear against the tibial component is a major concern with mobile-bearing designs and less with fixed designs. Attention to detail in the proper alignment of the prosthesis along the mechanical axis of the limb has been suggested to prevent excessive wear.

A multicenter study by Gaudot et al. comparing fixed-bearing with mobile-bearing implants found no significant differences in accuracy of positioning, clinical and

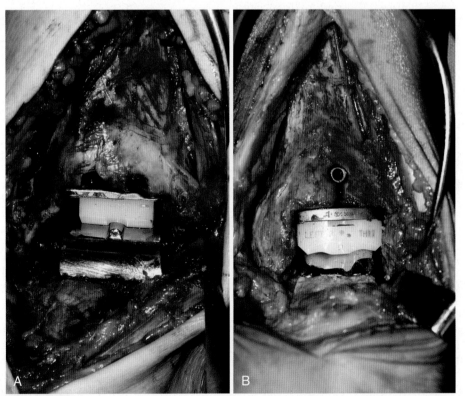

FIGURE 8.1 **A,** Mobile-bearing, three-component total ankle replacement; polyethylene is independent of tibial component. **B,** Fixed-bearing, two-component ankle replacement; polyethylene is fixed to tibial component. (From Easley ME, Adams SB Jr, Hembree C, DeOrio JK: Current concepts review: results of total ankle arthroplasty, *J Bone Joint Surg* 93A:1455, 2011.)

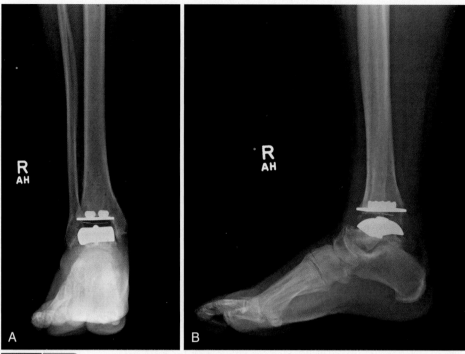

FIGURE 8.2   **A** and **B,** STAR arthroplasty in patient with good bone quality and minimal deformity. (Courtesy Dr. William C. McGarvey, Houston, TX.)

radiographic mobility, or morbidity. In a more recent randomized trial, Queen et al. also found no clinically meaningful differences in outcomes between the two implant types when examining gait mechanics and pain at 1-year follow-up. The most recent American Orthopaedic Foot and Ankle Society (AOFAS) scores were higher for patients with fixed-bearing implants than for those with mobile-bearing implants, and radiolucent lines and subchondral cysts were less frequent. In contrast, Currier et al. analyzed 70 retrieved ankle implants, most commonly for loosening and polyethylene fracture. Loosening occurred more frequently in fixed-bearing designs than in mobile-bearing designs. Lundeen et al. in a study of patients with a third-generation mobile-bearing TAA concluded that the multiplanar articulation in mobile-bearing TAA may reduce excessively high peak pressures during tibial and talar motion, which may have a positive effect on gait pattern, polyethylene wear, and implant longevity.

ALIGNMENT

Currently available implant systems are designed to be placed along the mechanical axis of the limb and depend on satisfactory alignment above and below the ankle joint. The most common method of obtaining correct alignment is an external alignment jig, using intraoperative fluoroscopy to judge the alignment. At least one system uses an intramedullary alignment rod (Fig. 8.3). One innovation is a tomography-produced customized cutting jig, such as those available for knee arthroplasty. Patient-specific instrumentation has been successfully used in arthroplasty of other joints (e.g., knee, shoulder, hip), but has rarely been described in TAA. Cadaver and clinical studies have shown this instrumentation to provide accuracy and reproducibility among multiple surgeons, implants, and facilities. Hamid et al. did not find a difference in postoperative alignment with patient-specific instrumentation or standard referencing; however, use of patient-specific

instrumentation significantly decreased operative time and, thus, costs. Another fairly recent system uses a lateral approach to more accurately reproduce the center of rotation of the ankle and minimize bone resection (Fig. 8.4).

INGROWTH VERSUS CEMENT FIXATION

In the United States, FDA-approved designs, except for the fourth-generation STAR ankle and the Hintermann Series2, are approved for use with cement and, although they are often porous coated similar to the cement-less implants of the hip or knee, implantation of the components without cement is considered off-label use. There are few reports comparing the use of cement with ingrowth fixation in the literature, and at this time, there does not appear to be a consensus on the issue.

METAPHYSEAL FIXATION

Distribution of the forces over as broad an area as possible is one goal of implant design. Tibial components should, if possible, rest flush on the cut surface of the metaphysis of the tibia and engage the anterior and posterior cortices without significant overhang. The use of stems of some type to help with the stability of the implant and broaden the weight-bearing surface seems prudent. Some designs have stems that are placed through a cut-out notch in the anterior cortex, and others are driven into the metaphysis in an intramedullary fashion. Changes in the geometry and depth of resection of the tibia and talus have been suggested to decrease aseptic component loosening. In a biomechanical study, standard flat-cut resections were compared to subject-specific, anatomic radius-based (round) resections to determine their effect on bony support. Statistically significant decreases in bony support for both the talus (8% to 19%) and tibia (8% to 46%) were seen with flat-cut resections. The authors concluded that biomechanical characteristics of TAA affected by bony support of the prostheses, including implant stability

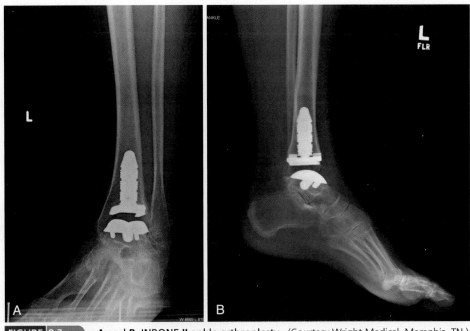

FIGURE 8.3   **A and B,** INBONE II ankle arthroplasty. (Courtesy Wright Medical, Memphis, TN.)

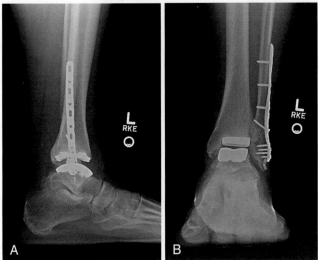

FIGURE 8.4   **A and B,** Trabecular metal total ankle (Zimmer, Warsaw, IN). (Courtesy Dr. Saltzman and Dr. Barg, University of Utah.)

and resistance to subsidence, may be improved with round resections compared to flat-cut resections.

TALAR COMPONENT DESIGN

Because the talar component is subjected to high forces during normal gait, talar components that cover the entire surface of the talus might have the advantage of better distribution of these forces and smaller chance of subsidence into the body of the talus. Balanced against this is the concern for wear or impingement in the medial and lateral ankle gutters. Fukuda et al. demonstrated that a talar component placed in a malrotated position had poor contact characteristics at the extremes of ankle motion, causing concern for increased polyethylene wear or talar component loosening. Evaluating the contact pressures with the Agility total ankle design, Nicholson et al. found pressures higher than those recommended for the talar component–polyethylene articulation. Although this design

has been modified since this study in 2004, the findings demonstrate the issue of talar component design regarding contact pressure and potential wear.

POLYETHYLENE WEAR

Wear debris of polyethylene within joint replacement systems has been shown to result in clinical complications, including osteolysis and component loosening. Highly cross-linked polyethylene (HXPE) was introduced to avoid these complications and has been shown to result in improved wear performance in total hip, knee, and shoulder implants. In a biomechanical study of bicondylar, fixed-bearing total ankle implants with either conventional polyethylene or HXPE, Bischoff et al. found that HXPE samples exhibited a wear rate reduction of 74% compared with conventional polyethylene articulating on metal. The extent to which these laboratory findings affect clinical outcomes has not been determined, and clinical outcomes studies are needed to clarify the benefits of HXPE in TAA implants.

PREOPERATIVE EVALUATION

A thorough understanding of the patient's medical history and review of systems are important in the decision-making process and the consideration of the patient for TAA. Systemic diseases such as diabetes, inflammatory arthritis, chronic obstructive pulmonary disease, and peripheral vascular or heart disease may adversely affect the outcome and healing of the incision. Conditions such as sleep apnea, malnutrition, vitamin D deficiency, and depression are associated with decreased functional outcomes and poor results. We do not perform elective TAA in active smokers. It must be clear that the ankle joint is indeed the cause of the patient's primary complaint. Many patients have adjacent joint disease that might also need to be treated before or at the time of surgery. Selective injections of lidocaine are helpful in accurately identifying the painful pathologic process. A complete assessment of the limb is important. A lumbar spine pathologic process with sciatica and radicular lower extremity pain or degenerative disease of the hip or knee may cause a change in the management plan. Patients with combined knee and ankle arthritis and deformity often are best managed by correction of the knee deformity first, followed by the ankle replacement.

A thorough evaluation of the neurovascular status of the limb is essential, and any concerns should prompt a formal vascular evaluation. The patient's gait should be evaluated for limp, and any alterations of knee or hip motion to compensate for the arthritic ankle and limb-length difference should be assessed. The standing evaluation is important for clinical assessment of ankle and hindfoot alignment. Is there a supramalleolar deformity that must be corrected? Is the hindfoot well aligned, or is there a component of varus or valgus? Clinical assessment of the gastrocsoleus complex and the Achilles tendon is important. The Silfverskiöld test for selective gastrocnemius tightness might reveal a contracture that is independent of ankle range of motion and that must be released intraoperatively. Coetzee and Castro demonstrated the inability to distinguish true range of motion of the tibiotalar joint on clinical examination and proposed a radiographic evaluation of the range of motion preoperatively. Nonetheless, an idea of sagittal plane range of motion is important. Overall hindfoot motion is important as well. A stiff, arthritic hindfoot might be the difference between choosing arthroplasty or arthrodesis. Strength testing of the leg motor groups should not reveal major deficits that would impair the outcome. The anterior skin should be stable and without lesions that would impair the healing of the surgical incision.

At a minimum, standing radiographs of the ankle in anteroposterior, lateral, and mortise views should be obtained. Any suspicion of proximal limb malalignment should be evaluated with standing lower extremity films. Because an accurate assessment of the alignment of the hindfoot is not possible with standing films of the ankle, Frigg et al. described a hindfoot alignment view (Fig. 8.5) that gives a better appreciation of overall alignment and helps to determine if an adjunctive procedure is needed to improve the alignment of the foot distal to the ankle joint.

Although coronal plane deformities usually are the focus of radiographic evaluation before TAA, sagittal plane deformities have been shown to alter the mechanics and joint reaction forces more than coronal plane deformities. Several methods for evaluating the lateral position of the talus on radiographs have been described. Veljkovic et al. described a sagittal talar position measurement that they named the lateral tibial station (LTS); the LTS defines the center of rotation of the talus as related to the anatomic tibial axis. In a study of 82 ankles, they showed that this measurement can be reliably obtained on preoperative weight-bearing lateral radiographs; the mean LTS measurement was 1.7 mm (normal range, 0.8076 to 3.1496 mm). The value of the LTS in evaluating ankle pathology remains to be established.

Radiographic evaluation should include assessment of the quality of the bone stock, coronal plane alignment of the ankle with supramalleolar deformities or joint incongruencies, the presence of osteophytes requiring removal, adjacent joint arthritis or malalignment that requires correction, calcaneal pitch angle as a predictor of gastrocsoleus contracture, and the presence of major cysts or defects that will need grafting.

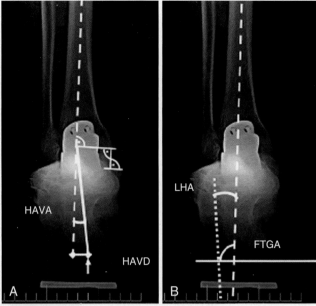

FIGURE 8.5 **A** and **B,** Hindfoot alignment view of right total ankle replacement. *FTGA,* Frontal tibial ground angle; *HAVA,* hindfoot alignment view angle; *HAVD,* hindfoot alignment view distance; *LHA,* lateral heel angle; *white line,* reconstruction of ankle joint based on length of medial malleolus. (From Frigg A, Nigg B, Hinz L, et al: Clinical relevance of hindfoot alignment view in total ankle replacement, *Foot Ankle Int* 31:871–879, 2010.)

The effect of bone mineral density (BMD) on outcomes of TAA has not been clearly delineated. Dual-energy x-ray absorptiometry (DEXA) scanning generally is not obtained to evaluate BMD before TAA because of the additional time and costs involved. CT scans are, however, often obtained before TAA, and Hounsfield units measured on CT have been shown to correlate well with DEXA T-scores. In a study of 198 ankles, BMD (Hounsfield units) was measured on preoperative CT scans and compared to outcomes at 2.4-year follow-up. After controlling for age, gender, and BMI, only tibial Hounsfield units of less than 200 were significantly associated with periprosthetic fracture. Prophylactic internal fixation of the medial malleolus may be considered for patients with tibial Hounsfield units of less than 200 as measured on CT scans. Severe osteoporosis often is listed as a contraindication to TAA, but newer implant designs and surgical techniques (e.g., noncemented fixation and patient-specific implants) have overcome some of the problems of TAA in osteoporotic bone, and outcomes have improved, especially in older, more sedentary patients with osteoporosis. DEXA scanning or BMD evaluation on CT scans is indicated in patients at risk for osteoporosis.

INDICATIONS

Although degenerative, inflammatory, and posttraumatic arthritic conditions of the ankle are the primary indications for TAA, there is little clinical evidence on which to base more specific indications and contraindications. The ideal candidate for ankle arthroplasty has been described as an older, thin, low-demand individual with minimal deformity and retained ankle range of motion. These descriptions, however, are vague and controversial. Some have defined "young" as younger than 50 years of age and "thin" as weighing less than 200 lb, but there is no clinical evidence to support these classifications. Commonly cited contraindications to TAA include age younger than 50 years, history of poor patient compliance, heavy industrial labor, heavy smoking, uncontrolled diabetes with neuropathy, significant ankle instability, angular deformity of more than 10 to 15 degrees, vascular insufficiency, obesity (over 250 lb), significant bone loss, osteonecrosis, and active or previous infection. More recently, however, a number of these contraindications have been questioned. Demetracopoulos et al. reviewed outcomes in 395 consecutive patients according to age (younger than 55, 55 to 70, and older than 70 years of age) and found no differences in pain relief or physical outcomes or in the incidences of wound complications, reoperations, or revisions. Tenebaum et al. compared clinical and gait outcomes in patients older than 70 years to those in patients between 50 and 60 years of age; improvements were equivalent in the two groups. Good results have been reported in both obese patients and diabetic patients (see sections on Obesity and Diabetes), as well as those with angular deformities of more than 20 degrees (see section on Deformity Correction).

Because TAA is generally considered a "motion-sparing" procedure rather than a "motion-producing" procedure, its use in individuals with ankle stiffness has been limited; however, Brodsky et al. compared outcomes to preoperative range of motion and found that, although a low preoperative range of motion was predictive of overall lower physical function, patients with stiff ankles had clinically greater improvements in function. These findings suggest that TAA can offer clinically meaningful improvements in gait function and should be considered for patients with end-stage tibiotalar arthritis, even with limited sagittal range of motion.

Reports are variable concerning the outcomes of TAA in arthritis of different etiologies; most studies, however, have not found etiology to significantly affect implant survival. Bennett et al. reviewed the outcomes of 173 TAAs of differing etiologies (osteoarthritis, rheumatoid arthritis, pilon fracture, ankle fracture, and posttraumatic arthritis without previous fracture) and found no major differences in any of the reported outcomes at 2-year follow-up. Whatever the etiology of the arthritis, severe involvement does not necessarily portend a poor result. In a group of 124 patients, Chambers et al. found no differences in Short-Form 36 (SF-36) scores regardless of Kellgren-Lawrence grade of arthritis severity. Those with the most severe arthritis (Kellgren-Lawrence grade 4) had the most improvement in all domains of the Foot and Ankle Outcome Score and were more satisfied (91%) with their outcomes than all other groups (50%); 94% of patients with severe arthritis thought their quality of life had been improved compared to 47% in those with severity grades of less than 4. Although radiographic severity is an important factor that should be considered, it does not appear to contradict TAA.

TOTAL ANKLE ARTHROPLASTY OR ANKLE ARTHRODESIS FOR ANKLE ARTHRITIS

Ankle arthrodesis (see chapter 9) has long been the gold standard for the surgical treatment of moderate to severe ankle arthritis. It is, therefore, reasonable to ask if there is a compelling reason to pursue TAA as a treatment option for patients with ankle arthritis. Although the patient satisfaction rate after ankle arthrodesis is fairly high, there are certainly circumstances in which arthrodesis might not be the best procedure, including preexisting subtalar or other hindfoot arthritis, contralateral hindfoot or ankle arthritis, and hip or knee impairment such that motion through the ankle joint may be beneficial to the overall limb and patient function.

No level I studies have directly compared the two procedures, and reports in the literature are contradictory (Table 8.1). The most recent reports seem to favor TAA with the latest-generation implants over arthrodesis, citing better functional outcomes, fewer complications, and better patient satisfaction. Some gait studies have noted no difference in gait patterns after arthroplasty and arthrodesis, whereas others report more nearly normal gait and better walking on uneven surfaces after arthroplasty; gait appears to be improved by either procedure. Daniels et al. compared intermediate outcomes (mean 5.5-year follow-up) of arthrodesis (107 patients) and arthroplasty (281 patients) in a diverse cohort of patients and found comparable clinical outcomes; however, rates of reoperation and major complications were higher after ankle arthroplasty. Norvell et al. found that ankle-specific adverse events were infrequent and only weakly associated with operative procedure. Careful patient selection is mandatory for the success of either of these procedures in the treatment of ankle arthritis.

OUTPATIENT TOTAL ANKLE ARTHROPLASTY

The success of outpatient total hip, knee, and shoulder arthroplasty, with no compromise of safety, satisfaction, or results, has prompted many surgeons to move TAA to an ambulatory surgical center. Although there are relatively few reports of the outcomes of this procedure, available reports cite good outcomes with few complications, in addition to cost savings and patient satisfaction. Two reviews of complications in outpatient TAA reported overall complication rates of 5% and 15%; most complications were minor, and readmissions and reoperation were infrequent. In a comparison of outpatient and inpatient TAA, Gonzales et al. found a 13% cost savings in the outpatient group, with a low complication rate and high patient satisfaction. The most important aspect of outpatient TAA, as with any outpatient arthroplasty, is careful patient selection. An algorithm developed by our surgeons for selecting patients for outpatient total joint arthroplasty is a helpful guide (Fig. 8.6). There is limited evidence to determine specific patient factors that may preclude outpatient TAA surgery; however, experience in arthroplasty of the foot and ankle and other joints has identified various patient factors that are associated with perioperative complications and a longer length of hospital stay, such as elevated HbA1c level, obesity, hypoalbuminemia, age greater than 64, increased operating room time, American Society of Anesthesiologists (ASA) score of 2 or higher, and presence of comorbidities. Taylor and Parekh formulated a detailed algorithm specifically for outpatient TAA based on a number of patient and procedure characteristics (Fig. 8.7).

In addition to selecting appropriate patients, appropriate use of a multimodal perioperative and postoperative pain management protocol is essential. The choice of pain management

TABLE 8.1

Reported Outcomes of Ankle Arthroplasty Compared With Ankle Arthrodesis

STUDY	PATIENTS	FOLLOW-UP	RESULTS
SooHoo et al. (2007)	4705 arthrodesis 480 TAA	5 years	Higher risk of complications in arthroplasty group but less frequent subtalar joint arthritis requiring fusion
Haddad et al. (2007)	852 arthroplasty 1262 arthrodesis	Literature review	Intermediate outcomes of arthroplasty and arthrodesis roughly equivalent
Saltzman et al. (2009)	224 patients	2 years	Arthroplasty group had better function and equivalent pain relief as ankles treated with arthrodesis
Slobogean et al. (2010)	107 patients	1 years	Significant improvements on preference-based quality of life measures in both; no significant differences
Schuh et al. (2011)	41 patients	3 years	No significant differences in activity levels, participation in sports scores, or UCLA and AOFAS scores
Krause et al. (2011)	161 patients	3 years	Significantly higher complication rate with arthroplasty (54%) than with arthrodesis (26%)
Flavin et al. (2013)	28 patients	Gait study	Arthroplasty produced a more symmetric vertical ground reaction force curve, which was closer to that of the controls that the curve of the arthrodesis group
Daniels et al. (2014)	388 patients	5.5 years	Intermediate-term clinical outcomes comparable; rates of reoperation and major complications higher after arthroplasty
Jiang et al. (2015)	12,250 arthrodesis 3002 arthroplasty	N/A	Arthroplasty independently associated with lower risk of blood transfusion, nonhome discharge, and overall complication rate; however, no significant difference in risk for the majority of medical perioperative complications
Jastifer et al. (2015)	77 patients	2 years (gait study)	Both had improved walking performance on uneven surfaces; arthroplasty patients had higher scores walking up stairs, down stairs, and uphill
Pedowitz et al. (2016)	47 arthroplasty 27 arthrodesis	Minimum 2 years	TAA preserves more anatomic movement, has better pain relief, and better patient-reported function
Stavrakis and SooHoo (2016)	1280 arthroplasty 8491 arthrodesis		Short-term complication rates low for both procedures; lower rates of readmission and periprosthetic joint/wound infection with TAA
DiGiovanni and Guss (2017)	273	3 years	Improvements in MFA and SF-36 scores significantly better with arthroplasty
Odum et al. (2017)	1574 arthroplasty 1574 arthrodesis	Data from NIS	Arthrodesis associated with a 1.8 times higher risk of a major complication, but a 29% lower risk of a minor complication
Kim et al. (2017)	Meta-analysis	TAA 6-67 months AA 6-62 months	Similar clinical outcomes; frequency of re-operation and major surgical complications significantly increased with TAA
Norvell et al. (2018)	494		Ankle-specific adverse events were infrequent and only weakly associated with operative procedure

AOFAS, American Orthopaedic Foot and Ankle Society; *MFA,* Musculoskeletal Function Assessment; *N/A,* not applicable; *NIS,* Nationwide Inpatient Sample; *SF-36,* Short-Form 36; *TAA,* total ankle arthroplasty; *UCLA,* University of California, Los Angeles.

protocols has shifted away from oral and intravenous administration of narcotics to peripheral nerve blocks and indwelling catheters as better options. Continuous popliteal sciatic nerve block is commonly used for major foot and ankle reconstructions. Liposomal bupivacaine (Exparel; Pacira Pharmaceuticals, Parsippany, NJ) administered as a periarticular injection has been shown to have marked benefits in postoperative pain control. Mulligan et al. compared liposomal bupivacaine to popliteal sciatic nerve block for TAA and found no significant differences between the groups with regard to complications, emergency department visits, readmissions, reoperations, visual analog scale (VAS) pain score, and narcotic use.

The management of perioperative blood loss, especially postoperative hemarthrosis, is another modifiable factor affecting patient recovery, complication rates, and costs. Tranexamic acid (TXA) has been shown to be effective for reducing perioperative blood loss with arthroplasty of other joints, but little information is available for determining its effectiveness in TAA. Nodzo et al. described 50 patients with uncemented TAA, 25 of whom received TXA and 25 who did not. Drain output and change in preoperative to postoperative hemoglobin levels were significantly less and the overall wound complication rate was lower in patients who received TXA. We do not routinely use TXA for TAA.

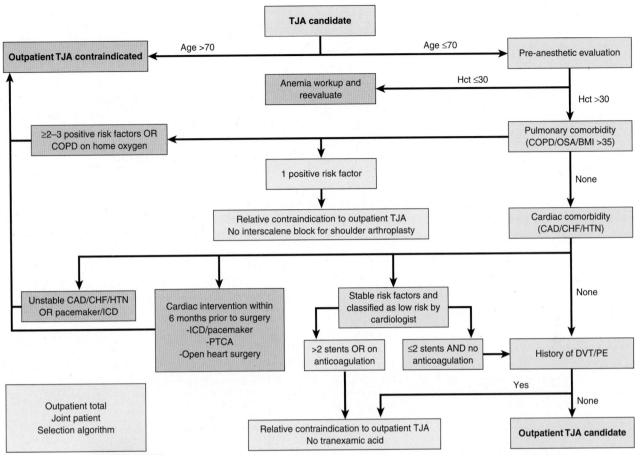

FIGURE 8.6 Algorithm for patient selection for outpatient total joint procedures. *BMI,* Body mass index; *CAD,* coronary artery disease; *CHF,* congestive heart failure; *COPD,* chronic obstructive pulmonary disease; *DVT,* deep vein thrombosis; *HTN,* hypertension; *ICD,* implantable cardiac defibrillator; *OSA,* obstructive sleep apnea; *PE,* pulmonary embolism; *PTCA,* percutaneous transluminal coronary angioplasty; *TJA,* total joint arthroplasty. (From Fournier MN, Stephens R, Mascioli AA, et al.: Identifying appropriate candidates for ambulatory outpatient total joint arthroplasty: validation of a patient selection algorithm, *J Shoulder Elbow Surg.* 28(1):65, 2019.)

TOTAL ANKLE ARTHROPLASTY

TECHNIQUE 8.1

PATIENT POSITIONING
- Most systems require an anterior approach to the ankle. Place the patient supine on the operating table with the foot near the end of the table. Place a small bump or lift under the ipsilateral hip to help place the ankle straight and avoid the tendency of the leg to externally rotate.
- After induction of general anesthesia, apply and inflate a thigh tourniquet to control bleeding and improve visualization.

APPROACH
- Any significant deformity above or below the ankle joint *must* be corrected before placement of the total ankle implants (see Technique 8.2).
- The approach is determined by the prosthesis design, and the reader is referred to the specific implant chosen; however, most systems require an anterior approach to the ankle.

- Make an incision from about 10 cm proximal to the ankle joint on the lateral side of the anterior tibial tendon, over the flexor hallucis tendon. This incision is medial to the most medial major branch of the superficial peroneal nerve, the dorsal medial cutaneous nerve. Often a very small medial branch of this nerve crosses the incision just distal to the ankle joint and must be incised for exposure. The patient should be warned before surgery that a small area of numbness may be present just medial to the incision.
- Open the flexor hallucis longus sheath and retract the tendon medially. Retract the neurovascular bundle containing the anterior tibial artery, vein, and deep peroneal nerve laterally with the extensor digitorum longus tendons.
- Make a straight incision in line with the skin incision in the ankle capsule and reflect the capsule medially until the medial ankle gutter is exposed and laterally until the lateral gutter is exposed.
- Expose the dorsal talonavicular joint and remove any anterior, medial, or lateral osteophytes. If better exposure of the joint line is needed, use an osteotome to perform a more aggressive removal of the anterior osteophytes.
- Prepare the bone for implant insertion according to the technique guide specific for the implant selected. Take

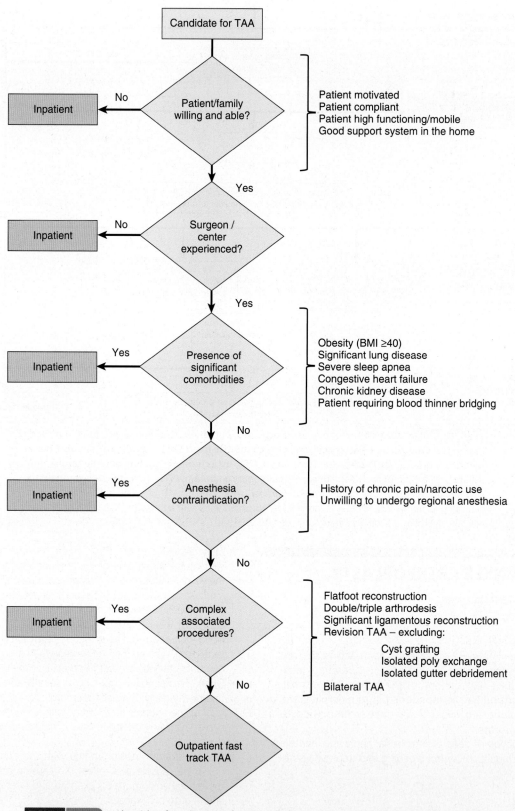

FIGURE 8.7 Algorithm for selection of patients for outpatient ambulatory total ankle arthroplasty. *BMI,* Body mass index; *TAA,* Total ankle arthroplasty. (From Taylor MA, Parekh SG: Optimizing outpatient total ankle replacement from clinic to pain management, *Orthop Clin N Am* 49:541–551, 2018.)

care to place the implant in proper alignment in all planes for sufficient bone coverage of the prosthesis and for proper tensioning of the soft tissues and ligamentous support after final implantation. There should be a balance between choosing a thicker polyethylene insert (better for wear characteristics) and excessive bone resection and joint motion and stability.

- Close the capsule over the prosthesis and insert a closed suction drain; close the superior extensor retinaculum over the flexor hallucis longus sheath and close the skin in layers.
- A popliteal block is routinely used for postoperative analgesia.

POSTOPERATIVE CARE At our institution, patients are typically kept overnight in the hospital and are seen by a physical therapist the following day for instruction in gait training with touch-down weight bearing. Patients with outpatient TAA have physical therapy instruction before surgery and carry out learned exercises at home. Therapy with antibiotics, binasal cannula oxygen, and deep venous thrombosis (DVT) prophylaxis with low-molecular-weight heparin is the normal postoperative protocol, although this is not typically continued after discharge unless the patient has risk factors for DVT; one aspirin daily after discharge may be beneficial. Different implants have different recommendations for postoperative care, but we typically delay weight bearing for 4 to 6 weeks and begin active ankle motion once the incision is healed, typically 2 weeks after surgery. Gradual progressive weight bearing, calf strengthening, proprioceptive training, and range-of-motion exercises are started at 4 to 6 weeks, with the ankle protected in a prefabricated walking boot. A light ankle brace is applied at 8 to 10 weeks, and full activities are allowed at 3 months, or when the calf muscles are fully rehabilitated. No restrictions are placed on the patients' activities or sports programs, but they are encouraged to avoid impact exercises for conditioning.

CONSIDERATIONS FOR ADJUNCTIVE PROCEDURES
DEFORMITY CORRECTION

Osteoarthritic ankles considered for arthroplasty should have minimal periarticular deformity, or this deformity should be correctable with osteotomy or arthrodesis.

Determination of the site of the deformity is mandatory. Bonasia et al. characterized deformities as varus or valgus, incongruent or congruent (Table 8.2). In the valgus ankle and hindfoot, the following procedures should be considered: medial displacement osteotomy of the calcaneus, Cotton osteotomy of the medial cuneiform or selective arthrodesis of the medial midfoot, subtalar arthrodesis with or without talonavicular arthrodesis, posterior tibial tendon reconstruction with tendon transfer, and closing wedge osteotomy of the distal tibia. Demetracopoulos et al. evaluated 80 patients with preoperative valgus deformities of at least 10 degrees (average of 15 degrees). After TAA, the average postoperative deformity was 1.2 degrees, with significant improvements in VAS, SF-36, American Orthopaedic Foot and Ankle Society (AOFAS), and Short Musculoskeletal Function Assessment (SMFA) scores.

TABLE 8.2

Ankle Joint Pathologies That Include Distal Tibial Articular Surface Malalignment, Talar Tilt due to Ligamentous Instability, or Both

DEFORMITY TYPE	ABNORMAL ANGLES
Varus tibial deformity-congruent joint	Increased LDTA, CORA at the level of tibial articular surface, normal tibial-talar angle
Valgus tibial deformity-congruent joint	Increased LDTA, CORA at the level of tibial articular surface, normal tibial-talar angle
Varus tibial deformity-incongruent joint	Decreased LDTA, CORA at the level of tibial articular surface, tibial-talar angle >10 degrees
Valgus tibial deformity-incongruent joint	Increased LDTA, CORA at the level of tibial articular surface, tibial-talar angle >10 degrees
Incongruent joint	Normal LDTA, tibial-talar angle >10 degrees

ADTA, Anterior distal tibial angle, sagittal plane—increased ADTA represents recurvatum deformity; *CORA*, center of rotation of angulation, at or proximal to joint line; *LDTA*, lateral distal tibial angle, coronal plane—decreased LDTA represents varus deformity; T-T angle—angle formed by tibial and talar articular surfaces: >10 degrees = incongruent joint.
Modified from Bonasia DE, Dettoni F, Femino JE, et al.: Total ankle replacement: When, why, and how?, *Iowa Orthop J* 30:119–130, 2010.

The authors concluded that correction of coronal alignment could be obtained and maintained in patients with moderate-to-severe preoperative valgus malalignment. Lee et al. compared intermediate and long-term outcomes of TAA in 144 ankles with preoperative varus, valgus, or neutral alignment. Outcomes similar to those in ankles with neutral alignment were obtained in ankles with varus or valgus malalignment of up to 20 degrees when neutral alignment was achieved with TAA.

For the varus ankle, procedures to consider include deltoid ligament release or sliding osteotomy of the medial malleolus, opening wedge osteotomy of the distal tibia (see Technique 9.1), Dwyer closing wedge osteotomy of the calcaneus, dorsiflexion osteotomy of the first metatarsal, and subtalar, double, or triple arthrodesis.

Varus deformity of the distal tibia above the level of the joint is best treated with supramalleolar osteotomy. Varus deformity of the tibial plafond at the joint from erosion of the medial malleolus or medial subchondral bone can be corrected by accurate placement of the tibial cut. Joo and Lee reported satisfactory clinical and radiographic outcomes in patients with moderate and severe varus deformities similar to those in patients with neutral alignment when postoperative neutral alignment was obtained, and special care was taken to correct causes of the varus malalignment with additional procedures.

For the varus unstable ankle with deformity below the level of the joint, sometimes an osteotomy of the hindfoot is required (Fig. 8.8). If instability persists intraoperatively, a lateral ligament reconstruction should be done. Judicious release of the deltoid ligament, especially the deep deltoid

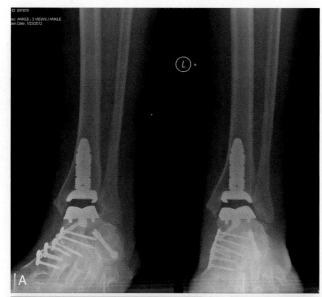

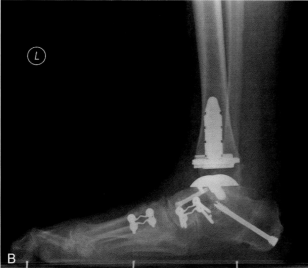

FIGURE 8.8 **A** and **B,** Calcaneal osteotomy and midfoot arthrodeses were required to correct pes planus deformity before total ankle arthroplasty.

ligament, may be wise in this setting. To avoid devascularization of the talus by injury to the deltoid branch of the posterior tibial artery, a sliding osteotomy of the medial malleolus has been described, with or without fixation. Reddy et al. reported correction of coronal plane deformity without osteotomy in ankles with an average of 18 degrees of varus. Deltoid release was necessary for all ankles with more than 18 degrees of varus deformity, and all ankles with more than 25 degrees of varus developed recurrent deformity. Hobson et al. suggested that TAA could be safely done with up to 30 degrees of coronal plane deformity. In their short-term follow-up of 103 patients with severe varus deformities, Sung et al. found that those with more than 20 degrees of varus deformity had outcomes similar to those with varus deformities of less than 20 degrees, with no significant differences in postoperative complications or implant failures. Adjunctive procedures, such as osteotomy, ligament release or lengthening, and tendon transfers, were done as needed. In the comparison study of Lee et al., adjunctive procedures were required in 71% of ankles with varus

deformities, in 56% of those with valgus deformities, and in 39% of those with neutral alignment. Percutaneous Achilles tendon lengthening and release of the medial deltoid ligament were the most frequently done concomitant procedures; calcaneal osteotomy was done in five ankles (three in the varus group and two in the valgus group).

Tan and Myerson divided varus ankle deformities into anatomic levels and described procedures for correction at each level. For extraarticular deformity above the ankle joint, they recommended a medial opening wedge osteotomy or, for severe ankle arthritis, a dome osteotomy. With a medial opening wedge osteotomy, they recommended a staged procedure in which total ankle replacement is done later. The dome osteotomy is useful for multiplanar supramalleolar deformity and can usually be done simultaneously with replacement (Fig. 8.9). For deformity at the level of the ankle joint and a congruent joint, a "neutralizing" distal tibial cut may be all that is needed for realignment. A wedge of the distal tibia is removed with minimal bone resection at the eroded medial plafond and a larger resection at the lateral plafond. For a severely tilted talus, additional procedures are required, including the removal of osteophytes from the lateral gutter and a lateral ankle stabilization procedure. Medial-side releases of the deltoid and posterior tibial tendon have been described, but Tan and Myerson recommended a lengthening medial malleolar osteotomy, as described by Doets et al. (Fig. 8.10), rather than soft-tissue releases, because it allows controlled lengthening of the medial side of the ankle and provides reliable bony healing. With more severe varus tilt of the talus with a markedly dysplastic medial malleolus and incongruent joint, a useful alternative osteotomy is the medial tibial plafondplasty, which is done as a separate, staged procedure before ankle replacement. Residual heel varus that remains after component implantation can be corrected with a lateralizing calcaneal osteotomy. Combined deformities are generally best treated with correction of the deformities, followed by a staged ankle arthroplasty. Supramalleolar deformities are corrected first, followed by correction of hindfoot and forefoot varus and any ligamentous reconstruction needed.

DOME OSTEOTOMY FOR CORRECTION OF VARUS DEFORMITY ABOVE THE ANKLE DEFORMITY

TECHNIQUE 8.2

(TAN AND MYERSON)

- Make an anterior midline incision, which also will be used for implantation of the total ankle prosthesis.
- Use cautery to carefully mark out the planned dome osteotomy, placing the center of the radius of curvature of the dome at the center of rotation of angulation.
- Make sure the cut will allow adequate room for the tibial prosthesis and its stem after internal fixation of the osteotomy.
- Drill multiple bicortical holes along the planned osteotomy and connect them with an osteotome to complete the osteotomy (Fig. 8.11A).

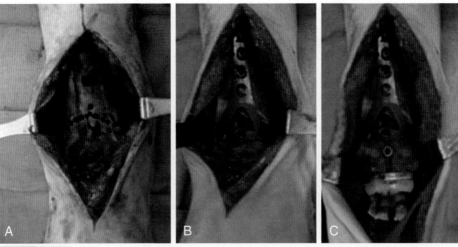

FIGURE 8.9   Dome osteotomy and ankle replacement done at the same time. **A,** Osteotomy is marked with electrocautery and completed. **B,** Osteotomy is then stabilized with an anterior plate placed superior to the tibial component. **C,** Total ankle components are then implanted in the usual fashion. (From Tan KJ, Myerson MS: Planning correction of the varus ankle deformity with ankle replacement, *Foot Ankle Clin N Am* 17:103–115, 2012.)

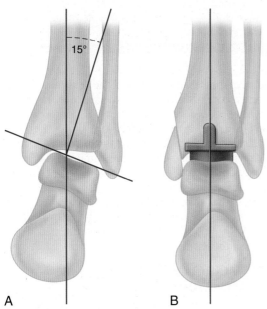

FIGURE 8.10   Medial malleolar lengthening osteotomy. **A,** Ankle with incongruent varus deformity. **B,** After implantation of a mobile-bearing prosthesis and correction of the deformity by medial malleolar osteotomy. (From Doets HC, van der Plaat LW, Klein JP: Medial malleolar osteotomy for the correction of varus deformity during total ankle arthroplasty: results in 15 ankles, *Foot Ankle Int* 29:171–177, 2008.)

- Manipulate the distal fragment in the coronal and sagittal planes to correct the deformity.
- Stabilize the osteotomy with an anterior plate and screws (Fig. 8.11B, C).
- Proceed with TAA in the usual fashion.
- Inflate the tourniquet after the arthrotomy and before preparation of the osseous surfaces.

MEDIAL TIBIAL PLAFONDPLASTY FOR VARUS DEFORMITY AT THE ANKLE JOINT

TECHNIQUE 8.3

(TAN AND MYERSON)

- Make a medial incision along the subcutaneous border of the tibia.
- Insert a guide pin in the medial tibia, aimed to exit at a point in the plafond just medial to the midpoint where the articular erosion ends. This acts as a guide for the planned osteotomy.
- Under fluoroscopic guidance, insert three additional Kirschner wires parallel to and 6 mm above the joint line in the subchondral bone of the distal tibia. These wires prevent violation of the articular surface by the oscillating saw used to make the osteotomy.
- Use an oscillating saw to make the osteotomy to the level of the three Kirschner wires and insert a broad osteotome to hinge open the osteotomy.
- Hinge the medial malleolar fragment downward to restore a more normal morphology of the ankle mortise.
- Debride the lateral gutter to facilitate realignment and to obtain lateral-sided stability, which may require an additional lateral-sided reconstruction.
- Hold the osteotomy open with a lamina spreader and pack it tightly with bone graft.
- Fix the osteotomy with a plate and screws.

LIGAMENT CONSIDERATIONS

Ligament stability is also imperative for optimal outcome, especially with less constrained designs. Some stability can be obtained intraoperatively by proper selection of implant and polyethylene thickness, but occasionally collateral ligament reconstruction should be done.

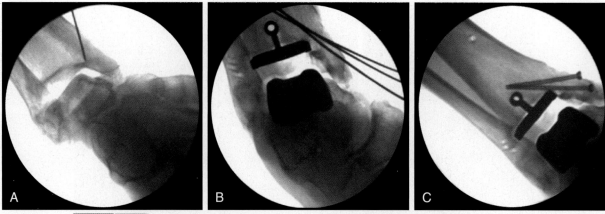

FIGURE 8.11   Intraoperative fluoroscopy views of medial malleolar osteotomy. **A,** Plane of the osteotomy is planned with a Kirschner wire and completed. **B,** Next, it is provisionally fixed with cannulated wires. **C,** The wires are replaced with cannulated screws after the prosthesis is implanted. (From Tan KJ, Myerson MS: Planning correction of the varus ankle deformity with ankle replacement, *Foot Ankle Clin N Am* 17:103–115, 2012. **SEE TECHNIQUE 8.2.**)

Techniques for the reconstruction of a chronically unstable ankle are discussed. Coetzee, however, reported that the usual "anatomic" lateral ligament reconstruction techniques were not satisfactory with TAA. He described a simple, nonanatomic reconstruction to provide a strong checkrein against inversion and to limit anterior translation of the ankle (Technique 8.4).

Medial reconstruction of the deltoid ligament with TAA is uncommon, but sometimes necessary, in late-stage posterior tibial tendon insufficiency. Correction of hindfoot valgus with osteotomy and/or arthrodesis may provide enough mechanical support to allow stability of the ankle prosthesis. Reconstruction of the deltoid ligament in this setting is an advanced procedure, and complications are not uncommon. Arthrodesis of the ankle may be advisable.

RECONSTRUCTION OF LATERAL ANKLE LIGAMENTS FOR CHRONIC INSTABILITY AS AN ADJUNCT TO TOTAL ANKLE ARTHROPLASTY

TECHNIQUE 8.4

(COETZEE)
- After implantation of the ankle components, perform a modified Broström reconstruction of the lateral ligaments.
- Make a separate incision to expose the lateral side of the ankle and the peroneal tendons. Harvest one half of the peroneus brevis tendon. If the tendon has signs of a pathologic process or a tear, harvest the entire tendon to ensure maximal strength. Leave the distal attachment intact and harvest the tendon as far proximal as possible.
- Route the peroneus brevis tendon over the modified Broström repair from the lateral side of the ankle to the anterolateral tibia.

- Secure the tendon under adequate tension to the tibia with a staple.
- Test the stability of the ankle to be sure that equal medial and lateral joint movements are possible.

Often, patients with arthritis of the ankle have a concomitant contracture of the triceps surae and may benefit from a lengthening procedure. Assessment of a contracture may be difficult in a stiff, arthritic ankle, but should be attempted after placement of the components. To regain ankle extension, either a smaller polyethylene component can be used, or a lengthening procedure can be done. Most patients with a significant contracture require a gastrocnemius recession (Vulpius) rather than a triple hemi-section; however, Queen et al. found equivalent outcomes with the two procedures. Patients with either lengthening procedure had better outcomes than those with TAA alone.

SPECIAL CIRCUMSTANCES
■ INFLAMMATORY ARTHRITIS

Patients with rheumatoid arthritis commonly have involvement of the foot and ankle, with severe pain and functional limitations. Arthrodesis has been the standard procedure for these patients, but more recently arthroplasty is being chosen because of the ability to preserve motion and decrease stress on the midfoot and subtalar joints. Early results of TAA in these patients were disappointing, with high complication rates and component loosening in as many as 75%. More recent studies, with the use of newer techniques and implants, report better outcomes. Kraal et al. had a cumulative incidence of failure at 15 years of 20% in 76 rheumatoid patients with mobile-bearing total ankle replacement. Pedersen et al. found similar outcomes in 50 patients with rheumatoid arthritis compared with a matched cohort of 50 patients with noninflammatory arthritis, although the noninflammatory arthritis group reported better function at final follow-up. Revision rates were 12% in the rheumatoid arthritis group and 10% in the noninflammatory arthritis group. Other studies have documented reliable pain relief and good functional results with uncemented prostheses and cemented two-piece and three-piece implants in patients with rheumatoid arthritis.

■ OBESITY

Obesity (body mass index [BMI] >30) is a growing problem that affects all types of orthopaedic surgery, including total joint replacement. Many patients with arthritis of the ankle are sedentary and obese, and this poses a dilemma for the surgeon, who must weigh the possibility of providing significant pain relief against the likelihood of implant failure caused by increased stress on the implant from extra weight. Outcomes of TAA in obese and morbidly obese (BMI >40) patients reported in the literature are varied. Schipper et al. compared outcomes in obese and nonobese patients and found that obese patients had an increased long-term risk of implant failure and a significantly decreased 5-year implant survivorship, whereas Bouchard et al. found no significant difference in the proportion of complications or revisions in a similar comparison study. Barg et al. also reported comparable survivorship (93% at 6 years), as well as significant pain relief and functional improvement in obese patients. In a series of 455 patients, including 266 with BMI of less than 30 (control), 116 with a BMI between 30 and 35, and 73 with a BMI of over 35, Gross et al. found no difference in complication, infection, or failure rates. Although obese patients had lower functional outcome scores, they did have significant functional and pain improvements after TAA. Although we have no definitive upper limit on weight for this procedure, a BMI over 40 is a reason for caution and careful patient counseling. Morbidly obese patients are strongly encouraged to use a bracing system to provide a measure of pain relief while they actively work on weight loss.

■ DIABETES

Perhaps no other medical condition affects decision making in foot and ankle surgery as much as diabetes. It has been shown to be a factor contributing to complications, particularly infection, after a variety of orthopaedic procedures. In their review of a national database, Schipper et al. found that diabetes was independently associated with a significantly increased risk of perioperative complications, nonhome discharge, and length of hospital stay after TAA and ankle arthrodesis. Gross et al., however, compared outcomes of TAA in 50 patients with diabetes with those in 55 patients without diabetes and found no significant differences in secondary operations, revisions, or failure rates. Although patients with diabetes were heavier and had worse ASA preoperative grades, they did not have significantly different rates of complications or infections, and all had pain relief and improved function. Findings that support the use of TAA in diabetic patients include hemoglobin A1C consistently less than seven, no evidence of peripheral neuropathy, normal vascular status, normal weight (or at least not morbid obesity), and no other target organ disease (retinopathy or nephropathy).

■ OSTEONECROSIS OF THE TALUS

Little has been written regarding the long-term results of TAA in patients with osteonecrosis of the talus. Certainly, a patient with an avascular, fragmented, and collapsed talar body is not a candidate for a total ankle prosthesis, and arthrodesis is recommended. However, a few patients with apparent osteonecrosis of the talus do not have collapse, and over a long period of time (minimum of 24 to 36 months) portions of the talus

may gradually revascularize, making the patient a better candidate for TAA (Fig. 8.12). A thorough evaluation with MRI or bone scanning may give clues as to whether or not a talus will accept and support a talar component. Lee et al. reported two successful total ankle arthroplasties after revascularization of the talus.

■ PANTALAR DISEASE; CONCOMITANT HINDFOOT ARTHRODESIS

Arthrodesis of arthritic adjacent joints, most often the subtalar and talonavicular joints, may be necessary with TAA. Mild to moderate arthritis in the adjacent joints, however, does not necessarily mean that arthrodesis is necessary. Often, the pain relief and improvement of motion after TAA are such that the stress on and pain from these joints are reduced significantly. Careful attention to the patient's examination may help determine the need for attention to these joints. Selective injections with or without fluoroscopy may also help with the diagnosis.

Timing of the procedures depends on the amount of deformity, extent of involvement of the arthritis, and the number of joints involved. Arthrodesis of the talonavicular joint through the same incision used for component implantation is fairly straight forward, and bone graft from the resection for the implant is available for use in the fusion. The subtalar joint is a different matter, and often a separate approach is necessary to fully prepare the joint for fusion. Extensive reconstructions may be best staged before the TAA procedure. At midterm follow-up, Lee et al. found similar results in ankles with and without hindfoot fusions and recommended fusion at the time of arthroplasty if indicated clinically. In contrast, Lewis et al. found that overall outcome and implant survivorship were slightly inferior with hindfoot fusion compared with TAA alone, although arthroplasty with ipsilateral hindfoot fusion resulted in significant improvements in pain and functional outcome. These authors also noted that, when indicated, hindfoot arthrodesis can be safely done in conjunction with TAA. Other authors have reported similar findings, noting that hindfoot fusions improved function and pain after TAA. Dekker et al. reviewed the outcomes of 140 TAAs at an average follow-up of 6.5 years and found only a minimal radiographic increase in adjacent subtalar and talonavicular arthritis, suggesting that motion preserved with TAA decreases the stresses and compensatory motion incurred with tibiotalar arthrodesis.

■ TAKEDOWN OF ANKLE ARTHRODESIS AND CONVERSION TO ANKLE ARTHROPLASTY

It has been almost an axiom over the years that one should never take down a successful ankle fusion. Some ankle fusions, however, have such a poor functional outcome that conversion to a TAA may be considered (Fig. 8.13). Hintermann et al. described conversion of 30 painful ankle arthrodeses to TAA, with 83% patient satisfaction; five ankles were completely pain free, 21 were moderately painful, and three remained painful. Several additional surgical procedures were required before takedown of the fusion, including subtalar or talonavicular joint fusion, fibular reconstruction, lateral or medial ligament reconstruction, calcaneal osteotomy, and Achilles tendon lengthening. More recently, Preis et al. reported conversion of 18 painful ankle arthrodeses to TAA. They concluded that this procedure is technically challenging

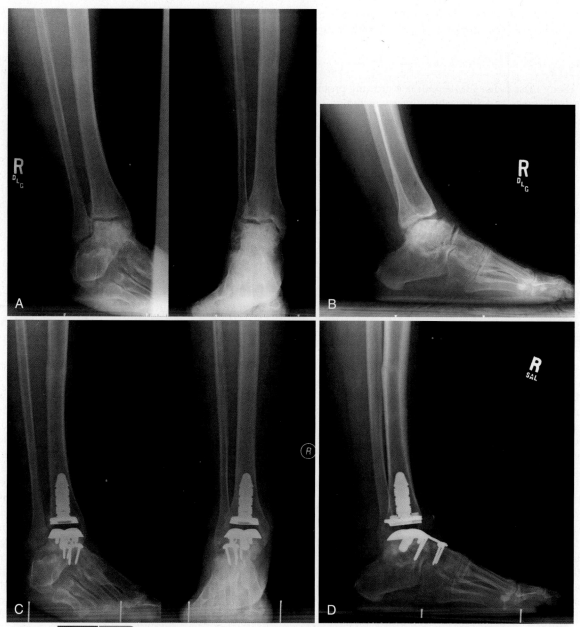

FIGURE 8.12 **A** and **B**, Osteonecrosis of ankle after talar fracture. **C** and **D**, After total ankle arthroplasty with INBONE II prosthesis.

and in their series, it was associated with frequent complications, including arthrofibrosis; however, pain and function did improve. Pellegrini et al. described conversion of tibiotalar arthrodesis to TAA for symptomatic adjacent hindfoot arthritis or tibiotalar or subtalar nonunion in 23 patients. Concomitant procedures were done in 18 ankles (78%), most commonly prophylactic malleolar fixation. Pain relief and function were improved in most patients; implant survival rate was 87% at an average 3-year follow-up. These authors recommended prophylactic malleolar fixation and did not recommend conversion to TAA for ankle arthrodeses that included distal fibulectomy. Although conversion of a nonunion of an attempted ankle fusion to an ankle arthroplasty has been done, to date we have no experience with the conversion of a well-healed ankle fusion.

TIBIOTALAR ARTHRODESIS CONVERSION TO TOTAL ANKLE ARTHROPLASTY

TECHNIQUE 8.5

(PELLEGRINI ET AL.)

PREOPERATIVE PLANNING

- Preoperative preparation and planning are similar to those for a primary TAA, and implants designed for primary TAA can be used in most patients.

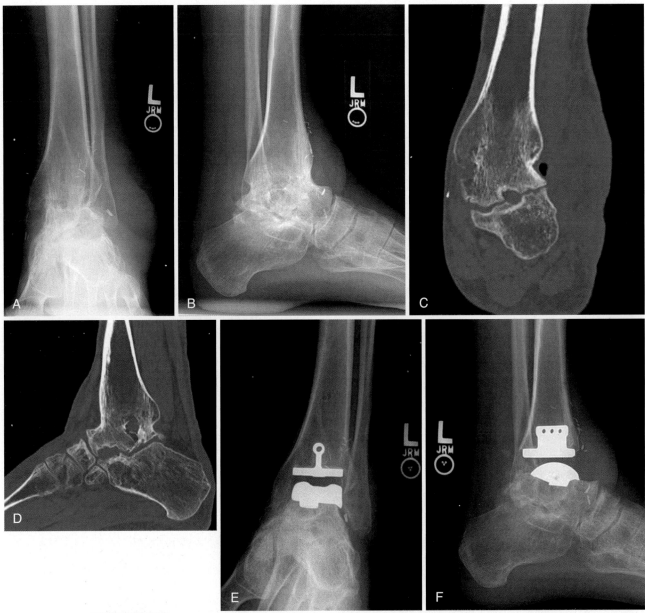

FIGURE 8.13 **A–D,** Despite well-healed, well-aligned ankle fusion, patient had persistent pain that necessitated takedown of fusion and total ankle arthroplasty with Salto Talaris implant (**E** and **F**). Eight months after total ankle arthroplasty, he returned to his full-time job as tactical agent with U.S. Border Patrol. (Courtesy Dr. Mark Casillas, San Antonio, TX.)

PATIENT POSITIONING AND PREPARATION
- Place the patient supine on the operating-room table with the heel over or near the edge of the table, with the foot resting at a right angle to the table.
- Place support under the ipsilateral hip.
- The anesthesia team routinely uses a popliteal catheter for regional anesthesia.
- Drape the extremity above the knee and use Esmarch and tourniquet control.

IMPLANT REMOVAL AND SCREW INSERTION
- Remove trans-articular screws or screws anticipated to interfere with implant positioning before inflating the tourniquet.

- Inflate the thigh tourniquet. In ankles in which arthrodesis was done with anterior plating, inflate the tourniquet before proceeding with an anterior approach to the ankle.
- Assuming that the malleoli have been stress-shielded in ankle arthrodesis, perform prophylactic fixation of both malleoli to avoid intraoperative fractures.
- Use percutaneous cannulated 3.5-mm diameter screws to preserve tourniquet time for the arthroplasty and improve stability. Place the screws as close to the cortex as possible in anticipation of gutter preparation.

RECREATE THE TIBIOTALAR JOINT

- Define the native articular line; this usually is straightforward when the ankle anatomy has been adequately preserved (Fig. 8.14A-C).
- Although the joint line can be identified clinically, place small-diameter Kirschner wires as a reference to define the joint line fluoroscopically.
- In some patients, re-establishing the tibiotalar joint line may be difficult, and radiographs of the contralateral, uninvolved ankle can serve as a reference for determining the joint line in the affected ankle; measure the distance from the medial malleolus to the natural joint line. The TAA implant also may serve as a reference for determining the ideal level for re-establishing the joint line; a particular screw or hole in a plate can serve as a useful reference point.
- Preserve the talar body. If necessary, make the joint line slightly more proximal to avoid leaving too little talus on which to rest the talar component. Avoid excessive proximal translation, however, because the more proximal the resection, the narrower the tibia and the greater risk for malleolar stress fracture.
- For implants with independent tibial and talar preparation, select the proper resection level, rotation, and slope as for primary TAA.
- Perform the initial tibial preparation with the same cutting guide used for a primary TAA.
- From the previous operation, the posterior soft tissue may be adhered to the posterior aspect of the tibia. Use a lateral fluoroscopic view to help confirm that the saw blade has not overcome the posterior tibial bone.
- Extract the resected bone from the joint.

SET THE OPTIMAL TALAR SLOPE

- To avoid excessive posterior talar slope, perform the initial talar preparation independent of the dedicated guide. This is particularly important when using a monoblock cutting guide to prepare the tibia and talus.
- After tibial preparation is complete, use a small reciprocating saw to recreate the gutters.
- Place the ankle in dorsiflexion, which will optimize the talar position for adequate preparation (Fig. 8.14D-I).

RECREATE THE MEDIAL AND LATERAL GUTTERS

- Place small-diameter Kirschner wires in the anticipated location of the native gutters and confirm fluoroscopically.
- Because monoblock instrumentation may be difficult for evaluating the malleoli and residual talar bone, use a smaller monoblock than may be suggested on intraoperative evaluation. An adequate intramedullary reference in this system is critical to placing the cutting guide in an optimal position.
- In a critical step of the surgical procedure, maintain the ankle in a stable position, regardless of the ankle system being used, until the gutters have been adequately recreated. Failure to achieve stability of the ankle may result in a malleolar fracture during distraction or mobilization.
- Recreate the gutters using a small reciprocating saw to remove approximately 2 to 3 mm of bone slightly more toward the malleoli rather than the talar bone (Fig. 8.15). This should ensure that sufficient talar dome will support the talar component.

MOBILIZE THE ANKLE AND USE BONE GRAFT IN DEFECTS FROM PREVIOUS IMPLANTS

- To avoid potential malleolar fractures, mobilize the ankle only after prophylactic malleolar screws have been placed, tibial and talar cuts have been completed, gutters have been reestablished, all resected bone has been removed, and scar tissue from the posterior aspect of the ankle has been excised; thereafter, conversion TAA is similar to primary TAA, with the exception of potential bone defects where implants were positioned.
- If the ankle remains locked, more release is needed.
- Apply distraction to assess whether the created joint space will accommodate the implant. Occasionally, further bone resection may be needed. Use a small reciprocating saw to remove incongruities of the bone surfaces.
- Despite adequate bone preparation and elevation of scar tissue, motion may be limited in an ankle arthrodesis takedown. Access to the posterior part of the ankle may be difficult.
- Use bone grafting in defects caused by previous implants to prevent later cyst formation or bone weakening.

TALAR PREPARATION

- Perform the routine steps for primary TAA, often ignoring bone defects from the ankle arthrodesis implants, but plan to repair the defects with bone-grafting before implanting the final talar component.
- Despite satisfactory bone preparation and elevation of scar tissue, note that access to the posterior aspect of the ankle joint can be challenging. This situation is less of a concern when a system designed for a flat-cut talus is used and more challenging when the talar preparation involves a posterior chamfer cut.
- Perform talar preparation in a manner similar to that for primary TAA. For this procedure, after milling the anterior chamfer, a bone defect can be obvious. Take the location of the bone defect into consideration when selecting the ankle design. If the bone defect is laterally based, use an ankle design with a medial talar stem and a lateral chamfer cut, thereby reducing the bone defect without compromising implant stability.
- At this point, the posterior capsule can be easily accessed and mobilized judiciously using an elevator to protect the neurovascular bundle and the malleoli (Figs. 8.16 and 8.17A-C).

TIBIAL PREPARATION AND DEFINITIVE COMPONENTS

- Perform tibial preparation in a manner similar to that for primary TAA.
- Plan for a talar component one size smaller than the tibial component to ensure (1) adequate gutter debridement and (2) sufficient bone support in anticipation of talar dome bone loss during arthrodesis takedown.
- The tibial component rarely has to be downsized unless there is concern for medial malleolar stress fracture in patients with relatively small ankles.
- After definitive components have been adequately implanted, assess ankle stability, ankle range of motion, and foot alignment.
- If concomitant ancillary procedures can be safely done during the same operation, do so. In general, hindfoot arthrodesis is staged to avoid jeopardizing talar blood supply and implant osseointegration.

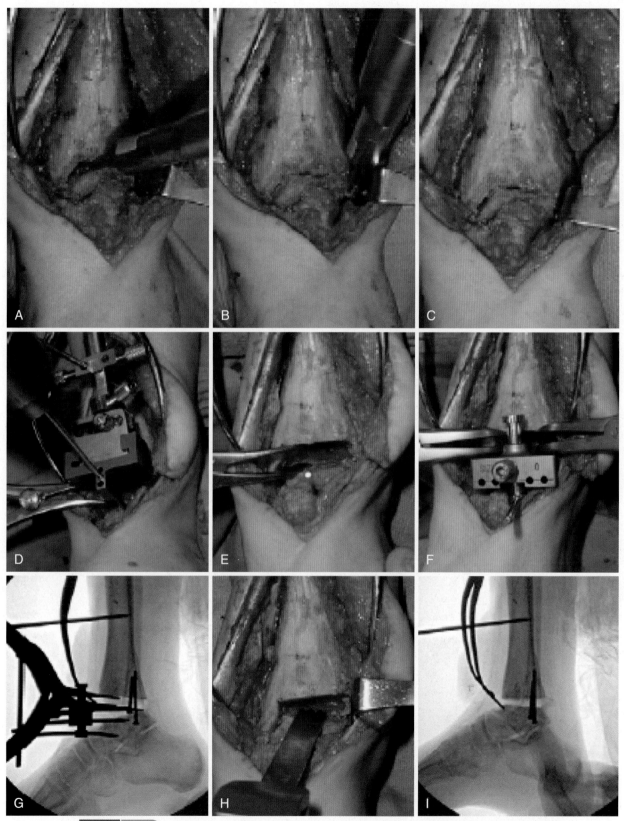

FIGURE 8.14 Pellegrini et al. technique for conversion of tibiotalar arthrodesis to total ankle arthroplasty (see text). **A-C,** Reestablishment of the native joint line. **D-I, Talar preparation.** (From Pellegrini MJ, Schiff AP, Adams SB Jr: Tibiotalar arthrodesis conversion to total ankle arthroplasty, *JBJS Essent Surg Tech* 6:e27, 2016.) **SEE TECHNIQUE 8.5.**

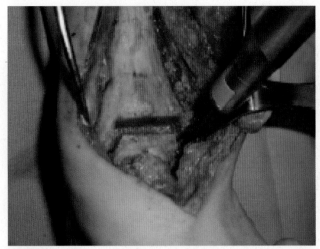

FIGURE 8.15 Pellegrini et al. technique for conversion of tibiotalar arthrodesis to total ankle arthroplasty (see text). Preparation of the medial and lateral gutters. (From Pellegrini MJ, Schiff AP, Adams SB Jr: Tibiotalar arthrodesis conversion to total ankle arthroplasty, *JBJS Essent Surg Tech* 6:e27, 2016.) **SEE TECHNIQUE 8.5.**

GOUT

Barg et al. reported low frequency of intraoperative or postoperative complications and high patient satisfaction and functional outcomes after bilateral total ankle arthroplasties in a subset of patients with the diagnosis of gouty arthritis.

BILATERAL TOTAL ANKLE ARTHROPLASTY

Barg et al. also reported outcomes of 23 patients with bilateral total ankle arthroplasties done at the same surgical setting and compared them with a cohort with unilateral replacement. At short-term follow-up, the unilateral group had better outcomes, but the differences disappeared by 1 and 2 years after surgery. More recently, Desai et al. compared outcomes in patients with unilateral and staged bilateral TAA and found that those with staged bilateral TAA benefited as much as patients with unilateral TAA, despite having a worse preoperative health status. Revision rates and implant survival times were similar. Bilateral replacements are not for the faint-hearted patient or surgeon, and patients should be warned of the lengthy recovery period.

OUTCOMES

As a preamble to the evaluation of outcomes reported in the literature, it may be important to turn a critical eye to the methods of reporting and the sources of the studies. Noting that patient-reported outcomes measures are designed to evaluate function or symptoms while missing ongoing

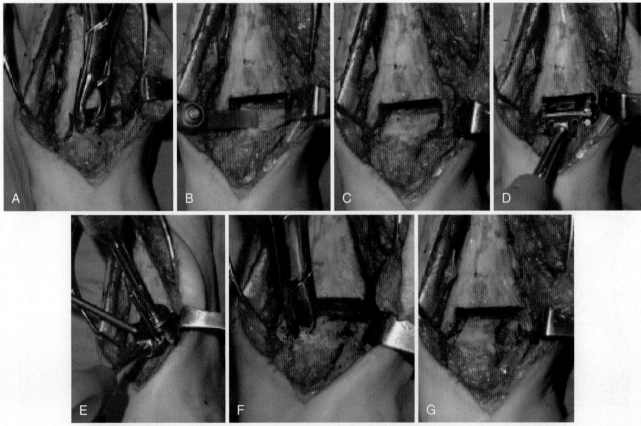

FIGURE 8.16 Pellegrini et al. technique for conversion of tibiotalar arthrodesis to total ankle arthroplasty (see text). Preparation of the anterior chamfer. **A,** Osteophytes removed from talar neck. **B,** Smoothing anterior chamfer. **C,** Anterior talar body prepared for anterior chamfer guide. **D,** Guide positioning. **E,** Anterior chamfer preparation. **F,** Note lateral talar defect from hardware placed during ankle arthrodesis. **G,** Defect requiring graft. (From Pellegrini MJ, Schiff AP, Adams SB Jr: Tibiotalar arthrodesis conversion to total ankle arthroplasty, *JBJS Essent Surg Tech* 6:e27, 2016.) **SEE TECHNIQUE 8.5.**

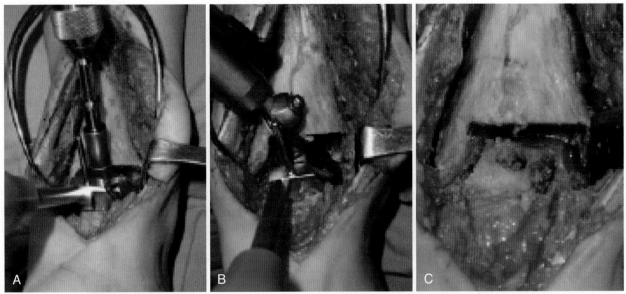

FIGURE 8.17 Pellegrini et al. technique for conversion of tibiotalar arthrodesis to total ankle arthroplasty (see text). Preparation of the lateral chamfer. **A,** Lateral chamfer guide flush on talus. **B,** Preparation of lateral chamfer with microsagittal saw. **C,** Prepared talus with lateral dome defect requiring bone grafting. (From Pellegrini MJ, Schiff AP, Adams SB Jr: Tibiotalar arthrodesis conversion to total ankle arthroplasty, *JBJS Essent Surg Tech* 6:e27, 2016.) **SEE TECHNIQUE 8.5.**

limitations with which patients must cope, Pinsker et al. proposed categorizing outcomes as "recovered-resolved" (better with no symptoms or residual effects), "recovered, not resolved" (better but with residual effects), or "not recovered" (not better). Most patients reported positive outcomes, but only 15% had resolution of all symptoms and limitations. Because patients' perceptions of satisfactory outcomes were not predicated on the resolution of all limitations, these authors suggested that the conventional definition of satisfactory outcomes should be expanded. Labek et al. noted that there is a significant difference in the revision rates in published sample series compared with those from national registries. They noted that implant developers represent about 50% of the published content and are likely overrepresented in the literature. Revision rates as collected in national registries have been reported to be approximately twice as high as in sample series, and the overall revision rates according to registry databases have been cited as 21.8% at 5 years and 43.5% at 10 years. A more recent review of National Joint Registry data, including 5152 primary and 591 revision total ankle arthroplasties, gave prosthesis survival rates of 94% at 2 years, 87% at 5 years, and 81% at 10 years. Another review of data from five national registers showed revision rates of approximately 10% at 5 years. According to a review of the literature by Easley et al., reported implant survivorship in 2240 total ankle arthroplasties ranged from 70% to 98% at 3 to 6 years and from 80% to 95% at 8 to 12 years; they also noted that most published reports have a fair-to-poor quality level of evidence. In their review of 90 patients with total ankle arthroplasties using both mobile-bearing and fixed-bearing implants, Queen et al. found improved function in all patients. In general, those with a fixed-bearing implant had more improvements in ankle moment and ground reaction forces, whereas those with mobile-bearing implants had more improvement in patient-reported pain. A more recent comparison study by Lefrancois et al. (451 TAAs) found more frequent metal component revisions with Mobility and Agility implants than with HINTEGRA and STAR systems.

For convenience, outcomes are reported for mobile-bearing prostheses and then fixed-bearing prostheses. Most, but not all, of the available literature reporting outcomes on third-generation, three-component, mobile-bearing prostheses come from outside the United States, where the implants have been in use for many years. Studies of the STAR, Salto, Mobility, and AES ankle systems report 5-year survivorship ranging from 83% to 97%, with 92% to 97% patient satisfaction (Table 8.3). Additional surgical procedures were required in 17% to 39% of patients. Frequent causes for revision included aseptic loosening, osteolysis and osteolytic cysts, implant failure, malleolar impingement, and malalignment.

Of the various fixed-bearing, two-component designs, the Agility total ankle has significant intermediate and long-term outcomes reported. Although relatively high rates of patient satisfaction have been reported, revision and reoperation rates also are high with this implant, and it is no longer available in the United States.

Currently, at our institution the most commonly used prosthesis is the INFINITY, most often with patient-specific guides. We have 5 years of experience with this implant. Recent reports by Cody et al. and Saito et al. have raised concerns regarding tibial component loosening, subsidence, and early revision; however, we have not encountered these problems in our patients. A prospective, multi-center trial is underway, and we hope to report early outcomes in the near future.

SPORTS PARTICIPATION

Two studies investigating the ability to participate in sports after TAA found rates of sports participation after surgery to be equal to or higher than those before surgery; however, activities did not include high-impact or contact sports and most often involved activities such as swimming, cycling, hiking, and fitness training.

TABLE 8.3

Results of Total Ankle Arthroplasty

STUDY	IMPLANT	NO. PATIENTS	FOLLOW-UP	RESULTS
Karantana et al. (2010)	STAR	45 (52 ankles)	8 years	Prosthesis survival at 5 years 90%, at 8 years 84% Revision rate 17%
Wood et al. (2010)	Mobility	96 (100 ankles)	4 years	Prosthesis survival at 3 years 97%, at 4 years 94% Patient satisfaction 97%
Skyttä et al. (2010)	STAR Biomet AES	645 (Finnish Arthroplasty Register)	7 years	Prosthesis survival at 5 years 83%, 7-year survival 78%
Mann et al. (2011)	STAR	76 (78 ankles)	9 years	Probability of prosthesis survival at 5 years 96%, at least 10 years 90% Patient satisfaction 92% Additional surgeries 17%
Bonnin et al. (2011)	Salto	96 (98 ankles)	11 years	Prosthesis survival at 10 years 65%; 85% when fusion or revision of any component used as criterion for failure Reoperation rate 35%
Nunley et al. (2012)	STAR	82 (82 ankles)	5 years	Prosthesis survival at 5 years 94%, projected 9 years 88% Additional surgeries 17%
Barg et al. (2013)	HINTEGRA	684 (722 ankles)	6 years	Prosthesis survival at 5 years 94%; projected 10-year 84%; 61 ankles (8%) had revision arthroplasties
Brunnerf et al. (2013)	STAR	72 (77 ankles)	12 years	Probability of implant survival 71% at 10 years, 46% at 14 years 29 (38%) required revision of at least one metallic component
Schweitzer et al. (2013)	Salto Talaris	67 (67 ankles)	3 years	Implant survival at 3 years 96% 8 patients (12%) had additional surgery after index procedure 15 patients (22%) with 23 complications
Sproule et al. (2013)	MOBILITY	85 (88 ankles)	3 years	Cumulative survival 90% at 3 years, 88% at 4 years Good pain relief and improved function in 82% 8 ankles (9%) required revision
Adams et al. (2014)	INBONE	194 (194 ankles)	4 years	Overall implant survival of 89% Revision rate of 6%
Ramaskandhan et al. (2014)	MOBILITY	106 (106 ankles)	2 years	53-point improvement in AOFAS scores 12% complication rate
Deleu et al. (2015)	HINTEGRA	50 (50 ankles)	4 years	AOFAS scores and ROM significantly improved Osteolysis identified in 24 ankles (48%)
Jastifer and Coughlin (2015)	STAR	18 (18 ankles)	10 years	Overall implant survival 94% Additional surgery required in 39% All patients reported their outcomes as good or excellent
Jung et al. (2015)	HINTEGRA, MOBILITY	52 (54 ankles)	2–3 years	Ankle impingement syndrome significantly more common with HINTEGRA; intraoperative malleolar fracture only with MOBILITY
Hsu and Haddad (2015)	INBONE	59 (59 ankles)	3 years	Estimated survival rate at 2 years 97% 14 patients (2%) required reoperation because of complication.
Daniels et al. (2015)	STAR	98 (111 ankles)	9 years	32 ankles (29%) required metal component revision and/or polyethylene bearing exchange
Zhou et al. (2016)	Unknown; 95 academic centers	2340 ankles	Unknown	Overall complication rate 1.4%, <0.5% after 2007 Readmission rate of 3%
META-ANALYSIS/SYSTEMATIC REVIEW				
Stengel et al. (2005)	Mobile bearing only	1107 ankles		Prosthesis survival at 5 years 91% Complication rates 2%-15% Secondary surgery in 12%, arthrodesis in 6%
Haddad et al.* (2007)	Mobile and fixed bearing	852 ankles		Excellent/good results ~70% 5-year implant survival 78% Revision rate 7%

TABLE 8.3				
Results of Total Ankle Arthroplasty—cont'd				
STUDY	**IMPLANT**	**NO. PATIENTS**	**FOLLOW-UP**	**RESULTS**
Gougoulias et al. (2010)	Mobile and fixed bearing	1105 ankles		Overall failure rate at 10 years 10% Deep infections 0%-5% Superiority of one implant design over another not supported by available data
Zhao et al. (2011)	Mobile bearing (STAR)	2088 ankles		5-year survival rate 86% 10-year survival rate 71%
Roukis (2012)	Mobile bearing (Agility)	2312 ankles		~10% revision rate
Zaidi et al. (2013)	STAR, Hintegra, TNK	7942 ankles		Overall survivorship 89% at 10 years
Roukis et al. (2015)	Mobile and fixed bearing (Salto)	1421 ankles		4% revision rate with mobile; 2.4% rate with fixed

*Comparison with arthrodesis (Table 8.1).
AOFAS, American Orthopaedic Foot and Ankle Society; *ROM*, range of motion.

ROLE OF EXPERIENCE AND NUMBERS OF CASES

TAA is not a procedure to be undertaken lightly. The risk of complications is not insignificant, and the instrumentation is, in general, complex. A thorough knowledge of the fundamental forces affecting the ankle and hindfoot is critical, and patient selection is paramount. Most studies show a definite learning curve, with improved outcomes related to experience, and implant designers require training with artificial bones and/or cadavers to become certified in the use of their equipment.

RANGE OF MOTION

Perhaps the only advantage the ankle joint has over the knee or hip joint in total joint replacement is the apparent range of motion necessary for gait and function. Although more extremes of motion are needed for activities such as jogging, running, or walking up or down an inclined surface, level ground walking requires only about 12 degrees of extension and 20 degrees of ankle flexion. Ajis et al. evaluated 119 patients and found no notable improvement in ankle range of motion at 6 months after TAA. Coetzee and Castro evaluated range of motion of the ankle joint on preoperative and postoperative radiographs and found that true tibiotalar motion improved from an average of 18.5 degrees before surgery to 23.4 degrees after surgery. They suggested that clinical assessments of range of motion are difficult to reproduce and likely to be invalid in the assessment of true improvements in ankle motion after TAA. Dekker et al. also determined that, because of increased midfoot and subtalar motion, actual ankle motion after TAA is approximately 12 degrees less than the total arc of motion that might be observed clinically.

BY DIAGNOSIS

The reported outcomes of TAA according to diagnosis are variable, with some reporting better results in inflammatory arthritis than in osteoarthritis or traumatic arthritis, others reporting better results in osteoarthritis, and still others reporting no difference in outcomes. Gramlich et al. reported that TAA in 60 patients with posttraumatic end-stage arthrosis was associated with a high revision rate (42%); frequent symptomatic periprosthetic bone cysts caused high rates of revision surgery and worse outcomes, which were not improved by secondary TAA. It appears that careful patient selection concerning other variables such as age, activity level, and joint alignment and stability is more important than the type of arthritis present.

COMPLICATIONS

Complications are relatively frequent after TAA and can range from minor to catastrophic. Glazebrook et al. classified complications into three grades:

High grade: deep infection, aseptic loosening, and implant failure; high failure rates (>50%)

Medium grade: technical error, postoperative fractures, and subsidence; moderate failure rates

Low grade: intraoperative fractures and wound healing problems; low failure rates

Gadd et al. reviewed complications in 212 total ankle arthroplasties and categorized them according to the Glazebrook classification. All complications recorded in their study except intraoperative fracture and wound healing, including those designated "medium grade" in the Glazebrook scheme (technical error, postoperative fracture, and subsidence), had a failure rate of at least 50%, prompting these authors to propose a simplified two-level classification: high risk and low risk for failure.

Younger et al. proposed a grading system for reoperations after TAA and ankle arthrodesis that was designed to capture all major adverse events for which reoperation is required. They suggested that future operations might be avoided if the cause of reoperation is identified and procedures or devices are modified accordingly.

IN-HOSPITAL COMPLICATIONS

Using data from the Nationwide Inpatient Sample (NIS), Odum et al. found an inpatient rate of major complications of 5% and a minor complication rate of 6% in 1574 patients with TAA; there were no in-hospital deaths. In their review of 905 patients with primary or revision TAA, Lai et al. identified older age, higher BMI, and revision procedures as associated with early complications. Cunningham et al., to the contrary, found that most common comorbidities did not reliably predict increased complications or costs. In-hospital TAA has been shown to be associated with more frequent complications than outpatient TAA. Although infrequent, blood transfusions during TAA have been found to be associated with increased in-hospital complications, including acute renal failure. Ewing et al. reported that blood transfusions were more likely to be needed in patients with congestive heart failure, peripheral vascular disease, hypothyroidism, coagulation disorder, or anemia. In a comparison of perioperative complications in patients who had TAA at an orthopaedic specialty hospital or academic teaching hospital, Beck et al. found that those treated at an orthopaedic specialty hospital had a significantly shorter length of stay, with no significant differences in readmission or reoperation rates.

WOUND HEALING COMPLICATIONS

One of the most unnerving complications in TAA is a postoperative wound dehiscence (Fig. 8.18). A careful preoperative evaluation may limit healing problems. If a healing problem is suspected, the patient should be evaluated for nutritional deficiencies, and we caution against surgery in active smokers. Although it is not known how long a patient should refrain from smoking before surgery, it seems prudent to be certain they are confident of not returning to smoking in the immediate postoperative period. Lampley et al. reported that tobacco cessation appeared to reverse the effects of smoking, decreasing the risk of wound complications. We routinely keep patients on binasal cannula oxygen while they are in the hospital after surgery. Other risk factors associated with wound dehiscence include peripheral vascular disease, cardiovascular disease, and a

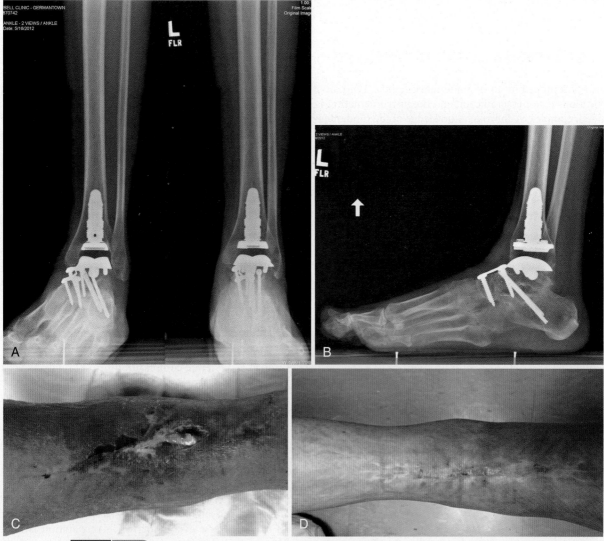

FIGURE 8.18 After total ankle arthroplasty (**A** and **B**), patient with rheumatoid arthritis developed wound dehiscence (**C**) because of nutritional deficiencies. With wound care, nutritional support, and secondary closure, wound eventually healed (**D**). No infection was present. It is important to have plastic surgery support in case of wound problems.

greater than 12 pack-year smoking history. In a series of 106 total ankle arthroplasties, Raikin et al. identified underlying inflammatory arthritis as the only significant risk factor for major wound complications. Although patients with inflammatory arthritis appear to be at higher risk for wound problems, evidence suggests that discontinuation of oral steroids or methotrexate is not beneficial and may in fact be detrimental, resulting in a postoperative flare of autoimmune disease. Antitumor necrosis factor-α medications such as Embrel, Arava, and Humira should be discontinued before surgery and should not be resumed until the wound is well healed.

Finding a significantly longer mean surgery time and a trend toward longer median tourniquet time in patients with wound problems, Gross et al. recommended limiting operative time and considering the staging of adjunctive procedures to decrease the risk of wound problems. Criswell et al., however, found no association between additional procedures requiring a separate incision and early complications.

Easley listed several suggestions to prevent wound problems: (1) use longer incisions that create less wound tension; (2) avoid direct skin retraction (retraction should be deep); (3) administer nasal oxygen in the immediate postoperative period; (4) maintain immobilization until the skin is healed; (5) leave the anterior tibial tendon in its sheath during exposure; and (6) use a drain. Matsumoto and Parekh compared wound healing with and without the use of negative pressure wound therapy (NPWT) in 74 patients and found healing problems in only 3% of the NPWT group compared with 24% of the control group.

Soft-tissue coverage of the prosthesis and tendons with a flap may prevent a catastrophic cascade leading to infection and implant failure. Gross et al. reviewed the outcomes and complications of flaps used to treat soft-tissue defects after TAA in 19 patients; four (21%) flaps failed resulting in two subsequent below-knee amputations.

OSTEOLYSIS, LOOSENING, AND SUBSIDENCE

Despite improvements in implants, instrumentation, and techniques, the longevity of TAA is not expected to approach that of knee and hip replacements at any time in the near future. At this time, it is difficult, if not impossible, to recommend one prosthesis over another because it is not yet known which designs will hold up and provide the best long-term results. The long-term success of most implants seems related to loosening and subsidence of the implant. It seems logical that improved coverage of bone by the implant should diminish peak pressures at the bone-implant interface. Wear debris and the lytic reaction to it may gradually create a lysis between the bone and implant. Small, nonprogressive cysts may be caused by stress shielding and bone remodeling after implant insertion, whereas large progressive lesions result from a macrophage-led immune response to polyethylene and metal wear particles in the periarticular tissues. A histologic analysis of 57 pathology samples by Schipper et al. showed that areas of osteolysis consisted of abundant polyethylene wear particles both intracellularly and extracellularly and appears to confirm that implant wear particles play a significant role in osteolysis.

Although some subsidence is common with most implants, the question about when to intervene is a difficult and open question. Asymptomatic subsidence in a stable,

well-aligned implant can be observed with annual radiographs. The same findings in a malpositioned implant are likely to only get worse with time, and earlier intervention may be well advised. With mobile-bearing designs, anterior translation of the talus under the tibia, as measured on the lateral view, has been associated with pain and worse outcomes. Yi et al. observed a significant correlation between the preoperative and postoperative talar position in the coronal plane at 36-month follow-up. Complications noted with talar translation included medial malleolar impingement, insert dislocation, and edge-loading. The diagnosis of implant loosening, or subsidence is suspected when more than 5 degrees or 5 mm of component movement is seen on serial radiographs.

Osteolysis is frequent after TAA but does not always correlate with component loosening or subsidence (Fig. 8.19). In one study, radiolucencies were present in 86% of ankles, but only 14% developed component subsidence or migration. Another study found periprosthetic osteolysis in 37 of 99 ankles, but no association was noted between the presence of osteolysis and clinical and radiographic outcomes. Asymptomatic focal osteolysis found on radiographs can simply be observed because it may not be progressive; however, Hsu et al. noted that, in their experience, most cysts do progress over time. Rapid cyst progression, particularly in symptomatic patients, warrants prompt intervention because it can progress to implant loosening and failure. Several studies have recommended adding CT imaging to postoperative follow-up for patients with suspected or known periprosthetic lucencies on radiographs.

Revision surgery decisions are based on structural constraints and typically involve the use of bone grafting procedures, exchange of implants to a more constrained design, and improved fixation and interference fit in the talus and distal tibia (see section on Revision Total Ankle Arthroplasty). Correction of the underlying deformity is critical, and the inability to do so may mean that it is necessary to convert to an arthrodesis. Gross et al. described 31 patients with bone cysts after TAA who were treated with a bone grafting procedure. The success rate was 91% at 24 months and 61% at 48 months. Four failures required three tibial and talar component revisions and one tibiotalocalcaneal fusion. The authors concluded that grafting without revision of the TAA is an effective and safe method for treating peri-prosthetic bone cysts. The techniques for conversion of an ankle arthroplasty to an arthrodesis are described in chapter 9.

MALALIGNMENT

Malalignment can be avoided by accurate bone cuts and proper soft-tissue balancing. Correction of malalignment may require calcaneal osteotomy and/or lateral ligament reconstruction for minor varus or valgus malalignment (see Fig. 8.5); supramalleolar osteotomy, subtalar arthrodesis, or triple arthrodesis for moderate to severe malalignment; or complete revision for severe malalignment.

■ POLYETHYLENE FAILURE

In a retrieval analysis of 70 total ankles, most commonly retrieved for loosening and polyethylene fracture, Currier et al. made several observations, including that loosening may be more of problem in fixed-bearing devices than in mobile-bearing devices. Gamma-sterilized polyethylene inserts oxidized at a higher rate than non–gamma sterilized inserts, and

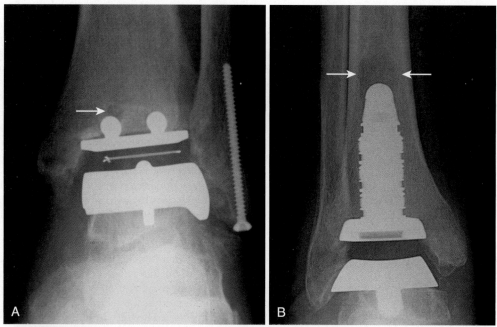

FIGURE 8.19 Periprosthetic lucencies may be related to technique and should not be misinterpreted as osteolysis. **A,** Postoperative radiograph shows mismatch between surgical drill hole *(arrow)* and medial cylindrical bar of tibial STAR component. **B,** Radiograph of INBONE device shows excessive medullary reaming *(arrows).* (From Bestic MJ, Bancroft LW, Peterson JJ, Kransdorf MJ: Postoperative imaging of the total ankle arthroplasty, *Radiol Clin North Am* 46:1003–1015, 2008.)

the presence of clinical fatigue (cracking and/or delamination) correlated with the amount of oxidation. Nine inserts, all gamma-sterilized, suffered fatigue damage or fracture in vivo.

FRACTURE

The most frequent intraoperative complication of TAA is fracture of the medial or lateral malleolus, which is reported to occur in about 10% of procedures in most series, although frequencies as high as 35% have been reported. The malleoli can be fractured if the saw blade cuts beyond the cutting block boundaries or if the bony resections leave so little bone that the force needed to seat the component is sufficient to cause a fracture. Medial malleolar fractures should be fixed with Kirschner wires (with or without a tension band), screws, a low-profile plate, or some combination of these because implant stability may rely on intact malleoli; lateral malleolar fractures can be fixed with a fibular plate. Some have recommended prophylactic Kirschner wire pinning of the medial malleolus or plate fixation of the lateral malleolus during TAA to prevent this complication. Calcaneal fractures also can be caused by excursion of the saw blade (Fig. 8.20).

Manegold et al. developed a classification system and treatment algorithm for periprosthetic fractures in TAA. The classification system is based on three sequentially assessed parameters: fracture cause, fracture location, and prosthesis stability (Table 8.4). The treatment algorithm is based on the classification system (Fig. 8.21). They identified 21 (4.2%) periprosthetic fractures in a group of 503 total ankle arthroplasties, 11 intraoperative and 10 postoperative; 14 of the 21 fractures were of the medial malleolus. The authors described fracture healing in all patients.

Postoperative malleolar fractures also have been reported, most often associated with patient noncompliance with postoperative weight-bearing restrictions. Many of these fractures

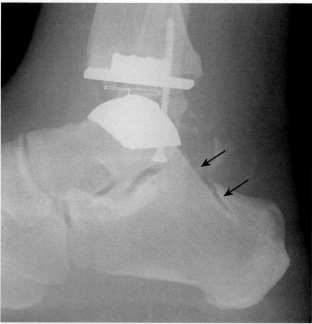

FIGURE 8.20 Postoperative radiograph shows linear defect through posterior calcaneus *(arrows)* caused by excessive excursion of oscillating saw during implant placement. (From Bestic MJ, Bancroft LW, Peterson JJ, Kransdorf MJ: Postoperative imaging of the total ankle arthroplasty, *Radiol Clin North Am* 46:1003–1015, 2008.)

can be treated nonoperatively, although open reduction and internal fixation may be required for some. Occasionally, a malleolar fracture can result in component loosening, requiring revision.

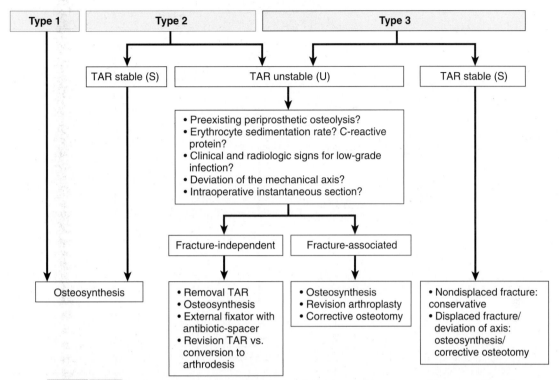

Periprosthetic fracture: decision-making

FIGURE 8.21 Classification based algorithm and decision-making protocol for treatment of periprosthetic ankle fractures. *TAR*, Total ankle replacement. (From Manegold S, Haas NP, Tsitilonis S, et al: Periprosthetic fractures in total ankle replacement: classification system and treatment algorithm, *J Bone Joint Surg* 95A:815–820, 2013.)

TABLE 8.4		
Classification of Periprosthetic Fractures		
FRACTURE TYPE	**FRACTURE LOCATION**	**PROSTHESIS STABILITY**
1 Intraoperative	A Medial malleolus	S Stable
2 Postoperative trauma	B Lateral malleolus	U Unstable
3 Postoperative, stress	C Tibia	
	D Talus	

From Manegold S, Haas NP, Tsitilonis S, et al.: Periprosthetic fractures in total ankle replacement: classification system and treatment algorithm, *J Bone Joint Surg* 95A:815, 2013.

INFECTION

Infection appears to be relatively infrequent after TAA. In systematic reviews of the literature, the rate of superficial infection ranges from 0% to 15%, with an average of 8%, and the rate of deep infection ranges from 0% to 5%, with an average of less than 1%. One report of causes of revision of TAA reported infection in less than 1% of 2198 ankles, whereas another large study by Althoff et al. reported infection in 4% of 6977 patients; independent risk factors for periprosthetic joint infections included age over 65 years, BMI over 30 kg/m² or under 19 kg/m², tobacco use, diabetes mellitus, inflammatory arthritis, peripheral vascular disease, chronic lung disease, and hypothyroidism. In a review of 966 ankle arthroplasties, Patton et al. found 29 infections (3%); operative intervention (irrigation and debridement, revision arthroplasty, or arthrodesis) resulted in limb salvage in 23 of the 29 (79%, 21% amputation rate). Risk factors identified included diabetes, prior ankle surgery, and wound healing problems more than 14 days after surgery. No significant difference was found between groups with respect to smoking, BMI, and operative time. Myerson et al. reported infections in 19 (3%) of 613 total ankle arthroplasties, 15 of which were late chronic infections. Only three of the 19 patients had successful revision with replacement implants, six had arthrodesis, seven had permanent antibiotic spacers, and three required transtibial amputation.

In their algorithm for evaluating painful ankles after TAA (Fig. 8.22), Vulcano and Myerson list two-stage revision, a permanent cement spacer, ankle fusion, and amputation as possible treatments for infection. They also listed some general guidelines for laboratory studies: elevated erythrocyte sedimentation rate (ESR) and C-reactive protein (CRP) + positive aspiration = infection until proved otherwise; elevated ESR and CRP + normal or inconclusive aspirate = infection cannot be ruled out; normal ESR and CRP + positive aspirate = infection until proved otherwise; normal ESR and CRP + negative aspirate = infection unlikely, consider mechanical causes of pain.

Lachman et al. reported their experience with irrigation and debridement and polyethylene exchange with component retention in the treatment of acute hematogenous periprosthetic joint infection in 14 patients. The long-term (3 years) failure rate was 54%. Two variables that were associated with failure of irrigation and debridement and polyethylene exchange were

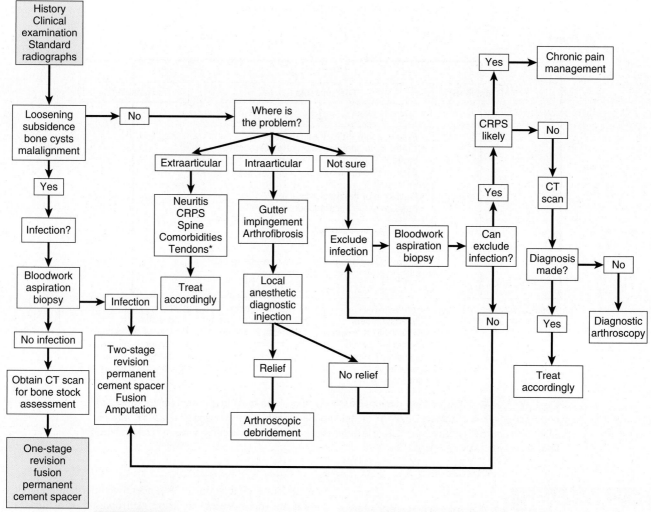

FIGURE 8.22   Diagnostic algorithm for the painful total ankle arthroplasty. *Lidocaine diagnostic injection: suspect posterior tibial tendon in neutral or flatfoot, peroneal tendons in cavus foot, and flexor hallucis longus if posterior impingement. *CRPS,* complex regional pain syndrome. (From Vulcano E, Myerson MS: The painful total ankle arthroplasty: a diagnostic and treatment algorithm, *Bone Joint J* 99-B:5–11, 2017.)

the time the patient was symptomatic prior to the procedure (average of 11 days) and the organism isolated on culture. The most common bacteria isolated in patients in whom the procedure failed was methicillin-resistant *Staphylococcus aureus*; the most common bacteria in patients who retained their implants were methicillin-sensitive *S. aureus*.

DEEP VENOUS THROMBOSIS

There is little information in the literature to give guidance to the decision of whether to treat patients with modalities or medication to lessen the chance of the development of DVT. Most series of TAA report a less than 1% frequency of DVT, with or without thromboprophylaxis. Saltzman et al., however, reported a 5% frequency, and Barg et al. reported symptomatic DVT in 4% of 701 total ankle arthroplasties. They identified the following as risk factors: obesity, previous venous thromboembolic event, and absence of full weight bearing postoperatively. Similar risk factors for infection were noted by Richey et al. in their cohort study of 22,486 patients with TAA, four of which were statistically significant: obesity, history of venous thromboembolism (VTE), use of hormone

replacement therapy, and postoperative non-weight-bearing immobilization for more than 6 weeks. Horne et al. reported DVT in only three (0.45%) of 637 patients. They concluded that chemoprophylaxis is not required in patients without identifiable risk factors for DVT. We routinely administer low-molecular-weight heparin in the immediate postoperative period and observe the patients closely at follow-up for signs and symptoms of this complication.

HETEROTOPIC OSSIFICATION

Reports in the literature are conflicting regarding the occurrence of postoperative heterotopic ossification after TAA, with reported frequencies ranging from 4% to 82% for different implant designs. The clinical consequences of heterotopic ossification also are controversial. Several authors have reported high frequencies of heterotopic ossification (42% to 82%) but with no association with clinical outcomes and no treatment required. Others have described limited dorsiflexion and plantarflexion and lower AOFAS in patients with heterotopic ossification. Most descriptions of heterotopic ossification after TAA place it in the posterior aspect of the ankle. Jung et al., however,

TABLE 8.5

Classification of Heterotopic Ossification After Total Ankle Arthroplasty

CLASS	CRITERIA
0	No heterotopic ossification
I	Islands of bone within the soft tissue about the ankle
II	Bone spurs from the tibia or talus, reducing the posterior joint space by <50%
III	Bone spurs from the tibia or talus, reducing the posterior joint space by ≥50%
IV	Bridging bone continuous between the tibia and the talus

From Lee KB, Cho YJ, Park JK, et al: Heterotopic ossification after primary total ankle arthroplasty, *J Bone Joint Surg* 93A:751, 2011.

reported that six of 13 developments of heterotopic ossification were in the anterior compartment and seven in the posterior compartment; heterotopic ossification in five of the six anterior compartments was in ankles with Mobility TAA components, likely because of the wide exposure of the cancellous bony surface at the talar neck. Associations have been reported between the development of heterotopic ossification and male sex, limited preoperative range of motion, previous heterotopic bone formation, posttraumatic osteoarthritis, ankylosing spondylitis, and infection. In their 80 patients, Lee et al. identified prolonged operative time as the only surgical factor found to significantly predispose patients to heterotopic ossification. These authors proposed a classification system for heterotopic ossification after TAA based on the Brooker classification of heterotopic ossification after total hip arthroplasty (Table 8.5) but made no treatment or prophylaxis recommendations based on the classification. To reduce the risk of heterotopic ossification, they recommended meticulous soft-tissue dissection, adequate implant size, and shortened operative time. Currently, nonsteroidal antiinflammatory drugs (NSAIDs) are the most frequently used method for prophylaxis against heterotopic ossification. We do not routinely administer NSAIDs before TAA, but prophylactic therapies (e.g., NSAIDs, radiation) may be used in patients who require excision of symptomatic heterotopic ossification. Noting the lack of a strong association between heterotopic ossification and postoperative ankle pain and functional limitation, Choi and Lee cautioned against attributing these symptoms to heterotopic ossification in the posterior ankle when considering its excision.

■ MEDIAL MALLEOLAR PAIN

The etiology and treatment of medial malleolar pain after TAA remain unclear. Suggested causes of medial pain include posterior tibial tendonitis, impingement, and stress fracture. Lundeen and Dunaway identified six patients (8%) with medial malleolar pain in 74 patients with TAA. All were treated with placement of two percutaneous medial malleolar screws, which relieved or reduced pain in all. These authors suggested that medial malleolar insufficiency fracture and placement of prophylactic medial malleolar screws should be considered in patients who present with new-onset medial malleolar pain with normal radiographs, especially if they are female or have medial malleolar thickness of less than 11 mm at the level of the tibial implant.

PROGRESSION OF ARTHRITIS IN ADJACENT JOINTS

The development or progression of arthritis in the subtalar or talonavicular joint after TAA has been described by several authors, whereas others found no subtalar arthritis. Wood et al. found worsening of subtalar arthritis in 15% of patients; Knecht et al., in 19%; and Mann et al., in 12%. It appears from these studies that TAA does not protect the adjacent hindfoot from the development or progression of arthritis.

OSTEOPHYTE FORMATION/IMPINGEMENT

Overgrowth of bone around the medial and lateral margins of the prosthesis (gutter impingement) is being more commonly recognized as a cause of pain after TAA (Fig. 8.23). The exact cause of impingement has not been clearly defined, but several inciting factors have been suggested: prosthesis design, oversized tibial and talar components, undersized talar components, uncontrolled varus or valgus thrust, component loosening, residual gutter debris, undersized polyethylene thickness, and talar subsidence. It is likely that no single factor is responsible and that the cause of impingement is multifactorial. Adequate resection of preexisting osteophytes and removal of all bone fragments from the joint margins can help prevent this complication. Aggressive gutter "clean-out" has been recommended as critical in reducing postoperative pain and gaining adequate postoperative motion. Schuberth et al. found symptomatic gutter impingement in 2% of 194 ankles with prophylactic gutter resection and in 7% of 295 ankles without gutter resection. They described using an open approach through a linear vertical incision directly over the involved gutter, which was debrided of all osseous and soft-tissue debris with power or hand instruments. Debridement was considered satisfactory when a 4.0-mm burr could be passed freely through the newly created corridor. Fluoroscopy was used to confirm adequate resection. Of 30 patients with postoperative impingement treated with only 1 gutter debridement procedure, 71% had excellent or good results. These authors caution, however, that radiographic determination of true gutter impingement often is obscure, subjective, and difficult to correlate with clinical examination. Postoperative symptomatic impingement may be relieved by local injection of cortisone and physical therapy; if symptoms persist, open or arthroscopic resection of the excess bone can be performed.

REVISION ANKLE ARTHROPLASTY

Decision-making in painful TAA is complex, and treatment is technically demanding. Pain is the primary symptom of early failure of TAA, and its location, quality, and onset can provide useful information about its etiology. Persistent pain after surgery may be indicative of a deep, indolent infection, whereas progressively worsening pain over time may indicate implant loosening and subsidence. Clinical examination should include evaluation of the surgical incision, tibiotalar and subtalar range of motion, ligamentous stability, alignment, gait, and tenderness to palpation about the medial and lateral gutters. Workup for periprosthetic infection should be done as a first step. If laboratory values are normal with

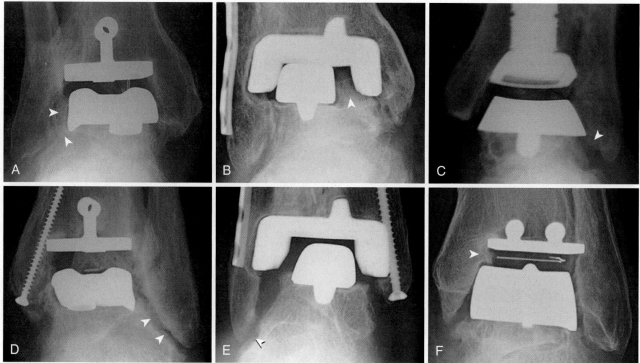

FIGURE 8.23 Radiographic examples of various gutter impingement morphologic features. **A,** Lateral impingement in a Salto Talaris implant. *Arrowheads* show areas of persistent arthrosis and hypertrophy of the talus after subsidence of the talar component. Note the proximity of the lateral component to the subtalar joint. **B,** Medial gutter impingement 7.5 years after implantation from a combination of polywear and talar subsidence. Note the talar bone mass in direct contact with the medial pillar of the tibial component *(arrowhead)*. **C,** Lateral talar impingement from an oversized talar component *(arrowhead)* 3 years after implantation. **D,** Lateral gutter impingement from residual lateral arthrosis from native bone *(arrowheads)*. **E,** Lateral impingement from the native distal fibular on the calcaneus *(arrowhead)*. **F,** Arrowhead shows site of overgrowth of bone at the medial gutter of a STAR prosthesis 2 years after implantation. Note that this bone growth allows the weight-bearing load to bypass the tibial component and is in direct contact with the poly layer. (From Schuberth JM, Babu NS, Richey JM, Christensen JC: Gutter impingement after total ankle arthroplasty, *Foot Ankle Int* 34:329–337, 2013.)

a negative or dry aspirate but pain persists, Hsu et al. recommended bone scan or single photon emission CT for further evaluation. If positive findings are seen on either radiographic study, they recommended reoperation to explore the joint for component osteolysis or infection. Croft et al. described the Ankle Arthritis Score (AAS) to evaluate functional impairment after TAA. They used this patient-reported outcome score to evaluate 509 patients (531 ankles). Revision surgery was associated with a higher postoperative AAS (higher level of functional impairment) and a longer follow-up.

Surgical management of failed TAA may require arthrodesis of the tibiotalar or tibiotalocalcaneal joints, revision arthroplasty, or below-knee amputation. Determining whether arthrodesis or revision arthroplasty is preferable is based on surgeon and patient preferences. Hsu et al. listed four situations in which they prefer revision with another prosthesis: (1) revision is technically achievable in the presence of a viable soft-tissue envelope; (2) there is adequate remaining bone stock; (3) good range of motion is present; and (4) the patient is compliant and requires early ambulation. In patients with stiff and painful ankles or massive bone loss associated with fractures, arthrodesis may be a better choice for definitive treatment. Meeker et al. listed their absolute and relative contraindications to revision TAA (Box 8.1).

BOX 8.1

Contraindications to Revision Total Ankle Arthroplasty

Absolute Contraindications
- Deep infection
- Neuropathic joint
- Insufficient bone stock
- Soft-tissue breakdown

Relative Contraindications
- Absence of the distal part of the fibula
- Instability resulting from incompetent ligaments
- Severe malalignment
- Peripheral vascular disease
- Significant bone loss
- Morbid obesity

From Meeker J, Wegner N, Francisco R, Brage M: Revision techniques in total ankle arthroplasty utilizing a stemmed tibial arthroplasty system, *Tech Foot Ankle Surg* 12:99–108, 2013.

Obtaining a plantigrade foot below the revision prosthesis may require osteotomies, ligament reconstructions, and tendon transfers in a combined or staged fashion to achieve solid tibial and/or talar fixation on residual bone stock without violating the subtalar joint, restoring ligamentous tensioning, and correcting hindfoot and forefoot alignment. Hsu et al. listed several key points to be considered in revision arthroplasty (Box 8.2).

The few available reports of the outcomes of revision TAA indicate that the procedure has a high rate of complications and variable functional outcomes. In their series of 41 patients with revision TAA, Ellington et al. reported that 28 patients (68%) had good to excellent results; however, only 18 (44%) were able to return to their previous levels of activity. Williams et al. described revision of 35 Agility total ankle arthroplasties (34 patients) to INBONE II prostheses, with a complication rate of 31% (Fig. 8.24). Thirty-one of the 34 patients had adjunctive procedures at the time of their final revision: curettage and grafting of cysts, subtalar fusion, Achilles lengthening, gastrocnemius recession, and realignment osteotomies, as well as internal fixation of pathologic fractures and gutter debridement. At final follow-up, only 13 patients (37%) had adequate range of motion; however, none of the patients complained of noteworthy pain, and none had been revised at a minimum of 6 months' follow-up. Of 29 patients with failed primary TAAs described by Lachman et al., the most common cause of revision was talar subsidence (52%), and the average time to revision was 4 years. A second revision or arthrodesis was required in 11%.

Ellington et al. described a classification of talar component subsidence—grade 1, no subsidence; grade 2, subsidence but not to the level of the subtalar joint; and grade 3, subsidence to the level of or interior to the subtalar joint—and noted that greater degrees of talar subsidence were associated with poor outcomes.

Failed TAA often is associated with bone loss, and custom-made talar components have been used to compensate for the bone loss as an alternative to arthrodesis. Wagener et al. reported good results in 11 of 12 ankles treated with custom talar components; all but one had improvements in the AOFAS hindfoot scores, and only one developed a deep infection that required arthrodesis.

Ali et al. and Kamrad et al. recommended salvage arthrodesis rather than revision TAA because of good results in their patients. At mean follow-up of 14 months, fusion had occurred in 22 (96%) of 23 ankles treated by Ali et al. with a hindfoot arthrodesis nail, and Kamrad et al. reported solid fusions in 90% of their 118 patients.

REVISION TOTAL ANKLE ARTHROPLASTY

TECHNIQUE 8.6

(MEEKER ET AL.)

PATIENT POSITIONING AND APPROACH
- Evaluate the existing ankle incision and determine if it is suitable for another operation. Although the optimal

---

approach for revision is through an anterior incision, whenever possible, modify this to incorporate previous incisions to minimize the risk of skin breakdown between narrow skin bridges.
- Place the patient supine on the operating table with a bump placed under the operative side so that the toes point vertical to the table.
- If an INBONE II prosthesis is selected for revision, place a radiolucent extension along the nonoperative side of the table so that the nonoperative leg can be abducted away from the operative field to make room for the leg holder.

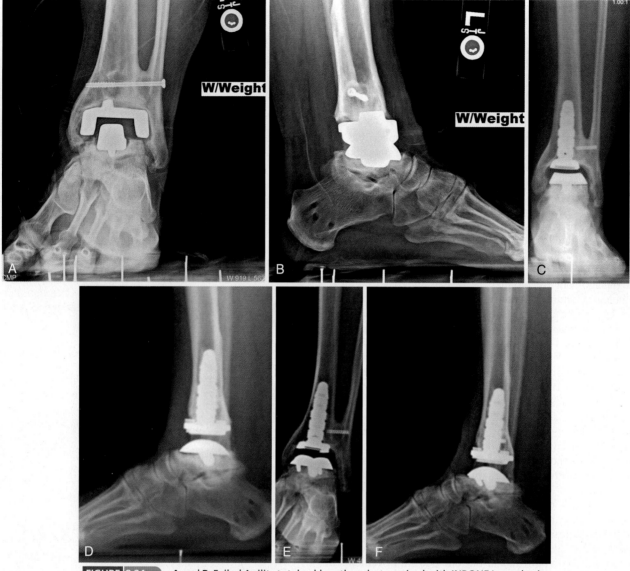

FIGURE 8.24   **A** and **B**, Failed Agility total ankle arthroplasty revised with INBONE I prosthesis. Talar component loosening **(C)** 2 years after implantation required revision with INBONE II talar component **(D)**.

- Place a thigh tourniquet and exsanguinate the operative limb with an Esmarch bandage after all incisions have been marked.
- Make an approximately 15-cm longitudinal incision through the skin over the anterior aspect of the ankle joint, centered midway between the medial and lateral malleoli. Approximately two thirds of the incision should extend proximal to the ankle joint, and the distal aspect should extend to the dorsum of the foot.
- Identify and retract laterally the superficial peroneal nerve where it crosses the incision at its distal extent.
- Incise the superficial fascia of the anterior compartment along with any remnants of the extensor fascia in line with the skin.
- Carefully develop the plane between the anterior tibial and extensor hallucis longus tendons, identifying the anterior tibial artery and the deep peroneal nerve. Retract the neurovascular bundle laterally with the extensor hallucis

longus as it crosses the ankle joint. Retract the anterior tibial tendon medially.
- Incise the anterior tibial periosteum and anterior ankle capsule longitudinally to expose the ankle joint and proximal portion of the talar neck.
- Continue dissection proximally and distally enough to expose the entire ankle joint and prosthesis.

IMPLANT REMOVAL
- After exposing the joint, debride any adherent soft tissue and bone obscuring the bone-implant interface.
- As the first step, disengage the polyethylene liner. This is simple when removing a mobile-bearing implant because it is free of any locking mechanism; however, most current TAA revisions in the United States are of two-component systems. It is important to know the locking mechanisms of the various implant systems.

AGILITY IMPLANT

- For removal of an Agility prosthesis, use fine chisels to make removal easier. Place a 5-mm chisel on each side of the polyethylene to shear off the hemicylindrical outcroppings from the polyethylene and lever the polyethylene out with a ¼ inch osteotome.
- Use tibial trial component from the Agility system to gauge the depth to which it is safe to introduce the chisel. Advance the chisel on either side of the keel to free the tibial component, taking care to avoid damaging posterior structures by plunging the chisels too deep.
- Because the Agility prosthesis has a porous coating on the medial and lateral aspects of the tibial component, use the chisel here as well. Take care to avoid malleolar fracture; consider prophylactic placement of Kirschner wires to stabilize malleoli that seem susceptible to fracture.
- Once the tibial component is freed, use the same chisels along the porous undersurface of the talus.
- If the central stem is customized to cross the subtalar joint, a retrograde approach may be necessary, accessing the tip through a calcaneal tuberosity approach. Open the outer cortex in line with the axis of the stem and use a combination of drills and gouges with small radii of curvature to free the stem from adherent bone. If the talar component still resists extraction, a tamp can be used on the tip of the stem to aid removal.

STAR IMPLANT

- Removal of a STAR implant is different because the mobile-bearing polyethylene is easily extracted.
- Use the fine chisels along the tibial component and to separate the porous undersurface of the talar component from bone. If the talus is firmly bonded to underlying bone, bone resection may be unavoidable.

SALTO TALARIS IMPLANT

- Again, use chisels to free the tibial component first.
- Because mobilizing the central keel of the tibial component risks bone loss, try to minimize this.
- Well-fixed talar components make bone loss a near certainty.

JOINT SPACE PREPARATION

- Once the components are removed, carefully assess the remaining joint space and bone quality.
- With the INBONE II prosthesis, bone cuts are guided with the use of an external leg holder. Keep lamina spreaders in the joint to preserve the alignment of the joint space when setting up the leg holder. Secure the hindfoot to the leg holder with pins in the calcaneus.
- The tibial cuts are guided with alignment rods that overlie the tibial canal. Confirm alignment in multiple planes.
- Access the tibial canal with a 6-mm drill through the plantar aspect of the foot, place the appropriately sized cutting guide on the leg-holder, and align it to allow appropriate bone cuts.
- Sequentially ream the tibia to a level necessary to obtain adequate placement of the tibial component. Place the appropriate number of modular stem pieces to provide adequate stability and affix the base plate through Morse taper impaction.
- Correct bony malalignment with improved bone cuts or with osteotomy of the distal tibia or calcaneus.

PROSTHESIS IMPLANTATION

- Fill bone voids with autograft or allograft. Trial the talar component with various thicknesses of polyethylene and assess for instability and hindfoot alignment.
- When the appropriate-sized components are selected, proceed with implantation.

INTRAOPERATIVE CONSIDERATIONS: LIGAMENTOUS INSTABILITY

- Before making bone cuts, evaluate the ligamentous stability and alignment of the ankle. Place lamina spreaders in the joint space and evaluate the hindfoot alignment by standing at the foot of the table while the leg is elevated for inspection.
- If severe medial or lateral instability exists, consider ligament reconstruction concomitant with the arthroplasty.

SUBTALAR JOINT

- If the patient has had a previous subtalar fusion, consider correcting malalignment with an opening or closing wedge osteotomy.
- If the subtalar joint remains but is arthritic or ankylosed, consider an arthrodesis to correct malalignment.
- For subtalar fusion, expose the joint through a separate sinus tarsi approach. If screw fixation is used, take care that the screws do not abut the talar component and are not in the path of the INBONE II fixation pegs, which may cause it to displace postoperatively.

BONE CYSTS

- Debride the areas where there are obvious cysts.
- Remove any lining of the cysts and perforate the sclerotic bone at the margin to allow adjacent bone ingrowth.
- If considerable bone loss exists, consider using allograft bone, bone graft substitute, or bone graft with iliac crest marrow aspirate.

JOINT BALANCING

- Once the trial components are in place, evaluate the joint for stability.
- Correct medial collateral tightness by performing a judicious deep deltoid release with a ½-inch curved osteotome.
- Correct lateral contracture by elevating the calcaneofibular ligament from its fibular attachment.
- If excess gapping occurs medially or laterally, consider allograft tendinous reconstruction either concomitantly or as a staged procedure.
- Once the appropriate insert has been selected that provides adequate stability, test ankle plantarflexion and dorsiflexion. If the ankle cannot be brought to neutral because of a posterior contracture, correct any posterior capsular tightness by careful release of scar tissue. If posterior tightness persists because of heel cord tightness, perform an Achilles lengthening or a gastrocnemius recession to improve dorsiflexion.

CLOSURE

- Debride any necrotic scar tissue and close in layers.
- Use absorbable suture to approximate the extensor retinaculum to prevent bowstringing of tendons.
- Close the skin carefully with interrupted or running nylon mattress sutures. Minimize skin ischemia that may result in wound breakdown. Place a drain if necessary.
- Place a plaster splint with the foot in neutral position.

POSTOPERATIVE MANAGEMENT

The patient remains non–weight bearing for 6 weeks to allow for osseous integration of the implants; this is followed by a period of protected weight bearing in a boot. The wound is checked every 2 weeks and, if there is no evidence of wound breakdown, the sutures are removed, and ankle range-of-motion exercises are begun. At 6 weeks, radiographs are obtained and, if there are no concerning findings, progressive weight bearing is allowed with the goal of full weight bearing at 10 to 12 weeks. If extensive bone grafting was necessary, the time to full weight bearing may be longer, as dictated by radiographic signs of osseous integration.

REFERENCES

GENERAL

Ajis A, Henriquez H, Myerson M: Postoperative range of motion trends following total ankle arthroplasty, *Foot Ankle Int* 34, 2013.

Bai LB, Lee KB, Song EK, et al.: Total ankle arthroplasty outcome comparison for post-traumatic and primary osteoarthritis, *Foot Ankle Int* 31:1048, 2010.

Besse JL, Colombier JA, Asencio J, et al.: Total ankle arthroplasty in France, *Orthop Traumatol Surg Res* 96:L291, 2010.

Easley ME, Adams SB, Hembree WC, DeOrio JK: Results of total ankle arthroplasty, *J Bone Joint Surg* 93A:1455, 2011.

Gougoulias NE, Khanna A, Maffulli N: How successful are current ankle replacements? a systematic review of the literature, *Clin Orthop Relat Res* 468:199, 2010.

Henricson A, Nilsson JA, Carlsson A: 10-year survival of total ankle arthroplasties: a report on 780 cases from the Swedish ankle register, *Acta Orthop* 82:655, 2011.

Labek G, Todorov S, Iovanescu L, et al.: Outcome after total ankle arthroplasty—results and findings from worldwide arthroplasty registers, *Int Orthop* 37:1677, 2013.

Law RY, Sabeh KG, Rosas S, et al.: Trends in total ankle arthroplasty and revisions in the Medicare database, *Ann Transl Med* 6:112, 2018.

Mercer J, Penner M, Wing K, Younger AS: Inconsistency in the reporting of adverse events in total ankle arthroplasty: a systematic review of the literature, *Foot Ankle Int* 37:127, 2016.

Pugely AJ, Lu X, Amendola A, et al.: Trends in the use of total ankle replacement and ankle arthrodesis in the United States Medicare population, *Foot Ankle Int* 35:207, 2014.

Queen RM, De Biassio JC, Butler RJ, et al.: Leonard Goldner Award 2011: changes in pain, function, and gait mechanics two years following total ankle arthroplaty performed with two modern fixed-bearing prostheses, *Foot Ankle Int* 33:535, 2012.

Raikin SM, Rasouli MR, Espandar R, Maltenfort MG: Trends in treatment of advanced ankle arthropathy by total ankle replacement or ankle fusion, *Foot Ankle Int* 35:216, 2014.

Reddy S, Koenig L, Demiralp B, et al.: Assessing the utilization of total ankle replacement in the United States, *Foot Ankle Int* 38:641, 2017.

Skyttä ET, Koivu H, Eskelinen A, et al.: Total ankle replacement: a population-based study of 515 cases from the Finnish arthroplasty registry, *Acta Orthop* 81:114, 2010.

Terrell RD, Montgomery SR, Pannell WC, et al.: Comparison of practice patterns in total ankle replacement and ankle fusion in the United States, *Foot Ankle Int* 34:1486, 2013.

Vakhshori V, Sabour AF, Alluri RK, et al.: Patient and practice trends in total ankle replacement and tibiotalar arthrodesis in the United States from 2007 to 2013, *J Am Acad Orthop Surg* 27:e77, 2019.

Yu JJ, Scheskier S: Total ankle replacement. evolution of the technology and future applications, *Bull Hosp Jt Dis* 71:120, 2014.

DESIGN RATIONALE, SURGICAL TECHNIQUE

Barg A, Elsner A, Anderson AE, Hintermann B: The effect of three-component total ankle replacement malalignment on clinical outcome: pain relief and functional outcome in 317 consecutive patients, *J Bone Joint Surg* 93A:1969, 2011.

Barg A, Elsner A, Chuckpaiwong B, Hintermann B: Insert position in three-component ankle replacement, *Foot Ankle Int* 31:754, 2010.

Barg A, Zwicky L, Knupp M, et al.: HINTEGRA total ankle replacement: survivorship analysis is 684 patients, *J Bone Joint Surg* 95A:1175, 2013.

Benich MR, Ledoux WR, m Orendurff MS, et al.: Comparison of treatment outcomes of arthrodesis and two generations of ankle replacement implants, *J Bone Joint Surg Am* 99:1782, 2017.

Bennett A, Ramaskandhan J, Siddique M: Total ankle replacement for osteoarthritis following pilon fracture of the tibia, *Foot Ankle Int* 39:1008, 2018.

Berlet GC, Penner MJ, Lancianese S, et al.: Total ankle arthroplasty accuracy and reproducibility using preoperative CT scan-derived, patient-specific guides, *Foot Ankle Int* 35:665, 2014.

Bishcoff JE, Fryman JC, Parcell J, et al.: Influence of crosslinking on the wear performance of polyethylene within total ankle arthroplasty, *Foot Ankle Int* 36:369, 2015.

Bischoff JE, Schon L, Saltzman C: Influence of geometry and depth of resections on bone support for total ankle replacement, *Foot Ankle Int* 38:1026, 2017.

Bonasia DE, Dettoni F, Femino JE, et al.: Total ankle replacement: when, why, and how?, *Iowa Orthop J* 30:119–130, 2010.

Bonnin M, Gaudot F, Laurent JR, et al.: The Salto total ankle arthroplasty: survivorship and analysis of failures at 7 to 11 years, *Clin Orthop Relat Res* 469:225, 2011.

Braito M, Dammerer D, Reinthaler A, et al.: Effect of coronal and sagittal alignment on outcome after mobile-bearing total ankle replacement, *Foot Ankle Int* 36:1029, 2015.

Brodsky JW, Kane JM, Taniguchi A, et al.: Role of total ankle arthroplasty in stiff ankles, *Foot Ankle Int* 38:1070, 2017.

Chambers S, Ramaskandhan J, Siddique M: Radiographic severity of arthritis affects functional outcome in total ankle replacement (TAR), *Foot Ankle Int* 37:351, 2016.

Cody EA, Lachman JR, Gausden EB, et al.: Lower bone density on preoperative computed tomography predicts periprosthetic fracture risk in total ankle arthroplasty, *Foot Ankle Int*, 2018. 1071100718799102. https://doi.org/10.1177/1071100718799102, Epub ahead of print.

Coetzee JC: Surgical strategies: lateral ligament reconstruction as part of the management of varus ankle deformity with ankle replacement, *Foot Ankle Int* 31:267, 2010.

Criswell BJ, Douglas K, Naik R, Thomson AB: High revision and reoperation rates using the agility™ total ankle system, *Clin Orthop Relat Res* 470:1980, 2012.

Currier BH, Hecht PJ, Nunley 2nd JA, et al.: Analysis of failed ankle arthroplasty components, *Foot Ankle Int* 40:131, 2019.

Daigre J, Berlet G, Van Dyke B, et al.: Accuracy and reproducibility using patient-specific instrumentation in total ankle arthroplasty, *Foot Ankle Int* 38:412, 2017.

Daniels TR, Mayich DJ, Penner MJ: Intermediate to long-term outcomes of total ankle replacement with the Scandinavian total ankle replacement (STAR), *J Bone Joint Surg* 97A:895, 2015.

Deleu PA, Devos Bevernage B, Gombault V, et al.: Intermediate-term results of mobile-bearing total ankle replacement, *Foot Ankle Int* 36:518, 2015.

Frigg A, Nigg B, Hinz L, et al.: Clinical relevance of hindfoot alignment view in total ankle replacement, *Foot Ankle Int* 31:871–879, 2010.

Fukuda T, Haddad SL, Ren Y, Zhang LQ: Impact of talar component rotation on contact pressure after total ankle arthroplasty: a cadaveric study, *Foot Ankle Int* 31:404, 2010.

Gaudot F, Colombier JA, Bonnin M, Judet T: A controlled, comparative study of a fixed-bearing versus mobile-bearing ankle arthroplasty, *Foot Ankle Int* 35:131, 2014.

Gauvain TT, Hames MA, McGarvey WC: Malalignment correction of the lower limb before, during, and after total ankle arthroplasty, *Foot Ankle Clin* 22:311, 2017.

Gross CE, Palanca AA, DeOrio JK: Design rationale for total ankle arthroplasty systems: an update, *J Am Acad Orthop Surg* 26:353, 2018.

Hamid KS, Matson AP, Nwachukwu BU, et al.: Determining the cost-savings threshold and alignment accuracy of patient-specific instrumentation in total ankle arthroplasty, *Foot Ankle Int* 38:49, 2017.

Hsu AR, Davis WH, Cohen BE, et al.: Radiographic outcomes of preoperative CT scan-derived patient-specific total ankle arthroplasty, *Foot Ankle Int* 36:1163, 2015.

Hsu AR, Haddad SL: Early clinical and radiographic outcomes of intramedullary-fixation total ankle arthroplasty, *J Bone Joint Surg* 97A:194, 2015.

Jastifer JR, Coughlin MJ: Long-term follow-up of mobile bearing total ankle arthroplasty in the United States, *Foot Ankle Int* 36:143, 2015.

Jung HG, Shin MH, Lee SH, et al.: Comparison of the outcomes between two 3-component total ankle implants, *Foot Ankle Int* 36:656, 2015.

Karantana A, Hobson S, Dhar S: The Scandinavian total ankle replacement: survivorship at 5 and 8 years comparable to other series, *Clin Orthop Relat Res* 468:951, 2010.

Knupp M: The use of osteotomies in the treatment of asymmetric ankle joint arthritis, *Foot Ankle Int* 38:220, 2017.

Lewis Jr JS, Green CL, Adams Jr SB, et al.: Comparison of a first- and second-generation fixed-bearing total ankle arthroplasty using a modular intramedullary tibial component, *Foot Ankle Int* 36:881, 2015.

Lundeen GA, Clanton TO, Dunaway LJ, et al.: Motion at the tibial and polyethylene component interface in a mobile-bearing total ankle replacement, *Foot Ankle Int* 37:848, 2016.

Nicholson JJ, Parks BG, Stroud CC, Myerson MS: Joint contact characteristics in Agility total ankle arthroplasty, *Clin Orthop Relat Res* 424:125, 2004.

Pellegrini MJ, Schiff AP, Adams Jr SB, et al.: Conversion of tibiotalar arthrodesis to total ankle arthroplasty, *J Bone Joint Surg* 97A:2004, 2015.

Queen RM, Franck CT, Schmitt D, et al.: Are there differences in gait mechanics in patients with a fixed versus mobile bearing total ankle arthroplasty? A randomized trial, *Clin Orthop Relat Res* 475:2599, 2017.

Queen RM, Grier A, Butler R, et al.: The influence of concomitant triceps surae lengthening at the time of total ankle arthroplasty on postoperative outcomes, *Foot Ankle Int* 35:863, 2014.

Ramaskandhan JR, Kakwani R, Kometa S, et al.: Two-year outcomes of mobility total ankle replacement, *J Bone Joint Surg* 96A:e53, 2014.

Rippstein PF, Huber M, Coetzee JC, Naal FD: Total ankle replacement with use of a new three-component implant, *J Bone Joint Surg* 93A:1426, 2011.

Schenk K, Lieske S, John M, et al.: Prospective study of a cementless, mobile-bearing, third generation total ankle prosthesis, *Foot Ankle Int* 32:755, 2011.

Schipper ON, Haddad SL, Fullam S, et al.: Wear characteristics of conventional ultrahigh-molecular-weight polyethylene versus highly cross-linked polyethylene in total ankle arthroplasty, *Foot Ankle Int* 39:1335, 2018.

Schipper ON, Hsu AR, Haddad SL: Reduction in wound complications after total ankle arthroplasty using a compression wrap protocol, *Foot Ankle Int* 36:1448, 2015.

Schweitzer KM, Adams SB, Viens NA, et al.: Early prospective clinical results of a modern fixed-bearing total ankle arthroplasty, *J Bone Joint Surg* 95A:1002, 2013.

INDICATIONS, ARTHROPLASTY VS ARTHRODESIS

Atkinson HD, Daniels TR, Klejman S, et al.: Pre- and postoperative gait analysis following conversion of tibiotalocalcaneal fusion to total ankle arthroplasty, *Foot Ankle Int* 31:927, 2010.

Courville XF, Hecht PJ, Tosteson AN: Is total ankle arthroplasty a cost-effective alternative to ankle fusion? *Clin Orthop Relat Res* 469:1721, 2011.

Dalat F, Trouillet F, Fessy MH, et al.: Comparison of quality of life following total ankle arthroplasty and ankle arthrodesis: retrospective study of 54 cases, *Orthop Traumatol Surg Res* 100:761, 2014.

Daniels TR, Mayich DJ, Penner MJ: Intermediate to long-term outcomes of total ankle replacements with the Scandinavian Total Ankle Replacement (STAR), *J Bone Joint Surg* 97A:895, 2015.

Daniels TR, Younger AS, Penner M, et al.: Intermediate-term results of total ankle replacement and ankle arthrodesis: a COFAS multicenter study, *J Bone Joint Surg* 96A:135, 2014.

Flavin R, Coleman SC, Tenebaum S, Bodsky JW: Comparison of gait after total ankle arthroplasty and ankle arthrodesis, *Foot Ankle Int* 34:1340, 2013.

Hintermann B, Barg A, Knupp M, Valderrabano V: Conversion of painful ankle arthrodesis to total ankle arthroplasty: surgical technique, *J Bone Joint Surg* 92A(Suppl 1, Pt 1):55, 2010.

Jastifer J, Coughlin MJ, Hirose C: Performance of total ankle arthroplasty and ankle arthrodesis on uneven surfaces, stairs, and inclines: a prospective study, *Foot Ankle Int* 36:11, 2015.

Jiang JJ, Schipper ON, Whyte N, et al.: Comparison of perioperative complications and hospitalization outcomes after ankle arthrodesis versus total ankle arthroplasty from 2002 to 2011, *Foot Ankle Int* 36:60, 2015.

Kim HJ, Suh DH, Yang JH, et al.: Total ankle arthroplasty versus ankle arthrodesis for the treatment of end-stage ankle arthritis: a meta-analysis of comparative studies, *Int Orthop* 41:101, 2017.

Kwon DG, Chung CY, Park MS, et al.: Arthroplasty versus arthrodesis for end-stage ankle arthritis: decision analysis using markov model, *Int Orthop* 35:1647, 2011.

Norvell DC, Shofer JB, Hansen ST, et al.: Frequency and impact of adverse events in patients undergoing surgery for end-stage ankle arthritis, *Foot Ankle Int* 39:1028, 2018.

Odum SM, Van Doren BA, Anderson RB, et al.: In-hospital complications following ankle arthrodesis versus ankle arthroplasty: a matched cohort study, *J Bone Joint Surg Am* 99:1469, 2017.

Pedowitz DI, Kane JM, Smith GM, et al.: Total ankle arthroplasty versus ankle arthrodesis: a comparative analysis of arc of movement and functional outcomes, *Bone Joint J* 98-B:634, 2016.

Schuh R, Hofstaetter J, Krismer M, et al.: Total ankle arthroplasty versus ankle arthrodesis: comparison of sports, recreational activities and functional outcomes, *Int Orthop* 36:1207, 2012.

Seo SG, Kim EJ, Lee DJ, et al.: Comparison of multisegmental foot and ankle motion between total ankle replacement and ankle arthrodesis in adults, *Foot Ankle Int* 38:1035, 2017.

Singer S, Klejman S, Pinsker E, et al.: Ankle arthroplasty and ankle arthrodesis: gait analysis compared with normal controls, *J Bone Joint Surg* 95A:e191, 2013.

Stavrakis AI, SooHoo NF: Trends in complication rates following ankle arthrodesis and total ankle replacement, *J Bone Joint Surg Am* 98:1453, 2016.

Veljkovic A, Norton A, Salat P, et al.: Lateral talar station: a clinically reproducible measure of sagittal talar position, *Foot Ankle Int* 34:1669, 2013.

Veljkovic A, Norton A, Salat P, et al.: Sagittal distal tibial articular angle and the relationship to talar subluxation in total ankle arthroplasty, *Foot Ankle Int* 37:929, 2016.

OUTCOMES

Adams SB, Demetracopoulos CA, Queen RM, et al.: Early to mid-term results of fixed-bearing total ankle arthroplasty with a modular-intramedullary tibial component, *J Bone Joint Surg* 96A:1983, 2014.

Barg A, Knupp M, Hintermann B: Simultaneous bilateral versus unilateral total ankle replacement: a patient-based comparison of pain relief, quality of life and functional outcome, *J Bone Joint Surg* 92B:1659, 2010.

Brag A, Bettin CC, Burstein AH, et al.: Early clinical and radiographic outcomes of trabecular metal total ankle replacement using a transfibular approach, *J Bone Joint Surg Am* 100:505, 2018.

Brodsky JW, Polo FE, Coleman SC, Bruck N: Changes in gait following the scandinavian total ankle replacement, *J Bone Joint Surg* 93A:1890, 2011.

Brunnerf S, Barg A, Knupp M, et al.: The Scandinavian total ankle replacement: long-term, eleven to fifteen-year, survivorship analysis of the prosthesis in seventy-two consecutive patients, *J Bone Joint Surg* 95A:711, 2013.

Chao J, Choi JH, Grear BJ, et al.: Early radiographic and clinical results of Salto total ankle arthroplasty as a fixed-bearing device, *Foot Ankle Surg* 21:91, 2015.

Cody EA, Bejarano-Pineda L, Lachman JR, et al.: Risk factors for failure of total ankle arthroplasty with a minimum five years of follow-up, *Foot Ankle Int*, 2018. 1071100718806474. https://doi.org/10.1177/1071100718806474, Epub ahead of print.

Cody EA, Scott DJ, Easley ME: Total ankle arthroplasty: a critical analysis review, *JBJS Rev* 6:e8, 2018.

Cody EA, Taylor MA, Nunley 2nd JA, et al.: Increased early revision rate with the infinity total ankle prosthesis, *Foot Ankle Int* 40:9, 2019.

Dekker TJ, Hamid KS, Easley ME, et al.: Ratio of range of motion of the ankle and surrounding joints after total ankle replacement: a radiographic cohort study, *J Bone Joint Surg Am* 99:576, 2017.

Demetracopoulos CA, Cody EA, Adams Jr SB, et al.: Outcomes of total ankle arthroplasty in moderate and severe valgus deformity, *Foot Ankle Spec*, 2018. 1938640018785953. https://doi.org/10.1177/1938640018785953, Epub ahead of print.

Desai SJ, Glazebrook M, Penner MJ, et al.: Quality of life in bilateral vs unilateral end-stage ankle arthritis and outcomes of bilateral vs unilateral total ankle replacement, *J Bone Joint Surg Am* 99:133, 2017.

DiGiovanni CW, Guss D: Ankle replacement or ankle fusion: who reigns supreme?: commentary on an article by Marisa R. Bench BS, et al.: Comparison of treatment outcomes of arthrodesis and two generations of ankle replacement implants, J Bone Joint Surg 99(21):2017.

Gramlich Y, Neun O, Klug A, et al.: Total ankle replacement leads to high revision rates in post-traumatic end-stage arthrosis, *Int Orthop* 42:2375, 2018.

Gross CE, Lampley A, Green CL, et al.: The effect of obesity on functional outcomes and complications in total ankle arthroplasty, *Foot Ankle Int* 37:137, 2016.

Harston A, Lazarides AL, Adams SB, et al.: Midterm outcomes of a fixed-bearing total ankle arthroplasty with deformity analysis, *Foot Ankle Int* 38:1295, 2017.

Hendy BA, McDonald EL, Nicholson K, et al.: Improvement of outcomes during the first two years following total ankle arthroplasty, *J Bone Joint Surg Am* 100:1473, 2018.

Hoffmann KJ, Shabin ZM, Ferkel E, et al.: Salto Talaris ankle arthroplasty: clinical results at a mean of 5.2 years in 78 patients treated by a single surgeon, *J Bone Joint Surg Am* 98:2036, 2016.

Joo SD, Lee KB: Comparison of the outcome of total ankle arthroplasty for osteoarthritis with moderate and severe varus malalignment and that with neutral alignment, *Bone Joint J* 99-B:1335, 2017.

Kerkhoff YR, Kosse NM, Metsaars WP, et al.: Long-term functional and radiographic outcome of a mobile bearing ankle prosthesis, *Foot Ankle Int* 37:1292, 2016.

Kim BS, Knupp M, Zwicky L, et al.: Total ankle replacement in association with hindfoot fusion: outcome and complications, *J Bone Joint Surg Br* 92:1540, 2010.

Lachman JR, Ramos JA, Adams SB, et al.: Patient-reported outcomes before and after primary and revision total ankle arthroplasty, *Foot Ankle Int* 40:34, 2019.

Lai WC, Arshi A, Ghorbanifaraizadeh A, et al.: Incidence and predictors of early complications following primary and revision total ankle arthroplasty, *Foot Ankle Surg* pii: S1268-7731(18)30325-4, 2018. https://doi.org/10.1016/j.fas.2018.10.009. Epub ahead of print.

Latham WC, Lau JT: Total ankle arthroplasty: an overview of the canadian experience, *Foot Ankle Clin* 21:267, 2016.

Lee GW, Wang SH, Lee KB: Comparison of intermediate to long-term outcomes of total ankle arthroplasty in ankles with preoperative varus, valgus, and neutral alignment, *J Bone Joint Surg Am* 100:835, 2018.

Lefrancois T, Younger A, Wing K, et al.: A prospective study of four total ankle arthroplasty implants by non-designer investigators, *J Bone Joint Surg Am* 99:342, 2017.

Lewis Jr JS, Adams Jr SB, Queen RM, et al.: Outcomes after total ankle replacement in association with ipsilateral hindfoot arthrodesis, *Foot Ankle Int* 35:535, 2014.

Mann JA, Mann RA, Jorton E: STAR(tm) ankle: long-term results, *Foot Ankle Int* 32:S473, 2011.

Nunley JA, Caputo AM, Ealey ME, Cook C: Intermediate to long-term outcomes of the star total ankle replacement: the patient perspective, *J Bone Joint Surg* 94A:43, 2012.

Oliver SM, Coetzee JC, Nilsson LJ, et al.: Early patient satisfaction results on a modern generation fixed-bearing total ankle arthroplasty, *Foot Ankle Int* 37:938, 2016.

Palanca A, Mann RA, Mann JA, et al.: Scandinavian total ankle replacement: 15-year follow-up, *Foot Ankle Int* 39:135, 2018.

Pangrazzi GJ, Baker EA, Shaheen PJ, et al.: Single-surgeon experience and complications of a fixed-bearing total ankle arthroplasty, *Foot Ankle Int* 39:46, 2018.

Pinsker E, Inrig T, Daniels TR, et al.: Symptom resolution and patient-perceived recovery following ankle arthroplasty and arthrodesis, *Foot Ankle Int* 37:1269, 2016.

Queen RM, Sparling TL, Butler RJ, et al.: Patient-reported outcomes, function, and gait mechanics after fixed and mobile-bearing total ankle replacement, *J Bone Joint Surg* 96A:987, 2014.

Raikin SM, Sandrowski K, Kane JM, et al.: Midterm outcome of the agility total ankle arthroplasty, *Foot Ankle Int* 38:662, 2017.

Roukis TS, Elliott AD: Incidence of revision after primary implantation of the salto® mobile version and salto talaris total ankle prostheses: a systematic review, *J Foot Ankle Surg* 54:311, 2015.

Roukis TS: Incidence of revision after primary implantation of the agility total ankle replacement system: a systematic review, *J Foot Ankle Surg* 51:198, 2012.

Saito GH, Sanders AE, de Cesar Netto C, et al.: Short-term complications, reoperations, and radiographic outcomes of a new fixed-bearing total ankle arthroplasty, *Foot Ankle Int* 39:787, 2018.

Schipper ON, Denduluri SK, Zhou Y, et al.: Effect of obesity on total ankle arthroplasty outcomes, *Foot Ankle Int* 37:1, 2016.

Slobogean GP, Younger A, Apostle KL, et al.: Preference-based quality of life of end-stage ankle arthritis treated with arthroplasty or arthrodesis, *Foot Ankle Int* 31(7):563, 2010.

Sproule JA, Chin T, Amin A, et al.: Clinical and radiographic outcomes of the mobility total ankle arthroplasty system: early results from a prospective multicenter study, *Foot Ankle Int* 34:491, 2013.

Stewart MG, Green CL, Adams Jr SB, et al.: Midterm results of the salto talaris total ankle arthroplasty, *Foot Ankle Int* 38:1215, 2017.

Tan EW, Maccario C, Talusan PG, et al.: Early complications and secondary procedures in transfibular total ankle replacement, *Foot Ankle Int* 37:835, 2016.

Tenenbaum S, Bariteau J, Coleman S, et al.: Functional and clinical outcomes of total ankle arthroplasty in elderly compared to younger patients, *Foot Ankle Surg* 23:102, 2017.

Usuelli FG, Maccario C, Granata F, et al.: Clinical and radiological outcomes of transfibular total ankle arthroplasty, *Foot Ankle Int* 40:24, 2019.

Usuelli FG, Maccario C, Manzi L, et al.: Posterior talar shifting in mobile-bearing total ankle replacement, *Foot Ankle Int* 37:281, 2016.

Usuelli FG, Pantalone A, Maccario C, et al.: Sports and recreational activities following total ankle replacement, *Joints* 5:12, 2017.

Wan DD, Choi WJ, Shim DW, et al.: Short-term clinical and radiographic results of the salto mobile total ankle prosthesis, *Foot Ankle Int* 39:155, 2018.

Wing K, Chapinal N, Coe MP, et al.: Measuring the operative treatment effect in end-stage ankle arthritis: are we asking the right questions? a COFAS multicenter study, *Foot Ankle Int* 38:1064, 2017.

Younger AS, Glazebrook M, Veljkovic A, et al.: A coding system for reoperations following total ankle replacement and ankle arthrodesis, *Foot Ankle Int* 37:1157, 2016.

Wood PL, Karski T, Watmough P: Total ankle replacement: the results of 100 Mobility total ankle replacements, *J Bone Joint Surg* 92B:958, 2010.

Zaidi R, Cro S, Gurusamy K, et al.: The outcome of total ankle replacement. a systematic review and meta-analysis, *Bone Joint J* 95B:1500, 2013.

OUTPATIENT TAA

Borenstein TR, Anand K, Li Q, et al.: A review of perioperative complications of outpatient total ankle arthroplasty, *Foot Ankle Int* 39:143, 2018.

Cunningham D, Karas V, DeOrio JK, et al.: Possible implications for bundled payment models of comorbidities and complications as drivers of cost in total ankle arthroplasty, *Foot Ankle Int* 40:210, 2019.

Fournier MN, Stephens R, Mascioli AA, et al.: Identifying appropriate candidates for ambulator outpatient total joint arthroplasty: validation of a patient selection algorithm, *J Shoulder Elbow Surg* 28(1):65, 2019.

Gonzalez T, Fisk E, Chiodo C, et al.: Economic analysis and patient satisfaction associated with outpatient total ankle arthroplasty, *Foot Ankle Int* 38:507, 2017.

Mulligan RP, Morash JG, DeOrio JK, et al.: Liposomal bupivacaine versus continuous popliteal sciatic nerve block in total ankle arthroplasty, *Foot Ankle Int* 38:1222, 2017.

Mulligan RP, Parekh SG: Safety of outpatient total ankle arthroplasty vs traditional inpatient admission or overnight observation, *Foot Ankle Int* 38:825, 2017.

Nodzo ST, Pavlesen S, Ritter C, et al.: Tranexamic acid reduces perioperative blood loss and hemarthrosis in total ankle arthroplasty, *Am J Orthop (Belle Mead NJ)* 47:8, 2018.

Taylor MA, Parekh SG: Optimizing outpatient total ankle replacement from clinic to pain management, *Orthop Clin North Am* 49:541, 2018.

Tedder C, DeBell H, Dix D, et al.: Comparative analysis of short-term postoperative complications in outpatient versus inpatient total ankle arthroplasty: a database study, *J Foot Ankle Surg* 58:23, 2019.

COMPLICATIONS AND REVISION

Ali AA, Forrester RA, O'Connor P, et al.: Revision of failed total ankle arthroplasty to a hindfoot fusion, *Bone Joint J* 100-B:475, 2018.

Alrashidi Y, Galhoum AE, Wiewiorski M, et al.: How to diagnose and treat infection in total ankle arthroplasty, *Foot Ankle Clin* 22:405, 2017.

Althoff A, Cancienne JM, Cooper MT, et al.: Patient-related risk factors for periprosthetic ankle joint infection: an analysis of 6977 total ankle arthroplasties, *J Foot Ankle Surg* 57:269, 2018.

Barg A, Henninger HB, Hintermann B: Risk factors for symptomatic deep-vein thrombosis in patients after total ankle replacement who received routine chemical thromboprophylaxis, *J Bone Joint Surg* 93B:921, 2011.

Beck DM, Padegimas EM, Pedowitz DI, et al.: Total ankle arthroplaslty: comparing perioperative outcomes when performed at an orthopaedic specialty hospital versus an academic teaching hospital, *Foot Ankle Spec* 10:441, 2017.

Berkowitz MJ, Clare MP, Walling AK, Sanders R: Salvage of failed total ankle arthroplasty with fusion using structural allograft and internal fixation, *Foot Ankle Int* 32:S493, 2011.

Besse JL, Brito N, Lienhart C: Clinical evaluation and radiographic assessment of bone lysis of the AES total ankle replacement, *Foot Ankle Int* 30:964, 2009.

Choi WJ, Lee JW: Heterotopic ossification after total ankle arthroplasty, *J Bone Joint Surg* 93B:1508, 2011.

Clough TM, Alvi F, Majeed H: Total ankle arthroplasty: what are the risks? *Bone Joint J* 100-B:1352, 2018.

Criswell B, Hunt K, Kim T, et al.: Association of short-term complications with procedures through separate incisions during total ankle replacement, *Foot Ankle Int* 37:1060, 2016.

Croft S, Wing KJ, Daniels TR, et al.: Association of ankle arthritis score with need for revision surgery, *Foot Ankle Int* 38:939, 2017.

Cunningham D, Karas V, DeOrio J, et al.: Patient risk factors do not impact 90-day readmission and emergency department visitation after total ankle arthroplasty: implications for the comprehensive care for joint replacement (CJR) bundled payment plan, *J Bone Joint Surg Am* 1001289, 2018.

Deforth M, Krähenbühl N, Zwicky L, et al.: Supramalleolar osteotomy for tibial component malposition in total ankle replacement, *Foot Ankle Int* 38:952, 2017.

Dekker TJ, Walton D, Vinson EN, et al.: Hindfoot arthritis progression and arthrodesis risk after total ankle replacement, *Foot Ankle Int* 38:1183, 2017.

Devos Bevernage B, Deleu PA, Birch I, et al.: Arthroscopic debridement after total ankle arthroplasty, *Foot Ankle Int* 37:142, 2016.

Ellington JK, Gupta S, Myerson MS: Management of failures of total ankle replacement with the agility total ankle arthroplasty, *J Bone Joint Surg* 95A:2112, 2013.

Ewing MA, Huntley SR, Baker DK, et al.: Blood transfusion during total ankle arthroplasty is associated with increased in-hospital complications and cost, *Foot Ankle Spec* 1938640018768093, 2018. https://doi.org/10.1177/1938640018768093. Epub ahead of print.

Gadd RJ, Barwick TW, Paling E, et al.: Assessment of a three-grade classification of complications in total ankle replacement, *Foot Ankle Int* 35(5):434, 2014.

Gross CE, Garcia R, Adams SB, et al.: Soft tissue reconstruction after total ankle arthroplasty, *Foot Ankle Int* 37:522, 2016.

Gross CE, Hamid KS, Green C, et al.: Operative wound complications following total ankle arthroplasty, *Foot Ankle Int* 38:360, 2017.

Gross CE, Huh J, Green C, et al.: Outcomes of bone grafting of bone cysts after total ankle arthroplasty, *Foot Ankle Int* 37:157, 2016.

Gross CE, Lewis JS, Adams SB, et al.: Secondary arthrodesis after total ankle arthroplasty, *Foot Ankle Int* 37:709, 2016.

Heida KA, Waterman B, Tatro E, et al.: Short-term perioperative complications and mortality after total ankle arthroplasty in the United States, *Foot Ankle Spec* 11:123, 2018.

Horne PH, Jennings JM, DeOrio JK, et al.: Low incidence of symptomatic thromboembolic events after total ankle arthroplasty without routine use of chemoprophylaxis, *Foot Ankle Int* 36:611, 2015.

Hsu AR, Haddad SL, Myerson MS: Evaluation and management of the painful total ankle arthroplasty, *J Am Acad Orthop Surg* 23:272, 2015.

Jung HG, Lee SH, Shin MH, et al.: Anterior heterotopic ossification at the talar neck after total ankle arthroplasty, *Foot Ankle Int* 37:703, 2016.

Kamrad I, Henricson A, Magnusson H, et al.: Outcome after salvage arthrodesis for failed total ankle replacement, *Foot Ankle Int* 37:255, 2016.

Kane JM, Costanzo JA, Raikin SM: The efficacy of platelet-rich plasma for incision healing after total ankle replacement using the Agility total ankle replacement system, *Foot Ankle Int* 37:373, 2016.

Kohonen Ia, Koivu H, Pudas T, et al.: Does computed tomography add information on radiographic analysis in detecting periprosthetic osteolysis after total ankle arthroplasty? *Foot Ankle Int* 34:180, 2013.

Krause FG, Windolf M, Bora B, et al.: Impact of complications in total ankle replacement and ankle arthrodesis analyzed with a validated outcome measurement, *J Bone Joint Surg* 93A:830, 2011.

Labek G, Klaus H, Schlichtherle R, et al.: Revision rates after total ankle arthroplasty in sample-based clinical studies and national registries, *Foot Ankle Int* 32:740, 2011.

Lachman JR, Ramos JA, DeOrio JK, et al.: Outcomes of acute hematogenous periprosthetic joint infection in total ankle arthroplasty treated with irrigation, debridement, and polyethylene exchange, *Foot Ankle Int* 39:1266, 2018.

Lampley A, Gross CE, Green CL, et al.: Association of cigarette use and complication rates and outcomes following total ankle arthroplasty, *Foot Ankle Int* 37:1052, 2016.

Lee KB, Cho YJ, Park JK, et al.: Heterotopic ossification after primary total ankle arthroplasty, *J Bone Joint Surg* 93A:751, 2011.

Lundeen GA, Dunaway LJ: Etiology and treatment of delayed onset medial malleolar pain following total ankle arthroplasty, *Foot Ankle Int* 37:822, 2016.

Manegold S, Haas NP, Tsitsilonis S, et al.: Periprosthetic fractures in total ankle replacement: classification system and treatment algorithm, *J Bone Joint Surg* 95A:815, 2013.

Matsumoto T, Parekh SG: Use of negative pressure wound therapy on closed surgical incision after total ankle arthroplasty, *Foot Ankle Int* 36:787, 2015.

Meeker J, Wegner NJ, Francisco R, Brage M: Revision techniques in total ankle arthroplasty utilizing a stemmed tibial arthroplasty system, *Tech Foot Ankle Surg* 12:99, 2013.

Myerson MS, Shariff R, Zonno AJ: The management of infection following total ankle replacement: demographic and treatment, *Foot Ankle Int* 35:855, 2014.

Noelle S, Egidy CC, Cross MB, et al.: Complication rates after total ankle arthroplasty in one hundred consecutive prostheses, *Int Orthop* 37:1789, 2013.

Odum SM, Van Doren BA, Anderson RB, et al.: In-hospital complications following ankle arthrodesis versus ankle arthroplasty: a matched cohort study, *J Bone Joint Surg Am* 99:1469, 2017.

Patton D, Kiewiet N, Brage M: Infected total ankle arthroplasty: risk factors and treatment options, *Foot Ankle Int* 36:626, 2015.

Pellegrini MJ, Schiff AP, Adams Jr SB, et al.: Tibiotalar arthrodesis conversion to total ankle arthroplasty, *JBJS Essent Surg Tech* 6:e27, 2016.

Preis M, Bailey T, Marchand LS, et al.: Conversion of painful tibiotalocalcaneal arthrodesis to total ankle replacement using a 3-component mobile bearing prosthesis, *Foot Ankle Int* pii: S1268-7731(17)31359-0, 2017. https://doi.org/10.1016/j.fas.2017.12.001. Epub ahead of print.

Rahm S, Klammer G, Benninger E, et al.: Inferior results of salvage arthrodesis after failed ankle replacement compared to primary arthrodesis, *Foot Ankle Int* 36:349, 2015.

Raikin SM, Kane J, Ciminiello ME: Risk factors for incision-healing complications following total ankle arthroplasty, *J Bone Joint Surg* 92A:2150, 2010.

Richey JM, Ritterman Weintraub ML, et al.: Incidence and risk factors of symptomatic venous thromboembolism following foot and ankle surgery, *Foot Ankle Int* 40:98, 2019.

Sagherian BH, Claridge R: Salvage of failed total ankle replacement using tantalum trabecular metal: case series, *Foot Ankle Int* 36:318, 2015.

Saito GH, Sanders AE, de Cesar Netto C, et al.: Short-term complications, reoperations, and radiographic outcomes of a new fixed-bearing total ankle arthroplasty, *Foot Ankle Int* 39:787, 2018.

Schipper ON, Haddad SL, Pytel P, et al.: Histological analysis of early osteolysis in total ankle arthroplasty, *Foot Ankle Int* 38:351, 2017.

Schuberth JM, Babu NS, Richey JM, Christensenn JC: Gutter impingement after total ankle arthroplasty, *Foot Ankle Int* 34:329, 2013.

Schuberth JM, Christensen JC, Seidensticker C: Takedown of ankle arthrodesis with insufficient fibular: surgical technique and intermediate-term follow-up, *J Foot Ankle Surg* 57:216, 2018.

Usuelli FG, Indino C, Maccario C, et al.: Infections in primary total ankle replacement: anterior approach versus lateral transfibular approach, *Foot Ankle Surg* 25:19, 2019.

Usuelli FG, Maccario C, Manzi L, et al.: Clinical outcome and fusion rate following simultaneous subtalar fusion and total ankle arthroplasty, *Foot Ankle Int* 37:696, 2016.

van Wijngaarden R, van der Plaat L, Nieuwe Weme RA, et al.: Etiopathogenesis of osteolytic cysts associated with total ankle arthroplasty, a histological study, *Foot Ankle Surg* 21:132, 2015.

Vulcano E, Myerson MS: The painful total ankle arthroplasty: a diagnostic and treatment algorithm, *Bone Joint J* 99-B:5, 2017.

Wagener J, Gross CE, Schweizer C, et al.: Custom-made total ankle arthroplasty for the salvage of major talar bone loss, *Bone Joint J* 99-B:231, 2017.

Whalen JL, Spelsberg SC, Murray P: Wound breakdown after total ankle arthroplasty, *Foot Ankle Int* 31:301, 2010.

Williams JR, Wenger N, Sangeorzan BJ, Brage ME: Intraoperative and perioperative complications during revision arthroplasty for salvage of a failed total ankle arthroplasty, *Foot Ankle Int* 36:135, 2015.

Yi Y, Cho JH, Kim JB, et al.: Change in talar translation in the coronal plane after mobile-bearing total ankle replacement and its association with lower-limb and hindfoot alignment, *J Bone Joint Surg Am* 99:e13, 2017.

Yoon HS, Lee J, Choi WJ, Lee JW: Periprosthetic osteolysis after total ankle arthroplasty, *Foot Ankle Int* 35:14, 2014.

Zhou H, Yakavonis M, Shaw JJ, et al.: In-patient trends and complications after total ankle arthroplasty in the United States, *Orthopedics* 39:e74, 2016.

COMORBIDITIES

Barg A, Knupp M, Anderson AE, Hintermann B: Total ankle replacement in obese patients: component stability, weight change, and functional outcome in 118 consecutive patients, *Foot Ankle Int* 32925, 2011.

Barg A, Knupp M, Kapron AL, Hintermann B: Total ankle replacement in patients with gouty arthritis, *J Bone Joint Surg* 93A:357, 2011.

Bouchard M, Amin A, Pinsker E, et al.: The impact of obesity on the outcome of total ankle replacement, *J Bone Joint Surg* 97A:904, 2015.

Choi WJ, Lee JS, Lee M, et al.: The impact of diabetes on the short- to mid-term outcome of total ankle replacement, *Bone Joint J* 96B:1674, 2014.

Demetracopoulos CA, Adams SB, Queen RM, et al.: Effect of age on outcomes in total ankle arthroplasty, *Foot Ankle Int* 36:871, 2015.

Gross CE, Green CL, DeOrio JK, et al.: Impact of diabetes on outcome of total ankle replacement, *Foot Ankle Int* 36:1144, 2015.

Gross CE, Lampley A, Green CL, et al.: The effect of obesity on functional outcomes and complications in total ankle arthroplasty, *Foot Ankle Int* 37:137, 2016.

Kraal T, van der Heide HJ, van Poppel BJ, et al.: Long-term follow-up of mobile-bearing total ankle replacement in patients with inflammatory joint disease, *Bone Joint J* 95B:1656, 2013.

Mayich DJ, Daniels TR: Total ankle replacement in ankle arthritis with varus talar deformity: pathophysiology, evaluation, and management principles, *Foot Ankle Clin* 17:127, 2012.

Pedersen E, Pinsker E, Younger AS, et al.: Outcome of total ankle arthroplasty in patients with rheumatoid arthritis and noninflammatory arthritis. A multicenter cohort study comparing clinical outcome and safety, *J Bone Joint Surg* 96A:1768, 2014.

Reddy SC, Mann JA, Mann RA, Mangold DR: Correction of moderate to severe coronal plane deformity with the STAR ankle prosthesis, *Foot Ankle Int* 32:659, 2011.

Ryssman D, Myerson MS: Surgical strategies: the management of varus ankle deformity with joint replacement, *Foot Ankle Int* 32:217, 2011.

Schipper ON, Denduluri SK, Zhou TY, Haddad SL: Effect of obesity on total ankle arthroplasty outcomes, *Foot Ankle Int* 37:1, 2016.

Schipper ON, Jiang JJ, Chen L, et al.: Effect of diabetes mellitus on perioperative complications and hospital outcomes after ankle arthrodesis and total ankle arthroplasty, *Foot Ankle Int* 36:258, 2015.

Sung KS, Ahn J, Lee KH, Chun TH: Short-term results of total ankle arthroplasty for end-stage ankle arthritis with severe varus deformity, *Foot Ankle Int* 35:225, 2014.

Tan KJ, Myerson MS: Planning correction of the varus ankle deformity with ankle replacement, *Foot Ankle Clin* 17:103, 2012.

Trajkovski T, Pinsker E, Cadden A, Daniels T: Outcomes of ankle arthroplasty with preoperative coronal-plane varus deformity of 10° or greater, *J Bone Joint Surg* 95A:1382, 2013.

The complete list of references is available online at Expert Consult.com.

ANKLE ARTHRODESIS

Clayton C. Bettin

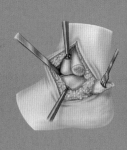

Ankle arthritis is a physically disabling condition, and its treatment can be both challenging and rewarding for the patient and the treating physician. Gait derangement is common in patients with ankle arthritis, and associated pain in the knee, hip, or back often contributes to general health problems. Arthrodesis, although not always perfect in outcome, can obtain a stable, pain-free ankle and dramatic improvement in the function and quality of life in appropriately selected patients. While the incidence of total ankle replacement is increasing, arthrodesis remains the procedure of choice for many patients with symptomatic ankle arthritis.

The biomechanical aspects of the ankle make it particularly suitable for arthrodesis. It is primarily a hinge joint and, although there is a continuously changing axis of rotation throughout the range of motion of the tibiotalar joint, fixation in a neutral position does not produce severe biomechanical consequences in the limb. The talus sits within a well-defined, stable architecture of the ankle mortise. It is supported by the medial malleolus, the congruent tibial plafond, and the lateral malleolus, all of which provide potential bone surfaces for healing of the arthrodesis. Since normal gait requires only 10 to 12 degrees of ankle extension and 20 degrees of ankle flexion, loss of some motion is not critical. This is in contrast to the knee or hip, where even modest loss of motion may be disabling for activities of daily living. Sagittal plane motion required for normal gait may be compensated for internally by a mobile transverse tarsal joint or externally by the application of a rocker sole shoe in a patient with ankle arthrodesis.

ALTERNATIVES TO ANKLE ARTHRODESIS
NONOPERATIVE TREATMENT

Surgical management of ankle arthritis is invasive, the recovery difficult, and the complications frequent. It is often best to think of the strategy in dealing with arthritis of the ankle as a *management* problem. It should be clear to the patient that returning the ankle to its prearthritic state is not possible, and conservative management may alleviate pain and restore function with little inherent risk. Conservative management will not improve pain and function to an acceptable level in all patients, but we routinely begin with several modalities before surgical intervention. This provides a measure of pain relief while giving the patient time to make intelligent, well-informed decisions regarding more invasive procedures.

Bracing to limit motion of the arthritic joint is a mainstay of conservative treatment. In our experience, the most effective brace is a double-upright, locked ankle brace with a steel shank and rocker sole in patients who are willing to accept the weight of the brace and shoewear limitations that accompany its use. It is durable and typically gives significant improvement in pain. It can accommodate deformity and changes in leg circumference from fluid shifts that may occur in this patient population. In other patients, an Arizona type brace, solid polypropylene ankle-foot orthosis, or lace-up ankle brace may be successful.

Nonsteroidal antiinflammatory agents are not without risks but may provide a measure of relief. Although glucosamine, chondroitin sulfate, and other dietary supplements are often tried, their efficacy is questionable. Intraarticular injections are a frequently used modality in these patients and, although hydrocortisone and a local anesthetic are a common combination, there may be a deleterious effect on viable cartilage and chondrocytes. Routine use of this modality outside of end-stage ankle arthritis is not recommended. Steroid injections are best used to aid in diagnosis and to temporarily alleviate pain in patients who are poor surgical candidates or who wish to delay elective surgical intervention until a time that better suits their schedule. The use of intraarticular hyaluronate preparations for viscosupplementation has been studied extensively in the knee. In the ankle, conflicting results have been found in well-designed studies. Sun et al. reported that in their 46 patients, three weekly intraarticular injections of hyaluronate provided pain relief and improved function, whereas DeGroot et al., in a randomized, double-blind, placebo-controlled study, found that a single intraarticular injection of hyaluronic acid was not demonstrably superior to a single intraarticular injection of saline solution

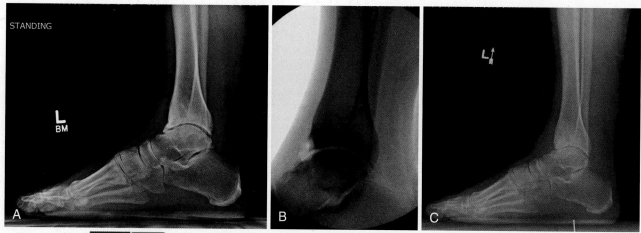

FIGURE 9.1 Joint debridement. **A,** Preoperative lateral radiograph. **B,** Intraoperative radiograph following anterior debridement of osteophytes. **C,** Postoperative lateral radiograph.

for the treatment of osteoarthritis of the ankle. More recent studies have confirmed that multiple injections of hyaluronic acid are more effective than single-injection protocols and that the use of fluoroscopy is indicated to ensure intraarticular infusion. In their prospective study, Lucas et al. found that neither etiology nor severity of the osteoarthritis was predictive of the response to viscosupplementation; however, Han et al. identified early stage disease and pain duration of less than 1 year as independent predictors of good outcomes. Viscosupplementation in the ankle is an off-label use, and insurance coverage issues should be discussed with the patient before proceeding with this treatment.

OPERATIVE TREATMENT

Although arthrodesis is a mainstay of treatment for ankle arthritis, it is not an optimal treatment for all patients due to the loss of joint motion and possible development of degenerative adjacent joint arthritis. Operative alternatives to ankle arthrodesis include open or arthroscopic debridement, realignment osteotomies, distraction arthroplasty, allograft replacement, and total ankle arthroplasty. Before ankle arthrodesis is chosen by a patient, alternative procedures should be considered and discussed.

■ JOINT DEBRIDEMENT

Arthroscopic or open debridement of the arthritic ankle can be effective in the overall management plan, but it must be used judiciously and with realistic expectations of the outcome (Fig. 9.1). Efficacy has been shown in several studies for the removal of anterior impingement osteophytes from the tibia and/or talus. Patients with mechanical locking of the ankle from a demonstrable loose body may also benefit from arthroscopic management, but it is likely that the debridement of more advanced arthritic ankles provides only short-term relief and is not recommended in most cases. Increased motion following removal of impinging osteophytes in a joint with irregular arthritic surfaces may lead to different or increased pain postoperatively and should be discussed with the patient before surgery. Aggressive removal of osteophytes also may lead to anterior extrusion of the talus postoperatively. Arthroscopic or open debridement can be done in combination with other procedures such as osteotomy and distraction arthroplasty.

■ PERIARTICULAR OSTEOTOMIES

Periarticular osteotomies of the tibia, fibula, or hindfoot, alone or in combination, are reasonable approaches to the management of localized arthritis of the ankle. The goal of realignment osteotomies is to unload the more arthritic portion of the joint and provide a more anatomic mechanical axis to the ankle to redistribute joint contact forces and loads. Realignment surgery can delay the need for arthrodesis or arthroplasty in younger active patients. Chondral loss primarily in the medial or lateral gutter of the ankle with minimal involvement of the superior surface of the talus, especially with supramalleolar deformity, seems best suited for this approach. The type of osteotomy is determined by the specific deformity, the condition of the surrounding soft tissues, the status of the articular surface, and leg-length considerations. Opening wedge osteotomy of the tibia for varus deformity and medial joint arthrosis is particularly effective as an alternative to more invasive treatment. Ahn et al. reported improvements in American Orthopaedic Foot and Ankle Society (AOFAS) scores, visual analogue scale (VAS) scores, and medial-distal tibial angle in 18 patients with medial ankle osteoarthritis and mortise widening after opening wedge distal osteotomy without fibular osteotomy. Although talar tilt was not corrected by this procedure, excellent clinical results were obtained in ankles with more than 7 degrees of talar tilt and good results in an ankle with 11 degrees of tilt. Before surgery, correction is planned by measuring the tibial-ankle surface angle and talar tilt on a weight-bearing anteroposterior radiograph and the tibial-lateral surface angle on a lateral weight-bearing radiograph (Fig. 9.2).

OPENING WEDGE OSTEOTOMY OF THE TIBIA FOR VARUS DEFORMITY AND MEDIAL JOINT ARTHROSIS

TECHNIQUE 9.1

- Through standard anteromedial and anterolateral portals, perform a full arthroscopic examination of the ankle.

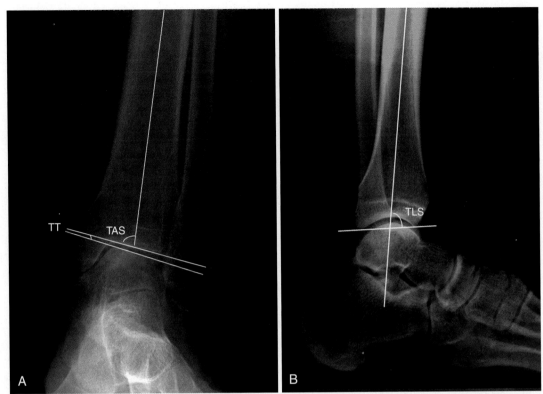

FIGURE 9.2 **A,** Anteroposterior weight-bearing radiograph showing measurement of tibial-ankle surface angle *(TAS)* and talar tilt angle *(TT)*. **B,** Lateral weight-bearing radiograph showing measurement of tibial-lateral surface angle *(TLS)*. (From Lee WC, Moon JS, Lee K, et al: Indications for supramalleolar osteotomy in patients with ankle osteoarthritis and varus deformity, *J Bone Joint Surg* 93A:1243–1248, 2011.)

■ Debride any impinging osteophytes, delaminated cartilage, and joint fibrosis.

■ For the fibular osteotomy, make a 2-cm lateral longitudinal incision 3 to 4 cm proximal to the articular surface of the medial malleolus.

■ Use a sagittal saw to make an oblique fibular osteotomy, placing a transfixing screw from anterior to posterior before completion of the osteotomy; do not tighten the screw.

■ For the tibial osteotomy, make a longitudinal incision beginning proximal to the tip of the medial malleolus to expose the anterior surface of the distal tibia; retain as much of the periosteum as possible.

■ Mark the osteotomy based on preoperative templating with a Kirschner wire and make the osteotomy with a water-cooled bone saw. Do not completely transect the tibia but leave several areas of cortex on the lateral side.

■ Carefully open the osteotomy with a Hintermann distractor or lamina spreader. Confirm on imaging that the deformity has been satisfactorily corrected and that the necessary size of autograft matches the preoperative templating. Insert the previously harvested iliac crest autograft.

■ Apply a contoured plate over the medial tibia to secure the autograft in place (Fig. 9.3).

■ Confirm alignment by observation and anteroposterior and lateral fluoroscopy.

■ Contour a plate and apply it across the fibular osteotomy.

■ Irrigate the wounds and close the fascial layer, subcutaneous tissue, and skin. Apply a sterile dressing and a short-leg splint.

POSTOPERATIVE CARE Non–weight-bearing ambulation is allowed the day after surgery, and flexion and extension exercises of the toes and knee are begun to prevent deep vein thrombosis and muscle weakness. A cast is worn for 4 to 6 weeks. After the cast is removed, active range-of-motion exercises of the ankle are begun. Weight bearing is gradually increased at 4 to 6 weeks in a fracture boot until full weight bearing out of the boot is allowed at 2 months after surgery.

INTRAARTICULAR OPENING MEDIAL WEDGE OSTEOTOMY (PLAFOND-PLASTY) OF THE TIBIA FOR INTRAARTICULAR VARUS ARTHRITIS AND INSTABILITY

Failure of traditional medial opening wedge and lateral closing osteotomy can occur because of persistence of the medial intraarticular tibial defect, resulting in recurrent

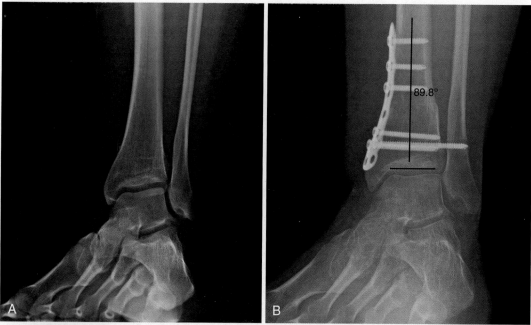

FIGURE 9.3 Medial closing wedge osteotomy for correction of supramalleolar deformity, preoperative (**A**) and postoperative (**B**) radiographs.

varus deformity. Becker and Myerson described a technique specifically for juxtaarticular varus ankle deformity associated with osteoarthritis and ankle instability. Mann et al. reported good results with this technique, along with lateral ligament reconstruction, in 19 patients. Four patients required ankle arthrodesis or ankle arthroplasty 7 to 48 months after the procedure; the other 15 patients were satisfied with their outcomes.

TECHNIQUE 9.2

(MANN, FILIPPI, AND MYERSON)

- After administration of general anesthesia and popliteal block for postoperative pain control, approach the ankle through a medial incision centered at the level of the deformity.
- Direct the apex of the osteotomy toward the intraarticular deformity from the medial aspect of the distal tibia.
- Use a Kirschner wire aimed at the apex of the deformity as a guide to the plane of the osteotomy (Fig. 9.4A).
- Insert three additional Kirschner wires parallel to the joint surface portion of the tibial plafond within the subchondral bone just under the articular cartilage at the apex of the plafond angulation to prevent penetration of the saw blade into the joint during the osteotomy and to act as a hinge during deformity correction (Fig. 9.4B).
- Make the osteotomy with a saw perpendicular to the anteroposterior axis of the tibia and in the same plane as the Kirschner wire, ending at the level of the three Kirschner wires, thereby keeping the bony bridge intact (Fig. 9.4C).
- Use the bony bridge and the three Kirschner wires as a hinge, and with a wide osteotome gradually bend the plafond until the medial tibial articular surface is parallel to the intact portion of the distal lateral tibia.

- Insert a lamina spreader into the cortical gap to hold the correction while allograft cancellous bone chips are inserted into the defect under fluoroscopic guidance to maintain a parallel joint surface (Fig. 9.4D).
- Secure the osteotomy with a locking plate to serve as a buttress to ensure that the allograft remains in place.
- If lateral ankle instability is present, correct it with a Broström or modified Chrisman-Snook procedure after ensuring that bone, osteophytes, and debris are removed from the lateral gutter.

POSTOPERATIVE CARE Patients are placed in a below-knee splint for the first 2 weeks, followed by application of a removable boot with instructions to remain non–weight bearing but to perform range-of-motion exercises. At 6 weeks, partial weight bearing is allowed, and at 8 weeks, full weight bearing is permitted. The boot is worn for a total of 10 to 12 weeks, depending on healing of the osteotomy.

■ DISTRACTION ARTHROPLASTY

With technical improvements to thin-wire external fixation for various deformity correction procedures, reports of using a thin-wire frame to provide distraction to the ankle joint for a period of time while allowing weight bearing seem to suggest some pain relief and functional improvement in carefully selected patients with ankle arthritis. Joint distraction arthroplasty is based on the concept that mechanical unloading of the joint and the intermittent flow of intraarticular synovial fluid encourage cartilage healing. Twenty-one (98%) of 23 patients reported by Tellisi et al. reported decreased pain after distraction arthroplasty; other series have reported good results in approximately 75%. In a randomized controlled trial, Saltzman et al. compared fixed distraction to motion

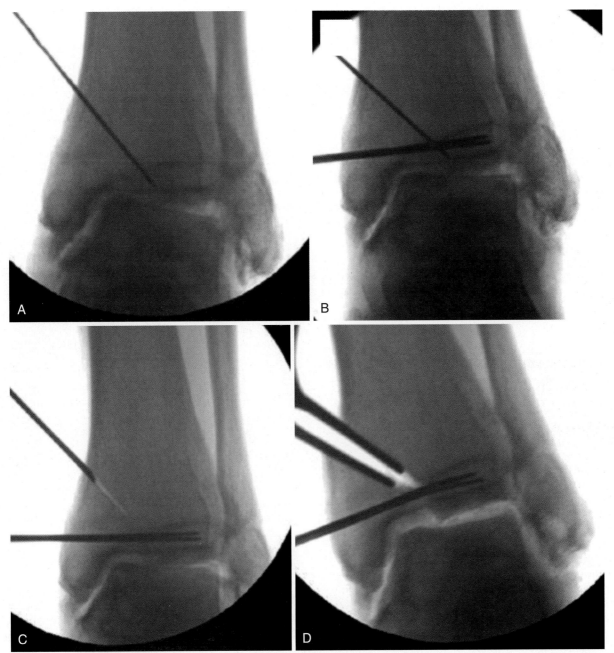

FIGURE 9.4 **A,** Guide pin inserted with tip positioned at the apex of the deformity. **B,** Kirschner wires inserted just proximal to the tibial plafond to prevent the saw from entering the joint. **C,** Osteotomy created with the saw aligned perpendicular to the coronal axis of the tibia. **D,** Displacement of the osteotomy with a lamina spreader for deformity correction.   (From Myerson MS, Zide JR: Management of varus ankle osteoarthritis with joint-preserving osteotomy, Foot Ankle Clin N Am 8:471, 2013.) **SEE TECHNIQUE 9.2.**

distraction in 36 patients and found that those with motion distraction had earlier and consistently better outcomes. Adverse events included 43 pin-track infections and eight neurapraxias.

The beneficial effects of distraction are not immediate and tend to occur over a long period of time, ranging from 6 months to 2 years. The ideal candidate for distraction arthroplasty is a young motivated patient whose symptoms are not relieved with conservative measures and who is unwilling to have an arthrodesis. Contraindications include active

infection, advanced coronal plane deformity, significant loss of bone stock, and patients who are poor frame candidates. Uncontrolled diabetes, tobacco use, chronic edema of the lower limb, severe ankle deformity, and severe ankle ankylosis are relative contraindications. In a randomized study, Herrera-Perez et al. showed similar functional outcomes and quality of life with debridement and a hinged distraction compared to debridement alone, although the rate of postoperative revision surgery was higher if distraction was not used. According to a comprehensive review of the literature by Smith et al., currently there is not enough high-level evidence to support ankle joint distraction for generally accepted indications. Tellisi et al. noted some key elements of the procedure and postoperative care that may improve outcomes:

1. Hinges should be placed along the axis of the ankle joint (Inman axis, line joining tips of the medial and lateral malleoli) to prevent uneven joint distraction through a range of motion and to preserve joint motion by evenly stretching the capsule.
2. Use of a forefoot wire should be avoided because this is very uncomfortable and discourages weight bearing.
3. No more than 5 to 6 mm of acute distraction should be applied in the operating room; if needed, more distraction can be applied gradually during the short postoperative hospital stay.
4. Range-of-motion exercises should be started early to preserve ankle mobility.
5. A circular fixator is superior to monolateral fixation because a monolateral frame delivers uneven distraction through cantilever mechanics and its simple hinge is difficult to place along the ankle axis.

DISTRACTION ARTHROPLASTY OF THE ANKLE

TECHNIQUE 9.3

PREOPERATIVE PLANNING
- On weight-bearing radiographs, measure the tibiotalar joint space and evaluate the degree of arthritis (Fig. 9.5A,B).
- Identify anterior osteophytes that might be sources of pain or blocks to dorsiflexion and need to be removed.
- Note the presence of any hardware in the ankle joint. Hardware generally does not need to be removed before distraction arthroplasty unless it inhibits application of the external fixator.
- Evaluate the ankle for periarticular deformity and determine if supramalleolar osteotomy is indicated in place of or in conjunction with distraction arthroplasty.

JOINT PREPARATION
- With arthroscopy or open arthrotomy, remove anterior osteophytes from the distal tibia and talus.
- Perform Achilles tendon lengthening or supramalleolar osteotomy as needed.

FRAME APPLICATION
- A tourniquet is not used during frame application because normal osseous and periosteal blood flow is needed to help cool passing wires and drills to avoid thermal necrosis.
- Usually a two-ring fixator is sufficient, comprising a distal tibial ring and a foot ring, with articulating hinges placed along the ankle joint axis between the rings. An additional ring may be needed if supramalleolar osteotomy was done or to enhance the stability of the construct in larger patients.

- Mount the proximal ring to the distal tibia with a combination of half-pins and tensioned wires. Place fixation in different planes to ensure adequate stability.
- Use of hydroxyapatite-coated pins is encouraged because of the enhanced bone ongrowth and stability for the extended duration that the frame will be used.
- Insert a smooth Kirschner wire immediately beneath the tip of the medial malleolus and check its position with anteroposterior and lateral fluoroscopy images to ensure proper placement (Fig. 9.6A).
- Attach two universal hinges with threaded rods, one on either side of the tibial ring. Place the hinges along the reference wire to approximate the true axis of rotation of the ankle joint. Check hinge placement with fluoroscopy.
- Secure the hinges to a foot ring that has been aligned to the foot (Fig. 9.6B). Insert a transverse midfoot wire through the cuneiform bones and tension it to the ring to establish alignment. Place two additional wires into the calcaneus and tension them (Fig. 9.6C). Insert a final wire into the talus, attach it to the foot ring, and gently tension it; this wire prevents inadvertent distraction of the subtalar joint.
- Place an anterior flexion-extension rod to control ankle motion.
- Distract the ankle approximately 5 mm (Fig. 9.5C,D) and, under fluoroscopic control, move it through a range of motion to check the amount of distraction and alignment.
- Place sterile dressings on the pin insertion sites.

POSTOPERATIVE CARE Patients usually are observed in the hospital overnight after surgery for pain control. Partial weight bearing is begun as soon as tolerated after surgery with ambulatory aids as needed (Fig. 9.6D). Deep venous thrombosis prophylaxis is implemented and continued until the patient is mobile. The patient is instructed in pin care, which consists of showering daily and cleaning any inflamed pin sites daily with diluted hydrogen peroxide or chlorhexidine gluconate. At 2 weeks, the sutures are removed, and distraction is evaluated. The goal at this time is 5 mm of distraction; if the joint space is less, additional distraction is applied in the office. At 12 weeks, the frame is removed in surgery with the patient sedated, a cam walker boot is applied, and weight-bearing ambulation is encouraged (Fig. 9.5E,F). In their recent review, Bernstein et al. suggested the addition of bone marrow aspirate to the ankle at the time of frame application, no more than 3 mm of acute distraction at time of surgery with additional distraction added later to maintain at least 5 mm, and no more than 12 weeks of distraction.

■ TOTAL ANKLE ARTHROPLASTY

A study looking at the Nationwide Inpatient Sample database from 2007 to 2013 showed the share of ankle replacement performed compared to arthrodesis increased markedly from 2007 (14%) to 2013 (45%), with arthrodesis patients continuing to have more comorbidities. The advantages and disadvantages of total ankle arthroplasty are discussed in detail in chapter 8. In general, arthrodesis has the advantage of predictable pain relief and the disadvantage of limited motion,

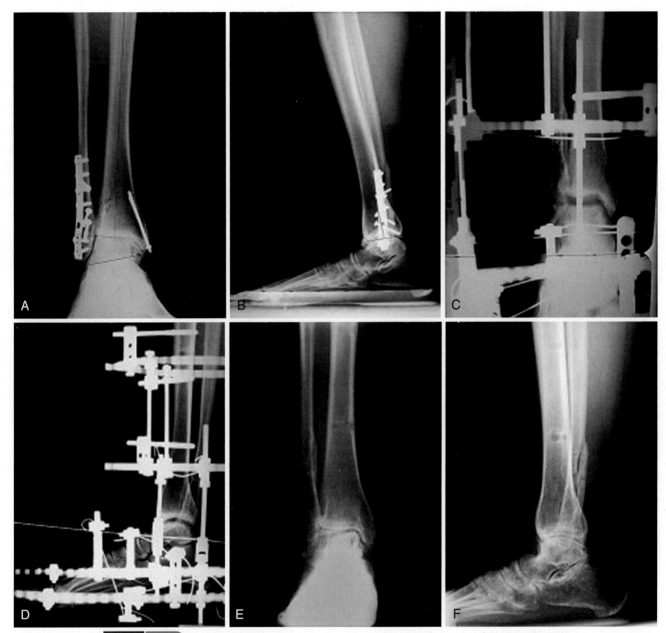

FIGURE 9.5   **A** and **B,** Posttraumatic arthritis and anterior osteophytes. **C** and **D,** Approximately 8 mm of ankle joint distraction obtained with hinged external fixation distraction device. **E** and **F,** Plantigrade foot at 3-year follow-up. (From Paley D, Lamm BM, Purohit RM, Specht SC: Distraction arthroplasty of the ankle—how far can you stretch the indications? *Foot Ankle Clin* 13:471–484, 2008.)
SEE TECHNIQUE 9.3.

whereas arthroplasty has the advantage of motion preservation and the disadvantage of more frequent complications. A study involving 114 ankle arthroplasties and 47 ankle arthrodeses reported no significant difference in the mean improvement in pain and function between the two groups at a minimum of 2 years postoperatively, but the complication rates were 54% after arthroplasty and 26% after arthrodesis. In a systematic review of the literature that included 1262 arthrodeses and 852 arthroplasties, Haddad et al. identified revision rates of less than 10% and infection rates of less than 5% after both procedures. Daniels et al., in a multicenter study involving 321 patients, reported that intermediate-term clinical outcomes of total ankle replacement and

ankle arthrodesis were comparable, although reoperation and major complications were more frequent after ankle replacement. More recently, Norvell et al. in a multisite prospective cohort study of 517 patients with arthrodesis or arthroplasty for ankle arthritis found no statistically significant difference in adverse events at 1 year after either procedure. Glazebrook et al. focused on survival and complication rates of total ankle arthroplasty and found that failure rates ranged from 1% to 32%, with an overall mean failure rate of 12%. Despite more costly implants, total ankle arthroplasty was determined to be a cost-effective alternative to ankle arthrodesis in a 60-year-old cohort with end-stage ankle arthritis. More recent comparisons have shown that patients with total ankle replacement

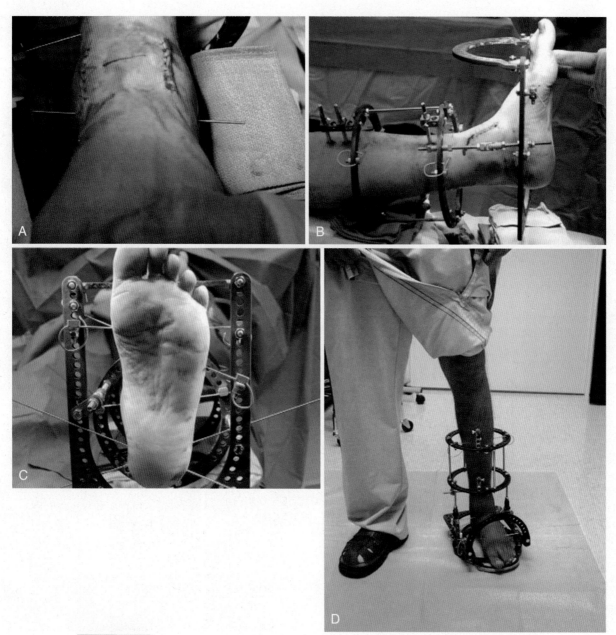

FIGURE 9.6 Distraction arthroplasty. **A,** Temporary guidewire inserted from tip of lateral malleolus to tip of medial malleolus as reference for ankle hinge placement. **B,** External fixator application. **C,** Wires placed in calcaneus and tensioned; note that foot is centered in fixator ring. **D,** Patient standing in frame with constrained ankle motion allowed through anatomically placed hinges. (From Beaman DN, Gellman RE, Trepman E: Ankle arthritis: deformity correction and distraction arthroplasty. In Coughlin MJ, Mann RA, Saltzman CL, editors: *Surgery of the foot and ankle*, ed 8, Philadelphia, 2007, Elsevier.) **SEE TECHNIQUE 9.3.**

have higher expectations before surgery than do patients with arthrodesis and are more likely to have their expectations met. Jasiter et al. found that patients with total ankle replacement had higher scores than ankle arthrodesis patients in walking on uneven surfaces, upstairs, downstairs, and uphill. Another study comparing 59 patients with total ankle arthroplasty to 46 with arthrodesis found that functional results were significantly better in those with arthroplasty; however, there was no difference in terms of quality of life (Dalat et al.). Studies that directly compare arthrodesis to arthroplasty must be carefully interpreted because of the inherent differences in patient

selection for each procedure. Many patients are better suited to either arthroplasty or arthrodesis, not both. In addition, each patient is different, and preexisting adjacent joint pathology may affect the long-term outcomes of both procedures. Gait analysis has shown that patients with total ankle replacement have a more normal gait pattern than those with arthrodesis; however, sports participation has been reported to be similar after both procedures, with approximately 76% in both groups active in sports after surgery.

The theoretical benefit of arthroplasty in preservation of adjacent joint cartilage compared to arthrodesis has yet to be demonstrated in the literature. In the first mid- to long-term outcome study of its kind, Dekker et al. reported a moderate radiographic increase in adjacent subtalar and talonavicular arthritis at a minimum of 5 years after arthroplasty. In 140 ankles averaging 6.5 years' follow-up, 40% and 34% of adjacent subtalar and talonavicular joints, respectively, showed progression of arthritic changes using the modified Kellgren Lawrence scale. In a separate study, Dekker et al. also demonstrated that 30% of the clinical motion observed after ankle arthroplasty occurs through the subtalar and talonavicular joints. This adjacent joint motion is similar to the numbers reported by Sealey et al. in their report of supraphysiologic adjacent joint motion after ankle arthrodesis. Sealey et al. reported 9.3 degrees of compensatory subtalar motion and 16.4 degrees of midfoot motion after ankle arthrodesis compared to Dekker's report of 6.7 degrees and 16.5 degrees for subtalar and midfoot compensatory motion after arthroplasty. These studies question whether arthroplasty can preserve adjacent joint motion and relieve adjacent joint stress long term. Pinsker et al. reported that only 15% of patients with arthroplasty or arthrodesis experienced resolution of all symptoms and limitations, which underscores that the procedure chosen should be tailored to the individual patient and realistic expectations should be managed by both the surgeon and patient.

INDICATIONS FOR ANKLE ARTHRODESIS

Ankle arthrodesis can be considered for patients who have painful limited motion of the ankle, in whom conservative measures have failed, and have any of the following diagnoses:

- Posttraumatic arthritis
- Osteoarthritis
- Arthritis from chronic instability of the ankle
- Rheumatoid or autoimmune inflammatory arthritis
- Gout
- Postinfectious arthritis
- Charcot neuroarthropathy
- Osteonecrosis of the talus
- Failure of total ankle arthroplasty
- Instability of the ankle from neuromuscular disorders

Absolute contraindications to ankle fusion include vascular impairment of the limb and infection of the skin through which the approach is planned. Relative contraindications include preexisting moderate-to-severe ipsilateral hindfoot arthrosis and contralateral ankle arthrosis likely to require surgical treatment in the foreseeable future. However, Houdek et al. reported that 31 patients with bilateral ankle arthrodesis rated their function as normal or nearly normal. In a retrospective cohort study comparing 10 bilateral to 10 unilateral ankle arthrodesis patients, Maenohara et al. reported that those with bilateral arthrodesis showed lower social functioning, but otherwise their outcomes did not appear inferior to those of patients with unilateral arthrodesis.

PATIENT EVALUATION
CLINICAL EVALUATION

A careful history is critical to an optimal outcome. Several questions should be considered before arthrodesis is chosen. What is the exact location of pain? Are there other existing orthopaedic issues with the limb, especially foot function, hip and knee function, and the presence or absence of back pain? What are the functional desires of the patient and what are his or her current impairments? Can the patient care for himself or herself, go to the store, exercise? What is the social support system? Who will help care for the patient after surgery?

Patient expectations must be determined and managed before surgery. Although pain relief is to be expected and functional activities will be substantially improved, some activity limitations will be present after ankle arthrodesis. In a study of 185 ankles at an average of 7 years after ankle arthrodesis, Kerkhoff et al. showed that participation in sports decreased slightly from 79.5% of patients before surgery to 68.9% after surgery; 73% of patients could hike an average of 40 minutes, 39.8% could kneel for 10 minutes, and 16.8% could run for 60 meters (Fig. 9.7). Patients are encouraged to engage in low-impact or nonimpact activities for conditioning postoperatively. Interestingly, cyclists may notice improved performance after ankle arthrodesis given the rigid lever arm created, which enhances energy transfer from the leg to the pedal. Shoewear limitations are common; low heels only for women and often a rocker sole shoe is needed for prolonged walking and hiking activities. Occasionally a brace is needed to support the hindfoot with more vigorous activities, especially if there is preexisting arthritis in these joints.

Assessment of medical comorbidities is important to prevent complications after surgery. In patients with diabetes, studies strongly suggest that good glycemic control, as manifested by a hemoglobin A1c level less than 7.0, should be obtained before major ankle or hindfoot reconstruction. Peripheral vascular disease should be identified and treated before surgery. Patients with a history of cardiac disease or pulmonary dysfunction also must have these conditions treated before surgery because of the increased functional demands in the immediate postoperative period as the patient mobilizes with crutches or a walker. Smoking tobacco directly interferes with the healing of the arthrodesis. In conjunction with a rheumatologist, patients with inflammatory arthritis should be taken off of antitumor necrosis factor-α medications preoperatively until the incisions are healed to decrease postoperative infection. Many patients have a vitamin D deficiency, and it is routine to supplement this pre- and postoperatively. Moderate-to-severe osteopenia found on plain radiographs should be investigated for a treatable cause before surgery. Patients in whom sleep apnea is suspected should be questioned about sleep habits, and this condition should be treated before surgery.

After a thorough history, assessment of the limb begins with evaluation of the patient's gait pattern. Two common mechanisms of decreasing motion through the ankle joint are "back-kneeing" and walking with an elevated foot progression angle (turning the foot outward to decrease the lever arm on the ankle). In some patients who back-knee, applying a small heel lift may improve symptoms. Limb-length discrepancy may be obvious in the gait assessment and may affect the type of arthrodesis chosen. The range of motion of the hip and knee should be assessed, as well as deformity of the knee in the coronal plane. Although every attempt is made to place the ankle perpendicular to the long axis of the tibia and parallel to the ground, varus or valgus deformity of the knee may affect outcome and should be considered before surgery. Range of motion through the tibiotalar joint

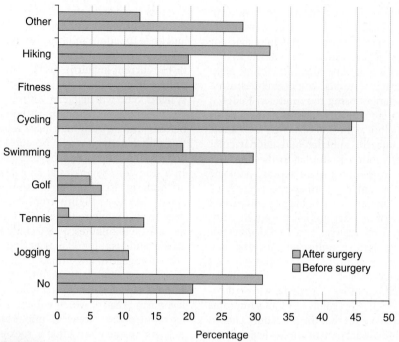

FIGURE 9.7 Participation in sports before the onset of disabling pain and after surgery. (From Kerkhoff YRA, Keijsers NLW, Louwerens JWK: Sports participation, functional outcomes, and complications after ankle arthrodesis: midterm follow-up, *Foot Ankle Int* 38:1085–1091, 2017)

is difficult to assess, but an effort should be made to isolate this joint and separately evaluate the hindfoot joints. The talonavicular joint, which will be responsible for most sagittal plane motion after surgery, should carefully be inspected for range of motion and pain. Overall flexibility of the hindfoot is important. A stiff, immobile, and irritable hindfoot may be a source of continued problems after tibiotalar arthrodesis, and deformity of the hindfoot must be identified and considered in preoperative planning. Although a few degrees of malalignment can be compensated for through the ankle arthrodesis, significant deformity will need to be corrected with a separate procedure. A thorough neurovascular examination is critical because approaches to the ankle are often placed near cutaneous nerves and any deficits should be noted preoperatively. Any suggestion of diminished pulses or patients with long-standing diabetes should prompt an in-depth assessment with arterial Doppler ultrasound. Selective injections of a local anesthetic, with or without the aid of fluoroscopy, can be helpful in patients with combined arthritis of the ankle and hindfoot. We give our patients a visual analog scale, with values of 0 (no pain) to 10 (worst pain imaginable) and ask them to check a location on the scale before and just after the injection is given. Stegeman et al., however, found that fluoroscopically guided anesthetic injections were not indicative of a successful outcome of arthrodesis. Based on the effect of the diagnostic injection and various clinical factors, patients were treated conservatively or with arthrodesis. Arthrodesis, regardless of the presence or absence of pain reduction after injection, resulted in improvements in pain and function, whereas conservative treatment resulted in worse pain and function.

RADIOGRAPHIC EVALUATION

Radiographic evaluation of the arthritic ankle begins with standing anteroposterior and lateral views. Typically, a long cassette is used to include as much of the distal tibia as possible

to help with the assessment of deformity and planning of correction if necessary. For more severe deformity, leg-length discrepancy should be evaluated on full standing lower limb films. The hindfoot alignment view can assist in assessing deformity distal to the ankle joint (Fig. 9.8). In addition to the amount of joint space loss on the anteroposterior view, coronal plane deformity should be assessed. Quality of bone stock and any cysts or other defects should be noted. On the lateral view, anteroposterior subluxation of the ankle should be noted, as well as any tilt of the tibial plafond, because this may affect the type of fusion and approach used.

Computed tomography, with or without weight bearing, can be used before ankle arthrodesis to further assess any defects in the region of the planned fusion and adjacent joint pathology. It may be helpful especially if a limited amount of joint space is lost and another procedure (e.g., arthroscopy or osteotomy) may be considered.

Nuclear medicine imaging can be helpful in determining if infection is present in patients with posttraumatic arthritis after open fracture, postinfectious arthritis, or previous infections. Gallium or technetium-labeled white blood cell imaging may add information to other forms of infection assessment (examination, white blood cell count, erythrocyte sedimentation rate, C-reactive protein).

TECHNIQUES OF ANKLE ARTHRODESIS

Common to all techniques is the desire to position the ankle in the proper orientation: neutral flexion/extension, external rotation of approximately 5 degrees, 5 degrees of valgus, and slight posterior translation of the talus under the tibia. Although slight flexion may be tolerated, extension is not and

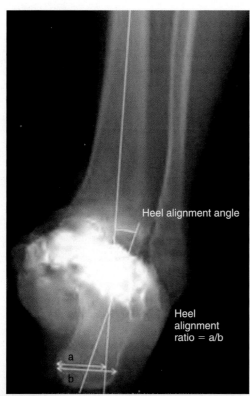

FIGURE 9.8   Hindfoot alignment view showing measurement of heel alignment angle and heel alignment ratio. Heel alignment angle is angle between tibial axis and calcaneal axis. Heel alignment ratio is calculated by dividing width of calcaneus medial to tibial axis by greatest width of calcaneus. (From Lee WC, Moon JS, Lee HS, Lee K: Alignment of ankle and hindfoot in early stage ankle osteoarthritis, *Foot Ankle Int* 32:693–699, 2011.)

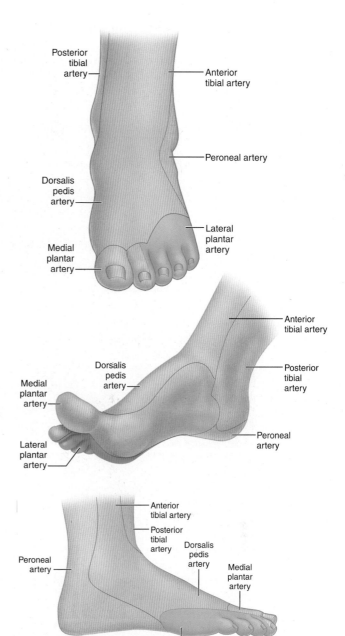

FIGURE 9.9   Angiosomes of the foot and ankle.

may result in excessive pressure and intractable pain under the heel. Other positions to avoid are any varus and anterior translation of the talus because this may lead to a "vaulting" type of gait pattern and knee pain. Every attempt is made to expose healthy, vascular bone and to remove or prepare the dense subchondral bone while respecting the soft tissues.

Many patients with ankle arthritis have prior injuries or surgeries, and the soft tissue abnormalities or scars should help direct the approach for the arthrodesis. Ankle arthrodesis can be done through a variety of approaches, so scarring should not limit access to the ankle joint in preparation for fusion. The use of previous incisions, if they are stable and well healed, is encouraged; however, skin in poor condition with minimal soft-tissue support or an incision that has been slow to heal should be avoided if possible. Knowledge of the angiosomes about the ankle (Fig. 9.9) and the vascular supply to the skin is important if wound complications are to be avoided. In their study of 215 patients with uncomplicated arthrodeses, Chalayon et al. found similar rates of nonunion regardless of surgical approach and technique, but higher rates of nonunion after prior subtalar arthrodesis for varus arthritis.

ARTHROSCOPIC ARTHRODESIS

The arthroscopic technique has several advantages over other techniques, including maintenance of malleolar congruency, which decreases the risk of malunion, gives more bone surface and anatomic support for fusion, and allows for possible take-down and conversion to arthroplasty in the future. In theory, there is less chance of disruption of the blood supply to the talus or distal tibia, which could complicate and delay healing of the fusion. Because of less soft tissue stripping, the postoperative pain after arthroscopic arthrodesis is generally less than open techniques. This technique is considered for patients with minimal coronal plane deformity or bone loss and those with osteonecrosis (Fig. 9.10). Jones et al. showed a 94% radiographic fusion rate at an average 7-year follow-up after arthroscopic arthrodesis in 120 ankles. In a systematic review of arthroscopic and open ankle arthrodesis, Park et al. showed similar rates of union, reoperations, and operative times between the two groups, with arthroscopic arthrodesis showing better clinical scores and fewer complications. The technique of arthroscopic ankle arthrodesis is described in other chapter.

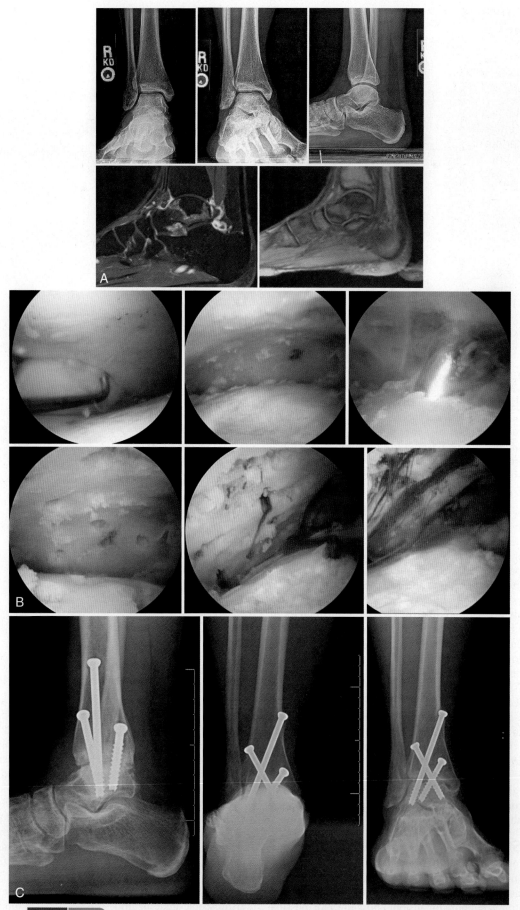

FIGURE 9.10 **A,** Preoperative radiographs and sagittal MRI in a 45-year-old patient with osteo-necrosis of the talus. **B,** Intraoperative arthroscopy: cartilage removal, subchondral bone penetration, and bleeding bone surfaces in preparation for arthrodesis. **C,** Radiographs 6 weeks after arthrodesis.

MINI-INCISION TECHNIQUE

When coronal plane deformity is minimal (<10 degrees of varus or valgus) and bone quality is satisfactory, a mini-incision technique can be used. The standard arthroscopic portals are enlarged slightly, the joint is directly observed and prepared, and fixation is inserted. Benefits similar to those of the arthroscopic technique are obtained with possibly a shorter operative time for surgeons not as familiar with arthroscopy. Miller et al. reported a fusion rate of 98% in two groups of patients with this procedure.

TECHNIQUE 9.4

- Place the patient supine on the operating room table with a lift under the ipsilateral hip so that the leg is oriented perpendicular to the floor. The foot should be near the end of the table and the table able to accept fluoroscopy.
- General and/or regional anesthesia can be used.
- Use a tourniquet to improve visualization and a headlight if available. Specialized instruments include Inge lamina spreaders, sharp curets, and osteotomes; a motorized burr may be desired.
- Make two 1.5-cm incisions, one just medial to the tibial tendon and one lateral to the peroneus tertius tendon (Fig. 9.11), taking care to identify the course of the dorsal intermediate cutaneous nerve near the lateral incision. It often can be seen by inverting the foot and plantar flexing the fourth toe.
- Incise the joint capsule in line with the skin and elevate it from the front of the ankle joint with an elevator.

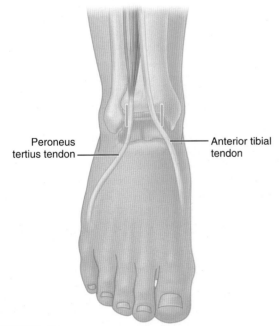

Peroneus tertius tendon —

Anterior tibial tendon

FIGURE 9.11   Mini-arthrotomy incisions, one just medial to tibial tendon and one lateral to peroneus tertius tendon. **SEE TECHNIQUE 9.4.**

- Inspect the joint and remove any periarticular osteophytes with a rongeur or osteotome to allow placement of the ankle in neutral and to allow evaluation of the joint.
- Place a periosteal elevator in one incision to lever the joint open slightly and place a lamina spreader in the other incision and open it to allow removal of the remaining cartilage and subchondral bone through the first incision. Use a curet first, then a high-speed burr or drill bit to penetrate the subchondral bone. Irrigate saline through the opposite incision as needed to prevent excessive heat build-up in the bone. Use a small osteotome to "fish scale" the bone.
- Prepare the medial gutter in a similar manner, switching the instruments between incisions to complete the preparation.
- There is no consensus regarding lateral gutter preparation for fusion. The extra motion of the fibula may lead to painful nonunion of this joint, but even without preparing this joint there occasionally is pain in this area after successful tibiotalar fusion. We generally do not formally prepare this joint and seldom have significant problems with it later.
- Autogenous bone graft typically is used and is inserted into the ankle joint at this time. The goal is to introduce biology into the fusion site and fill any defects while not inhibiting bone surface apposition.
- Insert large (typically 6.5- to 8.0-mm) cannulated screws over guidewires for fixation. Three screws are ideal, but sometimes only two are possible. We typically place the first two as partially threaded screws for compression followed by a fully threaded screw for stability. A desirable screw position is the so-called "home run" screw placed from the posterolateral tibia into the talar neck/head area distally (Fig. 9.12). A proximomedial screw directed into the posterior body of the talus usually is inserted next; this may be a fully-threaded screw to improve bone purchase on both sides of the arthrodesis site. This is followed by either a proximal anterolateral-to-distal medial screw or a distal lateral screw from the lateral process of the talus directed proximally, posteriorly, and medially.
- Close the joint capsule and the skin in a routine manner and apply a well-padded short-leg splint with the foot in neutral position.

POSTOPERATIVE CARE The dressing and sutures are removed at 2 weeks, and a short leg cast is applied. The patient is instructed to return for a cast change if the cast seems loose and is applying stress to the fusion site. The patient is kept non–weight bearing until the fusion seems healed, typically a minimum of 6 weeks. The use of a rolling walker, on which the patient rests the knee and propels himself or herself with the opposite limb (Fig. 9.13), has dramatically improved quality of life and increased postoperative compliance with the restricted weight-bearing status. Plain radiographs usually are sufficient to assess healing, but occasionally CT is necessary to be certain. A knee-high walking boot is applied when the fusion seems solid, and the patient can gradually wean from the boot to a shoe. For some patients, a shoe modified with a full-length steel shank and a rocker sole is beneficial for an improved gait pattern.

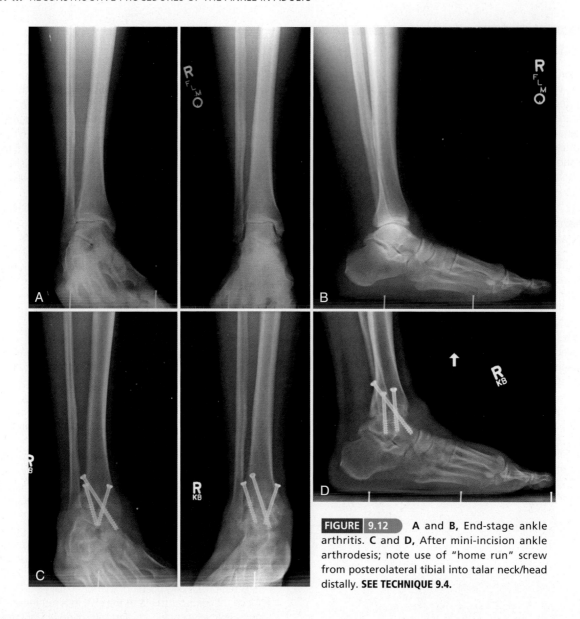

FIGURE 9.12 **A** and **B,** End-stage ankle arthritis. **C** and **D,** After mini-incision ankle arthrodesis; note use of "home run" screw from posterolateral tibial into talar neck/head distally. **SEE TECHNIQUE 9.4.**

TRANSFIBULAR (TRANSMALLEOLAR) ARTHRODESIS WITH FIBULAR STRUT GRAFT

The original technique of Mann has been modified to incorporate, if possible, a vascularized fibular strut graft. This graft brings an added measure of stability and vascular supply to the fusion site. Colman and Pomeroy reported a 96% fusion rate in 48 patients, with an average time to fusion of 82 days.

TECHNIQUE 9.5

- After induction of general anesthesia, position the patient supine on the operating table with a bump under the ipsilateral hip to allow easier access to the fibula. A ramp of bone foam or towels under the distal leg makes it easier to obtain correct positioning of the ankle and for intraoperative imaging.
- Administer a popliteal block, if not done preoperatively, and apply a thigh tourniquet.

- Center a longitudinal incision over the fibula and carry it distally approximately 2 cm past the tip of the fibula and then curve it along the course of the peroneal tendons. This allows access to the subtalar joint for debridement or arthrodesis if needed. Take care to protect the superficial peroneal nerve. Carry dissection onto the anterior surface of the tibia and place a deep retractor anteriorly.
- Use osteotomes and a mallet to remove large osteophytes on the anterior tibial plafond and talus.
- Use a sagittal saw to transect the fibula approximately 5 to 7 cm proximal to the tibial plafond and remove approximately 1 cm with a second parallel cut (Fig. 9.14A).
- Insert a lamina spreader between the fibula and tibia and spread them while incising the syndesmotic ligaments anteriorly. Alternatively, insert a curved osteotome into the incisura to release the fibula from the tibia anteriorly. Take care to preserve the posterior tibiofibular ligaments and blood supply to the fibula.
- While stabilizing the fibula with towel clips, make a cut in the sagittal plane to remove the medial half of the fibula, preserving the lateral half with its periosteal attachment.

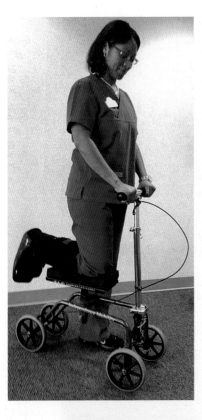

- While reflecting the fibula posteriorly, a Hintermann distractor can be placed on the tibia and talus with the handle pointing posteriorly, which will hold the residual fibula out of the way while opening the tibiotalar joint for preparation. Use of a laminar spreader to allow removal of residual joint contents also can be considered (Fig. 9.14B).
- If needed, make a separate medial incision to assist with medial gutter preparation. This is especially important in varus ankle arthritis.
- Preparation of the joint for fusion varies from "in situ" fusion, in which the normal articular surface topography is maintained for minimal deformity to flat cuts of the opposing tibial and talar surfaces for more severe deformity. Construct the fusion area to obtain neutral extension, slight external rotation relative to the tibial tubercle, and neutral to slight valgus, depending on the position and flexibility of the rest of the hindfoot and foot. If flat cuts are made, make a separate medial incision to expose the medial malleolus and to protect the posterior tibial tendon and neurovascular bundle before making the cut with a saw (Fig. 9.14C). The talus should be slightly translated posteriorly under the tibia. Obtain bleeding, healthy cancellous bone on all fusion surfaces. Take care to dorsiflex and plantarflex the ankle during joint preparation to make sure all remaining anterior and posterior talar cartilage is identified and removed.

FIGURE 9.13 Use of a rolling walker can dramatically improve patients' quality of life and increase compliance with weight-bearing restrictions.

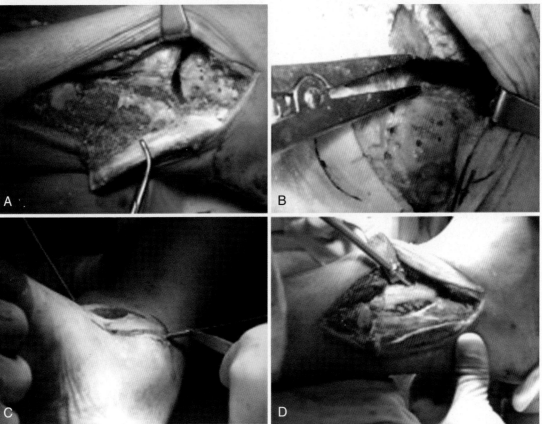

FIGURE 9.14 Transfibular (transmalleolar) arthrodesis with fibular strut graft (see text). **A,** Resection of fibula. **B,** Laminar spreader allows removal of residual joint contents. **C,** Separate anteromedial approach may be needed for deformity correction. **D,** Screw insertion from posteromedial side of tibia into talus. (From Saltzman CL: Ankle arthritis. In Coughlin MJ, Mann RA, Saltzman CL, editors: *Surgery of the foot and ankle*, ed 8, Philadelphia, 2007, Elsevier.) **SEE TECHNIQUE 9.5.**

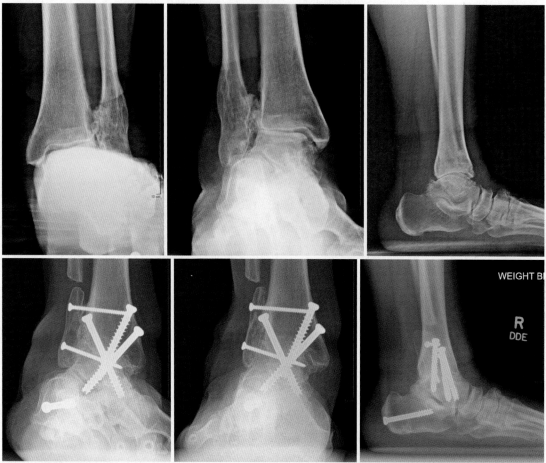

FIGURE 9.15 End-stage tibiotalar and tibiofibular arthritis with hindfoot valgus treated with transfibular arthrodesis with fibular onlay and calcaneal osteotomy.

- Lengthening of the heel cord may be necessary if residual equinus is noted; a triple hemisection technique typically is used. The distal cut is made medially proximal to the insertion of the tendon; the next is made 2.5 cm proximal to the first through the lateral half of the tendon; and the final one is made 2.5 cm proximal to the second through the medial half of the tendon. A dorsiflexion force is applied to correct any remaining equinus.
- Avoid extension, varus, or internal rotation at the ankle because these are poorly tolerated; also avoid anterior translation of the talus under the tibia, which can result in a gait pattern described as "vaulting" over the foot. Check the position of the ankle with fluoroscopy and careful visual inspection.
- If needed, add bone graft from the morselized resected medial fibula or from a remote location such as the proximal tibia or iliac crest.
- Insert multiple partially and fully threaded 6.5-mm or 7.0-mm cancellous screws from posterolateral in the tibia into the talar head and neck and from posteromedial into the talar body (Fig. 9.14D). Take care to protect tendons and neurovascular structures during screw insertion. An additional screw from the sinus tarsi into the tibia is helpful. Compression is obtained with the first two screws, which are partially threaded, and then a fully threaded screw is added for additional stability.
- The order of screw insertion depends on the pathology. For varus ankle arthritis, a laterally based screw typically is placed first to compress opposite the varus deformity, while a medial-screw-first construct is used for valgus arthritis.
- Remove any impinging osteophytes off of the subtalar joint with an osteotome and mallet.
- Remove residual cartilage from the lateral tibia and lateral talus in a similar fashion and manually appose the lateral fibula to this area. Take care to elevate the fibula slightly so as not to impinge on the subtalar joint and hold with a provisional Kirschner wire.
- Secure the residual fibula to the tibia and talus with two 3.5-mm lag screws (Fig. 9.15). Use of a low-profile plate with four to six screws spanning the fusion site also can be considered and may provide additional stability to the fusion site (Fig. 9.16).
- Close the wound in layers and apply a well-padded short-leg splint.

POSTOPERATIVE CARE At 10 to 14 days, the splint and sutures are removed and a non–weight bearing cast is applied. The cast is worn an additional 4 to 8 weeks until the ankle is healed clinically and radiographically. Care must be taken that the cast does not become loose because this would place stress on the fusion site. When the cast is removed, a walking boot is fitted and worn for an additional 4 weeks. Then a shoe can be modified with a shank and a rocker if needed, especially if there is concomitant hindfoot or midfoot disease.

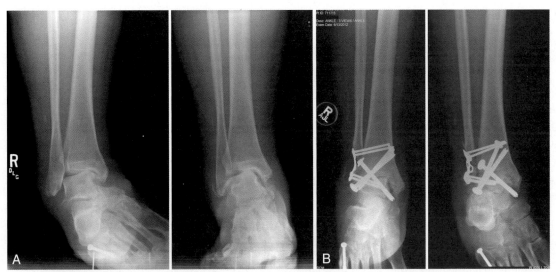

FIGURE 9.16 **A,** End-stage ankle arthritis with deformity. **B,** After transfibular arthrodesis with addition of low-profile plate to add stability to construct. **SEE TECHNIQUE 9.5.**

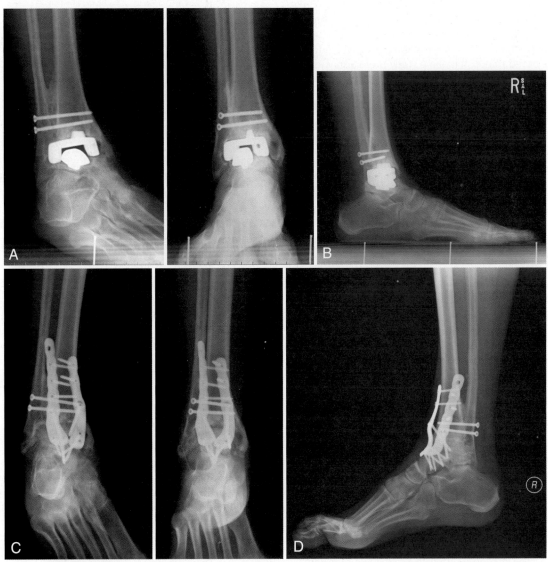

FIGURE 9.17 **A** and **B,** Total ankle arthroplasty with loosening, periarticular cyst, and medial and lateral anterior impingement. **C** and **D,** After arthrodesis with femoral head allograft and double-plate fixation. **SEE TECHNIQUE 9.6.**

ANTERIOR APPROACH WITH PLATE FIXATION

This approach is particularly appropriate for conversion of a failed total ankle arthroplasty to arthrodesis. Suggested advantages of plate fixation include less soft tissue disruption by using a single anterior incision, ease of deformity correction, early rehabilitation, and a high rate of union. Plaass et al. described an anterior double-plating technique (Fig. 9.17) for severe osteoarthritis, nonunion of ankle arthrodeses, and failed total ankle replacements; 27 (93%) of 29 patients were satisfied with their outcomes. More recently, Kestner et al., in a cadaver biomechanical study, showed that bending stiffness of a two-plate construct was 1.5 to 5 times greater than that of a single-plate construct and torsional stiffness was nearly double. They suggested that the stiffer two-plate system may improve clinical fusion rates, especially in patients with suboptimal bone quality. In a retrospective study of 65 ankles by a single surgeon, Mitchell et al. showed a trend toward a higher union rate with the addition of an anterior plate compared to a transfibular approach with screws only; however, a statistically significant difference was not detected. It should be noted that in this same study there also was a trend toward a higher infection rate in the anterior plate group. Similarly, Prissel et al. did not detect a significantly different union rate in their underpowered retrospective comparative study of 83 ankles.

TECHNIQUE 9.6

- After general anesthesia and a preoperative popliteal block are administered, place the patient supine on the operating table with a bump under the hip to hold the leg in neutral rotation. If desired, apply a tourniquet and exsanguinate the limb.
- Make a direct anterior approach to the ankle, taking care to protect the crossing branches of the superficial peroneal nerve. Develop the interval between the extensor hallucis longus and tibialis anterior with the neurovascular structures retracted laterally.
- Make an arthrotomy of the ankle and use a Cobb elevator to mobilize tissues medially and laterally in front of the tibial plafond such that retractors may be placed.
- Remove marginal osteophytes of the ankle. Use a lamina spreader or Hintermann distractor to distract the tibiotalar joint for cartilage removal.
- Remove cartilage from the dorsal talus and medial gutter. Typically, with the fibula intact, we do not prepare the lateral gutter. Take care to dorsiflex and plantarflex the ankle during joint preparation to make sure all remaining anterior and posterior talar cartilage is identified and removed.
- Penetrate the subchondral bone on the tibia and talus with a water-cooled drill bit. Place autogenous bone graft into the joint.
- Place the ankle into the appropriate position for fusion with slight valgus, external rotation, and neutral position in the sagittal plane. If equinus contracture limits the ability to

place the foot into the neutral position, perform a triple hemisection of the Achilles tendon.
- Provisionally hold the position of the talus relative to the tibia with a guide pin for a 6.5-mm cannulated screw placed from the medial tibia into the talus. If desired, a partially threaded screw can be placed over this wire to compress the talus medially and superiorly away from the unprepared fibula, possibly decreasing lateral gutter pain in the future. Alternatively, the wire can be removed after the plate is fixed to the tibia and before compression of the fusion site through the plate.
- A number of anterior ankle arthrodesis plates are available and implant-specific techniques are used. In general, apply the plate across the arthrodesis site and hold it in provisional position with Kirschner wires. A burr may be useful to clear off some of the dorsal talus and/or anterior tibia to allow the plate to sit flush on the bone.
- Use compression slots in the plate during screw insertion to generate compression at the arthrodesis site before placement of locking screws; alternatively use an external compression device.
- Place additional bone graft as needed, irrigate the wound, and close it in layers. Take care to repair the extensor retinaculum to avoid bowstringing of the extensor tendons. Meticulous soft-tissue technique is necessary because anterior wound complications can be devastating.
- Apply sterile dressings and a short leg splint.

POSTOPERATIVE CARE The sutures are removed at 2 to 3 weeks after surgery, and a new cast is applied. Transitioning into a fracture boot with progressive weight bearing is begun at 6 to 8 weeks postoperatively (Fig. 9.18).

LATERAL APPROACH WITH FIBULAR SPARING

This modification of the Mann lateral transfibular approach preserves the fibula. According to Smith et al., the intact fibula provides additional surface area for fusion, blocks valgus drift in cases of delayed union, and may serve as a guide to proper rotation and positioning. Preservation of the fibula also enables conversion to total ankle arthroplasty and maintains the native groove and restraints for the peroneal tendons.

TECHNIQUE 9.7

(SMITH, CHIODO, SINGH, WILSON)
- Position the patient supine with a bump under the ipsilateral hip to facilitate access to the lateral aspect of the ankle.
- Make an approximately 12-cm curvilinear incision directly lateral over the ankle, centered at the tip of the fibula and curving gently distally toward the base of the fourth metatarsal (Fig. 9.19A).
- Divide the anterior talofibular and calcaneofibular ligaments to allow the talus to be rotated out from underneath the mortise (Fig. 9.19B) and use a sharp curet to remove cartilage synovium and loose bodies.

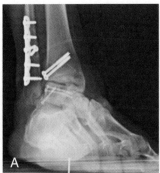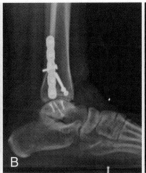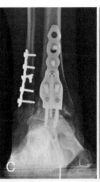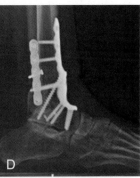

FIGURE 9.18   **A** and **B,** Graft collapse, broken implant, and posttraumatic arthritis of the ankle after fresh allograft implantation for talar osteonecrosis. **C** and **D,** After ankle fusion with an anterior fusion plate and locking screws. **SEE TECHNIQUE 9.6.**

- Fenestrate subchondral tibial and talar bone with a 4-mm powered burr at low speed (20,000 revolutions per minute) with continuous saline irrigation to prevent thermal necrosis (Fig. 9.19C).
- Harvest autogenous bone graft from the distal fibula through a fibular corticotomy created with the 4-mm burr or small saw (Fig. 9.19D) at the lateral fibula, preserving the fibular groove. Alternative graft sites such as the proximal tibia also can be used.
- Use a medium-sized curet to harvest 5 to 8 g of cancellous bone and pack the graft into the prepared tibial and talar surfaces.
- Under fluoroscopic guidance, pass two 6.5- or 7.3-mm screws from lateral to medial. Pass one screw with a washer in an anterior position from the base of the talar neck to the tibia. Start the second screw at the lateral process of the talus and direct it into the distal tibia posteriorly (Fig. 9.19E). Do not use a washer with the second screw to avoid impingement at the subtalar joint.

POSTOPERATIVE CARE Patients are kept non–weight bearing for 8 weeks, then partial weight bearing is begun in a pneumatic boot or walking cast. Unrestricted weight bearing is initiated 3 months after surgery if union is confirmed.

TIBIOTALOCALCANEAL ARTHRODESIS

In certain circumstances, arthrodesis of both the ankle and subtalar joints is necessary or advantageous. A lateral transfibular approach, with or without the onlay fibular graft, can be used. A posterior approach may be appropriate in some situations, such as patients with compromised skin and soft tissues in the area of a lateral approach. Numerous designs and constructs of compression screws, intramedullary nails, blade plates, and locking plates can be used, and a familiarity with the technique associated with the device is essential for a successful outcome. Blade plate and locking plate fixation (Fig. 9.20) are relatively recent techniques. Cadaver biomechanical studies have shown locking plate

fixation to have higher rigidity than intramedullary nails and to provide higher initial stiffness and higher torsional load to failure than blade plate fixation. Hamid et al. found no difference between compressive forces generated at the ankle and subtalar joint with a plate compared to a nail, although both were significantly higher than the compressive force generated by screws. Mulligan et al. compared intramedullary nailing with a posterior approach (38 patients) to a locked plate through a transfibular approach (28 patients) and found similar union, revision, and complication rates. The overall union rate was 71% in the nail group compared to 64% in the plate group, with revision because of symptomatic nonunion in 16% of the nail group and 7% of the plate group.

TECHNIQUE 9.8

- The position of the patient, lateral and medial skin incisions, soft-tissue dissection, and preparation of the tibiotalar joint are the same as described in Technique 9.5. A posterior approach can be used if wide exposure is necessary for removal of total ankle components or in patients with osteonecrosis of the talus or significant deformities that require correction.
- Distract the subtalar joint with a lamina spreader or Hintermann distractor and remove residual cartilage.
- If autogenous bone graft is being used, place it into the arthrodesis sites.
- After the arthrodesis site is prepared, determine the position by holding the patella straight up and placing the foot in neutral dorsiflexion-plantarflexion, 5 degrees of valgus at the heel, and slight posterior displacement of the calcaneus in relation to the tibia. Place provisional Kirschner wires and evaluate the foot position.
- If a lateral locking plate construct is to be used, follow the manufacturer's implant- specific procedures. In general, place cortical screws first to fix the plate to the bones using the compression slots to compress the joint surfaces, followed by locking screws to enhance the stability of the construct. If the cortical screws placed initially do not have good purchase in the bone, exchange them for locking screws. Additional cannulated or solid screws between the calcaneus, talus, and tibia can be inserted as desired.

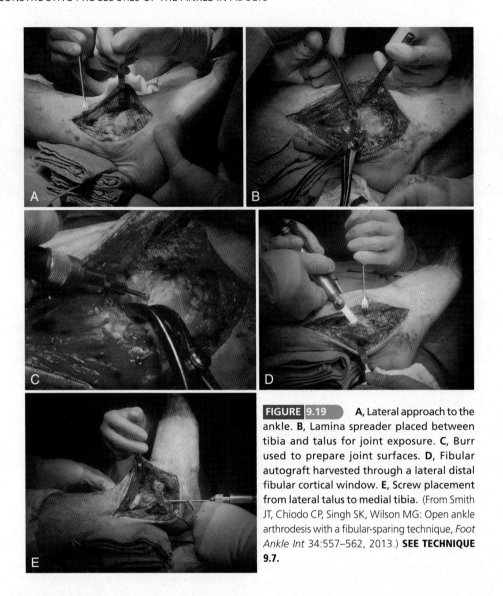

FIGURE 9.19 **A,** Lateral approach to the ankle. **B,** Lamina spreader placed between tibia and talus for joint exposure. **C,** Burr used to prepare joint surfaces. **D,** Fibular autograft harvested through a lateral distal fibular cortical window. **E,** Screw placement from lateral talus to medial tibia. (From Smith JT, Chiodo CP, Singh SK, Wilson MG: Open ankle arthrodesis with a fibular-sparing technique, *Foot Ankle Int* 34:557–562, 2013.) **SEE TECHNIQUE 9.7.**

- For intramedullary nailing, follow implant-specific procedures. Generally, determine the starting point on lateral fluoroscopy where the entry point on the calcaneus will allow the nail to pass into the center of the tibial diaphysis. In the coronal plane, the starting point must allow for the nail to pass into the diaphysis, which may be more medial on the calcaneus with a straight nail compared to more central in the calcaneus with a nail that has a valgus bend distally. A valgus bend nail may be useful in patients with severe hindfoot valgus because it can be difficult to get the calcaneus back over medially in line with the tibia for a straight nail to be confidently used. In cases of severe subtalar subluxation, a lateral locking plate may be a more appropriate choice of implant. The surgeon should be familiar with the implant chosen and the appropriate technique before the procedure.

- Take care not to enter the calcaneus through the sustentaculum tali because the calcaneus may fracture and drift into valgus.
- In the sagittal plane, draw a line from the second toe to the center of the heel; in the coronal plane, draw a line at the junction of the anterior and middle thirds of the heel pad (Fig. 9.21). The intersection of these lines approximately indicates the entry portal for the nail; however, this should be confirmed on fluoroscopy. Make a transverse or longitudinal incision in the heel and use a Kelly clamp to bluntly dissect down to the calcaneus.
- Insert the guide pin into the center of the medullary canal of the tibia using fluoroscopy.
- Take care not to aim too posterior into the tibia because when the nail follows this path it will move the foot into equinus.

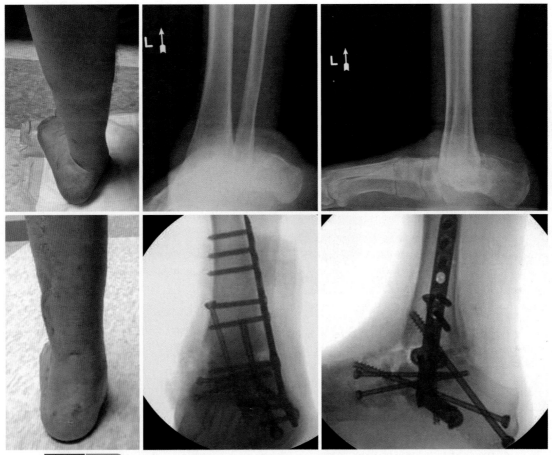

FIGURE 9.20 Preoperative and postoperative clinical and radiographic appearance after deformity correction with a lateral tibiotalocalcaneal locking plate.

- Use an entry reamer through a soft-tissue sleeve to enter the calcaneus and ream up to the tibia. Some implants, such as those with a valgus bend, now have the initial guide pin removed; a ball-tip guidewire is inserted into the tibia over which sequential reaming is done to the specifications of the specific nail size chosen. In general, we ream to 0.5 to 1.0 mm larger than the nail chosen. Larger diameter nails have more resistance to breakage, but care must be taken not to fracture the tibia during reaming or nail insertion if a larger nail size is chosen.
- If using a nail with a valgus bend, take care to have the bend oriented appropriately in the coronal plane; otherwise, unanticipated plantarflexion or dorsiflexion of the foot will result as the bend engages the bone.
- Seat the nail just inside the cortex of the calcaneus; as compression is applied, it will move to just outside the calcaneal cortex.
- Place interlocking screws in the calcaneus, talus, and tibia through outriggers or perfect-circle technique based on the specific implant; a variety of internal and external compression mechanisms are available with different implants.
- Place additional bone graft at the fusion sites if necessary. If desired, place supplemental cannulated or solid screws

between the calcaneus and tibia (Fig. 9.22). If a transfibular approach was used, fix the remnant lateral half of the fibula to the tibia and talus with two 3.5-mm lag screws.
- Close the wounds in layers, place sterile dressings, and apply a short-leg splint.

POSTOPERATIVE CARE Postoperative care is essentially the same as after compression arthrodesis (Technique 9.6). The short-leg cast is changed at 2 to 3 weeks. Weight bearing is allowed in a short-leg walking cast or fracture boot 6 to 8 weeks after surgery.

TIBIOCALCANEAL ARTHRODESIS

If the talar body has been removed and a tibiocalcaneal arthrodesis is being done, two modifications of the technique may be required. Because the calcaneus rests more laterally in relation to the ankle joint than does the talus, it may need to be translated medially 1 to 2 cm so that the lateral edge of the prepared surface of the tibia has no bony apposition with the calcaneus. Placing the pin in the

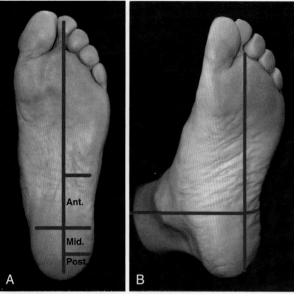

FIGURE 9.21 Method for estimating insertion site for retrograde intramedullary fixation of tibiocalcaneal arthrodesis. **A,** Line in sagittal plane drawn from tip of second toe to center of heel. **B,** Line can be drawn in coronal plane bisecting medial malleolus. Insertion of lines indicates correct entry portal for nail. (From Stephenson KA, Kile TA, Graves SC: Estimating the insertion site during retrograde intramedullary tibiotalocalcaneal arthrodesis, *Foot Ankle* 17:781–782, 1996.) **SEE TECHNIQUE 9.6.**

calcaneus anywhere but in the midline is difficult because of the contours of the plantar surface of the calcaneus. Consequently, moving the pin medially in the calcaneus and leaving it in its anatomic position is more difficult than placing the pin in the plantar midline surface of the calcaneus and translating the whole calcaneus slightly medially. This is done easily with both malleoli removed. We find a straight nail advantageous in these situations compared to a nail with a valgus bend distally (Fig. 9.23).

POSTERIOR APPROACH FOR ARTHRODESIS OF ANKLE AND SUBTALAR JOINTS

The posterior approach to the ankle is particularly useful in cases of osteonecrosis of the talus when the goal is tibiotalocalcaneal arthrodesis. Any of the aforementioned fixation techniques or external fixation can be used. Posterior arthrodesis permits lengthening of the Achilles tendon through the same incision and fusion of both the ankle and subtalar joints. The procedure also may be kept extraarticular. This technique is rarely used without fixation but may be appropriate when current instrumentation and equipment are not available.

TECHNIQUE 9.9

(CAMPBELL)
- Make a 7.5-cm longitudinal incision medial to and parallel with the Achilles tendon over the posterior aspect of the ankle.

- Retract the flexor hallucis longus medially and expose the posterior capsule of the ankle and subtalar joints. Protect the neurovascular bundle.
- Alternatively, make a direct midline posterior incision, followed by incising the Achilles tendon in the coronal plane and loosely suturing the proximal and distal stumps to the skin to aid in retraction. This allows lengthening of the tendon when it is repaired at the completion of the procedure.
- Incise the posterior capsule to expose the tibiotalar and subtalar cartilage. The same principles regarding joint distraction, cartilage removal, joint positioning, and fixation with either intramedullary nailing or a posterior tibiotalocalcaneal arthrodesis plate are applied.
- If the procedure is to be kept extraarticular, do not incise the capsule.
- With an osteotome, turn large flaps of bone distally from the posterior aspect of the tibia and proximally from the superior aspect of the calcaneus, overlapping them successively (Fig. 9.24A).
- Add additional autograft bone from the posterior iliac crest or allograft if necessary to make a large bony bridge across the ankle and subtalar joint (Fig. 9.24B and Fig. 9.25D).
- Fixation can be accomplished with an intramedullary nail (Fig. 9.25) or a posteriorly applied locking plate.

POSTOPERATIVE CARE The ankle is immobilized in a splint. Sutures are removed at 2 to 3 weeks and a cast is maintained for 8 to 10 weeks. Weight bearing is resumed at 10 to 12 weeks postoperatively. Posterior extraarticular arthrodeses usually require longer periods of immobilization than do other techniques. A shoe with a steel shank and rocker sole will assist the patient in having a more normal gait.

ARTHRODESIS WITH EXTERNAL FIXATION

For surgeons who do not routinely work with thin wire fixators in the design of Ilizarov or the Taylor spatial frame, external fixation of an otherwise uncomplicated ankle arthrodesis is probably more likely to lead to an increased complication rate, including nonunion and infection. There are times, however, when external fixation is necessary for either the primary fixation or as support of underlying internal fixation.

ARTHRODESIS WITH A THIN-WIRE EXTERNAL FIXATION

TECHNIQUE 9.10   *Figure 9.26*

- To prepare the ankle for arthrodesis, an anterior or transfibular approach can be used. In cases of ulceration, incising proximally and distally from the ulcer may allow exposure as well as permit possible ulcer closure at the completion of the procedure.
- Remove residual cartilage from the joint surfaces to be fused. Remove any necrotic or infected bone. With

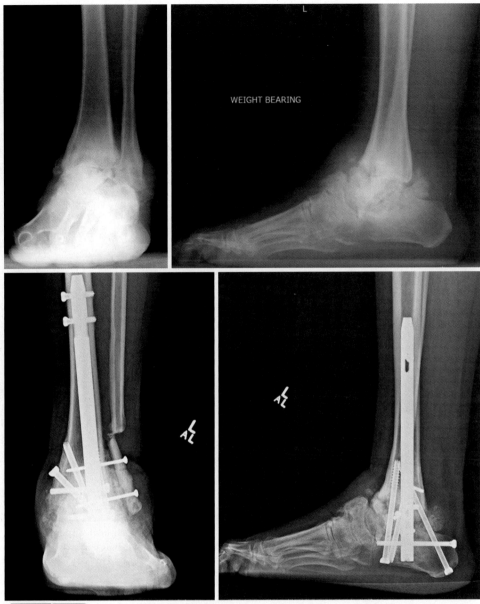

FIGURE 9.22 Preoperative and postoperative radiographs of intramedullary nail and supplemental screw fixation for Charcot ankle and hindfoot deformities. **SEE TECHNIQUE 9.8.**

significant deformity, flat cut osteotomies allow correction but will shorten the limb. This shortening can be accommodated later with a modified shoe.

- If the entire talus is removed, typically the medial malleolus should be excised to allow the calcaneus to be placed onto the tibia.
- Contour the calcaneus and tibia with a burr to allow conformity and apposition with the foot in appropriate position.
- Use large Kirschner wires or Steinmann pins from the calcaneus into the tibia for provisional fixation. This will permit the multiplanar external fixator to be applied around the ankle without the need to continue to hold it in appropriate position.
- Close the surgical wounds in a layered fashion.

EXTERNAL FIXATOR APPLICATION

- We typically use a static Ilizarov or Taylor spatial frame for external fixation. The main difference is that in a static frame, threaded rods connect the foot ring to the distal tibial ring compared to multiplanar adjustable struts in a Taylor spatial frame. Both are acceptable options, although the spatial frame struts come at significantly increased cost. The spatial frame allows multiplanar deformity correction postoperatively if needed; however, in most cases the deformity is corrected at the time of surgery, making a static Ilizarov frame perfectly acceptable. Significant compression at the arthrodesis site is achieved with either option, in our experience, although the threaded rods seem to provide more stability than the spatial frame struts. If desired, struts can be exchanged for threaded rods in the clinic after deformity is corrected.
- Apply the thin-wire fixation to the leg, beginning with ring fixators at the mid-tibia and supramalleolar region, initially anchored with tensioned wires; alternatively, use two half-pins or one half-pin and one wire at each level. Higher periprosthetic tibial fracture rates have been demonstrated

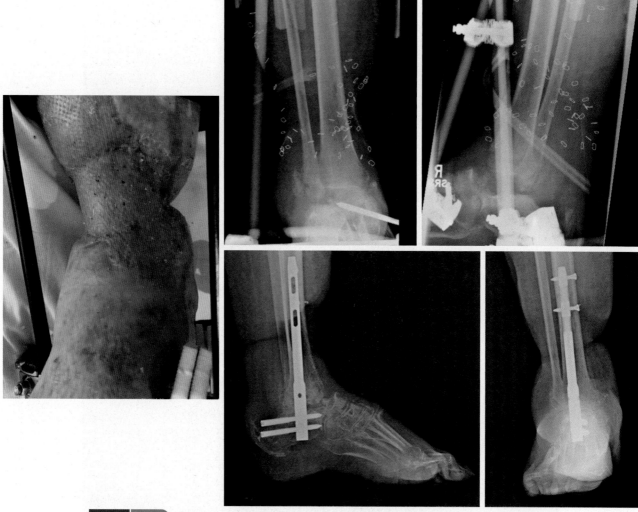

FIGURE 9.23 Preoperative and postoperative radiographs and clinical appearance of arthroscopic-assisted tibiocalcaneal arthrodesis after open extruded talar injury in a patient with compromised soft tissues. **SEE TECHNIQUE 9.8.**

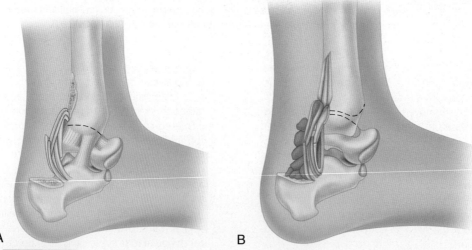

A   B

FIGURE 9.24 Posterior arthrodesis of ankle and subtalar joints. **A,** Flaps of bone from posterior tibia and superior calcaneus turned using osteotome. **B,** Bone graft added. **SEE TECHNIQUE 9.9.**

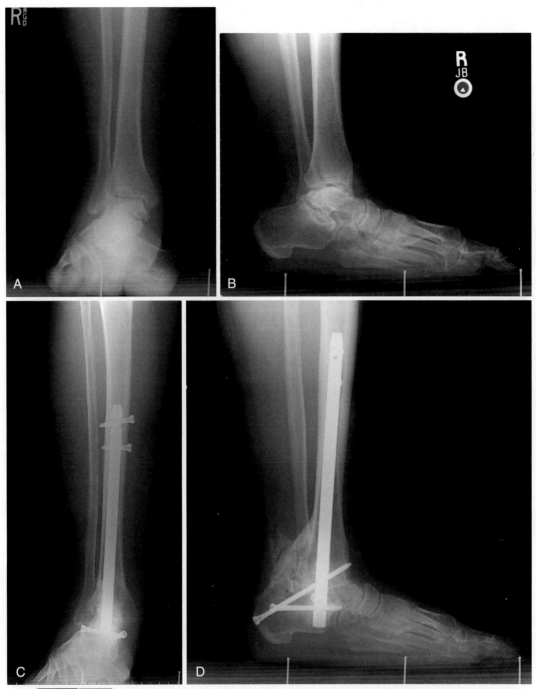

FIGURE 9.25 **A** and **B,** Osteonecrosis of the talus in 55-year-old man. **C** and **D,** After posterior approach arthrodesis of ankle and subtalar joints with intramedullary nail and onlay bone graft obtained with reamer-irrigator-aspirator (RIA) technique. **SEE TECHNIQUE 9.9.**

with the use of half-pins instead of tensioned wires in neuropathic patients.
- Add a calcaneal-forefoot extended half-ring and anchor it with tensioned wires through the calcaneus and through the metatarsals, or attach a half-pin and transfixing calcaneal wire to the half-ring.
- Verify correct positioning of the talus along the anteroposterior axis, juxtaposition, and coaptation of the surfaces visually and radiographically (see Fig. 9.26H-N).

- After the fixator is applied, dial in compression between the foot ring and distal tibial ring by sequentially turning the nuts superior to the distal tibial ring and then tightening the inferior distal tibial ring nuts when the desired compression is achieved. Remove the provisional Kirschner wire fixation before compressing.
- Apply sterile and/or silver-impregnated dressings around the pin sites and surgical wounds.

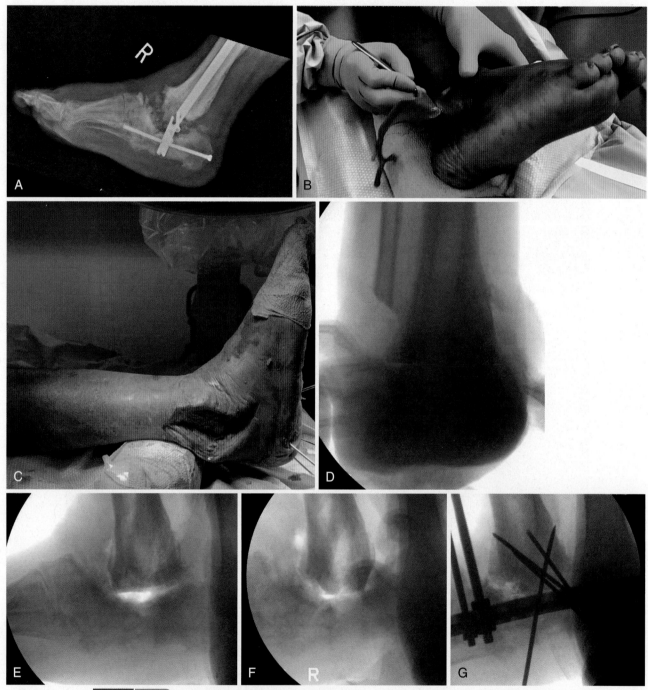

FIGURE 9.26   **A,** Infected tibiotalocalcaneal arthrodesis with broken implant. **B,** Purulent material found at time of initial debridement and implant removal. **C-G,** Extensile approach is made, followed by osteotomies and contouring of the remaining bone until surfaces are apposed with the foot plantigrade; provisional fixation is obtained with Kirschner wires.

Continued

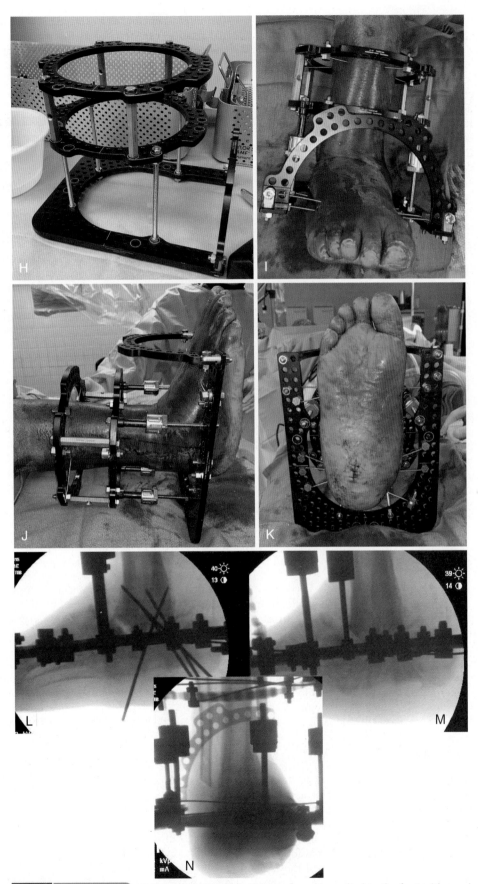

FIGURE 9.26, Cont'd   **H-K,** A pre-built, static Ilizarov frame is applied to the foot with provisional fixation in place. **L-N,** Provisional fixation is removed and compression is applied to the bone surfaces through the external fixator. **SEE TECHNIQUE 9.10.**

POSTOPERATIVE CARE Antibiotics (e.g., cefazolin) are administered perioperatively to all patients. The leg is elevated to 45 degrees for the first 2 days. Despite this, a large hematoma may develop between 24 and 72 h after surgery. These hematomas generally do not require drainage, and most heal uneventfully with no superficial or deep infections, slough, or dehiscence. On the third day, partial weight bearing is initiated with patients allowed to place the foot on the ground for balance while transferring or using a walker for ambulation. We typically leave the surgical dressings in place for 1 week to allow maturation of the pin-skin interfaces before removing dressings and beginning pin site care along with daily showering. Additional compression can be applied postoperatively at surgeon discretion. Patients are assessed clinically and radiographically weekly for the first month, biweekly for the second month, monthly until fusion, and then semiannually. Because the rings of the fixator are metal, finding the radiographic "window" that allows optimal visualization and assessment can be difficult, necessitating use of an image intensifier with the surgeon in attendance to judge fusion and alignment or using cross-sectional CT imaging. Interim radiographs are inspected for evidence of bone resorption or malalignment, which would require further compression or adjustments in the fixator. Alignment is "fine-tuned" as necessary, especially if dynamic struts were used. The fixator is maintained in place until signs of fusion are apparent. After the fixator is removed, the patient is placed in a below-knee walking cast for 4 weeks followed by a double upright brace with a rocker sole shoe to assist with ambulation.

SPECIAL CONSIDERATIONS
OSTEONECROSIS OF THE TALUS

Although osteonecrosis of the talus most often results from fracture of the neck or body of the talus, nontraumatic causes, such as the use of high-dose corticosteroids and sickle cell disease, may be the cause. Over a period of several years after fracture, creeping substitution of the necrotic bone by vascularized bone may occur; if there is not obvious collapse and fragmentation of the talus, evaluation of the vascularity by MRI or bone scan may find enough vascular supply to justify isolated tibiotalar arthrodesis. If the structure of the talus is sound, a tibiotalocalcaneal arthrodesis through a posterior approach is done with an onlay graft from the posterior iliac crest (Technique 9.6). If there is severe collapse with fragmentation, the body of the talus is removed, usually through a lateral or posterior approach, the space is filled with iliac crest strut bone graft, and a plate or intramedullary nail is used for fixation. We try to avoid tibiocalcaneal arthrodesis if possible because it shortens the leg and, if the malleoli are not removed, makes footwear difficult. In cases of infection and destruction of the talus where strut grafting may be contraindicated, tibiocalcaneal fusion is acceptable as a salvage procedure. Although internal fixation can be used as discussed earlier, described in the following technique is the method of preparation and external fixation for tibiocalcaneal fusion.

TIBIOTALAR ARTHRODESIS WITH A SLIDING BONE GRAFT

Blair described a procedure that fuses the distal tibia to the talar neck in situations in which the body of the talus has been lost or is osteonecrotic. This method uses an anterior tibial sliding graft, allows nearly normal appearance of the foot with little shortening of the extremity, and permits some flexion-extension motion of the foot on the leg. Morris et al. modified the technique and used a transcalcaneotibial pin for 6 weeks to improve stability. Klein et al. described a slot-graft inlay technique for arthrodesis in a group of high-risk patients and reported union in 13 of 17 feet, as well as low pain scores, high satisfaction scores, and a low complication rate.

TECHNIQUE 9.11

(BLAIR; MORRIS ET AL.)
- Make an anterior longitudinal incision beginning 8 cm proximal to the ankle and ending at the medial cuneiform (Fig. 9.27A).
- Dissect the interval between the extensor hallucis longus and extensor digitorum longus and retract the neurovascular bundle medially.
- Incise the capsule and periosteum in line with the skin incision.
- Remove the avascular talar body if present (Fig. 9.27B); morselize it if necessary. Do not damage the talar head or neck.
- Using a power saw, cut a rectangular graft 5.0 cm × 2.5 cm from the anterior aspect of the distal tibia.
- Make a transverse slot 2 cm deep in the superior aspect of the talar neck and slide the tibial graft into it (Fig. 9.27C).
- Hold the foot in 0 degrees of dorsiflexion, 5 degrees of valgus, and 10 degrees of external rotation, and fix the proximal part of the graft to the tibia with a screw (Fig. 9.27D).
- Insert a Steinmann pin vertically through the calcaneus and 3 to 10 cm into the distal tibia for added stability.
- Pack cancellous bone grafts around the fusion site.
- We typically apply a static Ilizarov external fixator at this point, but a long leg cast with the knee flexed 30 degrees can be applied instead.

POSTOPERATIVE CARE At 6 weeks, the cast and Steinmann pin are removed, and a short leg walking cast is applied; this cast is worn until fusion is solid.

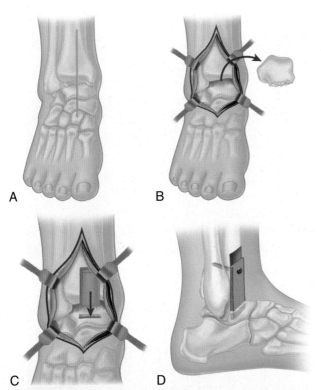

FIGURE 9.27 Blair fusion. **A,** Approach to the ankle. **B,** Excision of body of talus. **C,** Sliding bone graft. **D,** Graft in final position. **SEE TECHNIQUE 9.11.**

FAILED TOTAL ANKLE ARTHROPLASTY

With the rising popularity of total ankle arthroplasty comes the challenge of reconstructing the failed total ankle with arthrodesis if revision arthroplasty is not possible. Although some studies have shown that salvage arthrodesis after failed total ankle arthroplasty results in impaired life quality, reduction of function, and increased pain compared with primary arthrodesis, Deleu et al. reported that tibiotalar and tibiotalocalcaneal arthrodeses using massive cancellous allografts were effective procedures, resulting in fusion after the primary procedure in 14 of 17 patients; of the four nonunions, three united after a second procedure and one was asymptomatic. All patients were symptom free at the latest follow-up. In patients with no infection, a one-stage procedure was done: tibiotalar arthrodesis for patients with good bone stock and an intact subtalar joint or tibiotalocalcaneal arthrodesis for those with poor bone quality, subtalar joint arthritis, or severe bone loss. For patients with infection, extensive debridement and implant removal, insertion of an antibiotic-impregnated spacer, stabilization with a brace or external fixator, and intravenous antibiotic therapy were done before arthrodesis, which usually was possible within 6 weeks of infection treatment. The authors recommend the use of bulk allografts in combination with autografts. Laboratory and adjunctive studies may be necessary to evaluate for infection. Often a significant bone defect accompanies the failure, and extensive grafting is necessary. A key decision point in these cases is the presence or absence of subtalar arthritis. If the subtalar joint is to be preserved, we prefer arthrodesis through an anterior approach with grafting (autograft or allograft) and dual plating (see Fig. 9.17). This has the benefit of the use of the previous anterior incision, which makes removal of the implant easier. If the subtalar joint is

to be fused, the same anterior approach can be used with grafting as described, or a lateral transfibular approach gives improved access to the subtalar joint. Berkowitz et al. described salvage of 24 failed total ankle arthroplasties with isolated ankle or ankle-hindfoot fusions using structural allografts and internal fixation with anterior plates and screws, intramedullary nails, or a combination nail-plate construct. Fusion was eventually achieved in 23 of the 24 ankles, but several patients required multiple procedures and little functional improvement was noted in all patients. Results were worse and complications more frequent in patients with tibiotalocalcaneal fusions than in those with isolated ankle fusion. Ali et al. showed 95% and 87% union rates of the tibiotalar and subtalar joints, respectively, after single-stage tibiotalocalcaneal arthrodesis without the use of interposition grafts, although limb shortening averaged 2.4 cm and ranged from 1.3 to 3.5 cm in these 23 ankles. Kamrad et al. reported a 90% union rate in 118 cases of salvage arthrodesis for failed ankle arthroplasty; however, fewer than half of patients were satisfied, and functional scores were low. In a systematic review of the literature that included 193 patients, Gross et al. found that 81% of arthrodeses fused after the first procedure, patients with intercalary bone grafts, and those with blade plate fixation had the highest rates of fusion with low complication rates.

TIBIOTALAR OR TIBIOTALOCALCANEAL FUSION WITH STRUCTURAL ALLOGRAFT AND INTERNAL FIXATION FOR SALVAGE OF FAILED TOTAL ANKLE ARTHROPLASTY

TECHNIQUE 9.12

(BERKOWITZ ET AL.)

- Expose the ankle through the previous anterior approach.
- Debride associated synovitis. If infection is suspected, send synovial and bone biopsy specimens for pathologic evaluation and culture.
- Remove the polyethylene insert first, then the tibial and talar components. The talar implant usually is loose and relatively easy to dislodge, but the tibial component may be well fixed and require the use of flexible osteotomes to disrupt the bone-implant interface. If necessary, make a formal anterior cortical window in the distal tibia to loosen and remove the tibial component.
- Once the components are removed, debride all fibrinous material and necrotic bone until bleeding bone surfaces are seen. Evaluate the dimensions of the resulting bone defect and the integrity of the residual talus.
- If sepsis is detected, place an antibiotic-impregnated cement spacer within the defect and initiate a staged protocol.
- If no sepsis is detected and the residual talar bone is sufficient to achieve stable internal fixation and the subtalar joint is intact, proceed with tibiotalar fusion, choosing a suitable bone graft to fill the bone defect such that limb length can be preserved.

- Using either a nonstructural cancellous allograft or a structural graft such as autogenous iliac crest, distal tibial allograft, allograft iliac crest wedges, or allograft femoral head, fashion the graft to match the bone defect and to help restore neutral ankle alignment in the sagittal plane and 5 to 7 degrees of hindfoot valgus.
- Insert cannulated lag screws and an anterior plate for fixation.
- If the remaining talar bone is inadequate to obtain stability of tibiotalar fusion, or if the subtalar joint is degenerative or eroded by the total ankle arthroplasty, proceed with ankle-hindfoot arthrodesis and include the subtalar joint in the arthrodesis construct.
- Usually the subtalar joint is adequately exposed through the anterior incision, but if necessary for adequate debridement and preparation, make a separate lateral approach.
- If the size of the defect when ankle-hindfoot arthrodesis is required precludes the use of autograft bone, a bulk femoral head allograft or other structural allograft bone is used.
- If bulk femoral head allograft is chosen, use acetabular reamers to create a round, concentric bone defect. Use reverse acetabular reamers to fashion the femoral head to the exact size of the defect to allow an intimate fit between the host bone and the bone graft. Use cancellous allograft bone to augment the fusion and fill any residual bone defects.
- Fixation can be done with an intramedullary nail placed through the heel (see Technique 9.6), an anterior plate and lag screws, or a combined nail and plate construct (Fig. 9.28).

POSTOPERATIVE CARE The patient is immobilized in a non–weight-bearing cast for 10 to 12 weeks. Weight bearing is begun around 12 weeks after surgery when radiographs begin to demonstrate incorporation of the graft. After successful resumption of ambulation, patients are transitioned to a walking fracture boot and physical therapy is begun when indicated.

INFECTION/OSTEOMYELITIS

Ankle fusion in the presence of osteomyelitis is a daunting task and often must be accomplished in stages. External fixation is indicated for stabilization in most patients with infection; in more severe cases in which bone graft will be needed, the procedure is staged with the use of antibiotic methyl methacrylate bone cement and external fixation, followed by 6 weeks of intravenous antibiotics and removal of the cement, bone grafting, and compression with the external fixator until healed. Saltzman described treatment of eight patients with diffuse ankle osteomyelitis with resection of all infected tissue and hybrid-frame compression arthrodesis. One patient required below-knee amputation because of vascular insufficiency; none of the seven fused ankles required further surgery at an average 3-year follow-up.

CHARCOT NEUROARTHROPATHY

The pathology of Charcot arthropathy is discussed in other chapter. Timing of the surgery is important, because many of these

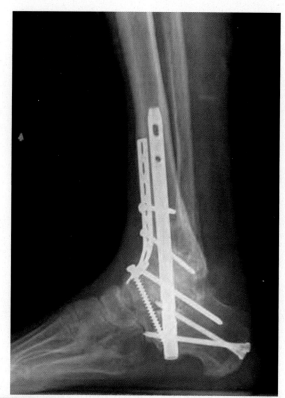

FIGURE 9.28 Ankle-hindfoot arthrodesis using combined nail-plate construct. (From Berkowitz MJ, Clare MP, Walling AK, Sanders R: Salvage of failed total ankle arthroplasty with fusion using structural allograft and internal fixation, *Foot Ankle Int* 32:S493–502, 2011.) **SEE TECHNIQUE 9.12.**

patients have severe, unbraceable deformities, and surgery is best done before a difficult deformity leads to skin breakdown and infection. Patients with a dense neuropathy and a history of Charcot arthropathy or other diabetic target organ disease (retinopathy, nephropathy) who sustain an ankle fracture may best be treated with arthrodesis at the time of fracture. This is especially true for the highly comminuted fractures of the ankle often seen in these patients. The techniques described earlier are recommended, with the idea that "overfixation" is often the goal. Internal fixation with the use of a supporting external fixator may be justified, although the external fixator does pose additional risks of infection and periprosthetic fracture. Siebachmeyer et al. described one-stage correction of deformity and fusion with a retrograde intramedullary hindfoot nail in 20 patients with Charcot neuroarthropathy, ulceration, and instability; seven patients had simultaneous midfoot fusion. Limb salvage was achieved in all patients, and all but one patient regained independent mobilization. The authors emphasized that a multidisciplinary care plan, including revascularization procedures, infection treatment, and an off-loading regimen when needed, is essential (see Fig. 9.1). Pantalar arthrodesis (fusion of the tibiotalar, subtalar, talonavicular, and calcaneocuboid joints) may be indicated as a salvage procedure in patients with neuroarthropathies to avoid amputation (Fig. 9.29). Although reported to provide pain relief, correct ankle and hindfoot malalignment, and improve function in some patients, pantalar arthrodesis, as either a single or staged procedure, is a difficult operation and major complications are frequent. Regardless of the

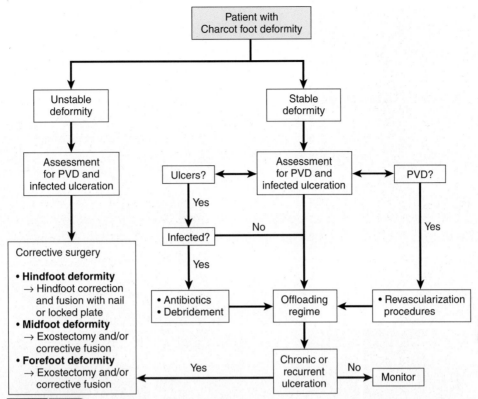

FIGURE 9.29 Management algorithm for patients with Charcot foot deformity. *PVD*, peripheral vascular disease. (Modified from Siebachmeyer M, Boddu K, Bilal A, et al: Outcome of one-stage correction of deformities of the ankle and hindfoot and fusion in Charcot neuroarthropathy using a retrograde intramedullary hindfoot arthrodesis nail, *Bone Joint J* 97-B:76–82, 2015. Copyright British Editorial Society of Bone and Joint Surgery.)

procedure chosen, tight glycemic control is imperative to obtain optimal results. A review of a national database that included over 12,000 patients with ankle arthrodesis found a complication rate of 16% in diabetic patients compared with 7% in nondiabetic patients.

BONE GRAFT/SUPPLEMENTATION

A variety of options exist for bone graft supplementation of the fusion site. Each technique lends itself to a particular type of graft. A valid question is whether supplemental bone graft is necessary. Certainly, for defects or gaps in the fusion site, bone graft of some type is advantageous. DiGiovanni et al. showed that a graft fill of over 50% of the cross-sectional area of the fusion space on a CT scan led to a higher fusion rate (81%) compared to when less than 50% graft fill was achieved (21%). In other cases, where healthy cancellous surfaces are apposed, often no supplementation is necessary. The simplest graft is that harvested from the resected fibula in the transfibular approach (Technique 9.5). If the fibula is not used as an onlay graft, a small acetabular reamer can be applied to the fibula before resection to produce a morselized graft. With the mini-incision technique (Technique 9.4), we generally supplement with bone graft harvested from the proximal tibia. Whitehouse et al. described bone graft harvest from the proximal tibia for foot and ankle arthrodesis. Suggested advantages of the proximal tibia as a bone graft source include its position in the operative field and under tourniquet control. In 131 patients with 148 procedures (primarily triple arthrodesis, 40%; subtalar

arthrodesis, 26%; and midfoot fusions, 23%) using proximal tibial autografts, 96% had no pain at the graft harvest site and 4% had only very mild pain with activities such as kneeling. Wheeler et al. described the use of a low-speed burr to create a bone "slurry" and found improved fusion rates in their patients. When intramedullary nail fixation is used, a reamer-irrigator-aspirator (RIA) can be used to harvest bone from the hindfoot or tibial shaft during reaming. A comparison of fusion and complication rates between iliac crest bone grafts and RIA bone grafts in 56 patients with tibiotalar arthrodesis found a significantly higher nonunion rate and an increased frequency of chronic pain at the graft site in those with iliac crest grafts. Use of an RIA system also avoids morbidity associated with graft harvest from the iliac crest. We have used RIA with good results (Fig. 9.30).

BONE GRAFT HARVEST FROM THE PROXIMAL TIBIA

TECHNIQUE 9.13

(WHITEHOUSE ET AL.)
- Prepare and drape the lower limb, leaving the proximal tibia exposed. Apply and inflate a thigh tourniquet unless contraindicated.

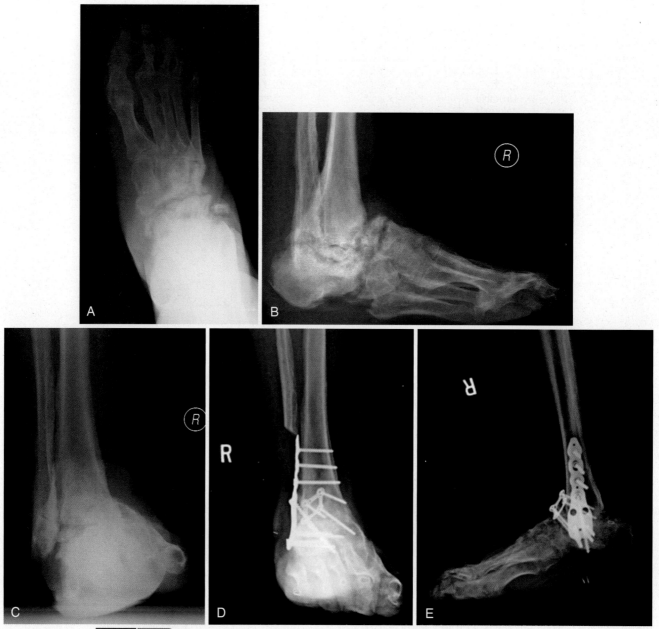

FIGURE 9.30   **A** and **B**, Severe varus deformity of hindfoot and ankle with Charcot arthropathy in a 55-year-old diabetic patient. **C-E**, After hindfoot pantalar arthrodesis fixed with lateral ankle fusion plate; tibial bone graft was obtained with reamer-irrigator-aspirator technique.

- Make a longitudinal or oblique incision just lateral to the tibial tuberosity directly over Gerdy's tubercle.
- Incise the fascia, separate the muscle by blunt dissection, and use a periosteal elevator to expose the underlying bone.
- Use a 1-cm osteotome to cut a rectangular window measuring approximately 2 cm × 1 cm and harvest cancellous bone with curets. Alternatively, use the 6.5-mm end of a 6.5/3.2-mm soft-tissue sleeve to manually penetrate the cortex over Gerdy's tubercle, and harvest additional bone with a large pituitary rongeur through this cortical window.
- Replace the bone window, if desired, and close the wound in a layered fashion.

Although the iliac crest is not used as often as a source of graft as in the past, it may be important if knee implants or a pathologic process around the knee prevents the use of the proximal tibia or in difficult cases when a strut autograft seems most appropriate. The variety of bone grafting techniques described in the literature can help in adapting ankle arthrodesis to many different situations. A tricortical block of iliac crest, split carefully between the two tables, can be wedged into a 2.5-cm wide trough in the tibia and talus with the cancellous side facing the tibia bed (Fig. 9.31A). A sliding graft, approximately 2 cm wide, 1 cm deep, and 8 to 10 cm long, can be taken from the anterior, lateral, or medial tibia and impacted into a tunnel created in the talar neck (Fig. 9.31B) or talar bed (Fig. 9.31C). A central bone graft was achieved in a shorter time (124 days compared with 161 days). Several articles by DiGiovanni et al. have described the use of purified recombinant human platelet–derived growth factor-BB (rhPDGF-BB) combined with an osteoconductive matrix (β-tricalcium phosphate) as an alternative to bone graft in hindfoot and ankle fusions and have reported comparable fusion rates, less pain, and fewer side effects, such as autograft harvest morbidity, compared with the use of autografts. Although the basic science behind many of these products is sound, it remains to be seen whether outcomes will support conversion from autograft to these products.

COMPLICATIONS

NONUNION

Nonunion rates vary widely in the literature, largely dependent on technique, underlying diagnosis, and patient selection. Factors that seem, in general, to improve results include arthroscopic or mini-incision technique, the use of more than two screws or an adjunct plate (or fibular strut), and a diagnosis of primary osteoarthritis (as opposed to inflammatory, postinfectious, or posttraumatic arthritis). With modern techniques, attention to detail, and management of concurrent medical conditions, fusion rates of better than 90% should be expected in standard, uncomplicated ankle arthrodesis.

In an extensive review of the literature, Thevendran et al. determined a number of risk factors for nonunion after ankle arthrodesis (Table 9.1); however, clinical evidence is insufficient for most of these factors to be definitely implicated in the development of nonunion. The authors did note that there is fair evidence (grade B) to advocate the use of internal fixation and evolving grade B evidence suggesting that minimally invasive techniques may be equivalent to open procedures in selected patients.

The presence of union may be, at times, difficult to establish. Physical findings of persistent swelling, pain at the fusion site, and difficulty with weight bearing should lead to careful scrutiny of the plain radiographs. Bridging callus across the fusion site on more than one view usually confirms successful fusion. In some cases, CT is necessary to establish that fusion has occurred or to evaluate the nonunion.

■ TREATMENT

Assessment of a patient with a delayed union or nonunion begins with an overall assessment for the medical issues as outlined earlier. We routinely draw 25-hydroxyvitamin D levels, albumin, prealbumin, parathyroid hormone, thyroid stimulating hormone, calcium, C-reactive protein, erythrocyte sedimentation rate, and hemoglobin A1c levels in the office in the workup of these patients. Satisfactory immobilization of a delayed union in a protected weight-bearing boot or cast is necessary. Although the US Food and Drug Administration has approved pulsed electronic magnetic field devices for stimulation of bone growth after failed arthrodesis, Saltzman et al. reported that the use of these devices with immobilization and limited weight bearing was successful in only five of 19 delayed unions of foot and ankle arthrodeses. Better results have been reported with revision arthrodesis: 75% to 94% successful fusion. Despite attention to detail in the management of these patients, some will require reoperation with bone grafting and more stable fixation.

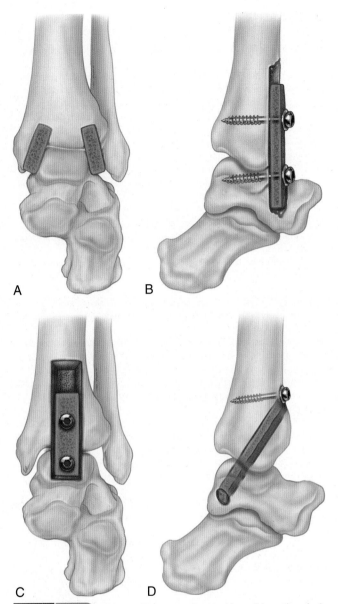

FIGURE 9.31 Types of bone grafts used in ankle arthrodesis. **A,** Tricortical block of iliac crest wedged between tibia and talus. **B** and **C,** Sliding graft impacted into tunnel in talar neck or head. **D,** Central bone graft inserted in hole bored across ankle.

(Fig. 9.31D) has been recommended for tubercular or rheumatoid ankles; the hole bored across the ankle also can be filled with cancellous bone graft from the iliac crest. The medial and lateral malleoli can be used as local bone grafts or placed as onlay grafts. Free vascularized autogenous bone grafts can be used for reconstruction of ankles with segmental bone loss caused by osteomyelitis, tumor, or trauma.

Bone graft substitutes have become widely used, and these groups of synthetic or allograft biocomposites are discussed in other chapter. There are, at present, no randomized level 1 studies that compare autograft to any commercially available product for use in ankle arthrodesis. Fourman et al., however, compared fusion rates with and without rhBMP-2 in 82 patients with comorbidities who required complex ankle arthrodesis. More patients with rhBMP-2 had fusion (93%) than did those without rhBMP-2 (53%), and fusion

TABLE 9.1

Risk Factors for Nonunion of Ankle Arthrodesis

RISK FACTOR	GRADE OF EVIDENCE
PATIENT FACTORS	
Systemic Factors	
Diabetes	B
Cigarette smoking	B
Alcohol	I
Osteoporosis	I
NSAIDs	C
Age	I
Obesity	I
Poor compliance with WB restrictions	C
Local Factors	
Infection	I
Vascularity and osteonecrosis	I
Soft-tissue injury and revision surgery	B
SURGICAL FACTORS	
Mechanical Factors	
Construct stability	I
Interfragmentary gaps	I
Surgeon Factors	
High-volume vs. low-volume surgeons	I

Grades of evidence: *A*, strong clinical evidence; *B*, fair clinical evidence; *C*, conflicting clinical evidence; *I*, insufficient clinical evidence
NSAIDs, Nonsteroidal antiinflammatory drugs; *WB*, weight bearing.
Modified from Thevendran G, Younger A, Pinney S: Current concepts review: risk factors for nonunions in foot and ankle arthrodesis, *Foot Ankle Int* 33:1031–1041, 2012.

ADJACENT JOINT PAIN AND ARTHRITIS

The development of adjacent joint arthritis, especially in the subtalar joint, has been noted by numerous authors, but whether these joints require treatment is debatable. In some patients, the development of adjacent joint arthritis is painful and requires bracing or surgical fusion; however, usually these joints are fairly asymptomatic and no further treatment is required. In their sports participation study of 185 ankles undergoing arthrodesis, Kerkhoff et al. found at an average 7 years after surgery only a 7% incidence of subtalar pain as confirmed by injection and a 2% incidence of ipsilateral subtalar arthrodesis. In patients with pantalar arthritis before ankle fusion, consideration should be given to alternative treatments, such as arthroplasty. Complicating the management of painful subtalar arthritis after ankle fusion is the loss of height with subtalar compression arthrodesis, which places the hindfoot in slight equinus. A small strut graft should be considered in these cases to prevent this complication, but this likely increases the nonunion rate which is already higher after adjacent joint ankle arthrodesis.

REFERENCES

Abicht BP, Roukis TS: Incidence of nonunion after isolated arthroscopic ankle arthrodesis, *Arthroscopy* 29:949, 2013.

Ahn TK, Yi Y, Cho JH, Lee WC: A cohort study of patients undergoing distal tibial osteotomy without fibular osteotomy for medial ankle arthritis with mortise widening, *J Bone Joint Surg* 97:381, 2015.

Ajis A, Tan KJ, Myerson MS: Ankle arthrodesis vs ttc arthrodesis: patient outcomes, satisfaction, and return to activity, *Foot Ankle Int* 34:657, 2013.

Akra GA, Middleton A, Adedapo AO, et al.: Outcome of ankle arthrodesis using a transfibular approach, *J Foot Ankle Surg* 49:508, 2010.

Ali AA, Forrester RA, O'Connor P, et al.: Revision of failed total ankle arthroplasty to a hindfoot fusion: 23 consecutive cases using the Phoenix nail, *Bone Joint J* 100-B:475, 2018.

Bai Z, Zhang E, He Y, et al.: Arthroscopic ankle arthrodesis in hemophilic arthropathy, *Foot Ankle Int* 34:1147, 2013.

Barg A, Amendola A, Beaman DN, Saltzman CL: Ankle joint distraction arthroplasty: why and how? *Foot Ankle Clin* 18:459, 2013.

Barg A, Pagenstert GI, Horisberger M, et al.: Supramalleolar osteotomies for degenerative joint disease of the ankle joint: indication, technique and results, *Int Orthop* 37:1683, 2013.

Berkowitz MJ, Clare MP, Walling AK, Sanders R: Salvage of failed total ankle arthroplasty with fusion using structural allograft and internal fixation, *Foot Ankle Int* 32:493, 2011.

Bernstein M, Reidler J, Fragomen A, et al.: Ankle distraction arthroplasty: indications, technique, and outcomes, *J Am Acad Orthop Surg* 25:89, 2017.

Chalayon O, Wang B, Blankenhorn B, et al.: Factors affecting the outcomes of uncomplicated primary open ankle arthrodesis, *Foot Ankle Int* 36:1170, 2015.

Chang KV, Hsiao MY, Chen WS, et al.: Effectiveness of intra-articular hyaluronic acid for ankle osteoarthritis treatment: a systematic review and meta-analysis, *Arch Phys Med Rehabil* 94:951, 2013.

Chopra S, Rouhani H, Assal M, et al.: Outcome of unilateral ankle arthrodesis and total ankle replacement in terms of bilateral gait mechanics, *J Orthop Res* 32:377, 2014.

Clare MP, Sanders RW: The anatomic compression arthrodesis technique with anterior plate augmentation for ankle arthrodesis, *Foot Ankle Clin* 16:91, 2011.

Cottino U, Collo G, Marino L, et al.: Arthroscopic ankle arthrodesis: a review, *Curr Rev Musculoskelet Med* 5:151, 2012.

Cuttica DJ, DeBries JG, Hyer CF: Togenous bone graft harvest using reamer irrigator aspirator (RIA) technique for tibiotalocalcaneal arthrodesis, *J Foot Ankle Surg* 49:571, 2010.

Dalat F, Trouillet F, Fessy MH, et al.: Comparison of quality of life following total ankle arthroplasty and ankle arthrodesis: retrospective study of 54 cases, *Orthop Traumatol Surg Res* 100:761, 2014.

Daniels TF, Younger AS, Penner MJ, et al.: Prospective randomized controlled trial of hindfoot and ankle fusions treated with rhPDGF-BB in combination with a ß-TCP-collagen matrix, *Foot Ankle Int* 36:739, 2015.

Daniels TR, Younger AS, Penner M, et al.: Intermediate term results of total ankle replacement and ankle arthrodesis: a COFAS multicenter study, *J Bone Joint Surg* 96:135, 2014.

Dannawi Z, Nawabi DH, Patel A, et al.: Arthroscopic ankle arthrodesis: are results reproducible irrespective or pre-operative deformity? *Foot Ankle Surg* 17:294, 2011.

DeGroot 3rd H, Uzunishvili S, Weir R, et al.: Intra-articular injection of hyaluronic acid is not superior to saline solution injection for ankle arthritis: a randomized double-blind, placebo-controlled study, *J Bone Joint Surg* 94(2), 2012.

Dekker TJ, Hamid KS, Easley ME, et al.: Ratio of range of motion of the ankle and surrounding joints after total ankle replacement. A radiographic cohort study, *J Bone Joint Surg Am* 99:576, 2017.

Dekker TJ, Walton D, Vinson EN, et al.: Hindfoot arthritis progression and arthrodesis risk after total ankle replacement, *Foot Ankle Int* 38:1183, 2017.

Deleu PA, Devos Beverage B, Maldague P, et al.: Arthrodesis after failed total ankle replacement, *Foot Ankle Int* 35:549, 2014.

Didomenico LA, Sann P: Posterior approach using anterior ankle arthrodesis locking plate for tibiotalocalcaneal arthrodesis, *J Foot Ankle Surg* 50:626, 2011.

DiGiovanni CW, Baumhauer J, Lin SS, et al.: Prospective, randomized, multi-center feasibility trial of rhPDGH-BB versus autologous bone graft in a foot and ankle fusion model, *Foot Ankle Int* 32:344, 2011.

DiGiovanni CW, Lin SS, Baumhauer JF, et al.: Recombinant human platelet-derived growth factor-bb and beta-tricalcium phosphate (rhPDGF-BB/ß-TCP): an alternative to autogenous bone graft, *J Bone Joint Surg* 95:1184, 2013.

DiGiovanni CW, Lin SS, Daniels TR, et al.: The importance of sufficient graft material in achieving foot or ankle fusion, *J Bone Joint Surg Am* 98:1260, 2016.

Doets HC, Zürcher AW: Salvage arthrodesis for failed total ankle arthroplasty, *Acta Orthop* 81:142, 2010.

Easley ME: Surgical treatment of the arthritic varus ankle, *Foot Ankle Clin* 17:665, 2012.

El-Alfy B: Arthrodesis of the ankle joint by Ilizarov external fixator in patients with infection or poor bone stock, *Foot Ankle Surg* 16:96, 2010.

Fitzgibbons TC, Hawks MA, McMullen ST, Inda DJ: Bone grafting in surgery about the foot and ankle: indications and techniques, *J Am Acad Orthop Surg* 19:112, 2011.

Fourman MS, Borst EW, Bogner E, et al.: Recombinant human BMP-2 increases the incidence and rate of healing in complex ankle arthrodesis, *Clin Orthop Relat Res* 472:732, 2014.

Fragomen AT, Borst E, Schachter L, et al.: Complex ankle arthrodesis using the Ilizarov method yields high rate of fusion, *Clin Orthop Relat Res* 470:2864, 2012.

Fuentes-Sanz A, Moya-Angeler J, López-Oliva F, Forriol F: Clinical outcome and gait analysis of ankle arthrodesis, *Foot Ankle Int* 33:819, 2012.

Glazebrook M: End-stage ankle arthritis: magnitude of the problem and solutions, *Instr Course Lect* 59:359, 2010.

Gross C, Erickson BJ, Adams SB, Parekh SG: Ankle arthrodesis after failed total ankle replacement: a systematic review of the literature, *Foot Ankle Spec* 8:143, 2015.

Guo C, Yan Z, Barfield WR, Hartsock LA: Ankle arthrodesis using anatomically contoured anterior plate, *Foot Ankle Int* 31:492, 2010.

Hamid KS, Glisson RR, Morash JG, et al.: Simultaneous intraoperative measurement of cadaver ankle and subtalar joint compression during arthrodesis with intramedullary nail, screws, and tibiotalcalcaneal plate, *Foot Ankle Int* 39:1128, 2018.

Han SH, Park do Y, Kim TH: Prognostic factors after intra-articular hyaluronic acid injection in ankle osteoarthritis, *Yonsei Med J* 55:1080, 2014.

Hendricks RP, Stufkens SA, de Bruijn EE, et al.: Medium- to long-term outcome of ankle arthroesis, *Foot Ankle Int* 32:940, 2011.

Henricson A, Rydholm U: Use of a trabecular metal implant in ankle arthrodesis after failed total ankle replacement, *Acta Orthop* 81:745, 2010.

Herrera-Perez M, Alrashidi Y, Galhoum AE, et al.: Debridement and hinged motion distraction is superior to debridement alone in patients with ankle osteoarthritis: a prospective randomized controlled trial, *Knee Surg Sports Traumatol Arthrosc*, 2018 Sep 27, https://doi.org/10.1007/s00167-018-5156-3, [Epub ahead of print].

Herscovici Jr D, Scaduto JM: Use of the reamer-irrigator-aspirator technique to obtain autograft for ankle and hindfoot arthrodesis, *J Bone Joint Surg* 94B:75, 2012.

Herscovici D, Sammarco GJ, Sammarco VJ, Scaduto JM: Pantalar arthrodesis for post-traumatic arthritis and diabetic neuroarthropathy of the ankle and hindfoot, *Foot Ankle Int* 32:581, 2011.

Hoover JR, Santrack RD, James 3rd WC: Ankle fusion stability: a biomechanical comparison of external versus internal fixation, *Orthopedics* 34:272, 2011.

Houdek MT, Wilke BK, Ryssman DB, Turner NS: Radiographic and functional outcomes following bilateral ankle fusions, *Foot Ankle Int* 35:1250, 2014.

Jasiter J, Coughlin MJ, Hirose C: Performance of total ankle arthroplasty and ankle arthrodesis on uneven surfaces, stairs, and inclines: a prospective study, *Foot Ankle Int* 36:11, 2015.

Jehan S, Hill SO: Operative technique of two parallel compression screws and autologous bone graft for ankle arthrodesis after failed total ankle replacement, *Foot Ankle Int* 33:767, 2012.

Jiang JJ, Schipper ON, Whyte N, et al.: Comparison of perioperative complications and hospitalization outcomes after ankle arthrodesis versus total ankle arthroplasty from 2002 to 2011, *Foot Ankle Int* 36:360, 2015.

Jones CR, Wong E, Applegate GR, et al.: Arthroscopic ankle arthrodesis: a 2-15 year follow-up study, *Arthroscopy* 34:1641, 2018.

Kamrad I, Henricson A, Magnusson H, et al.: Outcome after salvage arthrodesis for failed total ankle replacement, *Foot Ankle Int* 37:255, 2016.

Kerkhoff YRA, Keijsers NLW, Louwerens JWK: Sports participation, functional outcome, and complications after ankle arthrodesis: midterm follow-up, *Foot Ankle Int* 38:1085, 2017.

Kestner CJ, Glisson RR, DeOrio JK, Nunley 2nd JA: A biomechanical analysis of two anterior ankle arthrodesis systems, *Foot Ankle Int* 34:1006, 2013.

Khanfour AA: Versatility of Ilizarov technique in difficult cases of ankle arthrodesis and review of literature, *Foot Ankle Surg* 19:42, 2013.

Klein SE, Putnam RM, McCormick JJ, Johnson JE: The slot graft technique for foot and ankle arthrodesis in a high-risk patient group, *Foot Ankle Int* 32:686, 2011.

Krause FG, Windolf M, Bora B, et al.: Impact of complications in total ankle replacement and ankle arthrodesis analyzed with a validated outcome measurement, *J Bone Joint Surg* 93A:830, 2011.

Labib SA, Raikin SM, Lau JT, et al.: Joint preservation procedures for ankle arthritis, *Foot Ankle Int* 34:1040, 2013.

Lee WC, Moon JS, Lee K, et al.: Indications for supramalleolar osteotomy in patients with ankle osteoarthritis and varus deformity, *J Bone Joint Surg* 93A:1243–1248, 2011.

Lucas Y, Hernandez J, Abad J, et al.: Tibiotalocalcaneal arthrodesis using a straight intramedullary nail, *Foot Ankle Int* 36:539, 2015.

Lucas Y, Hernandez J, Darcel V, et al.: Viscosupplementation of the ankle: a prospective study with an average follow-up of 45.5 months, *Orthop Traumatol Surg Res* 99:593, 2013.

Maenohara Y, Taniguchi A, Tomiwa K, et al.: Outcomes of bilateral vs unilateral ankle arthrodesis, *Foot Ankle Int* 39:530, 2018.

Mann HA, Filippi J, Myerson MS: Intra-articular opening medial tibial wedge osteotomy (plafond-plasty) for the treatment of intra-articular varus ankle arthritis and instability, *Foot Ankle Int* 33:255, 2012.

McCoy TH, Goldman V, Fragomen AT, Rozbruch SR: Circular external fixator-assisted ankle arthrodesis following failed total ankle arthroplasty, *Foot Ankle Int* 33:947, 2012.

McKinley JC, Shortt N, Arthur C, et al.: Outcomes following pantalar arthrodesis in rheumatoid arthritis, *Foot Ankle Int* 32:681, 2011.

Mei-Dan O, Carmont M, Laver L, et al.: Intra-articular injections of hyaluronic acid in osteoarthritis of the subtalar joint: a pilot study, *J Foot Ankle Surg* 52:172, 2013.

Mitchell PM, Douleh DG, Thomson AB: Comparison of ankle fusion rates with and without anterior plate augmentation, *Foot Ankle Int* 38:419, 2017.

Mohamedean A, Said HG, El-Sharkawi M, et al.: Technique and short-term results of ankle arthrodesis using anterior plating, *Int Orthop* 34:833, 2010.

Mongon ML, Garcia Costa KV, Bittar CK, Livani B: Tibiotalar arthrodesis in posttraumatic arthritis using the tension band technique, *Foot Ankle Int* 34:851, 2013.

Mulligan RP, Adams Jr SB, Easley ME, et al.: Comparison of posterior approach with intramedullary nailing versus lateral transfibular approach with fixed-angle plating for tibiotalocalcaneal arthrodesis, *Foot Ankle Int* 38:1343, 2017.

Myers TG, Lowery NJ, Frykberg RG, Wukich DK: Ankle and hindfoot fusions: comparison of outcomes in patients with and without diabetes, *Foot Ankle Int* 33:20, 2012.

Myerson MS, Zide JR: Management of varus ankle osteoarthritis with joint-preserving osteotomy, *Foot Ankle Clin N Am* 8:471, 2013.

Nickisch F, Avilucea FR, Beals T, Saltzman C: Open posterior approach for tibiotalar arthrodesis, *Foot Ankle Clin* 16:103, 2010.

Nodzo SR, Kaplan NB, Hohman DW, Ritter CA: A radiographic and clinical comparison of reamer-irrigator-aspirator versus iliac crest bone graft in ankle arthrodesis, *Int Orthop* 38:1199, 2014.

Norvell DC, Shofer JB, Hansen ST, et al.: Frequency and impact of adverse events in patients undergoing surgery for end-stage ankle arthritis, *Foot Ankle Int* 39:1028, 2018.

O'Connor KM, Johnson JE, McCormick JJ, et al.: Clinical and operative factors related to successful revision arthrodesis in the foot and ankle, *Foot Ankle Int* 37:809, 2016.

Olson KM, Dairyko Jr GH, Toolan BC: Salvage of chronic instability of the syndesmosis with distal tibiofibular arthrodesis: functional and radiographic results, *J Bone Joint Surg* 93A:66, 2011.

Onodera T, Majima T, Kasahara Y, et al.: Outcome of transfibular ankle arthrodesis with Ilizarov apparatus, *Foot Ankle Int* 33:964, 2012.

Pakzad H, Thevendran G, Penner MJ, et al.: Factors associated with longer length of hospital stay after primary elective ankle surgery for end-stage ankle arthritis, *J Bone Joint Surg* 96:32, 2014.

Park JH, Km HJ, Suh DH, et al.: Arthroscopic versus open ankle arthrodesis: a systematic review, *Arthroscopy* 34:988, 2018.

Pinsker E, Inrig T, Daniels TR, et al.: Reliability and validity of 6 measures of pain, function, and disability for ankle arthroplasty and arthrodesis, *Foot Ankle Int* 36:617, 2015.

Pinsker E, Inrig T, Daniels TR, et al.: Symptom resolution and patient-perceived recovery following ankle arthroplasty and arthrodesis, *Foot Ankle Int* 37:1269, 2016.

Prissel MA, Simpson GA, Sutphen SA, et al.: Ankle arthrodesis: a retrospective analysis comparing single column, locked anterior plating to crossed lag screw technique, *J Foot Ankle Surg* 56:453, 2017.

Pugely AJ, Lu X, Amendola A, et al.: Trends in the use of total ankle replacement and ankle arthrodesis in the United States Medicare population, *Foot Ankle Int* 35:207, 2014.

Rahm S, Klammer G, Benninger E, et al.: Inferior results of salvage arthrodesis after failed ankle replacement compared to primary arthrodesis, *Foot Ankle Int* 36:349, 2015.

Saltzman CL, Kadoko RG, Suh JS: Treatment of isolated ankle osteoarthritis with arthrodesis or the total ankle replacement: a comparison of early outcomes, *Clin Orthop Surg* 2(1), 2010.

Schipper ON, Jiang JJ, Chen L, et al.: Effect of diabetes mellitus on perioperative complications and hospital outcomes after ankle arthrodesis and total ankle arthroplasty, *Foot Ankle Int* 36:258, 2015.

Schuh R, Hofstaetter J, Krismer M, et al.: Total ankle arthroplasty versus ankle arthrodesis: comparison of sports, recreational activities and functional outcome, *Int Orthop* 36:1207, 2012.

Shah KS, Younger AS: Primary tibiotalocalcaneal arthrodesis, *Foot Ankle Clin* 16:115, 2011.

Siebachmeyer M, Boddu K, Bilal A, et al.: Outcome of one-stage correction of deformities of the ankle and hindfoot and fusion in Charcot neuroarthropathy using a retrograde intramedullary hindfoot arthrodesis nail, *Bone Joint J* 97-B:76, 2015.

Singer S, Klejman S, Pinsker E, et al.: Ankle arthroplasty and ankle arthrodesis: gait analysis compared with normal controls, *J Bone Joint Surg* 95:e191, 2013.

Slobogean GP, Younger A, Apostle KL, et al.: Preference-based quality of life of end-stage ankle arthritis treated with arthroplasty or arthrodesis, *Foot Ankle Int* 31:563, 2010.

Smith JT, Chiddo CP, Singh SK, Wilson MG: Open ankle arthrodesis with a fibular-sparing technique, *Foot Ankle Int* 34:557, 2013.

Stegman M, van Ginneken BT, Boetes B, et al.: Can diagnostic injections predict the outcome in foot and ankle arthrodesis? *BMC Musculoskelet Disord* 15:11, 2014.

Strasser NL, Turner NS: Functional outcomes after ankle arthrodesis in elderly patients, *Foot Ankle Int* 33:699, 2012.

Strauss AC, Goldmann G, Wessling M, et al.: Total ankle replacement in patients with haemophilia and virus infection—a safe alternative to ankle arthrodesis? *Haemophilia* 20:702, 2014.

Sun SF, Hsu CW, Sun HP, et al.: The effect of three weekly intra-articular injections of hyaluronate on pain, function, and balance in patients with unilateral ankle arthritis, *J Bone Joint Surg* 93:1720, 2011.

Thevendran G, Younger A, Pinney S: Current concepts review: risk factors for nonunion in foot and ankle arthrodeses, *Foot Ankle Int* 33:1033, 2012.

Thiryayi WA, Naqui Z, Khan SA: Use of the Taylor spatial frame in compression arthrodesis of the ankle: a study of 10 cases, *J Foot Ankle Surg* 49:182, 2010.

Thomas RL, Sathe V, Habib SI: The use of intramedullary nails in tibiotalocalcaneal arthrodesis, *J Am Acad Orthop Surg* 20(1), 2012.

Townshend D, Di Silvestro M, Krause F, et al.: Arthroscopic versus open ankle arthrodesis: a multicenter comparative case series, *J Bone Joint Surg* 95:98, 2013.

Vakhshori V, Sabour AF, Alluri RK, et al.: Patient and practice trends in total ankle replacement and tibiotalar arthrodesis in the United States from 2007 to 2013, *J Am Acad Orthop Surg* 27:e77, 2019.

Witteveen AG, Kok A, Sierevelt IN, et al.: The optimal injection technique for the osteoarthritic ankle: a randomized, cross-over trial, *Foot Ankle Surg* 19:283, 2013.

Yoshimura I, Kanazawa K, Takeyama A, et al.: The effect of screw position and number on the time to union of arthroscopic ankle arthrodesis, *Arthroscopy* 28:1882, 2012.

Younger AS, Wing KJ, Glazebrook M, et al.: Patient expectation and satisfaction as measures of operative outcome in end-stage ankle arthritis: a prospective cohort study of total ankle replacement versus ankle fusion, *Foot Ankle Int* 36:123, 2015.

Yousry AH, Abdalhady AM: Management of diabetic neuropathic ankle arthropathy by arthrodesis using an Ilizarov frame, *Acta Orthop Belg* 76:821, 2010.

Zwipp H, Rammelt S, Endres T, Heineck J: High union rates and function scores at midterm followup with ankle arthrodesis using a four screw technique, *Clin Orthop Relat Res* 468:958, 2010.

The complete list of references is available online at Expert Consult.com.

PART IV

RECONSTRUCTIVE PROCEDURES OF THE SHOULDER AND ELBOW IN ADULTS

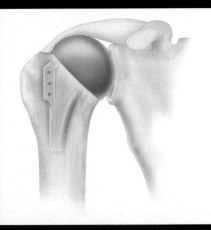

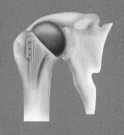

RECONSTRUCTIVE PROCEDURES OF THE SHOULDER

Prosthetic replacement of the glenohumeral joint has become accepted as a successful treatment for a variety of degenerative, traumatic, and posttraumatic conditions around the shoulder. Multiple studies with long-term follow-up have demonstrated improvements in pain and function with excellent longevity. As experience with primary arthroplasty has accumulated, improved techniques for revision surgery have evolved as well. In the past 2 decades, the emergence of the reverse total shoulder arthroplasty has added another option for the treatment of patients with advanced glenohumeral conditions associated with end-stage rotator cuff dysfunction and/or glenoid deformity. This chapter discusses the indications, surgical technique, outcomes, and complications of shoulder arthroplasty.

HISTORY

The earliest known report of shoulder arthroplasty dates back to 1893, when a French surgeon, Péan, substituted a platinum and rubber implant for a glenohumeral joint destroyed by tuberculosis. In the early 1950s, Neer introduced a humeral head prosthesis that he planned to use for complex shoulder fractures. In 1951, he reported his initial results of replacement of the humeral head with an unconstrained cobalt-chromium alloy (Vitallium) prosthesis. In 1974, the Neer II humeral prosthesis, which was modified to articulate with a glenoid component, was introduced. In the early 1990s, Paul Grammont introduced an improved design of a semiconstrained shoulder replacement using a metal sphere implanted into the glenoid and a polyethylene liner and stem into the humerus: the reverse total shoulder arthroplasty. Although implant design factors continue to evolve, the primary features of this prosthesis are retained in current iterations of reverse arthroplasty.

Glenoid components for anatomic total shoulder arthroplasty were initially designed for cementless fixation using screws and porous coating on metal backing with a polyethylene shell. But long-term studies have shown an unacceptably high complication rate, and as such these implants have been largely abandoned. Subsequently, more emphasis was placed on restoring normal kinematics with anatomic location and orientation of the glenoid joint surface, advanced soft-tissue balancing techniques, and physiologic stabilization of the joint. Most current glenoid implants are polyethylene and use cement for fixation with either a pegged or keeled configuration on the backside of the component. Use of anchor-pegged devices to improve glenoid fixation and encourage bony ingrowth also has become a popular implant design.

ANATOMY AND BIOMECHANICS

The anatomy of the shoulder joint permits more mobility than any other joint in the body. Although it often is described as a ball-and-socket joint, the large humeral head articulates against and not within the small glenoid cavity. The glenohumeral joint depends on the static and dynamic stabilizers for movement and stability, especially the rotator cuff, which not only stabilizes the glenohumeral joint while allowing greater freedom of motion but also fixes the fulcrum of the upper extremity against which the deltoid can contract and elevate the humerus. The rotator cuff must act simultaneously and synergistically, however, with the deltoid muscle for normal function.

Restoration of glenohumeral anatomy is essential for a good functional outcome in shoulder replacement. Anatomic studies have defined the humeral geometry further and suggested applications to shoulder arthroplasty prosthesis design and surgical techniques (Fig. 10.1 and Table 10.1). The articular surface of the humeral head is essentially spherical, with an arc of approximately 160 degrees covered by articular cartilage. The radius of curvature is approximately 25 mm and is slightly larger in men than in women. The glenoid articular surface radius of curvature is 2 to 3 mm larger than that of the humeral head. The average neck-shaft angle is 45 degrees (±5 degrees), with a range of 30 to 50 degrees. Murthi et al. found that arthritic shoulders have a flatter neck-shaft angle close to 50 degrees. CT studies found that the normal position of the glenoid surface in relation to the axis of the scapular body ranged from 2 degrees of anteversion to 7 degrees of retroversion.

The superior margin of the humeral head articular surface normally is superior to the top of the greater tuberosity by 8 to 10 mm (Fig. 10.2). Restoring the center of rotation for the humeral head in relation to the axis of the humeral diaphysis may play a role in prolonging glenoid fixation and decreasing polyethylene wear. The distance from the lateral base of the coracoid process to the lateral margin of the greater tuberosity is called the *lateral humeral offset*. Maintaining this distance is important because a significant decrease reduces the lever arms for the deltoid and supraspinatus muscles, which weakens abduction and impairs function. A significant increase causes excessive tension on the soft tissues ("overstuffing" of the joint), which results in loss of motion and also likely accelerates polyethylene wear. A biomechanical cadaver study determined that humeral articular malposition of more than 4 mm led to increased subacromial contact and that offset of 8 mm in any direction significantly decreased passive range of motion. The authors suggested that anatomic reconstruction

TABLE 10.1	
Anatomic Characteristics of the Shoulder Important for Prosthesis Design	
GLENOID DIAMETER	
Superior anteroposterior	18-30 mm
Inferior anteroposterior	21-35 mm
Superoinferior (height)	30-48 mm
INCLINATION	
Glenoid	Average 4.2 degrees (−7 to 20 degrees)
Humeral head	30-55 degrees
VERSION	
Glenoid	1.5 degrees retroversion (10.5-9.5 degrees anteversion)
Humeral head	0-55 degrees retroversion (dependent on measurement method; highly variable among individuals)
SURFACE AREA	
Glenoid	4-6 mm
Humeral head	11-19 mm
CARTILAGE THICKNESS	
Glenoid	2.16 mm
Humeral head	1.44 mm
RADIUS OF CURVATURE	
Glenoid	22-28 mm
Humeral head	23-28 mm (smaller in women than men)
HUMERAL OFFSET	
Medial (coronal)	4-14 mm
Posterior (transverse)	−2 to 10 mm
Head-shaft angle	30-55 degrees

of the humeral head/humeral shaft offset should be within 4 mm of normal to minimize subacromial contact and maximize glenohumeral motion.

Based on the clinical success of the Neer II implant, numerous modular designs were developed to improve implant fixation and durability. Detailed studies of shoulder anatomy found not only that normal shoulder anatomy aligned differently than the commonly used prostheses, but also that normal anatomy varied greatly among individuals. Modularity allows a better fit for individual patients because various stem and head sizes can be "mixed and matched" to an individual's anatomy. Biomechanical studies also showed that shoulder biomechanics are adversely affected by the use of a prosthetic head that is too thick, too thin, or shifted too far from its original position along the plane of the anatomic humeral neck. Other characteristics of shoulder anatomy that are important in prosthesis design are retroversion, head-shaft angle, offset, radius of curvature, and humeral head height. Proximal humeral retroversion is highly variable, ranging from 0 to 55 degrees, depending on the method used for measurement. The proximal and the distal axes used to

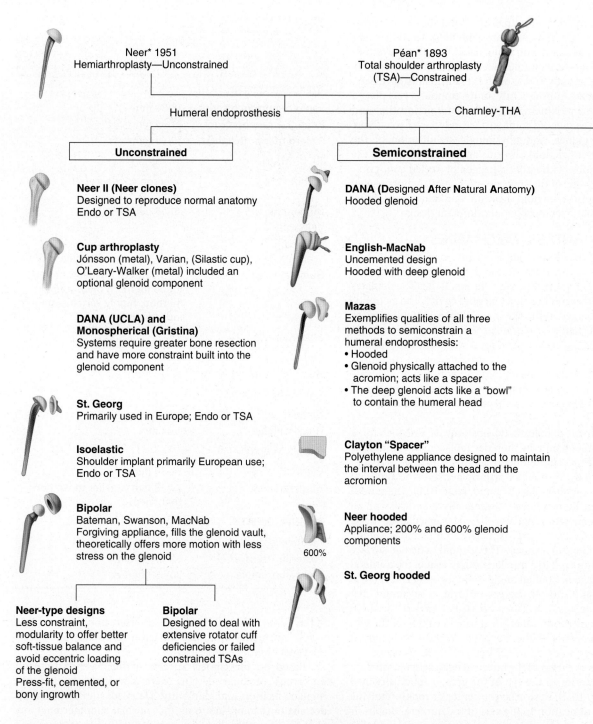

Neer* 1951
Hemiarthroplasty—Unconstrained

Péan* 1893
Total shoulder arthroplasty
(TSA)—Constrained

Humeral endoprosthesis

Charnley-THA

Unconstrained

Semiconstrained

Neer II (Neer clones)
Designed to reproduce normal anatomy
Endo or TSA

Cup arthroplasty
Jónsson (metal), Varian, (Silastic cup),
O'Leary-Walker (metal) included an
optional glenoid component

**DANA (UCLA) and
Monospherical (Gristina)**
Systems require greater bone resection
and have more constraint built into the
glenoid component

St. Georg
Primarily used in Europe; Endo or TSA

Isoelastic
Shoulder implant primarily European use;
Endo or TSA

Bipolar
Bateman, Swanson, MacNab
Forgiving appliance, fills the glenoid vault,
theoretically offers more motion with less
stress on the glenoid

DANA (Designed **A**fter **N**atural **A**natomy)
Hooded glenoid

English-MacNab
Uncemented design
Hooded with deep glenoid

Mazas
Exemplifies qualities of all three
methods to semiconstrain a
humeral endoprosthesis:
• Hooded
• Glenoid physically attached to the
  acromion; acts like a spacer
• The deep glenoid acts like a "bowl"
  to contain the humeral head

Clayton "Spacer"
Polyethylene appliance designed to maintain
the interval between the head and the
acromion

Neer hooded
Appliance; 200% and 600% glenoid
components

600%

St. Georg hooded

Neer-type designs
Less constraint,
modularity to offer better
soft-tissue balance and
avoid eccentric loading
of the glenoid
Press-fit, cemented, or
bony ingrowth

Bipolar
Designed to deal with
extensive rotator cuff
deficiencies or failed
constrained TSAs

In the end it appears that Neer's original design is
as similar to the "modern TSA" as Charnley's initial
THA is to the "modern THA."

Some of these appliances may still be available; however,
they would be hard to find. The benefit-to-risk ratio is poor
when weighing the functional improvement against the
increased complications.

*On display at the Smithsonian.

FIGURE 10.1 **Family tree of shoulder arthroplasty prostheses.** (Adapted from Gross RM: The
history of total shoulder arthroplasty. In Crosby LA, editor: *Total shoulder arthroplasty*, Rosemont, IL, 2000,
American Academy of Orthopaedic Surgeons.)

Constrained†

Ball and Socket

Trispherical TSA
Remarkably similar to Péan's original TSA
The extreme mobility of this appliance
minimizes stress at the bony fixation points
Floating fulcrum was a problem

Michael
Reese

BME

Stanmore

**Bickel, Michael Reese, Model
BME (Germany), and Stanmore (England)**
All four of these appliances are of the
"captured head" type
Breakage, dislocation, and glenoid
loosening were all too frequent
complications
Bickel, Michael Reese, and BME are
metal on polyethylene
Stanmore originally was metal on
metal and later converted to metal
on polyethylene

Reverse Ball and Socket

Floating socket TSA
Reverse bipolar and reverse ball
and socket

Fenlin TSA
The Fenlin and the Floating Socket are
both large-head reverse ball-and-socket
Large head design aimed at increasing
motion

Neer Mark III
Fixed fulcrum reverse ball-and-socket with
a rotating stem within the humeral shaft

Kessel
Large central screw fixation of the glenoid
component, no cement

Kölbel TSA
Screw fixation to glenoid similar to Péan's
original glenoid fixation

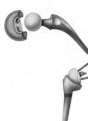

Liverpool TSA
Cemented mini "reverse THA"

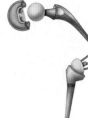

Delta III
Sole survivor, uncemented glenoid
surface mount

†Development, as well as failure, of the constrained TSA came as a result of two false
assumptions: (1) most arthritic patients would have deficient rotator cuffs and (2)
the function of the rotator cuff could effectively be replaced by a fixed fulcrum.

FIGURE 10.1, Cont'd

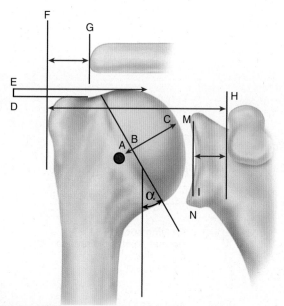

FIGURE 10.2 Normal glenohumeral relationships. Humeral offset is depicted by distance F to H, thickness of humeral head from B to C, and center of humeral head at C. Note superior position of humeral head proximal to greater tuberosity (D to E).

define retroversion have various definitions. For the proximal reference axis, the plane of the articular surface, a line connecting the center of rotation and the central point of the articular surface, and a line from the greater tuberosity to the central point of the articular surface have been used. For the distal reference axis, the trochlear axis, a line between epicondyles, and the forearm itself have been used. The inclination of the proximal humeral articular surface relative to the humeral shaft is the neck-shaft angle; it ranges from 30 to 55 degrees, depending on the method of measurement. The humeral offset defines the position of the proximal humeral articular surface relative to the humeral shaft; it is measured as the distance from the center of rotation of the proximal humeral articular surface to the central axis of the humeral canal. The medial offset (coronal plane) ranges from 4 to 14 mm, and the anteroposterior offset (transverse plane) ranges from −2 to 10 mm. Reported values for the radius of curvature of the proximal humeral articular surface range from 20 to 30 mm; smaller radii typically are reported in women, and some authors have reported that the radius of curvature is larger in the coronal plane than in the sagittal plane.

PROSTHESIS DESIGN

Most current systems are modular with varying humeral head diameters and neck lengths to allow more accurate coverage of the cut surface of the humeral neck and improve the ability to establish correct position of the joint line and rotator cuff tension. Some designs allow independent sizing of head thickness and head diameter to make soft-tissue balancing easier. Most stems are made of cobalt-chrome or titanium alloy and have proximal porous ingrowth coating to allow insertion without cement.

In an effort to match the proximal humeral anatomy as closely as possible, several implant systems offer concentric and offset humeral heads. In an anatomic dissection study, Boileau and Walch found that the center of the humeral head

was 2.6 mm posterior and 6.9 mm medial to the center of the humeral shaft, and Robertson et al., using CT, noted similar measurements of 2.2 and 7.4 mm.

Anatomic positioning of the humeral head prosthesis is best done with an eccentric locking position of the Morse taper, which allows adjustments to the variable medial offset and any posterior offset. Curiously, postoperative kinematics after total shoulder arthroplasty do not mimic those of the native shoulder. Massimini et al. found that the posterosuperior quadrant of the glenoid is the primary contact location and that the replaced shoulder is not subject to traditional kinematic conceptions. Nevertheless, positioning the head too far superiorly puts additional tension on the overlying supraspinatus tendon and can cause impingement between the head and the acromion. Positioning the head too far inferiorly may cause abutment of the greater tuberosity on the acromion or internal impingement on the rim of the glenoid. Positioning the head too far anteriorly or posteriorly can result in abutment of the uncovered humeral neck on the corresponding glenoid rim and excessive tension on the overlying subscapularis or posterior rotator cuff tendons. Most current systems offer humeral heads that are offset by 3 or 4 mm; some allow several discrete positions, and some allow free rotation around the taper.

Most stems can be inserted with a press-fit or cemented technique. In a cadaver study, micromotion was found to be significantly less with proximal cement than with press-fit; no difference was found between proximal cementation and full cementation, and full cementation did not increase rotational stability over proximal cementation. One study found a very low rate of radiolucencies around proximal porous-coated stems and no clinical signs of loosening. Clinically significant loosening of the humeral component in the absence of infection is uncommon regardless of fixation methods. Due to improved design concepts and ingrowth technology, the use of shorter stems and stemless implants to preserve proximal humeral bone also has become more popular.

Cemented all-polyethylene components remain the gold standard for glenoid component fixation, but designs remain in evolution. Both inlay and onlay glenoid components are available, and many systems now employ bone ingrowth technology to reduce reliance on the bone-cement-implant interface. Regardless of these design features, most components now have an increased radius of curvature (i.e., nonconforming glenoid components) compared with the humeral head (2 to 6 mm larger) to allow translation during movement and to decrease edge loading. Several studies have shown that translation accompanies glenohumeral rotation after total shoulder arthroplasty. Such translation in a perfectly congruent or conforming joint may have a potential for localized wear and loosening (rocking-horse effect); however, increased loosening and polyethylene wear have not been reported to occur when the radii of curvature of the glenoid component and the humeral head are matched within 2 mm. In a multicenter study of 319 total shoulder arthroplasties using the same type of prosthesis, Walch et al. noted fewer radiolucencies with mismatches between the glenoid and humeral head diameters of more than 5.5 mm (6 to 10 mm). Current opinion seems to suggest that a nonconforming glenoid with a radius curvature of 2 to 4 mm larger than the humeral head allows normal translation during rotation without rim loading or risk of loosening (Fig. 10.3).

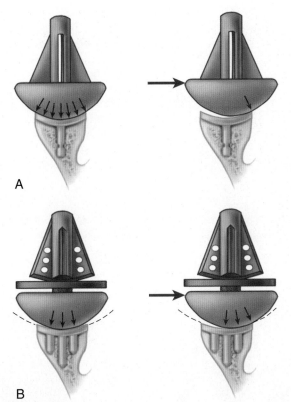

FIGURE 10.3 **A,** When radii of curvature of glenoid component and humeral head conform, translation results in glenoid component rim loading. **B,** Slight increase in diameter of curvature of glenoid component over that of humeral head allows some translation before rim loading occurs.

A larger glenoid component results in an increased risk for volumetric polyethylene wear similar to what is seen in hip and knee arthroplasty, but this risk has not been substantiated clinically. However, larger components have been linked with improved stability. In a biomechanical study, Tammachote et al. demonstrated improved stability with increasing sizes of glenoid components. Specifically, transverse plane stability improved 17% between the small and medium components and then improved 10% between the medium and large components.

All-polyethylene glenoid components generally are cemented into place. A biomechanical study found that cemented all-polyethylene designs had an overall stress pattern closer to that of an intact glenoid than did uncemented metal-backed components. In a report of 408 shoulder arthroplasties using a standard glenoid component and followed for more than 2 years, Neer reported that only three (0.07%) required reoperation because of glenoid loosening. More recently, Hopkins et al. found that bone quality was important in achieving solid glenoid component fixation. They also stressed the importance of proper implant positioning.

Polyethylene glenoid components generally have a central keel or multiple peripheral pegs for fixation into the glenoid vault. The preponderance of biomechanical evidence suggests an advantage to pegged designs, however. Lacroix et al., using a three-dimensional model and finite element analysis, found that bone stresses were not much affected by prosthesis design except at the tip of the central peg or keel. They did conclude, however, that pegged prostheses were

better for normal bone. As understanding of glenoid deformities has improved, augmented glenoid components also have been developed to accommodate commonly seen glenoid wear patterns. Although long-term studies are not yet available, short-term outcomes have been promising.

The biomechanics of reverse total shoulder arthroplasty revolve around recruitment of the deltoid to restore active motion in a rotator cuff-deficient shoulder. All reverse arthroplasty designs medialize the center of rotation to some degree and generally lengthen the deltoid to increase its lever arm to power forward elevation. The original Grammont style reverse total shoulder arthroplasty design medialized the center of rotation at the glenoid face and used a valgus neck-shaft angle of 155 degrees in the humeral component to provide straight line vertical pull of the deltoid. Although this implant improved loosening rates over prior designs and was reliable for the restoration of forward elevation, the return of external rotation was less reliable, and concerns developed over impingement between the polyethylene humeral bearing surface and glenoid neck with resultant scapular notching. Therefore, implant designers turned toward developing "lateralized" (i.e., less-medialized) components in which the center of glenohumeral rotation is placed lateral to the glenoid face. This can be done through the glenosphere or with bone graft (so-called medial humerus-lateral glenoid constructs) or the humeral bearing surface (lateral humerus-medial glenoid constructs). Because most current systems employ modular design concepts that often allow conversion between anatomic total shoulder arthroplasty and reverse total shoulder arthroplasty, constructs that employ a lateral humerus and lateral glenoid design are available, but uncommonly used. Nevertheless, these convertible systems offer an advantage in the revision setting because they often allow preservation of the humeral stem without the need for removal.

The biomechanical data on lateralization in reverse total shoulder arthroplasty suggest an improvement in remaining rotator cuff torque, which may be helpful for restoration of internal and external rotation. In addition, a systematic review concluded that lateralized constructs reduce scapular notching rates as well as improve external rotation. In general, larger glenospheres are thought to improve range of motion and decrease scapular notching as well. Additional investigation has focused on the position of the humeral component in reverse total shoulder arthroplasty. Placing the humeral stem in neutral version demonstrated the least amount of intraarticular and extraarticular impingement, but stems placed in 40 degrees of retroversion allowed the greatest range of motion in a simulator study. To balance these two priorities, most authorities recommend placing the humeral stem in 20 to 30 degrees of retroversion for reverse total shoulder arthroplasty.

CLINICAL PRESENTATION AND RADIOGRAPHIC EVALUATION

The clinical appearance of advanced glenohumeral degeneration was initially described by Neer. Patients typically present with global pain about the shoulder with difficulty performing overhead activities and, often, activities of daily living. On physical examination, diminished active and passive range of motion may be observed, and patients may have previously been diagnosed with adhesive capsulitis. In patients with intact rotator cuff tendons, strength is often preserved but may be diminished secondary to pain. Palpable crepitus often can be elicited with passive internal and external rotation of the glenohumeral joint and/or with strength testing. The acromioclavicular joint and biceps tendon should be carefully evaluated because symptomatic acromioclavicular degeneration and/or biceps tendinitis may also be present.

Standard radiographs include anteroposterior views with a 40-degree posterior oblique view in neutral position and internal and external rotation and an axillary lateral view. Radiographs of the opposite, uninvolved shoulder and humerus are helpful in unusual situations, such as when a custom implant is indicated for large humeral or glenoid deficiencies.

The radiographic appearance varies with the patient's pathologic process. Those with osteoarthritis reliably demonstrate subchondral sclerosis and a large osteophyte on the inferior aspect of the humeral head (Fig. 10.4). This so-called "goat's beard" is pathognomonic of advanced glenohumeral degeneration. These osteophytes can enlarge the humeral head to twice its normal size, resulting in capsular distention (Fig. 10.5). Joint space narrowing, which is so reliably seen in hip and knee osteoarthritis, is not commonly seen in the shoulder until very late in the disease process owing to the non-weight-bearing position of the shoulder under standard radiography. Axillary lateral radiographs typically demonstrate posterior subluxation of the humeral head on the glenoid, and a wear pattern in the posterior glenoid may be present (Fig. 10.6). Patients with capsulorrhaphy arthropathy have a similar radiographic appearance except that loose bodies and osteophytes tend to be more common and numerous (Fig. 10.7) than in standard osteoarthritis.

Malunions of proximal humeral fractures can make shoulder arthroplasty more difficult. A varus malunion between the head and shaft can complicate positioning of components, but osteotomy usually is unnecessary as newer short-stem and stemless designs allow accommodation of these deformities. Patients with inflammatory arthritis often do not have an inferior osteophyte on radiographs and, instead, demonstrate a more symmetrical pattern of joint space narrowing with periarticular osteopenia. The wear pattern is more commonly central in the glenoid, and posterior subluxation of the humeral head is less common. Cystic change is also common. Rotator cuff tears are more common in patients with rheumatoid arthritis than in patients with osteoarthritis: full-thickness rotator cuff tears have been identified in 25% to 50% of patients undergoing shoulder arthroplasty. Most of these tears are in the superior rotator cuff.

MRI can be a useful preoperative planning tool in this population. In patients with strength deficits that could be caused by either arthritic pain or a torn rotator cuff, MRI can help determine the status of the tendons. Whereas rotator cuff tendinopathy is common in this setting, full-thickness tears are uncommon and are seen in only about 10% of patients. MRI also typically demonstrates advanced cartilage degeneration and may show numerous other findings, including thinning of the subscapularis and degenerative changes in the biceps tendon. Increased capsular volume posteriorly and capsular contraction anteriorly are usual changes as well. Finally, in patients with precollapse osteonecrosis, MRI is useful for visualizing the area of dead bone and is often the best tool to make the diagnosis (Fig. 10.8).

CT is also a valuable asset in the evaluation and preoperative planning for patients with advanced glenohumeral degeneration. The scans give an excellent picture of the patient's glenoid bone stock and the pattern of glenoid wear,

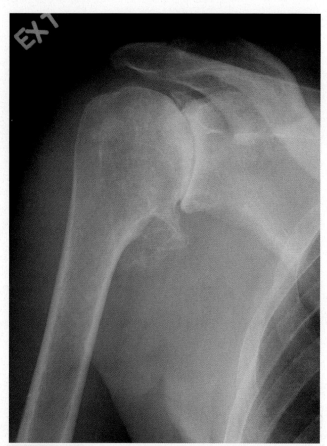

FIGURE 10.4 Subchondral sclerosis and large osteophyte on inferior aspect of humeral head.

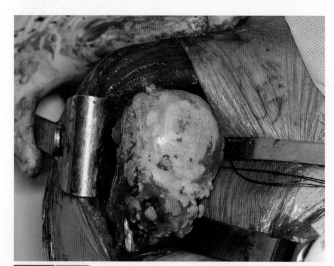

FIGURE 10.5 "Goat's beard" is pathognomonic of advanced glenohumeral degeneration.

which is essential for determining if standard glenoid components can be used or if a bone graft will be needed. Loose bodies may be seen in the axillary or subscapularis recess or attached to the synovium. In the case of malunions or nonunions, three-dimensional reconstruction helps to precisely show the bony deformities and defects before surgery. CT arthrography often is useful to evaluate both the bony architecture of the shoulder and the rotator cuff in patients with contraindications to MRI.

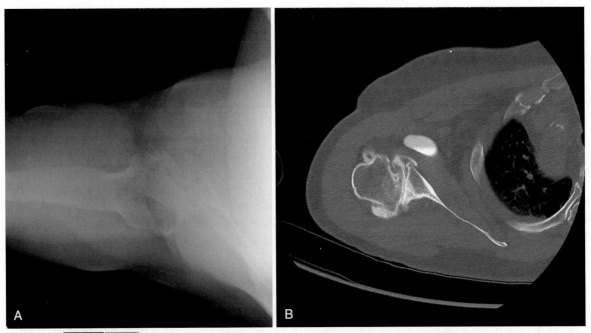

FIGURE 10.6 Axillary radiograph **(A)** and CT scan **(B)** showing severe degenerative arthritis.

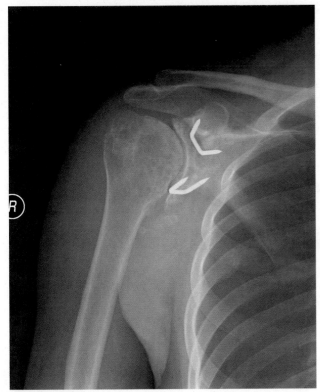

FIGURE 10.7 Radiograph showing capsulorrhaphy arthropathy; note numerous loose bodies and osteophytes.

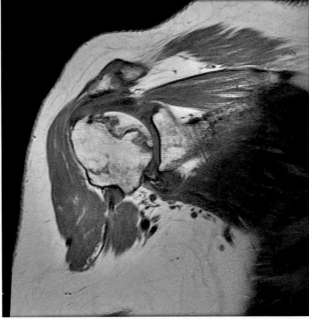

FIGURE 10.8 Magnetic resonance image showing precollapse osteonecrosis.

PREOPERATIVE PLANNING

Once the patient is determined to have advanced glenohumeral degeneration and has consented to a shoulder arthroplasty, preoperative planning includes careful evaluation of the radiographs and the CT scans, if obtained. As noted earlier, CT gives a clear view of the glenoid bone stock and wear pattern. Viewing these changes preoperatively allows the surgeon to prepare for the possibility that glenoid bone grafting, augmented components, or glenoid recontouring procedures may be necessary to correct the deformity. The role of preoperative planning based on three-dimensional CT scans to optimize implant position, size, and range of motion is an evolving area of investigation. Most reports have concluded that preoperative planning software using CT scans results in more accurate glenoid component placement with either conventional or patient-specific implants. In particular, shoulders with significant posterior glenoid erosion tend to benefit from implant reaming and targeting systems.

In patients who have had previous shoulder surgery, infection can be evaluated by laboratory tests including erythrocyte sedimentation rate (ESR), C-reactive protein (CRP), and complete blood cell count. Aspiration and culture of glenohumeral joint fluid, holding the culture for at least 14 days to isolate *Cutibacterium acnes* (formerly *Propionibacterium acnes*), is essential if infection is suspected. Electromyography and nerve conduction studies should be obtained preoperatively in patients with suspected deficits. Finally, preoperative medical clearance often is warranted in this typically elderly population.

HEMIARTHROPLASTY
■ INDICATIONS

The predominant indication for shoulder hemiarthroplasty is end-stage joint degeneration in a patient with a contraindication to glenoid resurfacing. The preponderance of evidence indicates that total shoulder arthroplasty is superior to hemiarthroplasty regarding pain, function, activity level, long-term survival, and revision rate and, therefore, the glenoid should be resurfaced if at all possible in patients with bipolar arthritis. However, young laborers, patients with glenoid bone stock insufficiency, patients with high activity levels, and those with preserved glenoid cartilage may benefit from hemiarthroplasty. Also, rotator cuff tears remain a contraindication to prosthetic glenoid resurfacing. Although excellent pain relief and moderate improvements in function and motion have been reported after total shoulder arthroplasty in patients with irreparable rotator cuff tears, some long-term follow-up studies noted an association between glenoid component loosening and irreparable rotator cuff tears. Eccentric loading of the glenoid caused by superior migration of the humeral component has been cited as a cause of glenoid loosening (the "rocking-horse effect").

Historically, hemiarthroplasty was recommended for patients in whom a massive, long-standing tear of the rotator cuff caused progressive degenerative changes of the glenohumeral joint (cuff tear arthropathy). However, reverse total shoulder arthroplasty has emerged as a more reliable option to reestablish shoulder level function in these patients.

Matsen et al. listed five situations in which hemiarthroplasty should be considered: (1) the humeral joint surface is rough, but the cartilaginous surface of the glenoid is intact, and there is sufficient glenoid arc to stabilize the humeral head; (2) there is insufficient bone to support a glenoid component; (3) there is fixed upward displacement of the humeral head relative to the glenoid (as in cuff tear arthropathy or severe rheumatoid arthritis); (4) there is a history of remote joint infection; and (5) heavy demands would be placed on the joint (anticipated heavy loading from occupation, sport, or lower extremity paresis).

Contraindications to hemiarthroplasty are recent sepsis, a neuropathic joint, a paralytic disorder of the joint, deficiencies in shoulder cuff and deltoid muscle function, and lack of patient cooperation. Remote infection may not be an absolute contraindication, but the operation should be undertaken only after thorough workup to document sterilization of the glenohumeral joint and careful consideration by the surgeon and the patient of all the potential hazards involved.

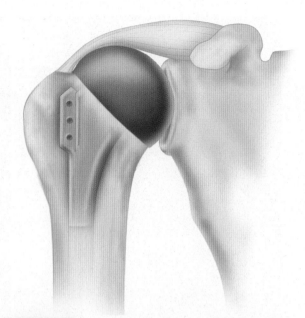

FIGURE 10.9 Use of humeral head component that is too large results in overstuffing of joint, which can limit range of motion and lead to rotator cuff failure.

■ SURGICAL TECHNIQUE

The goal of hemiarthroplasty is restoration of the humeral articular surface to its normal location and configuration. Because the glenoid is not replaced, the size, radius, and orientation of the prosthetic joint surface must duplicate that of the original biologic humeral head. Radiographs of the contralateral shoulder can provide information about a patient's normal humeral head anatomy. Care should be taken to avoid a "big head" humeral prosthesis that can "overstuff" the joint (Fig. 10.9).

HEMIARTHROPLASTY

TECHNIQUE 10.1

- Place the patient in the beach chair position to allow positioning of the patient at the top and edge of the table (Fig. 10.10A). Pad all bony prominences. The medial border of the scapula should be free and off the table, allowing full adduction to gain access to the intramedullary canal.
- Secure the patient's head to the headrest, holding the head in a position that avoids hyperextension or tilting of the neck, which can cause compression of the cervical roots.
- Prepare the arm and drape it widely. We recommend using occlusive dressings to cover the entire surgical field.
- Make an incision anteriorly, approximately one third to halfway between the coracoid and the lateral aspect of the acromion (Fig. 10.10B). Carry dissection down to the deltoid and raise medial and lateral flaps to mobilize the deltoid.
- Open the deltopectoral interval and allow the cephalic vein to fall medially.

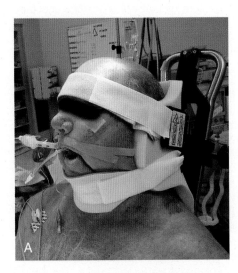
A

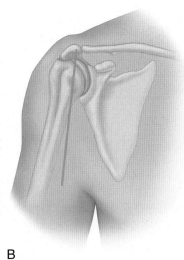
B

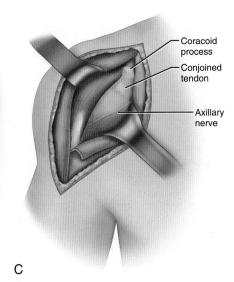
C

Coracoid process

Conjoined tendon

Axillary nerve

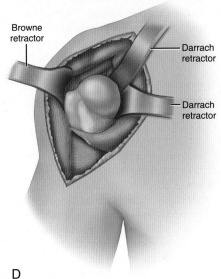
D

Browne retractor

Darrach retractor

Darrach retractor

FIGURE 10.10 Hemiarthroplasty technique (see text). **A,** Beach-chair position with arm extended off table. **B,** Incision. **C,** Axillary nerve is identified. **D,** Darrach retractor is used to lift head of humerus out of glenoid fossa. **SEE TECHNIQUE 10.1.**

- Perform subdeltoid, subcoracoid, and subacromial releases to release the proximal humerus. In the subcoracoid space, locate the axillary nerve by passing the volar surface of the index finger down along the anterior surface of the subscapularis muscle (Fig. 10.10C). If scarring and adhesions make identification of the nerve difficult, pass an elevator along the anterior surface of the subscapular muscle to create an interval between the muscle and the nerve. Great care must be taken in this step to avoid plunging into the brachial plexus. After the axillary nerve is identified, carefully retract and hold it out of the way, especially during the crucial steps of releasing the anteroinferior capsule.
- We prefer to perform a biceps tenodesis before incising the subscapularis. A figure-of-eight stitch is placed between the biceps and pectoralis major tendons. The

biceps is then divided, and the proximal portion is later resected before making the humeral head osteotomy.
- Incise the subscapularis 1 cm medial to the lesser tuberosity. Place two retention sutures in the subscapularis to be used as traction sutures when freeing the rest of the tendon from the underlying capsule and scar tissue. Some authors prefer either a lesser tuberosity osteotomy or a release of the subscapularis directly off of bone. If external rotation is markedly limited, the subscapularis also can be reattached to the proximal humerus more medially to allow increased external rotation. Alternatively, the tendon can be lengthened with a coronal Z-plasty technique.
- Incise the rotator interval, directing the cut medially toward the glenoid. Typically, a large amount of synovial fluid escapes as the joint is entered.

- Release the anteroinferior capsule from the humerus and externally rotate the arm to bring the inferior aspect of the shoulder capsule into view. Take care to stay directly on bone so as not to injure the axillary nerve during the capsular release. The importance of the inferior capsule release cannot be overstated and must be thoroughly carried out to at least the 7 o'clock position to dislocate the humeral head and gain access to the glenoid.
- Once the capsule is adequately released, place a large Darrach retractor in the joint and gently externally rotate, adduct, and extend the arm to deliver the humeral head up and out of the glenoid fossa (Fig. 10.10D). If the humeral head cannot be delivered in this fashion, the inferior capsule must be released further.
- Prepare the humeral canal, using the humeral axis to reference the osteotomy. Initially, open the canal with a high-speed burr at the base of the rotator cuff footprint and ream it to a size where appropriate fit is felt. Do not use motorized equipment for reaming, and be careful not to overream the canal, which could create a stress riser or cause a fracture.
- We prefer to use a cutting guide that employs extramedullary referencing, using the axis of the forearm as the reference point, with the cutting guide pinned into position at 30 degrees of retroversion. Other surgeons may prefer a free-hand, anatomic neck-cutting technique. Regardless of the cutting technique, care must be taken to avoid violating the rotator cuff.
- Complete the osteotomy with an oscillating saw. If any inferior humeral head osteophyte remains, remove it with a rongeur.
- After the head cut, broach the humeral canal to the same size as the reamed canal. It is imperative to confirm proper position of the broaches in 30 degrees of retroversion during this step to prevent component malposition.
- Inspect the glenoid to confirm there is enough glenoid cartilage to provide an adequate bearing surface for the metal humeral head. After this inspection, check the humeral trial stem to ensure it is seated securely within the humeral canal. If so, tap the component stem into position, taking care to keep the stem in 30 degrees of retroversion.
- If cementing is deemed necessary because of a previous surgical procedure, fracture, osteoporosis, rheumatoid arthritis, or degenerative cysts, place a cement restrictor or a cortical bone plug from the resected humeral head 2 cm inferior to the tip of the prosthesis.
- Place a trial humeral head and reduce the glenohumeral joint using internal rotation and gentle traction. With the arm in neutral rotation, check the height of the humeral head to confirm anatomic reconstruction. As a rule of thumb, the most superior aspect of the humeral head should be 1 cm superior to the greater tuberosity.
- Also check the version to confirm that the humeral head rests directly across from the glenoid. With a thumb on the lesser tuberosity, push the humeral head posteriorly and then release it: 50% posterior excursion with immediate "bounce back" of the humeral head is optimal. Evaluate forward elevation and internal rotation.
- Once the checks have been performed, thoroughly clean the Morse taper, impact the humeral head into position, and reduce the joint for the final time.

- Perform a tight closure of the rotator interval and the subscapularis with heavy nonabsorbable suture. Both transosseous and tendon-to-tendon repair techniques are reasonable. If the tendon was divided or lengthened, repair and secure it with heavy nonabsorbable sutures to allow immediate passive movement beginning the day after surgery. If a lesser tuberosity osteotomy is preferred, robust fixation of the bone back to the humeral shaft is critical. Place a drain in the deltopectoral interval and close it with No. 0 sutures. Close the skin in standard fashion and place the arm in a soft sterile dressing and a sling while the patient is still upright and before being aroused from anesthesia.

POSTOPERATIVE CARE Patients are instructed in a gentle home exercise program with passive forward elevation to 90 degrees and passive external rotation to neutral. Patients typically are discharged from the hospital on the morning after surgery and are encouraged to use a pillow behind the elbow while recumbent in the sling to support the extremity. Full-time sling immobilization continues for 6 weeks, followed by 6 weeks of sling use only in unprotected environments. Therapy progresses to full passive range of motion by 6 to 12 weeks and to isometric strengthening at 10 weeks.

OUTCOMES

Hemiarthroplasty has been reported to initially relieve pain in 75% to 95% of patients with glenohumeral arthritis and severe rotator cuff deficiency, with more modest improvements in range of motion and strength. However, long-term results have been compromised by persistent pain from glenoid arthrosis, anterosuperior instability, and progressive bone loss.

The best results of shoulder hemiarthroplasty are in patients with osteonecrosis, in whom hemiarthroplasty has been reported to provide consistently good pain relief in 90%, with an almost normal preoperative range of motion (Table 10.2). Results are not quite as good in patients with rheumatoid arthritis, osteoarthritis, glenoid dysplasia, or posttraumatic glenohumeral arthrosis but are satisfactory in most patients, although range of motion is decreased. In particular, one long-term report found that only 25% of patients were satisfied with stemmed hemiarthroplasty for shoulder osteoarthritis at an average of 17 years follow-up.

MODIFIED HEMIARTHROPLASTY: INTERPOSITION ARTHROPLASTY AND GLENOIDPLASTY (REAM AND RUN)

As it has become clear that glenoid arthritis continues to be a long-term concern for patients undergoing isolated shoulder hemiarthroplasty, some authors have explored various types of glenoid resurfacing procedures, particularly for younger, higher-demand patients. These interposition techniques aim to allow the metal humeral head to articulate with a cushioning surface rather than with the native glenoid in an effort to minimize arthritic progression and subsequent pain. Although most interposition procedures have demonstrated early success, intermediate-term outcome studies have been disappointing.

Fascial interposition hemiarthroplasty (biologic resurfacing) has been recommended for use in young, active

TABLE 10.2

Reported Results of Shoulder Hemiarthroplasty for Rotator Cuff Tear Arthropathy

STUDY	NO	MEAN AGE (RANGE)	MEAN FOLLOW-UP, YEARS (RANGE)	NO PAIN OR MILD POSTOPERATIVE PAIN	ACTIVE ELEVATION PREOPERATIVE/ POSTOPERATIVE MEAN, DEGREES (RANGE)	SUCCESSFUL RESULTS	COMMENTS
Arntz et al. (1993)	18	71 (54-84)	2 (2-10)	11 (61%)	66 (44-90)/112 (70-160)	NR	Two reoperations for symptomatic glenoid erosion, one for symptomatic instability, one for postoperative traumatic fracture of the acromion
Williams and Rockwood (1996)	21	72 (59-80)	4 (2-7)	18 (86%)	70 (0-155)/120 (15-160)	18 (86%)	No instability or reoperation reported
Field et al. (1997)	16	74 (62-83)	3 (2-5)	13 (81%)	60 (40-80)/100 (80-130)	10 (62%)	One intraoperative humeral shaft fracture; 4 patients with instability, 2 of whom required reoperation for subscapularis advancement (1) and resection arthroplasty (1)
Zuckerman et al. (2000)	15	73 (65-81)	2 (1-5)	7 (47%)	69 (20-140)/86 (45-140)	NR	Eleven of 15 patients satisfied with operation; 1 had anterior instability
Sanchez-Sotelo: Mayo Clinic series (2003)	33	69 (50-87)	5 (2-11)	24 (73%)	72 (30-150)/91 (40-165)	22 (67%)	One intraoperative humeral shaft fracture; 7 patients with anterosuperior instability
Goldberg et al. (2008)	34	72 (48-90)	4 (2-12)	26 (76%)	78 (20-165)/111 (40-180)	26 (76%)	One patient required reoperation for osteophyte removal; no problems related to implant failure, loosening, infection, or fracture

Modified from Sanchez-Sotelo J: Shoulder arthroplasty for cuff-tear arthropathy. In Morrey BF, editor: *Joint replacement arthroplasty*, ed 3, Philadelphia, 2003, Churchill Livingstone. *NR*, Not reported.
Copyright of Mayo Foundation.

patients with osteoarthritis. The glenoid is resurfaced using the anterior capsule sewn over the glenoid face, a free fascia lata graft, or commercially available patch devices. Good long-term outcomes have been reported with this biologic glenoid resurfacing technique. Other studies, however, have noted a high number of failures and poor outcomes using Achilles tendon allograft as a resurfacing material with hemiarthroplasty.

Lateral meniscal allografts also have been used as an interposition material. In this procedure, the anterior and posterior horns of the allograft are sewn to each other to form a circular surface for articulation with the humeral head. The allograft is laid onto the glenoid and secured, typically with suture anchors. Despite initially positive results, intermediate-term outcomes have been inferior to standard hemiarthroplasty.

A third technique that has been advanced involves concentric reaming of the glenoid combined with shoulder hemiarthroplasty, the "ream and run" procedure. Intermediate-term outcomes have demonstrated range-of-motion and Simple Shoulder Test scores to be significantly improved after this procedure, with a revision rate of 16%. However, it should be noted that strict patient selection criteria should be used and that an intensive and extended rehabilitation program is associated with this procedure.

■ RESURFACING HEMIARTHROPLASTY

In an attempt to preserve proximal humeral bone stock, shoulder resurfacing procedures have been developed. Resurfacing implants do not use a stem for intramedullary fixation but instead form a cap over the humeral articular surface and are typically stabilized with a smaller post in the metaphysis. This implant design has been reported to more closely replicate humeral head geometry and reduce eccentric glenoid loading compared with stemmed hemiarthroplasty (Fig. 10.11). Outcomes of humeral resurfacing have generally been successful, with patient satisfaction rates as high as 93% and overall results similar to that of stemmed prostheses. Several series have reported similar success in specific patient cohorts with rheumatoid arthritis, osteoarthritis, and cuff tear arthropathy; however, the reported revision rate of humeral head resurfacing is higher than that of stemmed hemiarthroplasty.

TOTAL SHOULDER ARTHROPLASTY

Total shoulder arthroplasty is a well-established procedure with an excellent long-term track record of pain relief and functional improvements. Long-term results have been reported that are equivalent to those after replacement of the knee and hip. In a meta-analysis of series that included 646 shoulder arthroplasties done for osteoarthritis, Wilde found that 89% had complete or nearly complete relief of pain; 91% of patients with rheumatoid arthritis reported satisfactory relief.

■ INDICATIONS

The primary indication for total shoulder arthroplasty is end-stage glenohumeral joint degeneration with an intact rotator cuff. This encompasses a number of conditions, including osteoarthritis, rheumatoid arthritis, osteonecrosis, posttraumatic arthritis, and capsulorrhaphy arthropathy. Contraindications to shoulder arthroplasty include active or recent infection and irreparable rotator cuff tears. Paralysis with complete loss of function of the deltoid is also a contraindication. Debilitating medical status and uncorrectable glenohumeral instability are additional contraindications to shoulder arthroplasty.

Other patient-specific factors should be considered before total shoulder arthroplasty: morbidly obese patients are known to have a higher rate of medical complications and to incur higher costs; diabetes is reported to correlate with a higher rate of perioperative medical complications; and hepatitis C also has been established as an independent factor correlating with increased complications, including infection and need for revision. Therefore, although perioperative mortality is only approximately 1%, careful medical optimization and patient selection are recommended before shoulder arthroplasty.

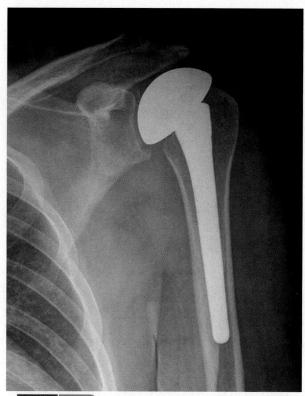

FIGURE 10.11 Stemmed shoulder hemiarthroplasty.

■ SURGICAL TECHNIQUE

TOTAL SHOULDER ARTHROPLASTY

TECHNIQUE 10.2

- Approach the glenohumeral joint as described in Technique 10.1. Once the trial broach is tapped into position, remove the retractors from about the humerus. Of note, stemless humeral components for total shoulder arthroplasty have been investigated and approved by the United States Food and Drug Administration (FDA).
- Expose the glenoid by placing a retractor on the posterior aspect of the glenoid to sublux the humerus posteriorly.
- Debride the glenoid vault of all remaining labral tissue and articular cartilage.
- Release the anterior capsule and place a flat Darrach retractor on the anterior glenoid neck to aid exposure.
- The glenoid is not adequately exposed until the anterior, posterior, superior, and inferior aspects of the glenoid can be seen. Once this is accomplished, inspect the glenoid for wear and bone defects. Typically, there is posterior erosion of the glenoid, and the anterior rim of the glenoid needs to be lowered to reestablish correct version (Fig. 10.12). This can be done by eccentric reaming. Alternatively, glenoid bone grafting or augmented glenoid components can elevate the posterior glenoid to re-establish version. A preoperative CT scan with or without planning software can aid in understanding glenoid orientation and morphology.
- Once the glenoid vault is debrided, make a centering hole, typically with a guide. It often is helpful to confirm adequate depth and position of the starting hole with a small curet. After the starting hole is made, proceed with glenoid reaming until the sclerotic bone of the arthritic glenoid is removed and the subchondral plate is seen. With the common posterior wear pattern of osteoarthritis, reaming typically is done in an eccentric fashion so that the anterior lip of the glenoid is planed down. If posterior rim wear is significant and the anterior rim has not been lowered, the component sits excessively retroverted, and anterior glenoid neck perforation is likely. Take care also not to ream too aggressively medially and thereby compromise the glenoid bone stock, as this may result in component subsidence.
- When reaming is complete, prepare the glenoid for the implant. Systems vary in their instrumentation but involve precise placement of the anchoring pegs or keel. To provide secure fixation and reduce the risk of loosening, the glenoid trial must sit securely against the subchondral bone of the glenoid without any rocking after the glenoid is prepared. Cement cannot be used to adjust for poor seating of the glenoid component.

- Prepare the glenoid vault for cementing with pulsed lavage to remove debris and blood. Thoroughly dry the peg holes or keel before cementation.
- Tuberculin syringes are helpful to pressurize the cement. Pack cement into the syringe and then inject it into the peg holes or into the keel.
- Next, insert the glenoid component and maintain thumb pressure until the cement has hardened. Most shoulder systems also come with an instrument to hold the glenoid component in place while the cement hardens. This method allows excellent pressurization and interdigitation of the cement into the cancellous bone of the glenoid vault, and postoperative radiolucent lines seen with other cementing techniques are minimized. Some systems use a polyethylene or metal ingrowth post to provide a press-fit of the glenoid component, which provides immediate stability so that the component does not rely solely on digital pressure while the cement is curing (Fig. 10.13). Although totally uncemented, metal-backed glenoid components exist, they are associated with higher revision and failure rates.
- After the cement has hardened, check the broach to ensure that it is still secure within the humeral canal. If so, insert the humeral prosthesis as described in Technique 10.1. Head height, range of motion, and soft-tissue balancing are critical to providing an optimal outcome. With posterior pressure on the lesser tuberosity, the ideal cuff tension allows the humeral head to translate approximately 50% of the glenoid component width and then recenter it when pressure is removed. If the humeral head dislocates posteriorly with this maneuver, it must be corrected with a larger and/or thicker head. Most current systems use modular heads with a variety of diameters and thicknesses to accomplish this goal.
- Once the appropriate head is selected, dry the Morse taper and tap the head into position. Reduce the glenohumeral joint and close the wound as described in Technique 10.1.

POSTOPERATIVE CARE Postoperative care and rehabilitation are essentially the same as after shoulder hemiarthroplasty (see Technique 10.1) and are governed by protection of the subscapularis repair.

■ OUTCOMES

The preponderance of evidence in randomized and nonrandomized studies suggests that, although hemiarthroplasty can provide pain relief and increased range of motion in patients with osteoarthritis and a concentric glenoid, total shoulder arthroplasty generally provides superior results in terms of patient satisfaction, function, and strength, especially at longer-term follow-up. A Cochrane Database systemic review of seven studies found that total shoulder arthroplasty is associated with better shoulder function than

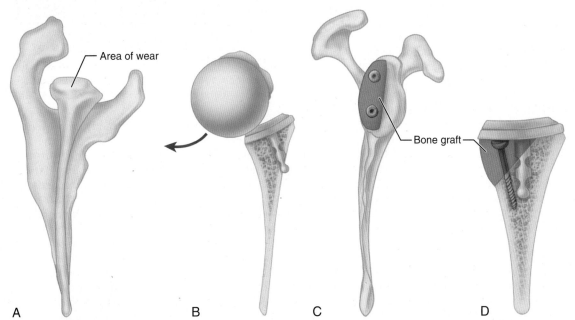

FIGURE 10.12 Problem of and solution for uneven wear and erosion of glenoid. **A,** Area of wear. **B,** If glenoid component is inserted without correction of slope, anchoring device passes out of medullary canal; tilt and loss of height also make implant unstable. **C** and **D,** Severe erosion is corrected by bone grafting. Piece of humeral head is secured to scapula with 4-mm AO navicular screw. Lesser erosion can be offset by building up low side with acrylic cement or lowering high side. Building up with cement is not recommended because of feared cement loosening. Lowering high side often requires shortening holding device of glenoid component and creates laxity between components, which can make implant temporarily unstable and requires special postoperative care. Alternatively, an augmented glenoid component can be used to correct glenoid version. **SEE TECHNIQUE 10.2.**

hemiarthroplasty but does not provide any other significant clinical benefits. Mather et al. found that in elderly patients (≥64 years) with osteoarthritis, total shoulder arthroplasty with a cemented glenoid component was more cost effective than hemiarthroplasty in improving quality of life. In addition, an economic decision model concluded that total shoulder arthroplasty was a more cost-effective intervention compared to hemiarthroplasty in young patients with shoulder arthritis.

Results after total shoulder arthroplasty have been predictable in producing pain relief and functional improvements for patients with a variety of degenerative glenohumeral conditions, with good results reported in 65% to 95% of patients. Loosening of the glenoid component, however, has been reported in almost half of shoulders at more than 10-year follow-up and is often associated with pain. The best functional results are obtained in patients with osteoarthritis because the rotator cuff usually is intact and of good quality and the bone stock is typically adequate. In patients with rheumatoid arthritis, the quality of the rotator cuff directly influences the functional result.

The durability of total shoulder replacement is similar to that of hip and knee replacements. Results at long-term follow-up in several series have reported 85% component retention at 20 years of follow-up and revision rates for all causes averaging less than 10%. Loosening of the glenoid component has been reported in almost half of shoulders at more than 10-year follow-up and often is associated with pain; however, glenoid component loosening has averaged 4.3% over multiple studies.

OSTEOARTHRITIS

Most total shoulder arthroplasties are done in patients with osteoarthritis or rheumatoid arthritis. Few (<10%) patients with osteoarthritis have complete rotator cuff tears, but contracture of the subscapularis tendon is common. A large multicenter study reported significant improvements in Constant scores and range of motion at 10-year follow-up. Glenoid component survivorship with revision as the end point was 94.5%. In patients older than 80 years, total shoulder arthroplasty remains a reliable option, with 80% attaining an excellent or satisfactory result at an average of 5.5 years, even though there is an increased risk for perioperative medical complications. In patients younger than 50 years, one report with a 20-year minimum follow-up found over 75% component retention, but clinical outcomes tended to decline, ultimately with a large number of unsatisfactory results. This and other similar studies, including a systematic review, suggest caution in performing total shoulder arthroplasty in younger patients.

INFLAMMATORY ARTHRITIS

Total shoulder replacement also is effective in patients with inflammatory arthritis, resulting in significant improvements in pain, range of motion, function, and quality of life. The frequency of perioperative complications in patients with rheumatoid arthritis is similar to that in patients who have total shoulder arthroplasty for other indications; in fact, patients with rheumatoid arthritis have been reported to have shorter average hospital stays and a higher likelihood of routine discharge. Satisfactory pain relief also was reported in 11 shoulders severely affected by juvenile rheumatoid arthritis, although improvements in range of motion were minor.

If shoulder and ipsilateral elbow replacements are necessary, the most painful joint should be replaced first.

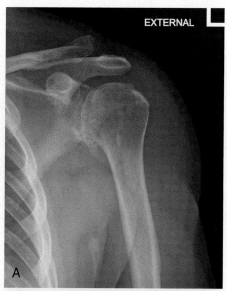
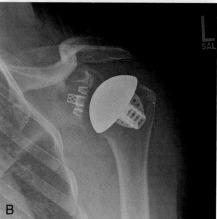

FIGURE 10.13 **A,** Degenerative joint disease of left shoulder. **B,** Anatomic total shoulder arthroplasty with a stemless humeral component and ingrowth glenoid implant. **SEE TECHNIQUE 10.2.**

Function may not be significantly improved in patients with severe rheumatoid arthritis until the second joint is replaced. If the shoulder is operated on first, and if a cemented prosthesis is chosen, a cement restrictor or canal plug must be used to prevent cement from entering the distal medullary canal. A stress riser can occur in the humeral diaphysis between the tips of the two humeral components. If shoulder arthroplasty is done first, a short-stem prosthesis should be used; if a long-stem component is in place at either joint, the cement column for the second arthroplasty should extend to and include the cement column of the first arthroplasty. If shorter components are used, a long length (~360 mm) of unfilled humerus should be left between the cement columns.

POSTTRAUMATIC ARTHRITIS AND POSTTRAUMATIC SEQUELAE

Shoulder arthroplasty for arthritis secondary to chronic displaced fractures and fracture-dislocations of the glenohumeral joint is particularly difficult because of contractures and scarring of the soft tissues, malunion or nonunion of the tuberosities, and possible nerve injuries. Axillary nerve injuries can significantly impair motion and strength due to loss of deltoid function.

Anatomic shoulder arthroplasty also has been described for proximal humeral malunions. In a mixed cohort of hemiarthroplasty and total shoulder arthroplasty, an average forward elevation of 109 degrees and improvements in pain were reported. However, postoperative instability because of rotator cuff dysfunction or capsular injury was a common complication.

OSTEONECROSIS

The most common causes of osteonecrosis of the humeral head are heavy corticosteroid use, sickle cell disease, and alcoholism; less common causes include dysbarism, Gaucher disease, and systemic lupus erythematosus. Idiopathic osteonecrosis also is fairly common. Cruess classified osteonecrosis of the humeral head into five stages of increasing severity (Fig. 10.14). Symptomatic progression of the osteonecrosis is almost certain in those with stage IV or stage V. Both total shoulder arthroplasty and hemiarthroplasty have been successful in obtaining subjective improvement in most patients with humeral head osteonecrosis.

Most patients with osteonecrosis are relatively young, with good bone quality, and secure press-fit fixation of the humeral component can be obtained. The need for a glenoid component (see section on hemiarthroplasty) is based on the condition of the glenoid fossa, the amount of deformity present, and the degree of articular cartilage loss. In many patients with intact glenoid cartilage, humeral head replacement alone is satisfactory, whereas most patients with stage V disease require a glenoid component because of extensive articular cartilage loss.

CAPSULORRHAPHY ARTHROPATHY AND ARTHROPATHY OF RECURRENT INSTABILITY

Advanced glenohumeral arthritis can be a late sequela of anterior instability surgery. It is more common after nonanatomic repairs and in younger patients than typical glenohumeral arthritis and is characterized by severe internal rotation contracture and a severely osteophytic arthritis. Excessive soft-tissue tension on the side of the dislocation may produce a fixed subluxation of the humeral head in the posterior direction, requiring release of the iatrogenic soft-tissue contracture to restore joint balance and mobility. Subscapularis lengthening, anterior capsular release, or posterior capsular plication may be required to correct soft-tissue contractures. Although total shoulder arthroplasty can improve function in patients with glenohumeral degeneration associated with shoulder instability or instability surgery, a complication rate of 40% has been reported, particularly subscapularis insufficiency, with 20% of patients requiring additional surgery.

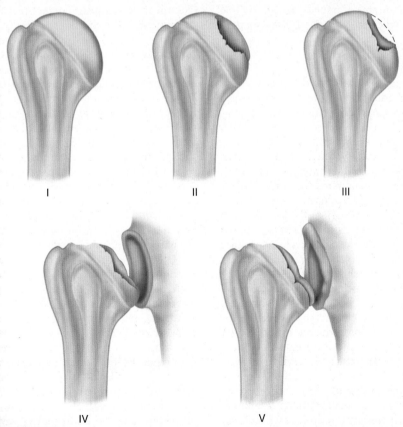

I

II

III

IV

V

FIGURE 10.14 Stages of osteonecrosis of humeral head. Stage I changes are invisible on plain radiographs, and they are not discernible on gross examination. Stage II is marked by sclerotic changes and evidence of bone remodeling, but shape and sphericity of humeral head are maintained. Stage III is differentiated from stage II by presence of subchondral bone collapse or fracture, resulting in loss of humeral head sphericity. In stage IV, humeral head has area of collapsed articular surface; fragment may become displaced intraarticularly. In stage V, there are osteoarthritic changes in the glenoid fossa.

Comparative studies have demonstrated equivalent functional outcomes but lower complication rates when reverse total shoulder arthroplasty is employed for this disorder.

REVERSE TOTAL SHOULDER ARTHROPLASTY

In 1983, Neer, Craig, and Fukuda described "cuff-tear arthropathy" as a distinct form of osteoarthritis associated with a massive chronic tear of the rotator cuff. Clinically, rotator cuff arthropathy is characterized by pain, poor active motion, near-normal passive motion, crepitus, weakness, and occasionally significant fluid buildup under the deltoid. Radiographic changes include elevation of the humeral head, formation of an acromiohumeral pseudoarticulation, and loss of joint space at the glenohumeral joint. The radiographic pattern of degenerative changes can vary, and not all patients with rotator cuff arthropathy have pain or limited motion.

The glenohumeral instability resulting from this condition is manifested as proximal migration of the humerus relative to the glenoid, resulting in erosion of the superior glenoid and the caudal surface of the acromion. Rotator cuff tears have been implicated in early glenoid component loosening in total shoulder replacements, and irreparable tears are a contraindication to traditional glenoid resurfacing. Until the introduction of reverse total shoulder arthroplasty, patients with cuff tear arthropathy were generally treated with hemiarthroplasty, which was a durable, if imperfect, solution that provided adequate pain relief but did not restore forward elevation.

■ INDICATIONS

The primary indication for reverse total shoulder arthroplasty is a nonfunctional rotator cuff. This encompasses a number of disease processes, including cuff tear arthropathy, pseudoparalysis caused by massive rotator cuff tear without arthritis, multiple failed rotator cuff repairs with poor function and anterosuperior instability, three- and four-part proximal humeral fractures in the elderly, proximal humeral nonunions, greater tuberosity malunions, and failed shoulder arthroplasty with rotator cuff insufficiency. Reverse total shoulder arthroplasty is most appropriate for patients with an intact deltoid, adequate bone stock to support the glenoid component, no evidence of infection, no severe neurologic deficiency (Parkinson disease, Charcot joints, syringomyelia), and no excessive demands on the shoulder joint (Box 10.1).

Contraindications generally include loss or inactivity of the deltoid and excessive glenoid bone loss that would not allow secure implantation of the glenoid component. Some authors have suggested that the procedure is unsuitable for patients younger than 70 years old; however, current opinion has moved more toward accepting use of the reverse prosthesis in younger patients for some end-stage disorders. Surgeon inexperience also is a relative contraindication to reverse total shoulder arthroplasty. One study demonstrated a volume-value relationship in which costs and hospital length of stay were minimized in specialized, high-volume shoulder arthroplasty centers.

■ SURGICAL TECHNIQUE

Biomechanically, the reverse prosthesis works by reestablishing a fulcrum around which the deltoid muscle

---

BOX 10.1

Indications for Reverse Total Shoulder Arthroplasty

- Cuff-tear arthropathy
- Massive rotator cuff tear with pseudoparalysis
- Severe inflammatory arthritis with a massive cuff tear
- Failed shoulder arthroplasty
  - Absence of tuberosities (failed hemiarthroplasty for fracture/nonunion)
  - Absence of cuff (failed hemiarthroplasty for cuff-tear arthropathy)
  - Instability
- Proximal humeral fracture
- Proximal humeral nonunion
- Reimplantation for deep periprosthetic infection
- Reconstruction after tumor removal

From Sanchez-Sotelo J: Reverse total shoulder arthroplasty. In Morrey BF, ed: *Joint replacement arthroplasty: basic science, elbow and shoulder*, Philadelphia, 2011, Wolters Kluwer, p 277.

---

can power shoulder motion. With standard prostheses, absence of the rotator cuff allows the humeral head to subluxate superiorly during deltoid muscle contraction. The reverse prosthesis corrects this by moving the center of rotation of the shoulder medially and distally and reestablishing a semiconstrained fulcrum around that fixed point (Fig. 10.15).

Because the reverse prosthesis places high shear stresses across the glenoid, several investigators have sought to define the factors most important in maximizing glenoid fixation. Parsons et al. stressed that proper orientation of the baseplate and placement of the screws in optimal position were important for fixation. Others have found that the inferior screw faces the highest shear stress and is key to prevent loosening, whereas others have recommended screw placement in areas with the highest quality bone: the coracoid base, the scapular spine, or the inferior pillar. A device with a lateralized center of rotation was shown to obtain adequate fixation despite a 69% greater moment at the baseplate-glenoid interface.

Glenoid wear is common in rotator cuff-deficient conditions. Frankle et al. (2009) studied 216 glenoids with plain radiographs and CT scans before operative intervention and found that 37.5% of the glenoids had abnormal morphology. They classified the wear patterns as posterior (17.6%), superior (9.3%), global (6.5%), and anterior (4.2%). These wear patterns were found to affect surgical technique, often requiring placement of the center screw along an alternate center line along the scapular spine. In a later follow-up study of 143 of these patients, all 56 shoulders with abnormal glenoids had center screw placement along the alternative center line, and 22 had bone grafting procedures; larger glenospheres also were used more often than in shoulders with normal glenoids. Outcomes were not significantly different between the two groups. Augmented glenoid components and bone grafting procedures also are available to treat glenoid deficiency.

REVERSE TOTAL SHOULDER ARTHROPLASTY

TECHNIQUE 10.3

- Approach the proximal humerus and prepare it for stem implantation as described in Technique 10.1. Some authors recommend a superior approach, but we prefer the deltopectoral approach because of its versatility and easily extensive nature. However, there are some important differences in humeral preparation from a total shoulder arthroplasty or hemiarthroplasty. First, because of the common superior subluxation deformity of rotator cuff-deficient shoulders, a larger humeral head cut is often required. Second, some authors advocate placing the stem in less retroversion (~20 degrees) to prevent impingement and maximize rotation; however, we believe that stem placement in 30 degrees of retroversion is not only acceptable but also preferable to prevent the more common instability in adduction and extension seen with the reverse prosthesis. Although stems were initially cemented in reverse total shoulder arthroplasty, the use of uncemented and shorter stems has been reported with clinical success. Once the glenoid vault is adequately debrided and all four borders are visible, identify the centering point. Move the starting point inferiorly 1 to 2 mm to allow inferior placement of the baseplate to prevent scapular notching. Most authors recommend placing the baseplate with the inferior aspect flush with the inferior surface of the bony glenoid.
- Place a guide pin through this centering hole using a guide. Take care to place the guide pin in 10 to 15 degrees of inferior tilt, again to prevent scapular notching.
- Ream the glenoid until the "smiley face" is achieved, with bleeding cancellous bone inferiorly and hard sclerotic bone superiorly (Fig. 10.16). This confirms adequate inferior tilt of the baseplate.
- Impact the baseplate and secure it with screws. The peripheral screws are ideally placed in the "pillars" of densest cortical bone—the coracoid base, inferior pillar, and scapular spine. We have found screw placement to be inconsistent in the scapular spine; however, fixed-angle locking screws can be reliably positioned in the coracoid base and inferior pillar by internally rotating a circular baseplate approximately 10 degrees.
- Dry the Morse taper and impact the glenosphere into position.
- Place the humeral stem as described in Technique 10.1, using trial components to test for stability and motion. Reduction and dislocation of the glenohumeral joint typically are more difficult than with standard shoulder arthroplasty. Reduction involves a combination of longitudinal traction and forward elevation on the arm. The deltoid tension should be slightly greater than before joint relocation, but take care not to overlengthen the deltoid, which can result in dehiscence and/or acromial fracture. There can be 2 to 3 mm of gapping in the glenohumeral articulation once the joint is reduced without loss of stability.
- To dislocate the glenohumeral joint, place the dislocation instrument between the bearing surface and glenosphere to disrupt the articulation. Then pull the humerus anteriorly (shoulder extension) to deliver the bearing surface.
- Once the proper bearing surface is chosen, dry the Morse taper and impact it into position. Reduce the glenohumeral joint for a final time. Close the wound as described in Technique 10.1. The importance of subscapularis repair after reverse total shoulder arthroplasty remains controversial. One study found no correlation between subscapularis integrity and outcome. Another large study found that outcomes were not inferior when the subscapularis was left free compared to when it was repaired. However, closure of the subscapularis has been found to correlate with improved stability in traditional Grammont style prostheses but is likely less important for lateralized designs.

POSTOPERATIVE CARE Postoperative care is as described for Technique 10.1.

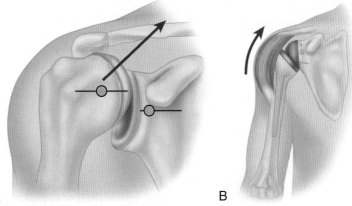

A, In a shoulder with no rotator cuff tendons there are few restraints to antero-superior subluxation of the humeral head when patient attempts to raise the arm. Pull of the deltoid muscle worsens this by pulling superiorly and medially *(arrow)*. **B,** With reverse arthroplasty, deltoid muscle lever arm is restored, providing a fulcrum around which the deltoid can pull to restore forward elevation *(arrow)*.

FIGURE 10.15

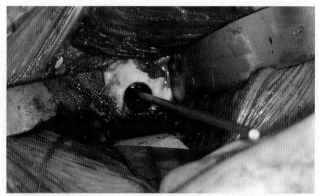

FIGURE 10.16 Some authorities prefer reaming the glenoid to create an "inferior smile," with bleeding cancellous bone at the bottom of glenoid to provide inferior tilt of baseplate. **SEE TECHNIQUE 10.3.**

OUTCOMES

In the past decade, multiple authors have reported the outcomes of reverse total shoulder arthroplasty done for a number of indications. In general, outcomes vary by etiology, with posttraumatic conditions and revision procedures having worse outcomes and a higher complication rate. Fatty infiltration or absence of the teres minor has also been shown to compromise outcomes. Overall, good and excellent results have been reported in 67% to 82% of patients, with significant increases in functional scores and average forward elevation between 100 and 138 degrees. Longer-term survivorship studies are emerging with implant survival rates of over 90% at 10 years and 87% at 15 years of follow-up. Survivorship for glenoid loosening has been reported at 84% over the same period. Although the acceptable postoperative activity level that the reverse prosthesis can tolerate is unknown, a high percentage of patients nevertheless report medium- and high-demand use of the operative limb after surgery.

CUFF TEAR ARTHROPATHY

Several large studies have reported good results for reverse total shoulder arthroplasty done for rotator cuff arthropathy. In a multicenter study of 80 shoulders observed for an average of 44 months, 96% of patients reported no or minimal pain, and there was an increase in active forward elevation from 73 to 138 degrees. Forty-nine patients (64%) had medial component encroachment and scapular notching, however, without evidence of loosening. Another study reported that 78% of 45 patients were satisfied with their results at midterm follow-up (average 40 months); 67% had no or slight pain. Results were significantly better in patients who had primary arthroplasty for cuff tear arthropathy than in patients who had revision of a failed standard arthroplasty. Frankle et al. (2006) reported their results with reverse total shoulder arthroplasty at an average 33-month follow-up of 60 patients who had severe rotator cuff deficiency. Significant improvements were found in pain and function scores; 41 (68%) of the 60 patients rated their outcomes as excellent or good, 16 (27%) were satisfied, and three (5%) were dissatisfied. Seven patients required revision surgery to another reverse total shoulder arthroplasty (five patients) or hemiarthroplasty (two patients). Finally, comparative studies have found reverse total shoulder arthroplasty to be superior to hemiarthroplasty for the treatment of cuff tear arthropathy.

ROTATOR CUFF DYSFUNCTION WITHOUT ARTHRITIS

More recently, indications have been expanded from cuff tear arthropathy to include other conditions of rotator cuff insufficiency. Mulieri et al. reported 90% implant survivorship at a little over 4 years after surgery of 72 shoulders with rotator cuff dysfunction without glenohumeral arthritis; 20% of patients had a complication. Ek et al. and Ernstbrunner et al. have reported similar series of younger patient cohorts with clinical improvements that were maintained up to 10 years after surgery; however, the complication rate remains high as in the series reported by Mulieri et al.

PROXIMAL HUMERAL FRACTURES

Several authors have reported the use of reverse total shoulder arthroplasty to treat proximal humeral fractures in the elderly. Results have been satisfactory, with average forward elevation of approximately 100 degrees but a high rate of scapular notching. A growing body of evidence supports the use of reverse total shoulder arthroplasty over hemiarthroplasty in the treatment of comminuted proximal humeral fractures in elderly patients; two meta-analyses have found reverse total shoulder arthroplasty to be superior to hemiarthroplasty for proximal humeral fractures in this population. One survey study demonstrated a consensus that reverse total shoulder arthroplasty is the preferred surgical treatment for four-part fractures in the older population. Other studies have compared the results of reverse total shoulder arthroplasty with nonoperative treatment for comminuted proximal humeral fractures in the elderly and reported mixed results with no clear advantage to reverse total shoulder arthroplasty. However, in one study functional outcomes were reported to be slightly better with reverse total shoulder arthroplasty.

RHEUMATOID ARTHRITIS WITH ROTATOR CUFF TEAR

Two studies have reported the use of reverse total shoulder arthroplasty in patients with rheumatoid arthritis. At an average follow-up of 2 years, John et al. reported improvements in all outcomes scores in 17 patients. Scapular notching occurred in roughly one fourth of patients, but there were no radiologic signs of loosening. Holcomb et al. also reported significant improvements in all outcomes measurements in 21 shoulders observed for an average of 3 years. The complication rate was 14%, and 18 patients rated their results as either good or excellent. Young et al. found similar clinical results but noted a high rate of intraoperative and postoperative fractures in this population.

SALVAGE PROCEDURES

In general, the outcomes of reverse total shoulder arthroplasty for revision of failed shoulder arthroplasty have been less satisfactory than those for primary reverse total shoulder arthroplasty for other conditions. Cuff et al. reported the outcomes of reverse total shoulder arthroplasty in the treatment of 22 shoulders that had either one- or two-staged irrigation, debridement, and conversion to reverse total shoulder arthroplasty. There were no recurrent infections and motion was significantly improved; however, the average forward elevation was only 80 degrees. Boileau et al. reported that, although results were not as good as for primary reverse total shoulder arthroplasty, 93% of 40 patients were satisfied with their results. Average forward elevation was 123 degrees at final follow-up, and the complication rate was 12%. The authors stressed that reverse total shoulder arthroplasty in patients with more than 90 degrees of forward elevation before surgery risks loss of motion in this plane and decreased patient satisfaction.

GLENOID BONE LOSS

Much of the recent debate and investigation surrounding degenerative shoulder conditions has centered on the concept of glenoid wear patterns. Although glenoid defects are more common in revision situations than in primary arthroplasties, they may be present at primary surgery. These wear patterns have been classified by several authors (Table 10.3; Fig. 10.17).

Central bone loss is most common in patients with rheumatoid arthritis. Placing a centering hole and evaluating the depth of the glenoid neck are recommended. A depth of less than 1 cm generally does not allow for adequate fixation and typically precludes the use of a glenoid component without bone grafting. Central cavitary defects usually can be filled with local bone graft from the humeral head.

Because the glenohumeral joint tends to sublux posteriorly with osteoarthritis, posterior wear patterns are common and can progress to severe bone loss, the so-called B2 and B3 glenoids. These eccentric glenoid wear patterns result in a twofold increase in the glenoid component loosening rate compared with concentric wear patterns (A1 and A2 glenoids). Some authorities have advocated placing the glenoid component without bone grafting and compensating for the increased retroversion by anteverting the humeral component so that the sum of the two versions is 30 to 40 degrees; however, a cadaver study determined that compensatory humeral component anteversion does not contribute to stability in the setting of a retroverted glenoid.

Alternatively, eccentric reaming of the glenoid has been recommended to correct excess retroversion. Multiple studies have concluded that glenoid retroversion of more than 17 to 18 degrees cannot be corrected with eccentric reaming and that defects of more than 20 degrees typically do not allow placement of a glenoid component.

In situations in which eccentric reaming cannot correct abnormal glenoid version, bone grafting or component augmentation is recommended (Figs. 10.18 and 10.19). There are multiple reports of both techniques used in an attempt to correct glenoid version in anatomic total shoulder arthroplasty. Although no consensus exists regarding the best technique to restore glenoid version, other areas of investigation have centered on the use of patient-specific or re-usable guides to correct these difficult wear patterns, and improved component positioning has been reported (Fig. 10.20). Finally, in elderly patients with severe posterior glenoid bone loss, reverse total shoulder arthroplasty, with or without bone grafting, has been advocated as an alternative to anatomic arthroplasty (Fig. 10.21).

For bony defects present at primary or revision reverse total shoulder arthroplasty, placement of the center screw down an alternate scapular spine center line improves the amount of bone stock available for fixation.

ACTIVITIES AFTER SHOULDER ARTHROPLASTY

With mid-term and long-term outcomes studies of anatomic and reverse shoulder arthroplasty demonstrating excellent durability and function, attention has focused on return to sports and other high-level activities. Multiple studies have demonstrated predictable improvements in activities of daily living but also successful return to sport activities such as weightlifting, swimming, and golf. Rates of return are slightly higher after anatomic total shoulder arthroplasty than after reverse shoulder arthroplasty and are more predictable for noncontact athletics. Curiously, despite conventional wisdom that suggests younger patients will be more active and place greater stress on their implants, survey data indicate that older patients are at least as active as their younger peers after reverse arthroplasty.

COMPLICATIONS OF SHOULDER ARTHROPLASTY

The overall complication rate after total shoulder arthroplasty is estimated to be approximately 15% (Table 10.4). The most commonly reported complications, in order of frequency, are component (primarily glenoid) loosening, glenohumeral instability, rotator cuff tear, periprosthetic fracture, infection, implant failure including dissociation of modular prostheses, and deltoid weakness or dysfunction. A study of over 400 total shoulder arthroplasties done with cemented all-polyethylene glenoid components between 1990 and 2000 found a 12% complication rate, and only one reoperation was required because of component loosening. The most frequent complications in this review were rotator cuff tearing, glenohumeral instability, and periprosthetic humeral fracture.

Complications after total shoulder arthroplasty tend to occur late in the postoperative course (5 to 10 years after surgery); component loosening has been reported to occur approximately 8 years after surgery, infection at 12 years, and periprosthetic fractures at 6 years.

Reverse total shoulder arthroplasty initially resulted in relatively high complication rates (50%) and some unique complications. In the past decade, with improved techniques and better understanding of the device, the complication rate has fallen (6% recently reported). The most common complications after reverse total shoulder arthroplasty are scapular

TABLE 10.3			
Classification of Glenoid Wear Patterns			
WALCH ET AL.	**SPERLING ET AL.**	**ANTUNA ET AL.**	**BERCIK ET AL. MODIFICATION OF WALCH CLASSIFICATION**
Type A (central) Type B (posterior) Type C (excessive glenoid retroversion >25°)	None Mild (erosion into subchondral bone) Moderate (hemispheric deformation and medialization of subchondral bone) Severe (bone loss extending to the coracoid base)	Defects caused by osteolysis/loosening of polyethylene glenoid implants: Central Peripheral Combined	Type A1 same as Walch et al. Type A2 glenoid in which line drawn from anterior to posterior rims of native glenoid transects humeral head (see Fig. 10.17) B1 and B2 same as Walch et al. B3 monoconcave, posterior wear, 15° retroversion, 70% humeral head subluxation Type C same as Walch et al. Type D any level glenoid anteversion or humeral head subluxation less than 40% (anterior subluxation)

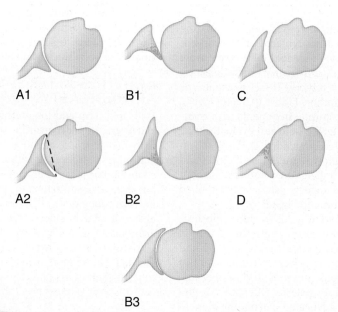

FIGURE 10.17 Bercik et al. modification of the Walch classification, with the addition of B3 and D glenoids. (Redrawn from Bercik M, Kruse K, Yalizis M, et al: A modification to the Walch classification of the glenoid in primary glenohumeral osteoarthritis using three-dimensional imaging, *J Shoulder Elbow Surg* 25:1601, 2016.)

notching, hematoma formation, glenoid dissociation such as baseplate failure or aseptic loosening, glenohumeral dislocation, acromial and scapular spine fractures, infection, loosening or dissociation of the humeral component, and nerve injury.

■ INTRAOPERATIVE COMPLICATIONS

The most common intraoperative complications in shoulder arthroplasty are fracture, usually of the humeral shaft in the mid to distal diaphysis (Fig. 10.22); nerve injury, most often to the axillary nerve; and malpositioning of components.

Most often, intraoperative periprosthetic fractures of the humerus or glenoid are caused by errors in surgical technique, such as inadvertent reaming, overzealous impaction, or manipulation of the upper extremity during exposure of the glenoid. Spiral fractures of the humerus usually are caused by excessive external rotation of the shoulder during attempts to improve exposure. Complete anterior and inferior capsular releases and the use of a bone hook to deliver the proximal humerus out of the glenoid fossa may help minimize torsion forces on the humeral shaft and thereby minimize the risk of fracture.

A humeral shaft fracture is most likely at two points in the surgical procedure. During the reaming process, when resistance is met, and if the assistant has a firm hold of the patient's arm, excessive torque can be generated that generates a spiral fracture. The assistant should be instructed to hold the arm loosely in a supportive position at the elbow. Further, if any resistance is felt, releasing the grip on the patient's arm and allowing it to rotate with the hand reamer is advisable. The second critical period is during the reduction and dislocation maneuver to test implant stability. Longitudinal distraction must be used, and manual assistance to lift the prosthetic humeral head from the joint cavity prevents the force from being transferred inferiorly into the humeral shaft.

Simple cerclage wiring of the proximal end of the humerus and implantation of a standard-size prosthesis usually are

sufficient for fractures proximal to the tip of the humeral prosthesis. We prefer to convert to a longer-stem prosthesis for unstable intraoperative humeral fractures in which standard length stem fixation is compromised. The use of a longer stem prosthesis, extending at least two humeral cortical diameters beyond the most distal extent of the fracture, has several advantages over dynamic compression plating or cerclage wiring alone: the need for secure screw purchase in bone that often is of poor quality is obviated, bending and torsional loads are better tolerated and decrease the risk of implant failure, a rigid and biomechanically sound surgical construct usually can be obtained, the extensile exposure and soft-tissue dissection required for plate fixation are avoided, and stress shielding is minimized.

Fractures of the glenoid are extremely rare and usually occur in osteopenic bone. Most often, this complication occurs after the glenoid has been reamed to subchondral bone and the canal has been prepared to receive a keeled prosthesis. Retraction on the anterior or posterior glenoid cortex can produce cortical bone failure. Stable fixation of the fracture is essential to prevent instability of the glenoid component. Good preoperative axillary radiographs or CT scans can help determine if posterior wear of the glenoid is present. Reaming of the glenoid to its neutral version and tilt restores alignment for proper orientation before canal preparation is started. If the cortex is penetrated, the defect can be bone grafted to prevent cement extrusion.

Although permanent nerve injury during total shoulder arthroplasty is rare, it is devastating when it does occur. Most reported instances of permanent axillary nerve injury involved revision surgery or primary surgery in a shoulder that had multiple previous operations. The radial nerve can be injured by an intraoperative humeral shaft fracture and internal fixation of the fracture. Extrusion of cement through a defect in the humeral canal has been reported to result in radial nerve injury; nerve function returned after removal

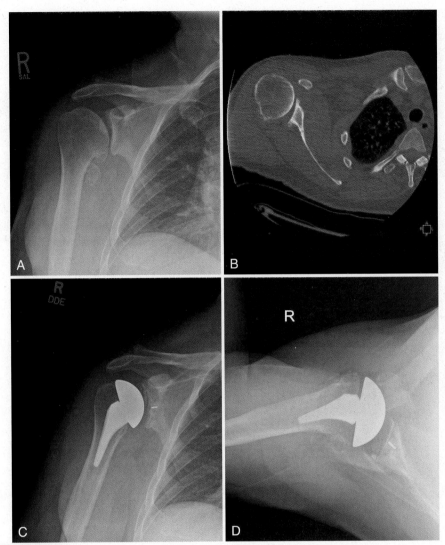

FIGURE 10.18 **A** and **B,** Patient with advanced osteoarthritis and B3 glenoid wear pattern treated with augmented glenoid component to restore glenoid version and recenter the humeral head (**C** and **D**).

TABLE 10.4

Complications After Unconstrained Total Shoulder Arthroplasties Reported in 33 Series (2540 Shoulders)

COMPLICATION	% ALL SHOULDERS	NO. SHOULDERS	% ALL COMPLICATIONS
COMPONENT LOOSENING	6.31	161	39
Glenoid	5.3	134	32
Humerus	1.1	27	6.5
INSTABILITY	4.9	124	30
Superior	3	77	19
Posterior	1	25	6
Anterior	0.9	22	5
PERIPROSTHETIC FRACTURE	1.8	46	11
Intraoperative	1.1	27	6.5
Postoperative	0.7	19	4.6
ROTATOR CUFF TEAR	1.3	32	7.7
NEURAL INJURY	0.8	20	4.8
INFECTION	0.7	19	4.6
DELTOID DETACHMENT	0.08	2	0.5

Modified from Bohsali KI, Wirth MA, Rockwood CA Jr: Complications of total shoulder arthroplasty, *J Bone Joint Surg* 88A:2279, 2006.

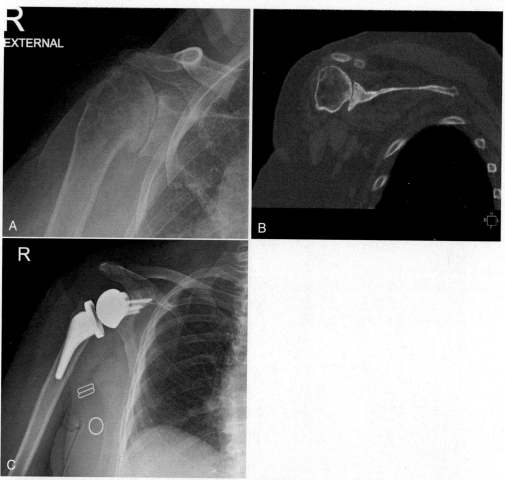

FIGURE 10.19 **A** and **B,** Cuff-deficient patient with B2 glenoid wear pattern treated with reverse total shoulder arthroplasty using augmented glenoid baseplate **(C).**

of the cement near the nerve. However, most nerve injuries are neurapraxias that recover with time. A complete neurologic examination should be done early in the postoperative period to document any nerve deficits. If no recovery is noted after 6 weeks, an electromyographic examination should be obtained and should be repeated at 3 months. If no recovery has occurred as evident by electromyography at 3 months, exploration of the nerve should be considered.

If malposition of the humerus is noted with an uncemented component, it can typically be disimpacted and repositioned. If a cemented component is used, an offset humeral head prosthesis can be used to attempt to correct version. The offset humeral head allows 5 to 7 degrees of version correction in the anterior or posterior direction. However, in reality, a malpositioned cemented humeral stem often requires a lengthy and difficult revision procedure to remove the well-fixed component and replace it in an appropriate position.

POSTOPERATIVE COMPLICATIONS

Postoperative complications include glenoid loosening, glenohumeral instability, rotator cuff tears, periprosthetic fracture, infection, deltoid rupture, tuberosity nonunion or malunion, humeral loosening, impingement, heterotopic bone formation, mechanical failure of components, and loss of motion.

GLENOID LOOSENING

Symptomatic loosening of glenoid or humeral components is the most common problem encountered in total shoulder arthroplasty, accounting for one third of all complications. Loosening of the glenoid component is significantly more common than loosening of the humeral component. Radiographic lucent lines at the cement-bone interface of the glenoid component have been observed in varying degrees in up to 96% of patients in some studies. One meta-analysis found that asymptomatic radiolucent lines occur at a rate of 7% per year, with symptomatic loosening occurring at 1.2% per year, and resultant revision occurring at 0.8% per year. Although some have found no association between radiographic changes and clinical results, progression of the lines has been correlated with a decrease in function and an increase in pain in most patients. A shift in the position of the glenoid component or circumferential radiolucent lines at least 1.5 mm wide are evidence of a loose glenoid component. Injection of the cement under pressurization provided by a syringe and application of cement on the back side of the glenoid component has been reported to improve glenoid component fixation by providing more complete cementation. Radiolucencies tend to evolve late (after 5 years), indicating the need for further technical and prosthetic innovation to improve long-term component durability. Indeed, one report on loosening of pegged, cemented,

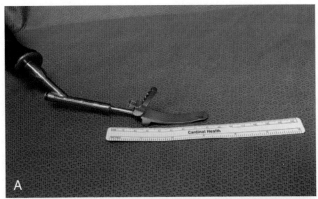

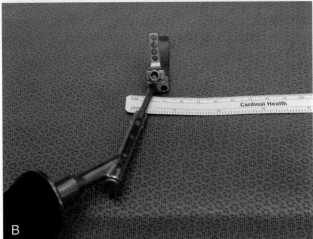

FIGURE 10.20 **A and B,** Commercially available, noncustom, reusable targeting guide. (From: Mulligan RP, Azar FM, Throckmorton TW: Generic targeting guides place revision glenoid components in more anatomic version than traditional techniques, *J Shoulder Elbow Surg* 26:786, 2017.)

all-polyethylene components found a marked increase in radiographic loosening between 5 and 10 years, increasing 8% to nearly 60%.

Polyethylene debris from glenoid wear has been reported in approximately 20% of revision shoulder arthroplasty cases. In a retrieval study of 52 shoulders undergoing revision surgery after total shoulder arthroplasty, osteolysis was more common when screws had been used for glenoid component fixation and was highly associated with third body wear. Radiolucent lines also were significantly associated with osteolysis. No significant differences were found regarding the presence of particulate debris, however. Another analysis of 78 retrieved glenoid components found that scratching, pitting, and burnishing were the most common modes of glenoid polyethylene wear, mostly in the inferior quadrant, and that radiographic analysis underestimates the amount of clinical glenoid loosening. Others have postulated that the functional malcentering of the humeral head associated with the common posterior subluxation pattern in osteoarthritis can contribute to glenoid wear postoperatively if not corrected at the time of joint replacement.

One controversy has been the relative clinical and radiographic performances of pegged glenoid designs and those that use a keel. Multiple authors have concluded that the biomechanical data support pegged glenoid components. Although a randomized controlled trial by Edwards et al. found a significantly higher rate of radiolucencies in keeled implants (46%) than in pegged components (15%), other clinical data have been somewhat mixed. Whereas one radiostereometric analysis found that keeled components demonstrated more migration than pegged implants, another prospective randomized trial using radiostereometric analysis found no difference between pegged and keeled implant micromigration at 2 years of follow-up. More recently, we found no significant differences in clinical or radiographic outcomes between pegged and keeled components at intermediate-term follow-up, indicating that glenoid lucencies develop over time, most likely as a result of the stresses placed across the bone-cement-polyethylene interface.

Improvements in material and component design have led to the evolution of cementless ingrowth and hybrid ingrowth-cemented glenoid components. Although long-term studies are not yet available, early and intermediate-term follow-up studies suggest a low rate of radiolucency and mechanical failure in these implants.

Arthroscopy has been reported to be useful in evaluating glenoid component loosening. If glenoid loosening is present in an asymptomatic patient, only observation is indicated; however, if loosening is present in a patient who has symptoms of pain, decreased range of motion, and functional disability, further investigation is warranted to determine if implant replacement is appropriate. A painful "clunking" sensation with forward elevation of the arm has been described as a sign of symptomatic glenoid loosening.

HUMERAL LOOSENING

Humeral radiolucent lines are not nearly as common as radiolucent lines around the glenoid component. Radiolucent lines may progress over time to component loosening, which typically is diagnosed by a change in implant position or progression to circumferential radiolucent lines, and is now thought to often indicate indolent infection. Raiss et al., however, suggested that polyethylene wear from the anatomic glenoid component is associated with proximal humeral osteolysis around the humeral component. Although early studies reported humeral radiolucent lines in up to 61% of implants, mostly at the distal stem tip, actual loosening of the component was much less frequent, and few components required revision because of symptomatic loosening. In a more recent study, we found essentially no evidence of loosening and minimal (1 mm) radiolucent lines in 6.5% of proximally coated ingrowth humeral stems at an average of approximately 4 years of follow-up. These results are mirrored in a study of reverse total shoulder arthroplasty, where humeral stem loosening was reported to be less than 1%.

INSTABILITY

Instability is the second leading cause of complications associated with shoulder arthroplasty, with a reported prevalence of 4% and accounting for 30% of all complications. It can occur in any direction and in variable degrees of subluxation and dislocation. In a meta-analysis of 11 series of total shoulder arthroplasties that included 838 patients, Wilde reported a 1.2% incidence of postoperative dislocation over a follow-up period of 20 to 54 months.

Approximately 80% of instability complications after total shoulder arthroplasty involve anterior or superior instability, and most are the result of soft-tissue deficiency. Key to

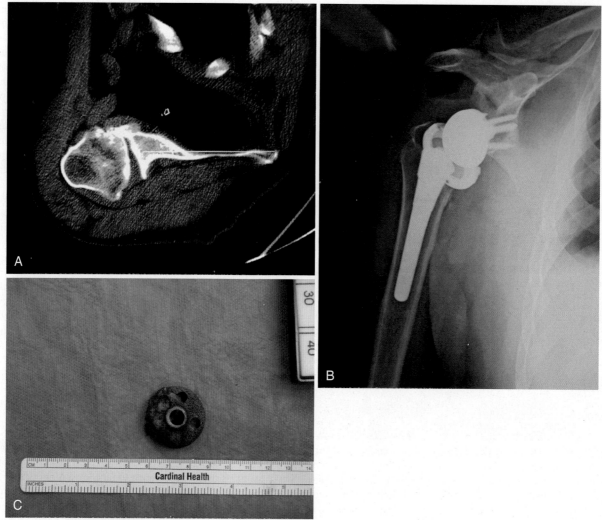

FIGURE 10.21 Patient with osteoarthritis and B2 glenoid wear pattern **(A)** treated with reverse total shoulder arthroplasty **(B)**. Impaction bone grafting technique was employed to enhance baseplate support **(C)**.

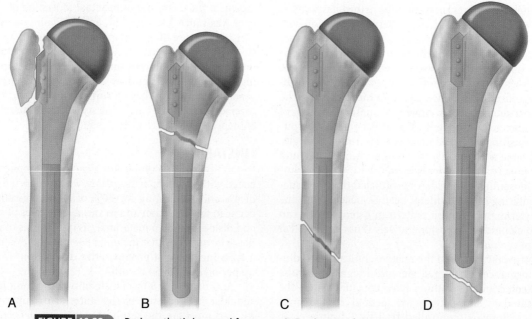

FIGURE 10.22 Periprosthetic humeral fractures. **A,** Region 1, tuberosity. **B,** Region 2, proximal metaphysis. **C,** Region 3, proximal diaphysis. **D,** Region 4, middiaphysis and distal diaphysis.

designing treatment for this problem is isolating and understanding the exact cause of the instability. Anterior instability most commonly is associated with subscapularis failure, glenoid anteversion, malrotation of the humeral component, or anterior deltoid dysfunction. Anterior instability secondary to subscapularis rupture generally is a consequence of operative technique, tissue quality, inappropriate physical therapy, or the use of oversized components. Anterior instability also can be caused by the use of a humeral head that is too small for the joint volume (Fig. 10.23). Replacement of the humeral head with an appropriate-size implant, which also can be an offset-type component, can be done to regain stability. If abnormal humeral version is found to be the cause of anterior instability, revision of the stem should be considered. A torn subscapularis tendon is likely to be underreported and will not correlate with the postoperative physical examination; however, it can contribute to anterior instability and must be repaired to regain joint stability. However, often the subscapularis is irreparable, necessitating a revision to reverse arthroplasty. Platform systems that allow conversion from anatomic to reverse replacement without removal of the humeral stem have simplified the process with a lower complication rate.

Concerns about postoperative subscapularis integrity have resulted in a multitude of techniques in addition to subscapularis tenotomy to prevent this complication. One such technique is a lesser tuberosity osteotomy (LTO), in which the bone-tendon unit is reflected to access the glenohumeral joint and then fixed at the end of the procedure. Overall, the biomechanical evidence has favored LTO over other techniques. A systematic review of cadaver studies concluded that LTO is biomechanically more secure than soft-tissue repair, but clinical series, including a randomized controlled trial and a systematic review, have not demonstrated superiority of one technique over another for subscapularis management. One report suggested that LTO failure may be an underreported complication.

Progressive superior migration of the humeral head has been reported in association with dynamic muscle dysfunction, attenuation of the supraspinatus, failed rotator cuff repairs, and frank rupture of the rotator cuff. Asymptomatic patients should be encouraged to continue rehabilitation and do not require operative intervention; however, long-term superior migration of the humeral head can result in loosening of the glenoid component, and repair of rotator cuff tears at the time of arthroplasty can help prevent this complication. Symptomatic patients may require revision to reverse arthroplasty.

Posterior instability has been attributed most often to malpositioning of the components but may be multifactorial as well. Posterior glenoid erosion with excessive component retroversion and soft-tissue imbalance has been implicated in the development of posterior instability. If the glenoid or humeral component is placed in too much retroversion, posterior instability may occur and revision is recommended. If the capsule is stretched from long-standing posterior wear on the glenoid, it may require imbrication to gain stability. Patients with posterior glenohumeral subluxation associated with long-standing osteoarthritis or a history of chronic posterior instability, whether recurrent or fixed, are at increased risk for posterior instability after shoulder arthroplasty. Proper use of eccentric reaming, with or without bone grafting or augmented components, and accurate placement of the humeral and glenoid components has been shown to minimize the risk of this complication, but soft-tissue balancing, as described in the surgical technique for total shoulder arthroplasty, is a critical component of the operation. In most such patients, external rotation is restricted, with tight and contracted anterior structures and an attenuated and stretched posterior capsule. Thus proper attention to component position in addition to soft-tissue balancing is a crucial step in preventing posterior instability.

Inferior instability is related to the loss of normal humeral height and is most common after hemiarthroplasty for proximal humeral fractures. Removal of too much of the proximal humerus, with resultant inferior placement of the humeral head, can lead to inferior instability. Patients usually have difficulty elevating the arm past the horizontal plane because of weakness of the deltoid caused by shortening of the humerus. Revision surgery usually is necessary to restore humeral length and regain deltoid strength.

PERIPROSTHETIC FRACTURE

The reported prevalence of postoperative periprosthetic humeral shaft fractures ranges from 0.5% to 2%. Postoperative humeral shaft fractures are most frequent in women and in patients with rheumatoid arthritis.

Wright and Cofield classified periprosthetic humeral shaft fractures into three types. Type A fractures extend proximally from the tip of the prosthesis, type B fractures are centered at the tip of the prosthesis, and type C fractures involve the humeral shaft distal to the prosthesis. Treatment of type A postoperative periprosthetic fractures often require revision arthroplasty and fracture stabilization if the fracture disrupts a large portion of the bone-implant interface and leads to implant loosening. Type B fractures can be treated with a fracture brace if acceptable alignment can be obtained. If union is delayed, open reduction and internal fixation with a plate and screws and cerclage wiring, without prosthesis removal, is recommended; however, it should be stressed that these fractures take an average of 5 to 9 months to heal and the patient should be counseled regarding the extended treatment course from this complication. Type C fractures usually heal with immobilization and can be managed as other fractures of the humeral shaft. Again, extended healing times should be anticipated.

Initial nonoperative management has been recommended for fractures proximal to the stem tip and for fractures with acceptable alignment at the tip of a well-fixed humeral stem. For fractures with unacceptable alignment at the stem tip, open reduction and internal fixation has been advocated, particularly if the fracture extends distally. Revision with a long stem is recommended for similar fractures when the humeral component was loose.

ROTATOR CUFF FAILURE

Rotator cuff failure is becoming more recognized as a common complication after shoulder arthroplasty than was originally thought. Although the historically reported incidence was 1% to 2%, analysis of complications reported to the US Food and Drug Administration indicates that rotator cuff failure is the second most common complication after anatomic shoulder arthroplasty, representing 15% of the reported problems. Rupture of the subscapularis tendon is involved in most rotator cuff tears. Factors reported to be associated with postoperative tears of the subscapularis tendon include multiple operations, overstuffing of the joint, overly aggressive therapy involving external rotation during the early postoperative period, and tendon compromise by lengthening techniques.

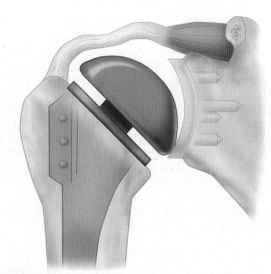

FIGURE 10.23 Humeral head component that is too small can result in anterior or posterior instability.

Secondary rotator cuff dysfunction increases over time and is associated with functional decline of the prosthesis. Preoperative fatty infiltration of the infraspinatus and a glenoid component placed in superior tilt are risk factors for subsequent rotator cuff failure. Symptomatic tears can be repaired in the standard fashion with care to preserve the coracoacromial ligament but may require revision to reverse prosthesis. Recurrent tears of the superior rotator cuff may result in little improvement in function and motion, however, after operative repair. Large tears cause superior subluxation and eventual loosening of the glenoid component from compression forces on the superior rim of the glenoid (the so-called rocking horse glenoid). Repair of large or massive tears may be impossible. One treatment for this difficult problem involves removing the glenoid component, bone grafting of the glenoid cavity defect, and allowing the humeral prosthesis to migrate superiorly. A competent coracoacromial ligament must be present to provide superior stability if this salvage procedure is done. More recently, conversion to reverse total shoulder arthroplasty has been described, with satisfactory results, although the outcomes of this conversion are not as favorable as those for primary rotator cuff arthropathy.

INFECTION

Infection is rare after both primary anatomic and reverse total shoulder arthroplasty (~1% to 2%); male sex and younger age at the time of arthroplasty are risk factors. As with all joint replacements, several factors contribute to the predilection for bacterial seeding, including bacterial adhesion, glycoprotein encapsulation, bacterial resistance to antibiotics, physical properties of the implant such as chemical composition and surface texture, and inhibiting factors from ion elution. The literature also suggests an increased risk of infection in patients with diabetes mellitus, rheumatoid arthritis, systemic lupus erythematosus, remote sites of infection, and those undergoing shoulder injection within 3 months of surgery. Other factors implicated in an increased susceptibility to infection include immunosuppressive chemotherapy, systemic corticosteroids, multiple steroid injections, and previous shoulder surgery. Several reports have linked infection around total joint prostheses to transient bacteremia secondary to dental

manipulation, urinary tract infection, pneumonia, and genitourinary instrumentation. As in patients with other total joint arthroplasties, prophylactic antimicrobial coverage should be individualized for each patient and procedure.

Cutibacterium acnes (formerly known as Propionibacterium acnes) is the most commonly isolated organism after shoulder arthroplasty but has a protean presentation and is very difficult to diagnose. A gram-positive, aerotolerant anaerobic rod that lives in the skin (not on the skin), *C. acnes* has a different behavior and profile than other organisms such as *Staphylococcus aureus*. Typical inflammatory indices (white blood cell count [WBC], CRP, ESR) often are not revealing, and even cultures are not uniformly reliable. The most common symptom is unexplained pain. Because of the organism's slow-growing nature, cultures should not be discarded in 3 to 5 days, but should be held for at least 2 weeks to isolate this organism. More recent work has centered on the use of nontraditional testing to identify *C. acnes* infection. Among the reported tests, synovial interleukin (IL)-6 measurement, with or without combined synovial cytokine profiles, alpha-defensin, hemolysis in certain *C. acnes* strains, and polymerase chain reaction with restricted fragment length polymorphism, all have demonstrated varied success. Implant sonication, which has been used successfully in the detection of hip and knee periprosthetic joint infections, showed no benefit over standard cultures. Further, no gold standard laboratory or culture values have been identified to reliably constitute a clinically significant *C. acnes* infection. Thus, the diagnosis of periprosthetic shoulder infection remains largely a clinical one. Further complicating the picture, *C. acnes* is a common contaminant that can be identified during primary shoulder arthroplasty even in those with no previous surgery.

Intraoperative findings of humeral loosening, turbid fluid, and membrane formation all correlate with the likelihood of a positive culture for *C. acnes*. Intraoperative histopathology has been reported to have very high specificity but only approximately 50% sensitivity for *C. acnes* infection. A threshold of 10 polymorphonuclear leukocytes per high-power field (rather than five) to diagnose infection has been suggested to increase the sensitivity of intraoperative pathology without affecting specificity. Multiple cultures (at least five) are recommended and held a minimum of 10 to 14 days to isolate the organism. In revision arthroplasty when there is a low clinical suspicion for infection, cultures may return positive (the so-called unexpectedly positive culture [UPC]). In these patients reinfection rates are low (~1%), and they require either a 6-week course of postoperative intravenous antibiotics or an empiric 2-week course.

If the infection is identified early (3 to 6 weeks after surgery) and the organism is susceptible, retention of the components can be considered. One-stage irrigation and debridement with replacement components, along with appropriate parenteral antibiotic therapy, has been shown to be effective treatment. If the organism is resistant or the infection occurs late, removal of the implants and all cement generally is recommended. Placement of an antibiotic-impregnated spacer helps to sterilize the soft-tissue envelope, and a 6-week course of parenteral antibiotics can be followed by implantation of revision components with the use of antibiotics in the cement.

Much investigation has centered on the use of one- or two-stage procedures for the treatment of periprosthetic shoulder infection. Several series have demonstrated effectiveness of both approaches; a meta-analysis found no difference between one- and two-stage protocols but noted the retrospective nature of the analyzed studies. Some authors noted that infection with more virulent organisms such as *Staphylococcus aureus* generally necessitates a two-stage approach, whereas more indolent organisms such as *C. acnes* respond well to a one-stage reconstruction. In clear cases of gross or chronic infection, particularly with difficult organisms, such as methicillin-resistant *S. aureus* (MRSA), we routinely remove all components, perform a thorough debridement, place an antibiotic cement spacer, administer intravenous antibiotics, and follow inflammatory indices (complete blood cell count, ESR, CRP) with the plan for component replantation if the infection is cleared. We obtain an aspiration and culture of glenohumeral joint fluid before replantation. In patients with less robust infectious organisms such as *C. acnes*, we often employ a one-stage reconstruction. In selected patients who either refuse or are medically unfit for a revision arthroplasty, use of a functional antibiotic spacer has been reported to obtain satisfactory outcomes.

DELTOID MUSCLE DYSFUNCTION

Deltoid muscle dysfunction caused by axillary nerve injury or detachment of the deltoid muscle can result in a catastrophic loss of shoulder function. Deltoid degeneration after reverse total shoulder arthroplasty has been attributed to an increase in the moment arm in the anterior and middle heads of the deltoid, which reduces the muscle effort required for most activities but can result in attritional stretching of the deltoid with later loss of function. Postoperative fatty infiltration of the deltoid, thought to be secondary to the altered biomechanics of the device, also has been reported to result in inferior clinical outcomes.

HETEROTOPIC OSSIFICATION

Heterotopic ossification has been noted to occur after shoulder arthroplasty in 10% to 45% of patients. Male gender and osteoarthritis are risk factors. Bridging heterotopic bone of the glenohumeral joint or glenoacromial space can occur in extreme situations. No correlation is evident, however, between heterotopic ossification and the development of shoulder pain. Heterotopic ossification after total shoulder arthroplasty usually is low grade, is present early in the postoperative period, is nonprogressive, and does not adversely affect clinical results.

STIFFNESS

Many patients who are dissatisfied with the outcomes of their total shoulder arthroplasties cite stiffness as the reason. Postoperative stiffness, typically manifested by loss of forward elevation or external rotation, usually results from oversizing of components, shortening or overtightening of the subscapularis, or insufficient rehabilitation. Treatment involves soft-tissue balancing procedures to completely mobilize the subscapularis in anatomic arthroplasty. Excision of the anterior capsule and release of the rotator interval and coracohumeral ligament may be required to accomplish this. If the subscapularis is still tight, a Z-plasty lengthening in the frontal plane may be required. A general rule is that 1 cm of lengthening equals approximately 20 degrees of increased external rotation.

COMPLICATIONS OF REVERSE TOTAL SHOULDER ARTHROPLASTY

Because of its unique configuration, reverse shoulder arthroplasty can result in complications other than those usually associated with total shoulder arthroplasty. Notching of the scapula is unique to this prosthesis but has variable incidences in the literature; it has been reported in 10% to 96% of reverse arthroplasties. Notching is thought to be an osteolytic reaction caused by impingement of the polyethylene humeral bearing surface, mainly in adduction and external rotation. Nerot classified this notching into four grades, ranging from none to notching severe enough to cause glenoid loosening (Fig. 10.24). In most patients, the notching stabilizes at grade 2 at about 12 months after implantation; however, notching has been shown to result in inferior clinical outcomes and higher rates of radiolucencies.

Surgical techniques to decrease the rate of scapular notching have been extensively studied. Several factors have been implicated and technical changes have included placing the baseplate in an inferior position with inferior tilt, usually about 10 to 15 degrees. Levigne et al. found that superior tilt of the glenosphere correlated with scapular notching in their study of 448 shoulders observed for an average of approximately 4 years. Other studies have focused on increasing glenosphere size and lateral offset. Review of the available evidence indicates that inferior placement of the baseplate with inferior tilt are the two most important factors to decrease notching. Kelly et al. recommended placing the initial drill hole 11.5 mm superior to the inferior glenoid rim to optimize baseplate positioning. Use of a more varus stem with a neck-shaft angle of 135 degrees (rather than 155 degrees) and a lateralized glenosphere has been reported to result in lower notching rates as well. Another study noted that a longer scapular neck is associated with a lower notching rate, suggesting that some patient-specific anatomic factors may have a role in this complication.

Instability after reverse total shoulder arthroplasty also is a known complication; it occurs primarily in extension and adduction at a rate of approximately 5%. Muscle forces across the joint appear to be the primary determinant of implant stability, and an irreparable subscapularis tendon has been reported to correlate with a higher dislocation rate in traditional Grammont-style prostheses. This is less important with lateralized constructs. Additional factors that contribute to instability include male gender, history of prior open shoulder surgery, and operative indication of fracture sequelae. Technical factors that can improve stability include placing the baseplate in inferior tilt, use of an inferior offset glenosphere and, when necessary, a constrained polyethylene bearing surface. Interestingly, the use of constrained liners has been reported to result in a comparable level of scapular notching as with unconstrained surfaces.

Acromial stress fractures are thought to be caused by increased stress placed on the acromion by the configuration of the prosthesis and resultant increased deltoid tension. A meta-analysis concluded that these fractures occur in 4% of reverse total shoulder arthroplasty procedures but that surgical treatment is not typically helpful. Overlengthening of the deltoid at the time of reverse total shoulder arthroplasty is thought to be an important contributing factor. Scapular spine fractures are more common in osteoporotic patients and are associated with the use of a baseplate that relies on a center screw for fixation.

As outcomes studies for reverse total shoulder arthroplasty extend into the second decade, there has been concern about polyethylene wear from the semiconstrained articulation. This is particularly true with the use of retentive liners, which have been shown to have increased wear compared with nonretentive bearing surfaces. Future longitudinal studies examining in vivo wear rates and the possible evolution of aseptic loosening patterns will aid in understanding this topic.

REVISION SHOULDER ARTHROPLASTY

The rate of revision of primary shoulder arthroplasties, as reported in the earlier literature, ranged from 0% to 12.5%; however, with longer follow-up, more recently reported revision rates for constrained and unconstrained implants range from 5% to 42%.

■ INDICATIONS

Revision surgery is technically demanding, and the causes of failure of the primary procedure often are multifactorial, involving soft tissues, bony structures, and the implant. Determining the results of revision arthroplasty is difficult because many reported series of total shoulder arthroplasties include limited patient numbers. Nevertheless, the main indication and goal for revision shoulder arthroplasty is pain relief. Restoration of motion, strength, and function are secondary goals because they are less reliably obtained.

Dense scarring from previous operations commonly complicates the surgical approach in revision shoulder arthroplasty. Exposure is typically quite difficult, making component implantation less predictable. Foruria et al. described an anteromedial approach to the shoulder in which the anterior deltoid is taken down from the clavicle and acromion, allowing full access to the underlying structures. Meticulous transosseous repair of the deltoid is required at the end of the procedure to prevent dehiscence.

Failed hemiarthroplasty due to glenoid arthritis is an increasingly common indication for revision arthroplasty. Anatomic glenoid component implantation is reliable to relieve pain and improve range of motion, but some authors have noted that preexisting instability or subscapularis deficiency, or both, often is not correctable with an anatomic revision arthroplasty. In case of instability, revision to reverse arthroplasty is more likely to be successful, although the recurrent instability risk remains approximately 14%. The overall results of revision to reverse total shoulder arthroplasty for failed hemiarthroplasty demonstrate improvements in pain and function, with a 7% revision rate and 93% component survival at 5 years.

Symptomatic loosening of the glenoid component is a common reason for revision surgery and usually is treated by removal, with or without replacement of the component. Loosening, polyethylene wear or dissociation, and component malposition are the most common causes of glenoid failure. A new component can be cemented in place if adequate glenoid bone stock is available, and the deltoid and rotator cuff muscles are functional. In general, the goal of revision arthroplasty should be to resurface the glenoid to maximize pain relief, but recurrent glenoid loosening has historically been reported in 67% of patients. However, a more recent series demonstrated 10-year survival free of reoperation to be 79% after revision glenoid resurfacing. Concentric reaming and bone grafting can help provide adequate fixation of the new prosthesis as well. Reimplantation usually is impossible if bone loss is severe, but removal of the glenoid component also may provide satisfactory pain relief, and bone grafting

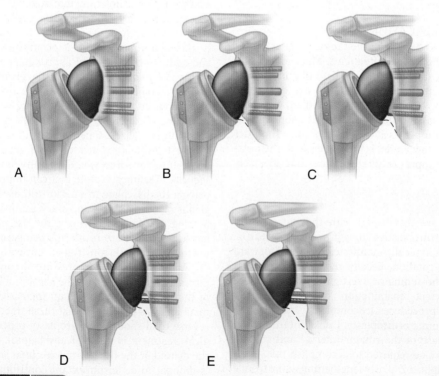

FIGURE 10.24 Nerot classification of progressive scapular notching. **A,** Grade 0, no notch. **B,** Grade 1, small notch. **C,** Grade 2, notch with condensation (stable). **D,** Grade 3, evolutive notch (erosion of inferior screw). **E,** Grade 4, first glenoid loosening.

can improve bone stock for later implantation. Another alternative reported to be successful in these situations is conversion to reverse total shoulder arthroplasty. Both structural and nonstructural bone grafting procedures have been successful for revision to reverse total shoulder arthroplasty in shoulders with significant glenoid deficiency.

Revision of the humeral stem for loosening is uncommon and depends on the type of fixation used. As noted previously, indolent infection should be suspected in cases of isolated humeral stem loosening. In uncemented prostheses, disruption of the remaining ingrowth surface and removal of the component followed by replacement with a cemented or uncemented stem (based on the remaining humeral bone stock) is recommended. Interestingly, conversion to a shorter stem in these situations has been reported as a bone-preserving solution with good results. When a cemented humeral stem is loose, component removal followed by a cement-within-cement technique can be used. Alternatively, complete removal of the cement mantle may be accomplished with subsequent placement of an ingrowth stem, if adequate bone stock remains. When a well-fixed stem must be removed, humeral windowing and longitudinal split techniques have been described with high healing and low complication rates.

Another potential consequence of revision arthroplasty is massive (>4 cm) proximal humeral bone loss. Causes include trauma, bone loss from revision surgery, and prior infection. In these patients, the rotator cuff obviously is deficient, and alternative methods are needed to restore proximal humeral stability. Both allograft-prosthesis composites and endoprosthetic reconstruction techniques have been described for these deficiencies.

◼ OUTCOMES

Outcomes after revision of unconstrained shoulder arthroplasties generally are inferior to the outcomes after primary arthroplasty, and the clinical data remain somewhat mixed. Dines et al. reviewed the results of 78 revision total shoulder replacements and found that results were significantly better for component revisions than for soft-tissue reconstructions. When revising failed hemiarthroplasty to anatomic total shoulder replacement, Hattrup reported 70% good and excellent results at an average of 4.5 years, and Sheth et al. demonstrated 86% component survival at 5 years after the same procedure. However, Carroll et al. found a high rate (47%) of unsatisfactory outcomes at 5.5 years of follow-up in a similar group of patients and concluded that this procedure is a salvage situation with outcomes inferior to those of primary total shoulder arthroplasty. Similarly, although revision of resurfacing hemiarthroplasty is attractive because it is technically less demanding than a stemmed replacement, the results are often unsatisfactory; almost 60% of patients achieve an unacceptable outcome.

The versatility of reverse total shoulder arthroplasty makes it an attractive option for revision situations in which the rotator cuff often is not functional. Although a reverse replacement may be the only reasonable option in some patients, the complication rate of revision reverse total shoulder arthroplasty has been reported to be higher than that of primary reverse total shoulder arthroplasty and is typically over 50%; patient satisfaction remains high, however. Although most of these complications are minor, we nevertheless urge caution when undertaking a revision shoulder arthroplasty. When a reverse arthroplasty requires revision, patients should be cautioned that multiple procedures often are necessary but that the prosthesis usually can be salvaged.

OTHER SURGICAL OPTIONS FOR FAILED SHOULDER ARTHROPLASTY
◼ HEMIARTHROPLASTY

Hemiarthroplasty is discussed earlier in this chapter and has been described as a salvage procedure for failed reverse total shoulder replacement.

◼ RESECTION ARTHROPLASTY

Resection arthroplasty may be considered for failed shoulder arthroplasties in patients with resistant infection, intractable pain, or extensive loss of bone or soft tissue that precludes reimplantation of a prosthesis. Successful eradication of recalcitrant shoulder infection has been reported after resection arthroplasty with and without the use of antibiotic spacers. Although the procedure is reliable for pain relief, range of motion and function are generally poor because the fulcrum of the shoulder is lost.

◼ GLENOHUMERAL ARTHRODESIS

Glenohumeral arthrodesis rarely is indicated as a primary procedure for arthritic shoulder conditions but may be appropriate for failed shoulder arthroplasty in patients with severe bone loss, chronic low-grade infection, multiple failed revision arthroplasties, intractable instability, or extensive deficiencies of the deltoid. Techniques for and results of shoulder arthrodesis are discussed in chapter 11.

REHABILITATION AFTER SHOULDER ARTHROPLASTY

Little comparative data exist regarding rehabilitation protocols after shoulder arthroplasty. Most surgeons have their own protocols, but, in general, the goals for rehabilitation are restoration of function and motion (Box 10.2). Recovering motion and strengthening the anterior deltoid and external rotators are of greatest importance. Of particular importance in anatomic replacements is protecting the subscapularis repair, and most protocols are governed by this premise. Patients with

---

BOX 10.2

Rehabilitation Protocol After Shoulder Arthroplasty

POD 1 to 6 weeks—AA/PROM only
- Forward elevation—in the plane of the scapula as tolerated, up to 90 degrees
- Internal rotation, with upper arm at side, to chest
- External rotation, with upper arm at side, 0-20 degrees
- Pendulum exercises five times per day
- AA→AROM for elbow, wrist, and hand

6-12 weeks—continue AA/PROM
- Forward elevation to full
- External rotation to 30 degrees
- Wand and overhead pulley
- Isometric strengthening for flexion, extension, external rotation, and abduction *in neutral position only*

At 12 weeks—start AROM/dynamic strengthening
- Continue AROM, stretches, and TheraBand strengthening
- Progress strengthening
- Progress to home program

AAROM, Active-assisted range of motion; *AROM,* active range of motion; *POD,* postoperative day; *PROM,* passive range of motion.

poorly functioning deltoid and rotator cuff muscles are placed in the limited-goals category and are given an exercise program aimed at achieving a more modest range of motion.

A sling or immobilizer is applied immediately after surgery and is worn for the first 6 weeks when not performing physical therapy. Most patients begin early passive and active-assisted range of motion, including pendulum, isometric elbow, and wrist and hand exercises. At 6 weeks, the sling or immobilizer is removed and gentle activities in front of the body are permitted. Pulley exercises for overhead motion and exercises for external rotation are initiated at this point as well. Passive forward elevation, internal rotation, and external rotation should be maximized before isometric strengthening is initiated at 10 weeks. Active internal rotation and passive external rotation are limited to protect the subscapularis repair for 12 weeks. Patients should be cautioned to avoid using their arm to push themselves up in bed or from a chair because this requires forceful contraction of the subscapularis. Unrestricted activity is permitted at 12 weeks, but patients are cautioned not to participate in contact sports or do any aggressive weight training. If any residual tightness is present at 12 to 16 weeks, aggressive stretching should be started. Range of motion usually is approximately two thirds to three quarters of normal after completion of a rehabilitation program. The rehabilitation protocol should be modified as necessary in circumstances requiring rotator cuff repair or revision.

A home-based program of rehabilitation after total shoulder arthroplasty also can be effective (Table 10.5). Patients are instructed in the first sequence of exercises while in the hospital, and these are practiced with a relative or friend in three or four sessions with a physical therapist. At 5 weeks, patients return for a single physical therapy session for instruction in the newer exercises. Serial radiographs are made annually to ensure that no signs of component failure are present. Patients with rheumatoid arthritis, traumatic arthritis, or osteonecrosis may be at risk for failure to regain motion and for complications with tendon, particularly subscapularis, healing.

RECONSTRUCTIVE PROCEDURES OF THE ELBOW

Elbow arthroplasty has been described in multiple forms over time. Debridement procedures, soft-tissue interposition, and prosthetic arthroplasty have all been reported. Semiconstrained total elbow arthroplasty, in particular, has a well-studied track record of pain relief and restoration of function for activities of daily living in low-demand patients. However, the procedure is associated with a relatively high complication rate and is not as durable as replacements of the hip, knee, or shoulder. In particular, the excessive loads placed on the device by high-demand patients is a common cause of failure.

ANATOMY AND BIOMECHANICS

In the normal elbow joint, stability is maintained by the combination of highly congruent joint geometry, capsuloligamentous integrity, and balanced intact musculature. The biceps, brachialis, anconeus, and triceps muscles are especially important. The medial collateral ligament complex consists of anterior, posterior, and transverse components (Fig. 10.25A). The anterior bundle is the most easily identifiable and is the

TABLE 10.5

Home-Based Exercise Program for Rehabilitation After Total Shoulder Arthroplasty

EXERCISE	DAYS AFTER SURGERY	WEEKS AFTER SURGERY
Active hand, forearm, elbow motion	1	
Passive shoulder motion	1	
Assisted pulley for elevation	21	3
Active-assisted motion and stretching with wand/cane: flexion-extension, elevation-adduction	35	5
Isometrics for light strengthening	35	5
Strengthening with TheraBand*		10

*The Hygenic Corp., Akron, Ohio.
From Boardman ND III, Cofield RH, Bengtson KA, et al: Rehabilitation after total shoulder arthroplasty, *J Arthroplasty* 6:483, 2001.

major portion of the medial collateral ligament complex. The anterior bundle inserts along the medial aspect of the coronoid process (sublime tubercle) and is taut with the elbow in flexion and extension. The posterior bundle is taut during flexion.

The lateral ligament complex consists of the radial collateral ligament, the lateral ulnar collateral ligament, the accessory lateral collateral ligament, and the annular ligament (Fig. 10.25B). The radial collateral ligament arises from the lateral epicondyle and inserts into the annular ligament along with fibers of the capsule. The lateral ulnar collateral ligament consists of the posterior fibers of the radial collateral ligament, which extend superficially to and across the annular ligament, inserting on the crista supinatoris (supinator crest) of the ulna. The accessory lateral collateral ligament arises from the lateral epicondyle and inserts into the inferior margin of the annular ligament. It is taut when the elbow is stressed in varus. The annular ligament arises and inserts on the anterior and posterior margins of the lesser sigmoid notch of the ulna and stabilizes the radial head adjacent to the ulna. Of these, the lateral ulnar collateral ligament is most crucial to maintaining elbow stability.

In extension, the anterior capsule provides approximately 70% of soft-tissue restraint to distraction. Valgus stress in extension is divided equally among the medial collateral ligament, capsule, and joint surface. Varus stress in extension is limited equally by the joint articulation, lateral ulnar collateral ligament, and capsule. In flexion, the medial collateral ligament complex provides a soft-tissue restraint to distraction and is the prime stabilizing structure resisting valgus stress, with the radial head providing a secondary restraint. The joint articulation provides about 75% of the stability and resistance to varus stressing with the elbow flexed.

Many activities involving the elbow produce valgus forces. An intact medial collateral ligament and intact radial head are essential to prevent dislocation of the normal elbow joint. The ulnohumeral joint maintains stability as the elbow flexes and extends, whereas the radiocapitellar joint resists valgus stress and transmits vertical loading forces of pushing and lifting.

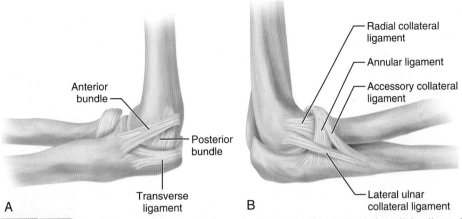

FIGURE 10.25 Collateral ligaments of elbow. **A,** Classic representation of medial collateral ligament complex consisting of anterior and posterior oblique bundle and transverse component. **B,** Typical pattern of more variable radial collateral ligament complex consists of contribution from humerus to ulna, which O'Driscoll and Morrey termed *lateral ulnar collateral ligament.*

The elbow is composed of three joints. One is the ulno-humeral joint, which is a hinged, or ginglymoid, joint. The others consist of the radiocapitellar and proximal radioulnar articulations, which are pivoted, or trochoid, joints, allowing 2 degrees of freedom. This articulation has been termed a *trochoginglymoid joint,* or "sloppy" hinge.

Motion in the elbow involves rotation of the ulna around the humerus during flexion and extension and rotation of the radius around the ulna during supination and pronation. The instant center of flexion and extension for the elbow is at the center of concentric circles formed by the lateral projection of the capitellum and trochlea of the distal humerus. It is 2 to 3 mm in diameter and is located in the center of the trochlea when viewed from the lateral aspect (Fig. 10.26). The axis of rotation of the elbow lies anterior to the humeral midline and on a line drawn along the anterior cortex of the humerus. The carrying angle of the elbow varies from 11 degrees of valgus with the elbow in full extension to 6 degrees of varus with the elbow in full flexion (Fig. 10.27). The joint surfaces slide until the extremes of full flexion and extension are reached, and then bony impingement occurs. The transverse axis of rotation of the radiocapitellar joint coincides with the ulno-humeral axis. The longitudinal axis of the forearm passes through the radial head proximally and the ulnar head distally and is oblique to the longitudinal axes of the radius and ulna. The normal range of motion of the elbow is from 0 degrees (full extension) to approximately 150 degrees (full flexion).

The anatomic restraints of elbow motion include the geometry of the joint; the surrounding bone, capsule, ligaments, and muscles; impaction of the olecranon process on the olecranon fossa, impaction of coronoid against the coronoid fossa, and impaction of the radial head against the radial fossa. Pronation-supination is limited by passive resistance of the stretched muscles and the ligaments and impingement of the flexor pollicis longus against the finger flexors.

The contact surfaces of the elbow change with different elbow positions. In full extension, the contact surfaces are on the inferomedial aspect of the ulna. In other positions, most of the joint contact occurs along the trochlear notch, which passes from posterolateral to anteromedial. Electromyographic studies of elbow muscle activity show that the brachialis is active in most ranges of elbow motion and is the "workhorse" of flexion.

The forces around the elbow joint also have been extensively studied. Static analyses of the muscle and joint reaction forces suggest that the joint forces are greatest in extension, the flexed elbow being able to tolerate higher loads than the extended elbow. Joint forces also are found to be greatest in pronation. Twisting moments around the humeral axis can be quite high, especially when loads are applied to the hand with the elbow flexed (Fig. 10.28).

Maximal elbow flexion strength occurs at 90 degrees, whereas about one third to one half the maximal lifting force can be generated with the elbow in an extended or a 30-degree flexed position. A force three times the body weight can be developed in the elbow joint during strenuous lifting. As the forces on the elbow are directed toward the anterior or the posterior margins of the joint, the weight-bearing surfaces decrease, maximal compressive forces are elevated, and the stress distribution becomes uneven. For the most part, joint compression forces along the mediolateral plane that cause valgus or varus stress are small compared with the forces in the sagittal plane directed anteriorly or posteriorly. Forces at the distal humerus are greatest in a posterior and proximal direction, causing anterior tilting of a distal humeral component and resorption of the anterior cortex of the humerus when prostheses loosen or when anterior bone grafting is not used. With the elbow extended and axially loaded, approximately 40% of the stress is on the ulnohumeral joint, with 60% on the radiocapitellar joint.

Considerable rotatory torque is developed at the distal humerus when the elbow is flexed to 90 degrees and force is applied to the hand from the side. Tensile forces on the medial collateral ligament can approach two times the body weight, and compressive forces on the radial head can approach three times the body weight. If the radial head is excised, radiocapitellar force is transmitted to the ulna, and the medial collateral ligament tension adds to the ulnohumeral force, which may concentrate the entire load on the lateral edge of the coronoid articular surface (Fig. 10.29). This may apply a force of nine times the body weight to the medial collateral ligament and is associated with progression of ulnohumeral joint degeneration. These forces are applied to the ulnar and

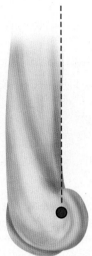

FIGURE 10.26 Axis of rotation of elbow in flexion and extension is through center of trochlea, collinear with distal anterior cortex of humerus.

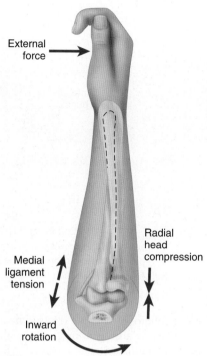

FIGURE 10.28 Forces at elbow during inward rotation.

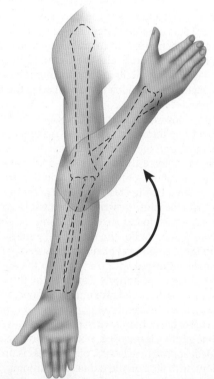

FIGURE 10.27 Carrying angle of elbow changes from valgus angle in full extension to varus angle in full flexion. (Redrawn from Morrey BF, Chao EYS: Passive motion of the elbow joint, *J Bone Joint Surg* 58A:501, 1976.)

humeral components of a prosthetic arthroplasty if the radial head is resected and not replaced.

Goals for the ideal elbow arthroplasty include a painless, stable, mobile, durable, revisable, and reproducible prosthesis. It should preserve the olecranon, have a carrying angle, sacrifice as little bone as possible, provide stable fixation on the supporting bone, be free of moving or multiple parts, be durable

and biologically inert, leave minimal dead space, be relatively easy to implant, be readily available without need for custom implants, and provide joint stability and a good range of movement. The main problems in design have been achievement of long-term bony fixation without loosening, minimization of polyethylene wear, and the development of satisfactory materials able to withstand high loads in active patients.

TYPES OF ARTHROPLASTY

Three types of arthroplasties are discussed in this chapter: debridement, interpositional, and prosthetic. Depending on the rigidity of humeral component fixation to the ulnar component, the implant arthroplasties are designated as constrained, semiconstrained, and unconstrained. Constrained, metal-to-metal prostheses include the Stanmore, Dee, McKee, GSB I (Gschwend, Scheier, and Bähler), and Mazas designs and generally have a metal-to-metal hinge with polymethyl methacrylate bone cement fixation. These implants have been largely abandoned, and the technique of their implantation is not described here.

The semiconstrained prostheses are two-part or three-part prostheses that have a metal-to-high-molecular weight polyethylene articulation, which may be connected with a locking pin or with a snap-fit device. The semiconstrained hinged prostheses have built-in laxity to provide for dissipation of forces. The GSB III, HSS-Osteonics, Coonrad-Morrey, Nexel, and Discovery prostheses are examples of semiconstrained devices (Fig. 10.30). The linked prostheses are highly versatile because they do not depend on intact ligamentous structures for stability. As such, they can be applied to a number of end-stage pathologies, including posttraumatic arthritis, chronic instability, and tumor reconstruction.

The unconstrained prostheses are two- or three-part devices consisting of metal articulating with high-molecular weight polyethylene. They usually do not have a snap-fit,

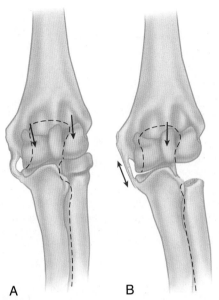

FIGURE 10.29 **A,** Forearm bones in equilibrium against humerus during flexion, no collateral tension. **B,** Forces concentrate on lateral edge of coronoid process after radial head excision. Medial ligament tension prevents valgus deformity.

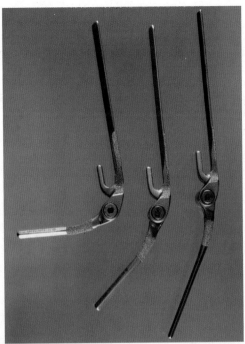

FIGURE 10.30 Coonrad-Morrey total elbow prostheses in different sizes. (*Right* from Herren DB, O'Driscoll SW, An KN: Role of collateral ligaments in the GSB-linked total elbow prosthesis, *J Shoulder Elbow Surg* 10:260, 2001; *middle* from Kraay MJ, Figgie MP, Inglis AE, et al: Primary semiconstrained total arthroplasty: survival analysis of 113 consecutive cases, *J Bone Joint Surg* 76B:636, 1994.)

link, or pin connection. Some designs consist of a resurfacing device, and some have stems for the humeral component. The unconstrained implant arthroplasties include the capitellocondylar (Ewald), London, Kudo, Ishizuki, Lowe-Miller, Wadsworth, Souter-Strathclyde, and Latitude designs. Of note, the Latitude is a hybrid device that can be converted to a semiconstrained articulation with a locking ring. Outcomes and overall complication rates are comparable with other implants, but loosening or disengagement of the radial head component has been a persistent concern. Most of these prostheses represent an attempt to anatomically duplicate the articular surfaces of the elbow. They restore the joint's anterior offset from the humerus and have a single center of rotation. All resurfacing or unconstrained prostheses require normal intact ligaments and anterior capsule as well as appropriate static alignment. If bone loss or capsuloligamentous destruction is extensive, an unconstrained prosthesis generally cannot be used.

Early clinical reports of experience with many of the prosthetic designs were preliminary evaluations of small numbers of patients, with no standardized method of assessment. Some reports mixed different prostheses and included patients with posttraumatic arthritis, osteoarthritis, and rheumatoid arthritis. These factors have limited the objective comparison of the different implants. More recent reports allow better understanding of the advantages and limitations of the various prosthetic designs.

■ DEBRIDEMENT ARTHROPLASTY

Debridement arthroplasty for degenerative elbow conditions is recommended for younger, higher-demand patients who may not be able to comply with the lifting restrictions associated with total elbow replacement. A lateral approach or combined medial and lateral approaches can be used to remove loose bodies and to debride osteophytes in a painful, stiff osteoarthritic elbow. A medial approach has been

recommended because of the frequent concomitant ulnar nerve symptoms and the importance of evaluating for and removing osteophytes from the medial edge of the coronoid and olecranon rather than their respective processes (see Technique 10.4). Arthroscopic debridement also has been described; this is discussed more fully in other chapter.

DEBRIDEMENT ARTHROPLASTY

TECHNIQUE 10.4

(WADA ET AL.)

■ With the patient supine and the involved extremity on an arm board, make a curved posteromedial incision along the distal border of the pronator teres, passing 1 cm posterior to the medial epicondyle and extending 4 cm proximal to the olecranon process (Fig. 10.31A,B). Protect the sensory branches before ulnar nerve isolation and decompression.

■ Elevate the flexor-pronator origin and anterior capsule to expose the anterior humeroulnar and radiocapitellar joints (Fig. 10.31C).

■ Use rongeurs or chisels to remove osteophytes from the coronoid process, the medial edge of the coronoid, the coronoid fossa, and the radial fossa. If needed for osteophyte excision, retract the anterior band of the medial collateral ligament medially, but preserve it (Fig. 10.31D).

■ Elevate the ulnar nerve, excise the posterior bundle of the medial collateral ligament, and elevate the triceps posteriorly for debridement of the posterior humeroulnar joint and the olecranon fossa (Fig. 10.31E).

■ Dissect between the triceps and the brachioradialis to expose the lateral condyle and joint capsule (Fig. 10.31F).

■ Expose the radial head by opening longitudinally the radial collateral ligament.

■ Elevate the anterior joint capsule subperiosteally and remove any osteophytes.

■ Alternatively, carefully elevate the muscular fibers of the brachioradialis, extensor carpi radialis longus, and brachialis off the anterior joint capsule before excising the capsule and performing the joint debridement.

■ Preserve the lateral ulnar collateral ligament by keeping the capsular dissection anterior to a line connecting the midpoint of the lateral epicondyle to the midportion of the radiocapitellar joint.

■ Carry the dissection posterior to the lateral epicondyle and proximally along the anterior border of the triceps laterally to expose the posterior fat pad and the olecranon fossa (Fig. 10.31G). Loose bodies and osteophytes often are encountered posteriorly, and dissection distal to the lateral epicondyle into the posterior radiocapitellar joint is required for completion of the lateral debridement.

■ Copiously irrigate the joint after satisfactory motion has been obtained.

■ Obtain hemostasis as much as possible and cover raw cancellous bone surfaces with paraffin.

■ If the flexor-pronator group has been detached, approximate it to a soft-tissue cuff or to bone through drill holes.

■ Manage the ulnar nerve according to its behavior through the elbow range of motion achieved. If there is minimal tension on the nerve throughout the motion arc and the

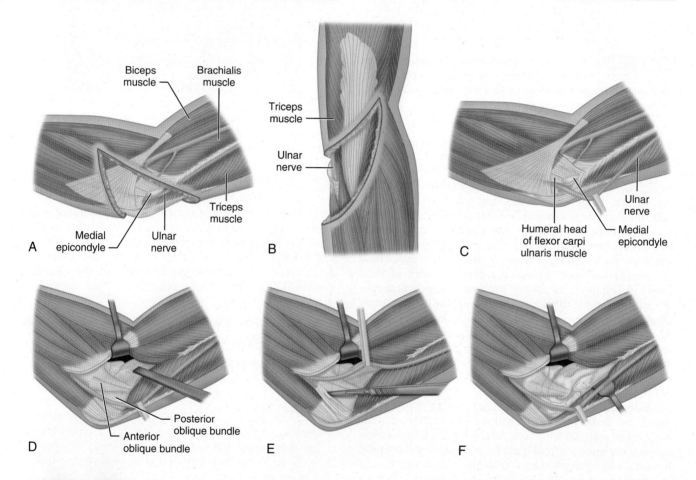

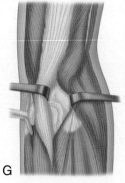

FIGURE 10.31 Debridement arthroplasty of elbow (see text). **A** and **B,** Incision. **C,** Elevation of flexor-pronator origin. **D,** Exposure of anterior elbow compartment. **E,** Excision of posterior oblique bundle and posterior capsule. **F,** Exposure of anterior, medial, and posterior aspects of ulnohumeral joint. **G,** Exposure and excision of osteophytes on medial aspect of olecranon and olecranon fossa. **SEE TECHNIQUE 10.4.**

nerve is not forcefully subluxing over the medial epicondyle, simply leave it decompressed in situ. If ulnar nerve subluxation is forceful or nerve tension is excessive with elbow flexion, perform an anterior transposition procedure.

- Place suction drains and close the incisions in routine fashion.

POSTOPERATIVE CARE Physical therapy is begun on postoperative day 1, and the drains are removed. Static splints frequently are used to prevent the recurrence of an elbow flexion contracture.

More recently, some authors have advocated arthroscopic elbow debridement for degenerative conditions. Adams et al. reported 42 elbows followed for a minimum of 2 years after arthroscopic debridement and capsular release for osteoarthritis. The authors reported significant gains in flexion, extension, supination, pain, and Mayo Elbow Performance

Scores. Complications were uncommon, and 81% of patients achieved good or excellent results. Although these early reports have been promising with this so-called osteocapsular arthroplasty, further study is needed to determine the long-term effectiveness of this procedure.

■ INTERPOSITION (FASCIAL) ARTHROPLASTY

Interposition arthroplasty is another intervention to treat degenerative elbow conditions in patients who have a contraindication to implant placement. The primary indication may be loss of motion or incapacitating pain or both. Loss of motion can be caused by inflammatory or degenerative arthritis, sepsis, burns, or trauma. Ankylosis can be bony or fibrous. Incapacitating pain in a young, active patient may be the most compelling indication. If the pain and restriction of motion are the results of sepsis, a careful preoperative evaluation must determine that the infection is under control. The best indication for interposition arthroplasty is painful, post-traumatic loss of motion in the absence of infection. Because interposition arthroplasty does not inherently contribute to

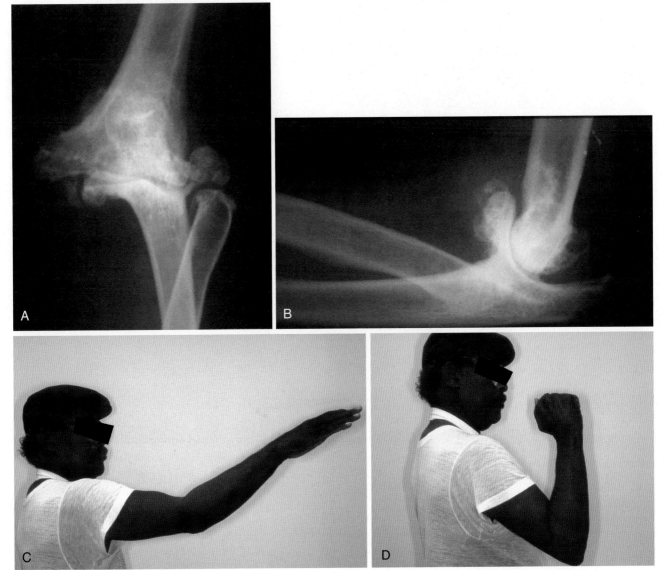

FIGURE 10.32 **A** and **B,** After interposition fascial arthroplasty. **C,** Extension 20 years after surgery. **D,** Flexion 20 years after surgery.

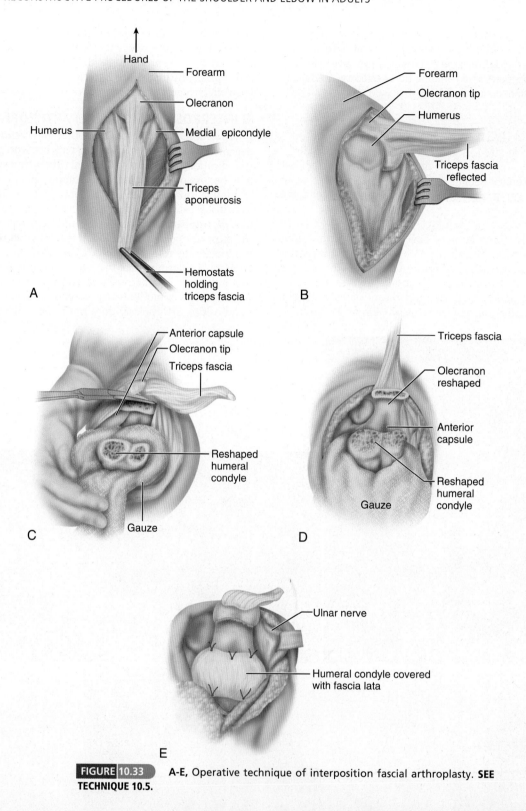

FIGURE 10.33 A-E, Operative technique of interposition fascial arthroplasty. **SEE TECHNIQUE 10.5.**

elbow stability, instability is not a good indication for this procedure.

Identification of appropriate patients for interposition arthroplasty is difficult and involves an evaluation of the underlying pathologic process and the motivation of the patient. To achieve success, the condition of the soft tissues surrounding the elbow must be as normal as possible. Weak, atrophic muscles; thin, delicate skin; and extensive scarring or adherence of skin to underlying bone may prevent a satisfactory result. The forearm musculature must be in good condition so that postoperative strength and stability can be achieved through the rehabilitation of these muscles. Furthermore, it is important to preserve as much bone stock as possible and to maintain the integrity of the capsuloligamentous and muscular soft tissues surrounding the elbow joint.

Interposition arthroplasty can be considered in younger patients with posttraumatic, degenerative, or inflammatory arthritis (Fig. 10.32). It can be effective in these patients and remains an alternative to total elbow arthroplasty.

INTERPOSITION ARTHROPLASTY
TECHNIQUE 10.5

- Beginning proximal to the elbow joint, make an incision 15 to 20 cm long on the posterior aspect of the arm and forearm just medial to the midline of the limb.
- Elevate the deep fascia laterally 2 to 3 cm and expose the broad aponeurosis of the triceps muscle (Fig. 10.33A).
- To approach the joint, one of two methods can be used. In the first, enter the Kocher interval and carry the dissection along the lateral head of the triceps, taking care not to proceed so proximally as to endanger the radial nerve.
- In the second method, a triceps-splitting midline approach can be used.
- After either approach, with a periosteal elevator, strip the periosteum from the distal third of the posterior surface of the humerus, retract it medially and laterally, and expose the radial head and olecranon (Fig. 10.33B).
- If the joint is fused, osteotomize the fusion between the olecranon and humerus and between the radial head and humerus, carefully protecting the ulnar nerve.
- Flex the joint and displace the radius and ulna medially.
- Fashion the distal end of the humerus into one condyle convex from anteriorly to posteriorly (Fig. 10.33C). Although no attempt is made to reproduce the contours of the capitellum and trochlea, some mediolateral stability can be achieved if the distal humerus is shaped into an inverted V.
- With a curved chisel, excise superficial bone to deepen and lengthen the trochlear notch of the ulna and cut away the head of the radius to the level of the distal part of this notch (Fig. 10.33D).
- Smooth all surfaces with a rasp.
- Prepare an Achilles tendon allograft by folding it in half crosswise with its smooth surface on the inside and anchor its folded edge to the anterior part of the capsule with three sutures, one on each side and one in the middle. Other authors prefer to use an acellular dermis matrix patch, which can be prepared in a similar way.
- Place the proximal half of the fascia over the newly fashioned hu\meral condyle and with interrupted sutures fasten the medial and lateral edges of this half to the adjacent soft tissues well over the medial and lateral borders of the humerus; if the soft tissues are insufficient, secure the fascia by sutures passed through holes drilled in these borders.
- As an alternative, use suture anchors to expedite the attachment of the fascia to the humerus and olecranon and the attachment of the capsuloligamentous tissues to the humerus.
- Place the distal half of the fascia over the trochlear notch and suture it in place (Fig. 10.33E). (In the presence of synostosis between the proximal radius and ulna, excise enough bone to permit free rotation of the radius.)
- Insert a fold of the same fascia between the radius and ulna and invest the radial head, or place a separate sheet of fascia around the head and fix it with a purse-string suture.
- Reduce the joint and, with the elbow flexed to 90 degrees, close the capsule from distally to proximally. Apply a long-arm posterior splint or cast with the elbow in 90 degrees of flexion.

POSTOPERATIVE CARE The elbow is immobilized in 90 degrees of flexion on an elbow splint or in a cast for 10 to 14 days to prevent rotation. When the wound has healed completely, a hinged elbow brace is applied. The brace is removed for 1 to 2 hours three or four times a day for active exercises to develop the flexors and extensors of the elbow and the flexors of the fingers. At 6 weeks after surgery, the brace can be discarded during the day and a sling used as necessary for support, but the splint should be worn at night until a useful range of motion in the elbow and good strength in the muscles have been regained; this usually is at 12 weeks after surgery. The patient must continue active exercises for at least 6 months. Maximal strength and motion usually are regained within 2 years after surgery.

The prognosis after elbow interposition remains guarded. Larson and Morrey reported that only 29% of 45 patients achieved a good or excellent result on 45 elbows at 6-year follow-up, although there were significant improvements in pain, motion, and functional scores. Preoperative instability was associated with worse functional outcomes.

The functional results and the radiographic appearance of the elbow after interpositional arthroplasty correlate poorly (see Fig. 10.32). In general, the fair and poor results of fascial arthroplasty have been caused by persistent pain, loss of motion (reankylosis), and excessive instability.

Complications of interposition arthroplasty in the elbow include bony resorption, triceps rupture, heterotopic bone formation, instability, infection, and seroma formation in the thigh donor site if fascia lata is used for interposition material. Bony resorption may occur at the distal humeral condyles and may contribute to instability. Triceps rupture, which may be related to the surgical exposure, is an uncommon complication. It can be minimized or prevented by using approaches that preserve the triceps insertion, such as those described above. Excessive heterotopic bone formation limits motion. Although excision of the heterotopic bone may improve motion, bone formation may recur, regardless of most methods used to prevent it.

Treatment of infection after fascial arthroplasty of the elbow should be prompt and aggressive. If the infection is superficial or if cellulitis develops, oral antibiotics, elevation of the elbow, and immobilization may allow resolution. In the event of deep infection, open drainage and debridement or excision of the fascial graft may be required. If autogenous fascia lata is used as a graft material, hematoma and seroma formation in the thigh donor site frequently resolve over weeks and rarely require drainage. If drainage is required, aseptic technique is used and needle aspiration may be sufficient. Pain, reankylosis, or instability may cause the procedure to fail. Deterioration may also occur with time. Revision of the fascial arthroplasty may be helpful if the exact nature of the failure can be identified and reasonable success has been reported with revision.

◼ RESECTION AND IMPLANT ARTHROPLASTY OF THE RADIAL HEAD

Radial head resection is a commonly used procedure for symptomatic radiocapitellar dysfunction. The typical indications for radial head resection include isolated radiocapitellar arthritis, mechanical block to pronation-supination in the posttraumatic elbow, and inflammatory arthritis in association with a debridement procedure. Radial head resection also has been described for acute comminuted radial head fractures. Although clinical outcomes at 15 to 17 years of follow-up were good to excellent, posttraumatic changes including elbow and wrist arthrosis, proximal radial migration, and a valgus carrying angle were noted. The radial head is an important secondary stabilizer to valgus stress; therefore we recommend ensuring the lateral collateral ligament complex is intact when considering radial head resection to mitigate postoperative instability and ulnohumeral arthrosis.

Because of the high incidence of associated injury to the lateral collateral ligament complex, radial head replacement is most often used in the treatment of comminuted radial head fractures, but it also can be used for other disorders of the radial head, such as elbow instability and deformity. Silicone (Silastic) implants were introduced in the early 1980s but have been abandoned. Most currently used radial head prostheses are metal, which have been reported to be more durable and help to maintain valgus stability of the elbow after radial head replacement. For patients who are not candidates for radial head arthroplasty, radiocapitellar disc arthroplasty has been described to reduce contact pressure on the lateral coronoid after radial head resection.

▌RADIAL HEAD ARTHROPLASTY

Radial head fractures associated with elbow dislocations frequently are comminuted and cannot be reconstructed. In this situation, the lateral ulnar collateral ligament is injured with concomitant elbow instability, and a radial head replacement is recommended to help stabilize the joint and facilitate early mobilization (Fig. 10.34). These complex injury patterns may include either a coronoid fracture and/or a medial collateral ligament rupture. If the radial head is fractured and the distal radioulnar joint is dislocated (the Essex-Lopresti lesion), proximal migration of the radius after simple radial head excision may be mitigated by a radial head implant.

Attempts to prevent recurrent elbow dislocation, proximal migration of the radius, and excessive instability after certain elbow and forearm axis injuries have led to an evolution of radial head prosthetic designs. Although prosthetic replacement of the radial head after acute fractures of the radial head and after radial head excision with or without elbow synovectomy is controversial, it is reasonable to consider this procedure after injury or disease has caused significant instability of the elbow joint, radial forearm axis, and distal radioulnar joint. In particular, outcomes of comminuted radial head fractures treated with radial head arthroplasty have been reported to be superior to open reduction internal fixation at short-term follow-up. Many types of radial head implants have evolved from a monoblock design to modular prostheses, some of which

incorporate bipolar features and different materials that may lessen the likelihood of capitellar wear from the prosthesis. Both cemented and uncemented designs are available.

The results of complex radial head fractures treated with a variety of monoblock and bipolar prostheses are encouraging. A systematic review concluded that there was no evidence to support one type of radial head implant design over others, with the exception of silicone prostheses that have been abandoned. Mid-term results are emerging that suggest preserved good outcomes of a smooth-stemmed modular implant at an average follow-up of over 8 years. In general, the results are good to excellent in approximately 80% of patients, with a 10% to 20% reduction in strength. Pain relief is typically excellent, elbow extension-flexion and pronation-supination arcs are within 10 to 20 degrees of normal values, and maintenance of ulnohumeral joint stability generally is successful. However, return to a high-level of function, such as a sport or military duties, is mixed with a more guarded prognosis.

One mid-term to long-term concern is a lack of implant durability because of loosening of the stem with either ingrowth or cemented components. Reported in one third or more of press-fit radial head arthroplasties, the loosening causes significant proximal radial osteolysis and generally necessitates removal. Additionally, rigid implant fixation in the proximal radius has been linked to increased complications and revision rates, particularly loosening. Smooth stemmed implants have demonstrated lower rates of proximal radial osteolysis compared with porous ingrowth designs.

Investigation into radial head arthroplasty has focused on implant sizing. An oversized radial head implant can increase tension on the interosseous membrane with subsequent risk of stiffness and pain, and one report found that more than 2 mm of lengthening can increase radiocapitellar contact pressures. Therefore, a radial head replacement should be close to an anatomic substitute. Generally, the proximal edge of the radial head is 0.9 mm distal to the lateral coronoid edge, but patient variability might make imaging of the contralateral elbow useful for sizing purposes. To prevent overstuffing the radiocapitellar joint, the proximal edge of the prosthesis should be level with the lateral coronoid edge (Fig. 10.35). Moon et al. found that overstuffing the radial head implant can decrease the ipsilateral ulnar variance, an indicator that can be used during surgery to judge correct sizing, and Athwal et al. reported that gapping in the lateral ulnohumeral joint line is a reliable indicator of radial head overlengthening. Changes in the medial ulnohumeral joint line, however, were apparent only after 6 mm of overlengthening. After correctly sizing the implant, appropriate reattachment of the lateral ligamentous complex also is necessary to prevent edge binding of the radial head prosthesis (Fig. 10.36).

To correct subtle radiocapitellar malalignment and to reduce stresses at the bone-implant interface, bipolar radial head implants have been described. Both cemented and uncemented bipolar designs have demonstrated favorable results at mid-term follow-up. Comparative studies between unipolar and bipolar radial head replacements have mixed results, with some suggesting higher rates of loosening in bipolar implants. However, two systematic reviews concluded that there are no major differences in clinical outcomes or revision rates among radial head implant designs.

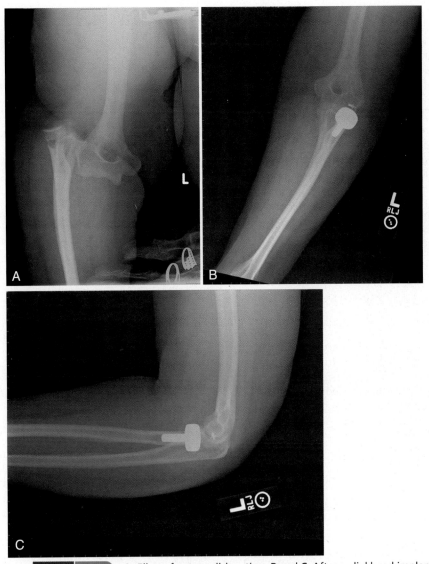

FIGURE 10.34 **A,** Elbow fracture-dislocation. **B** and **C,** After radial head implant.

RADIAL HEAD ARTHROPLASTY

TECHNIQUE 10.6

- Position the patient supine or in the lateral position with the affected elbow up. Prepare and drape the arm to expose the elbow with the arm across the chest. Use a pneumatic tourniquet.
- Begin the incision superior to the lateral epicondyle and extend it distally approximately 6 cm across the joint in the interval between the extensor carpi ulnaris and the anconeus.
- Develop the interval between these two muscles and expose the lateral capsule of the elbow. Often the lateral capsular structures are stripped from the lateral epicondyle, and the interval created from the trauma should allow removal of bone fragments and exposure of the radial neck.

- Incise the annular ligament transversely and cut the radial neck just proximal to the fracture site (Fig. 10.37).
- Prepare the proximal radial medullary canal with burrs or rasps to accept the implant stem.
- Cut the surface of the proximal radius evenly so that contact between it and the collar of the prosthesis is complete.
- Achieve a tight fit of the stem in the medullary canal if using a press-fit implant and ensure that contact with the capitellum is satisfactory. Avoid excessive compression of the implant.
- Carry the forearm through a range of flexion, extension, and rotation to observe the relationship between the capitellum and the implant in anteroposterior and lateral projections.
- After the use of a trial prosthesis has shown satisfactory contact between the capitellum and the prosthesis and a good fit in the radial medullary canal, insert the final prosthesis.

- Make drill holes or use a suture anchor at the capitellar rotation center to reattach lateral capsular structures, including the lateral ulnar collateral ligament to its isometric point with the ulnohumeral joint held reduced.
- Close the wound in layers and protect the elbow with a compression dressing in 90 degrees of flexion.

POSTOPERATIVE CARE The dressing is removed 3 to 5 days after surgery, and gentle passive motion of the elbow is begun immediately after surgery. Aggressive physical therapy should be avoided. If other injuries are present, including distal radioulnar dislocation, ligamentous injuries, or elbow instability, immobilization of the elbow is continued for 2 weeks with gentle passive range of motion thereafter. Mobilization after radioulnar disruption depends on the management of the distal radioulnar joint and its temporary fixation with pins. Active motion is begun under supervision approximately 6 weeks after surgery.

BOX 10.3

Mayo Elbow Performance Score

Pain (45 points)
- None (45 points)
- Mild (30 points)
- Moderate (15 points)
- Severe (0 points)

Range of Motion (20 points)
- Arc > 100 degrees (20 points)
- Arc 50 to 100 degrees (15 points)
- Arc < 50 degrees (5 points)

Stability (10 points)
- Stable (10 points)
- Moderately unstable (5 points)
- Grossly unstable (0 points)

Function (25 points)
- Able to comb hair (5 points)
- Able to feed oneself (5 points)
- Able to perform personal hygiene tasks (5 points)
- Able to put on shirt (5 points)
- Able to put on shoes (5 points)
- Maximal total = 100 points

Outcomes classification: 90-100 = excellent, 75-89 = good, 60-74 = fair, <60 = poor.

TOTAL ELBOW ARTHROPLASTY

Total elbow arthroplasty is among the best studied procedures in orthopaedic surgery. Multiple authors have reported their outcomes with various implant types. The method of evaluating the results of elbow implant arthroplasty is becoming standardized, and rating systems have been established by Morrey et al., the American Shoulder and Elbow Surgeons (ASES), Inglis and Pellicci, and Ewald. The Mayo Elbow Performance Score, which takes into account pain, motion, stability, and daily function, is most commonly used to compare various operative procedures on the elbow (Box 10.3).

■ INDICATIONS

The goals of reconstructive elbow surgery are to restore function through pain relief and restoration of motion and stability. When evaluating candidates for elbow arthroplasty, two factors must be considered: patient selection and implant selection. A stable, painless elbow with preservation of motion in the middle or functional range usually does not require arthroplasty.

Although many indications and relative indications have been reported, deformity and dysfunction without pain are not indications for surgery. Rather, the primary indications for total elbow arthroplasty are pain and/or instability. In particular, an unreconstructible distal humeral fracture in an elderly patient is an increasingly common indication for total elbow arthroplasty. Rheumatoid arthritis with radiographic evidence of joint destruction, which is too far advanced to benefit from radial head excision and synovectomy, especially in patients with painful instability and painful stiffness that limit activities, is generally considered to be an indication. However, the emergence of immunomodulating disease-remitting agents for rheumatoid arthritis has been largely responsible for a decrease in the number of total elbow arthroplasties performed for this indication. Elderly patients with end-stage posttraumatic sequelae also are acceptable candidates for total elbow replacement. Bony or fibrous ankylosis with the elbow in a poorly functioning position is another indication for elbow arthroplasty. In patients with rheumatoid arthritis, arthroplasty should be considered only after medical treatment has failed and the disease has advanced to show bony changes, which is beyond the stage at which synovectomy would be beneficial.

The best candidate for total elbow replacement has been described as a patient with severely painful and disabling rheumatoid arthritis with altered articular architecture; however, the decision to proceed with arthroplasty must be made cautiously because of the high complication rate. Patients with rheumatoid arthritis who have limitation of motion, ankylosis, instability, or incapacitating pain generally do better after implant arthroplasty than do patients with posttraumatic arthritis.

Selection of the type of prosthetic implant depends to a great extent on the state of the capsuloligamentous structures around the elbow and the integrity of the musculature and the amount of bone remaining at the elbow joint. Generally, the more bone remaining and the more stable the joint, the more suitable the joint is for replacement with a resurfacing or unconstrained prosthetic implant. More constrained prosthetic designs should be selected for patients with injury to the stabilizing ligaments and capsule of the joint, atrophic musculature, and loss of considerable bone stock.

Ewald suggested that one absolute contraindication to prosthetic elbow implant arthroplasty is a history of previous elbow sepsis. Because of the design of his capitellocondylar implant, he also considered a previous fascial or other interpositional arthroplasty and previous hinged arthroplasty to be

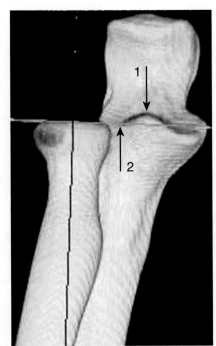

FIGURE 10.35   Radial head implant (see text). Three-dimensional CT scans used to determine plane defined by distal margins of articular surface of radial head. *Arrow 1,* Central ridge of coronoid process. *Arrow 2,* Lateral edge of coronoid process. (From Doornberg JN, Linzel DS, Zurakowski D, et al: Reference points for radial head prosthesis size, *J Hand Surg* 31A:53, 2006.)

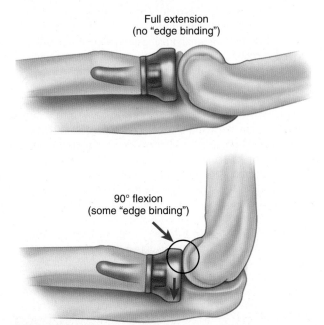

Full extension
(no "edge binding")

90° flexion
(some "edge binding")

FIGURE 10.36   Radial head implant (see text). Implant should be checked for stability during elbow motion to ensure that any potential edge binding of implant and capitellum does not occur.

absolute contraindications to the use of the capitellocondylar device. Relative contraindications to the use of an unconstrained resurfacing arthroplasty included excessive bone loss, as in giant rheumatoid cysts, deficiency of the trochlear notch of the ulna, and posttraumatic or degenerative arthritis.

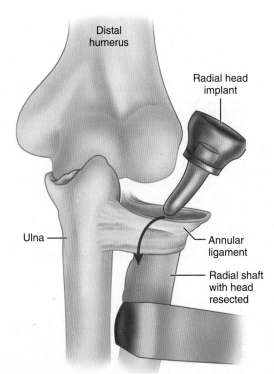

FIGURE 10.37   Radial head arthroplasty (see text). Annular ligament is incised transversely to allow end-on view of canal for implant placement. **SEE TECHNIQUE 10.6.**

Coonrad and Morrey considered infection, excessive use of the elbow, ankylosis of the ipsilateral shoulder, and the presence of neurotrophic joints to be contraindications. Kudo et al. concluded that extensive bone loss on either side of the joint and poorly functioning flexor and extensor mechanisms were contraindications. Morrey et al. reported that no consistently reliable total prosthetic arthroplasty is available for patients with posttraumatic degenerative arthritis in the elbow. However, in these salvage situations this does not always represent an absolute contraindication to total elbow arthroplasty.

■ SURGICAL TECHNIQUE
▌SEMICONSTRAINED (LINKED) TOTAL ELBOW ARTHROPLASTY

Most semiconstrained hinged prostheses use a high-molecular-weight polyethylene bushing and titanium humeral and ulnar components. They are designed with 7 degrees of rotary and side-to-side laxity. Humeral and ulnar stems match the shapes of the medullary canals. The triangular humeral stem is flattened near the base at the inferior flatter and wider portion of the medullary canal of the humerus. The large medullary stem enhances rigid fixation. The stem contour and distal anterior flange increase resistance to torque. Careful bone removal in the intercondylar area of the humerus is necessary to allow a tight fit of the humeral prosthesis. The humeral and ulnar components typically are joined with a linking mechanism that, if necessary, can be disarticulated. The axis of rotation of these prostheses are near the anatomic center when the device is properly implanted. Because the components are relatively large, a disadvantage in smaller patients is that they occasionally require manufacture of custom components.

COONRAD-MORREY PROSTHESIS

TECHNIQUE 10.7

- Place the patient supine with the affected arm in front of the chest and with a sandbag beneath the ipsilateral shoulder (Fig. 10.38A). Alternatively, the patient can be placed in the lateral decubitus position. When preparing and draping the arm, leave the entire elbow area and forearm exposed so that the prosthesis can be inserted properly. Use a sterile tourniquet and exsanguinate the limb before inflating the tourniquet.
- Use a straight posteromedial incision.
- Identify the ulnar nerve, gently mobilize and protect it, and transpose it anteriorly after the operation.
- Carefully elevate the triceps mechanism in continuity with the periosteum over the proximal ulna and olecranon to avoid transection or separation of the triceps mechanism (Fig. 10.38B).
- Reflect the triceps mechanism to the radial side of the olecranon to expose the proximal ulna. Some authors prefer to keep the triceps insertion intact to avoid the risk of weakness and rupture after surgery—the so-called *triceps-on* approach. These techniques include either a Kocher approach with partial elevation of the triceps insertion or the para-olecranon approach described by Studer et al. One comparative report found that total elbow arthroplasty performed with the triceps-on technique resulted in similar outcomes and cement mantle quality as the triceps-off approach and with no risk of tendon rupture. As such, we prefer a triceps-on technique when performing total elbow arthroplasty.
- Release the collateral ligaments on each side of the elbow.
- Rotate the forearm laterally to dislocate the elbow and allow exposure of the distal humerus.
- Remove the midportion of the trochlea with an oscillating saw to allow access to the medullary canal of the humerus (Fig. 10.38C). Identify the canal with a burr applied to the roof of the olecranon fossa (Fig. 10.38D).
- Remove the cortex of the olecranon fossa and open the medullary canal to a size sufficient to allow a twist reamer (Fig. 10.38E).
- Preserve the medial and lateral portions of the supracondylar columns during the preparation of the distal humerus. Use the medial and lateral supracondylar columns for reference during the bone preparation to ensure satisfactory orientation and alignment.
- Place the alignment stem down the medullary canal with a T-handle (Fig. 10.38F).
- Remove the handle and apply the cutting block with the appropriate right or left placement of the side arm of the cutting block. Allow the side arm to rest on the capitellum to provide for the proper depth of the cut (Fig. 10.38G).
- Use an oscillating saw to remove the trochlear and capitellar bone to correspond with the size of the appropriate cutting block. If the bone is osteoporotic, score the cortex with electrocautery, using the cutting block as a guide.

- Remove any remaining bone after the cut with a rongeur. Avoid injury to the medial and lateral supracondylar columns to avoid fracture. Remove the bone carefully, small amounts at a time, repeatedly inserting the trial prosthesis until the margins of the prosthesis are exactly level with the epicondylar articular surface margins on the capitellar and trochlear sides. Also ensure that the rotational center of the trial prosthesis corresponds to the native center of rotation of the elbow.
- Hollow the flattened areas of the distal humerus to allow a precise fit of the shoulders of the humeral stem by curettage of cancellous bone from the epicondylar and distal flaring portions of the humerus. This should allow satisfactory cement fixation (Fig. 10.38H).
- Remove the tip of the olecranon.
- Use a high-speed burr and remove subchondral and cancellous bone to allow identification of the ulnar medullary canal.
- Remove additional bone from the tip of the olecranon to form a notch for placement of the serial reamers to be introduced down the medullary canal of the ulna (Fig. 10.38I). Use the appropriate right or left ulnar rasps as needed.
- Select the appropriate size rasp and use a burr to remove the subchondral bone gently around the coronoid process (Fig. 10.38J).
- After the proximal ulna and distal humerus have been prepared, insert a trial prosthesis and evaluate the elbow for complete flexion and extension.
- If there is a limitation to full extension, release the anterior capsule and evaluate the trial components again until the elbow can be straightened.
- Before inserting the final prosthesis with cement, use the trial prosthesis to determine if the radial head impinges on the prosthesis. If it is present, resect the radial head.
- Fashion a bone graft from the previously cut trochlea to be placed behind the anterior humeral flange during component implantation. The graft usually is 2 to 3 mm thick, 1.5 cm long, and 1 cm wide. Elevate the brachialis from the anterior humerus to provide a bed for placement of the bone graft.
- Clean the medullary canals of the humerus and ulna with a pulsatile lavage irrigating system and dry the canals.
- Place cement restrictors in the humeral and ulnar canals.
- Use a cement gun with flexible tubing to insert the cement into the canals (Fig. 10.38K). Inject the cement early in the polymerization process. Inject the cement into the ulna, leaving 1 to 2 cm of medullary canal unfilled to allow for back flow of the cement.
- Insert the ulnar component first as far distally as the coronoid process. Align the center of the ulnar component with the center of the greater sigmoid notch (Fig. 10.38L). Remove the excess cement from around the ulnar component.
- Insert cement into the humeral canal, leaving about 1 cm of canal unfilled to allow for back flow of cement (Fig. 10.38M).
- While the cement is still soft, place the humeral component down to a point that allows articulation of the device and the placement of the axis pin. Place the bone graft against the distal humerus beneath the soft tissue (Fig. 10.38N). At this point, the bone graft is partially covered by the anterior flange of the humeral component.

- Articulate the humeral device by placing the axis pin through the humerus and ulna. Secure it with a split locking ring (Fig. 10.38O). There will be a confirmatory click when the locking device engages.
- Impact the humeral component into the humerus so that the axis of rotation of the prosthesis is at the level of the normal anatomic axis of rotation (Fig. 10.38P,Q). This usually is accomplished when the base of the anterior flange is flush with the anterior bone of the olecranon fossa.
- Check the bone graft to ensure that it is still behind the anterior humeral flange and secure between it and humerus.
- Place the arm in maximal extension while the cement hardens. While this occurs, carefully remove excess cement.
- Deflate the tourniquet and obtain hemostasis. Leave a drain in the depths of the wound.
- If the triceps was released during the approach, drill holes in an X configuration through the olecranon to accept the sutures to repair the triceps mechanism with a locking running stitch (Fig. 10.38R). Also place a transverse suture through the olecranon and tie it over the top of the approximated triceps to provide additional fixation. Close the remainder of the triceps with absorbable suture.
- Apply a compression dressing with the elbow in full extension and a long anterior splint to minimize pressure on the posterior incision.

POSTOPERATIVE CARE The extremity is elevated overnight with the elbow above the shoulder. The drain and compressive dressing are removed the day after surgery. If the triceps was released during the approach, we limit elbow flexion past 90 degrees for the first 6 weeks, and active elbow extension must be avoided for 3 months. In patients who had a triceps-on approach, passive range of motion can be initiated early through a comfortable arc as tolerated. In either approach a sling is used and instructions in activities of daily living are provided by an occupational therapist. Strengthening exercises are avoided, and the patient is encouraged to avoid lifting more than 5 lb with the involved arm for the first 3 months after surgery. Thereafter, lifting is restricted to 10 pounds. Despite these recommendations, most patients, particularly young men and those with posttraumatic disorders, have been shown to engage in higher demand activities, despite receiving these instructions.

■ OUTCOMES

Long-term (10 to 20 years) outcomes of semiconstrained and unconstrained total elbow implant arthroplasty are now available; 5- and 10-year survival rates have been reported at 90% and 81%, respectively, in a study of the Norwegian joint arthroplasty database. However, the survival rate dropped to 71% at 15 years and 61% at 20 years. A separate study similarly found a 67% survival rate at 20 years. In the review of results for implant arthroplasty, several generalizations seem appropriate. If the available published reports of semiconstrained and unconstrained arthroplasties are considered, an average of 75% satisfactory results have been achieved, but

implant survival and complication rates lag behind those for other forms of total joint arthroplasty. Furthermore, quality of life indices have been reported to be improved after total elbow arthroplasty. If reports of the earlier hinged designs are excluded, the satisfactory results approach 90%. The best results from total elbow arthroplasty are obtained when the procedure is done for rheumatoid arthritis, where satisfactory results average about 90%. In contrast, total elbow arthroplasty for posttraumatic sequelae is generally less successful. Caution is warranted when considering total elbow arthroplasty for younger, more active patients, especially if younger than 50 years old, because of the very high complication rate.

■ UNCONSTRAINED TOTAL ELBOW ARTHROPLASTY

Numerous unconstrained total elbow implants have been in use, most with various modifications. With unconstrained "surface replacement" arthroplasties, an overall average of nearly 85% satisfactory results has been reported, and 90% of patients may achieve satisfactory results when patient selection and surgical techniques are satisfactory.

Patients with rheumatoid arthritis constitute the largest group treated with unconstrained prostheses. Aseptic loosening was found in 10% of 522 Souter-Strathclyde implants used in patients with inflammatory arthritis at average follow-up of 6.6 years. Aside from aseptic loosening, the survivorship was 96% and 84% at 5 and 10 years. Trail et al., after their experience with 309 Souter-Strathclyde total elbow arthroplasties in rheumatoid patients, recommended that a longer humeral component be used because 25 of their 32 revisions were for humeral component loosening. Despite lucency rates of 100% and 8.9% for humeral and ulnar components, a 90% survival rate at 16 years with an average Mayo score improvement from 43 to 77 was reported with the use of Kudo type 3 total elbow implants.

Ulnar nerve palsy, deep infection, wound complications, stiffness, and instability are common problems encountered with all these devices. The more prevailing concern underlying all these implants and other unlinked implants more recently introduced into the market is the high rate of radiographic lucencies around the humeral and ulnar components. Multiple recent reports have found that a semiconstrained device demonstrated better longevity than unconstrained replacements.

■ SEMICONSTRAINED TOTAL ELBOW ARTHROPLASTY

Semiconstrained total elbow replacement for rheumatoid arthritis has been well studied. Early reports indicated good results in about 85% of patients, with implant survival of 92%, although complication rates were relatively high (14% to 26%). A more recent comparison of the outcomes of unconstrained and semiconstrained total elbow arthroplasties for rheumatoid arthritis reported a 93% survivorship at 5 years and 76% at 10 years for the unconstrained device. In contrast, 5-year retention of the semiconstrained device has been reported to be 97% to 100%, and 10- and 20-year survival rates of 92% and 68%, respectively, have been published. The unconstrained device had high rates of loosening (18%) and instability (9%) that accounted for the inferior survival rate. Other reports also have found an advantage to semiconstrained designs over unconstrained implants.

Total elbow arthroplasty for distal humeral fractures in the elderly has been shown to be effective in properly selected patients. Patients older than age 65 years with small

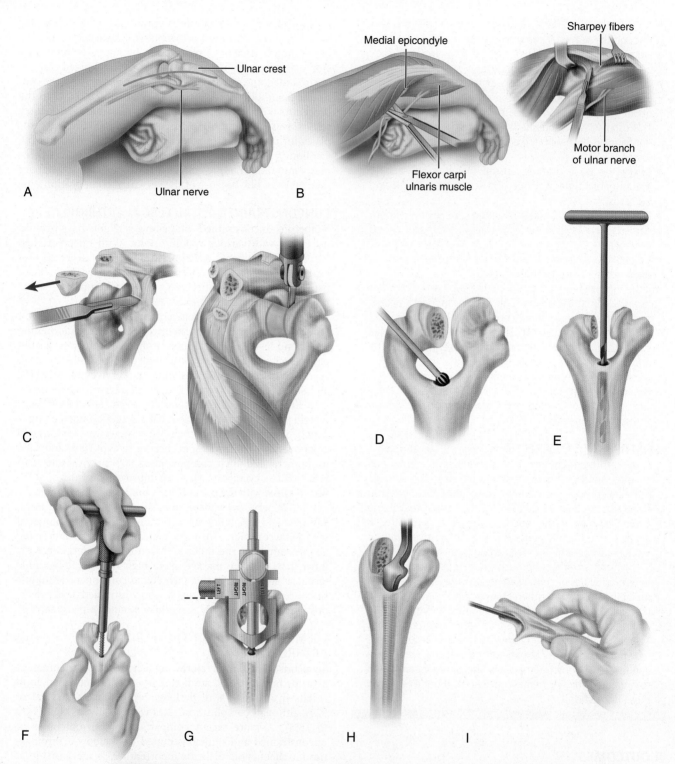

FIGURE 10.38   **A-R,** Coonrad-Morrey total elbow arthroplasty. (Redrawn from Coonrad RW, Morrey BJ: *Coonrad/Morrey total elbow: surgical technique*, Warsaw, IN, 1988, Zimmer USA.) **SEE TECHNIQUE 10.7.**

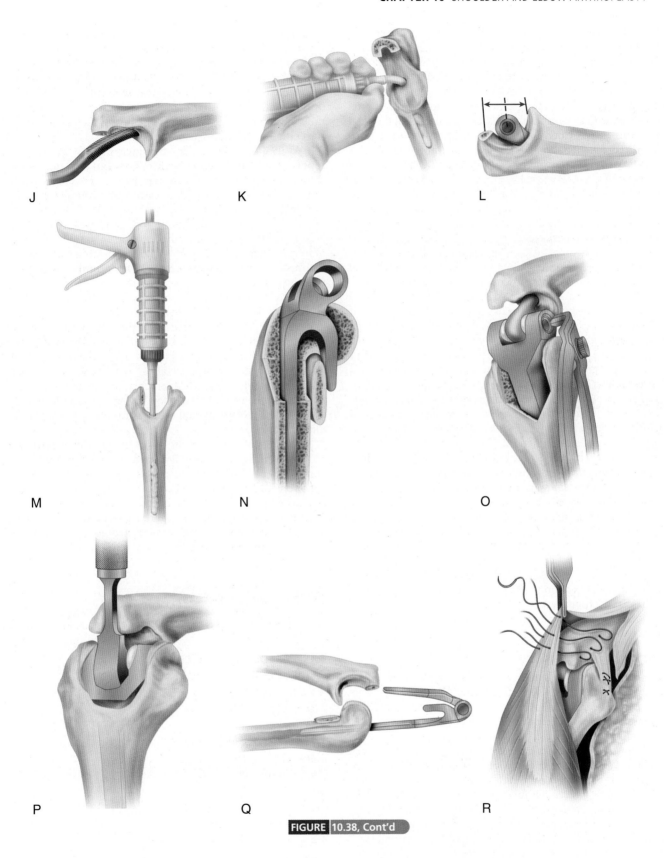

bone fragments or poor bone quality and significant comorbid factors, such as rheumatoid arthritis, osteoporosis, diabetes mellitus, and conditions requiring steroids, have had superior outcomes at short-term follow-up with total elbow replacement as opposed to fixation. A multicenter, randomized prospective study comparing internal fixation with total elbow arthroplasty for displaced intraarticular distal humeral fractures in the elderly found that arthroplasty resulted in improved functional outcomes at 2 years; however, inferior results were reported in younger patients (average age, 23 years) with fractures caused by gunshot wounds. Longer-term follow-up studies are now available, demonstrating 10-year implant survival rates of approximately 90% in this population. Curiously, survival rates were lower when total elbow arthroplasty was performed for distal humeral fractures in patients with rheumatoid arthritis. Although off-label and not typically available in the United States, use of distal humeral hemiarthroplasty for these fractures also has been reported.

Posttraumatic arthritis also is an indication for total elbow arthroplasty that has been expanding. At an average of 68 months after total elbow arthroplasty, 83% of 41 patients with posttraumatic arthritis had good or excellent results. Failures were typically attributed to overuse of the implant in this younger, more active population. An update on this series with an average follow-up of 9 years found 70% component retention at 15 years; 68% of patients had good or excellent results. Other authors have reported their experiences with total elbow arthroplasties for posttraumatic sequelae. In general, a stable and functional elbow can be achieved, but implant longevity, particularly when performed in younger patients, remains a concern; caution is recommended when considering total elbow arthroplasties for this condition in patients under 60 years of age.

Failed elbow procedures of any type may be an indication for implant arthroplasty as a revision. Suggested indications for arthroplasty include intractable pain with radiographic evidence of destruction of the radiohumeral and humeroulnar joints, instability, failed synovectomy with radial head excision, and loss of bone stock caused by tumor, hemophilic arthropathy, trauma, or infection. Patients with primary tumors generally have better results than patients with metastatic lesions.

■ COMPLICATIONS

An overall complication rate in total elbow arthroplasty of up to 43% has been reported, including an 18% revision rate and 15% "permanent" complications. However, a recent meta-analysis reported a 13.5% revision rate, with aseptic loosening, infection, and periprosthetic fracture as the most common indications for reoperation. In contrast, the most commonly encountered complications include ulnar neuritis and triceps insufficiency. Perioperative mortality has been reported to be 0.6% and is most commonly caused by cardiac complications. Patients with rheumatoid arthritis have higher infection rates than those with posttraumatic sequelae; however, total elbow arthroplasty performed for posttraumatic arthritis is more likely to require reoperation.

Infection is a dreaded complication of total elbow arthroplasty, with a reported incidence of 0% to 11.5% and an average of 5% to 6%. In particular, persistent wound drainage is highly indicative of deep infection and predicts the likelihood

of subsequent component resection. Although one-stage revision is possible in some circumstances, two-stage revision generally is recommended, with reports indicating an acceptable level of eradication. Well-fixed components may be retained at the time of initial debridement and placement of local antibiotics. After completion of a course of intravenous antibiotics, a repeat debridement with re-articulation of the components can be successful.

Wear of the polyethylene bearing surface has also been reported after total elbow arthroplasty but accounts for a minority of revision procedures. Factors associated with the development of bushing wear were younger patient age, male sex, posttraumatic arthritis, preoperative elbow deformity, supracondylar nonunion, and high activity levels. Implant malalignment has also been implicated in a biomechanical model. Biomechanical testing of vitamin E-infused polyethylene indicates it is a promising alternative to reduce bearing surface wear, but it is not yet supported by clinical data.

Osteolytic reaction similar to that seen in total hip and knee replacements has been found in total elbow replacement. In a retrieval study of 16 elbows, multiple modes of wear were observed, including asymmetric thinning of the humeral and ulnar bearing surfaces and metal-on-metal debris. In another study, polyethylene particles, cement, and metal debris were all found at the time of total elbow revision. The authors suggested that osteolysis in total elbow arthroplasty is therefore a multifactorial process.

A principal complication of unconstrained total elbow arthroplasty has been loosening, usually of the humeral component (Table 10.6). For semiconstrained prostheses, loosening of the humeral component, previously the most common cause for revision, has been reduced with improvements in prosthesis design, changes in operative technique, and better understanding of the anatomy and function of the elbow. In particular, one study noted that use of a shorter (4 inch) stem

TABLE 10.6

Complications of Implant Elbow Arthroplasty

	AVERAGE (%)
RARELY REQUIRING SURGERY	
Nerve paresthesias	11
Wound problems	14
Fracture, humerus	5
Fracture, ulna	5
USUALLY REQUIRING SURGERY	
Nerve entrapment*	3
Triceps problems	4
Ankylosis*	4
USUALLY REQUIRING REVISION	
Loosening (semiconstrained)	5
Instability (unconstrained)	9
Infection	7
Fracture and loosening*	5

*Rarely reported by most authors.
Average percentage from published reports.

in semiconstrained total elbow arthroplasty resulted in earlier time to revision than longer (6 inch) stems. Nevertheless, humeral stem loosening remained uncommon at a rate of approximately 2% at an average of 7 years of follow-up. Ulnar component loosening and osteolysis increased with the addition of a polymethylmethacrylate precoat in the 1990s but has decreased since the surface finish was changed to a plasma spray preparation.

Instability in the form of dislocation or subluxation is the most common complication requiring revision of unconstrained prostheses and has been reported to occur in between 9% and 10% of total elbow arthroplasties. True dislocation occurs in fewer than 5% of unlinked implants and is dependent on surgical technique. Appropriate tensioning of the medial and lateral ligament complexes and preservation of the anterior capsule and triceps can help avoid this complication.

A number of measures have been recommended to minimize the occurrence of other complications of elbow implant arthroplasty, especially infection and problems with the triceps, ulnar nerve, and wound healing. These include the use of a straight incision medial to the olecranon tip, detachment of the triceps in continuity from the olecranon without division of the tendon or the use of a triceps-on approach, anterior transposition of the ulnar nerve, drainage of the wound with at least one suction drain, and initial splinting of the elbow in full extension.

SALVAGE
■ REVISION ELBOW ARTHROPLASTY

Initial results of revision elbow arthroplasty were poor with a high complication rate and an equally high rate of unsatisfactory outcomes; however, with improved surgical technique and understanding of the failure modes of these implants, more recent outcomes have been more promising. Nevertheless, revision total elbow arthroplasty remains a difficult salvage situation and patients should be counseled as to the end-stage nature of their disorders before intervention so that expectations are properly set.

Wolfe et al. identified preoperative risk factors for infection after total elbow arthroplasty, including previous elbow surgery or infection, psychiatric illness, and class IV rheumatoid arthritis. Postoperative risk factors included wound drainage, spontaneous drainage after 10 days, and reoperation for any reason. For deep infection after elbow implant arthroplasty, removal of the implant has been recommended, although more recent recommendations allow for retention of well-fixed components. For superficial infection, Wolfe et al. recommended debridement with salvage of the implant, resection arthroplasty, or elbow arthrodesis. In patients with gross loosening of the implant, salvage attempts were not worthwhile. In patients with no implant loosening, however, salvage was possible. Aggressive measures were used to stabilize the soft tissues, including excision of sinus tracts; debridement of thinned skin and exposed bone; and the use of skin grafts, rotation flaps, and muscle pedicle flaps. Salvage of an infected elbow prosthesis by serial debridement and antibiotic therapy has been described, and successful single-stage exchange arthroplasty.

In a later report by Yamaguchi, Adams, and Morrey, 25 patients with postoperative infections were grouped according to the treatment they received. In group I, the implant was retained using antibiotics and serial debridement, which included exchange of the polyethylene bushings. In group II, the implant was removed and reimplantation was done either immediately or as a delayed procedure. In group III, resection arthroplasty was done. The infection was successfully treated in seven of the 14 patients in group I. The results depended on the causative organism. Less satisfactory outcomes were seen in patients infected with *Staphylococcus epidermidis.* In group II, four of six patients had successful reimplantation of a prosthesis. In group III, none of the five patients had signs of infection at latest follow-up. Resection arthroplasty had a more predictable outcome in medically "frail" patients and in patients with reduced demands for the elbow. More recent reports have found success with a two-stage revision technique of initial resection followed by delayed component replantation. Infection can be eradicated in 72% to 88% of patients with fair to good results.

Advancements in design and improvements in cementing techniques should help to minimize loosening. Selection of appropriate patients for elbow implant arthroplasty (who have a low level of activity, such as patients with rheumatoid arthritis) also may help to minimize loosening. Prosthetic designs that allow valgus and varus and rotational motion at the coupling of the semiconstrained devices help to dissipate the forces at the elbow. Symptomatic loosening of an elbow prosthesis can be treated by revision using a different type of prosthesis, removal of the prosthesis creating a resection arthroplasty, revision of the remaining bone to create an interposition arthroplasty, or arthrodesis. Because of scarring, contractures, and poor bone quality, revision surgery for elbow prostheses can be exceedingly difficult. Of particular concern when revising the humeral component is the proximity of the radial nerve. When proximal dissection is warranted, typically to remove a well-fixed humeral stem, we recommend formally identifying and protecting the radial nerve over simple palpation.

Various types of bone grafting procedures have been used in revisions for component loosening, including impaction grafting, strut allografts, and allograft-prosthesis constructs. Eight of 12 implants revised with impaction bone grafting were reported to be intact at 6 years in one series and good to excellent results were found in 15 of 16 patients in another. Strut allograft reconstruction improved Mayo Elbow Performance scores in 21 patients, but complications were frequent (36%), and allograft-prosthesis constructs were reported to be successful in relieving pain in approximately 70% of patients, although functional gains were minimal. Graft healing and incorporation occurred in 92% of cases, with a similar complication rate as strut grafting procedures.

Periprosthetic fractures have also been reported after total elbow arthroplasty: humeral component fractures occur in 0.65% of implants and ulnar component fractures in 1.2%. Athwal and Morrey reported 26 elbows that had revision because of component fracture. At 5-year follow-up, the average Mayo Elbow Performance score was 82 but complications were frequent (62%).

Dislocation of the prosthetic components, uncoupling of the articulating device, or fracture of a prosthetic component can cause failure of an implant elbow arthroplasty. If the coupling device of a prosthesis fails, it should be revised by replacement of the polyethylene component.

Similarly, if a component fractures or dislocates, it should be replaced by revision surgery. Revision surgery requires careful handling of the soft tissues and bone. Gaps in bone may require the use of custom prostheses or allografts to achieve satisfactory results. In the absence of infection, satisfactory results can be achieved in as many as 85% of revisions in patients without documented infection and with "sufficient bone stock" and adequate soft tissues.

Revision elbow arthroplasty is a salvage procedure that, when successful, is superior functionally to resection arthroplasty or arthrodesis.

■ RESECTION ARTHROPLASTY

Resection arthroplasty is rarely indicated except for end-stage elbow disorders that cannot be treated with salvage techniques. Resection of the elbow joint may cause nearly incapacitating instability, and, if bone resorption occurs at the sites of resection, the instability is worsened. Resection arthroplasty has been used in the treatment of refractory sepsis, elbow ankylosis after infection or trauma, and rheumatoid arthritis. Impressive improvement may be seen in some patients when the joint is resected for ankylosis. Currently, the indications for resection arthroplasty include refractory joint sepsis (either primary infection or after elbow arthroplasty), and salvage of a failed implant elbow arthroplasty. Although disability scores remain high after the procedure, reports of resection arthroplasty indicate it is an acceptable solution to a persistently infected total elbow replacement.

ELBOW RESECTION ARTHROPLASTY

TECHNIQUE 10.8

(CAMPBELL)
- With the patient supine, make a longitudinal posterior incision curving to the radial side of the olecranon.

- Dissect the subcutaneous tissues and mobilize skin flaps from the triceps aponeurosis.
- Elevate and invert a V-shaped tongue or flap of the triceps aponeurosis, leaving the triceps tendon attached distally to the tip of the olecranon (Fig. 10.39A). As in total elbow arthroplasty, a triceps-on approach may also be considered.
- Split the triceps muscle longitudinally and expose the distal humerus subperiosteally.
- With a rongeur, remove the distal end of the humerus to form a convex surface when seen from the lateral side. Some stability can be preserved if the lower end of the humerus is shaped into an inverted V. Remove the articular surface from the semilunar notch of the ulna, forming a concave recess. If this is left with a slight convexity to fit the humeral inverted V, the joint has more mediolateral stability.
- Resect a small portion of the coronoid process. In total, remove approximately 2 cm of bone from the distal humerus and 1 cm from the articular surface of the olecranon.
- If the radiocapitellar joint is normal, do not debride it. If the joint is diseased, excise the radial head and reshape the capitellum, leaving the proximal radioulnar joint intact.
- Attach the triceps muscle to the anterior capsule as an interposition material (Fig. 10.39B) and close the triceps aponeurosis (Fig. 10.39C).
- If an extension contracture is present before surgery, advance triceps aponeurosis distally to release this contracture and close the wound in a V-Y configuration.
- Release the tourniquet and obtain hemostasis.
- Close the remainder of the wound in layers. Leave suction drainage tubes in the depths of the wound as necessary, depending on the amount of bleeding on the muscle surface.
- Apply a posterior splint or long arm cast.

POSTOPERATIVE CARE The elbow is immobilized for approximately 3 weeks. Active range-of-motion exercises are begun and increased as pain and swelling permit.

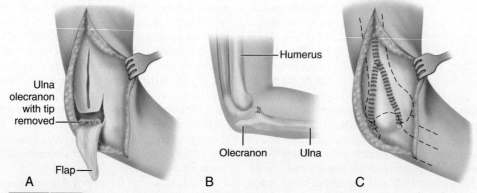

FIGURE 10.39   Campbell technique for elbow resection arthroplasty. **A,** Distally based triceps tongue is left attached to olecranon. **B,** Triceps muscle is interposed between reshaped surfaces. **C,** Closure of triceps tongue in V-Y position to release posterior contracture. **SEE TECHNIQUE 10.8.**

REFERENCES

RECONSTRUCTIVE PROCEDURES OF THE SHOULDER

HISTORY, ANATOMY, PROSTHESIS DESIGN

Boutsiadis A, Lenoir H, Denard PJ, et al.: The lateralization and distalization shoulder angles are important determinants of clinical outcomes in reverse shoulder arthroplasty, *J Shoulder Elbow Surg* 27(7):1226, 2018.

Hendel MD, Bryan JA, Barsoum WK, et al.: Comparison of patient-specific instruments with standard surgical instruments in determining glenoid component position: a randomized prospective clinical trial, *J Bone Joint Surg* 94A:2167, 2012.

Hoenecke Jr HR, Hermida JC, Flores-Hernandez C, D'Lima DD: Accuracy of CT-based measurements of glenoid version for total shoulder arthroplasty, *J Shoulder Elbow Surg* 19:166, 2010.

Hoenecke Jr HR, Tibor LM, Elias DW, et al.: A quantitative three-dimensional templating method for shoulder arthroplasty: biomechanical validation in cadavers, *J Shoulder Elbow Surg* 21:1377, 2012.

Iannotti J, Baker J, Rodriguez E, et al.: Three-dimensional preoperative planning software and a novel information transfer technique technology improve glenoid component positioning, *J Bone Joint Surg* 96A:e71, 2014.

Iannotti JP, Weiner S, Rodriguez E, et al.: Three-dimensional imaging and templating improve glenoid implant positioning, *J Bone Joint Surg* 97A:651, 2015.

Karelse A, Leuridan S, Van Tongel A, et al.: A glenoid reaming study: how accurate are current reaming techniques? *J Shoulder Elbow Surg* 23:1120, 2014.

Laver L, Garrigues GE: Avoiding superior tilt in reverse shoulder arthroplasty: a review of the literature and technical recommendations, *J Shoulder Elbow Surg* 23:1582, 2014.

Levy JC, Everding NG, Frankle MA, Keppler LJ: Accuracy of patient-specific guided glenoid baseplate positioning for reverse shoulder arthroplasty, *J Shoulder Elbow Surg* 23:1563, 2014.

Massimini DF, Li G, Warner JP: Glenohumeral contact kinematics in patients after total shoulder arthroplasty, *J Bone Joint Surg* 92A:916, 2010.

Throckmorton TW, Gulotta LV, Bonnarens FO, et al.: Patient-specific targeting guides compared with traditional instrumentation for glenoid component placement in shoulder arthroplasty: a multi-surgeon study in 70 arthritic cadaver specimens, *J Shoulder Elbow Surg* 24:965, 2015.

Throckmorton TW, Zarkadas PC, Sperling JW, Cofield RH: Radiographic stability of ingrowth humeral stems in total shoulder arthroplasty, *Clin Orthop Relat Res* 468:2122, 2010.

Venne G, Rasquinha Bj, Pichora D, et al.: Comparing conventional and computer-assisted surgery baseplate and screw placement in reverse shoulder arthroplasty, *J Shoulder Elbow Surg* 24:1112, 2015.

Werner BS, Chaoui J, Walch G: The influence of humeral neck shaft angle and glenoid lateralization on range of motion in reverse shoulder arthroplasty, *J Shoulder Elbow Surg* 26(10):1726, 2017.

HEMIARTHROPLASTY

Al-Hadithy N, Domos P, Sewell MD, et al.: Cementless surface replacement arthroplasty of the shoulder for osteoarthritis: results of fifty Mark III Copeland prosthesis from an independent center with four-year mean follow-up, *J Shoulder Elbow Surg* 21:1776, 2012.

Bonnevialle N, Mansat P, Mansat M, Bonnevialle P: Hemiarthroplasty for osteoarthritis in shoulder with dysplastic morphology, *J Shoulder Elbow Surg* 20:378, 2011.

Duan X, Zhang W, Dong X, et al.: Total shoulder arthroplasty versus hemiarthroplasty in patients with shoulder osteoarthritis: a meta-analysis of randomized controlled trials, *Semin Arthritis Rheum* 43:297, 2013.

Gadea F, Alami G, Pape G, et al.: Shoulder hemiarthroplaslty: outcomes and long-term survival analysis according to etiology, *Orthop Traumatol Surg Res* 98:659, 2012.

Hammond G, Tibone JE, McGarry MH, et al.: Biomechanical comparison of anatomic humeral head resurfacing and hemiarthroplasty in functional glenohumeral positions, *J Bone Joint Surg* 94A:68, 2012.

Hammond LC, Lin EC, Harwood DP, et al.: Clinical outcomes of hemiarthroplasty and biological resurfacing in patients aged younger than 50 years, *J Shoulder Elbow Surg* 22:1345, 2013.

Lebon J, Delclaux S, Bonnevialle N, et al.: Stemmed hemiarthroplasty versus resurfacing in primary shoulder osteoarthritis: a single-center retrospective series of 78 patients, *Orthop Traumatol Surg Res* 100(Suppl 6):S327, 2014.

Levine WN, Fischer CR, Nguyen D, et al.: Long-term follow-up of shoulder hemiarthroplasty for glenohumeral osteoarthritis, *J Bone Joint Surg* 94A:e164, 2012.

Mather 3rd RC, Watters TS, Orlando LA, et al.: Cost effectiveness analysis of hemiarthroplasty and total shoulder arthroplasty, *J Shoulder Elbow Surg* 19:325, 2010.

Sandow MJ, David H, Bentall SJ: Hemiarthroplasty vs total shoulder replacement for rotator cuff intact osteoarthritis: how do they fare after a decade? *J Shoulder Elbow Surg* 22:877, 2013.

Shukla DR, McAnany S, Kim J, et al.: Hemiarthroplasty versus reverse shoulder arthroplasty for treatment of proximal humeral fractures: a meta-analysis, *J Shoulder Elbow Surg* 25(2):330, 2016.

Singh JA, Sperling J, Buchbinder R, McMaken K: Surgery for shoulder osteoarthritis: a Cochrane systematic review, *J Rheumatol* 38:598, 2011.

Somerson JS, Matsen 3rd FA: Functional outcomes of the ream-and-run shoulder arthroplasty: a concise follow-up of a previous report, *J Bone Joint Surg Am* 99(23):1999, 2017.

Somerson JS, Neradilik MB, Service BC, et al.: Clinical and radiographic outcomes of the ream-and-run procedure for primary glenohumeral arthritis, *J Bone Joint Surg Am* 99(15):1291, 2017.

TOTAL SHOULDER ARTHROPLASTY

Ahmadi S, Lawrence TM, Sahota S, et al.: Significance of perioperative tests to diagnose the infection in revision total shoulder arthroplasty, *Arch Bone Jt Surg* 6(5):359, 2018.

Bartelt R, Sperling JW, Schleck DC, Cofield RH: Shoulder arthroplasty in patients aged fifty-five years of younger with osteoarthritis, *J Shoulder Elbow Surg* 20:123, 2011.

Baumgarten KM, Osborn R, Schweinle Jr WE, Zens MJ: The influence of anatomic total shoulder arthroplasty using a subscapularis tenotomy on shoulder strength, *J Shoulder Elbow Surg* 27(1):82, 2018.

Bhat SB, Lazarus M, Getz C, et al.: Economic decision model suggests total shoulder arthroplasty is superior to hemiarthroplasty in young patients with end-stage shoulder arthritis, *Clin Orthop Relat Res* 474(11):2482, 2016.

Boileau P, Moineau G, Morin-Salvo N, et al.: Metal-backed glenoid implant with polyethylene insert is not a viable long-term therapeutic option, *J Shoulder Elbow Surg* 24:1534, 2015.

Cadet ER, Kok P, Greiwe RM, et al.: Intermediate and long-term follow-up of total shoulder arthroplasty for the management of postcapsulorrhaphy arthropathy, *J Shoulder Elbow Surg* 23:1301, 2014.

Choate WS, Kwapisz A, Momaya AM, et al.: Outcomes for subscapularis management techniques in shoulder arthroplasty: a systematic review, *J Shoulder Elbow Surg* 27(2):363, 2018.

Christensen J, Brockmeier S: Total shoulder arthroplasty in the athlete and active individual, *Clin Sports Med* 37(4):549, 2018.

Churchill RS: Stemless shoulder arthroplasty: current status, *J Shoulder Elbow Surg* 23:1409, 2014.

Clitherow HD, Frampton CM, Astley TM: Effect of glenoid cementation on total shoulder arthroplasty for degenerative arthritis of the shoulder: a review of the New Zealand National Joint Registry, *J Shoulder Elbow Surg* 23:775, 2014.

Daly CA, Hutton WC, Jarrett CD: Biomechanical effects of rotator interval closure in shoulder arthroplasty, *J Shoulder Elbow Surg* 25(7):1094, 2016.

Farng E, Zingmond D, Krenek L, Soohoo NF: Factors predicting complication rates after primary shoulder arthroplasty, *J Shoulder Elbow Surg* 20:557, 2011.

Foruria AM, Sperling JW, Ankem HK, et al.: Total shoulder replacement for osteoarthritis in patients 80 years of age and older, *J Bone Joint Surg* 92B:970, 2010.

Gallinet D, Ohl X, Decroocq L, et al.: Is reverse total shoulder arthroplasty more effective than hemiarthroplasty for treating displaced proximal humeral fractures in older adults? A systematic review and meta-analysis, *Orthop Traumatol Surg Res* 104(6):759, 2018.

Griffin JW, Novicoff WM, Browne JA, Brockmeier SF: Morbid obesity in total shoulder arthroplasty: risk, outcomes, and cost analysis, *J Shoulder Elbow Surg* 23:1444, 2014.

Harmer L, Throckmorton T, Sperling JW: Total shoulder arthroplasty: are the humeral components getting shorter? *Curr Rev Musculoskelet Med* 9(1):17, 2016.

Huguet D, DeClercq G, Rio B, et al.: Results of a new stemless shoulder prosthesis: radiologic proof of maintained fixation and stability after a minimum of three years' follow-up, *J Shoulder Elbow Surg* 19847, 2010.

Jacobson JA, Duquin TR, Sanchez-Sotelo J, et al.: Anatomic shoulder arthroplasty for treatment of proximal humerus malunions, *J Shoulder Elbow Surg* 23:1232, 2014.

Johnson DJ, Johnson CC, Gulotta LV: Return to play after shoulder replacement surgery: what is realistic and what does evidence tell us, *Clin Sports Med* 37(4):585, 2018.

Kany J, Jose J, Katz D, et al.: The main cause of instability after unconstrained shoulder prosthesis is soft tissue deficiency, *J Shoulder Elbow Surg* 26(8):e243, 2017.

Kilian CM, Morris BJ, Sochacki KR, et al.: Radiographic comparison of finned, cementless central pegged glenoid component and conventional cemented pegged glenoid component in total shoulder arthroplasty: a prospective randomized study, *J Shoulder Elbow Surg* 27(6S):S10, 2018.

Kirsch JM, Khan M, Thornley P, et al.: Platform shoulder arthroplasty: a systematic review, *J Shoulder Elbow Surg* 27(4):756, 2018.

Lehmann L, Magosch P, Mauermann E, et al.: Total shoulder arthroplasty in dislocation arthropathy, *Int Orthop* 34:1219, 2010.

Lenart BA, Namdari S, Williams GR: Total shoulder arthroplasty with an augmented component for anterior glenoid bone deficiency, *J Shoulder Elbow Surg* 25(3):398, 2016.

Liu JN, Garcia GH, Mahony G, et al.: Sports after shoulder arthroplasty: a comparative analysis of hemiarthroplasty and reverse total shoulder replacement, *J Shoulder Elbow Surg* 25(6):920, 2016.

Mulligan RP, Azar FM, Throckmorton TW: Is a generic targeting guide useful for glenoid component placement in shoulder arthroplasty, *J Shoulder Elbow Surg* 25(4):e90, 2016.

Nelson CG, Brolin TJ, Ford MC, et al.: Five-year minimum clinical and radiographic outcomes of total shoulder arthroplasty using a hybrid glenoid component with a central porous titanium post, *J Shoulder Elbow Surg* 279(8):1462, 2018.

Ponce BA, Menendez ME, Oladeji LO, Soldado F: Diabetes as a risk factor for poorer early postoperative outcomes after shoulder arthroplasty, *J Shoulder Elbow Surg* 23:671, 2014.

Power I, Throckmorton TW: Treating humeral bone loss in shoulder arthroplasty: modular humeral components for allografts, *Am J Orthop (Belle Mead NJ)* 47(2), 2018, https://doi.org/10.12788/ajo.2018.0011.

Ramkumar PN, Navarro SM, Haeberle HS, et al.: Evidence-based thresholds for the volume-value relationship in shoulder arthroplasty: outcomes and economies of scale, *J Shoulder Elbow Surg* 26(8):1399, 2017.

Roberson TA, Bentley JC, Griscom JT, et al.: Outcomes of total shoulder arthroplasty in patients younger than 654 years: a systematic review, *J Shoulder Elbow Surg* 26(7):1298, 2017.

Schoch BS, Barlow JD, Schleck C, et al.: Shoulder arthroplasty for post-traumatic osteonecrosis of the humeral head, *J Shoulder Elbow Surg* 2015, [Epub ahead of print].

Schoch B, Schleck C, Cofield RH, Sperling JW: Shoulder arthroplasty in patients younger than 50 years: minimum 20-year follow-up, *J Shoulder Elbow Surg* 24:705, 2015.

Schumann K, Flury MP, Schwyzer HK, et al.: Sports activity after anatomic total shoulder arthroplasty, *Am J Sports Med* 38:2097, 2010.

Shrock JB, Kraeutler MJ, Houck DA, et al.: Lesser tuberosity osteotomy and subscapularis tenotomy repair techniques during total shoulder arthroplasty: a meta-analysis of cadaveric studies, *Clin Biomech (Bristol, Avon)* 40:33, 2016.

Somerson JS, Stein BA, Wirth MA: Distribution of high-volume shoulder arthroplasty surgeons in the United States: data from the 2014 Medicare provider utilization and payment data release, *J Bone Joint Surg Am* 98(18):e77, 2016.

Throckmorton TW, Zarkadas PC, Sperling JW, Cofield RH: Radiographic stability of ingrowth humeral stems in total shoulder arthroplasty, *Clin Orthop Relat Res* 468:2122, 2010.

Wang J, Popchak A, Giugale J, et al.: Sports participation is an appropriate expectation for recreational athletes undergoing shoulder arthroplasty, *Orthop J Sports Med* 6(10):2325967118800666, 2018.

Waterman BR, Dunn JC, Bader J, et al.: Thirty-day morbidity and mortality after elective total shoulder arthroplasty: patient-based and surgical risk factors, *J Shoulder Elbow Surg* 24:24, 2015.

Werthel JD, Lonjon G, Jo S, et al.: Long-term outcomes of cemented versus cementless humeral components in arthroplasty of the shoulder: a propensity score-matched analysis, *Bone Joint J* 99-B(5):666, 2017.

Willemot LB, Elhassan BT, Sperling JW, et al.: Arthroplasty for glenohumeral arthritis in shoulders with a previous Bristow or Laterjet procedure, *J Shoulder Elbow Surg* 27(9):1607, 2018.

Wong JC, Schoch BS, Lee BK, et al.: Culture positivity in primary total shoulder arthroplasty, *J Shoulder Elbow Surg* 27(8):1422, 2018.

Wright TW, Bryant TL, Stevens CG, et al.: Midterm follow-up of divergent peg glenoid components in total shoulder arthroplasty, *J Surg Orthop Adv* 27(1):6, 2018.

Young A, Walch G, Boileau P, et al.: A multicentre study of the long-term results of using a flat-back polyethylene glenoid component in shoulder replacement for primary osteoarthritis, *J Bone Joint Surg* 93B:210, 2011.

REVERSE SHOULDER ARTHROPLASTY

Bacle G, Nové-Josserand L, Garaud P, Walch G: Long-term outcomes of reverse total shoulder arthroplasty: a follow-up of a previous study, *J Bone Joint Surg Am* 99(6):454, 2017.

Bercik MJ, Kruse K, Yalizis M, et al.: A modification to the Walch classification of the glenoid in primary glenohumeral osteoarthritis using three-dimensional imaging, *J Shoulder Elbow Surg* 25:1601, 2016.

Boyle MJ, Youn SM, Frampton CM, Ball CM: Functional outcomes of reverse shoulder arthroplasty compared with hemiarthroplasty for acute proximal humeral fractures, *J Shoulder Elbow Surg* 22:32, 2013.

Chan K, Langohr GDG, Mahaffy M, et al.: Does humeral component lateralization in reverse shoulder arthroplasty affect rotator cuff torque? Evaluation in a cadaver model, *Clin Orthop Relat Res* 475:2564, 2017.

Chivot M, Lami D, Bizzozero P, et al.: Three- and four-part displaced proximal humeral fractures in patients older than 70 years: reverse shoulder arthroplasty or nonsurgical treatment?, *J Shoulder Elbow Surg* piiS1058-2746(18)30546-9, 2018.

Cuff DJ, Pupello DR: Comparison of hemiarthroplasty and reverse shoulder arthroplasty for the treatment of fractures in elderly patients, *J Bone Joint Surg* 95A:2050, 2013.

Dedy NJ, Gouk CJ, Taylor FJ, et al.: Sonographic assessment of the subscapularis after reverse shoulder arthroplasty: impact of tendon integrity on shoulder function, *J Shoulder Elbow Surg* 27(6):1051, 2018.

Distefano JG, Park AY, Nguyen TQ, et al.: Optimal screw placement for base plate fixation in reverse total shoulder arthroplasty, *J Shoulder Elbow Surg* 20:467, 2011.

Drake GN, O'Connor DP, Edwards TB: Indications for reverse total shoulder arthroplasty in rotator cuff disease, *Clin Orthop Relat Res* 468:1526, 2010.

Ek ET, Neukom L, Catanzaro S, Gerber C: Reverse total shoulder arthroplasty for massive irreparable rotator cuff tears in patients younger than 65 years old: results after five to fifteen years, *J Shoulder Elbow Surg* 22:1199, 2013.

Ernstbrunner L, Suter A, Catanzaro S, et al.: Reverse total shoulder arthroplasty for massive, irreparable rotator cuff tears before the age of 60 years: long-term results, *J Bone Joint Surg Am* 99(20):1721, 2017.

Ernstbrunner L, Werthel JD, Wagner E, et al.: Glenoid bone grafting in primary reverse total shoulder arthroplasty, *J Shoulder Elbow Surg* 26(8):1441, 2017.

Favre P, Sussmann PS, Gerber C: The effect of component positioning on intrinsic stability of the reverse shoulder arthroplasty, *J Shoulder Elbow Surg* 19:550, 2010.

Ferrell JR, Trinh TQ, Fischer RA: Reverse total shoulder arthroplasty versus hemiarthroplasty for proximal humeral fractures: a systematic review, *J Orthop Trauma* 29:60, 2015.

Friedman RJ, Flurin PH, Wright TW, et al.: Comparison of reverse total shoulder arthroplasty outcomes with and without subscapularis repair, *J Shoulder Elbow Surg* 26(4):662, 2017.

Giuseffi SA, Streubel P, Sperling J, Sanchez-Sotelo J: Short-stem uncemented primary reverse shoulder arthroplasty: clinical and radiological outcomes, *Bone Joint J* 96-B:526, 2014.

Helmkamp JK, Bullock GS, Amilo NR, et al.: The clinical and radiographic impact of center of rotation lateralization in reverse shoulder arthroplasty, *a systematic review* 27(11):2099, 2018.

Ho JC, Amini MH, Entezari V, et al.: Clinical and radiographic outcomes of a posteriorly augmented glenoid component in anatomic total shoulder arthroplasty for primary osteoarthritis with posterior glenoid bone loss, *J Bone Joint Surg Am* 100(22):1934, 2018.

Holcomb JO, Hebert DJ, Mighell MA, et al.: Reverse shoulder arthroplasty in patients with rheumatoid arthritis, *J Shoulder Elbow Surg* 19:1076, 2010.

Hussey MM, Steen BM, Cusick MC, et al.: The effects of glenoid wear patterns on patients with osteoarthritis in total shoulder arthroplasty: an assessment of outcomes and value, *J Shoulder Elbow Surg* 24:682, 2015.

John M, Pap G, Angst F, et al.: Short-term results after reverse shoulder arthroplasty (Delta III) in patients with rheumatoid arthritis and irreparable rotator cuff tear, *Int Orthop* 34:71, 2010.

Klika BJ, Wooten CW, Sperling JW, et al.: Structural bone grafting for glenoid deficiency in primary total shoulder arthroplasty, *J Shoulder Elbow Surg* 23:1066, 2014.

Kontaxis A, Chen X, Berhouet J, et al.: Humeral version in reverse shoulder arthroplasty affects impingement in activities of daily living, *J Shoulder Elbow Surg* 26(6):1073, 2017.

Lawrence TM, Ahmadi S, Sanchez-Sotelo J, et al.: Patient reported activities after reverse shoulder arthroplasty: part II, *J Shoulder Elbow Surg* 21:1464, 2012.

Leung B, Horodyski M, Struk AM, Wright TW: Functional outcome of hemiarthroplasty compared with reverse total shoulder arthroplasty in the treatment of rotator cuff tear arthropathy, *J Shoulder Elbow Surg* 21:319, 2012.

Lévigne C, Garret J, Boileau P, et al. Scapular notching in reverse shoulder arthroplasty: is it important to avoid it and how? *Clin Orthop Relat Res* 469:2512, 2011.

Mahylis JM, Puzzitiello RN, Ho JC, et al.: Comparison of radiographic and clinical outcomes of revision reverse total shoulder arthroplasty with structural versus nonstructural bone graft, *J Shoulder Elbow Surg* Pii:S1058-2746(18)30497-X, 2018.

Mizuno N, Denard PJ, Raiss P, Walch G: Reverse total shoulder arthroplasty for primary glenohumeral osteoarthritis in patients with a biconcave glenoid, *J Bone Joint Surg* 95A:1297, 2013.

Mollon B, Mahure SA, Roche CP, Zuckerman JD: Impact of scapular notching on clinical outcomes after reverse total shoulder arthroplasty: an analysis of 476 shoulders, *J Shoulder Elbow Surg* 26(7):1253, 2017.

Mulieri P, Dunning P, Klein S, et al.: Reverse shoulder arthroplasty for the treatment of irreparable rotator cuff tear without glenohumeral arthritis, *J Bone Joint Surg* 92A:2544, 2010.

Nolan BM, Ankerson E, Wiater JM: Reverse total shoulder arthroplasty improves function in cuff tear arthropathy, *Clin Orthop Relat Res* 469:2476–2482, 2011.

Roche CP, Diep P, Hamilton MA, et al.: Impact of inferior glenoid tilt, humeral retroversion, bone grafting, and design parameters on muscle length and deltoid wrapping in reverse shoulder arthroplasty, *Bull Hosp Jt Dis* 71:284, 2013.

Sabesan V, Callanan M, Ho J, Iannotti JP: Clinical and radiographic outcomes of total shoulder arthroplasty with bone graft for osteoarthritis with severe glenoid bone loss, *J Bone Joint Surg* 95A:1290, 2013.

Sabesan V, Callanan M, Sharma V, Iannotti JP: Correction of acquired glenoid bone loss in osteoarthritis with a standard versus an augmented glenoid component, *J Shoulder Elbow Surg* 23:964, 2014.

Sanchez-Sotelo J: Reverse total shoulder arthroplasty. In Morrey BF, ed.: Joint replacement arthroplasty: basic science, elbow and shoulder, *Philadelphia* 2011, Wolters Kluwer, p 277.

Sanchez-Sotelo J, Wagner ER, Sim FH, Houdek MT: Allograft-prosthetic composite reconstruction for massive proximal humeral bone loss

in reverse shoulder arthroplasty, *J Bone Joint Surg Am* 99(24):2069, 2017.

Savin DD, Zamfirova I, Iannotti J, et al.: Survey study suggests that reverse total shoulder arthroplasty is becoming the treatment of choice for four-part fractures of the humeral head in the elderly, *Int Orthop* 40(9):1919, 2016.

Sebastiá-Forcada E, Cebrián-Gómez R, Lizaur-Utrilla A, Gil-Guillén V: Reverse shoulder arthroplasty versus hemiarthroplasty for acute proximal humeral fractures. A blinded, randomized, controlled, prospective study, *J Shoulder Elbow Surg* 23:1419, 2014.

Shrock JB, Kraeutler MJ, Crellin CT, et al.: How should I fixate the subscapularis in total shoulder arthroplasty? A systematic review of pertinent subscapularis repair biomechanics, *Shoulder Elbow* 9(3):153, 2017.

Stechel A, Fuhrmann U, Irlenbusch L, et al.: Reverse shoulder arthroplasty in cuff tear arthritis, fracture sequelae, and revision arthroplasty, *Acta Orthop* 81:367, 2010.

Stephens SP, Paisley KC, Giveans MR, Wirth MA: The effect of proximal humeral bone loss on revision reverse total shoulder arthroplasty, *J Shoulder Elbow Surg* 24:1519, 2015.

Tashjian RZ, Martin BI, Ricketts CA, et al.: Superior baseplate inclination is associated with instability after reverse total shoulder arthroplasty, *Clin Orthop Relat Res* 476(8):1622, 2018.

Vourazeris JD, Wright TW, Struk AM, et al.: Primary reverse total shoulder arthroplasty outcomes in patients with subscapularis repair versus tenotomy, *J Shoulder Elbow Surg* 26(3):450, 2017.

Wagner ER, Houdek MT, Hernandez NM, et al.: Cement-within-cement technique in revision reverse shoulder arthroplasty, *J Shoulder Elbow Surg* 26(8):1448, 2017.

Wagner ER, Statz JM, Houdek MT, et al.: Use of a shorter humeral stem in revision reverse shoulder arthroplasty, *J Shoulder Elbow Surg* 26(8):1454, 2017.

Walch G, Boileau P, Noel E: Shoulder arthroplasty: evolving techniques and indications, *Joint Bone Spine* 77:501, 2010.

Walters JD, Barkoh K, Smith RA, et al.: Younger patients reports similar activity levels to the older patients after reverse total shoulder arthroplasty, *J Shoulder Elbow Surg* 25(9):1418, 2016.

Wang J, Zhu Y, Zhang F, et al.: Meta-analysis suggests that reverse shoulder arthroplasty in proximal humerus fractures is a better option than hemiarthroplasty in the elderly, *Int Orthop* 2015, [Epub ahead of print].

Werner BS, Chaoui J, Walch G: Glenosphere design affects range of movement and risk of friction-type scapular impingement in reverse shoulder arthroplasty, *Bone Joint J* 100-B(9):1182, 2018.

Werner BS, Jacquot A, Molé D, Walch G: Is radiographic measurement of acromiohumeral distance on anteroposterior view after reverse shoulder arthroplasty reliable? *J Shoulder Elbow Surg* 25(9):e276, 2016.

Young AA, Smith MM, Bacle G, et al.: Early results of reverse shoulder arthroplasty in patients with rheumatoid arthritis, *J Bone Joint Surg* 93A:1915, 2011.

Young SW, Zhu M, Walker CG, Poon PC: Comparison of functional outcomes of reverse shoulder arthroplasty with those of hemiarthroplasty in the treatment of cuff-tear arthropathy: a matched-pair analysis, *J Bone Joint Surg* 95A:910, 2013.

COMPLICATIONS AND REVISION

Ackland DC, Roshan-Zamir S, Richardson M, Pandy MG: Moment arms of the shoulder musculature after reverse total shoulder arthroplasty, *J Bone Joint Surg* 92A:1221, 2010.

Ahsan ZS, Somerson JS, Matsen 3rd FA: Characterizing the Propionibacterium load in revision shoulder arthroplasty: a study of 137 culture-positive cases, *J Bone Joint Surg Am* 99(2):150, 2017.

Aibinder WR, Schoch B, Schleck C, et al.: Revisions for aseptic glenoid component loosening after anatomic shoulder arthroplasty, *J Shoulder Elbow Surg* 26(3):443, 2017.

Assenmacher AT, Alentorn-Geli E, Dennison T, et al.: Two-stage reimplantation for the treatment of deep infection after shoulder arthroplasty, *J Shoulder Elbow Surg* 26(11):1978, 2017.

Boileau P, Melis B, Duperron D, et al.: Revision surgery of reverse shoulder arthroplasty, *J Shoulder Elbow Surg* 22:1359, 2013.

Bonnevialle N, Melis B, Neyton L, et al.: Aseptic glenoid loosening or failure in total shoulder arthroplasty: revision with glenoid reimplantation, *J Shoulder Elbow Surg* 22:745, 2013.

Buchalter DB, Haure SA, Mollon B, et al.: Two-stage revision for infected shoulder arthroplasty, *J Shoulder Elbow Surg* 26(6):939, 2017.

Buckley T, Miller R, Nicandri G, et al.: Analysis of subscapularis integrity and function after lesser tuberosity osteotomy versus subscapularis tenotomy in total shoulder arthroplasty using ultrasound and validated clinical outcome measures, *J Shoulder Elbow Surg* 23:1309, 2014.

Cancienne JM, Dempsey IJ, Holzgrefe RE, et al.: Is hepatitis C infection associated with a higher risk of complications after total shoulder arthroplasty, *Clin Orthop Relat Res* 474(12):2664, 2016.

Carpenter S, Pinkas D, Newton MD, et al.: Wear rates of retentive versus nonretentive reverse total shoulder arthroplasty liners in an in vitro wear simulation, *J Shoulder Elbow Surg* 24:1372, 2015.

Cheung EV, Sarkissian EJ, Sox-Harris A, et al.: Instability after reverse total shoulder arthroplasty, *J Shoulder Elbow Surg* 27(11):1946, 2018.

Clouthier AL, Hetzler MA, Fedorak G, et al.: Factors affecting the stability of reverse shoulder arthroplasty: a biomechanical study, *J Shoulder Elbow Surg* 22:439, 2013.

Crosby LA, Wright TW, Yu S, Zuckerman JD: Conversion to reverse total shoulder arthroplasty with and without humeral stem retention: the role of a convertible-platform stem, *J Bone Joint Surg Am* 99(9):736, 2017.

de Wilde LF, Poncet D, Middernacht B, Ekelund A: Prosthetic overhang is the most effective way to prevent scapular conflict in a reverse total shoulder prosthesis, *Acta Orthop* 81:719, 2010.

Edwards TB, Labriola JE, Stanley RJ, et al.: Radiographic comparison of pegged and keeled glenoid components using modern cementing techniques: a prospective randomized study, *J Shoulder Elbow Surg* 19:251, 2010.

Erickson BJ, Frank RM, Harris JD, et al.: The influence of humeral head inclination in reverse total shoulder arthroplasty: a systematic review, *J Shoulder Elbow Surg* 24:988, 2015.

Falconer TM, Baba M, Kruse LM, et al.: Contamination of the surgical field with Propionibacterium acnes in primary shoulder arthroplasty, *J Bone Joint Surg Am* 98(20):1722, 2016.

Fishman MP, Budge MD, Moravek Jr JE, et al.: Biomechanical testing of small versus large lesser tuberosity osteotomies: effect on gap formation and ultimate failure load, *J Shoulder Elbow Surg* 23:470, 2014.

Florschütz AV, Lane PD, Crosby LA: Infection after primary anatomic versus primary reverse total shoulder arthroplasty, *J Shoulder Elbow Surg* 24:1296, 2015.

Foruria AM, Oh LS, Sperling JW, Cofield RH: Anteromedial approach for shoulder arthroplasty: current indications, complications, and results, *J Shoulder Elbow Surg* 19:734, 2010.

Fox TJ, Foruria AM, Klika BJ, et al.: Radiographic survival in total shoulder arthroplasty, *J Shoulder Elbow Surg* 22:1221, 2013.

Frangiamore SJ, Saleh A, Grosso MJ, et al.: Neer Award 2015: analysis of cytokine profiles in the diagnosis of periprosthetic joint infections of the shoulder, *J Shoulder Elbow Surg* 26(2):186, 2017.

Gilot G, Alvarez-Pinzon AM, Wright TW, et al.: The incidence of radiographic aseptic loosening of the humeral component in reverse total shoulder arthroplasty, *J Shoulder Elbow Surg* 24:1555, 2015.

Giuseffi SA, Wongtriratanachai P, Omae H, et al.: Biomechanical comparison of lesser tuberosity osteotomy versus subscapularis tenotomy in total shoulder arthroplasty, *J Shoulder Elbow Surg* 21:1087, 2012.

Glanzmann MC, Kolling C, Schwyzer HK, Audigé L: Conversion to hemiarthroplasty as a salvage procedure for failed reverse shoulder arthroplasty, *J Shoulder Elbow Surg* 25(11):1795, 2016.

Greiner SH, Back DA, Herrmann S, et al.: Degenerative changes of the deltoid muscle have impact on clinical outcome after reversed total shoulder arthroplasty, *Arch Orthop Trauma Surg* 130:177, 2010.

Groh GI, Groh GM: Complication rates, reoperation rates, and the learning curve in reverse shoulder arthroplasty, *J Shoulder Elbow Surg* 23:388, 2014.

Grosso MJ, Frangiamore SJ, Ricchetti ET, et al.: Sensitivity of frozen section histology for identifying Propionibacterium acnes infections in revision shoulder arthroplasty, *J Bone Joint Surg* 96A:442, 2014.

Grosso MJ, Frangiamore SJ, Yakubek G, et al.: Performance of implant sonication culture for the diagnosis of periprosthetic shoulder infection, *J Shoulder Elbow Surg* 27(2):211, 2018.

Grubhofer F, Imam MA, Wieser K, et al.: Staged revision with antibiotic spacers for shoulder prosthetic joint infections yields high infection control, *Clin Orthop Relat Res* 476(1):146, 2018.

Hernandez NM, Chalmers BP, Wagner ER, et al.: Revision to reverse total shoulder arthroplasty restores stability for patients with unstable shoulder prostheses, *Clin Orthop Relat Res* 475(11):2716, 2017.

Hoffelner T, Moroder P, Auffarth A, et al.: Outcomes after shoulder arthroplasty revision with glenoid reconstruction and bone grafting, *Int Orthop* 38:775, 2014.

Holmes S, Pena Diaz AM, Athwal GS, et al.: Neer Award 2017: a rapid method for detecting Propionibacterium acnes in surgical biopsy specimens from the shoulder, *J Shoulder Elbow Surg* 26(2):179, 2017.

Hsu JE, Bumgarner RE, Matsen 3rd FA: Propionibacterium in shoulder arthroplasty what we think we know today, *J Bone Joint Surg Am* 98(7):597, 2016.

Hsu JE, Gorbaty JD, Whitney IJ, Matsen 3rd FA: Single-stage revision is effective for failed shoulder arthroplasty with positive cultures for Propionibacterium, *J Bone Joint Surg Am* 98(24):2047, 2016.

Jackson JC, Cil A, Smith J, Steinmann SP: Integrity and function of the subscapularis after total shoulder arthroplasty, *J Shoulder Elbow Surg* 19:1085, 2010.

Kelly 2nd JD, Zhao JX, Hobgood ER, Norris TR: Clinical results of revision shoulder arthroplasty using the reverse prosthesis, *J Shoulder Elbow Surg* 21:1516, 2012.

Kempton LB, Ankerson E, Wiater JM: A complication-based learning curve from 200 reverse shoulder arthroplasties, *Clin Orthop Relat Res* 469:2496, 2011.

Kempton LB, Balasubramaniam M, Ankerson E, Wiater JM: A radiographic analysis of the effects of prosthetic design on scapular notching following reverse total shoulder arthroplasty, *J Shoulder Elbow Surg* 20:571, 2011.

Klein SM, Dunning P, Mulieri P, et al.: Effects of acquired glenoid bone defects on surgical technique and clinical outcomes in reverse shoulder arthroplasty, *J Shoulder Elbow Surg* 92A:1144, 2010.

Kowalsky MS, Galatz LM, Shia DS, et al.: The relationship between scapular notching and reverse shoulder arthroplasty prosthesis design, *J Shoulder Elbow Surg* 21:1430, 2012.

Lévigne C, Garret J, Boileau P, et al.: Scapular notching in reverse shoulder arthroplasty: is it important to avoid it and how? *Clin Orthop Relat Res* 469:2512–2520, 2011.

Levy JC, Triplet J, Everding N: Use of a functional antibiotic spacer in treating infected shoulder arthroplasty, *Orthopedics* 38:e512, 2015.

Mahylis JM, Entezari V, Karichu J, et al.: Hemolytic strains of Propionibacterium acnes do not demonstrate greater pathogenicity in periprosthetic shoulder infection, *J Shoulder Elbow Surg* 27(6):1097, 2018.

Mayne IP, Bell SN, Wright W, Coghlan JA: Acromial and scapular spine fractures after reverse total shoulder arthroplasty, *Shoulder Elbow* 8(2):90, 2016.

McLendon PB, Schoch BS, Sperling JW, et al.: Survival of the pegged glenoid component in shoulder arthroplasty: part II, *J Shoulder Elbow Surg* 26(8):1469, 2017.

Melis B, Bonnevialle N, Neyton L, et al.: Glenoid loosening and failure in anatomical total shoulder arthroplasty: is revision with a reverse shoulder arthroplasty a reliable option? *J Shoulder Elbow Surg* 21:342, 2012.

Merolla G, Wagner E, Sperling JW, et al.: Revision of failed shoulder hemiarthroplasty to reverse total arthroplasty: analysis of 157 revision implants, *J Shoulder Elbow Surg* 27(1):75, 2018.

Muh Sj, Streit JJ, Lenarz CJ, et al.: Resection arthroplasty for failed shoulder arthroplasty, *J Shoulder Elbow Surg* 22:247, 2013.

Nam D, Kepler CK, Neviaser AS, et al.: Reverse total shoulder arthroplasty: current concepts, results, and wear analysis, *J Bone Joint Surg* 92A(Suppl 2):23, 2010.

Nam D, Kepler CK, Nho SJ, et al.: Observations on retrieved humeral polyethylene components from reverse total shoulder arthroplasty, *J Shoulder Elbow Surg* 19:1003, 2010.

Nicholson GP, Strauss EJ, Sherman SL: Scapular notching: recognition and strategies to minimize clinical impact, *Clin Orthop Relat Res* 469:2521–2530, 2011.

Nowark DD, Gardner TR, LU Bigliani, et al.: Interobserver and intraobserver reliability of the Walch classification in primary glenohumeral arthritis, *J Shoulder Elbow Surg* 19:180, 2010.

Otto RJ, Virani NA, Levy JC, et al.: Scapular fractures after reverse shoulder arthroplasty: evaluation of risk factors and the reliability of a proposed classification, *J Shoulder Elbow Surg* 22:1514, 2013.

Padegimas EM, Lawrence C, Narzikul AC, et al.: Future surgery after revision shoulder arthroplasty: the impact of unexpected positive cultures, *J Shoulder Elbow Surg* 26(6):975, 2017.

Paisley KC, Kraeutler MJ, Lazarus MD, et al.: Relationship of scapular neck length to scapular notching after reverse total shoulder arthroplasty by use of plain radiographs, *J Shoulder Elbow Surg* 23:882, 2014.

Papadonikolakis A, Neradilek MB, Matsen 3rd FA: Failure of the glenoid component in anatomic total shoulder arthroplasty: a systematic review of the English-language literature between 2006 and 2012, *J Bone Joint Surg* 95A:2205, 2013.

Patterson DC, Chi D, Parsons BO, Cagle Jr PJ: Acromial spine fracture after reverse total shoulder arthroplasty: a systematic review, *J Shoulder Elbow Surg* 28(4):792, 2019.

Pottinger P, Butler-Wu S, Neradilek MB, et al.: Prognostic factors for bacterial cultures positive for Propionibacterium acnes and other organisms in a large series of revision shoulder arthroplasties performed for stiffness, pain, or loosening, *J Bone Joint Surg* 94A:2075, 2012.

Raiss P, Edwards TB, Deutsch A, et al.: Radiographic changes around humeral components in shoulder arthroplasty, *J Bone Joint Surg* 96A:e54, 2014.

Rasmussen JV, Olsen BS, Al-Hamdani A, Brorson S: Outcome of revision shoulder arthroplasty after resurfacing hemiarthroplasty in patients with glenohumeral osteoarthritis, *J Bone Joint Surg Am* 98(19):1631, 2016.

Sahota S, Sperling JW, Rh Cofield: Humeral windows and longitudinal splits for component removal in revision shoulder arthroplasty, *J Shoulder Elbow Surg* 23:1485, 2014.

Saltzman BM, Chalmers PN, Gupta AK, et al.: Complication rates comparing primary with revision reverse total shoulder arthroplasty, *J Shoulder Elbow Surg* 23:1647, 2014.

Sassoon AA, Rhee PC, Schleck CD, et al.: Revision total shoulder arthroplasty for painful glenoid arthrosis after humeral head replacement: the nontraumatic shoulder, *J Shoulder Elbow Surg* 21:1484, 2012.

Scalise JJ, Ciccone J, Iannotti JP: Clinical, radiographic, and ultrasonographic comparison of subscapularis tenotomy and lesser tuberosity osteotomy for total shoulder arthroplasty, *J Bone Joint Surg* 92A:1627, 2010.

Schmidt CC, Jarrett CD, Brown BT, et al.: Effect of lesser tuberosity osteotomy size and repair construct during total shoulder arthroplasty, *J Shoulder Elbow Surg* 23:117, 2014.

Sheth MM, Sholder D, Abboud J, et al.: Revision of failed hemiarthroplasty for painful glenoid arthritis to anatomic total shoulder arthroplasty, *J Shoulder Elbow Surg* 27(10):1884, 2018.

Shi LL, Jiang JJ, Ek ET, Higgins LD: Failure of the lesser tuberosity osteotomy after total shoulder arthroplasty, *J Shoulder Elbow Surg* 24:203–209, 2015.

Shields MV, Abdullah L, Namdari S: The challenge of Propionibacterium acnes and revision shoulder arthroplasty: a review of current diagnostic options, *J Shoulder Elbow Surg* 25(6):1034, 2016.

Somerson JS, Hsu JE, Neradilek MB, Matsen 3rd FA: Analysis of 4063 complications of shoulder arthroplasty reported to the US Food and Drug Administration from 2012 to 2016, *J Shoulder Elbow Surg* 27(11):1978, 2018.

Stone GP, Clark RE, O'Brien KC, et al.: Surgical management of periprosthetic shoulder infections, *J Shoulder Elbow Surg* 26(7):1222, 2017.

Throckmorton TW, Zarkadas PC, Sperling JW, Cofield RH: Pegged versus keeled glenoid components in total shoulder arthroplasty, *J Shoulder Elbow Surg* 19:726, 2010.

Throckmorton TW, Zarkadas PC, Sperling JW, Cofield RH: Radiographic stability of ingrowth humeral stems in total shoulder arthroplasty, *Clin Orthop Relat Res* 468:2122, 2010.

Trappey 4th GJ, O'Connor DP, Edwards TB: What are the instability and infection rates after reverse shoulder arthroplasty? *Clin Orthop Relat Res* 469:2505, 2011.

Verhelst L, Stuyck J, Bellemans J, Debeer P: Resection arthroplasty of the shoulder as a salvage procedure for deep shoulder infection: does the use of a cement spacer improve outcome? *J Shoulder Elbow Surg* 20:1224, 2011.

Young AA, Walch G, Pape G, et al.: Secondary rotator cuff dysfunction following total shoulder arthroplasty for primary glenohumeral osteoarthritis: results of a multicenter study with more than five years of follow-up, *J Bone Joint Surg* 94A:685, 2012.

RECONSTRUCTIVE PROCEDURES OF THE ELBOW

IMPLANT ARTHROPLASTY

Agyeman KD, Damodar D, Watkns I, Dodds SD: Does radial head implant fixation affect functional outcomes? A systematic review and meta-analysis, *J Shoulder Elbow Surg* Pii: S1058-2746(18)30568-8, 2018.

Athwal GS, Frank SG, Frewal R, et al.: Determination of correct implant size in radial head arthroplasty to avoid overlengthening: surgical technique, *J Bone Joint Surg* 92A(Suppl 1 Pt 2):250, 2010.

Barco R, Streubel PN, Morrey BF, Sanchez-Sotelo J: Total elbow arthroplasty for distal humeral fractures: a ten-year-minimum follow-up study, *J Bone Joint Surg Am* 99(18):1524, 2017.

Barlow JD, Morrey BF, O'Driscoll SW, et al.: Activities after total elbow arthroplasty, *J Shoulder Elbow Surg* 22:787, 2013.

Barthel PY, Mansat P, Sirveaux F, et al.: Is total elbow arthroplasty indicated in the treatment of traumatic sequelae? 19 cases of Coonrad-Morrey(*) reviewed at a mean follow-up of 5.2 years, *Orthop Traumatol Surg Res* 100:113, 2014.

Brownhill JR, Pollock JW, Ferreira LM, et al.: The effect of implant malalignment on joint loading in total elbow arthroplasty: an in vitro study, *J Shoulder Elbow Surg* 21:1032, 2012.

Chen H, Wang Z, Shang Y: Clinical and radiographic outcomes of unipolar and bipolar radial head prosthesis in patients with radial head fracture: a systemic review and meta-analysis, *J Invest Surg* 31(3):178, 2018.

Cohn M, Glait SA, Sapienza A, Kwon YW: Radiocapitellar joint contact pressures following radial head arthroplasty, *J Hand Surg Am* 39:1566, 2014.

Dachs RP, Fleming MA, Chivers DA, et al.: Total elbow arthroplasty: outcomes after triceps-detaching and triceps-sparing approaches, *J Shoulder Elbow Surg* 24:339, 2015.

Day JS, Baxter RM, Ramsey ML, et al.: Characterization of wear debris in total elbow arthroplasty, *J Shoulder Elbow Surg* 22:924, 2013.

De Vos MJ, Wagener ML, Hannink G, et al.: Short-term clinical results of revision elbow arthroplasty using the latitude total elbow arthroplasty, *Bone Joint J* 98-B(8):1086, 2016.

Dunn JC, Kusnezov NA, Koehler LR, et al.: Radial head arthroplasty in the active duty military service member with minimum 2-year follow-up, *J Hand Surg Am* 42(8):660, 2017.

Ernstbrunner L, Hingsammer A, Imam MA, et al.: Long-term results of total elbow arthroplasty in patients with hemophilia, *J Shoulder Elbow Surg* 27(1):126, 2018.

Flinkkilä T, Kaisto T, Sirniö K, et al.: Short- to mid-term results of metallic press-fit radial head arthroplasty in unstable injuries of the elbow, *J Bone Joint Surg* 94B:805, 2012.

Goodman AD, Johnson JP, Kleiner JE, et al.: The expanding use of total elbow arthroplasty for distal humerus fractures: a retrospective database analysis of 56379 inpatients from 2002-2014, *Phys Sportsmed* 46(4):492, 2018.

Gramlich Y, Krausch EL, Klug A, et al.: Complications after radial head arthroplasty: a comparison between short-stemmed bipolar and monopolar long-stemmed osteointegrative rigidly fixed prostheses, *Int Othop* 2018, [Epub ahead of print].

Heijink A, Kodde IF, Mulder PGH, et al.: Cemented bipolar radial head arthroplasty: midterm follow-up results, *J Shoulder Elbow Surg* 25(11):1829, 2016.

Heijink A, Kodde IF, Mulder PG, et al.: Radial head arthroplasty: a systematic review, *JBJS Rev* 4(10): pii:01874474-201610000-0001 2016.

Jenkins PJ, Watts AC, Norwood T, et al.: Total elbow replacement:outcome of 1,146 arthroplasties from the Scottish Arthroplasty Project, *Acta Orthop* 84:119, 2013.

Jeon JH, Morrey BF, Anakwenze OA, Tran NV: Incidence and implications of early postoperative wound complications after total elbow arthroplasty, *J Shoulder Elbow Surg* 20:857, 2011.

Jeon JH, Morrey BF, Sanchez-Sotelo J: Ulnar component surface finish influenced the outcome of primary Coonrad-Morrey total elbow arthroplasty, *J Shoulder Elbow Surg* 21:1229, 2012.

Kachooei AR, Heesakkers NAM, Heijink A: The B, Eygendaal D: Radiocapitellar prosthetic arthroplasty: short-term to midterm results of 19 elbows, *J Shoulder Elbow Surg* 27(4):726, 2018.

Kodde IF, Heijink A, Kaas L, et al.: Press-fit bipolar radial head arthroplasty, midterm results, *J Shoulder Elbow Surg* 25(8):1235, 2016.

Krukhaug Y, Hallan G, Dybvik E, et al.: A survivorship study of 838 total elbow replacements: a report from the Norwegian Arthroplasty Register 1994-2016, *J Shoulder Elbow Surg* 27(2):260, 2018.

Kupperman ES, Kupperman AI, Mitchell SA: Treatment of radial head fractures and need for revision procedures at 1 and 2 years, *J Hand Surg Am* 43(3):241, 2018.

Kusnezov N, Eisenstein E, Dunn JC, et al.: Operative management of unstable radial head fractures in a young active population, *Hand* 13(4):473, 2018.

Laflamme M, Grenier-Gautheir PP, Leclerc A, et al.: Retrospective cohort study on radial head replacements comparing results between smooth and porous stem designs, *J Shoulder Elbow Surg* 26(8):1316, 2017.

Lanting BA, Ferreira LM, Johnson JA, et al.: Radial head implant diameter: a biomechanical assessment of the forgotten dimension, *Clin Biomech (Bristol, Avon)* 30:444, 2015.

Larson AN, Adams RA, Morrey BF: Revision interposition arthroplasty of the elbow, *J Bone Joint Surg* 92B:1273, 2010.

Laumonerie P, Reina N, Ancelin D, et al.: Mid-term outcomes of 77 modular radial head prostheses, *Bone Joint J* 99-B(9):1197, 2017.

Laumonerie P, Reina N, Kerezoudis P, et al.: The minimum follow-up required for radial head arthroplasty: a meta-analysis, *Bone Joint J* 99-B(12):1561, 2017.

Li N, Chen S: Open reduction and internal-fixation versus radial head replacement in treatment of Mason type III radial head fractures, *Eur J Orthop Surg Traumatol* 24:851, 2014.

Lott A, Broder K, Goch A, et al.: Results after radial head arthroplasty in unstable fractures, *J Shoulder Elbow Surg* 27(2):270, 2018.

Mansat P, Bonnevialle N, Rongieres M, et al.: Experience with the Coonrad-Morrey total elbow arthroplasty: 78 consecutive total elbow arthroplasties reviewed with an average 5 years of follow-up, *J Shoulder Elbow Surg* 22:1461, 2013.

Marsh JP, Grewal R, Faber KJ, et al.: Radial head fractures treated with modular metallic radial head replacement: outcomes at a mean follow-up of eight years, *J Bone Joint Surg Am* 98(7):527, 2016.

Mehta SS, Watts AC, Talwalkar SC, et al.: Early results of latitutde primary total elbow replacement with a minimum follow-up of 2 years, *J Shoulder Elbow Surg* 26(10):1867, 2017.

Moon JG, Hong JH, Bither N, Shon WY: Can ulnar variance be used to detect overstuffing after radial head arthroplasty? *Clin Orthop Relat Res* 472:727, 2014.

Morrey BF, Sanchez-Sotelo J: Approaches for elbow arthroplasty: how to handle the triceps, *J Shoulder Elbow Surg* 20(Suppl 2):S90, 2011.

Morrey ME, Sanchez-Sotelo J, Abdel MP, Morrey BF: Allograft-prosthetic composite reconstruction for massive bone loss including catastrophic failure in total elbow arthroplasty, *J Bone Joint Surg* 95A:1117, 2013.

Mukka S, Berg G, Hassany HR, et al.: Semiconstrained total elbow arthroplasty for rheumatoid arthritis patients: clinical and radiological results of 1-8 years follow-up, *Arch Orthop Trauma Surg* 135:595, 2015.

Nestorson J, Rahme H, Adolfsson L: Arthroplasty as primary treatment for distal humeral fractures produces reliable results with regards to revisions and adverse events: a registry-based study, *J Shoulder Elbow Surg* pii:S1058-2746(18)30620-7, 2018.

Park SE, Kim JY, Cho SW, et al.: Complications and revision rate compared by type of total elbow arthroplasty, *J Shoulder Elbow Surg* 22:1121, 2013.

Peach CA, Nicoletti S, Lawrence TM, Stanley D: Two-stage revision for the treatment of the infected total elbow arthroplasty, *Bone Joint J* 95-B:1681, 2013.

Parretta D, van Leeuwen WF, Dyer G, et al.: Risk factors for reoperation after total elbow arthroplasty, *J Shoulder Elbow Surg* 26(5):824, 2017.

Phadnis J, Watts AC, Bain GI: Elbow hemiarthroplasty for the management of distal humeral fractures: current technique, indications, and results, *Shoulder Elbow* 8(3):171, 2016.

Pham TT, Delclaux S, Huguet S, et al.: Coonrad-Morrey total elbow arthroplasty for patients with rheumatoid arthritis: 54 prostheses reviewed at 7 years' average follow-up (maximum, 16 years), *J Shoulder Elbow Surg* 27(3):398, 2018.

Plaschke HC, Thillemann TM, Brorson S, Olsen BS: Implant survival after total elbow arthroplasty: a retrospective study of 324 procedures performed from 1980 to 2008, *J Shoulder Elbow Surg* 23:829, 2014.

Prasad N, Ali A, Stanley D: Total elbow arthroplasty for non-rheumatoid patients with a fracture of the distal humerus: a minimum ten-year follow-up, *Bone Joint J* 98-B(3):381, 2016.

Prkic A, Welsink C, The B, et al.: Why does total elbow arthroplasty fail today? A systematic review of recent literature, *Arch Orthop Trauma Surg* 137(6):761, 2017.

Puskas GJ, Morrey BF, Sanchez-Sotelo J: Aseptic loosening rate of the humeral stem in the Coonrad-Morrey total elbow arthroplasty. Does size matter? *J Shoulder Elbow Surg* 23:76, 2014.

Qureshi F, Draviaraj KP, Stanley D: The Kudo 5 total elbow replacement in the treatment of the rheumatoid elbow: results at a minimum of ten years, *J Bone Joint Surg* 92B:1416, 2010.

Rajaee SS, Lin CA, Moon CN: Primary total elbow arthroplasty for distal humeral fractures in elderly patients: a nationwide analysis, *J Shoulder Elbow Surg* 25(11):1854, 2016.

Ramazanian T, Müller-Lebschi JA, Chuang MY, et al.: Effect of radiocapitellar Achilles disc arthroplasty on coronoid and capitellar contact pressures after radial head excision, *J Shoulder Elbow Surg* 27(10):1785, 2018.

Rhee YG, Cho NS, Parke CS: Impaction grafting in revision total elbow arthroplasty due to aseptic loosening and bone loss, *J Bone Joint Surg* 95A:e741, 2013.

Sanchez-Sotelo J, Morrey BF: Total elbow arthroplasty, *J Am Acad Orthop Surg* 19:121, 2011.

Rudge WBJ, Eseonu K, Brown M, et al.: The management of infected elbow arthroplasty by two-stage revision, *J Shoulder Elbow Surg* 27(5):879, 2018.

Sanchez-Sotelo J, Baghdadi YM, Morrey BF: Primary linked semiconstrained total elbow arthroplasty for rheumatoid arthritis: a single-institution experience with 461 elbows over three decades, *J Bone Joint Surg Am* 98(20):1741, 2016.

Schoch B, Wong J, Abboud J, et al.: Results of total elbow arthroplasty in patients less than 50 years old, *J Hand Surg Am* 42(10):797, 2017.

Schöni M, Drerup S, Angst F, et al.: Long-term survival of GSB III elbow prostheses and risk factors for revisions, *Arch Orthop Trauma Surg* 133:1415, 2013.

Spormann C, Achermann Y, Simmen BR, et al.: Treatment strategies for periprosthetic infections after primary elbow arthroplasty, *J Shoulder Elbow Surg* 21:992, 2012.

Streubel PN, Simone JP, Morrey BF, et al.: Infection in total elbow arthroplasty with stable components: outcomes of a staged surgical protocol with retention of the components, *Bone Joint J* 98-B(7):976, 2016.

Studer A, Athwal GS, McDermid JC, et al.: The lateral para-olecranon approach for total elbow arthroplasty, *J Hand Surg Am* 38:2219, 2013.

Throckmorton TW, Zarkadas PC, Sanchez-Sotelo J, Morrey BF: Radial nerve palsy after humeral revision in total elbow arthroplasty, *J Shoulder Elbow Surg* 20:199, 2011.

Throckmorton TW, Zarkadas P, Sanchez-Sotelo J, Morrey B: Failure patterns after linked semiconstrained total elbow arthroplasty for posttraumatic arthritis, *J Bone Joint Surg* 92A:1432, 2010.

Toulemonde J, Ancelin D, Azoulay V, et al.: Complications and revisions after semi-constrained total elbow arthroplasty: a mono-centre analysis of one hundred cases, *Int Orthop* 40(1):73, 2016.

Triplet JJ, Kurowicki J, Momoh E, et al.: Trends in total elbow arthroplasty in the Medicare population: nationwide study of records from 2005 to 2012, *J Shoulder Elbow Surg* 25(11):1848, 2016.

Wagener ML, de Vos M, Hannink G, et al.: Mid-term clinical results of a modern convertible total elbow arthroplasty, *Bone Joint J* 97-B:681, 2015.

Welsink CL, Lambers KTA, van Deurzen DFP, et al.: Total elbow arthroplasty: a systematic review, *JBJS Rev* 5(7):e4, 2017.

Zmistowski B, Pourjafari A, Padegimas EM, et al.: Treatment of periprosthetic joint infection of the elbow: 15-year experience at a single institution, *J Shoulder Elbow Surg* 27(9):1636, 2018.

RESECTION ARTHROPLASTY

Chauhan A, Palmer BA, Baratz ME: Arthroscopically assisted elbow interposition arthroplasty without hinged external fixation: surgical technique and patient outcomes, *J Shoulder Elbow Surg* 24:947, 2015.

Iftimie PP, Calmet Garcia J, de Loyola Garcia Forcada I, et al.: Resection arthroplasty for radial head fractures: long-term follow-up, *J Shoulder Elbow Surg* 20:45, 2011.

Larson AN, Adams RA, Morrey BF: Revision interposition arthroplasty of the elbow, *J Bone Joint Surg* 92B:1273, 2010.

Rhee YG, Cho NS, Park JG, Song JH: Resection arthroplasty for periprosthetic infection after total elbow arthroplasty, *J Shoulder Elbow Surg* 25:105, 2016.

Yalcinkaya M, Bagatur AE, Erdogan S, Zorer G: Resection arthroplasty for Mason type III radial head fractures yield good clinical but poor radiological results in the long term, *Orthopedics* 36:e1358, 2013.

Zarkadas PC, Cass B, Throckmorton T, et al.: Long-term outcome of resection arthroplasty for the failed total elbow arthroplasty, *J Bone Joint Surg Am* 92:2576, 2010.

The complete list of references is available online at Expert Consult.com.

CHAPTER 11

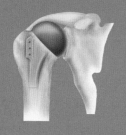

SALVAGE OPERATIONS FOR THE SHOULDER AND ELBOW

Tyler J. Brolin

This chapter discusses the indications and techniques for arthrodesis of the shoulder and elbow joints as well as the most common tendon transfers performed around the shoulder. Because of the limited function and morbidity after shoulder and elbow arthrodesis, as well as the development of more reliable alternatives, the indications for arthrodesis are becoming increasingly rare. Unlike arthrodesis, tendon transfers around the shoulder continue to be viable alternatives in young, high-demand patients with irreparable rotator cuff tears for which arthroplasty may not be an option.

SHOULDER ARTHRODESIS

Historically, shoulder arthrodesis was a relatively common procedure. Indications in the past were mainly upper extremity paralysis caused by poliomyelitis or arthropathy caused by tuberculosis. Because of the success of the procedure, the list of indications grew over the next several decades. The earliest techniques did not use internal or external fixation devices. A purely extraarticular technique of shoulder arthrodesis was recommended for tuberculous infection to prevent systemic dissemination from the infected joint. With the advent of antitubercular drugs, however, this technique became unnecessary. Later procedures placed various types of bone grafts into the beds of the decorticated glenohumeral or acromiohumeral joints, or both. These procedures all required prolonged spica casting.

External fixation has been used to apply compression across the fusion site, with the external fixator removed at 6 weeks and a spica cast worn for 3 months. Although fusion rates with external fixation alone are generally poor, it is still useful in carefully selected patients, especially if infection is present or trauma has occurred with significant soft-tissue injury.

With the advancement of internal fixation techniques, shoulder arthrodesis has continued to evolve because external support alone is unable to provide adequate compression and stabilization of the contact surfaces to promote fusion. Also, if rigid internal fixation is obtained, the use of prolonged immobilization is avoided, allowing early functional use. Various techniques of internal fixation have been described, including isolated screw fixation, external fixation combined with screws, as well as single and double plating (Fig. 11.1). A biomechanical study of fixation techniques used for shoulder arthrodesis found that double plating using 4.5-mm dynamic compression plates had the highest bending strength and torsional stiffness, followed by (in order of decreasing strength) single plating, external fixation combined with screws, external fixation alone, and screws alone. Conversely, a cadaver study comparing various six-screw configurations with a reconstruction plate found that certain screw configurations were as mechanically stable as a 16-hole reconstruction plate, with no significant difference in construct strength between the two groups. The use of a pelvic reconstruction plate instead of a dynamic compression plate has the advantages of greater intraoperative contouring and less implant prominence and is a more common technique performed today. This also allows excellent intraarticular (glenohumeral) and extraarticular (acromiohumeral) stabilization. Advantages of screw-only fixation over plate fixation include less soft-tissue dissection, a lower infection rate, a decreased rate of postoperative humeral fractures, and less frequent need to remove painful implants. Disadvantages of screw fixation are a higher nonunion rate and a greater need for postoperative immobilization.

Recently, all-arthroscopic and arthroscopically assisted techniques for shoulder arthrodesis have been described. These techniques are minimally invasive, decreasing the morbidity associated with large dissection and with fusion rates, outcomes, and complications that are comparable to traditional open procedures.

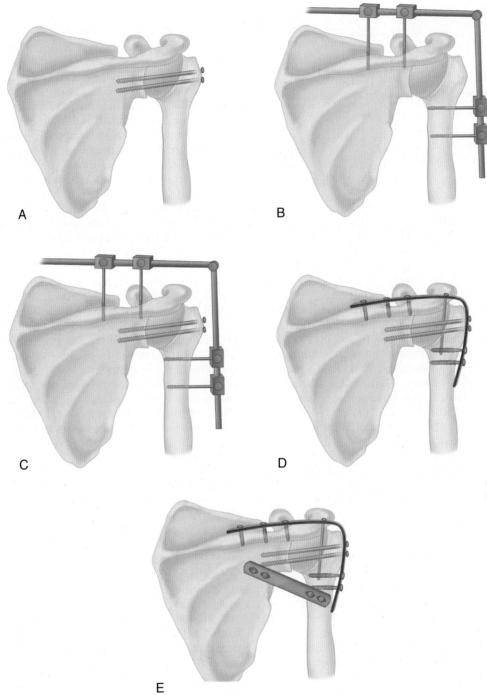

FIGURE 11.1 Fixation techniques for shoulder arthrodesis (posterior view). **A,** Screws alone. **B,** External fixation alone. **C,** External fixation with screws. **D,** Single-plate fixation. **E,** Double-plate fixation. (Redrawn from Miller BS, Harper WP, Gillies RM, et al.: Biomechanical analysis of five fixation techniques used in glenohumeral arthrodesis, *Aust N Z J Surg* 73:1015, 2003.)

INDICATIONS

The goal of shoulder arthrodesis is to give the humerus stability in a functional position that allows optimal use of the distal upper extremity. The indications for shoulder arthrodesis have declined over time given the success with shoulder arthroplasty to treat a wide variety of end-stage shoulder conditions as well as the near eradication of poliomyelitis and tuberculosis, and improved techniques to treat shoulder fractures and instability.

However, shoulder arthrodesis remains a successful treatment option for certain conditions including paralytic conditions, combined insufficiency of the rotator cuff and deltoid, recalcitrant instability, and chronic infections. Given the advancements in shoulder arthroplasty, other less common indications include failed shoulder arthroplasty, arthritic conditions in young, active patients unsuitable for arthroplasty, and neoplastic lesions. Current indications are listed in Box 11.1.

BOX 11.1

Indications for Glenohumeral Arthrodesis

Indications
- Paralytic disorders
- Deficiency of the rotator cuff and deltoid
- Recalcitrant instability
- Chronic Infection

Relative Indications
- Failed shoulder arthroplasty
- Arthritic conditions in patients unsuitable for arthroplasty
- Neoplastic lesions

One of the most common indications, currently, for shoulder arthrodesis is paralytic disorders of the upper extremity, including obstetrical brachial plexus injuries and traumatic brachial plexus injuries. When nerve repair, nerve grafting, and tendon transfers have failed or are contraindicated, shoulder arthrodesis may be indicated. Obstetrical brachial plexus injuries can be treated with arthrodesis near skeletal maturity when growth arrest and position changes are less of a concern. Some authors recommend combining shoulder arthrodesis with transhumeral amputation and prosthetic fitting in patients with complete brachial plexus palsy. Although a minimum age of 10 to 12 years has been suggested, in a review of shoulder arthrodesis in 102 patients, significant growth arrest occurred in only one child. Early arthrodesis has been advocated for children older than 6 years of age who have an irreversible flail shoulder with adequate scapulothoracic muscles, intact elbow flexors, and a functional hand with skin sensation. Finally, shoulder arthrodesis can be used in adult patients with flail limbs caused by persistent traumatic brachial plexus injuries. Wong et al. reported glenohumeral arthrodesis using a reconstruction plate in 6 patients, all of whom achieved fusion, with 5 reporting satisfactory pain relief. Ruhmann et al. reported 77 patients with persistent brachial plexus palsies treated with either trapezius transfer or shoulder arthrodesis. In the 14 patients who had arthrodesis, average abduction improved from 9.6 to 59.3 degrees and average forward elevation improved from 11.4 to 50.7 degrees postoperatively. Complications that necessitated multiple revisions and ultimately led to a poor outcome occurred in 1 patient.

In patients with combined deltoid and rotator cuff paralysis or insufficiency, arthrodesis is indicated over arthroplasty. With deltoid deficiency, the muscle power required to achieve adequate function after arthroplasty is lacking and complication rates are high. In patients with chronic infections, arthroplasty is contraindicated, and arthrodesis with limited internal fixation, with or without external fixation, often is the preferred salvage option. In these patients, though, it is important to adequately debride the shoulder of any infected tissue or bony sequestra in an attempt to minimize the infectious load and increase the chance of successful union. Patients with persistent shoulder instability after multiple failed procedures generally have deficiency of all capsulolabral structures with or without deltoid deficiency. These patients generally have

inferior subluxation of the humeral head leading to painful instability, and arthrodesis in these patients gives a stable shoulder with low levels of pain.

Shoulder arthrodesis may be indicated after malignant tumor resection when soft tissues do not allow endoprosthetic reconstruction. Bone graft is required, and Bilgin et al. described the use of a vascularized free fibular autograft to augment bony healing in this situation. Massive bone loss also may be encountered in arthrodesis following failed shoulder arthroplasty when revision is impossible. Scalise and Iannotti described the use of different bone graft techniques to achieve shoulder arthrodesis. Additional procedures frequently are required to obtain union, and caution should be used in these complex patients. Others have reported acceptable outcomes with resection arthroplasty, which may be preferable to arthrodesis because of the technical difficulties associated with that procedure. In general, a physical laborer who is not required to routinely perform overhead lifting is the ideal candidate for shoulder arthrodesis.

Success after shoulder arthrodesis requires a functional scapulothoracic articulation. Given this, functional scapular stabilizers, including the trapezius, serratus anterior, and levator scapulae, are paramount, and paralysis of this musculature is a contraindication to shoulder arthrodesis. In particular, the trapezius and levator scapulae are responsible for shoulder abduction and the serratus anterior is responsible for forward elevation after shoulder arthrodesis. Other contraindications include ipsilateral elbow arthrodesis or contralateral shoulder arthrodesis, which produce significant functional deficits with activities of daily living, and Charcot arthropathy, which has an unacceptable nonunion rate.

POSITION

The proper position of the arm at the time of arthrodesis (Fig. 11.2) remains controversial (Table 11.1). Currently, most authors prefer 10 to 20 degrees of abduction, 10 to 20 degrees of flexion, and 35 to 45 degrees of internal rotation. This position allows the patient to reach the mouth, waist, back pocket, and contralateral shoulder, facilitating activities of daily living. The position of rotation is the most crucial factor in obtaining optimal function. One study found that more than 15 degrees of flexion and rotation of either less than 40 degrees or more than 60 degrees constituted a malposition that required operative treatment. Another study suggested that abduction of approximately 35 degrees and forward elevation of 30 degrees provided optimal functional results, but that internal rotation of more than 45 degrees should be avoided to prevent problems with hand-to-face activities.

Abduction can be determined at the time of surgery by clinically measuring the angle formed by the body and the humerus. Alternatively, this angle can be determined by obtaining an anteroposterior radiographic view using the spine rather than the border of the scapula as a landmark. Flexion is determined by observing the angle that the humerus forms with the horizontal plane in a supine patient. After the positions of abduction and flexion have been determined, the elbow is flexed to 90 degrees. The hand is positioned over the ipsilateral area of the chest between the sternum and axilla so that further flexion of the elbow allows the top of the thumb to touch the chin (Fig. 11.3).

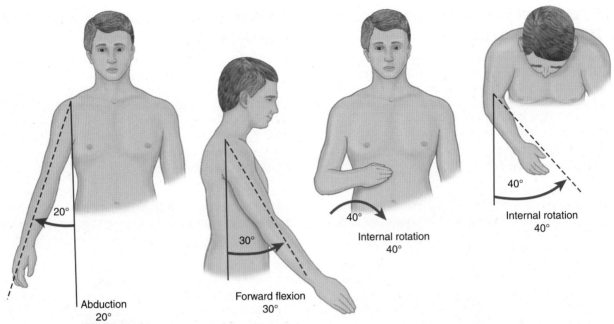

FIGURE 11.2   Position of arm for arthrodesis of shoulder as recommended by Rowe: 20 degrees of abduction (clinical measurement), 30 degrees of forward flexion, and 40 to 50 degrees of internal rotation.

TABLE 11.1

Recommended Positions for Shoulder Arthrodesis

AOA committee (1942)	50 degrees abduction 15-25 degrees flexion 25 degrees internal rotation
Rowe (1974)	20-25 degrees abduction and flexion ~40 degrees internal rotation
Cofield and Briggs (1979)	45 degrees abduction 25 degrees flexion 21 degrees internal rotation
Hawkins and Neer (1987)	25-40 degrees abduction 20-30 degrees flexion 25-30 degrees internal rotation
Richards et al. (1988)	~30 degrees abduction, forward flexion, internal rotation
Jónsson et al. (1989)	20-30 degrees abduction, forward flexion, internal rotation
Groh et al. (1997)	10-15 degrees abduction 10-15 degrees flexion 45 degrees internal rotation
Matsen et al. (2004)	~15 degrees abduction, forward flexion 40 degrees internal rotation
Clare et al. (2001)	10-15 degrees abduction 10-15 degrees flexion 45 degrees internal rotation
Nagy et al. (2004)	15-30 degrees of flexion 35-45 degrees of abduction 30-40 degrees internal rotation
Safran and Iannotti (2006)	20 degrees flexion 20 degrees abduction 40 degrees internal rotation
Scalise and Iannotti (2009)	10-20 degrees abduction 10-20 degrees flexion 35-45 degrees internal rotation

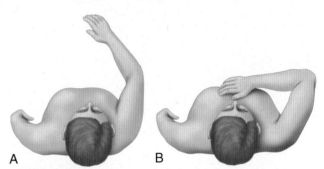

FIGURE 11.3   Method of determining appropriate internal rotation for arthrodesis of shoulder. **A,** Hand positioned midway between sternum and axilla. **B,** Further flexion of elbow should allow tip of thumb to strike chin.

SURGICAL TECHNIQUES

Fusion of the glenohumeral joint, as well as between the humeral head and undersurface of the acromion, should be attempted, and numerous techniques have been described. Stable internal fixation can reduce the need for bone grafting, external fixation, or prolonged immobilization. Postoperative use of a premade custom orthosis to hold the position of the arm until fusion has been achieved is generally well tolerated by most patients and can be used for any of these techniques.

Shoulder arthrodesis without implants is primarily of historical interest. The techniques of Watson-Jones, Putti, Steindler, Brett, and Gill are not included in this edition because they are rarely indicated. For details of these techniques, the reader may refer to earlier editions of this textbook or the original articles.

EXTERNAL FIXATION

Charnley originally described a procedure to accomplish shoulder arthrodesis by applying external compression. External fixation, preferably with screw supplementation, should be considered when an arthrodesis is indicated in a patient with significant soft-tissue loss or deficiency. This technique is also useful in patients with recalcitrant infections.

TECHNIQUE 11.1

(CHARNLEY AND HOUSTON)

- Preoperatively, fit a prefabricated shoulder orthosis to the patient in the intended position of fusion. Adjustments can be made in the operating room while the patient is still under anesthesia. Alternatively, before the operation, apply the trunk portion of a shoulder spica cast with the patient awake, allow it to harden, and then bivalve it and save it for use later.
- Position the patient in a semireclining or beach-chair posture and make a "saber cut" incision centered over the lateral border of the acromion.
- Using electrocautery, take down the anterior and lateral deltoid muscle and then tag and retract this muscle.
- Excise the soft tissue from the subacromial space. Denude the upper half of the glenoid fossa of articular cartilage and the undersurface of the acromion to bleeding bone. Remove the articular cartilage from the humeral head and reduce the joint.
- With an osteotome or oscillating saw, resect the greater tuberosity and humeral head bone to allow articulation superiorly against the undersurface of the acromion and the superior part of the glenoid fossa. Use the resected bone as graft material around the fusion. Insert a 4-mm pin from the posterior superior aspect of the acromion into the scapular neck deep to the glenoid fossa (Fig. 11.4). Another pin can be placed in the base of the coracoid process. Alternatively, 3 pins can be placed into the scapular spine.
- Insert a second set of 2 or 3 similar pins into the surgical neck of the humerus posterolaterally perpendicular to the shaft of the humerus.
- Additionally, 6.5-mm cannulated screws can be placed intraarticularly and extraarticularly to augment compression and fixation.
- Construct an external frame of adjustable pin clamps and bars and connect it to the pins for application of compression with the arm in the desired position for arthrodesis.
- Reattach the deltoid to the acromion and close the wound in layers over a drain.
- Apply the external shoulder orthosis or previously made shoulder spica cast with the patient still under anesthesia, incorporating the external fixator.

POSTOPERATIVE CARE The pins and external fixator are removed after 6 to 8 weeks. Immobilization is continued until the arthrodesis is solid.

PLATE FIXATION

The AO group described a double plating technique for rigid stabilization in glenohumeral arthrodesis. This is particularly useful in humeral head resection in which a second plate significantly aids stability. The disadvantage of this technique is the possible need for a second procedure to remove symptomatic implants after the arthrodesis is solid.

TECHNIQUE 11.2

(AO GROUP)

- Place the patient in the lateral decubitus position.
- Make an incision along the spine of the scapula, over the acromion, and along the proximal third of the humerus. Expose the scapular spine, glenoid fossa, and proximal third of the humerus.
- Denude the glenoid fossa and humeral head of all cartilage.
- Decorticate the undersurface of the acromion and the lateral portion of the humerus for contact with the acromion.
- An osteotomy of the acromion may be necessary to increase surface contact between the plate and bones.
- Position the humeral head in the desired position in the glenoid fossa.
- Use a malleable template to determine the contour for a standard broad AO plate and contour the plate with bending press and irons. The plate is to lie along the scapular spine, over the acromion, and against the proximal third of the humerus (Fig. 11.5).
- Fasten the plate initially with a long cortical screw inserted vertically into the scapular neck. Insert the remaining proximal screws into the scapula using standard AO technique.
- Displace the humerus superiorly and medially to lie against the acromion and glenoid fossa in the desired position for arthrodesis.
- Fix the plate distally with two screws that pass through it and the humeral head and into the glenoid fossa and scapular neck. Insert at least two more screws to fix the plate to the humerus. If the plate does not achieve complete stability at the arthrodesis site, apply a second plate posteriorly from the scapular spine to the humerus (see Fig. 11.5).
- Apply bone grafts as desired. Close the wound in layers over drains.

POSTOPERATIVE CARE A Velpeau dressing is applied. The sutures are removed at 2 weeks if nonabsorbable. Active rehabilitation of the elbow, wrist, and hand is begun within the first few days after surgery, but care should be taken not to place stress on the fusion site.

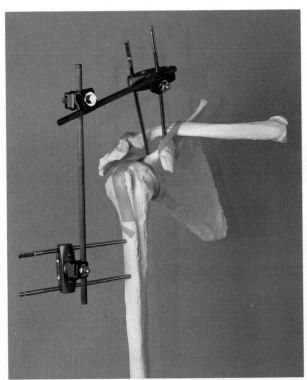

FIGURE 11.4 Arrangement of pins and compression clamps in compression arthrodesis of shoulder. Pins penetrate from lateral aspect and do not transfix shoulder, requiring only two skin perforations. (From Charnley J, Houston JK: Compression arthrodesis of the shoulder, *J Bone Joint Surg* 46B:614, 1964.) **SEE TECHNIQUE 11.1.**

PELVIC RECONSTRUCTION PLATE

To overcome the technical difficulties of contouring the AO plate and the occasional problems caused by prominent screws, Richards et al. used a malleable pelvic reconstruction plate, obtaining successful fusion in 11 patients without the need for plate removal. Chun and Byein also reported success with this technique in eight patients followed for approximately 4 years. This is our preferred method to achieve shoulder fusion.

TECHNIQUE 11.3

(MODIFICATION OF RICHARDS ET AL.)

- Place the patient in a modified beach-chair position with the head of the bed approximately at 45 degrees and drape the arm free. Ensure the entire ipsilateral scapula is exposed.
- Make an incision extending from the spine of the scapula to the midpoint on the lateral aspect of the acromion and distally on the lateral aspect of the humeral shaft.
- Split the deltoid muscle and extend dissection distally to ensure adequate exposure for the entire length of the intended plate.
- Resect the rotator cuff. Decorticate the glenoid fossa, the undersurface of the acromion, and the head of the humerus. While the humeral head is dislocated, glenoid reamers can aid in decorticating the glenoid.

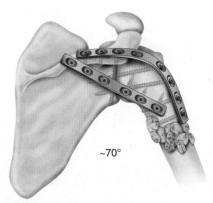

~70°

FIGURE 11.5 Müller et al. technique of shoulder arthrodesis. (Redrawn from Müller ME, Allgower M, Willenegger H: *Manual of internal fixation: techniques recommended by the AO group*, ed 2, Berlin, 1979, Springer.) **SEE TECHNIQUE 11.2.**

- Support the shoulder in 30 degrees of flexion, 30 degrees of abduction, and 30 degrees of internal rotation, and measure abduction from the side of the body. Bring the head of the humerus proximally to appose the decorticated undersurface of the acromion. Abducting and flexing the humerus 30 degrees apposes the head of the humerus to the undersurface of the acromion and the glenoid fossa. Make sure adequate bony contact between all intended fusion sites is obtained.
- Maintain the position by supporting the arm with folded sterile sheets and have an assistant maintain this position while the plate is contoured. Alternatively, the use of an arm positioner can aid in this process.
- Use hand-held bending irons to contour a 4.5-mm reconstruction plate along the spine of the scapula, over the acromion, and down onto the shaft of the humerus. This generally requires a 12- to 16-hole plate. Bend the plate gently 60 degrees over the acromion and twist it 20 to 25 degrees just distal to the bend to appose the shaft of the humerus (Fig. 11.6).
- Two independent partially threaded 6.5-mm cancellous screws with washers can be placed through the lateral aspect of the humeral head and into the glenoid vault to achieve compression of the glenohumeral joint. This aids in provisional fixation while positioning the plate.
- Place the plate onto the scapular spine and onto the lateral aspect of the humerus. Place 4.5-mm cortical or locking screws through the plate and into the scapular spine as well as the humerus. Direct a cortical screw from the spine of the scapula into the base of the coracoid process. Place a 6.5-mm cancellous screw across the acromiohumeral site of fusion and an additional screw across the glenohumeral joint.
- Do not osteotomize the acromion because it is used to augment the fixation of the scapula to the humerus.
- Pack the residual space with corticocancellous bone chips to augment fusion.
- Close the wound in layers over a drain.

POSTOPERATIVE CARE The operative extremity is placed into a "gunslinger" orthosis in the intended fusion position for 6 weeks, with elbow, wrist, and hand range of motion exercises only. If there are no signs of implant loosening, the arm is transitioned to a simple sling. Strenuous activity is delayed for at least 16 weeks after surgery.

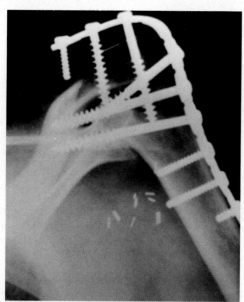

FIGURE 11.6 Richards et al. technique of arthrodesis of shoulder. Pelvic reconstruction plate is bent at fourth hole and twisted slightly distally to appose shaft of humerus with shoulder in 30 degrees of abduction, 30 degrees of flexion, and 30 degrees of internal rotation. (From Richards RR, Sherman RMP, Hudson AR, et al: Shoulder arthrodesis using a pelvic-reconstruction plate: a report of eleven cases, *J Bone Joint Surg* 70A:416, 1988.) **SEE TECHNIQUE 11.3.**

SHOULDER ARTHRODESIS AFTER FAILED PROSTHETIC SHOULDER ARTHROPLASTY

Although not a common indication for shoulder arthrodesis, the combination of a failed shoulder arthroplasty with rotator cuff and deltoid dysfunction has few other reconstructive options. Because of proximal humeral bone loss, soft-tissue deficiencies, and multiple previous operations, shoulder arthrodesis in this situation is associated with high rates of nonunion and revision surgery, but it does represent a salvage option for selected patients for whom other reconstruction options are unlikely to be of benefit.

TECHNIQUE 11.4

(SCALISE AND IANNOTTI)

- Before surgery, determine whether a bone graft will be needed and, if so, what type of bone graft will be most appropriate. Large segmental defects may require a vascularized autogenous fibular graft. If the volume of bone graft needed cannot be obtained from the patient, allografts such as a femoral head should be available.
- Place the patient in a modified beach-chair position that allows the involved extremity to be fully adducted and extended and provides full access to the posterior aspect of the shoulder.
- After induction of general anesthesia and administration of an interscalene block, make an incision over the spine of the scapula and curve it anteriorly toward the midportion of the acromion lateral to the acromioclavicular joint

and then distally to the level of the deltoid tuberosity, incorporating deltopectoral incisions from previous surgeries if present (Fig. 11.7A).
- Develop the deltopectoral interval and identify the atrophic or detached deltoid. Resect this sclerotic tissue from the distal end of the clavicle and the anterolateral aspect of the acromion.
- Retract the detached deltoid tissue distally to expose the entire proximal end of the humerus.
- Typically, much of the rotator cuff envelope is deficient. Release any remaining inferior portion of the subscapularis from its humeral insertion.
- Place a large Darrach retractor in the glenohumeral joint and a bent Hohmann retractor in the subacromial space behind the humeral head. Dislocate the proximal end of the humerus anterosuperiorly with adduction, extension, and external rotation, and remove the prosthetic components. If the humeral bone is thin and osteopenic, take care to avoid fracture.
- If implant removal is difficult, use an oscillating saw to create a unicortical longitudinal osteotomy. Place a broad osteotome in this gap to gently expand the diameter of the diaphysis to loosen osseous on-growth or disrupt the bone-cement interface.
- For removal of the glenoid implant, circumferentially excise the scar and devitalized tissue surrounding the glenoid, as well as any within the glenoid vault.
- With the entire glenoid rim and vault exposed, use a high-speed burr to plane the undersurface of the acromion flat to determine the best placement of the bone graft to maximize osseous contact.
- With the proximal end of the humerus apposed to the glenoid and the underside of the acromion, place two 3-mm Steinmann pins to provide temporary fixation while the optimal position of the fusion is determined. Place one pin laterally from the humerus into the glenoid and one superiorly through the acromion into the humerus (Fig. 11.7B).
- Remove and replace the Steinmann pins as needed while the position of the humerus is adjusted to obtain optimal fusion position.
- When the appropriate position is determined, use an oscillating saw to cut the medial portion of the proximal end of the humerus parallel to the glenoid face to maximize osseous contact. If necessary, temporarily remove the Steinmann pin during this step. Save the resected bone for graft material.
- Replace the Steinmann pins with 6.5-mm partially threaded screws, compressing the humerus to the glenoid first, followed by screw fixation of the humerus to the acromion.
- Contour a 4.5-mm pelvic reconstruction plate to the spine of the scapula, the lateral surface of the acromion, and the lateral aspect of the proximal end of the humerus. The plate should extend far enough proximally to allow placement of at least three bicortical screws in the scapula. Distally, the plate should have at least three bicortical screws in the humeral shaft.
- Compression of the humerus to the glenoid results in relative medialization of the humeral shaft. Shape the femoral head allograft to fit the gap between the undersurface of the plate and the lateral cortex of the proximal end of the humerus. Stabilize the graft with interfragmentary compression screws.
- Secure the neutralization plate to the spine of the scapula and to the humerus with screws, transfixing the graft, humerus, and glenoid (Fig. 11.7C).

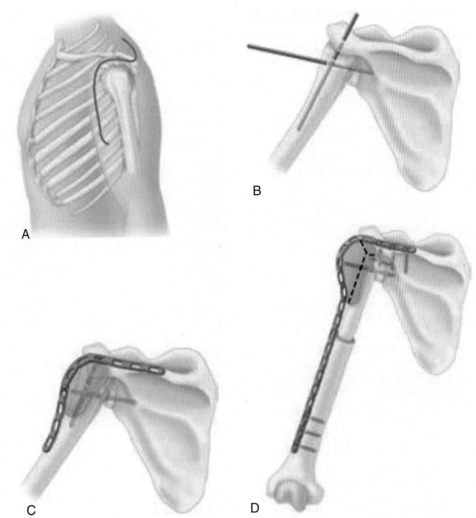

FIGURE 11.7 Arthrodesis with autograft or allograft (Scalise and Iannotti). **A,** Skin incision. **B,** Provisional Steinmann pin fixation. **C,** Application of contoured 4.5-mm pelvic reconstruction plate and bulk allograft. **D,** Use of fibular autograft secured with large-fragment reconstruction plate. (Redrawn from Scalise JJ, Iannotti JP: Glenohumeral arthrodesis after failed prosthetic shoulder arthroplasty: surgical technique, J Bone Joint Surg 91A[Suppl 2 pt 1]:30, 2009.) **SEE TECHNIQUE 11.4.**

- If a vascularized fibular autograft is to be used to span a large humeral defect, harvest a length of fibula that is 6 cm longer than the defect.
- Strip the fibular graft of its soft tissue so that it can be inserted in the canal of the remaining part of the humerus. Provisionally fix the graft with one or two interfragmentary 4.5-mm lag screws.
- To maximize contact with the glenoid, use a high-speed burr to create a slot on the face of the glenoid to allow the fibula to be recessed at the proper orientation to provide the appropriate humeral position.
- Place the bulk allograft and secure it laterally to the fibular graft with interfragmentary screws.
- Contour a large-fragment reconstruction plate and secure it to the surface of the scapula, acromion, fibular graft, and distal humerus (Fig. 11.7D).
- For a vascularized graft, revascularization of the fibula is done by the microvascular team once the graft is stabilized, using end-to-side anastomosis of the peroneal artery and either an end-to-side or end-to-end venous anastomosis.

- Use either an autologous iliac crest bone marrow aspirate mixed with an allograft matrix or a traditional iliac crest cancellous autograft to pack around both the proximal and distal osteosynthesis sites.
- Repair any remaining deltoid to the acromion through bone tunnels to maximize soft-tissue coverage.
- Place a drain in the deep space, close the soft tissue in layers, and apply a hinged shoulder immobilizer that maintains the position of the arthrodesis. As an alternative, a shoulder spica cast can be used.

POSTOPERATIVE CARE The shoulder is immobilized for 12 to 16 weeks or until union is verified radiographically. Range of motion of the hand, wrist, and elbow is allowed immediately. Scapulothoracic range-of-motion exercises, with progression to strengthening of the scapular stabilizers, are begun after union has been obtained, typically by 8 to 12 weeks. If union is not established by 12 weeks, bone grafting of the fusion site should be considered to prevent failure of the implants.

ARTHROSCOPIC SHOULDER ARTHRODESIS FOR BRACHIAL PLEXUS INJURY

Lenoir et al. described arthroscopic shoulder arthrodesis with external fixation in eight patients; glenohumeral fusion was achieved in all eight at a mean of 3 months. Two 6.5-mm cannulated screws are placed for intraarticular compression. If bone quality is poor, a third 6.5-mm cannulated screw can be placed from the acromion to the humeral head under imaging. The only two complications, a superficial wound infection and migration of an acromiohumeral screw, did not compromise the final outcome.

TECHNIQUE 11.5

(LENOIR)

- Place the patient in the beach-chair position. Obtain fluoroscopic anteroposterior and Bernageau profile views of the glenoid before the start of surgery.
- Place three pins of the external fixator percutaneously in the scapular spine and three pins in the humeral shaft (Fig. 11.8).
- Establish standard anterior and posterior arthroscopic portals, and remove the glenohumeral ligament and labral complex with radiofrequency ablation. Remove the glenoid and humeral head cartilage and subchondral bone with a 5-mm arthroscopic bur.
- Place the arm in 30 degrees of forward flexion, 30 degrees of abduction, and 30 degrees of internal rotation and assemble the external fixator. Check the position by placing the patient's hand at the forehead and ipsilateral buttock.
- Debride the rotator cuff by enlarging the percutaneous screw incisions. The humeral head can be moved up to directly contact the acromion or alternatively bone graft can be used in the subacromial space.
- Place 2 parallel guidewires percutaneously through the humeral head into the glenoid under fluoroscopic imaging. Place 26.5-mm cannulated screws for intraarticular compression. If bone quality is poor, a third 6.5-mm cannulated screw can be placed from the acromion to the humeral head under imaging.

POSTOPERATIVE CARE The shoulder is immobilized with an abduction pillow for 4 weeks. After immobilization, active-assisted exercises are performed to mobilize the scapulothoracic joint. The external fixator is removed 2 months postoperatively.

COMPLICATIONS

Complications associated with shoulder arthrodesis are listed in Box 11.2. Immediate postoperative complications are uncommon and mainly involve wound problems, such as infection, skin breakdown, and wound hematoma. The surgeon must also be mindful of pressure sores if a spica cast is used. Loss of elbow motion has been reported but is usually temporary as long as the elbow is not immobilized for more than 2 weeks.

Later postoperative complications are more prevalent. Malunion has been reported in up to a third of patients with

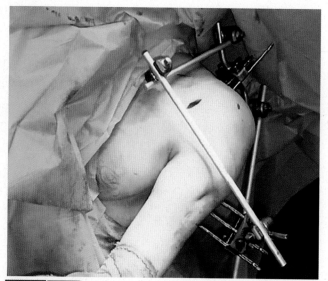

FIGURE 11.8 Arthrodesis with screw fixation only. External fixator in place. Two partially threaded cannulated screws are placed across the glenohumeral joint and one across the acromiohumeral interval to achieve arthrodesis. (From Lenoir H, Williams T, Giffart A, et al: Arthroscopic arthrodesis of the shoulder in brachial plexus palsy, *J Shoulder Elbow Surg* 26:e115, 2017.) **SEE TECHNIQUE 11.5.**

shoulder arthrodesis. Malposition can lead to a traction neuritis or periscapular muscle strain, especially when the arm is positioned in too much abduction. A recent study reported an overall complication rate of 28%. Specifically, pseudarthrosis was more common when screw fixation was used, whereas infection, periprosthetic fracture, and symptomatic implants were more common when plates were used.

Nonunion rates in most modern series are less than 10%. Union is generally achieved with autologous bone grafting. Secondary degenerative arthritis of the acromioclavicular joint is common. If any signs of acromioclavicular arthritis are present preoperatively, a concurrent distal clavicle excision should be performed.

Ipsilateral humeral fractures after shoulder fusion have been reported in 25% of patients in some series. Most authors recommend nonoperative treatment with a shoulder spica or orthosis in these patients.

OUTCOMES

There has been a paucity of literature detailing the long-term outcomes of shoulder arthrodesis. Dimmen and Madsen reported 18 patients who had shoulder fusion using plate fixation. All obtained full or partial arthrodesis, and at an average 8-year follow-up the mean Oxford shoulder score was 32 and the mean American Shoulder and Elbow Surgeons (ASES) score was 59. Complications were uncommon: one patient required reoperation because of severe pain and one for a postoperative humeral shaft fracture; one patient had complex regional pain syndrome. In 21 patients who had shoulder arthrodesis as a primary or secondary procedure after tumor resection, Fuchs et al. found no local recurrences and no metastatic disease at an average 11-year follow-up. The average Toronto Extremity Salvage Score was 81% and the average Musculoskeletal Tumor Society score was 23. However, 43% of patients developed a complication that required additional surgical intervention. Another study by Miller et al. (2011) reported the outcomes of shoulder arthrodesis in 11 children (13 procedures) with flail shoulders caused by polio. At an average follow-up of 41 months, all patients were satisfied and pain free with improved shoulder function. Six patients underwent implant removal, and two shoulders required humeral osteotomy for malrotation. In a larger series of 54 patients undergoing shoulder arthrodesis for brachial plexus palsy, Atlan et al. reported an ultimate fusion rate of 94% and average active abduction of 59 degrees at an average follow-up of approximately 3 years. Arthrodesis rates were improved with the use of a subacromial bone graft.

ELBOW ARTHRODESIS

INDICATIONS

Although total elbow arthroplasty has become an accepted treatment for a variety of degenerative and traumatic elbow conditions, concerns regarding its durability in young and/or high-demand patients make elbow arthrodesis an acceptable alternative in this population. Although partially mitigated by the ability of adjacent joints to compensate for lack of elbow motion, significant functional disability, particularly with self-care and activities of daily living, is common. As a result, total elbow arthroplasty, fascial arthroplasty, or even resection arthroplasty in the presence of functional musculature often provides better function of the upper extremity than does elbow arthrodesis.

Indications for elbow arthrodesis are listed in Box 11.3. In general, elbow arthrodesis is reserved for patients with painful arthritis who are not candidates for total elbow arthroplasty, especially individuals who place high demands on the upper extremities, such as manual laborers. Elbow fusion also is indicated for persistent infection, including tuberculosis, which historically was the main indication for this procedure. More recently, elbow arthrodesis has also become recognized as the optimal treatment for massive upper extremity trauma seen on the battlefield. Typically, a combined internal and external fixation technique is recommended because of the extensive soft-tissue injury that is usually associated with such injuries.

For unilateral arthrodesis of the elbow, a position of 90 to 100 degrees of flexion is desirable to provide the most powerful grip strength. There is no ideal fusion position for all patients; the optimal position depends on whether occupational activity or self-care is the primary goal, as well as on the mobility of the contralateral arm. Simulation of arthrodesis by use of preoperative splints or casts set at varying degrees of flexion has been recommended.

Bilateral elbow arthrodesis rarely is indicated because of resultant functional limitations. If indicated, one elbow should be placed in 110 to 120 degrees of flexion to permit the patient to reach the mouth, and the other should be placed in 45 to 65 degrees to aid in personal hygiene. These positions can be varied to meet the requirements of the patient's occupation.

Arthrodesis of the elbow joint is difficult because of the unique bony anatomy of the elbow and the long lever arm of the upper extremity distal to the elbow. For successful elbow arthrodesis, adequate bone stock must be present, although resection of the radial head may be necessary to preserve pronation and supination, and internal or external fixation with bone grafting is typically required.

SURGICAL TECHNIQUES

In an early technique of arthrodesis reported by Hallock in 1932, the olecranon was osteotomized and wedged into the posterior distal humerus. Steindler (1944) used a tibial graft wedged into the olecranon tip and secured it into the posterior distal humerus with screws.

ELBOW ARTHRODESIS

In 1952, Staples devised a technique for arthrodesis of the elbow in which the bony surfaces are extensively exposed for contact with an iliac graft and fixed to the humerus and ulna by screws.

TECHNIQUE 11.6

(STAPLES)
- Approach the elbow through a posterior longitudinal incision and isolate and retract the ulnar nerve (Fig. 11.9A).
- Osteotomize the olecranon as shown in Figure 11.9B.
- Split the triceps tendon medially and laterally and raise it proximally as a flap, along with the attached fragment of the olecranon.
- Denude the elbow joint of cartilage and cut the distal posterior surface of the humerus down to a flat surface in line with the surface of the remaining proximal end of the ulna.
- Pack iliac bone chips into the joint and apply an iliac graft to the posterior surface of the humerus and the proximal surface of the ulna. Anchor the graft above with one screw (Fig. 11.9C).
- Replace the olecranon process and fasten it with a second screw that passes through the olecranon and the lower end of the graft and into the upper end of the ulna.

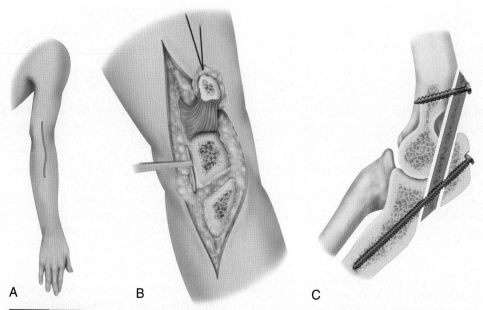

A   B   C

FIGURE 11.9 Staples arthrodesis of elbow. **A,** Incision. **B,** Tip of olecranon osteotomized to form bed for graft. Ulnar nerve is protected. **C,** Graft fixed to humerus and ulna. **SEE TECHNIQUE 11.5.**

ELBOW ARTHRODESIS

The AO group recommended combined internal and external fixation for arthrodesis of the elbow. In this technique, an external compression device is used with a cancellous screw securing the olecranon to the distal humerus.

TECHNIQUE 11.7

(MÜLLER ET AL.)
- Expose the elbow posteriorly as described in the previous technique.
- Resect all cartilage and synovium from the olecranon and distal humerus.
- Fashion a squared-off shelf in the proximal ulna and resect the distal end of the humerus to fit it (Fig. 11.10).
- Resect the radial head at the level of the biceps tuberosity.
- Insert a Steinmann pin from the olecranon into the medullary canal of the humerus to stabilize the arthrodesis temporarily in the desired position. Insert a Steinmann pin transversely through the olecranon in line with the anterior cortex of the humerus. Remove the transfixing medullary pin and replace it with a cancellous screw and washer. Insert another transverse Steinmann pin through the humerus and use an external fixator to apply compression across the arthrodesis.
- Close the wound in layers over drains.

POSTOPERATIVE CARE The fixator and pins are removed at 6 to 8 weeks, and a long arm cast is worn until the arthrodesis is clinically and radiographically solid.

ELBOW ARTHRODESIS

More recently, Spier reported successful fusion in 4 patients using internal fixation with a broad AO type of plate bent to 90 degrees. He also recommended resection of the radial head and osteotomy of the humerus and olecranon to fit in a manner similar to the AO technique. McAuliffe et al. reported 15 elbow arthrodeses using the AO compression plate technique. The most common indication was a high-energy, open, infected injury with associated bone loss. Arthrodesis was successful in all but one elbow, in which a severe, deep infection necessitated amputation.

TECHNIQUE 11.8

(SPIER)
- Expose the elbow posteriorly as described previously, debride the joint, and resect the radial head.
- Osteotomize the olecranon and humerus to fit as in the AO technique (see Technique 11.7).
- Contour an 8- to 12-hole AO plate to achieve the desired degree of flexion at the elbow and secure it to the posterior humerus.
- Secure a tensioning device to the ulna and the distal end of the plate and apply compression to the arthrodesis site. Secure the plate to the ulna with screws in the standard fashion (Fig. 11.11). Accessory cancellous screws can be used for additional stability if needed.
- Apply bone graft around the fusion as necessary, close the wound in layers over drains, and apply a long arm cast.

POSTOPERATIVE CARE The sutures are removed at 2 weeks, and the cast is changed. Support is continued until the arthrodesis is solid. The plate and screws should not be removed earlier than 1 year after surgery. Some authors have reported that postoperative immobilization is not necessary with compression plate fixation.

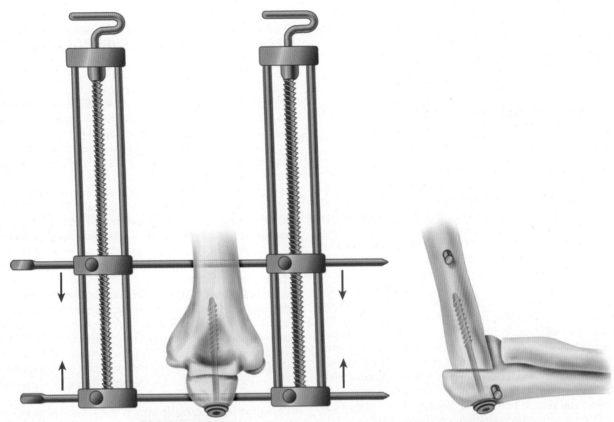

FIGURE 11.10 Müller et al. technique of elbow arthrodesis. **SEE TECHNIQUE 11.6.**

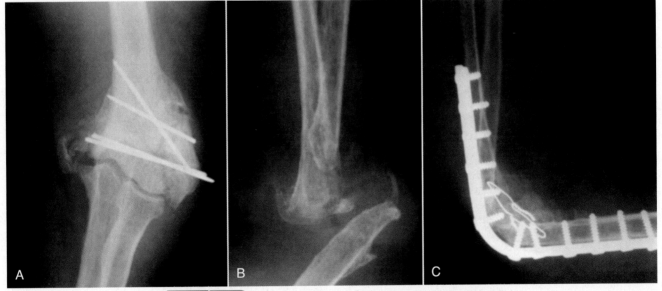

FIGURE 11.11 A–C, Spier arthrodesis of elbow. **SEE TECHNIQUE 11.7.**

COMPLICATIONS

Complications of elbow arthrodesis include neurovascular injury, wound infection, delayed union, nonunion, and malunion. Painful prominent implants and skin breakdown can occur over the posterior aspect of the elbow where subcutaneous tissue is minimal. Repeat surgery for painful implants is common. We recommend waiting at least 18 months after radiographic fusion before considering implant removal. The elbow should be protected with a brace or cast for several weeks after implant removal to prevent fracture.

OUTCOMES

Long-term follow-up studies of elbow arthrodesis have been infrequently reported in the literature, and most report small numbers of patients. The three largest series, involving a total of almost 50 patients, reported fusion rates ranging from 56% to 100% with the use of compression plating and external fixation. Koller et al. reported an average 5-year follow-up of 14 patients, all of whom achieved bony fusion with no pain in eight elbows and moderate pain in six; however, postoperative complications required revision surgeries in six patients. Finally, in a series of five failed total elbow arthroplasties undergoing arthrodesis, Otto et al. concluded that the procedure is not recommended for this indication because of the high nonunion and reoperation rates. In these instances, resection arthroplasty has been shown to be modestly more successful, although the complication rate remains high.

TENDON TRANSFERS FOR IRREPARABLE ROTATOR CUFF TEARS

Massive, irreparable rotator cuff tears present a unique challenge for surgeons. Multiple treatment strategies have been described, including debridement with biceps tenotomy or tenodesis, partial rotator cuff repair, superior capsular reconstruction, tendon transfer, and reverse total shoulder arthroplasty. Selecting the appropriate operation for each patient requires a thorough understanding of patient factors, including age, activity level, major complaints, preoperative function, and expectations after surgery. Rotator cuff debridement with management of the biceps tendon has been shown to provide pain relief, but restores little function to the shoulder. Reverse total shoulder arthroplasty has revolutionized the treatment of rotator cuff-deficient conditions, but concerns over long-term survivorship and durability make this a less desirable option in young, active patients. Tendon transfers have been advocated for the treatment of irreparable rotator cuff tendons to provide pain relief and restore function to the shoulder in patients in whom a joint-preserving operation is preferred.

INDICATIONS

The goal of a tendon transfer for an irreparable rotator cuff tear is to provide balance and stability, restore compressive forces, and correct abnormal kinematics of the glenohumeral joint. For a tendon transfer to be successful, standard tendon transfer rules must be followed (Box 11.4). General indications for tendon transfer for massive irreparable rotator cuff tears include a younger, active patient with minimal glenohumeral arthritis, absence of pseudoparalysis, and adequate intact rotator cuff musculature opposite the tear who desires improved strength and function as well as pain relief. Adequate intact rotator cuff musculature generally is considered to be an intact subscapularis in tendon transfers for irreparable posterior superior rotator cuff tears and an intact teres minor and a portion of the infraspinatus for tendon transfers for irreparable subscapularis tears.

BOX 11.4

Tendon Transfer Rules

- Transferred and recipient muscles should have similar excursion and tension.
- Transferred muscle must be expendable.
- Transferred and recipient tendons should have similar lines of pull.
- Transferred muscle should be designed to replace only one function of the recipient muscle.

From Elhassan BT, Wagner ER, Werthel JD: Outcome of lower trapezius transfer to reconstruct massive irreparable posterior-superior rotator cuff tear, *J Shoulder Elbow Surg* 25:1346, 2016.

SURGICAL TECHNIQUES

■ LATISSIMUS DORSI TENDON TRANSFER FOR IRREPARABLE POSTERIOR SUPERIOR ROTATOR CUFF TEARS

The latissimus dorsi is a large muscle originating from T7 to T12, the thoracolumbar fascia, iliac crest, lower three or four ribs, and the inferior angle of the scapula. Its tendinous insertion is flat and attaches to the floor of the bicipital groove. The neurovascular pedicle comprises the thoracodorsal nerve and artery and has been shown previously to have sufficient length needed for transfer. The axillary and radial nerves are in close proximity and have been shown to penetrate the latissimus dorsi tendon 6% of the time. Also, the latissimus dorsi and teres major are intimately associated and fascial connections are seen in 10% of patients.

Given its success in the treatment of brachial plexus palsies, Gerber et al. proposed a latissimus dorsi transfer for the treatment of irreparable posterior superior rotator cuff tears in 1988. The transferred tendon was thought to act as a humeral head depressor and restore active external rotation or in part act as an external rotation tenodesis to restore function lost from irreparable supraspinatus and infraspinatus tears. Whether the transferred tendon acts synergistically with abduction and external rotation through muscle contractions or passively through a tenodesis effect is debatable. Iannotti et al. reported that only one of 14 patients had electrical activity on EMG with forward elevation, none of 14 during external rotation in 90 abduction, and six of 14 during external rotation with the arm at the side. Synchronous in-phase contraction of the transferred latissimus dorsi was associated with a better clinical outcome. Henseler et al., however, showed that using surface EMG the transferred latissimus tendon functioned synergistically in abduction and external rotation as compared to a more antagonistic role prior to transfer and concluded that the clinical improvements associated with latissimus transfer are not based solely on the tenodesis effect.

The optimal fixation point also has been investigated, with one study showing it to be just posterior to the long head of the biceps if the major gain of external rotation with the arm at the side is desired, and at the infraspinatus footprint if external rotation in the abducted position is desired. Generally performed as an open technique, recently arthroscopically assisted techniques have been described, negating the need to violate the deltoid, with similar results.

LATISSIMUS DORSI TRANSFER, OPEN TECHNIQUE

TECHNIQUE 11.9

(GERBER ET AL.)
- Place the anesthetized patient in the lateral decubitus position.
- Make an 8-cm superolateral skin incision in the Langer lines immediately lateral to the acromioclavicular joint and release the lateral deltoid from the acromion (Fig. 11.12A).
- Excise the bursa and inspect the rotator cuff footprint. Attempt to mobilize and repair the torn rotator cuff tendons; if irreparable, proceed to latissimus dorsi transfer.

- Make a 12- to 15-cm incision lateral to the latissimus dorsi border extending to the posterior axillary crease (Fig. 11.12B). With the arm in an abducted and internally rotated position, release the latissimus dorsi from the humeral shaft (Fig. 11.12C). Take care to protect the radial and axillary nerves, which are in close proximity, as well as to identify and protect the neurovascular pedicle, which allows for safe release of deep fascial attachments.
- Place No. 2 nonabsorbable sutures into the latissimus dorsi tendon in a Krackow fashion. With blunt dissection create a tunnel deep to the deltoid and between the infraspinatus and teres minor (Fig. 11.12D,E). Bring the latissimus tendon over the top of the humeral head and repair it to the greater tuberosity transosseously over the lateral aspect of the lesser tuberosity. Repair the remaining rotator cuff stump medially to the transferred tendon if possible (Fig. 11.12F).

LATISSIMUS DORSI TRANSFER, ARTHROSCOPICALLY ASSISTED TECHNIQUE

TECHNIQUE 11.10

(CASTRICINI ET AL.)
- Place the patient in the lateral decubitus position with the arm under longitudinal traction and the patient under general anesthesia.
- Perform diagnostic arthroscopy using standard posterior and lateral portals to confirm the indication for latissimus dorsi transfer.
- Remove the traction and place the arm in the abducted position with use of an armrest. Make a 6- to 8-cm incision

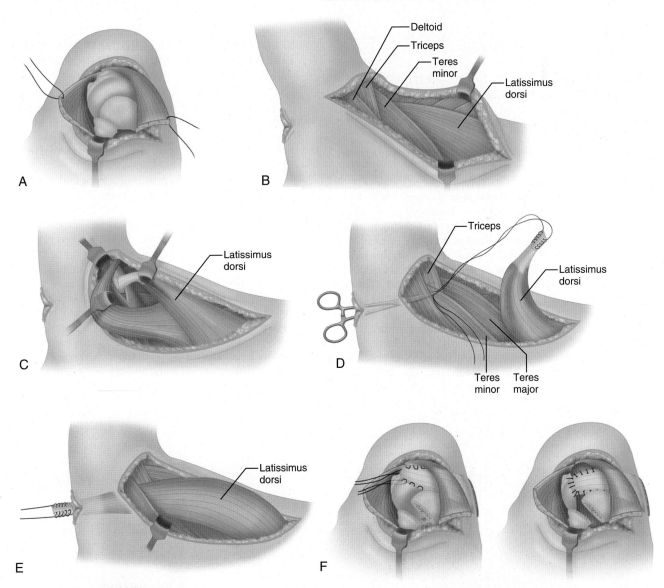

FIGURE 11.12 Gerber et al. technique of latissimus dorsi transfer for irreparable posterior superior rotator cuff. **A,** Exposure of greater tuberosity and rotator cuff footprint. **B,** Incision for latissimus dorsi tendon harvest. **C,** Exposure of latissimus dorsi footprint. **D,** Transfer of tendon deep to deltoid. **E,** Excursion needed for transfer. **F,** Repair of latissimus dorsi to greater tuberosity with repair of residual rotator cuff to medial tendon.

just anterior to the posterior axillary crease along the lateral margin of the latissimus dorsi. Identify the latissimus dorsi tendon and, with the arm in internal rotation, detach it from the humeral shaft. Place No. 2 nonabsorbable sutures in the tendon in a Krackow fashion. Perform tendon mobilization, which ideally should allow the tendon to pass at least 2 cm over the posterior border of the acromion (Fig. 11.13A).

- Resume the arthroscopic procedure and prepare the greater tuberosity. Insert a Wissinger rod through the posterior portal underneath the deltoid and exiting the open incision between the triceps and deltoid (Fig. 11.13B). Insert a dilator over the rod from distal to proximal and pass sutures through the dilator, allowing the latissimus dorsi tendon to be passed into the subacromial space (Fig. 11.13C). Retrieve the sutures through an anterior portal and fix them to the greater tuberosity with two knotless suture anchors (one on the anterior aspect of the greater tuberosity and another in a more lateral position) (Fig. 11.13D).

POSTOPERATIVE CARE Postoperatively, an orthosis is used to keep the arm in an abducted and externally rotated position for 6 weeks. After 6 weeks the orthosis is discontinued and active range of motion is begun. Strengthening begins at week 12 and progresses to 6 months postoperatively.

OUTCOMES

Reports of outcomes after latissimus dorsi tendon transfer for posterior superior irreparable rotator cuff tears have demonstrated improvements in pain, function, and range of motion. A systematic review by Namdari et al. showed that the mean adjusted Constant score improved from 45.9 preoperatively to 73.2 postoperatively, mean active forward elevation improved from 101.9 to 137.4 degrees, and mean active external rotation improved from 16.8 to 26.7 degrees. The authors concluded that patients and surgeons should not expect complete pain relief or normal shoulder function after latissimus transfer. Gerber et al. reported long-term (147 months) results following latissimus transfers in 46 shoulders. Pain and function showed improvements from preoperative values, including mean subjective shoulder value (SSV), which improved from 29% to 70%; relative Constant score, which improved from 56% to 80%; and pain, which improved from 7 to 13. Modest improvements in range of motion were seen, including forward elevation from 118 to 132

degrees, abduction from 112 to 123 degrees, and external rotation from 18 to 33 degrees. Overall, progression in osteoarthritis was seen as well as a decrease in the acromial-humeral index. Studies by Castricini et al. and Kany et al. showed similar results with arthroscopically assisted latissimus dorsi transfer and open technique, with mean postoperative forward elevation ranging from 157.8 to 160 degrees, mean external rotation 43 degrees, and Constant score 68.7 to 69.5.

Given the inconsistent results seen postoperatively, multiple studies have identified risk factors for lower postoperative patient satisfaction and poor outcomes following latissimus dorsi transfer for posterior superior rotator cuff tears, including previous surgery, subscapularis insufficiency, advanced teres minor atrophy, pseudoparalysis, and acromiohumeral index less than 6 mm. The ideal indication for latissimus dorsi transfer is a patient with an irreparable supraspinatus and infraspinatus rotator cuff tear with an intact teres minor and subscapularis, forward elevation of more than 90 degrees of active forward elevation, and no history of prior surgery.

■ LOWER TRAPEZIUS TENDON TRANSFER FOR IRREPARABLE POSTERIOR SUPERIOR ROTATOR CUFF TEARS

The lower trapezius tendon most commonly originates from T2 to T10 and inserts on the dorsum of the medial scapular spine with an average tendon footprint length of 29.4 mm. The lower trapezius is innervated by the spinal accessory nerve, which courses an average of 58 mm medial to the tip of the tendon, but can be as close as 23 mm.

Elhassan et al. first described transferring the lower and middle trapezius tendons to restore shoulder external rotation in a patient with a brachial plexus injury in 2009. With initial success seen with brachial plexus injuries, the indications have expanded to include the treatment of massive irreparable posterior superior rotator cuff tears. The lower trapezius transfer has been advocated due to its line of pull that closely mimics that of the infraspinatus tendon. Several biomechanical studies have demonstrated superiority of the lower trapezius tendon compared to the latissimus dorsi tendon in the treatment of posterior superior rotator cuff tears due to its increased abduction and external rotation moment arms, better ability to provide anterior to posterior balance, restoration of compressive forces, and correction of abnormal shoulder kinematics.

Initially described using an acromial osteotomy for exposure of the humeral head and greater tuberosity footprints, the

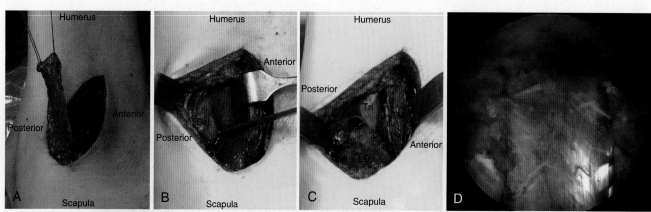

FIGURE 11.13 Arthroscopically assisted latissimus dorsi tendon transfer for irreparable posterior superior rotator cuff tear. **A,** Tendon harvest. **B,** Wissinger rod to aid passage of tendon. **C,** Latissimus dorsi tendon passed deep to deltoid into subacromial space. **D,** Arthroscopic fixation of latissimus dorsi tendon.

technique has evolved with the use of a deltoid split approach or arthroscopically assisted techniques to avoid significant violation of the deltoid attachment.

LOWER TRAPEZIUS TRANSFER, OPEN TECHNIQUE

TECHNIQUE 11.11

(ELHASSAN ET AL.)

■ Place the patient in the lateral decubitus position under general anesthesia. Prepare the entire upper extremity, making sure that adequate exposure medial to the scapula is obtained.

TENDON HARVEST

■ Make a 5-cm vertical incision from the upper to lower borders of the lower trapezius approximately 1 cm medial to the medial border of the scapula. Alternatively, make a 4- to 5-cm transverse incision along Langer lines just inferior to the scapular spine starting 1 cm medial to 3 cm lateral to the medial border of the spine of the scapula.

■ Identify the lateral border of the trapezius and dissect the tendon free from the deep fascial tissues. Dissect the lower trapezius tendon up to its insertion on the medial scapular spine and release it. Carry dissection medial to free the tendon from the middle trapezius. Take care to avoid vigorous dissection on the deep surface of the musculature because the spinal accessory nerve runs 2 cm medial to the medial border. Once adequate mobilization is complete, place non-absorbable sutures in the lower trapezius tendon and place the tendon back into the wound (Fig. 11.14A, B).

GREATER TUBEROSITY EXPOSURE

■ Make a saber incision just medial to the lateral acromion. Remove soft tissue from the acromion and use an oscillating saw to perform an acromial osteotomy of the middle deltoid origin. Alternatively, a deltoid split just off the posterior acromion that avoids deltoid detachment can be used. Attempt to repair as much of the rotator cuff as possible with some of the infraspinatus usually able to be repaired. Prepare the greater tuberosity with a bur.

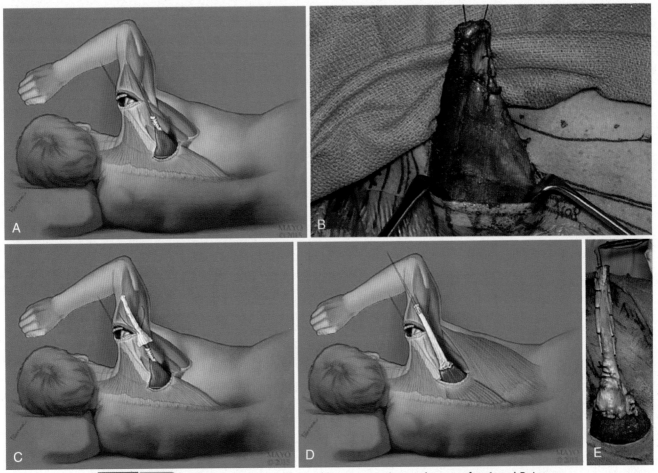

FIGURE 11.14 Elhassan et al. technique of lower trapezius tendon transfer. **A** and **B,** Lower trapezius tendon harvest and adequate excursion. **C-E,** Achilles allograft to augment lower trapezius tendon. (From Elhassan BT, Wagner ER, Werther JD: Outcome of lower trapezius transfer to reconstruct massive irreparable posterior-superior rotator cuff tear, *J Shoulder Elbow Surg* 25:1346, 2016.)

ALLOGRAFT PREPARATION AND PASSAGE

- Use an Achilles tendon allograft to prolong the lower trapezius tendon (Fig. 11.14C). Place two No. 2 nonabsorbable sutures in the thick portion of the graft in a Krackow configuration; this will serve as the main fixation of the graft to the greater tuberosity (Fig. 11.14D, E).
- Create a tunnel between the medial and lateral wounds deep to the posterior deltoid by opening the fascia of the infraspinatus musculature. Use a large grasping instrument to shuttle the Achilles tendon from the medial wound and pass it laterally.

GRAFT FIXATION

- Place the arm in 60 degrees of external rotation and 50 degrees of abduction and fix the Achilles tendon to the infraspinatus and supraspinatus footprints with knotless suture anchors. If poor bone quality is encountered, cortical button fixation can be used.
- Cycle the tendon through shoulder range of motion and place the arm back in external rotation and abduction. Secure the graft to the lower trapezius tendon with nonabsorbable No. 2 sutures while maintaining adequate medial tension on the Achilles tendon allograft and lateral tension on the lower trapezius tendon. A Pulvertaft weave can be used as well.
- Close the wound and repair the acromial osteotomy with No. 2 nonabsorbable sutures.

LOWER TRAPEZIUS TRANSFER, ARTHROSCOPICALLY ASSISTED TECHNIQUE

TECHNIQUE 11.12

(ELHASSAN ET AL.)

- Place the patient in the beach-chair position under general anesthesia with the entire ipsilateral back exposed.
- Perform lower trapezius harvest as previously described. A horizontal incision is generally used because it allows easier graft passage.
- Prepare the Achilles tendon allograft as previously described (see Technique 11.11).
- Perform diagnostic arthroscopic examination through a standard posterior portal and then insert the arthroscope into the subacromial space and establish a standard lateral portal.
- Perform a complete subacromial bursectomy and prepare the greater tuberosity to bleeding subchondral bone.
- Before graft passage, place two anchors into the posterior aspect of the greater tuberosity for incorporation into double-row fixation.
- Through the medial incision identify the infraspinatus and open the fascia to allow graft passage. Additionally, a switching stick can be placed through the medial wound into the subacromial space, and a dilator can be used over the switching stick to ensure adequate room for graft passage.
- Insert a large clamp through a lateral or anterolateral portal toward the medial incision and use it to pull the Achilles tendon graft into the subacromial space by the previously placed Krackow sutures (Fig. 11.15A). Marking the sides and surfaces of the graft allows easy identification of appropriate orientation after graft passage.
- Once the graft is passed, pass the sutures from the two previously placed anchors into the allograft with a self-retrieving suture passer. Fix the graft onto the tuberosity incorporating the Krackow sutures as well as the sutures from the posterior anchors into knotless anchors placed in the anteromedial and anterolateral positions on the greater tuberosity.
- Once the graft is securely fixed onto the greater tuberosity, move the arm through a range of motion, and securely fix the Achilles tendon graft to the lower trapezius tendon as previously described (Fig. 11.15B).

POSTOPERATIVE CARE The patient is immobilized in a custom external rotation orthosis for 6 to 8 weeks. No internal rotation is allowed for 4 weeks. Active-assisted range of motion is begun after immobilization with strengthening beginning at 12 weeks postoperatively. Unrestricted activity is allowed after 6 months postoperatively.

| OUTCOMES

Elhassan et al. reported 33 patients who had lower trapezius transfers with Achilles tendon allografts for massive irreparable posterior superior rotator cuff tears. At an average of 47 months follow-up, the mean SSV improved from 54% to 78% and the mean DASH score improved from 52 to 18. Pain and range of motion also improved, and patients had on average 120 degrees of forward flexion, 90 degrees of abduction, and 50 degrees of external rotation. Importantly, patients with less than 60 degrees of preoperative flexion and abduction had less improvement in motion compared to those with more preserved motion preoperatively.

■ PECTORALIS MAJOR TENDON TRANSFER FOR IRREPARABLE SUBSCAPULARIS TEARS

The pectoralis major arises from the medial clavicle, sternum, ribs 2 through 7, and the aponeurosis of the external oblique muscle. The two primary muscle bellies are the clavicular and sternal heads, in which the clavicular head forms 61% of the total muscle bulk. Both tendons insert just lateral to the biceps tendon on the anterior humerus. The sternal and clavicular lamellae rotate 180 degrees so that the sternal head inserts superior and posterior to the clavicular head. The lateral pectoral nerve innervates the clavicular head at a mean of 12.5 cm medial to its humeral insertion, whereas the medial pectoral nerve innervates the sternal head at an average of 6.3 cm medial to the humeral insertion. Limiting medial dissection to 8.5 cm medial to the humeral insertion of the pectoralis major limits neurologic injury to the pectoral nerves. The musculocutaneous nerve is in close proximity and enters the coracobrachialis at a point between 5.4 and 6.1 cm distal to the coracoid tip.

Transfer of the pectoralis major for irreparable subscapularis ruptures was first described by Wirth and Rockwood in 1997. The authors described transferring the pectoralis major, pectoralis minor, or both over the conjoint tendon. At an average of 5 years follow-up, 10 of the 13 patients were deemed a success using the Neer classification with an average forward

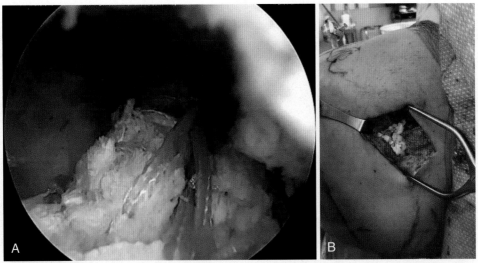

FIGURE 11.15 Arthroscopically assisted lower trapezius tendon transfer. **A,** Arthroscopic view of Achilles allograft being passed into the subacromial space. **B,** Achilles allograft has been securely fixed to lower trapezius tendon.

elevation of 143 degrees. Given the pectoralis major is anterior to the chest wall, Resch et al. described their technique of transferring the upper one half to two thirds of the pectoralis major beneath the conjoint tendon in 12 patients to better replicate the line of pull of the subscapularis as well as provide interposition between the humeral head and coracoid process. The transferred tendon was sutured to the lesser tuberosity in those with isolated subscapularis tears and to the lesser tuberosity/anterior greater tuberosity in those with combined tears of the subscapularis and supraspinatus. At final follow-up patients had significant pain relief and forward elevation improved from 9 to 129 degrees and abduction from 85 to 113 degrees, and 5 of 12 had a negative belly press.

A biomechanical study by Konrad et al. confirmed that pectoralis major transfer under the conjoint tendon better restored glenohumeral kinematics because it is a closer line of action to the subscapularis tendon compared to transfer above the conjoint tendon. There remains concern over the proximity of the musculocutaneous nerve to the transferred pectoralis major in a subcoracoid position. Klepps et al. found that transferring the pectoralis major subcoracoid but superficial to the musculocutaneous nerve creates less tension on the nerve compared to a transfer deep to the nerve. Debulking of the pectoralis major may be required as 6 of 20 specimens had compression of the musculocutaneous nerve with complete transfer, suggesting the need for split tendon transfer.

PECTORALIS MAJOR TRANSFER

TECHNIQUE 11.13

(MODIFICATION OF RESCH ET AL.)
- Place the patient in the beach-chair position and make a standard deltopectoral approach.
- Tenotomize the biceps tendon and tag it for later tenodesis.

- Expose the lesser tuberosity, remove the anterior scar from the humeral head, and attempt to mobilize the subscapularis for repair (Fig. 11.16A). If repair is not possible, proceed with pectoralis tendon transfer.
- Expose the entire length of the pectoralis major insertion and isolate the sternal head deep and superior to the clavicular head (Fig. 11.16B–D). If the sternal head is inadequate, a portion of the clavicular head can be transferred as well. Release adhesions between the two heads to ensure adequate excursion, but limit dissection to 8.5 cm medial to humeral insertion. Place a standard four-strand Krackow suture in the pectoralis tendon (Fig. 11.16E).
- Enter the space between the conjoint tendon and pectoralis minor and identify the location of the musculocutaneous nerve. Make a path deep to the conjoint tendon as well as superficial and superior to the musculocutaneous nerve.
- Pass the sutures with a large, curved forceps and secure them to the lesser tuberosity by either transosseous technique or suture anchors (Fig. 11.16F). If the supraspinatus tendon is also ruptured, the transfer can be placed onto the anterior greater tuberosity as well.

POSTOPERATIVE CARE The shoulder is immobilized in internal rotation for 6 weeks. Gentle passive range of motion is begun with limiting external rotation to neutral and forward elevation to 90 degrees. After 6 weeks, active-assisted and active range of motion is initiated. Strengthening begins at 12 weeks.

▌OUTCOMES
Gavriilidis et al. reported on 15 patients with an average follow-up of 37 months who had subcoracoid transfer in conjunction with posterior superior rotator cuff tears, 70% of which were intact on MRI imaging. The average Constant score improved from 71.7 to 68.1, with significant improvements in pain and ADLs, but with no improvement in strength or ROM. Galatz et al. published their experience with

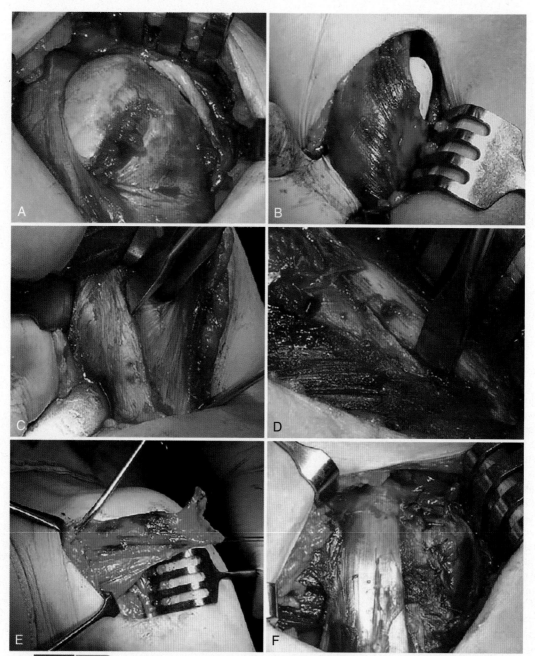

FIGURE 11.16 Pectoralis major transfer. **A,** Exposure of lesser tuberosity. **B,** Isolation of entire pectoralis major. **C,** Exposure of sternal head. **D,** Removal of sternal head of pectoralis major subperiosteally from humerus. **E,** Mobilization of pectoralis major. **F,** Final pectoralis major transfer underneath coracoid process. (From Moroder P, Schulz E, Mitterer M et al: Long-term outcome after pectoralis major transfer for irreparable anterosuperior rotator cuff tears, *J Bone Joint Surg Am* 99:239, 2017.)

pectoralis transfer in patients with anterior-superior subluxation and showed significant improvements in pain but modest improvement in ROM and function. There is a paucity of long-term follow-up of pectoralis major transfer. Moroder et al. followed 22 patients for an average of 10 years following subcoracoid transfer; 91% were either very satisfied or rather satisfied and 95% would undergo the same procedure again. Adjusted Constant score improved from 54% preoperatively to 83% at last follow-up. Pain was improved and maintained at

long-term follow-up. Range of motion decreased from short-term follow-up but was improved compared to preoperative levels; however, internal rotation strength decreased to preoperative levels. Overall, two thirds of patients had progression of their Hamada grades. Jost et al. described transferring the complete pectoralis major superficial to the conjoint tendon in 30 shoulders. At an average of 32 months of follow-up the adjusted Constant score improved from 47% to 70%, with 83% excellent or good results. Poorer outcomes were seen with irreparable supraspinatus tears: adjusted Constant score 49% compared to 79%.

A systematic review by Shin et al. showed mean Constant score improvement from 37.8 to 61.3 postoperatively. Overall, better functional outcomes were seen with subcoracoid transfer compared to transfer of the pectoralis major superficial to the conjoint tendon. Lift-off tests were negative in 56%, and belly-press tests were negative in 51% of patients. There were two neurologic complications in 195 cases (one axillary nerve, one musculocutaneous nerve). Outcomes following pectoralis major for irreparable subscapularis tendon tears have shown success given the salvage nature of the operation. Reliable pain relief can be expected with less predictable functional gains, especially in patients with irreparable supraspinatus tears and those with anterior-superior instability.

■ LATISSIMUS DORSI TENDON TRANSFER FOR IRREPARABLE SUBSCAPULARIS TEARS

Transfer of the latissimus dorsi tendon has been described for the management of irreparable subscapularis tears. As described above, the results of pectoralis major tendon transfer have been inconsistent, given it originates anterior to the chest wall and has a line of pull almost 90 degrees to the subscapularis. In contrast, the latissimus dorsi tendon originates posterior to the chest wall and has a line of pull that better mimics that of the subscapularis, making it a better potential option for irreparable subscapularis tears, especially where anterior instability is present. Elhassan et al. described the feasibility of isolated or combined transfers of the latissimus dorsi and teres major to the lesser tuberosity. They advocated latissimus dorsi transfer because it is a more feasible transfer and has a lower risk of compression of the radial or axillary nerves.

LATISSIMUS DORSI TENDON TRANSFER

TECHNIQUE 11.14

(MUN ET AL.)

- Place the patient in the beach-chair position under general anesthesia.
- Make a standard deltopectoral approach, release the biceps, and tag it for latter tenodesis.
- Expose the lesser tuberosity, and identify and mobilize the subscapularis tendon. Attempt tendon repair; if repair is not possible, perform latissimus dorsi tendon transfer.
- Detach the upper one third of the pectoralis major tendon at its humeral insertion and tag it for later repair. Isolate the latissimus dorsi tendon and release it directly from its humeral attachment and separate it from the underlying teres major (Fig. 11.17A).
- Place nonabsorbable sutures in a Krackow fashion and mobilize the tendon until adequate excursion is obtained (Fig. 11.17B).
- Clear the lesser tuberosity of soft tissue and lightly decorticate it to augment tendon-to-bone healing. Transfer the latissimus dorsi tendon to the proximal portion of the lesser tuberosity and secure it with knotless suture anchors (Fig. 11.17C).

POSTOPERATIVE CARE The shoulder is immobilized in internal rotation for 6 weeks. At 6 weeks after surgery, passive shoulder exercises are initiated and gradual return to daily activities is allowed. At 3 months postoperatively, gentle strengthening exercises are begun and slowly progressed.

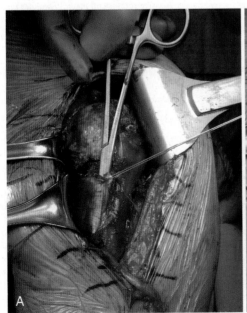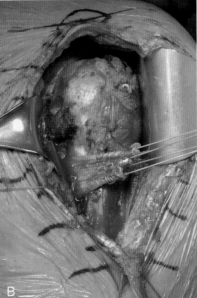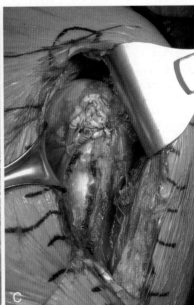

FIGURE 11.17 Latissimus dorsi tendon transfer for irreparable subscapularis tear. **A,** Expose entire length of latissimus tendon attachment. **B,** Four-strand Krackow repair placed into latissimus dorsi tendon. **C,** Completion of latissimus dorsi tendon transfer to lesser tuberosity secured with suture anchors.

OUTCOMES

There is a paucity of literature regarding latissimus dorsi tendon transfers for irreparable subscapularis tears. Mun et al. evaluated 24 patients with irreparable subscapularis tendon tears treated with latissimus dorsi tendon transfer. At an average 27.8 months of follow-up, improvements were seen in the Constant score from 46 to 69, ASES from 40 to 70, and VAS from 6 to 2. Improvements were seen in forward elevation from 135 to 166 degrees and internal rotation from L5 to L1. Overall, the belly press was negative in 18 of 24 and lift-off was negative in 16 of 24 patients, which compared favorably to pectoralis major tendon transfer. Kany et al. reported success using an arthroscopically assisted technique in five patients. A 5- to 7-cm axillary based incision was used to harvest the latissimus dorsi, which was arthroscopically fixed to the anterosuperior humeral head with cortical button fixation. One patient developed a postoperative infection with graft rupture; excluding this patient, the SSV improved from 18.75 to 63.75 and the Constant score from 32.5 to 68. Overall, the belly press test improved to negative in 2, equivocal in 2, and positive in 1.

COMPLICATIONS

Complications following tendon transfer around the shoulder are primarily wound complications, including infection and hematoma formation, as well as deltoid-related complications following deltoid detachment or acromial osteotomy for open techniques. Neurologic injuries have been described, particularly axillary and radial nerve injury following latissimus dorsi transfers and musculocutaneous nerve injury following pectoralis major transfer. Rupture of the transferred tendon also has been described, and in one series of arthroscopically assisted latissimus transfer for posterior superior rotator cuff tears rupture occurred in 38%, most often at the bone-tendon interface.

REFERENCES

ARTHRODESIS OF THE SHOULDER

Atlan F, Durand S, Fox M, et al.: Functional outcome of glenohumeral fusion in brachial plexus palsy: a report of 54 cases, *J Hand Surg [Am]* 37:683–688, 2012.

Bilgin SS: Reconstruction of proximal humeral defects with shoulder arthrodesis using free vascularized fibular graft, *J Bone Joint Surg* 94:e94, 2012.

Esenyel CZ, Oztürk K, Imren Y, et al.: Shoulder arthrodesis with plate fixation, *Acta Orthop Traumatol Turc* 45:412, 2011.

Irlenbusch U, Rott O, Irlenbusch L: Indication, technique and long-term results after shoulder arthrodesis performed with plate fixation, *Z Orthop Unfall* 156:53, 2018.

Jiménez-Martin A, Pérez-Hidalgo S: Arthroscopic arthrodesis of the shoulder: fourteen-year follow-up, *Int J Shoulder Surg* 5:54, 2011.

Kovack TJ, Jacob PB, Mighell MA: Elbow arthrodesis: a novel technique and review of the literature, *Orthopedics* 37:313, 2014.

Legato JM, O'Connell M, Fuller DA: Shoulder arthrodesis, *J Orthop Trauma* 32(Suppl 1):54, 2018.

Lenoir H, Williams T, Griffart A, et al.: Arthroscopic arthrodesis of the shoulder in brachial plexus palsy, *J Shoulder Elbow Surg* 26:e115, 2017.

Lerch S, Keller S, Kirsch L, et al.: Biomechanical analysis for primary stability of shoulder arthrodesis in different resection situations, *Clin Biomech* 28:618, 2013.

Miller JD, Pinero JR, Goldstein R, et al.: Shoulder arthrodesis for treatment of flail shoulder in children with polio, *J Pediatr Orthop* 31:679, 2011.

Porcellini G, Savoie 3rd FH, Campi F, et al.: Arthroscopically assisted shoulder arthrodesis: is it an effective technique? *Arthroscopy* 30:1550, 2014.

Puskas GJ, Lädermann A, Hirsiger S, et al.: Revision rate after screw or plate arthrodesis of the glenohumeral joint, *Orthop Traumatol Surg Res* 103:875, 2017.

Sousa R, Pereira A, Massada M, et al.: Shoulder arthrodesis in adult brachial plexus injury: what is the optimal position? *J Hand Surg Eur* 36:541, 2011.

Wagner ER, McLaughlin R, Sarfani S, et al.: Long-term outcomes of glenohumeral arthrodesis, *J Bone Joint Surg Am* 100:598, 2018.

Wieser K, Modaressi K, Seeli F, et al.: Autologous double-barrel vascularized fibula bone graft for arthrodesis of the shoulder after tumor resection, *Arch Orthop Trauma Surg* 133:1219, 2013.

ARTHRODESIS OF THE ELBOW

Jen CL, Tan JC: Neuropathic arthropathy of the elbow treated with double-plate arthrodesis and resection site bone graft, *Shoulder Elbow* 8:48, 2016.

Koller H, Kolb K, Assuncao A, et al.: The fate of elbow arthrodesis: indications, techniques, and outcomes in fourteen patients, *J Shoulder Elbow Surg* 17:293, 2008.

Kovack TJ, Jacob PB, Mighell MA: Elbow arthrodesis: a novel technique and review of the literature, *Orthopedics* 37:313, 2014.

Otto RJ, Mullieri PJ, Cottrell BJ, Mighell MA: Arthrodesis for failed total elbow arthroplasty with deep infection, *J Shoulder Elbow Surg* 23:302, 2014.

Reichel LM, Wiater BP, Friedrich J, Hanel DP: Arthrodesis of the elbow, *Hand Clin* 27:179, 2011.

Sala F, Catagni M, Pili D, et al.: Elbow arthrodesis for post-traumatic sequelae: surgical tactics using the Ilizarov frame, *J Shoulder Elbow Surg* 24:1757, 2015.

Sheean AJ, Tennent DJ, Hsu JR, et al.: Elbow arthrodesis as a salvage procedure for combat-related upper extremity trauma, *Mil Med* 181:773, 2016.

Zarkadas PC, Cass B, Throckmorton T, et al.: Long-term outcome of resection arthroplasty for the failed total elbow arthroplasty, *J Bone Joint Surg* 92:2576, 2010.

TENDON TRANSFERS

Bargoin K, Boissard M, Kany J, et al.: Influence of fixation point of latissimus dorsi tendon transfer for irreparable rotator cuff tear on glenohumeral rotation: a cadaver study, *Orthop Traumatol Surg Res* 102:971, 2016.

Castricini R, De Benedetto M, Famillari F, et al.: Functional status and failed rotator cuff repair predict outcomes after arthroscopic-assisted latissimus dorsi transfer for irreparable massive rotator cuff tears, *J Shoulder Elbow Surg* 25:658, 2016.

Castricini R, Longo UG, De Benedetto M, et al.: Arthrosopic-assisted latissimus dorsi transfer for the management of irreparable rotator cuff tears: short-term results, *J Bone Joint Surg Am* 96:e119, 2014.

Elhassan BT, Alentorn-Geli E, Assenmacher AT, et al.: Arthroscopic-assisted lower trapezius tendon transfer for massive irreparable posterior-superior rotator cuff tears: surgical technique, *Arthrosc Tech* 5:e981, 2016.

Elhassan BT, Cox RM, Shukla DR, et al.: Management of failed rotator cuff repair in young patients, *J Am Acad Orthop Surg* 25:e261, 2017.

Elhassan BT Wagner ER, Werthel JD: Outcome of lower trapezius transfer to reconstruct massive irreparable posterior-superior rotator cuff tear, *J Shoulder Elbow Surg* 25:1346, 2016.

Ernstbrunner L, Wieser K, Catanzaro S, et al.: Long-term outcomes of pectoralis major transfer for the treatment of irreparable subscapularis tears: results after a mean follow-up of 20 years, *J Bone Joint Surg Am* 101:2091, 2019.

Galasso O, Mantovani M, Muraccini M, et al.: The latissimus dorsi tendon functions as an external rotator after arthroscopic-assisted transfer for massive irreparable posterosuperior rotator cuff tears, *Knee Surg Sports Traumatol Arthrosc*, 2019, [Epub ahead of print].

Gavriilidis I, Kircher J, Majosch P, et al.: Pectoralis major transfer for the treatment of irreparable anterosuperior rotator cuff tears, *Int Orthop* 34:689, 2010.

Gerber C, Rahm SA, Catanzaro S, et al.: Latisssmus dorsi tendon transfer for treatment of irreparable posterosuperior rotator cuff tears: long-term results at a minimum follow-up of ten years, *J Bone Joint Surg Am* 95:1920, 2013.

Gibon E, El Hajj F, Ouaknine M: Arthroscopic transfer of the pectoralis major for irreparable tear of the subscapularis: a preliminary report, *Arthrosc Tech* 3:e61, 2013.

Greenspoon JA, Millett PJ, Moulton SG, et al.: Irreparable rotator cuff tears: restoring joint kinematics by tendon transfers, *Open Orthop J* 10:266, 2016.

Hartzler RU, Barlow JD, An KN, et al.: Biomechanical effectiveness of different types of tendon transfers to the shoulder for external rotation, *J Shoulder Elbow Surg* 21:1370, 2012.

Kany J: Tendon transfers in rotator-cuff surgery, *Orthop Traumatol Surg Res* 106(1S):S43, 2020.

Kany J, Guinand R, Croutzet P, et al.: Arthroscopic-assisted latissimus dorsi tendon transfer for subscapularis deficiency, *Arthroscopy* 26:L329, 2016.

Kany J, Sekaran P, Grimberg J, et al.: Risk of latissimus dorsi tendon rupture after arthroscopic transfer for posterior superior rotator cuff tear: a comparative analysis of 3 humeral head fixation techniques, *J Shoulder Elbow Surg* 29:282, 2020.

Kany J, Selim HA: Combined fully arthroscopic transfer of latissimus dorsi and teres major for treatment of irreparable posterosuperior rotator cuff tears, *Arthrosc Tech* 9:e147, 2019.

Kany J, Grimberg J, Amaravathi RS, et al.: Arthroscopically-assisted latissimus dorsi transfer for irreparable rotator cuff insufficiency: modes of failure and clinical correction, *Arthroscopy* 34:1139, 2018.

Miyazaki AN, Checcia CS, de Castro Lopes W, et al.: Latissimus dorsi tendon transfer using tendinous allograft for irreparable rotator cuff lesions: surgical technique, *Rev Bras Ortop (Sao Paulo)* 54:99, 2019.

Moroder P, Schulz E, Mitterer M, et al.: Long-term outcome after pectoralis major transfer for irreparable anterosuperior rotator cuff tears, *J Bone Joint Surg Am* 99:239, 2017.

Mun SW, Ksim JY, Yi SH, et al.: Latissimus dorsi transfer for irreparable subscapularis tendon tears, *J Shoulder Elbow Surg* 27:1057, 2018.

Namdari S, Voleti P, Baldwin K, et al.: Latissimus dorsi tendon transfer for irreparable rotator cuff tears: a systematic review, *J Bone Joint Surg Am* 94:891, 2012.

Nelson GN, Namdari S, Galatz L, et al.: Pectoralis major tendon transfer for irreparable subscapularis tears, *J Shoulder Elbow Surg* 23:909, 2014.

Omid R, Cavallero MJ, Granholm D, et al.: Surgical anatomy of the lower trapezius tendon transfer, *J Shoulder Elbow Surg* 24:1353, 2015.

Reddy A, Gulotta LV, Chen X, et al.: Biomechanics of lower trapezius and latissimus dorsi transfers in rotator cuff-deficient shoulders, *J Shoulder Elbow Surg* 28:1257, 2019.

Shin JJ, Saccomanno MF, Cole BJ, et al.: Pectoralis major transfer for treatment of irreparable subscapularis tear: a systematic review, *Knee Surg Sports Traumatol Arthrosc* 24:1951, 2016.

Wagner ER, Woodmass JM, Welp KM, et al.: Novel arthroscopic tendon transfers for posterosuperior rotator cuff tears: latissimus dorsi and lower trapezius transfers, *JBJS Essent Surg Tech* 8:e12, 2018.

Werthel JD, Wagner ER, Sperling JW, et al.: Tendon transfer options for trapezius paralysis: a biomechanical study, *J Am Acad Orthop Surg* 27:e235, 2019.

Yamakado K: Arthroscopic-assisted pectoralis minor transfer for irreparable anterosuperior massive rotator cuff tear, *Arthrosc Tech* 7:e193, 2018.

The complete list of references is available online at expertconsult.inkling.com.